PHARMACOTHERAPY HANDBOOK

Second Edition

PSYCHIATRIC DISORDERS

Edited by Barbara G. Wells, PharmD, FASHP, FCCP, BCPP

RENAL DISORDERS

Edited by Cindy W. Hamilton, PharmD

RESPIRATORY DISORDERS

Edited by Terry L. Schwinghammer, PharmD, FCCP, BCPS

APPENDICES

Edited by Barbara G. Wells, PharmD, FASHP, FCCP, BCPP

PREFACE

This second edition of the pocket companion to *Pharmacotherapy: A Pathophysiologic Approach*, Fourth Edition, is designed to provide practitioners and students with critical information that can be easily used to guide drug therapy decision-making in the clinical setting. To ensure brevity and portability, the bulleted format provides the user with essential textual information, key tables and figures, and treatment algorithms.

Corresponding to the major sections in the main text, disorders are alphabetized within the following sections which appear as a tabbing guide on the back of the book: Bone and Joint Disorders; Cardiovascular Disorders; Dermatologic Disorders; Endocrinologic Disorders; Gastrointestinal Disorders; Gynecologic and Obstetric Disorders; Hematologic Disorders; Infectious Diseases; Neurologic Disorders; Nutritional Disorders; Oncologic Disorders; Ophthalmic Disorders; Psychiatric Disorders; Renal Disorders; and Respiratory Disorders. Drug-induced conditions associated with allergic and pseudoallergic reactions, hematologic disorders, liver disease, pulmonary disorders, skin disorders, and renal disease appear in six tabular appendices (three more than in the first edition). In the second edition, pharmacoeconomic considerations are added when appropriate.

Carrying over a popular feature from *Pharmacotherapy*, each chapter is organized in a consistent format:

- Disease state definition
- Concise review of relevant pathophysiology
- Clinical presentation
- Diagnosis
- Desired outcome
- Treatment and monitoring

The treatment section may include nonpharmacologic therapy, drug selection guidelines, dosing recommendations, adverse effects, pharmacokinetic considerations, and important drug–drug interactions. More treatment algorithms are included in this edition than in the previous edition. If more in-depth information is required, the reader is encouraged to refer to the primary text, *Pharmacotherapy: A Pathophysiologic Approach*, Fourth Edition.

It is our sincere hope that students and practitioners find this book helpful as they continuously strive to deliver the highest quality care to patients. We invite your comments on how we may improve subsequent editions of this work.

Barbara G. Wells
Joseph T. DiPiro
Terry L. Schwinghammer
Cindy W. Hamilton

ACKNOWLEDGMENTS

The editors wish to express our sincere appreciation to the authors whose chapters in the fourth edition of *Pharmacotherapy: A Pathophysiologic Approach* served as the basis for this book. The dedication and professionalism of these outstanding practitioners, teachers, and clinical scientists are evident on every page of this work. The authors of the chapters from the fourth edition are acknowledged at the end of each respective *Handbook* chapter. Cheryl Mehalik, our Editor-in-Chief at Appleton & Lange, deserves special recognition for her creativity, her unique ideas, and for shepherding the book to production. Thanks also to Lisa Guidone, Production Editor, for guiding the production process of this book and Eve Siegel, Art Manager. We also wish to thank our spouses, Richard Wells, Cecily DiPiro, Donna Schwinghammer, and Raleigh Hamilton for their love, encouragement, and patience.

TO THE READER

Basic and clinical research provide a continuous flow of biomedical information that enables practitioners to use medications more effectively and safely. The editors, authors, and publisher of this book have made every effort to ensure accuracy of information provided. *However, it is the responsibility of all practitioners to assess the appropriateness of published drug therapy information, especially in light of the specific clinical situation and new developments in the field.* The editors and authors have taken care to recommend dosages that are consistent with current published guidelines and other responsible literature. However, when dealing with new and unfamiliar drug therapies, students and practitioners should consult several appropriate information sources.

Chapter Cross-Reference

Pharmacotherapy Handbook	*Pharmacotherapy: A Pathophysiologic Approach: 4/E*
1	85
2	84
3	82
4	83
5	14
6	9
7	11
8	19
9	10
10	12
11	13
12	21 & 22
13	18
14	17
15	88
16	88
17	70
18	71
19	35
20	34
21	34
22	30
23	38
24	32
25	33
26	37
27	31
28	76
29	78
30	74
31	91
32	93
33	96
34	97
35	101
36	110
37	103
38	114
39	104
40	98

Chapter Cross-Reference

Pharmacotherapy Handbook	*Pharmacotherapy: A Pathophysiologic Approach: 4/E*
41	99
42	109
43	107
44	100
45	112
46	102
47	106
48	113
49	52
50	57
51	56
52	55
53	53
54	126
55	129
56	132
57	128
58	116
59	118
60	122
61	123
62	117
63	120
64	119
65	86
66	61
67	67
68	66
69	65
70	64
71	69
72	62 & 63
73	49
74	44
75	47
76	48
77	41
78	42
79	87
80	24
81	25

Bone and Joint Disorders

Edited by Terry L. Schwinghammer, PharmD, FCCP, BCPS

Chapter 1

▶ GOUT AND HYPERURICEMIA

▶ DEFINITIONS

- The term gout describes a disease spectrum including hyperuricemia, recurrent attacks of acute arthritis associated with monosodium urate crystals in leukocytes found in synovial fluid, deposits of monosodium urate crystals in tissues (tophi), interstitial renal disease, and uric acid nephrolithiasis.
- Hyperuricemia may be an asymptomatic condition, with an increased serum uric acid as the only apparent abnormality. A urate concentration >7.0 mg/dL is abnormal and associated with an increased risk for gout.

▶ PATHOPHYSIOLOGY

- In humans, uric acid is the product of the degradation of purines. It serves no known physiologic purpose and therefore is regarded as a waste product. The size of the urate pool is increased severalfold in individuals with gout. This excess accumulation may result from either overproduction or underexcretion.
- The purines from which uric acid is produced originate from three sources: dietary purine, conversion of tissue nucleic acid to purine nucleotides, and *de novo* synthesis of purine bases.
- Abnormalities in the enzyme systems that regulate purine metabolism may result in overproduction of uric acid. An increase in the activity of phosphoribosyl pyrophosphate (PRPP) synthetase leads to an increased concentration of PRPP, a key determinant of purine synthesis and thus uric acid production. A deficiency of hypoxanthine–guanine phosphoribosyl transferase (HGPRT) may also result in overproduction of uric acid. HGPRT is responsible for the conversion of guanine to guanylic acid and hypoxanthine to inosinic acid. These two conversions require PRPP as the cosubstrate and are important reutilization reactions involved in the synthesis of nucleic acids. A deficiency in the HGPRT enzyme leads to increased metabolism of guanine and hypoxanthine to uric acid and more PRPP to interact with glutamine in the first step of the purine pathway. Complete absence of HGPRT results in the childhood Lesch–Nyhan syndrome, characterized by choreoathetosis, spasticity, mental retardation, and markedly excessive production of uric acid.

- Uric acid may also be overproduced as a consequence of increased breakdown of tissue nucleic acids such as occurs with myeloproliferative and lymphoproliferative disorders.
- Dietary purines play an unimportant role in the generation of hyperuricemia in the absence of some derangement in purine metabolism or elimination.
- About two-thirds of the uric acid produced each day is excreted in the urine. The rest is eliminated through the gastrointestinal tract, after enzymatic degradation by colonic bacteria. A decline in the urinary excretion of uric acid to a level below the rate of production leads to hyperuricemia and an increased miscible pool of sodium urate.
- Drugs that decrease renal clearance of uric acid through modification of filtered load or one of the tubular transport processes include diuretics, salicylates (<2 g/day), pyrazinamide, ethambutol, nicotinic acid, ethanol, levodopa, and cytotoxic drugs.
- Normal individuals produce 600–800 mg of uric acid daily and excrete less than 600 mg in urine. Individuals who excrete more than 600 mg on a purine-free diet may be considered overproducers. Hyperuricemic individuals who excrete less than 600 mg of uric acid per 24 hours on a purine-free diet may be defined as underexcretors of uric acid. On a regular diet, excretion of >1000 mg per 24 hours reflects overproduction; less than this is probably normal.
- Deposition of urate crystals in synovial fluid results in an inflammatory process involving chemical mediators that cause vasodilation, increased vascular permeability, and chemotactic activity for polymorphonuclear leukocytes. Phagocytosis of urate crystals by the leukocytes results in rapid lysis of cells and a discharge of proteolytic enzymes into the cytoplasm. The inflammatory reaction that ensues is associated with intense joint pain, erythema, warmth, and swelling.
- Uric acid nephrolithiasis occurs in 10–25% of patients with gout. Factors that predispose individuals to uric acid nephrolithiasis include excessive urinary excretion of uric acid, an acidic urine, and a highly concentrated urine.
- In acute uric acid nephropathy, acute renal failure occurs as a result of blockage of urine flow secondary to massive precipitation of uric acid crystals in the collecting ducts and ureters. This syndrome is a well-recognized complication in patients with myeloproliferative or lymphoproliferative disorders and is a result of massive malignant cell turnover, particularly after initiation of chemotherapy. Chronic urate nephropathy is caused by the long-term deposition of urate crystals in the renal parenchyma.
- Tophi (urate deposits) are uncommon in the general population of gouty subjects and are a late complication of hyperuricemia. The most common sites of tophaceous deposits in patients with recurrent acute gouty arthritis are the base of the great toe, the helix of the ear, olecranon bursae, Achilles tendon, knees, wrists, and hands.

► CLINICAL PRESENTATION

- Acute attacks of gouty arthritis are characterized by rapid onset of excruciating pain, swelling, and inflammation. The attack is typically monoarticular at first, most often affecting the first metatarsophalangeal joint (podagra), and then, in order of frequency, the insteps, ankles, heels, knees, wrists, fingers, and elbows. Attacks commonly begin at night with the patient awakening from sleep with excruciating pain. The affected joints are erythematous, warm, and swollen. Fever and leukocytosis are common. Untreated attacks may last from 3–14 days before spontaneous recovery.
- Although acute attacks of gouty arthritis may occur without apparent provocation, attacks may be precipitated by stress, trauma, alcohol ingestion, infection, surgery, rapid lowering of serum uric acid by ingestion of uric acid–lowering agents, and ingestion of certain drugs known to elevate serum uric acid concentrations.

► DIAGNOSIS

- The definitive diagnosis is accomplished by aspiration of synovial fluid from the affected joint and identification of intracellular crystals of monosodium urate monohydrate in synovial fluid leukocytes.
- When joint aspiration is not a viable option, a presumptive diagnosis of acute gouty arthritis may be made on the basis of the presence of the characteristic signs and symptoms as well as the response to treatment.

► DESIRED OUTCOME

The goals in the treatment of gout are to terminate the acute attack, prevent recurrent attacks of gouty arthritis, and prevent complications associated with chronic deposition of urate crystals in tissues.

► TREATMENT

ACUTE GOUTY ARTHRITIS

Indomethacin

- Indomethacin is as effective as colchicine in the treatment of acute gouty arthritis and is preferred because acute GI toxicity occurs far less frequently than with colchicine (Figure 1–1). It is customary to start with a relatively large dose for the first 24–48 hours and then taper the therapy over 3–4 days to minimize the risk of recurrent attacks. For example, 75 mg of indomethacin may be given initially, followed by 50 mg every 6 hours for 2 days, then 50 mg every 8 hours for 1 or 2 days.
- Side effects unique to indomethacin include headache and dizziness. All nonsteroidal anti-inflammatory drugs (NSAIDs) have been impli-

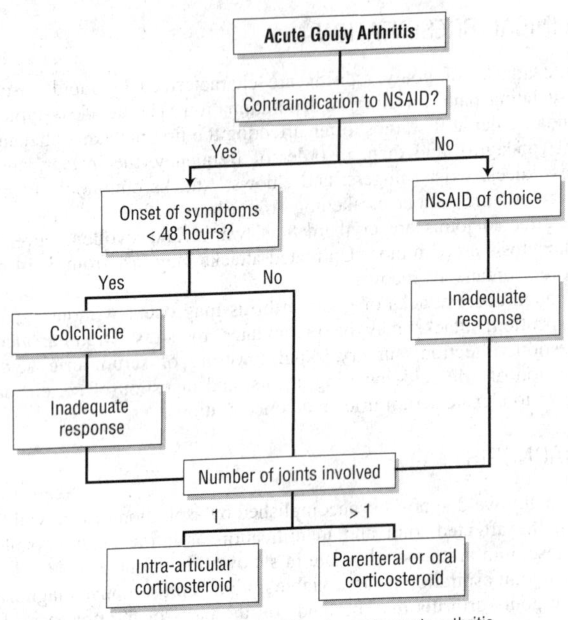

Figure 1–1. Treatment algorithm for acute gouty arthritis.

cated in causing gastric ulceration and bleeding, but this is unlikely with short-term therapy.

Other NSAIDs

- Other NSAIDs are also effective in relieving the inflammation of acute gout (Table 1–1). NSAIDs should be used with caution in individuals with a history of acid peptic disease, heart failure, chronic renal failure, or coronary artery disease.

Colchicine

- The usual oral dose is 1 mg initially, followed by 0.5 mg every 2 hours until the joint symptoms subside, the patient develops abdominal discomfort, or diarrhea, or a total dose of 8 mg has been given. About 75–90% of patients with acute gouty arthritis respond favorably to colchicine when ingestion of the drug is begun within 24–48 hours of the onset of joint symptoms. Gastrointestinal (GI) toxicity occurs in 50–80% of patients before the relief of the attack. Elderly patients may become severely dehydrated and incur serious electrolyte losses.
- This high incidence of GI toxicity may be circumvented by administering colchicine intravenously. The initial intravenous (IV) dose of colchicine is 2 mg. If relief is not obtained, an additional 1-mg dose may

TABLE 1–1. Dosage Regimens of Nonsteroidal Anti-inflammatory Drugs (NSAIDs) for Treatment of Acute Gouty Arthritis

Generic (Brand) Name	Dosage and Frequency
Fenoprofen (Nalfon)	800 mg q 6 h
Flurbiprofen (Ansaid)	100 mg qid for 1 day, then 50 mg qid
Ibuprofen (Motrin)	600–800 mg qid
Ketoprofen (Orudis)	50 mg qid or 75 mg tid
Meclofenamate (Meclomen)	100 mg tid-qid
Naproxen (Naprosyn)	750 mg initially, then 250 mg q 8 h
Piroxicam (Feldene)	40 mg qd
Sulindac (Clinoril)	200 mg bid
Tolmetin (Tolectin)	400 mg tid-qid

be given at 6 and at 12 hours to a total dose of 4 mg for a specific attack. The colchicine should be diluted with 20 mL of normal saline before administration to minimize sclerosis of the vein. IV colchicine subjects patients to the risk of local extravasation, which can cause inflammation in and necrosis of the surrounding tissue. Very small, difficult-to-inject veins and renal impairment are relative contraindications to IV colchicine therapy. Colchicine should not be used intravenously in individuals who are neutropenic, have severe renal impairment (creatinine clearance <10 mL/min), or have combined renal and hepatic insufficiency.

Corticosteroids

- Corticosteroids may be used to treat acute attacks of gouty arthritis, but they are reserved primarily for resistant cases or for patients with a contraindication to colchicine and NSAID therapy. **Prednisone** may be administered orally in doses of 30–60 mg daily in patients with multiple-joint involvement. Because rebound attacks may occur upon steroid withdrawal, the dose should be gradually tapered in 5-mg increments over 10–14 days and discontinued.
- Doses of 40–80 USP units of **ACTH gel** are given intramuscularly (IM) every 6–8 hours for 2–3 days and then the doses are reduced in stepwise fashion and discontinued.
- Intra-articular administration of **triamcinolone hexacetonide** in a dose of 20–40 mg may be useful in treating acute gout limited to a single joint.

PROPHYLACTIC THERAPY

General Principles

- If the first episode of acute gouty arthritis was mild and responded promptly to treatment, the patient's serum urate concentration was only minimally elevated, and the 24-hour urinary uric acid excretion was not excessive (<1000 mg/24 hours on a regular diet), then prophylactic treatment can be withheld.

- If the patient had a severe attack of gouty arthritis, a complicated course of uric acid lithiasis, a substantially elevated serum uric acid (>10 mg/dL), or a 24-hour urinary excretion of uric acid of more than 1000 mg, then prophylactic treatment should be instituted immediately after resolution of the acute episode.
- Prophylactic therapy is also appropriate for patients with frequent (i.e., more than two or three per year) attacks of gouty arthritis even if the serum uric acid concentration is normal or only minimally elevated.

Colchicine

- Prophylactic therapy with low-dose oral colchicine, 0.5–0.6 mg twice daily, may be effective in preventing recurrent arthritis in patients with no evidence of visible tophi and a normal or slightly elevated serum urate concentration. Patients do not become resistant to or tolerant of daily colchicine, and if they sense the beginning of an acute attack, they should increase the dose to 1 mg every 2 hours; in most instances, the attack aborts after 1 or 2 mg of colchicine.

Uric Acid Lowering Therapy

- Patients with a history of recurrent acute gouty arthritis and a significantly elevated serum uric acid concentration are probably best managed with uric acid lowering therapy.
- Colchicine at a dose of 0.5 mg twice daily should be administered during the first 6–12 months of antihyperuricemic therapy to minimize the risk of acute attacks that may occur during initiation of uric acid lowering therapy.
- The therapeutic objective of antihyperuricemic therapy is to reduce the serum urate concentration below 6 mg/dL, well below the saturation point.

Uricosuric Drugs

- Uricosuric drugs **(probenecid, sulfinpyrazone)** increase the renal clearance of uric acid by inhibiting the renal tubular reabsorption of uric acid. Therapy with uricosuric drugs should be started at a low dose to avoid marked uricosuria and possible stone formation. The maintenance of adequate urine flow and alkalinization of the urine with sodium bicarbonate or Shohl's solution during the first several days of uricosuric therapy further diminish the possibility of uric acid stone formation.
- Probenecid is given initially at a dose of 250 mg twice a day for 1–2 weeks, then 500 mg twice a day for 2 weeks. Thereafter, the daily dose is increased by 500-mg increments every 1–2 weeks until satisfactory control is achieved or a maximum dose of 2 g is reached.
- The initial dose of sulfinpyrazone is 50 mg twice a day for 3–4 days, then 100 mg twice a day, increasing the daily dose by 100-mg increments each week up to 800 mg/day.

- The major side effects associated with uricosuric therapy are GI irritation, rash and hypersensitivity, precipitation of acute gouty arthritis, and stone formation. These drugs are contraindicated in patients who are allergic to them and in patients with impaired renal function (i.e., creatinine clearance <50 mL/min).

Xanthine Oxidase Inhibitor

- Both **allopurinol** and its major metabolite, oxypurinol, are xanthine oxidase inhibitors and thus impair the conversion of hypoxanthine to xanthine and xanthine to uric acid. Allopurinol also lowers the intracellular concentration of PRPP. Because of the long half-life of its metabolite, allopurinol can be given once daily. An oral daily dose of 300 mg is usually sufficient. Occasionally, as much as 600–800 mg/d may be necessary.
- Allopurinol is the antihyperuricemic drug of choice in patients with a history of urinary stones or impaired renal function, in patients who have lymphoproliferative or myeloproliferative disorders and need pretreatment with a xanthine oxidase inhibitor before initiation of cytotoxic therapy to protect against acute uric acid nephropathy, and in patients with gout who are overproducers of uric acid.
- The major side effects of allopurinol are skin rash, leukopenia, occasional GI toxicity, and increased frequency of acute gouty attacks with the initiation of therapy.

▶ EVALUATION OF THERAPEUTIC OUTCOMES

- Patients should be monitored for symptomatic relief of joint pain as well as potential adverse effects and drug interactions related to drug therapy. The acute pain of an initial attack of gouty arthritis should begin to ease within about eight hours of treatment initiation. Complete resolution of pain, erythema, and inflammation usually occurs within 48 to 72 hours.

See Chapter 85, Gout and Hyperuricemia, authored by David W. Hawkins, PharmD, and Daniel W. Rahn, MD, for a more detailed discussion of this topic.

Chapter 2

▶ OSTEOARTHRITIS

▶ DEFINITION

Osteoarthritis (OA) is a common, slowly progressive disorder affecting primarily the weight-bearing diarthrodial joints of the peripheral and axial skeleton. It is characterized by progressive deterioration and loss of articular cartilage resulting in osteophyte formation, pain, limitation of motion, deformity, and progressive disability. Inflammation may or may not be present in the affected joints.

▶ PATHOPHYSIOLOGY

- An initial biochemical change in cartilage appears to be an increase in water content of the cartilage matrix despite a reduction in hydrophilic proteoglycans. This initial change results in a thickened articular cartilage but one less able to withstand mechanical forces.
- Soon after these changes in water content occur, the glycosaminoglycan composition changes, reflecting changes in keratan sulfate and the ratio of chondroitin 4-sulfate to chondroitin 6-sulfate. These changes may result in decreased proteoglycan–collagen interaction in the cartilage. The collagen content does not appear to change until severe disease is present. Increases in collagen synthesis and in the distribution and diameter of the fibers have been noted.
- The net effect of these biochemical changes is the failure of the cartilage to repair itself, resulting in loss of cartilage, eburnation of bone, and pain.
- Pathologic changes in the cartilage and bone also occur. There is an initial thickening of the articular cartilage, reflecting the damage to the collagen network and increase of water content. Joint synovial lining may show moderate degrees of inflammation. Fibrillation, a splitting of the noncalcified cartilage, exposes the underlying bone, which may ultimately lead to microfractures of the subchondral bone. With continued progression, the cartilaginous layer is completely eroded, leaving denuded subchondral bone that becomes dense, smooth, and glistening (eburnation).
- Microfractures result in the production of callus and increased amounts of osteoid. New bone (osteophytes) forms at the joint margins, away from the area of cartilage destruction. Osteophytes may be an attempt to stabilize the joints and may not be part of the destructive aspects of osteoarthritis.
- Inflammation, such as synovitis, is seen and may result from the release of inflammatory mediators such as prostaglandins secreted by the chondrocytes.

▶ CLINICAL PRESENTATION

- In the United States, both sexes tend to be affected equally; potential risk factors include obesity, repetitive use through work or leisure activities, and heredity.
- The clinical presentation depends on the duration of disease, joints affected, and severity of joint involvement. The predominant symptom is a localized deep, aching pain associated with the affected joint. Early in the course of the disease, pain occurs when the joint is first used and becomes relieved by rest or removal of weight from the affected joint. Later, the pain occurs with minimal motion or activity and may be present even during rest.
- The joints most commonly affected are the distal and proximal interphalangeal (DIP and PIP) joints of the hand, the first carpometacarpal (CMC) joint, knees, hips, cervical and lumbar spine, and the first metatarsophalangeal (MTP) joint of the toe.
- In addition to pain in the affected joint, limitation of motion, stiffness, crepitus, and deformities may be present. A sense of weakness or instability may be associated with this limitation of motion in patients with lower extremity involvement.
- The joint stiffness lasts less than 30 minutes and often occurs after sitting or resting for some time. Joint enlargement typically is related to bony proliferation or, in some cases, thickening of the synovium and joint capsule. The presence of a warm, red, tender joint may suggest an inflammatory synovitis.
- Joint deformity may be present in the later stages and is the result of subluxation, collapse of subchondral bone, formation of bone cysts, or bony overgrowths.
- Physical examination of the affected joint or joints reveals pain, tenderness, crepitus, and possible joint enlargement. Heberden's and Bouchard's nodes are bony enlargements (osteophytes) of the DIP and PIP joints, respectively.

▶ DIAGNOSIS

- The diagnosis of osteoarthritis is strongly dependent on an evaluation of the patient's history, clinical examination of the affected joint(s), and radiologic findings.
- Radiologic evaluation is necessary for the accurate diagnosis of OA. In early, mild OA, radiographic changes may be normal. With the progression of degenerative changes in cartilage, the joint space may begin to narrow, subchondral bony sclerosis occurs, and marginal osteophyte and cyst formation may develop. Late in the disease process, subluxation and deformity may be apparent. Osteoporosis and joint erosions are not usually seen but may occur in some patients with erosive OA.

- Joint arthroscopic examination also can confirm the diagnosis or extent of OA present in a particular joint, but few clinical situations require this procedure to establish the diagnosis.
- No specific clinical laboratory abnormalities occur in primary OA. The erythrocyte sedimentation rate (ESR) may be slightly elevated in patients with generalized or erosive inflammatory OA. The rheumatoid factor test is negative. Analysis of the synovial fluid reveals fluid with high viscosity. This fluid demonstrates a mild leukocytosis (<2000 WBC/mm^3) with predominantly mononuclear cells.

▶ DESIRED OUTCOME

The major goals for the management of osteoarthritis are to: (1) educate the patient, caregivers, and relatives; (2) relieve symptoms such as pain and stiffness; (3) preserve the joint motion and function by limiting disease progression; and (4) minimize the disability.

▶ TREATMENT

NONPHARMACOLOGIC TREATMENT

- The first step is to educate the patient about the extent, degree of involvement, prognosis, and management approach. For the patient who is overweight, dietary counseling is an important recommendation.
- Physical therapy—with heat or cold treatments and an exercise program—helps to maintain and regain joint range of motion, relieve pain, and reduce muscle spasms. Transcutaneous electrical nerve stimulation (TENS) may provide some relief of acute pain, but it is cumbersome and expensive. Exercise programs using isometric techniques are designed to strengthen the muscles and improve joint function and motion.
- Various assistive devices—including splints, canes, walkers, and braces—can be used during exercise or daily activities. Other orthotic devices such as heel cups or insoles may also be tried to help relieve pain and improve the patient's ability to walk.
- Surgical procedures (e.g., osteotomy, joint debridement, osteophyte removal, partial or total arthroplasty, joint fusion) are indicated for patients who have severe disease or who have substantial pain or marked functional disabilities and in whom conservative therapy has not been effective.

PHARMACOLOGIC THERAPY

General Principles

- Drug therapy in OA is directed at the symptomatic relief of pain and inflammation when present.
- Because OA often occurs in older individuals who may also have other preexisting medical conditions, a conservative approach to the use of medications is warranted.

- An individualized approach to treatment is necessary (Figure 2–1). Some patients with mild symptoms may require simple topical or oral analgesics; patients who receive no relief from the analgesics or who have signs of active inflammation may benefit from the use of an anti-inflammatory medication.

Analgesics

Acetaminophen

- The major oral analgesic of choice is acetaminophen in doses of 325–650 mg four times daily. The maximum dose is 4 g/d. Several recent reports have demonstrated the comparable efficacy of acetaminophen (2.6–4 g/d) to either ibuprofen at doses of 1200 or 2400 mg/d or naproxen 750 mg/d in relieving the pain symptoms associated with OA of the knee. Practice guidelines by the American College of Rheumatology recommend the use of acetaminophen in doses less than 4 g/d as first-line therapy for the short-term symptomatic relief of OA pain.
- Acetaminophen is usually well tolerated by patients, but hepatic and renal toxicity have been reported when it has been taken in excess, for prolonged periods of time, or by at-risk populations.

Salicylates

- Aspirin in doses of 325–650 mg four times daily also provides analgesia; doses greater than 3.6 g/d are necessary to achieve anti-inflammatory activity.
- Salicylates can cause adverse gastrointestinal (GI) effects ranging from mild discomfort to gastric ulcers. To minimize these effects, the salicylates should be taken with food or milk. Enteric-coated products cause less gastric mucosal injury compared with buffered or plain aspirin. The nonacetylated salicylate products also produce less GI irritation and bleeding than plain aspirin but are considerably more expensive. Aspirin products may cause impaired renal function and increases in serum transaminases.

Capsaicin

- Topical administration of capsaicin, an extract of red peppers that produces release of and ultimately depletion of substance P, has been beneficial in providing pain relief in OA.
- When used alone or as an adjunct to oral analgesics or nonsteroidal anti-inflammatory drugs (NSAIDs), capsaicin may help to avoid or minimize the systemic effects associated with those medications.
- Capsaicin is administered two to four times a day by gently rubbing the cream around the affected joint. Several weeks of *consistent* application may be required before maximal pain relief is achieved.
- Capsaicin is generally well tolerated, but some patients report a burning or stinging sensation when it is first applied.

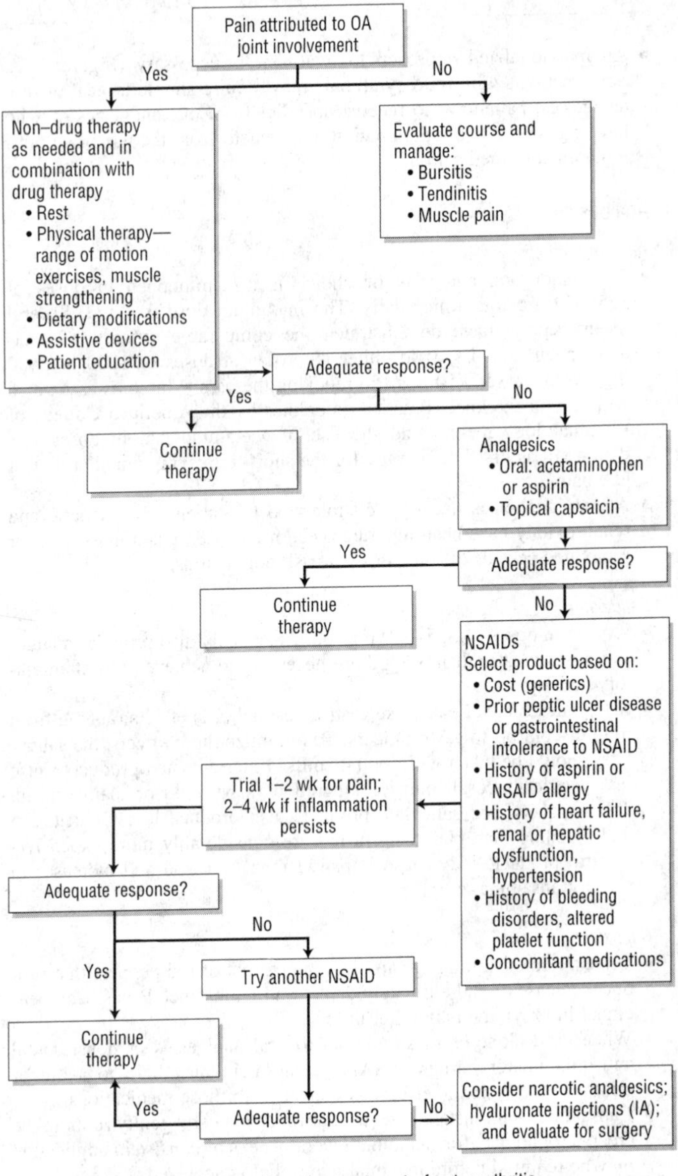

I

Pain attributed to OA joint involvement

Yes → Non–drug therapy as needed and in combination with drug therapy
- Rest
- Physical therapy—range of motion exercises, muscle strengthening
- Dietary modifications
- Assistive devices
- Patient education

No → Evaluate course and manage:
- Bursitis
- Tendinitis
- Muscle pain

Adequate response?

Yes → Continue therapy

No → Analgesics
- Oral: acetaminophen or aspirin
- Topical capsaicin

Adequate response?

Yes → Continue therapy

No → NSAIDs
Select product based on:
- Cost (generics)
- Prior peptic ulcer disease or gastrointestinal intolerance to NSAID
- History of aspirin or NSAID allergy
- History of heart failure, renal or hepatic dysfunction, hypertension
- History of bleeding disorders, altered platelet function
- Concomitant medications

Trial 1–2 wk for pain; 2–4 wk if inflammation persists

Adequate response?

Yes → Continue therapy

No → Try another NSAID

Adequate response?

Yes → Continue therapy

No → Consider narcotic analgesics; hyaluronate injections (IA); and evaluate for surgery

Figure 2–1. Algorithm for treatment of osteoarthritis.

Other Analgesics

- **Tramadol, propoxyphene,** or opioids such as **codeine** are usually reserved for patients who have failed single- or multiple-agent therapy with simple analgesics, topical agents, or NSAIDs.
- Patients should be instructed to use these products primarily for severe pain and for the shortest duration possible. Ideally, prescriptions should be written for a limited quantity with only one or two refills to minimize the potential for abuse and assist with assessing the degree of pain relief obtained.

Nonsteroidal Anti-Inflammatory Drugs

- In general, the NSAIDs are indicated after simple analgesics have failed to relieve pain, toxic effects have developed, or inflammation is present.
- As a class, the NSAIDs are comparably effective in reducing pain and modifying the inflammatory process (Table 2–1). NSAIDs are as effective as aspirin and cause fewer GI complaints.
- The choice of a particular NSAID is frequently a matter of prescriber preference based on past treatment, cost, patient preference, toxic effects, and compliance.
- A patient may respond well to one drug in a particular chemical class but experience little or no benefit from another NSAID in the same class. Therefore, other NSAIDs may be used in a selective manner after an adequate trial (2–3 weeks) at an adequate dose (either anti-inflammatory or analgesic) of other NSAIDs in the same or another chemical class.
- Combination of NSAIDs with other NSAIDs or aspirin increases toxic effects while providing no added benefit.
- Gastrointestinal complaints are the most common adverse effects observed with NSAIDs, and administration with food or milk should be encouraged, except for the enteric-coated products (milk or antacids may destroy the enteric coating and cause increased GI symptoms in some patients). Diarrhea can occur but is more commonly observed with meclofenamate than the other NSAIDs.
- All NSAIDs have the potential to cause GI bleeding through a variety of mechanisms related to direct topical or systemic effects of the NSAIDs. Several factors increase the risk of ulcers and ulcer complications related to NSAIDs. These include patient age above 65 years; prior ulcer disease or complications; therapy with high-dose or multiple NSAIDs; concomitant corticosteroid therapy; NSAID therapy duration of less than 3 months, and cardiovascular disease. Concomitant therapy with a mucosal protective agent (e.g., misoprostol) should be considered in patients who are considered to be at high risk.
- NSAIDs may also cause renal complications, hepatitis, platelet dysfunction, hypersensitivity reactions, rash, or central nervous system (CNS) complaints such as drowsiness, dizziness, headaches, depression, confusion, and tinnitus.

TABLE 2–1. Medications Commonly Used in the Treatment of Osteoarthritis

Medication	Dosage and Frequency	Maximum Dosage (mg/d)
Oral Analgesics		
Acetaminophen	325–650 mg every 4–6 h or 1 g 3 or 4 times per day	4000
Tramadol	50–100 mg every 4–6 h	400
Topical Analgesics		
Capsaicin 0.025% or 0.075%	Apply to affected joint 3 or 4 times per day	—
Nonsteroidal Anti-inflammatory Drugs (NSAIDs)		
Carboxylic acids		
Acetylated salicylates		
Aspirin, plain, buffered or enteric coated	325–650 mg every 4–6 h for pain Anti-inflammatory doses start at 3600 mg/d in divided doses	3600[a]
Nonacetylated salicylates		
Salsalate	500–1000 mg 2 or 3 times per day	3000[a]
Diflunisal	500–1000 mg in 2 divided doses	1500
Choline salicylate[b]	500–1000 mg 2 or 3 times per day	3000[a]
Choline magnesium salicylate	500–1000 mg 2 or 3 times per day	3000[a]
Acetic acids		
Etodolac	800–1200 mg/d in divided doses	1200
Diclofenac	100–150 mg/d in divided doses	200
Indomethacin	25 mg 2 or 3 times a day; 75 mg SR once daily	200; 150
Ketorolac[c]	10 mg every 4–6 h	40
Nabumetone[d]	500–1000 mg 1 or 2 times a day	2000
Propionic acids		
Fenoprofen	300–600 mg 3 or 4 times per day	3200
Flurbiprofen	200–300 mg/d in 2–4 divided doses	300
Ibuprofen	1200–3200 mg/d in 3 or 4 divided doses	3200
Ketoprofen	150–300 mg/d in 3 or 4 divided doses	300
Naproxen	250–500 mg twice per day	1500
Naproxen sodium	275–550 mg twice per day	1375
Oxaprozin	1200 mg/d	1800
Fenamates		
Meclofenamate	200–400 mg/d in 3 or 4 divided doses	400
Mefenamic acid[e]	250 mg every 6 h	1000
Oxicams		
Piroxicam	20 mg/d	20

[a]Monitor serum salicylate levels over 3–3.6 g/d.
[b]Only available as a liquid; 870 mg salicylate/5 mL.
[c]Not FDA approved for treatment of OA for more than 5 days.
[d]Nonorganic acid but metabolite is an acetic acid.
[e]Not FDA approved for treatment of OA.

- The most potentially serious drug interactions include the concomitant use of NSAIDs with lithium, warfarin, oral hypoglycemics, methotrexate, antihypertensives, angiotensin-converting enzyme (ACE) inhibitors, β blockers, and diuretics.

Corticosteroids

- Systemic corticosteroid therapy is not recommended in the treatment of OA, as side effects associated with prolonged use outweigh any potential benefits of therapy.
- The use of intra-articular corticosteroids (IAC) may temporarily be helpful in patients with knee effusions, but their long-term benefit remains controversial. If used, IAC should be administered infrequently at intervals of 4–6 months for any given joint and not to exceed 3–4 injections per month. If no improvement occurs from one or two injections, then further treatment is not likely to succeed. After injection, the patient should be instructed to minimize joint activity and the joint stress load for several days. Injection into the ligaments or pericapsular areas can be beneficial and is associated with reduced risks relative to IAC administration.

Hyaluronate Injections

- Hyaluronic acid assists in the reconstitution of the synovial fluid, thereby improving its elasticity and viscosity and enhancing joint function. It also plays an important role in cartilage matrix formation through its role in aggregation with proteoglycan.
- Two intra-articular agents containing hyaluronic acid are available for the treatment of pain associated with OA of the knee: **sodium hyaluronate (Hyalgan)** and **hylan G-F 20 (Synvisc).** A treatment cycle consists of a 2-mL intra-articular injection into the affected knee once weekly for 3 (hylan G-F 20) or 5 (sodium hyaluronate) consecutive weeks.
- Based on current information, these products may be of value in patients who have failed to respond adequately to conservative nonpharmacologic therapy and simple analgesics (e.g., acetaminophen). However, further long-term trials and clinical experience will ultimately determine the value of these modestly expensive therapies.
- Hyaluronic acid products are relatively well tolerated; adverse effects include injection site pain and local skin reactions (e.g., rash, ecchymoses, or pruritus). There is a risk of infection with repeated knee injections.

▶ EVALUATION OF THERAPEUTIC OUTCOMES

- The monitoring plan for assessing therapeutic efficacy consists of establishing the patient's baseline pain through the use of a pain visual analog scale (VAS) and identifying the range of motion for the affected joint (flexion, extension, abduction, or adduction).

- Depending on the joint affected, measurement of grip strength may aid in the measurement of hand OA; measuring the time needed to walk 50 feet may aid in the assessment of hip and knee OA.
- Baseline radiographs of the respective joint are often performed to assist with establishing the degree and/or extent of joint involvement; these may be repeated when the clinical course indicates a worsening of symptoms.
- Other measures include the clinician's global assessment based on the patient's history of activities and limitations caused by the OA as well as documentation of analgesic or NSAID use.
- Disease-specific quality of life (QOL) questionnaires for arthritis provide another valuable tool for assessing a patient's clinical response to various therapeutic interventions.
- Patients should be questioned directly to determine if they are having adverse effects from their medications. They should also be monitored for any signs of drug-related effects, such as skin rash, headaches, drowsiness, weight gain, or alterations in blood pressure from NSAIDs.
- Baseline serum creatinine determinations, hematology profiles, and serum transaminases with repeat levels as needed are useful in identifying specific toxicities to the kidney, liver, GI tract, or bone marrow.

See Chapter 84, Osteoarthritis, authored by Larry E. Boh, MS, RPh, for a more detailed discussion of this topic.

Chapter 3

▶ OSTEOPOROSIS

▶ DEFINITION

Osteoporosis is a heterogeneous disease characterized by a gradual reduction in bone mass. The World Health Organization defines osteoporosis as bone density ≥2.5 standard deviations (SD) below the average young adult peak bone mass. Severe osteoporosis includes fractures with minimal trauma. Osteopenia, the precursor condition to osteoporosis, is defined as bone density of 1 to <2.5 SD below the average young adult peak bone mass. Three categories of osteoporosis have been described. *Postmenopausal osteoporosis* affects primarily trabecular bone in women within 5–15 years after menopause. *Senile osteoporosis* affects women and men (2-to-1 ratio) older than age 70. *Secondary osteoporosis* is caused by other diseases or medications and occurs in either gender at any age.

▶ PATHOPHYSIOLOGY

- Estrogen deficiency is associated with an increase in bone resorption without an increase in bone formation.
- In women, cortical bone loss proceeds at a rate of 3% per decade until menopause, at which time it accelerates to about 9% per decade. The rate returns to age-related rates 10–20 years after menopause.
- Age-related bone loss results from decreases in osteoblast function, calcium intake and absorption, sex hormone concentrations, and mechanical bone stress and remodeling. Concomitant diseases and medications may also play a role.
- The lower osteoporosis incidence in men may result from higher peak bone mass at skeletal maturity, shorter life expectancy, lower bone loss rate during aging, fewer falls, and/or a gradual (versus a distinct) cessation of hormone production.
- Drug-induced osteoporosis may result from glucocorticoids (prednisone doses ≥7.5 mg/d), heparin (>15–30,000 units/d for more than 3–6 months), thyroid hormones, and anticonvulsants.

▶ CLINICAL PRESENTATION

- The usual presentation of osteoporosis is shortened stature, kyphosis, lordosis, bone pain, or a fracture, most commonly of a vertebra, hip, or forearm. Fractures can occur after minor trauma, such as bending, lifting, or falling. Vertebral fractures are the most common and are frequently recurrent.
- Chest wall changes can lead to pulmonary and cardiovascular complications.
- Collapsed vertebrae rarely lead to spinal cord compression.
- Acute fracture pain usually resolves in 2–3 months. Chronic fracture pain may be manifested as a nagging, deep, dull pain localized to the general area of the fracture.

▶ DIAGNOSIS

- A comprehensive patient history and physical examination should be obtained to identify risk factors for osteoporosis.
  - Genetic factors include Caucasian or Asian ethnicity, family history of osteoporosis or fractures, and small body frame (tall, thin, low body mass index).
  - Lifestyle and dietary factors include sedentary lifestyle with minimal exercise, smoking, excessive alcohol ingestion, minimal sun exposure, low calcium intake at any time in life, lactose intolerance, high caffeine intake, high phosphorus intake, high animal protein intake, weight loss >10% after age 50, and anorexia nervosa.
  - Gynecologic factors include late menarche, surgical or early natural menopause, oophorectomy without estrogen replacement therapy, nulliparity, and amenorrhea.
  - Chronic illnesses that may increase risk include hyperthyroidism, Cushing's syndrome, and diabetes mellitus.
  - As described above, medications increasing risk include excessive thyroid replacement, glucocorticoids, long-term high-dose heparin therapy, and anticonvulsants.
- Regular chest radiographs are not helpful for diagnosing osteoporosis because 30–40% of bone loss is required before visualization. However, radiographs are helpful in diagnosing acute fracture.
- Several noninvasive measurements of bone mineral density are available. Single-photon absorptiometry (SPA) is recommended for the forearm, and dual-energy x-ray absorptiometry (DEXA) is best for the spine and hip. Using bone densitometry, for every 1 SD below average young adult peak bone mass, the fracture risk increases 1.5–2.5 times. Computed tomography provides a three-dimensional picture and directly measures both trabecular and cortical bone densities, but it is expensive and has the highest radiation exposure. Ultrasound evaluation of the heel is feasible for clinic use, involves no radiation, is inexpensive, portable, and can predict hip and vertebral fracture risk.
- The initial routine screen for osteoporosis includes a complete blood count, chemistry panel, and urinalysis.
- A bone biopsy can provide information on bone quality, quantity, and turnover rate, thereby differentiating osteoporosis from osteomalacia.
- Various serum and urinary markers of bone resorption, formation, and turnover are sometimes used to identify bone remodeling problems or responses to therapy but do not quantify bone mass. Markers for bone resorption are hydroxyproline; total, free, or peptide-bound deoxypyridinoline; and C-terminal or N-terminal telopeptides. Markers for bone formation include total and bone-specific alkaline phosphatase and C-terminal and N-terminal procollagen extension peptides. A marker of bone turnover is intact, fragmented, carboxylated, or undercarboxylated osteocalcin.

▶ DESIRED OUTCOME

- Osteoporosis prevention begins with increasing peak bone mass in children, adolescents, and young adults. In women and men under the age of 35–40 years, maintenance of bone mass is critical. In older men and postmenopausal women, prevention focuses on eliminating or decreasing bone loss and preventing falls and fractures. Pain control may be important for patients with new fractures or severe osteoporosis.

▶ PREVENTION AND TREATMENT (Table 3–1)

NONPHARMACOLOGIC APPROACHES

- Because caffeine increases urinary calcium excretion, restricting caffeine ingestion to less than 2 cups of coffee daily in both genders is recommended.
- Women and men should stop smoking, as smoking is associated with lower bone mass, increased fracture rates, and earlier menopause.
- Increased weight-bearing aerobic and strengthening exercises may prevent bone loss and decrease falls and fractures.
- Prevention of falls in the elderly is critical. Home environments may need to be redesigned. Sedatives should be discontinued or switched to short-acting agents, diuretics should be given during the day, and orthostatic blood pressure problems should be resolved.

ANTIRESORPTIVE APPROACHES

Calcium

- Supplemental calcium can significantly slow the rate of bone loss and may decrease fractures. Calcium works better to prevent bone loss in cortical bones, in women with the lowest dietary or life history of calcium intake, and in women before or after the first 5 years of menopause. Its effect is enhanced when combined with other osteoporosis medications and exercise; calcium alone is insufficient to prevent osteoporosis.
- All patients should meet the National Institutes of Health (NIH) consensus conference recommendations for calcium intake (Table 3–2). Table 3–3 lists foods with high calcium content. Calcium absorption from milk is about 25–35%.
- Table 3–4 lists common forms of calcium supplementation and their calcium content. Calcium carbonate contains the most elemental calcium by weight (40%).
- Calcium carbonate should be ingested with meals to enhance absorption from meal-stimulated acid secretion. Calcium carbonate has acid-dependent absorption, whereas calcium citrate has acid-independent absorption. The citrate salt may therefore have particular usefulness in elderly patients who may have decreased acid secretion. Because the fraction of calcium absorbed decreases as tablet strength increases, divided doses (no more than 500–600 mg/dose) should be used to enhance the amount absorbed.

TABLE 3–1. Osteoporosis Prevention and Treatment Guidelines for Children, Women, and Men

Age (years)	0–18	19–45	45^a – < 65			≥ 65		
Goal	Increase bone mass	Maintain bone mass	Prevent bone loss			Prevent bone loss and falls		
Exercise	Yes	Yes	Yes			Yes, may need physical assessment		
Lifestyle changes[b]	Yes	Yes	Yes			Yes		
Calcium[c]	Adequate intake	Adequate intake	Adequate intake			Adequate intake		
Vitamin D[d]	Adequate intake	Adequate intake	Adequate intake			Adequate intake		
Bone density[e]			< 1 (P)	1–2.5 (P/T)	>2.5 (T)	<1 (P)	1–2.5 (P/T)	>2.5 (T)
ERT/HRT[f]		OC[h] if amenorrheic	Yes, especially if risks[i]	Yes	Yes	Yes, especially if risks[i]	Yes	Yes
Alendronate (A)			OK	OK, especially if no ERT	Yes[j]	OK, especially if no ERT	Yes[j]	Yes[j]
Nasal calcitonin[g]				Bone pain	Bone pain or if ERT & A contraindicated		Bone pain	Bone pain, if ERT & A contraindicated

[a]Beginning age for women is postmenopausal age.
[b]Lifestyle changes—stop smoking, increase calcium and vitamin D in diet, decrease caffeine and phosphates in diet, minimize alcohol use.
[c]See National Institutes of Health and Institute of Medicine Recommendations in Table 3–2.
[d]Daily adequate intakes for vitamin D (cholecalciferol): birth to 50 years is 200 IU, 51 to 70 years is 400 IU, older than 70 years is 600 IU.
[e]Standard deviation below young adult peak bone mass, <1 = prevention (P), 1-2.5 = prevention or treatment (P/T), > 2.5 = treatment (T).
[f]ERT, estrogen replacement therapy; HRT, hormonal (estrogen and progestin) replacement therapy; for women as long as no absolute contraindications exist; if intact uterus, need concomitant progestin or annual endometrial biopsy.
[g]May consider sooner for treatment of acute fracture or chronic bone pain.
[h]Oral contraceptives.
[i]Risks include cardiovascular disease, family history of Alzheimer's (investigational), urogenital disorders.
[j]Combination therapy with ERT or HRT under investigation, use in patients with ongoing bone loss or fracture while on ERT/HRT (non–FDA-approved indications).

TABLE 3–2. Optimal Calcium Requirements Recommended by the National Institutes of Health Consensus Panel

Age Group	Optimal Daily Intake of Calcium (mg)
Infant	
Birth–6 mo	400
6 mo–1 yr	600
Children	
1–5 yr	800
6–10 yr	800–1200
Adolescents/young adults	
11–24 yr	1200–1500
Women	
19–24 yr	1200–1500
Pregnant or nursing	1200–1500
Premenopause (25–50 yr)	1000
51–70 yr	
Postmenopause without estrogens	1500
Postmenopause with estrogens	1000
Women well beyond menopause >70 yr	1500
Men	
19–24 yr	1200–1500
25–65 yr	1000
over 65 yr	1500

- The most common side effect is constipation. Calcium should not be administered with fiber laxatives. Calcium can decrease the absorption of iron, tetracycline, fluoroquinolones, alendronate, etidronate, phenytoin, and fluoride when given concomitantly.

Diuretics

- Thiazide diuretics promote a decrease in renal calcium excretion, whereas loop diuretics increase renal calcium excretion. Concurrent thiazides and estrogens result in greater bone mineral density than do thiazides alone.

Vitamin D and Its Metabolites

- Vitamin D is obtained by dietary intake and created by ultraviolet light's effect on 7-dehydrocholesterol. Vitamin D is metabolized in the liver to 25-hydroxyvitamin D and then to the active metabolite 1,25-dihydroxyvitamin D in the kidney.
- 1,25-dihydroxyvitamin D (**calcitriol**) increases calcium absorption and stimulates osteoblasts and osteoclasts. The increased calcium concentration decreases PTH release, thereby decreasing bone resorption.
- Vitamin D supplementation should be given to patients with inadequate sun exposure or ingestion of less than the recommended daily vitamin D intake. Infants, children, adolescents, premenopausal women, and men up to the age of 50 years should receive 200 IU daily. Both men and post-

TABLE 3–3. Dietary Sources of Calcium

Food	Serving Size	Elemental Calcium Content (mg)
Whole milk	1 cup	291
Skim milk	1 cup	302
Ice cream	1 cup	200
Yogurt (low-fat)	1 cup	345–415
American cheese	1 oz	150
Cheddar cheese	1 oz	211
Swiss cheese	1 oz	250
Cottage cheese (low-fat)	1 cup	154
Sardines	3 oz	372
Salmon with bones	3 oz	167
Bokchoy	1/2 cup	126
Broccoli	1 cup	100–136
Collards, raw	1/2 cup	179
Soybeans	1 cup	131
Spinach	1/2 cup	113
Tofu	4 oz	106
Turnip greens	1/2 cup	126
Figs, dried	5 medium	126
Cheese pizza	1 slice	150
Macaroni and cheese	1 cup	362

menopausal women age 51–70 years should receive 400 IU daily, and men and women over the age of 70 years should receive 600 IU daily.
- Vitamin D in high doses can cause hypercalcemia and hypercalciuria.

Hormonal Therapy

- Estrogens decrease bone resorption, increase calcitriol concentrations, and increase intestinal calcium absorption and retention.
- In 1993, the Osteoporosis Consensus Development Conference stated that estrogen replacement therapy (ERT) is the treatment of choice for preventing osteoporosis in postmenopausal women.
- A significant increases in bone mass (2–3% per year) may occur if estrogen therapy is initiated within the first 3–6 years after menopause.
- Continuous hormone replacement therapy (HRT) (estrogens and progesterones) is similar to cyclic HRT in preserving bone mass at cortical and trabecular bone sites.
- ERT decreases osteoporotic fracture incidence, but the effect varies by bone type, age, onset of therapy, and duration of ERT.
- Because transdermal ERT bypasses the liver, less positive lipid effects, which occur after about 6 months of therapy, are achieved compared with oral ERT. Combination therapy with progesterones and androgens can minimize or eliminate the positive ERT lipid effect.

TABLE 3–4. Calcium Product Selection[a]

Product	Calcium Content %	Calcium (mg)	Tablets for 1 g[b]
Calcium Carbonate	40		
Generic		200–600	2–6
Generic + Vit D (125 IU)		600	2
Generic suspension		500/5 mL	10 mL
Calcilyte + Vit D (200 IU)		500	2[c]
Calel-D + Vit D (200 IU)		500	2
Caltrate		600	2
Caltrate + Vit D (125 IU)		600	2
OsCal		500	2
OsCal + Vit D (125 IU)		500	2
Titralac Chewable		168	5
Extra Strength		300	4
Liquid		400/5 mL	12.5 mL
Tums		200	5
E-X		300	4
Ultra		500	2
Calcium Citrate	24		
Citracal 950		200	5
Citracal Liquitab		500	2
Citracal + Vit D (200 IU)		316	4
Calcium Lactate	18		
Generic		42–84	12–24

[a]Not all calcium products listed, only those with 500–600 mg per tablet or with an alternative dosage form (i.e., chewable, liquid, dissolvable tablet).
[b]When using a combination product, determine if total vitamin D ingestion is appropriate for the age of the person.
[c]Tablet for solution.

- The suggested doses of ERT for osteoporosis prevention and treatment are **conjugated estrogens** 0.625 mg, **ethinyl estradiol** 0.02 mg, **estropipate** 0.625 mg, **esterified estrogens** 0.625 mg, **micronized estradiol** 1 mg, **estrone sulfate** 1 mg, and **transdermal estradiol** 0.05 mg/day.
- ERT is usually administered continuously with continuous or cyclic progestin. Continuous HRT is usually started because 60–80% of women will be amenorrheic within 6–12 months after starting therapy and fewer women will have hyperplasia. Until then, random spotting and bleeding will occur. If amenorrhea does not develop after 1 year, predictable patterns with cyclic therapy may be preferred. Unopposed ERT increases the risk of endometrial cancer in women with an intact uterus. Concomitant progestin therapy for at least 12–14 days a month usually eliminates or reduces this risk and may even be protective. Continuous ERT alone is usually used only for women with a hysterectomy.
- For continuous therapy, conjugated estrogens 0.625 mg or equivalent is administered daily, and **medroxyprogesterone acetate** 5–10 mg is administered for 12–14 days at the beginning of the month or 2.5–5.0 mg is administered daily. For the cyclic regimen, conjugated estrogens 0.625 mg or equivalent is administered for 3 or 4 weeks, with medroxy-

progesterone acetate 5–10 mg administered for the last 12–14 days of ERT.

- The duration of therapy is for at least 10 years and potentially for life. Response, tolerance, and other ERT benefits such as cardiovascular protection influence the duration of therapy.
- Common adverse reactions of HRT include vaginal spotting and bleeding, breast tenderness and enlargement (especially in older women), pedal edema, and weight gain. Uncommon adverse reactions are facial hair growth, bloating, nausea, vomiting, leg pain, headache, increase or decrease in sexual desire, dizziness, and mood changes. A 2.5-fold increase in cholelithiasis exists with ERT.
- Absolute contraindications to ERT include active or suspected estrogen-dependent cancer, abnormal vaginal bleeding, severe liver disease, and active vascular thrombosis. Relative contraindications include migraine headaches, history of thromboembolic disease (especially with pregnancy or past oral contraceptive use), hypertriglyceridemia, uterine fibroids, endometriosis, gallbladder disease, strong family history of breast cancer, and chronic hepatic dysfunction.

Selective Estrogen Receptor Modulators (SERMs)

- **Tamoxifen,** the first SERM, is both an estrogen antagonist in breast tissue and an agonist in bone and uterine tissue. Small but significant increases in bone density occur with doses of 20 mg/d. It may also reduce the incidence of fatal myocardial infarction but has been associated with endometrial cancer, requiring routine follow-up and sometimes endometrial biopsy.
- **Raloxifene** (Evista) and **droloxifene** (investigational) are SERMs that have estrogen-like effects on bone (increased bone mineral density) and lipid metabolism (decreased total and LDL cholesterol levels). Unlike tamoxifen, these agents are antagonists in breast and uterine tissue. Raloxifene has been shown to increase bone mineral density by about 2% and improve lipid metabolism with no endometrial changes. Raloxifene is indicated for prevention of osteoporosis in postmenopausal women and may be preferred in those with a personal history of current or past breast cancer or a strong family history of breast cancer. The drug is contraindicated in women with current or past thromboembolic events. The recommended dose is 60 mg daily, which may be taken any time of day without regard to meals. The most common adverse reaction is hot flashes.

Testosterone and Anabolic Steroids

- Anabolic steroids enhance osteoblastic activity, but their predominant effect in clinical trials is decreased bone resorption. Their effect may be more related to increased muscle mass and strength.
- **Methyltestosterone** 1.25 or 2.5 mg and **testosterone transdermal patches** are sometimes co-administered with ERT or HRT in women with depression or decreased libido, sexual function, or energy level. **Nandrolone decanoate** 50 mg IM every 3–4 weeks has also been used.

These drugs have either no effect or an additive effect on bone density, but they reverse the increased HDL and cause virilizing side effects such as hirsutism, acne, and hoarseness. Liver function abnormalities may also occur.

Bisphosphonates

- Bisphosphonates bind to bone hydroxyapatite, later becoming a permanent part of bone structure. They are resistant to enzymatic hydrolysis, resulting in estimated half-lives that are similar to bone (1–10 years). When osteoclasts bind to the bisphosphonate-contained bone surface, their structure and function are altered, preventing adherence and resorption. **Etidronate** (but not **alendronate**) also inhibits bone mineralization, which can cause osteomalacia.
- Alendronate 10 mg/d may produce greater effects on bone mineral density than HRT, increasing the density of the lumbar spine by 5–10%, femoral neck by 1–5%, trochanter by 7%, and distal forearm by 0.3–2%. Vertebral and nonvertebral fractures have been shown to be decreased. The effect is greatest in the first year but continues in subsequent years. After discontinuation, the rate of bone loss eventually returns to average age-related losses but bone density remains higher than for nonusers.
- Intermittent administration of etidronate (400 mg/d for 2 weeks) followed by calcium and vitamin D for 13 weeks was shown to continually increase vertebral bone density and decrease vertebral fracture rates. Intermittent cyclical administration for up to 4 years had an additive effect with HRT on vertebral and hip bone densities with no reported osteomalacia, but 33% of those on etidronate alone developed osteomalacia.
- Alendronate is the preferred bisphosphonate because it does not inhibit bone mineralization. It is indicated for the prevention (5 mg/d) and treatment (10 mg/d) of osteoporosis. Because of its poor absorption (1–5%), it should be taken in the morning 30–120 minutes before the first food, beverage, or medication of the day with a full glass of plain water (not coffee, juice, or milk). The patient should then remain in an upright position for at least 30 minutes to prevent esophageal irritation and ulceration. Calcium and, when needed, vitamin D should also be used but taken at different times. The most common side effects of alendronate are nausea and diarrhea.

Calcitonin

- **Salmon calcitonin** causes stimulation of calcitonin osteoclastic receptors, resulting in decreased osteoclast bone attachment, motility, life span, and numbers; altered osteoclastic cellular structure; and decreased renal tubular reabsorption of sodium and calcium.
- Calcitonin increases lumbar spine bone density by 1–3%, with less effect on cortical bone. Nasal calcitonin has been shown to decrease vertebral fractures. Neutralizing antibodies develop in 40–70% of patients treated with subcutaneous calcitonin, which can minimize its

effect or cause tolerance with continuous long-term treatment. Intermittent dosing regimens have been investigated to overcome this effect but are usually less effective than daily administration. The rate of bone loss reverts to age-related losses after discontinuation.

- Calcitonin provides pain relief within days to weeks for many patients with osteoporotic bone pain.
- Calcitonin is FDA-approved for the treatment of postmenopausal osteoporosis, but it is not as effective as other medications and is generally reserved for patients with acute fractures or chronic osteoporotic pain and for those patients in whom hormonal or bisphosphonate therapy is contraindicated, not tolerated, or refused.
- The intranasal dose is 200 IU daily, alternating nares each day. The subcutaneous dose is 100 IU daily. Concomitant calcium and, when needed, vitamin D should be used. If the primary reason for use is pain control, a reduction in the weekly dose can be attempted after pain is controlled.
- Adverse effects of subcutaneous administration include nausea, anorexia, diarrhea, stomach discomfort, abdominal pain, salty taste, injection site pain, and flushing; these decrease with nighttime administration and duration of use. Nasal administration produces fewer side effects, which include rhinitis, epistaxis, and nasal irritation.

INVESTIGATIONAL BONE FORMATION THERAPY

Fluoride

- Fluoride ions serve as hydroxy radicals in the hydroxyapatite crystals, forming fluorapatite. This compound alters the size and structure of crystals, resulting in increased bone crystallinity and a decrease in solubility. Adequate calcium concentrations are required. Fluoride also produces an uncoupling of the remodeling process and prolongs the remodeling cycle, which favors formation over resorption. Bone density increases with lower doses, but with larger doses the increased bone density has altered structure, leading to decreased strength and more microfractures.
- **Sodium fluoride** and **monofluorophosphate** are being investigated for treatment of osteoporosis. Rapid-release fluoride products have been associated with microfractures and nonvertebral fractures. Sustained-release sodium fluoride 25 mg twice daily administered with calcium citrate has been shown to increase lumbar and femoral bone density, but it produced no effect on radial bone density or fracture rate. Results with monofluorophosphate and enteric-coated sodium fluoride are not as favorable as with sustained-release products.
- Adverse effects with sustained-release sodium fluoride include gastrointestinal and musculoskeletal complaints.

▶ GLUCOCORTICOID–INDUCED OSTEOPOROSIS

- Bone loss begins within the first 6–12 months on glucocorticoid therapy, and trabecular bone has the greatest loss. Daily doses of 7.5 mg or more of **prednisone** cause substantial loss of bone in most patients. Men and women are equally affected.

- Long-term effects of inhaled steroids are still unknown but are probably minimal unless high doses are used.
- Glucocorticoids decrease bone formation and increase bone resorption. Decreased calcium gastrointestinal absorption and increased renal excretion leads to a negative calcium balance and secondary hyperparathyroidism.
- Osteonecrosis, also called aseptic necrosis, and muscle wasting are serious complications of steroid therapy. This usually involves the femoral and humeral heads and causes intense pain and decreased mobility.
- Glucocorticoids should be used in the lowest possible doses and for the shortest period of time. Alternate day therapy does not appear to lessen bone loss. Inhaled steroids have less effect on bone than oral therapy.
- Some of the medications used to prevent and treat osteoporosis (e.g., supplemental calcium, thiazides, vitamin D, ERT, calcitonin, alendronate, nandrolone decanoate) may be of some benefit.
- All patients should receive follow-up bone density measurements after 6–12 months of glucocorticoid therapy.

► EVALUATION OF THERAPEUTIC OUTCOMES

- Patients receiving prevention or treatment with ERT/HRT, alendronate, or calcitonin should be examined at least annually. For women on ERT/HRT, this includes an annual breast and pelvic examination, mammography, and Pap smear. Excessive bleeding should be evaluated with an endometrial biopsy, transvaginal ultrasonography, or dilation and curettage if needed.
- Medication adherence and tolerance should be evaluated at each visit.
- Bone mineral density measurements are recommended every 2–3 years if the baseline T score was more than −1.5. For prevention programs, bone density should be assessed every 1–2 years until the density is stabilized and then every 2–3 years thereafter. For treatment programs, bone density should be measured every year for 3 years. If stable, measurements can be done every 2 years; otherwise, annual determinations should continue until stable.
- The role of biochemical markers of bone remodeling for routine patient monitoring and evaluation of medications is still being defined.
- Serum calcium and sometimes urinary calcium concentrations should be monitored in patients receiving calcitriol because hypercalcemia and hypercalciuria can occur with high doses.

See Chapter 82, Osteoporosis and Osteomalacia, authored by Mary Beth O'Connell, PharmD, BCPS, FASHP, FCCP, for a more detailed discussion of this topic.

Chapter 4

▶ RHEUMATOID ARTHRITIS

▶ DEFINITION

Rheumatoid arthritis (RA) is a chronic and usually progressive inflammatory disorder of unknown etiology characterized by polyarticular symmetrical joint involvement and systemic manifestations.

▶ PATHOPHYSIOLOGY

- Although the precise etiology is unknown, RA results from a dysregulation of the humoral and cell-mediated components of the immune system.
- Most patients produce antibodies called rheumatoid factors; these seropositive patients tend to have a more aggressive course than do patients who are seronegative.
- In the initial cell-mediated process, macrophages engulf and process antigens and present them to T lymphocytes. The processed antigen is recognized by the major histocompatibility complex (MHC) proteins on the lymphocyte surface, resulting in T-cell activation and production of cytotoxins and cytokines that result in joint damage.
- Activated B lymphocytes produce plasma cells that form antibodies that, in combination with complement, result in accumulation of polymorphonuclear leukocytes (PMNs). PMNs release cytotoxins, free oxygen radicals, and hydroxyl radicals that promote cellular damage to synovium and bone.
- Vasoactive substances (histamine, kinins, prostaglandins) are released at the site of inflammation, increasing blood flow and vascular permeability; this causes edema, warmth, and pain.
- Chronic inflammatory changes may result in loss of joint space, loss of joint motion, bony fusion (ankylosis), joint subluxation, tendon contractures, and chronic deformity.

▶ CLINICAL PRESENTATION

- Nonspecific prodromal symptoms may include fatigue, weakness, low-grade fever, loss of appetite, and joint pain. Stiffness and myalgias may precede development of synovitis.
- Joint involvement tends to be symmetric and involve the small joints of the hands, wrists, and feet; the elbows, shoulders, hips, knees, and ankles may also be affected.
- Joint stiffness typically is worse in the morning and usually lasts at least 1 hour before maximal improvement is seen for the day.
- On examination, joint swelling may be visible or may be apparent only by palpation. The tissue feels soft and spongy and may appear erythematous and warm, especially early in the course of the disease.

- Chronic joint deformities commonly involve subluxations of the wrists, metacarpophalangeal (MCP) joints, and proximal interphalangeal (PIP) joints (swan-neck deformity, boutonniere deformity, ulnar deviation).
- Extra-articular involvement may include subcutaneous nodules, vasculitis, pleural effusions, pulmonary fibrosis, ocular manifestations, pericarditis, cardiac conduction abnormalities, bone marrow suppression, and lymphadenopathy.

▶ DIAGNOSIS

- The American Rheumatism Association criteria for the classification of RA are included in Table 4–1.
- Additional laboratory abnormalities that may be seen include normocytic, normochromic anemia; thrombocytosis or thrombocytopenia;

TABLE 4–1. American Rheumatism Association Criteria for Classification of Rheumatoid Arthritis—1987 Revision

Criteria[a]	Definition
1. Morning stiffness	Morning stiffness in and around the joints lasting at least 1 hour before maximal improvement.
2. Arthritis of three or more joint areas simultaneously	At least three joint areas have had soft tissue swelling or fluid (not bony overgrowth alone) observed by a physician. The 14 possible joint areas are (right or left): PIP, MCP, wrist, elbow, knee, ankle, and MTP joints.[b]
3. Arthritis of hand joints	At least one joint area swollen as above in wrist, MCP, or PIP joint.
4. Symmetric arthritis	Simultaneous involvement of the same joint areas (as in 2) on both sides of the body (bilateral involvement of PIP, MCP, or MTP joints is acceptable without absolute symmetry).
5. Rheumatoid nodules	Subcutaneous nodules, over bony prominences, or extensor surfaces, or in juxtaarticular regions, observed by a physician.
6. Serum rheumatoid factor	Demonstration of abnormal amounts of serum "rheumatoid factor" by any method that has been positive in less than 5% of normal control subjects.
7. Radiographic changes	Radiographic changes typical of RA on posterior–anterior hand and wrist x-rays, which must include erosions or unequivocal bony decalcification localized to or most marked adjacent to the involved joints (osteoarthritis changes alone do not qualify).

[a]For classification purposes, a patient is said to have rheumatoid arthritis (RA) if he or she has satisfied at least four of the above seven criteria. Criteria 1 through 4 must be present for at least 6 weeks. Patients with two clinical diagnoses are not excluded. Designation as classic, definite, or probable rheumatoid arthritis is not to be made.
[b]PIP, proximal interphalangeal; MCP, metacarpophalangeal; MTP, metatarsophalangeal.

leukopenia; elevated erythrocyte sedimentation rate (ESR); positive rheumatoid factors (60–70% of patients); and positive antinuclear antibodies (ANA) (25% of patients).

- Examination of aspirated synovial fluid may reveal turbidity, leukocytosis, reduced viscosity, and normal or low glucose relative to serum concentrations.
- Radiologic findings include soft tissue swelling and osteoporosis near the joint (periarticular osteoporosis). Erosions occurring later in the disease course are usually seen first in the MCP and PIP joints of the hands and metatarsophalangeal (MTP) joints of the feet.

▶ DESIRED OUTCOME

- The ultimate goal of RA treatment is to induce a complete remission, which is only rarely achievable.
- The primary objectives are to reduce symptoms of joint stiffness and pain, decrease joint swelling, preserve range of motion and joint function for essential activities of daily living, maximize quality of life, prevent systemic complications, and slow the rate of joint damage.

▶ TREATMENT

GENERAL PRINCIPLES

- There is no known cure for RA and no known method to prevent it.
- Early diagnosis and prompt therapeutic intervention are necessary to reduce the likelihood and severity of irreversible joint damage.
- Aggressive treatment early in the disease course may slow progression and delay development of joint damage and erosions.
- Disease-modifying antirheumatic drugs (DMARDs) should be used in all patients except those with limited disease or those with class IV disease in whom little reversibility of disease is expected.
- Combination drug therapy with two or more DMARDs is frequently beneficial but results in increased cost and toxicity.
- Regular follow-up is essential to assess disease activity and detect adverse drug effects.
- Patient education about the nature of the disease and the potential benefits and limitations of drug therapy is critical to the success of pharmacotherapy for RA.
- An algorithm for the treatment of RA is included in Figure 4–1.

NONPHARMACOLOGIC TREATMENT

- Adequate rest, weight reduction if obese, occupational therapy, physical therapy, and use of assistive devices may improve symptoms and help maintain joint function.
- Patients with severe disease may benefit from surgical procedures such as tenosynovectomy, tendon repair, and joint replacements.

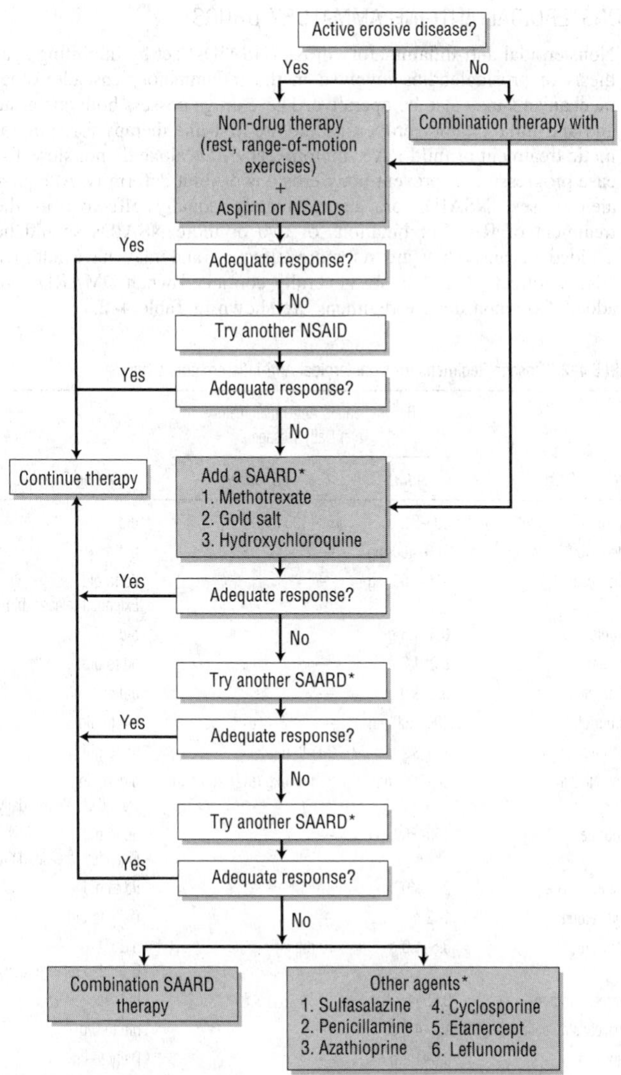

Figure 4–1. Algorithm for treatment of rheumatoid arthritis. *Corticosteroids may be necessary for patients with severe inflammatory disease in any of these phases to enable the patient to be more functional while awaiting the beneficial effects of therapy or in patients with partial responses to therapy. SAARD, slow-acting antirheumatic drug.

NONSTEROIDAL ANTI-INFLAMMATORY DRUGS

- Nonsteroidal anti-inflammatory drugs (NSAIDs) act by inhibiting synthesis of prostaglandins involved in the inflammatory cascade; other mechanisms may also be operative. These drugs possess both analgesic and anti-inflammatory properties and are first-line therapy for symptomatic treatment of mild RA symptoms. NSAIDs alone do not slow disease progression or prevent bony erosions or joint deformity. At equivalent doses, NSAIDs are approximately equally effective in the treatment of RA. Combinations of two or more NSAIDs should be avoided because they are no more effective and may have additive adverse effects. NSAIDs are generally continued when DMARDs are added. Common dosage regimens are shown in Table 4–2.

TABLE 4–2. Dosage Regimens for Nonsteroidal Anti-inflammatory Drugs

	Recommended Anti-inflammatory Total Daily Dosage		
Drug	*Adult*	*Children*	Dosing Schedule
Aspirin	2.6–5.2 g	60–100 mg/kg	qid
Celecoxib	200–400 mg	—	bid
Diclofenac	150–200 mg	—	tid to qid Extended release, bid
Diflunisal	0.5–1.5 g	—	bid
Etodolac	0.2–1.2 g	—	tid to qid
Fenoprofen	0.9–3.0 g	—	qid
Flurbiprofen	200–300 mg	—	bid to qid
Ibuprofen	1.2–3.2 g	20–40 mg/kg	tid to qid
Indomethacin	50–200 mg	2–4 mg/kg (max 200 mg)	bid to qid Extended release, daily
Ketoprofen	150–300 mg	—	tid to qid Extended release, daily
Meclofenamate	200–400 mg	—	tid to qid
Nabumetone	1–2 g	—	Daily to bid
Naproxen	0.5–1.0 g	10 mg/kg	bid Extended release, daily
Naproxen sodium	0.55–1.1 g	—	bid
Nonacetylated salicylates	1.2–4.8 g	—	bid to 6/d
Oxaprozin	0.6–1.8 g	—	Daily to tid
Piroxicam	10–20 mg	—	Daily
Sulindac	300–400 mg	—	bid
Tolmetin	0.6–1.8 g	15–30 mg/kg	tid to qid

DISEASE-MODIFYING ANTIRHEUMATIC DRUGS

General Principles

- Patients with active RA despite adequate NSAID treatment should be considered for DMARD therapy because these drugs have the potential to reduce or prevent joint damage, preserve joint function, and potentially reduce health care costs and improve the economic productivity of patients. Early initiation of therapy is crucial for optimal benefit.
- All DMARDs are relatively slow-acting (onset delay of 1–6 months), but the majority of patients ultimately achieve benefit from these drugs.
- Effective contraception is required for women of childbearing potential when most DMARDs are prescribed.
- Common dosage regimens and laboratory monitoring parameters for DMARDs are contained in Table 4–3.

Methotrexate

- **Methotrexate** is often selected as the initial DMARD, especially for patients with more severe disease. It may have the best long-term outcome because it is less toxic and less likely to be discontinued than other DMARDs. Its onset is relatively rapid (as early as 2–3 weeks), and 45–67% of patients continued it in studies ranging from 5 to 7 years. Sustained efficiency is reported in patients receiving methotrexate for up to 15 years.
- Toxicities are gastrointestinal (stomatitis, diarrhea, nausea, vomiting), hematologic (thrombocytopenia, leukopenia), pulmonary (fibrosis, pneumonitis), and hepatic (elevated enzymes, rare cirrhosis). Concomitant folic or folinic acid may reduce some adverse effects without loss of efficacy. Liver function must be monitored periodically, but a liver biopsy is recommended only in patients with persistently elevated hepatic enzymes.

Gold Preparations

- Intramuscular or oral gold preparations are effective but the onset may be delayed for 3 to 6 months. **Aurothioglucose** (suspension in oil) and **gold sodium thiomalate** (aqueous solution) require weekly injections for about 22 weeks before a less frequent maintenance regimen may be initiated. Oral gold **(auranofin)** is more convenient than IM gold, but it is less effective.
- Adverse effects are gastrointestinal (nausea, vomiting, diarrhea), dermatologic (rash, stomatitis), renal (proteinuria, hematuria), and hematologic (anemia, leukopenia, thrombocytopenia). Gold sodium thiomalate is associated with nitritoid reactions (flushing, palpitations, hypotension, tachycardia, headache, blurred vision). Patients receiving IM gold may experience a postinjection disease flare for 1 to 2 days after an injection.

TABLE 4–3. Usual Doses and Laboratory Monitoring Parameters for Antirheumatic Drugs

Drug	Usual Dose	Monitoring Parameters	
		Initial	*Maintenance*
NSAIDs	See Table 4–2	Scr or BUN, CBC q 2–4 weeks after starting therapy for 1–2 months	Same as initial plus stool guaiac q 6–12 months
Methotrexate	Oral or IM: 7.5–15 mg q week	Baseline: AST, ALT, alk phos, alb, t. bili, hep B & C studies, CBC w/plt, Scr	CBC w/plt, AST, alb q 1–2 months
Gold			
Auranofin	Oral: 3 mg daily to bid	Baseline: UA, CBC w/plt	Same as initial q 1–2 months
Gold sodium thiomalate or aurothioglucose	IM: 10-mg test dose, then weekly dosing 25–50 mg, after response may increase dosing interval	Baseline and until stable: UA, CBC w/plt preinjection	Same as initial every other dose
Hydroxychloroquine	Oral: 200–300 mg bid, after 1–2 months may decrease to 200 mg bid or daily	Baseline: color fundus photography and automated central perimetric analysis	Ophthalmoscopy q 9–12 months and Amsler grid at home q 2 weeks
Sulfasalazine	Oral: 500 mg bid, then increase to 1 g bid max	Baseline: CBC w/plt, then q week for 1 month	Same as initial q 1–2 months
Azathioprine	Oral: 50–150 mg daily	CBC w/plt, AST q 2 weeks for 1–2 months	Same as initial q 1–2 months
D-Penicillamine	Oral: 125–250 mg daily, may increase by 125–250 mg q 1–2 months, max: 750 mg daily	Baseline: UA, CBC w/plt, then q week for 1 month	Same as initial q 1–2 months, but q 2 weeks if dose change
Cyclosporine	Oral: 2.5 mg/kg/d	Scr, blood pressure q month	Same as initial
Corticosteroids	Oral, IV, IM, IA, and soft-tissue injections: variable	Glucose, blood pressure q 3–6 months	Same as initial
Leflunomide	Oral: 100 mg daily × 3d, then 200 mg daily	AST or ALT q month	AST or ALT periodically
Etanercept	SC: 25 mg twice weekly	None	None

Alb, albumin; alk phos, alkaline phosphatase; ALT, alanine aminotransferase; AST, aspartate aminotransferase; BUN, blood urea nitrogen; CBC, complete blood count; hep, hepatitis; IA, intra-articular; IM, intramuscular; IV, intravenous; plt, platelet; q, every; SC, subcutaneous; Scr, serum creatinine; t. bili, total bilirubin; UA, urinalysis.

Hydroxychloroquine

- The antimalarial hydroxychloroquine is a good initial choice for patients with mild disease because of its safety, convenience, and low cost. It lacks the myelosuppressive, hepatic, and renal toxicities seen with some other DMARDs, simplifying its monitoring. Its onset may be as early as 6 weeks, but it may take as long as 6 months in some cases.
- Short-term toxicities include gastrointestinal (nausea, vomiting, diarrhea), ocular (accommodation defects, benign corneal deposits, blurred vision scotomas, night blindness, rare retinopathy), dermatologic (rash, alopecia, skin pigmentation), and neurologic (headache, vertigo, insomnia) effects. Periodic ophthalmologic examinations are necessary for early detection of reversible retinal toxicity (see Table 4–3).

Sulfasalazine

- This sulfonamide derivative is also effective for mild disease and is relatively safe and inexpensive. Its onset of action may occur in 1–2 months.
- Adverse effects include gastrointestinal (anorexia, nausea, vomiting, diarrhea), dermatologic (rash, urticaria), hematologic (leukopenia, rare agranulocytosis), and hepatic (elevated enzymes) effects. GI symptoms may be minimized by starting with low doses and taking the medication with food. Complete blood counts should be monitored periodically.

Penicillamine

- This chelating agent is effective and its effects may be seen in 1–3 months. Its use is limited by its infrequent but potentially serious induction of autoimmune diseases (e.g., Goodpasture's syndrome, myasthenia gravis).
- Other adverse effects include skin rash, metallic taste, hypogeusia, stomatitis, anorexia, nausea, vomiting, dyspepsia. Glomerular nephritis, manifested as proteinuria and hematuria, may also occur.

Azathioprine

- This potent immunosuppressive is reserved for patients unresponsive to or intolerant of other DMARDs.
- The effects of azathioprine may be seen in 3–4 weeks but may take as long as 12 weeks at maximal dosages.
- Its major adverse effects are bone marrow suppression (leukopenia, macrocytic anemia, thrombocytopenia, pancytopenia), stomatitis, GI intolerance, infections, hepatotoxicity, and oncogenic potential.

Cyclosporine

- This drug is an effective immunosuppressive agent with an onset in 1–3 months. Its use is limited by drug cost and the occurrence of frequent toxicities (hypertension, hyperglycemia, nephrotoxicity, tremor, GI intolerance, hirsutism, gingival hyperplasia). Hypertension and nephrotoxicity are usually reversible after drug discontinuation.

- Because therapy for rheumatoid arthritis is long-term and is commonly administered to older patients, cyclosporine should be reserved for patients refractory to or intolerant of other DMARDs. It should be avoided in patients with current or past malignancy, uncontrolled hypertension, renal dysfunction, immunodeficiency, low white blood cell or platelet counts, or elevated liver function tests.

Glucocorticoids

- Glucocorticoids have anti-inflammatory and immunosuppressive properties, and they may reduce the progression of erosive joint changes if given early in the course of the disease.
- In low oral doses (<10 mg/d of **prednisone** equivalent), they may be used as "bridging therapy" during the period before a DMARD has gained its full effect or for continuous therapy in patients whose disease is difficult to control with an NSAID and one or more DMARDs.
- High-dose oral or intravenous bursts may be used to suppress disease flares. High doses are sustained for several days until symptoms are controlled, followed by a taper to the lowest effective dosage.
- The intramuscular route may be used in patients with compliance problems. Depot forms **(triamcinolone acetonide, triamcinolone hexacetonide, methylprednisolone acetate)** provide 2–8 weeks of symptomatic control. The onset of effect may be delayed by several days. The depot effect provides a physiologic taper, avoiding hypothalamic-pituitary axis suppression.
- Intra-articular injections may be useful when only a few joints are involved. The same joint should not be injected more frequently than once every 3 months. No one joint should be injected more than 2 or 3 times per year.
- The adverse effects of systemic glucocorticoids limit their long-term use. Dosage tapering and eventual discontinuation should be considered at some point in patients receiving chronic therapy.

Other Therapies

- **Leflunomide (Arava)** inhibits pyrimidine synthesis by inhibiting dihydroorotate dehydrogenase (DHODH), thereby inducing arrest of activated lymphocytes and reducing the autoimmune response. It has been shown to reduce the progression of erosions in RA. The drug is indicated for active RA in adults to reduce signs and symptoms and to retard structural damage as evidenced by x-ray erosions and joint space narrowing. Information on dosing and monitoring is included in Tables 4–3 and 4–4. Adverse effects include diarrhea, skin rash, alopecia, and elevated liver function tests. The drug is teratogenic and should be avoided during pregnancy.
- **Etanercept (Enbrel)** is a human tumor necrosis factors (TNF) receptor p75-Fc fusion protein. It competitively binds to the cytokine TNF, preventing its binding to inflammatory cell surface receptors. Consequently, the agent neutralizes the proinflammatory activity of TNF and reduces RA activity. It is indicated for moderate to severe RA in

patients not responding adequately to DMARDs. It may be used alone or in combination with methotrexate. No dose-limiting toxicities have been identified, and the drug requires no laboratory monitoring. Information on dosing and monitoring is included in Tables 4–3 and 4–4. Mild injection site reactions (erythema, itching, pain, swelling) at subcutaneous injection sites have been reported. Patients with life-threatening infections or who are at high risk for sepsis should discontinue etanercept because blocking TNF activity may increase risk of mortality in patients who develop sepsis.

- **Minocycline** has been shown to have antirheumatic therapy and may benefit some patients. Its role in the management of rheumatoid arthritis remains to be determined.
- Although **cyclophosphamide** has been used in the past for severe rheumatoid arthritis when vasculitis is present, its potential risks (oncogenic potential, hematologic complications, immunosuppression) outweigh its benefits in most cases.
- Investigational agents that may ultimately prove to be beneficial include monoclonal antibodies directed against the T-cell receptor or adhesion molecules, type II collagen, and omega-3 fatty acids.

▶ EVALUATION OF THERAPEUTIC OUTCOMES

- Patients with quiescent disease may be seen twice yearly, with the frequency of laboratory and clinical monitoring determined by the particular drug regimen; patients with active disease should be seen more frequently until disease control is achieved.
- Clinical signs of improvement include reduction in joint swelling, decreased warmth over actively involved joints, and decreased tenderness to joint palpation.
- Symptom improvement includes reduction in joint pain and morning stiffness, longer time to onset of afternoon fatigue, and improvement in ability to perform daily activities.
- Laboratory monitoring is of little value in monitoring individual patient response to therapy but is essential for detecting and preventing adverse drug effects (Table 4–3).
- Functional status may be assessed with the Arthritis Impact Measurement Scale or the Health Assessment Questionnaire.
- Patients should be questioned about the presence of symptoms that may be related to adverse effects of their particular regimen (see Table 4–4).
- Joint radiographs may be of some value in assessing disease progression.

See Chapter 83, Rheumatoid Arthritis, authored by Arthur A. Schuna, MS, FASHP, Michael J. Schmidt, PharmD, and Denise Walbrandt Pigarelli, PharmD, for a detailed discussion of this topic.

TABLE 4–4. Clinical Monitoring of Drug Therapy in Rheumatoid Arthritis

Drug	Toxicities Requiring Monitoring	Symptoms to Inquire About[a]
NSAIDs and salicylates	GI ulceration and bleeding, renal damage	Blood in stool, black stool, dyspepsia, N/V, weakness, dizziness, abdominal pain, edema, weight gain, SOB
Corticosteroids	Hypertension, hyperglycemia, osteoporosis[b]	Blood pressure, polyuria, polydipsia, edema, SOB, visual changes, weight gain, headaches, broken bones or bone pain
Azathioprine	Myelosuppression, hepatotoxicity, lymphoproliferative disorders	Symptoms of myelosuppression (extreme fatigue, easy bleeding or bruising, infection), jaundice
Gold (Intramuscular or oral)	Myelosuppression, proteinuria, rash, stomatitis	Symptoms of myelosuppression, edema, rash, oral ulcers, diarrhea
Hydroxychloroquine	Macular damage, rash, diarrhea	Visual changes including a decrease in night or peripheral vision, rash, diarrhea
Methotrexate	Myelosuppression, hepatic fibrosis, cirrhosis, pulmonary infiltrates or fibrosis, stomatitis, rash	Symptoms of myelosuppression, SOB, N/V, lymph node swelling, coughing, mouth sores, diarrhea, jaundice
Penicillamine	Myelosuppression, proteinuria, stomatitis, rash, dysgeusia	Symptoms of myelosuppression, edema, rash, diarrhea, altered taste perception, oral ulcers
Sulfasalazine	Myelosuppression, rash	Symptoms of myelosuppression, photosensitivity, rash, N/V
Leflunomide	Hepatotoxicity	Jaundice
Etanercept	Sepsis	Chills, fever, infection

[a]Altered immune function increases infection, which should be considered particularly in those patients taking azathioprine, methotrexate, and corticosteroids or other drugs as a symptom of myelosuppression.
[b]Osteoporosis is not likely to manifest itself early in treatment but all patients should be taking appropriate steps to prevent bone loss.
N/V, nausea/vomiting; SOB, shortness of breath.
From American College of Rheumatology Ad Hoc Committee on Clinical Guidelines. Guidelines for monitoring drug therapy in rheumatoid arthritis. Arthritis Rheum *1996;39:723–731.*

Cardiovascular Disorders

Edited by Terry L. Schwinghammer, PharmD, FCCP, BCPS

Chapter 5

▶ ARRHYTHMIAS

▶ DEFINITION

Arrhythmia is defined as loss of cardiac rhythm, especially irregularity of heartbeat. This chapter covers the group of conditions caused by any abnormality in the rate, regularity, or sequence of cardiac activation.

▶ PATHOPHYSIOLOGY

SUPRAVENTRICULAR TACHYCARDIA

- Common supraventricular tachycardias requiring drug treatment are atrial fibrillation or atrial flutter, paroxysmal supraventricular tachycardia, and automatic atrial tachycardias. Other common supraventricular arrhythmias that usually do not require drug therapy (e.g., premature atrial complexes, wandering atrial pacemaker, sinus arrhythmia, sinus tachycardia) are not included in this chapter.

Atrial Fibrillation and Atrial Flutter

- Atrial fibrillation is characterized as an extremely rapid (400–600 atrial beats/min) and disorganized atrial activation. There is a loss of atrial contraction (atrial kick), and supraventricular impulses penetrate the atrioventricular (AV) conduction system in variable degrees, resulting in irregular ventricular activation and irregularly irregular pulse (120–180 beats/min).
- Atrial flutter is characterized by rapid (270–330 atrial beats/min) but regular atrial activation. The ventricular response usually has a regular pattern. This arrhythmia occurs less frequently than atrial fibrillation, but it has similar precipitating factors, consequences, and drug therapy.
- The predominant mechanism of atrial fibrillation and atrial flutter is reentry, which is usually associated with organic heart disease that causes atrial distention (e.g., ischemia or infarction, hypertensive heart disease, valvular disorders). Additional associated disorders include acute pulmonary embolus and chronic lung disease, resulting in pulmonary hypertension and cor pulmonale; and states of high adrenergic tone such as thyrotoxicosis, alcohol withdrawal, sepsis, or excess physical exertion.

Paroxysmal Supraventricular Tachycardia

- Paroxysmal supraventricular tachycardia (PSVT) arising by reentrant mechanisms includes arrhythmias caused by AV nodal reentry and AV reentry incorporating an anomalous AV pathway, and, less commonly, sinoatrial (SA) nodal reentry, and intra-atrial reentry.

Automatic Atrial Tachycardias

- Automatic atrial tachycardias such as multifocal atrial tachycardia appear to arise from supraventricular foci with enhanced automatic properties. Severe pulmonary disease is the underlying precipitating disorder present in 60–80% of patients.

VENTRICULAR ARRHYTHMIAS

Ventricular Premature Beats

- Ventricular premature beats (VPBs) are very common ventricular rhythm disturbances that occur in patients with or without heart disease and may be elicited experimentally by abnormal automaticity, triggered activity, or reentrant mechanisms.

Ventricular Tachycardia

- Ventricular tachycardia (VT) is defined by three or more repetitive VPBs occurring at >100 beats/min. The most common precipitating factor for an acute episode is acute myocardial infarction; other causes are severe electrolyte abnormalities (e.g., hypokalemia), hypoxemia, and digitalis toxicity. The chronic recurrent form is almost always associated with underlying organic heart disease (e.g., idiopathic dilated congestive cardiomyopathy or remote myocardial infarction with left ventricular aneurysm).
- Sustained VT is that which requires therapeutic intervention to restore a stable rhythm or that lasts a relatively long time (usually >30 seconds). Nonsustained VT (NSVT) self-terminates after a brief duration (usually <30 seconds). Incessant VT refers to VT occurring more frequently than sinus rhythm so that VT becomes the dominant rhythm. Exercise-induced VT occurs during high sympathetic tone (e.g., physical exertion). Monomorphic VT has a consistent QRS configuration, whereas polymorphic VT has varying QRS complexes.

Proarrhythmia

- Proarrhythmia refers to development of a significant new arrhythmia (such as VT, VF, or torsades de pointes) or worsening of an existing arrhythmia. Proarrhythmia results from the same mechanisms that cause other arrhythmias or from an alteration in the underlying substrate due to the antiarrhythmic agent (e.g., development of an accelerated tachycardia due to flecainide, which decreases conduction velocity without significantly altering the refractory period). Antiarrhythmic drugs cause proarrhythmia in 5–20% of patients. Although initially thought to occur within several days of drug initiation, risk may persist throughout treatment.
- Definite patient risk factors are underlying ventricular arrhythmias, ischemic heart disease, and poor left ventricular function; less well-

defined risk factors are elevated antiarrhythmic serum concentrations (and rapid dosage escalation), recent therapy with a type Ia antiarrhythmic, and underlying ventricular conduction delays.

Torsades de Pointes

- Torsades de pointes (TdP) is a rapid form of polymorphic VT associated with evidence of delayed ventricular repolarization due to blockade of potassium conductance. TdP may be hereditary or acquired. Acquired forms are associated with many clinical conditions and drugs, especially type Ia antiarrhythmics. Quinidine-induced TdP or quinidine syncope occurs in 4–8% of patients treated with this agent.

Ventricular Fibrillation

- VF is electrical anarchy of the ventricle resulting in no cardiac output and cardiovascular collapse. VF, often preceded by VT, is the most frequently documented rhythm in patients who die suddenly during electrocardiographic (ECG) monitoring. Sudden cardiac death occurs most commonly in patients with ischemic heart disease and primary myocardial disease.

BRADYARRHYTHMIAS

- Asymptomatic sinus bradyarrhythmias (heart rate <60 beats/min) are common especially in young athletes. However, some patients have sinus node dysfunction or sick sinus syndrome because of underlying organic heart disease and the normal aging process, which results in symptomatic sinus bradycardia, periods of sinus arrest, or both. Sinus node dysfunction is usually representative of diffuse conduction disease, which may be accompanied by AV block and by paroxysmal tachycardias such as atrial fibrillation. Alternating bradyarrhythmias and tachyarrhythmias are referred to as the tachy–brady syndrome.
- AV block is caused by conduction delay or block, which may occur in any area of the AV conduction system. AV block may be found in patients without underlying heart disease, such as trained athletes, or it may occur during sleep when vagal tone is high. AV block may be transient where the underlying etiology is reversible (e.g., myocarditis, myocardial ischemia, after cardiovascular surgery, during drug therapy) or irreversible. Beta blockers, digitalis, or calcium antagonists may cause AV block, primarily in the AV nodal area. Type I antiarrhythmic agents may exacerbate conduction delays below the level of the AV node.

► CLINICAL PRESENTATION

- Supraventricular tachycardias may cause a variety of clinical manifestations ranging from no symptoms to minor palpitations and/or irregular pulse to severe and even life-threatening symptoms. Patients may experience dizziness or acute syncopal episodes; symptoms of heart failure; anginal chest pain; or, more often, a choking or pressure sensation during the tachycardia episode. Symptoms such as palpitations and even syncope correlate poorly with documented recurrences of tachycardia.

- Atrial fibrillation or flutter may be manifested by the entire range of symptoms associated with other supraventricular tachycardias, but syncope is not a common presenting symptom. An additional complication of atrial fibrillation is arterial embolization resulting from atrial stasis and poorly adherent mural thrombi, which accounts for the most devastating complication, embolic stroke. In patients with atrial fibrillation, risk factors for cerebral embolism are concurrent mitral stenosis or severe systolic heart failure.
- Ventricular arrhythmias may yield manifestations ranging from no symptoms or only mild palpitations to a life-threatening situation associated with hemodynamic collapse. Consequences of proarrhythmia range from no symptoms to worsening of symptoms to sudden death. VF, by definition, is an acute medical emergency resulting in no cardiac output, cardiovascular collapse, and death, if effective treatment measures are not taken.
- Patients with bradyarrhythmias experience symptoms associated with hypotension such as dizziness, syncope, fatigue, and confusion. If left ventricular dysfunction exists, symptoms of congestive heart failure may be exacerbated. Except for recurrent syncope, these symptoms are often subtle and nonspecific.

► DIAGNOSIS

- Surface ECG is the cornerstone of diagnostic tools for cardiac rhythm disturbances.
- Less sophisticated methods are often the initial tools for detecting qualitative and quantitative alterations of heartbeat. For example, direct auscultation can reveal the irregularly irregular pulse that is characteristic of atrial fibrillation.
- Proarrhythmia can be difficult to diagnose because of the variable nature of underlying arrhythmias. Flecainide and encainide have been known to cause a rapid, sustained, monomorphic VT with a characteristic sinusoidal QRS pattern.
- TdP is characterized by long QT interval or prominent U waves on surface ECG.
- Specific maneuvers may be required to delineate the etiology of syncope associated with bradyarrhythmias. Diagnosis of carotid sinus hypersensitivity can be confirmed by performing carotid sinus massage with ECG and blood pressure monitoring. Vasovagal syncope can be diagnosed using the upright body tilt test. β blockers may be administered IV to predict response to oral therapy.
- AV block is usually categorized into three different types based on surface ECG findings (Table 5–1).

TABLE 5–1. Forms of Atrioventricular Block

Type	Criteria
First-degree block	Prolonged PR interval (> 0.2 s), 1:1 AV conduction
Second-degree block	
Mobitz I	Progressive PR prolongation until QRS is dropped, < 1:1 AV conduction
Mobitz II	Random nonconducted beats (absence of QRS), < 1:1 AV conduction
Third-degree block	AV dissociation, absence of AV conduction

▶ DESIRED OUTCOME

The desired outcome depends on the underlying arrhythmia. For example, the ultimate treatment goals of treating atrial fibrillation or flutter are restoring sinus rhythm, preventing thromboembolic complications, and preventing further recurrences.

▶ TREATMENT

GENERAL PRINCIPLES

- The Cardiac Arrhythmia Suppression Trial (CAST) revealed that proarrhythmia is an important side effect of antiarrhythmic drugs and has a potential negative effect on patient mortality.
- Technical advances in non-drug therapies (e.g., interrupting reentry circuits by radiofrequency ablation) may ultimately render long-term antiarrhythmic therapy obsolete in certain arrhythmias.
- Internal cardioverter/defibrillators are becoming first-line treatment for many serious, recurrent ventricular arrhythmias because of technologic advances combined with the now known hazards of drugs.
- For these reasons, the volume of antiarrhythmic drug usage has declined over the past several years.

MECHANISMS OF ANTIARRHYTHMIC DRUGS

- Drugs may have antiarrhythmic activity by directly altering conduction in several ways. Drugs may depress the automatic properties of abnormal pacemaker cells by decreasing the slope of phase 4 depolarization and/or by elevating threshold potential. Drugs may alter the conduction characteristics of the pathways of a reentrant loop.
- Although often criticized, the most frequently used classification system was first proposed by Vaughan Williams (Table 5–2). Type Ia drugs slow conduction velocity, prolong refractoriness, and decrease the automatic properties of sodium-dependent (normal and diseased) conduction tissue. Clinically, type Ia drugs are broad-spectrum antiarrhythmics, being effective for both supraventricular and ventricular arrhythmias.

II

TABLE 5–2. Classification of Antiarrhythmic Drugs

Type	Drug	Conduction Velocity[a]	Refractory Period	Automaticity	Ion Block
Ia	Quinidine Procainamide Disopyramide	↓	↑	↓	Sodium (intermediate)
Ib	Lidocaine Mexiletine Tocainide	0/↓	↓	↓	Sodium (fast on–off)
Ic	Flecainide Propafenone[c] Moricizine[d]	↓↓	0	↓	Sodium (slow on–off)
II[b]	β blockers	↓	↑	↓	Calcium (indirect)
III	Amiodarone[c,e] Bretylium[c] Sotalol[c] Ibutilide	0	↑↑	0	Potassium
IV[b]	Verapamil Diltiazem	↓	↑	↓	Calcium

[a]Variables for normal tissue models in ventricular tissue.
[b]Variables for SA and AV nodal tissue only.
[c]Also has type II, β-blocking actions.
[d]Classification controversial.
[e]Amiodarone also blocks calcium and sodium channels (fast on–off).

- Although categorized separately, type Ib drugs probably act similarly to type Ia drugs (i.e., accentuated effects in diseased tissues leading to bidirectional block in a reentrant circuit), except that type Ib agents are considerably more effective in ventricular than supraventricular arrhythmias.
- Type Ic drugs profoundly slow conduction velocity while leaving refractoriness relatively unaltered. Although effective for both ventricular and supraventricular arrhythmias, their use for ventricular arrhythmias has been limited by the risk of proarrhythmia.
- Collectively, type I drugs can be referred to as sodium channel blockers. Antiarrhythmic sodium channel receptor theories account for additive (e.g., quinidine and mexiletine) and antagonistic (e.g., flecainide and lidocaine) drug combinations, as well as potential antidotes to excess sodium-channel blockade (e.g., sodium bicarbonate, propranolol).
- Type II drugs include β-adrenergic antagonists; clinically relevant mechanisms result from their antiadrenergic actions. β blockers are most useful in tachycardias in which nodal tissues are abnormally auto-

matic or are a portion of a reentrant loop. These agents are also helpful in slowing ventricular response in atrial tachycardias (e.g., atrial fibrillation) by their effects on the AV node.

- Type III drugs specifically prolong refractoriness in atrial and ventricular fibers and include very different drugs that share the common effect of delaying repolarization by blocking potassium channels.
  - Bretylium prolongs repolarization by blocking potassium conductance independent of the sympathetic nervous system, increases the VF threshold, and seems to have selective antifibrillatory but not antitachycardic effects. Bretylium can be effective in VF but is often ineffective in ventricular tachycardia.
  - In contrast, amiodarone and sotalol are effective in many tachycardias. Amiodarone displays electrophysiologic characteristics consistent with each type of antiarrhythmic drug. It is a sodium-channel blocker with relatively fast on–off kinetics, has nonselective β-blocking actions, blocks potassium channels, and has slight calcium antagonist activity. Amiodarone seems to be the most effective antiarrhythmic agent, but it also has the most impressive side-effect profile. Sotalol is a potent inhibitor of outward potassium movement during repolarization and also possesses β-blocking actions. Ibutilide activates a slow, inward sodium current and blocks the potassium-delayed rectifier current.
- Type IV drugs inhibit calcium entry into the cell, which slows conduction, prolongs refractoriness, and decreases SA and AV nodal automaticity. Calcium channel antagonists are effective for automatic or reentrant tachycardias, which arise from or use the SA or AV nodes.
- In addition to exhibiting different mechanisms, antiarrhythmic agents are distinguished by their pharmacokinetic (Table 5–3) and safety profiles (Table 5–4).

ATRIAL FIBRILLATION OR ATRIAL FLUTTER

- Many methods are available for restoring sinus rhythm, preventing thromboembolic complications, and preventing further recurrences (Figure 5–1); however, treatment selection depends in part on onset and severity of symptoms.
- If symptoms are severe and of recent onset, patients may require direct-current cardioversion (DCC) to restore sinus rhythm immediately.
- If symptoms are tolerable, drugs that slow conduction and increase refractoriness in the AV node should be used as initial therapy. Type Ia and III antiarrhythmic agents should not be administered initially because they may paradoxically increase ventricular response in the absence of drugs that slow AV nodal conduction. **Digoxin's** place in therapy has been questioned because it is sometimes ineffective and often slow in onset. Many clinicians prefer calcium antagonists (e.g., IV **verapamil, diltiazem**). If a high adrenergic state is the precipitating factor, IV β blockers (e.g., **propranolol, esmolol**) can be highly effective and should be considered first.

II

TABLE 5–3. Pharmacokinetics of Antiarrhythmic Drugs

Drug	Bioavail-ability (%)	Primary Route of Elimination[a]	$V_{D,ss}$ (L/kg)	Protein Binding (%)	$t_{1/2}$	Therapeutic Range (mg/L)
Quinidine	70–80	H	2.0–3.5	80–90	5–9 h	2–6
Procainamide	75–95	H/R	1.5–3.0	10–20	2.5–5.0 h	4–15
Disopyramide	70–95	H/R	0.8–2.0	50–80	4–8 h	2–6
Lidocaine	20–40	H	1–2	65–75	1–3 h	1.5–5.0
Mexiletine	80–95	H	5–12	60–75	6–12 h	0.8–2.0
Tocainide	90–95	H	1.5–3.0	10–30	12–15 h	4–10
Moricizine	34–38	H	6–11	92–95	1–6 h	—
Flecainide	90–95	H/R	8–10	35–45	13–20 h	0.3–2.5
Propafenone[b]						
Poor	11–39	H	2.5–4.0	85–95	12–32 h	—
Extensive					2–10 h	
Amiodarone	22–88	H	70–150	95–99	15–100 d	1.0–2.5
Sotalol	90–95	R	1.2–2.4	30–40	12–20 h	—
Ibutilide	—	H	6–12	40–50	3–6 h	—
Bretylium	15–20	R	4–8	Negligible	5–10 h	0.5–2.0
Verapamil	20–40	H	1.5–5.0	95–99	4–12 h	>0.05
Diltiazem	35–50	H	3–5	70–85	4–10 h	>0.05

[a] H, hepatic; R, renal.
[b] Variables for parent compound (not 5-OH propafenone).

- After treatment with AV nodal blocking agents and a subsequent decrease in ventricular response, the patient should be evaluated for the possibility of restoring sinus rhythm.
- If sinus rhythm is restored, anticoagulation should be initiated because return of atrial contraction increases risk of thromboembolism. Current recommendations are **warfarin** treatment (INR 2.0–3.0) for at least 3 weeks prior to cardioversion and continuing for about 1 month after effective cardioversion. Exceptions in which anticoagulation may not be necessary are atrial flutter (unless concurrent risks for thrombosis are present); lone atrial fibrillation; atrial fibrillation of less than 48 hours' duration; and absence of atrial thrombus or severe stasis on transesophageal echocardiography (TEE).
- After prior anticoagulation, methods for restoring sinus rhythm in patients with atrial fibrillation or flutter are pharmacologic cardioversion and DCC. The time-honored method for pharmacologic cardioversion is oral **quinidine** therapy beginning with maintenance dosages; IV **procainamide,** oral **flecainide,** oral **propafenone, sotalol,** and IV **ibutilide** are suitable alternatives. Advantages of initial drug therapy are

TABLE 5–4. Side Effects of Antiarrhythmic Drugs

Quinidine	Cinchonism, diarrhea, GI,[a] hypotension, torsades de pointes, aggravation of underlying heart failure, conduction disturbances or ventricular arrhythmias, hepatitis, thrombocytopenia, hemolytic anemia
Procainamide	Systemic lupus erythematosus, GI, torsades de pointes, aggravation of underlying heart failure, conduction disturbances or ventricular arrhythmias, agranulocytosis
Disopyramide	Anticholinergic symptoms, GI, torsades de pointes, heart failure, aggravation of underlying conduction disturbances and/or ventricular arrhythmias, hypoglycemia, hepatic cholestasis
Lidocaine	CNS,[b] seizures, psychosis, sinus arrest, aggravation of underlying conduction disturbances
Mexiletine	CNS, psychosis, GI, aggravation of underlying conduction disturbances or ventricular arrhythmias
Tocainide	CNS, psychosis, GI, aggravation of underlying conduction disturbances or ventricular arrhythmias, rash, arthralgias, pulmonary infiltrates, agranulocytosis, thrombocytopenia
Moricizine	Dizziness, headache, GI, aggravation of underlying conduction disturbances or ventricular arrhythmias
Flecainide, propafenone	Blurred vision, dizziness, headache, GI, bronchospasm,[c] aggravation of underlying heart failure, conduction disturbances or ventricular arrhythmias
Amiodarone	CNS, corneal microdeposits/blurred vision, optic neuropathy/neuritis, GI, aggravation of underlying ventricular arrhythmias, torsades de pointes, bradycardia or AV block, bruising without thrombocytopenia, pulmonary fibrosis, hepatitis, hypothyroidism, hyperthyroidism, photosensitivity, blue-gray skin discoloration, myopathy, hypotension and phlebitis (IV use)
Sotalol	Fatigue, GI, depression, torsades de pointes, bronchospasm, aggravation of underlying heart failure, conduction disturbances or ventricular arrhythmias
Ibutilide	Torsades de pointes, hypotension
Bretylium	Hypotension, GI

[a]GI, nausea, anorexia.
[b]CNS, confusion, paresthesias, tremor, ataxia, etc.
[c]Propafenone only.

that an effective agent may be determined in case long-term therapy is required and there is little to lose with a short trial; disadvantages are significant side effects such as drug-induced TdP, drug–drug interactions, and lower cardioversion rate for drugs compared with DCC. Although DCC is quick and more often successful, it has the disadvantages of the need for prior sedation/anesthesia and a small risk of serious complications, such as sinus arrest or ventricular arrhythmias.

II

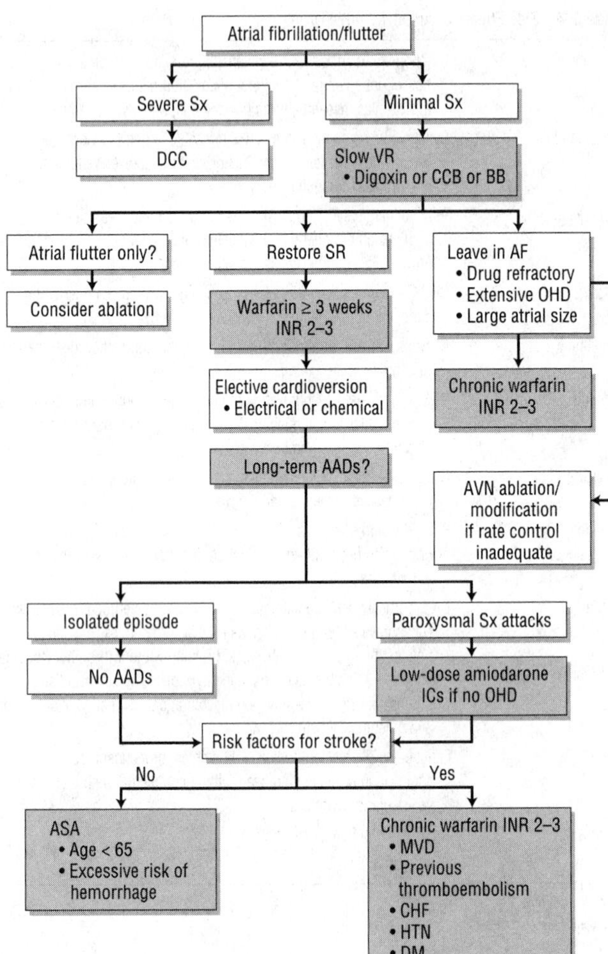

Figure 5–1. Algorithm for the treatment of atrial fibrillation and atrial flutter. Sx, symptoms; AVN, AV node; DCC, direct-current cardioversion; CCB, calcium channel antagonist (verapamil or diltiazem); BB, β blocker; ASA, aspirin; OHD, organic heart disease; AADs, antiarrhythmic drugs; INR, International Normalized Ratio; MVD, mitral valve disease; CHF, congestive heart failure; HTN, hypertension; DM, diabetes mellitus; VR, ventricular rate.

- Maintenance medications after sinus rhythm is restored may consist of digoxin, antithrombotic therapy, and antiarrhythmic drugs.
- Digoxin is often continued because of underlying ventricular dysfunction, but this practice has been questioned because digoxin may occasionally be profibrillatory.
- Warfarin significantly reduces the incidence of stroke in patients with atrial fibrillation (not associated with prior thromboembolic episodes or mitral valve disease) with an acceptable risk of bleeding complications. The American College of Chest Physicians Consensus Conference on antithrombotic therapy recommends chronic warfarin treatment (INR 2.0–3.0) for all patients with atrial fibrillation except for young (<60 years of age) patients with "lone" atrial fibrillation, patients with only atrial flutter, and patients who are unreliable or whose compliance is poor. Aspirin (325 mg/d) should generally be considered second-line treatment for those who are poor candidates for warfarin and for those without risk factors for thromboembolic complications (i.e., hypertension, recent heart failure, and prior thromboembolism).
- Atrial fibrillation usually recurs after initial cardioversion because most patients have irreversible underlying heart disease. A meta-analysis confirmed that quinidine maintained sinus rhythm better than placebo; however, 50% of patients had recurrent atrial fibrillation within a year, and more importantly, quinidine increased mortality, presumably due in part to proarrhythmia. Newer type Ic (e.g., flecainide, propafenone) and type III (e.g., amiodarone, sotalol) antiarrhythmic agents may provide alternatives to quinidine; however, these agents are also associated with proarrhythmia. Consequently, chronic antiarrhythmic drugs should be reserved for patients with symptomatic recurrences or symptomatic paroxysmal atrial fibrillation.

PAROXYSMAL SUPRAVENTRICULAR TACHYCARDIA DUE TO REENTRY

- The choice between pharmacologic and nonpharmacologic methods for treating PSVT depends on symptom severity (Figure 5–2). Synchronized DCC is the treatment of choice if symptoms are severe (e.g., syncope, near syncope, anginal chest pain, severe heart failure). Non-drug measures (e.g., carotid massage, valsalva maneuver) can be used for mild to moderate symptoms. If these methods fail, drug therapy is the next option.
- The choice among drugs is based on the QRS complex (Figure 5–2). Drugs can be divided into three broad categories: those that directly or indirectly increase vagal tone to the AV node (e.g., edrophonium, vasopressors, and digoxin); those that depress conduction through slow, calcium-dependent tissue (e.g., adenosine, β blockers, calcium channel blockers); and those that depress conduction through fast, sodium-dependent tissue (e.g., quinidine, procainamide, disopyramide, flecainide).
- **Adenosine** has been recommended as the drug of first choice in patients with PSVT because its short duration of action will not cause

Symptoms

Severe

Mild

Narrow QRS, regular

Wide QRS, regular

Wide QRS, irregular

AVNRT or othrodromic AVRT?

VT or antidromic AVRT?

AF with AP?

DCC

Verapamil, diltiazem, or adenosine

Adenosine or procainamide

Procainamide

Acute termination

AVNRT or AVRT

Definitive diagnosis (ECG, EPS)

Mild and infrequent episodes

Severe or frequent episodes

No therapy

PRN AAD

AVN modification or AP ablation

Chronic prevention

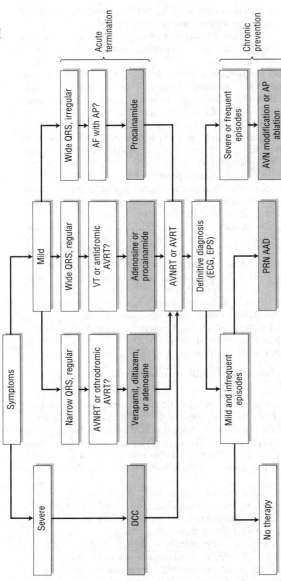

Figure 5–2. Algorithm for the treatment of acute (top portion) PSVT and chronic prevention of recurrences (bottom portion). DCC, direct current cardioversion; AVNRT, AV nodal reentrant tachycardia; AVRT, AV reentrant tachycardia; AVRT, AV reentrant tachycardia VT, ventricular tachycardia; AF, atrial fibrillation; AP, accessory pathway; ECG, electrocardiographic monitoring; EPS, electrophysiologic studies; PRN, as needed; AAD, antiarrhythmic drugs; AVN, AV node.AVN, AV node.

Note: For empiric bridge therapy prior to radiofrequency ablation procedures, calcium antagonists (or other AV nodal blockers) should not be used if the patient has AV reentry with an accessory pathway.

prolonged hemodynamic compromise in patients with wide QRS complexes who actually have VT rather than PSVT.

- After acute PSVT is terminated, long-term preventive treatment is indicated if frequent episodes necessitate therapeutic intervention, or episodes are infrequent but severely symptomatic. Serial testing of antiarrhythmic agents can be evaluated in the ambulatory setting via ambulatory ECG recordings (Holter) or telephonic transmissions of cardiac rhythm (event monitors), during hospitalization with Holter monitoring or telemetry, or by invasive electrophysiologic techniques in the laboratory. II
- Chronic antiarrhythmic drug treatment in young, otherwise healthy patients is problematic because of possible necessity of life-long daily medication, poor tolerability, occasionally severe side effects, and frequent lack of efficacy.
- Transcutaneous catheter ablation using radio frequency (rf) current on the PSVT substrate should be considered in any patient who would have previously been considered for chronic antiarrhythmic drug treatment. It is highly effective and curative, rarely results in complications, and obviates the need for chronic antiarrhythmic drug therapy.

AUTOMATIC ATRIAL TACHYCARDIAS

- Underlying precipitating factors should be corrected by ensuring proper oxygenation and ventilation, and by correcting acid–base or electrolyte disturbances.
- If tachycardia persists, the need for additional treatment is determined by symptoms. Patients with asymptomatic atrial tachycardia and relatively slow ventricular response usually require no drug therapy.
- If patients are symptomatic, medical therapy can be tailored either to control ventricular response or to restore sinus rhythm. Calcium antagonists (e.g., verapamil) are considered first-line drug therapy. Intravenous magnesium (independent of serum magnesium) can also be effective. Both probably act by suppressing calcium-mediated triggered activity.

VENTRICULAR PREMATURE BEATS

- In apparently healthy individuals, drug therapy is unnecessary because VPBs without associated heart disease carry little or no risk. If drug therapy is necessary, β blockers are the drugs of choice because they are generally better tolerated than type I agents and decrease mortality, particularly after myocardial infarction.

VENTRICULAR TACHYCARDIA

Acute Ventricular Tachycardia

- Initial management of an acute episode of VT requires a quick assessment of the patient's status and symptoms. If severe symptoms are present, then DCC should be instituted to restore sinus rhythm immediately. Precipitating factors should be corrected. If VT is an isolated electrical event associated with a transient initiating factor (e.g., acute myocardial ischemia, digitalis toxicity), then lidocaine should be administered and continued for 24–48 hours or until the patient is stable. There is no need for long-term antiarrhythmic therapy after precipitating factors are corrected.

- Patients with mild or no symptoms can be treated initially with antiarrhythmic drugs. Lidocaine (1–2 mg/kg loading dose followed by 2 mg/min infusion) is usually the drug of choice because of effectiveness, quick onset, and ease of administration. If lidocaine fails to terminate tachycardia, IV procainamide (loading dose and infusion) can be tried. DCC should be instituted or a transvenous pacing wire should be inserted if the patient's status deteriorates, VT degenerates to VF, or drug therapy fails.

Sustained Ventricular Tachycardia

- Chronic recurrent sustained VT deserves attention because of the high risk of death; trial-and-error attempts are unwarranted. Neither electrophysiologic studies nor Holter monitoring is ideal. These findings and the side-effect profiles of antiarrhythmic agents have led to non-drug approaches.
- The implantable automatic cardioverter defibrillator (ICD) is becoming popular because it is highly effective in preventing sudden death due to recurrent VT or VF and because technologic advances have been introduced that, for example, obviate the need for thoracotomy. Limitations include high cost of the device and of implantation, ultimate need for antiarrhythmic drugs (usually amiodarone) in up to 50% of patients, and lack of clear evidence of decrease in overall mortality.
- Patients with complex ventricular ectopy should not be treated with traditional (type I or III) antiarrhythmic drugs.

Nonsustained Ventricular Tachycardia

- The approach to NSVT is controversial. Obviously, patients with long symptomatic episodes require drug therapy, but most are asymptomatic. Epidemiologic data indicate that patients with NSVT and coronary disease are at risk for sudden death, particularly if they have inducible sustained tachycardias on invasive electrophysiologic studies. Serial drug testing can be used to stratify patients at increased risk. Noninvasive tools are an alternate approach to risk stratification; abnormal signal-averaged ECG is a significant risk factor for subsequent arrhythmia (sustained VT) or sudden death. Large prospective trials are necessary and ongoing to discern the proper approach to NSVT.

PROARRHYTHMIA

- Proarrhythmia is resistant to resuscitation with cardioversion or overdrive pacing. Some clinicians have had success with IV lidocaine or sodium bicarbonate.

TORSADES DE POINTES

- For an acute episode, most patients require and respond to DCC. However, TdP tends to be paroxysmal and often recurs rapidly after countershock.
- IV magnesium sulfate is considered the drug of choice for preventing recurrences of TdP. If that is ineffective, strategies to increase heart rate and shorten ventricular repolarization should be instituted (i.e., temporary transvenous pacing at 105–120 beats/min or pharmacologic pacing with isoproterenol or epinephrine infusion). Agents that prolong QT interval should be discontinued and exacerbating factors corrected. Drugs that further prolong repolarization (e.g., procainamide) are contraindicated. Lidocaine is usually ineffective.
- In heritable TdP, propranolol has been shown to prevent recurrences and sudden death. Because β blockers may not prevent all episodes of TdP, they are commonly employed with an ICD.
- In acquired long-QT syndromes, correction of underlying cause is crucial for successful preventive therapy. No drugs need be used chronically. In quinidine syncope, type Ia agents should be avoided as future treatment.

VENTRICULAR FIBRILLATION

- VF should be managed according to the American Heart Association's recommendations for advanced cardiac life support; additional details can be found in Chapter 6, Cardiopulmonary Resuscitation.

BRADYARRHYTHMIA DUE TO SINUS NODE DYSFUNCTION

- Treatment of sinus node dysfunction involves elimination of symptomatic bradycardia and possibly managing alternating tachycardias such as atrial fibrillation. Asymptomatic sinus bradyarrhythmias usually do not require therapeutic intervention.
- In general, long-term therapy of choice for patients with significant symptoms is a permanent ventricular pacemaker.
- Drugs commonly employed to treat supraventricular tachycardias should be used with caution, if at all, in the absence of a functioning pacemaker.
- Carotid-sinus hypersensitivity can also be treated with permanent pacemaker therapy. Patients who remain symptomatic may benefit from adding α-adrenergic stimulants (e.g., ephedrine), sometimes with β blockers to maximize α-sympathetic stimulation.
- Vasovagal syncope can usually be treated successfully with oral β blockers to inhibit the sympathetic surge that causes forceful ventricular contraction and precedes the onset of hypotension and bradycardia. Other drugs that have been used successfully (with or without β blockers) include scopolamine patches, α-adrenergic agonists, theophylline, dipyridamole, and disopyramide.

ATRIOVENTRICULAR BLOCK

- Temporary transvenous pacing is the cornerstone for acute treatment of symptomatic bradycardia or AV block. Until the right ventricular lead can be inserted, bridge therapy may include transcutaneous pacing devices or drugs that improve sinus and AV nodal conduction (e.g., atropine, epinephrine infusion). Atropine or sympathomimetics may improve symptoms and conduction in sinus bradycardia/arrest and AV nodal block, but they will not help if AV block is below the AV node (Mobitz II or trifascicular AV block).
- Chronic symptomatic AV block should be treated by inserting a permanent pacemaker.
- Patients without symptoms usually can be followed closely without a pacemaker.

▶ EVALUATION OF THERAPEUTIC OUTCOMES

- The most important monitoring parameters fall into the following categories: (1) mortality (total and arrhythmic), (2) arrhythmia recurrence (duration, frequency, and symptoms), (3) hemodynamic consequences (rate, blood pressure, and symptoms), and (4) treatment complications (need for alternative or additional drugs, devices, or surgery).
- Presence or recurrence of any arrhythmia can be documented by ECG means (e.g., surface ECG, Holter monitor, event monitor).
- Some therapeutic outcomes are unique to certain arrhythmias. For instance, patients with atrial fibrillation or flutter need to be monitored for thromboembolism and for complications of anticoagulation therapy (bleeding or drug interactions).

See Chapter 14, Arrhythmias, authored by Jerry L. Bauman, PharmD, BCPS, FCCP, FACC and Marieke Dekker Schoen, PharmD, BCPS, for a more detailed discussion of this topic.

Chapter 6

▶ CARDIOPULMONARY RESUSCITATION

▶ DEFINITION

Cardiopulmonary arrest occurs when spontaneous and effective ventilation and circulation abruptly terminate following a cardiac or respiratory event.

▶ PATHOPHYSIOLOGY

- Cardiac arrhythmias, such as ventricular tachycardia (VT) and ventricular fibrillation (VF), are the usual cause of sudden cardiac death. Other presenting arrhythmias include bradyarrhythmias, asystole, and pulseless electrical activity (PEA).
- Although approximately 80–90% of nontraumatic cardiac arrests are initiated by either VT or VF, only 35–55% of patients with out-of-hospital cardiac arrests are actually found to be in VF or VT. These statistics are relevant because the survival rate to hospital discharge is higher for patients found initially in VF or VT versus that of patients in asystole or PEA (20% versus 1–7%).
- Two theories exist regarding the mechanism of blood flow in cardiopulmonary resuscitation (CPR). The initial theory, known as the cardiac pump theory, explains forward blood flow based on active compression of the heart between the sternum and vertebrae. After the discovery of cough CPR, the thoracic pump theory was founded on the belief that blood flow during CPR results from intrathoracic pressure alterations induced by chest compressions. In reality, components of both theories may operate during CPR.
- Acid–base imbalances result from decreased perfusion and ineffective ventilation. Despite CPR, which raises cardiac output to approximately 30% of baseline, anaerobic metabolism predominates and raises P_{CO_2} concentrations. Elimination of P_{CO_2} is hampered by diminished blood flow.

▶ CLINICAL PRESENTATION

- Termination of spontaneous and effective ventilation and circulation may be preceded by cardiac symptoms, easy fatigability, or nonspecific complaints lasting days to months.
- The onset of cardiac arrest may be characterized by typical symptoms of an acute cardiac event (e.g., prolonged angina or pain of myocardial infarction), acute dyspnea or orthopnea, palpitations, or light-headed-

ness. Alternatively, the onset may occur without warning. Loss of consciousness and pulse are sine qua nons in cardiac arrest.

▶ DIAGNOSIS

- Rapid diagnosis is vital to the success of CPR. Patients must receive early intervention to prevent cardiac rhythms from degenerating into less treatable arrhythmias.
- Cardiac arrest is diagnosed initially by observation of clinical manifestations consistent with cardiac arrest. The diagnosis is confirmed by evaluating vital signs, especially heart rate and respirations.
- Electrocardiography (ECG) is useful for determining the cardiac rhythm, which in turn determines drug therapy.

▶ DESIRED OUTCOME

- Successful CPR comprises restoration of effective ventilation and stable heart rate, cardiac rhythm, and blood pressure [systolic blood pressure (SBP) >70 mm Hg]. To truly be successful, patients should remain neurologically intact with minimal morbidity.
- After successful resuscitation, the primary goals include optimizing tissue oxygenation, identifying the precipitating cause(s) of arrest, and preventing subsequent episodes.

▶ TREATMENT (Figure 6–1)

GENERAL PRINCIPLES

- The philosophies for providing CPR and emergency cardiac care have been organized and updated by the American Heart Association (AHA). The following guidelines are taken primarily from the 1997 update (see Figure 6–1).
- Factors proven to enhance prehospital survival include occurrence of a witnessed arrest, presence of VT or VF, rapid implementation of bystander CPR, early administration of defibrillation therapy for VF, and early application of prehospital advanced cardiac life support (ACLS).
- Basic life support is based on the assessment and application of the ABCs: airway, breathing, and circulation. If spontaneous breathing is absent, the airway should be opened and rescue breathing attempted. If the victim is pulseless, closed-chest compressions should be combined with rescue breathing. Basic life support should be continued until spontaneous circulation returns, ACLS is obtained, or exhaustion prohibits continued efforts.
- ACLS incorporates CPR, electrical defibrillation, airway management, ECG monitoring, and drug administration.

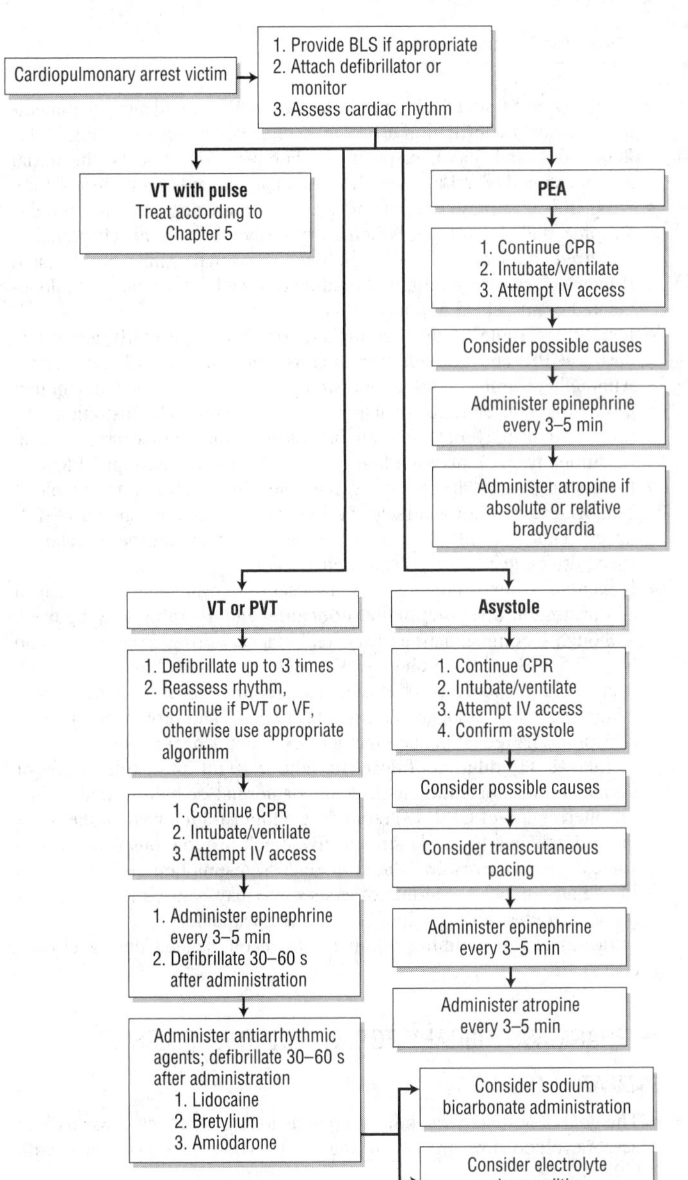

Figure 6–1. Treatment algorithm for adult cardiopulmonary arrest. *(Adapted from 1997–1999 Emergency Cardiovascular Care Programs, Advanced Cardiac Life Support. American Heart Association, 1997.)*

- Adult patients found in either pulseless VT or VF should receive immediate electrical defibrillation using up to three countershocks using 200 J, 200–300 J, and 360 J, respectively. For pediatric patients, the initial attempt should be 2 J/kg, and all subsequent attempts should use 4 J/kg.
- Drug therapy may consist of sympathomimetics, antiarrhythmics, atropine, and electrolytes, which are described later in this chapter. The preferred intravenous (IV) solution is normal saline or lactated Ringer's. Dextrose solutions should be reserved for patients with documented or suspected hypoglycemia.
- Ideally, the route of drug administration should be easily accessible during CPR and provide rapid entry into the central circulation. Although central venous administration results in earlier and higher peak drug concentrations than peripheral venous administration, the former route may not be available early in the cardiac arrest event. Additionally, attempts to obtain central access may interrupt CPR.
- Peripheral venous access, using the antecubital vein, is acceptable if central access is not available. Peripheral IV injections should be followed with a 20-mL fluid bolus; the extremity should be elevated to speed drug entry into the central circulation.
- If neither central nor peripheral access is available, endotracheal administration of **epinephrine, lidocaine,** and **atropine** may be used. Although recommendations vary, endotracheal doses in adults should be 2–2.5 times corresponding IV doses. Increased drug effects may occur when spontaneous circulation returns because endotracheal administration is associated with delayed onset and prolonged duration of action. The recommended method for endotracheal administration is as follows: (1) dilution of dose (for adults: 10 mL of distilled water or normal saline; for children: 1–2 mL of normal or half-normal saline, (2) interruption of CPR, (3) rapid drug administration beyond the tip of the endotracheal tube, (4) three to five quick insufflations using a bag-valve device to aerosolize the drug, and (5) resumption of CPR.
- In pediatric patients, the intraosseous route may be used temporarily if no other routes of drug administration are available.
- Intracardiac drug administration is not recommended during closed-chest CPR.

▶ PHARMACOTHERAPY FOR VF AND PULSELESS VT

SYMPATHOMIMETICS

- The goal of adrenergic agonist therapy is to augment both coronary and cerebral blood flow present during the low-flow state associated with CPR.
- Although the optimal adrenergic agent has not been identified, **epinephrine** (an α_1, α_2, β_1, and β_2 agonist) is recommended as first-line pharmacologic therapy in the treatment of VF, pulseless VT, asystole, and PEA.

- The standard adult dose of epinephrine is 1 mg (10 mL of 1:10,000 solution) administered by intravenous push (IVP) every 3–5 minutes. If the initial 1-mg dose is unsuccessful, alternative doses are 2–5 mg IVP every 3–5 minutes; 1 mg, 3 mg, 5 mg IVP given 3 minutes apart; or 0.1 mg/kg IVP every 3–5 minutes.
- The standard initial pediatric dose of epinephrine is 0.01 mg/kg (0.1 mL of a 1:10,000 solution). If the initial dose is unsuccessful, alternative doses are 0.1 mg/kg (0.1 mL/kg of a 1:1000 solution) up to a maximum of 0.2 mg/kg (0.2 mL/kg of a 1:1000 solution).
- Although higher doses may increase the initial resuscitation success rate, they do not improve survival to hospital discharge or neurologic outcome.
- **Norepinephrine** (an α_1, α_2, β_1 agonist) improves myocardial oxygen balance and regional cerebral blood flow compared with **epinephrine** in animals, but human studies have not confirmed this benefit.

ANTIARRHYTHMICS

- Antiarrhythmic agents are administered in the treatment of persistent pulseless VT or VF following unsuccessful defibrillation with initial epinephrine administration. The first-line antiarrhythmic agent is **lidocaine,** followed by **bretylium.** The selection of lidocaine over bretylium is based on the increased familiarity and preferred adverse effect profile of lidocaine, not on clinical trial evidence. Procainamide is no longer used due to the excessive time necessary for drug administration.
- Successive doses of antiarrhythmic agents should be administered at more frequent intervals during cardiac arrest to increase circulating blood concentrations and improve efficacy.

Lidocaine

- The initial adult dose of lidocaine is 1.5 mg/kg by IVP. If defibrillation is unsuccessful, an additional 1.5-mg/kg bolus can be administered in 3–5 minutes for a total dose of 3 mg/kg. A continuous lidocaine infusion of 2–4 mg/min should be started after the arrhythmia is suppressed.
- The recommended pediatric dose is 1 mg/kg. There are no recommendations for subsequent bolus doses if defibrillation is unsuccessful. If the arrhythmia is suppressed, a continuous infusion should be started at a rate of 20–50 μg/kg/min.
- **Lidocaine** may reduce arrhythmia recurrence following successful defibrillation. Plasma concentrations >6 μg/mL were necessary for antifibrillatory effects in an animal model.

Bretylium Tosylate

- For those patients nonresponsive to lidocaine, early administration of bretylium is desirable to increase the chance of successful defibrillation.

- The antiarrhythmic actions of bretylium result from a complex combination of direct myocardial and indirect adrenergic effects. Initially, bretylium administration potentiates norepinephrine release, which can be manifested clinically by increases in blood pressure, heart rate, and cardiac output, which may facilitate return of spontaneous circulation. Approximately 15–20 minutes after administration, bretylium blocks further release of norepinephrine, which may lead to hypotension and the need for fluids and vasopressors.
- In both adult and pediatric patients, the initial dose of bretylium is 5 mg/kg by IVP. The drug should be allowed to circulate for 1 or 2 minutes before defibrillation. If defibrillation is unsuccessful in pediatric patients, an additional bolus dose of 10 mg/kg may be administered. If defibrillation is unsuccessful in adults, subsequent bolus doses of 10 mg/kg may be administered at 5-minute intervals up to a total dose of 30–35 mg/kg. After the arrhythmia is suppressed, a continuous infusion may be initiated at 1–2 mg/min. If VT persists, 5–10 mg/kg should be diluted in 50 mL of fluid and infused over 8–10 minutes. Intravenous infusions should be used in conscious patients to avoid peak serum concentrations, which may induce nausea and vomiting.

Amiodarone

- **Amiodarone** is not currently included in the AHA treatment algorithm for VF or pulseless VT. However, once more experience is gained with its use in these situations, amiodarone may well replace bretylium as the preferred second-line agent based on its preferable side-effect profile.
- The initial adult dose is 150 mg given over 10 minutes, followed by a maintenance infusion given at a rate of 1 mg/min. After completing 6 hours of the maintenance infusion, the rate should be decreased to 0.5 mg/min. Supplemental rapid infusions (150 mg in 100 mL D_5W over 10 min) can be given for recurrent VT or VF. Infusions with concentrations exceeding 2 mg/mL should be given centrally to avoid phlebitis.
- The most frequently reported adverse events associated with IV amiodarone are hypotension (18–27%) and bradycardia (4–6%). Other acute effects include fever, elevated liver function tests, confusion, nausea, and thrombocytopenia. Amiodarone may elevate serum concentration of lidocaine and cyclosporine.

ALTERNATIVES FOR REFRACTORY VF OR VT

- Refractory ventricular arrhythmias may be associated with electrolyte abnormalities, primarily hyperkalemia, hypokalemia, and hypomagnesemia.
- **Calcium chloride** solution 10% should be administered IV at 4 mg/kg for known or suspected hyperkalemia (K^+ >6.0 mEq/L). **Sodium bicarbonate** 1 mEq/kg may also be given to drive potassium intracellularly.
- **Potassium** 10 mEq should be administered IV over 30 minutes for refractory VF and known or suspected hypokalemia.

- **Magnesium sulfate** 1–2 g should be diluted in 10 mL of fluid and administered IV over 1–2 minutes for refractory VF and known or suspected hypomagnesemia (Mg^{+2} <1.4 mEq/L). Caution should be used because rapid magnesium supplementation may produce significant hypotension or asystole.

▶ PHARMACOTHERAPY FOR ASYSTOLE AND PEA

- Patients with asystole should receive CPR, intubation, and IV access. Defibrillation should be avoided because it may increase parasympathetic tone, which, in turn, may worsen survival in patients with asystole. The primary pharmacologic agents are epinephrine and atropine.
- For the treatment of PEA, epinephrine should be administered after unsuccessful attempts to correct potential underlying disorders (hypoxia, hypovolemia, cardiac tamponade, tension pneumothorax, hypothermia, pulmonary embolism, drug overdose, hyperkalemia, acidosis, and acute myocardial infarction). Atropine may be used in the presence of absolute bradycardia (heart rate <60 beats/min).
- Recommended **epinephrine** doses are identical to those for VF and pulseless VT.
- **Atropine** should be initiated at a dose of 1 mg, which can be repeated at 3- to 5-minute intervals up to a total dose of 0.04 mg/kg (approximately 3 mg in a 70-kg adult). This recommendation differs from that for bradycardia, which begins with 0.5–1 mg up to a total dose of 0.03–0.04 mg/kg (approximately 2–3 mg in a 70-kg adult). In either case, doses <0.5 mg should be avoided in adults because of a potential paradoxical vagotonic effect. For pediatric patients with asystole, atropine should be initiated with a single dose of 0.02 mg/kg (recommended dosage range 0.1–0.5 mg in children; maximum dose 1 mg in adolescents). Doses may be repeated in 5-minute intervals to a maximum dose of 1 mg in children or 2 mg in adolescents.
- **Calcium** is only recommended for hyperkalemia, hypocalcemia, and calcium antagonist toxicity.

ACID–BASE MANAGEMENT DURING CPR

- **Sodium bicarbonate** has a limited role during CPR because it did not improve survival in clinical trials and may worsen acidosis. Selected patients may benefit from bicarbonate therapy if the following conditions are present: (1) known bicarbonate-responsive acidosis, (2) hyperkalemia, or (3) tricyclic antidepressant or phenobarbital overdose. Sodium bicarbonate may also be useful in cases with prolonged arrest times (i.e., >10 minutes); these patients should first receive adequate CPR, intubation, ventilation, and multiple epinephrine doses before sodium bicarbonate.
- The initial recommended dose of sodium bicarbonate for adults and children is 1 mEq/kg. Subsequent doses of 0.5 mEq/kg can be administered at 10-minute intervals.

▶ LONG-TERM STRATEGIES

- Education plays a pivotal role in long-term strategies to optimize CPR. All health care professionals should be proficient in current CPR procedures. Public awareness of the prevention of cardiovascular and cerebrovascular disease should be increased. Patients should be educated to identify early warning signs and symptoms so that medical care could be accessed earlier.

▶ EVALUATION OF THERAPEUTIC OUTCOMES

- To gauge the success of CPR, therapeutic outcome should be monitored throughout the attempt, after each intervention, and during the postresuscitation phase. Respiratory rate, heart rate, cardiac rhythm, and blood pressure should be assessed.
- The pharmacokinetic disposition of lidocaine may be altered because the primary determinant of clearance, hepatic blood flow, declines during cardiac arrest. In addition, the percentage of unbound lidocaine (free fraction) may be reduced. Toxicity may occur because of the aggressive lidocaine loading recommended by the AHA. Dosage reductions are suggested for maintenance infusions in patients with reduced cardiac output, hepatic dysfunction, or >70 years of age. Plasma lidocaine concentrations should be monitored during prolonged maintenance infusions. Patients should be assessed for adverse effects such as slurred speech, altered consciousness, muscle twitching, and seizures.
- Serum concentration monitoring is not useful with bretylium therapy because antifibrillatory activity correlates better with myocardial concentrations.
- Patients with persistent or recurrent VT or VF following antiarrhythmic administration should be assessed for electrolyte abnormalities.
- Blood gas analysis should be performed to guide administration of sodium bicarbonate.
- During the postresuscitation period, patients should receive a 12-lead ECG, chest x-ray, arterial blood gas, blood chemistry determinations, frequent vital signs, continuous ECG monitoring, and ventilatory support if necessary.
- Assessments of neurologic function that should be completed include (1) Glasgow Coma Scale determined at 24-hour postrecovery of spontaneous circulation, 6 months postevent, and 1 year postevent; and (2) Cerebral Performance Category recorded at hospital discharge, 6 months postevent, and 1 year postevent.

See Chapter 9, Cardiopulmonary Resuscitation, authored by Lori A. Jones, PharmD, for a more detailed discussion of this topic.

Chapter 7

▶ HEART FAILURE

▶ DEFINITION

Heart failure (HF) is a pathophysiologic state in which the heart is unable to pump blood at a rate sufficient to meet the metabolic needs of the body. The term heart failure is preferred over congestive heart failure because patients can have the clinical syndrome of heart failure without symptoms of congestion.

▶ PATHOPHYSIOLOGY

- HF can result from many cardiac diseases or disorders that alter systolic function, diastolic function, or both.
  - Causes of systolic dysfunction (i.e., decreased contractility) are dilated cardiomyopathies, ventricular hypertrophy, and reduction in muscle mass (e.g., myocardial infarction). Ventricular hypertrophy can be caused by pressure overload (e.g., systemic or pulmonary hypertension, aortic or pulmonic valve stenosis) or volume overload (e.g., valvular regurgitation, shunts, high-output states).
  - Causes of diastolic dysfunction (i.e., restricted ventricular filling) are increased ventricular stiffness, mitral or tricuspid valve stenosis, and pericardial disease (e.g., pericarditis, pericardial tamponade). Ventricular stiffness can be caused by ventricular hypertrophy, infiltrative diseases, and myocardial ischemia and infarction.
- The most common underlying etiologies are ischemic heart disease, hypertension, or both.
- As cardiac function decreases, the heart relies on the following compensatory mechanisms: (1) tachycardia and increased contractility through sympathetic nervous system activity; (2) the Frank–Starling mechanism, whereby increased preload increases stroke volume; (3) vasoconstriction; and (4) ventricular hypertrophy and remodeling. Although these compensatory mechanisms initially maintain cardiac function, they initiate vicious cycles that lead to continued worsening of HF.
- Neurohormones and autocrine/paracrine factors also play a role in compensatory responses. These substances include angiotensin II, norepinephrine, natriuretic peptides, arginine vasopressin, endothelin-1, and perhaps cytokines such as tumor necrosis factor α.
- Common precipitating factors that may cause a previously compensated patient to decompensate include noncompliance with diet or drug therapy, uncontrolled hypertension, administration of inappropriate or inadequate HF therapy, and arrhythmias.
- Drugs may precipitate or exacerbate HF because of negative inotropic or cardiotoxic effects, or because of sodium and water retention.

▶ CLINICAL PRESENTATION

- Clinical manifestations result from congestion developing behind the failing ventricle and therefore depend on whether failure is left or right sided (Table 7–1). Most patients initially have left ventricular failure, but both ventricles eventually fail because ventricles share a septal wall and because left ventricular failure increases right ventricular workload.
- Left ventricular failure causes signs and symptoms of pulmonary congestion. Associated signs and symptoms include dyspnea on exertion, orthopnea, paroxysmal nocturnal dyspnea, dyspnea at rest, and pulmonary edema.
- Right ventricular failure causes signs and symptoms consistent with systemic congestion. Peripheral edema is a cardinal finding in right-sided heart failure.

▶ DIAGNOSIS

- A diagnosis of HF should be considered in patients exhibiting characteristic signs and symptoms (Table 7–1).
- Ventricular hypertrophy can be demonstrated on chest x-ray or electrocardiogram (ECG).

TABLE 7–1. Signs and Symptoms of Heart Failure

Symptoms	Signs
Right ventricular dysfunction	
Abdominal pain	Peripheral edema
Anorexia	Jugular venous distension
Nausea	Hepatojugular reflux
Bloating	Hepatomegaly
Constipation	
Ascites	
Left ventricular dysfunction	
Dyspnea on exertion	Bibasilar rales
Paroxysmal nocturnal dyspnea	Pulmonary edema
Orthopnea	S_3 gallop
Tachypnea	Pleural effusion
Cough	Cheyne–Stokes respiration
Hemoptysis	
Nonspecific findings	
Exercise intolerance	Tachycardia
Fatigue	Pallor
Weakness	Cyanosis of digits
Nocturia	Cardiomegaly
CNS symptoms	

- The chest x-ray also provides a relatively specific but insensitive measure of the degree of pulmonary congestion.
- The most widely used classification system is the New York Heart Association (NYHA) Functional Classification System. Functional class (FC)-I patients have no limitation of physical activity, FC-II patients have slight limitation of physical activity, FC-III patients have marked limitation of physical activity, and FC-IV patients are unable to carry on physical activity without discomfort.

▶ DESIRED OUTCOME

Goals for the pharmacologic management of HF include improved symptoms and quality of life, reduced mortality, altered natural history of HF after symptoms are present, and prevention of progression to severe HF and cardiogenic shock. The treatment approach depends on the severity of HF and whether it is acute or chronic.

▶ TREATMENT OF ACUTE OR SEVERE HF

GENERAL PRINCIPLES

- Initial stabilization may require oxygen, mechanical ventilatory support, direct current cardioversion, or antiarrhythmic drugs if sustained tachyarrhythmias are present (see Figure 7–1). Temporary transvenous pacing may be necessary for significant bradyarrhythmias. Echocardiography is useful if physical examination cannot exclude structural abnormalities (e.g., tamponade, valvular insufficiency, intracardiac shunt).
- If the patient is manifesting inadequate systemic perfusion without pulmonary edema, intravascular volume expansion to increase preload is usually the first maneuver attempted to raise cardiac output. If this is ineffective, inotropic agents or vasodilators will be needed to improve perfusion.
- If systemic perfusion is adequate but the primary manifestation is pulmonary edema, careful reduction in end-diastolic pressure with venodilators is indicated. Short-acting, titratable agents (e.g., IV nitroglycerin) are preferable to avoid precipitous drops in filling pressure and further reduction in cardiac performance.
- If obstructive pathology is present (e.g., cardiac tamponade, mitral stenosis), volume expansion as tolerated and positive inotropes with vasoconstricting actions (if needed) are used to stabilize the patient until definitive therapy can be performed.
- If arterial impedance is high due to reflex vasoconstriction, small doses of arterial vasodilators often improve cardiac output. In the absence of high peripheral resistance, the response to vasodilators will be minimal and may critically reduce systemic perfusion pressure.

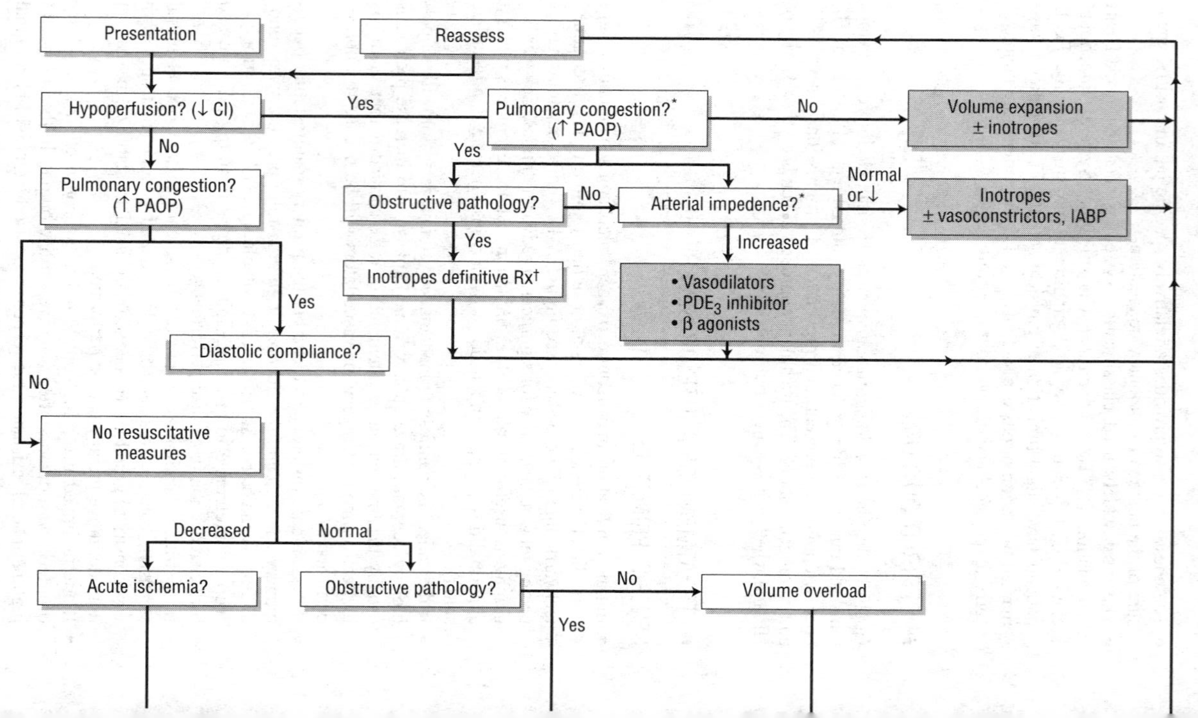
Presentation
Reassess
Hypoperfusion? (↓ CI)
Yes
No
Pulmonary congestion?*
(↑ PAOP)
No
Volume expansion
± inotropes
Yes
Pulmonary congestion?
(↑ PAOP)
Obstructive pathology?
No
Arterial impedence?*
Normal
or ↓
Inotropes
± vasoconstrictors, IABP
Yes
Increased
Inotropes definitive Rx†
• Vasodilators
• PDE3 inhibitor
• β agonists
Yes
Diastolic compliance?
No
No resuscitative
measures
Decreased
Normal
Acute ischemia?
Obstructive pathology?
No
Volume overload
Yes

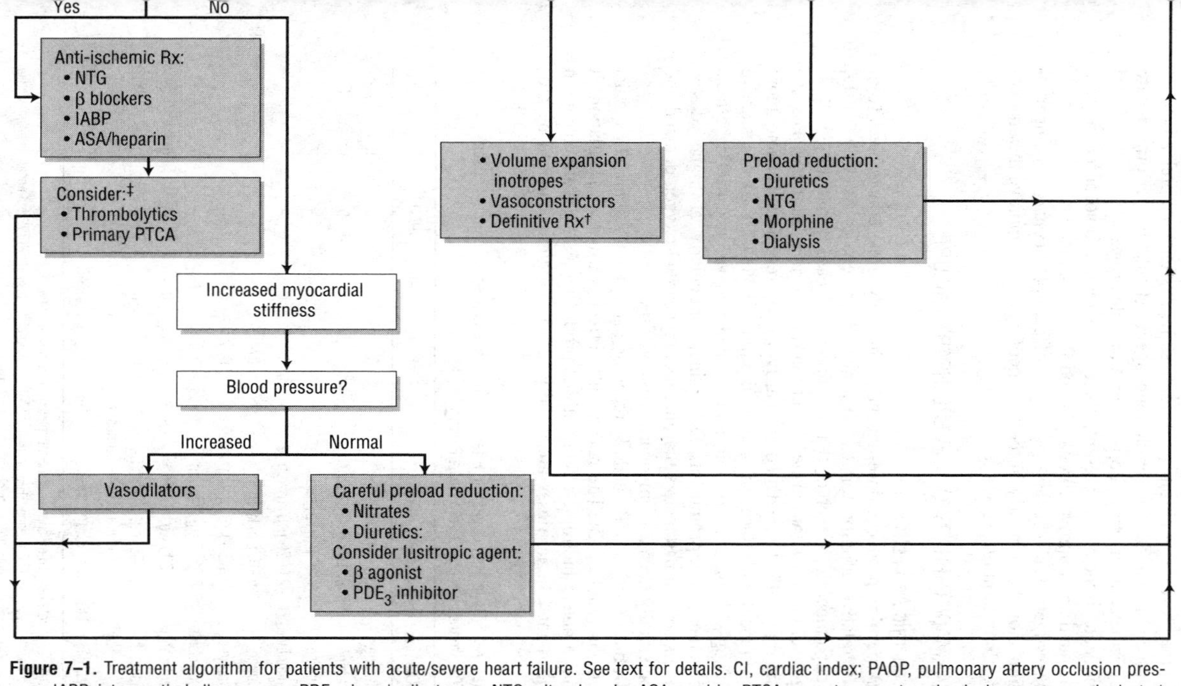

Figure 7–1. Treatment algorithm for patients with acute/severe heart failure. See text for details. CI, cardiac index; PAOP, pulmonary artery occlusion pressure; IABP, intra-aortic balloon pump; PDE, phosphodiesterase; NTG, nitroglycerin; ASA, aspirin; PTCA, percutaneous transluminal coronary angioplasty.* Evaluation for contributory ischemia is indicated.† See text for details or diagnostic methods/differential.‡ See chapter for indications.

- In the presence of chronic, severe diastolic dysfunction, preload reduction with venodilating or diuretic agents should be performed with extreme caution using short-acting, titratable drugs.
- If acute ischemia is present, therapy to reduce myocardial oxygen demand and improve coronary blood flow is paramount.
- Investigation of reversible etiologies of cardiopulmonary decompensation should begin early in the treatment course to improve the chances for long-term recovery.

PHARMACOTHERAPY OF SEVERE HEART FAILURE

Adrenergic Agonists

- **Dopamine** produces dose-dependent hemodynamic effects because of its relative affinity for α_1, β_1, and β_2 receptors as well as D_1 (dopaminergic) receptors. Low doses increase renal blood flow, glomerular filtration, urine output, natriuresis, and kaliuresis. Positive inotropic effects mediated primarily by β_1 receptors become more prominent with doses of 3–10 μg/kg/min (Table 7–2). At doses above 10 μg/kg/min, chronotropic and α_1-mediated vasoconstricting effects become more prominent. Dopamine, particularly at higher doses, alters several parameters that increase myocardial oxygen demand and potentially decreases myocardial blood flow.
- **Dobutamine** is a β_1 and β_2 receptor agonist with some α_1 agonist effects (Table 7–2). The net vascular effect is usually vasodilation. It has a potent inotropic effect without producing a significant change in heart rate. Initial doses are usually 2.5–5 μg/kg/min and can be pro-

TABLE 7–2. Usual Hemodynamic Effects of Intravenous Agents Commonly Used for Treatment of Acute/Severe Heart Failure[a]

Drug	Dose	HR	MAP	PAOP	CO	SVR
Dopamine	0.5–3 μg/kg/min	0	0	0	0/+	–
Dopamine	3–10 μg/kg/min	+	+	0	+	0
Dopamine	> 10 μg/kg/min	+	+	+	+	+
Dobutamine	2.5–20 μg/kg/min	0/+	0	–	+	–
Amrinone	5–10 μg/kg/min	0/+	0/–	–	+	–
Milrinone	0.375–0.75 μg/kg/min	0/+	0/–	–	+	–
Nitroprusside	0.25–3 μg/kg/min	0/+	0/–	–	+	–
Nitroglycerin	5–200 μg/min	0/+	0/–	–	0/+	0/–
Furosemide	20–80 mg, repeated as needed up to 4–6 times/d	0	0	–	0	0
Enalaprilat	1.25–2.5 mg q6–8h	0	0/–	–	+	+

[a]See text for a more detailed description of the interpatient variability in response.
+, increase; –, decrease; 0, no change; HR, heart rate; MAP, mean arterial pressure; PCWP, pulmonary capillary wedge pressure; CO, cardiac output; SVR, systemic vascular resistance.

gressively increased to 20 μg/kg/min or higher based on clinical and hemodynamic responses.

- There are hemodynamic differences between dopamine and dobutamine because of differences in their binding affinities for adrenergic receptors. Dobutamine increases cardiac index because of inotropic stimulation, arterial vasodilation, and a variable increase in heart rate. Dobutamine increases heart rate and mean arterial pressure less than dopamine.
- Attenuation of dobutamine's hemodynamic effects has been reported after 72 hours of continuous infusion.
- Some patients have sustained hemodynamic and clinical benefits for several days or months after a treatment course of dobutamine despite its 2.5-minute half-life. The potential for increased mortality, however, raises serious concerns about the chronic use of intermittent dobutamine infusions.

- **Norepinephrine** displays primary β_1 and α_1 agonist effects, with little or no β_2 effect. It is a suboptimal agent in most patients with severe HF because it has virtually no vasodilatory effect, and the combination of profound arteriolar constriction and tachycardia can result in excessive afterload reduction and arrhythmias when used alone. It should be reserved for profoundly hypotensive patients, preferably in combination with a vasodilating drug. The drug is given in doses of 0.1 to 1 μg/kg/min, titrated to the desired effect.
- **Epinephrine** has both α and β effects. It is rarely used in patients with HF.

Phosphodiesterase Inhibitors

- Phosphodiesterase inhibitors have positive inotropic and vasodilating effects and are sometimes called inodilators.
- The bipyridine derivatives **amrinone** and **milrinone** have similar pharmacologic and hemodynamic effects after IV administration. In patients with heart failure, their hemodynamic effects generally resemble those of dobutamine. The most consistent difference is a greater increase in heart rate with dobutamine.
- After IV administration, amrinone or milrinone increases cardiac index primarily because of an increase in stroke volume with little change in heart rate (Table 7–2). Amrinone and milrinone also decrease PAOP and thus are particularly useful in patients with a low cardiac index and an elevated end-diastolic pressure. This decrease in preload, however, can be hazardous for patients without excessive filling pressure, leading to a decrease in cardiac index.
- Amrinone and milrinone should not be used as single agents in patients with heart failure who have severe hypotension because these drugs will not increase, and may even decrease, arterial blood pressure.
- The mean terminal half-life of milrinone in patients with heart failure is 2.3 hours, whereas that of amrinone ranges from 2 to 4 hours in healthy subjects and up to 12 hours in patients with severe heart failure.

- The usual loading dose of amrinone is 0.75 mg/kg over 2–3 minutes, followed by a continuous infusion of 5–10 μg/kg/min. If the therapeutic response is inadequate, an additional loading dose of 0.75 mg/kg may be repeated after 30 minutes. Maintenance doses >20 μg/kg/min do not produce additional hemodynamic benefits and clearly enhance toxicity.
- The recommended loading dose of milrinone is 50 μg/kg over 10 minutes, followed by a continuous infusion of 0.5 μg/kg/min (range: 0.375–0.75 μg/kg/min).
- Other than undesirable hemodynamic effects, adverse events associated with these drugs are arrhythmias and a dose-dependent, reversible thrombocytopenia. Milrinone is preferred over amrinone because of its better side effect profile (thrombocytopenia <0.5% vs. 2.4%). Patients receiving either drug should be monitored for signs of bleeding and have platelet counts determined before and during therapy.
- Generally, milrinone or amrinone should be considered for patients who have not responded adequately to dobutamine, dopamine, IV vasodilators, or a combination of these agents, or when hypertension is present.
- A combination of amrinone or milrinone with dopamine or dobutamine may be helpful in patients with dose-limiting adverse effects to single-day therapy.

Vasodilators

- Arterial vasodilators (e.g., hydralazine) act as impedance-reducing agents and typically increase cardiac output. Venous vasodilators (e.g., nitroglycerin) act as preload reducers by increasing venous capacitance, reducing symptoms of pulmonary congestion in patients with high cardiac filling pressures. Mixed vasodilators (e.g., nitroprusside, angiotensin-converting enzyme inhibitors) act on both arterial resistance and venous capacitance vessels, reducing congestive symptoms and increasing cardiac output.

Nitroprusside

- **Sodium nitroprusside** is a mixed arterial–venous vasodilator that acts directly on vascular smooth muscle to increase cardiac index and decrease venous pressure. Despite its lack of direct inotropic activity, nitroprusside exerts hemodynamic effects that are qualitatively similar to those of dobutamine, amrinone, and milrinone (Table 7–2); however, nitroprusside generally decreases PAOP, SVR, and blood pressure more than dobutamine.
- Hypotension is an important dose-limiting adverse effect of nitroprusside and other vasodilators. Therefore, nitroprusside is primarily used in patients who have a significantly elevated SVR.
- The combination of nitroprusside and dopamine or dobutamine is useful for patients with pulmonary edema and cardiogenic shock who fail to respond to either agent alone.

- Generally, nitroprusside will not adversely affect, and may improve, the balance between myocardial oxygen demand and supply. However, an excessive decrease in systemic arterial pressure can decrease coronary perfusion and worsen ischemia.
- Nitroprusside has a rapid onset and a duration of action of <10 minutes, which necessitates use of continuous IV infusions. Nitroprusside should be initiated at a low dose (i.e., 0.1–0.25 μg/kg/min) to avoid excessive hypotension, and then increased by small increments (i.e., 0.1–0.2 μg/kg/min) every 5–10 minutes as needed and tolerated. Usually effective doses range from 0.5–3.0 μg/kg/min. Because of a rebound phenomenon after abrupt withdrawal of nitroprusside in patients with heart failure, doses should be tapered slowly when stopping nitroprusside therapy. Nitroprusside-induced cyanide and thiocyanate toxicity are unlikely when doses <3 μg/kg/min are administered for <3 days.

Nitroglycerin

- The major hemodynamic effects of **nitroglycerin** are decreased preload and PAOP due to its venous vasodilation. Nitroglycerin also has mild arterial vasodilating effects, which generally lead to a relatively small increase in cardiac index compared to that of inotropic agents. Combination therapy with nitroglycerin and dobutamine or dopamine is appealing because of complementary effects to increase cardiac index and decrease PAOP.
- Nitroglycerin should be initiated at 5–10 μg/min (0.1 μg/kg/min) and increased progressively every 5–10 minutes as necessary and tolerated. Maintenance doses usually vary from 35–200 μg/min (0.5–3.0 μg/kg/min). Some tolerance develops in most patients over 12–72 hours.

Enalaprilat

- Like other ACE inhibitors, IV **enalaprilat** is a mixed arterial–venous dilator but has a faster onset of action than oral drugs in this class. It should be used mainly for the short-term management of relatively stable patients who cannot take oral medication or to initiate ACE inhibitor therapy later in a treatment course to facilitate weaning from nitroprusside or inodilator therapy. The usual dose is 1.25–2.5 mg every 6–8 hours.

Diuretics

- **Furosemide** is the most widely used and studied IV loop diuretic for acute or severe HF. Others are ethacrynic acid, bumetanide, and torsemide.
- Bolus administration of diuretics decreases preload by functional venodilation within 5–15 minutes and later (>20 min) via salt and water excretion, thereby improving pulmonary congestion. However, acute reductions in venous return may severely compromise effective preload in patients with significant diastolic dysfunction or intravascular depletion.

- Because diuretics can cause excessive preload reduction, they must be used judiciously to obtain the desired improvement in congestive symptoms while avoiding a reduction in cardiac output.
- Diuresis may be improved by adding a second diuretic with a different mechanism of action (e.g., combining a loop diuretic with a distal tubule blocker such as **metolazone** or **hydrochlorothiazide**). Combination therapy should generally be reserved for inpatients who can be closely monitored for the development of severe sodium, potassium, and volume depletion. Very low doses of the thiazide-type diuretic should be used in the outpatient setting to avoid serious adverse events.

MECHANICAL CIRCULATORY SUPPORT

- The intra-aortic balloon pump (IABP) is the most widely used form of mechanical circulatory assistance and is typically used in patients with acute/severe HF who do not respond adequately to positive inotropic agents and vasodilators.
- IABP support increases cardiac index and coronary perfusion with decreased myocardial oxygen demand.
- IV vasodilators and inotropic agents are generally used in conjunction with the IABP to maximize hemodynamic and clinical benefits.

SURGICAL THERAPY

- Orthotopic cardiac transplantation is the best therapeutic option for patients with chronic irreversible NYHA Class IV HF, with a 5-year survival of approximately 75% in well-selected patients.
- New surgical techniques, including ventricular aneurysm resection, ventricular myoplasty, and latissimus dorsi wraps have shown variable degrees of symptomatic improvement.

▶ TREATMENT OF CHRONIC HF

GENERAL PRINCIPLES

- The first step in management of chronic HF is to determine the etiology or precipitating factors so that underlying disorders can be treated.
- Important nonpharmacologic interventions include cardiac rehabilitation and restriction of dietary sodium.
- An algorithm for treatment of chronic heart failure is shown in Figure 7–2.

VASODILATORS

- Because they have been shown to positively impact all therapeutic goals in HF, all patients with symptomatic HF should receive either an ACE inhibitor or hydralazine/nitrate combination.

Angiotensin-Converting Enzyme Inhibitors

- ACE inhibitors cause arterial and venous dilatation, thus reducing both preload and afterload (Table 7–3). Hemodynamic effects observed with

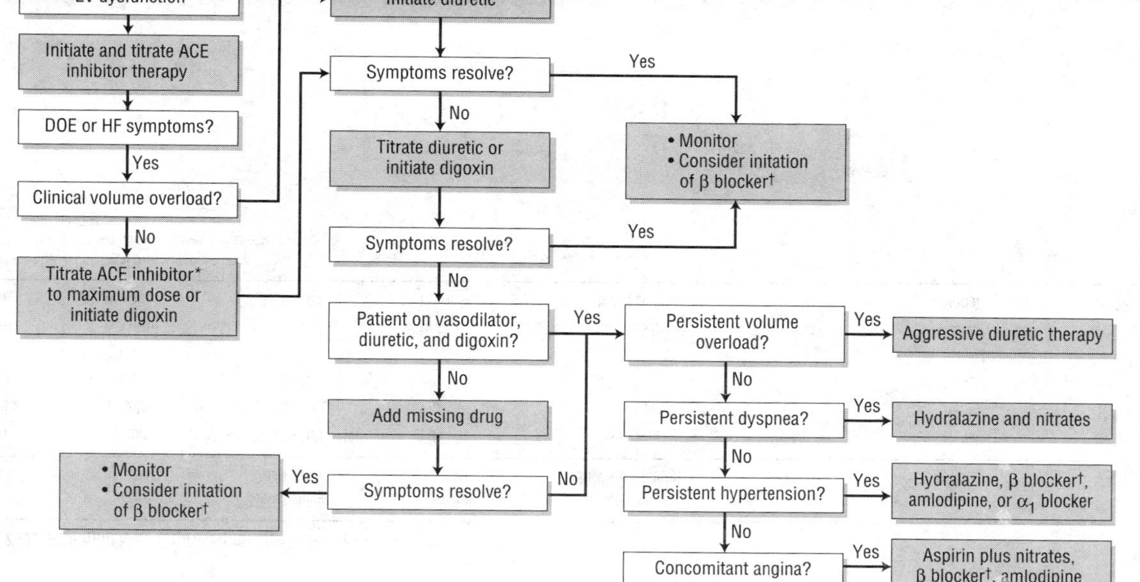

Figure 7–2. Treatment algorithm for patients with chronic heart failure. See text for details. Abbreviations: LV, left ventricular; ACE, angiotensin-converting enzyme; DOE, dyspnea on exertion; HF, heart failure. *If ACEI not started when LV dysfunction recognized, start now. If ACEI not started previously due to contraindication or patient intolerance, initiate hydralazine and nitrates now. †Initiation of ß blocker should be with appropriately low doses with slow, upward titration.

TABLE 7–3. ACE Inhibitors Approved for Use in Heart Failure

Generic Name	Brand Name	Usual Daily Dose (mg)	Dosing Frequency	Target Dosing—Survival Benefit[a]	Prodrug	Elimination[b]	$t_{1/2}$ (h)
Captopril	Capoten	18.75–150	tid	50 mg tid	No	Renal	2
Enalapril	Vasotec	2.5–40	bid	10 mg bid	Yes	Renal	10[c]
Lisinopril	Zestril Prinivil	5–40	qd	10 mg qd	No	Renal	12[c]
Quinapril	Accupril	5–80	bid	No data	Yes	Renal	25[c]
Ramipril	Altace	1.25–20	qd or bid	5 mg bid	Yes	Renal	9–18[c]

tid, three times daily; bid, twice daily; qd, once daily.

[a]Target doses associated with survival benefits in clinical trials.

[b]Primary route of elimination.

[c]Half-life of active metabolite.

long-term therapy include significant increases in cardiac index, stroke work index, and stroke volume index, as well as significant reductions in left ventricular filling pressure, SVR, MAP, and heart rate. II

- In clinical studies, ACE inhibitors significantly improved clinical status, functional class, exercise tolerance, left ventricular size, and mortality.
- ACE inhibitors may also prevent the development of HF in properly selected, high-risk patients, such as the recovery phase after acute myocardial infarction.

Nitrates and Hydralazine

- The predominant hemodynamic effect of nitrates is to reduce preload, although a slight reduction in SVR may be seen.
- **Isosorbide dinitrate (ISDN)** is the most extensively studied nitrate product for HF. The usual dose of ISDN is 40 mg (range: 20–80 mg) every 6 hours.
- The best alternative for minimizing nitrate tolerance appears to be 8- to 12-hour nitrate-free intervals.
- **Hydralazine** is a direct-acting vasodilator that acts predominantly on arterial smooth muscle and reduces SVR with resultant increases in stroke volume index and cardiac index; effects on preload are minimal. Average doses range from 200–300 mg/d, but doses as high as 3000 mg have been used.
- To achieve both preload and afterload reduction, the two vasodilators are frequently combined. Hydralazine 300 mg/d plus ISDN 160 mg/d (both given in divided doses) significantly reduced mortality in NYHA FC-II and FC-III patients in the Veterans Administration Cooperative Study (Vasodilators in Heart Failure Trial, VHeFT-I).
- Adverse effects to both nitrates and hydralazine are common, which limits use of this combination in many patients.
- The hydralazine–nitrate combination should be considered in the management of HF in two situations: (1) patients with symptomatic HF who are unable to take ACE inhibitors; and (2) patients who remain symptomatic despite optimal doses of an ACE inhibitor.

DIURETICS

- Diuretics decrease edema and pulmonary congestion by reducing preload. Diuretic therapy is indicated for all patients with evidence of fluid retention.
- Thiazide diuretics are relatively weak diuretics and are used infrequently in HF.
- Loop diuretics (e.g., **furosemide, bumetanide**) are the most widely used diuretics for HF. In addition to acting in the thick ascending limb of the loop of Henle, loop diuretics induce a prostaglandin-mediated increase in renal blood flow. Coadministration of nonsteroidal anti-inflammatory drugs (NSAIDs) blocks this effect and can diminish diuretic response.

- Diuretic dosages are titrated according to symptoms and body weight. Typical daily doses of furosemide range from 40 to 240 mg given in one or two doses. Unlike thiazide diuretics, loop diuretics maintain their effectiveness in the presence of impaired renal function, although higher doses are often necessary.
- Hypokalemia, the most common metabolic disturbance associated with both thiazide and loop diuretics, may be exacerbated by hyperaldosteronism. Hypokalemia is especially worrisome because it can precipitate ventricular arrhythmias in HF patients, especially if they are also taking digoxin.
- Hypomagnesemia is also common with diuretic therapy; it also increases the risk of arrhythmias.
- Resistance to diuretic therapy may be mediated by pharmacokinetic or pharmacodynamic mechanisms, or both.
  - Absorption of furosemide from the gut may be reduced or delayed, which can be overcome by giving the diuretic orally in larger doses or intravenously.
  - Although the pharmacodynamic mechanism is not clear, suppressed responses may be related to increased proximal and distal tubular sodium reabsorption. Maneuvers to overcome this resistance include treating the primary disease by other strategies (i.e., afterload reduction), giving low-dose dopamine to enhance diuresis, using larger IV bolus or continuous IV doses of furosemide, and adding a second diuretic with a different mechanism of action. Although the loop diuretic–thiazide combination is synergistic, this approach is generally reserved for the inpatient setting where the patient can be monitored closely because of the risk of profound diuresis and severe sodium, potassium, and volume depletion. Very low doses or only occasional doses of the thiazide-type diuretic should be used in the outpatient setting.

DIGITALIS GLYCOSIDES

- Questions about the role of **digitalis** in heart failure have been raised by flaws in and inconsistent results of controlled trials of digoxin, the controversy over the long-term use of positive inotropes, and the documented benefits of vasodilators. **Digoxin** appears to reduce hospitalizations and symptoms, but the Digitalis Investigation Group (DIG) trial showed neither beneficial nor adverse effects on all cause mortality.
- Digoxin therapy should be considered for two patient groups. First, in patients with left ventricular systolic dysfunction and supraventricular tachyarrhythmias such as atrial fibrillation, it should be considered early in therapy to help control ventricular response rate. Second, digoxin is indicated for patients in sinus rhythm who remain symptomatic after optimization of therapies known to improve survival. Digoxin is not first-line therapy for all patients in normal sinus rhythm because it does not improve survival.

- Most of the benefit from digoxin is achieved at low plasma concentrations. For most patients, the target plasma digoxin concentration should be approximately 1.0 ng/mL. Most patients can achieve this level with doses of 0.125–0.25 mg/d, although lower doses may be necessary in patients with significant renal impairment. In the absence of tachyarrhythmias, a loading dose is not indicated, because digoxin produces gradual effects over several hours, even after loading.

β BLOCKERS

- There is mounting evidence that stable patients initiated on low doses of a β blocker with upward dose titration over several weeks may derive significant benefits. Potential mechanisms proposed to explain these beneficial effects include blockade of detrimental effects of sympathetic stimulation, decreased sympathetic stimulation due to decreased plasma norepinephrine, and antiarrhythmic actions. They may also improve diastolic dysfunction by prolonging diastolic filling time.
- **Carvedilol** carries FDA approval for patients with NYHA FC-II or FC-III HF, added to standard therapy, to reduce disease progression and cardiovascular death, hospitalizations, and the need for upward titration of other HF medications. **Acebutolol, bisoprolol, labetalol, metoprolol,** and other β blockers have also been studied.
- β blockers have been documented to increase ejection fraction (EF) by 5–10 units (e.g., from an EF of 20% to 25–30%) without impairing exercise tolerance. Global assessments by physicians and patients also suggest symptomatic improvement. The drugs have positive effects on markers of HF progression, such as decreasing hospitalizations, need for increased HF medications, and heart transplantation. Although current data are inconclusive, several trials suggest that β blockers can improve survival in chronic HF.
- The recommended initial dose of carvedilol is 3.125 mg twice daily, with doubling of the dose every 2 weeks to the highest level tolerated or a target dose of 25 mg twice daily for those weighing up to 85 kg or 50 mg twice daily if over 85 kg.
- Current data suggest that β blockers should be strongly considered for patients with symptomatic HF with the primary goal of slowing disease progression.

ANGIOTENSIN II RECEPTOR ANTAGONISTS

- The angiotensin II receptor antagonists (e.g., **losartan, candesartan, irbesartan, valsartan**) block the angiotensin II receptor subtype AT_1, preventing the effects of angiotensin II, regardless of its origin. Thus, they offer a theoretical advantage over ACE inhibitors by more complete block of the effects of angiotensin II. However, their superiority in further reducing morbidity and mortality remains unproven.
- Until the results of ongoing trials are completed, these agents may be most useful in patients intolerant to ACE inhibitors due to severe cough

or those with persistent HF symptoms and/or hypertension despite maximal ACE inhibitor doses.

ANTIARRHYTHMIC THERAPY

- Antiarrhythmic therapy is appealing because sudden cardiac death, presumably due to ventricular arrhythmias, is the mode of death in up to 50% of HF patients.
- Class I antiarrhythmics should be avoided in all patients with left ventricular dysfunction.
- In contrast to other antiarrhythmic drugs, **amiodarone** does not appear to increase mortality, making it the first-line agent when antiarrhythmic therapy is needed (e.g., maintenance of sinus rhythm in HF patients with atrial fibrillation). However, the lack of proven benefit on survival and the potential for serious adverse effects argues against its routine use in this population.

▶ EVALUATION OF THERAPEUTIC OUTCOMES

- Patients should be monitored for signs and symptoms of HF caused by excess fluid retention (Table 7–1).
- Body weight should be monitored, especially in patients with chronic HF who receive diuretic therapy, because change in body weight is a sensitive marker of fluid status that reflects excess fluid retention or fluid loss.
- Critically ill patients should receive monitoring with ECG, continuous pulse oximetry, and automated sphygmomanometric blood pressure recording. Peripheral or femoral arterial catheters provide more accurate assessment of arterial pressure than cuff pressures in patients with severely depressed cardiac output.
- Initial stabilization in critically ill HF patients requires achievement of adequate arterial oxygen saturation and content ($SaO_2 \geq 90$, $CaO_2 \geq 18$ mL/dL).
- Adequate organ perfusion may be assessed by alert mental status, creatinine clearance sufficient to prevent metabolic azotemic complications, hepatic function adequate to maintain synthetic and excretory functions, a stable heart rate (generally between 50 and 110 beats/min) and rhythm, absence of ongoing myocardial ischemia or infarction, skeletal muscle and skin blood flow sufficient to prevent ischemic injury, and normal arterial pH (7.34–7.47) with a normal serum lactate concentration. These goals are most often achieved with a cardiac index >2.2 L/min/m^2, a mean arterial blood pressure >60 mm Hg, and PAOP ≤25 mm Hg.
- Invasive hemodynamic monitoring using a balloon-tipped, flow-directed pulmonary artery catheter has become a critically important tool in the management of patients with severe HF because the results can be used to guide selection of appropriate medical therapy.

- Improved peripheral perfusion can be evaluated by increased urine output, decreased peripheral vasoconstriction, and stronger peripheral pulses.

See Chapter 11, Heart Failure, authored by Julie A. Johnson, PharmD, BCPS, FCCP, Robert B. Parker, PharmD, FCCP, and Stephen A. Geraci, MD, for a more detailed discussion of this topic.

Chapter 8

▶ HYPERLIPIDEMIA

▶ DEFINITION

Hyperlipidemia is defined as an elevation of one or more of the following: cholesterol, cholesterol esters, phospholipids, or triglycerides. Abnormalities of plasma lipids can result in a predisposition to coronary artery disease, pancreatitis, xanthomas, and neurologic disease.

▶ PATHOPHYSIOLOGY

- Cholesterol, triglycerides, and phospholipids are transported as complexes of lipid and specialized proteins (apolipoproteins) known as lipoproteins. Elevated total and low density lipoprotein cholesterol (LDL-C) and reduced high density lipoprotein cholesterol (HDL-C) are associated with the development of coronary heart disease (CHD).
- The response-to-injury hypothesis states that risk factors such as oxidized LDL, mechanical injury to the endothelium, excessive homocysteine, immunologic attack, or infection-induced changes in endothelial and intimal function lead to endothelial dysfunction and a series of cellular interactions that culminate in atherosclerosis and eventually angina and myocardial infarction. Atherosclerotic lesions are thought to arise from transport and retention of plasma LDL-C through the endothelial cell layer into the extracellular matrix of the subendothelial space. Once in the artery wall, LDL is oxidized by various oxidative products produced locally. Mildly oxidized LDL then recruits monocytes into the artery wall. These monocytes then become transformed into macrophages that accelerate LDL oxidation.
- Oxidized LDL provokes an inflammatory response mediated by a number of chemoattractants and cytokines (e.g., monocyte colony-stimulating factor, intercellular adhesion molecule, platelet-derived growth factor, transforming growth factors, interleukin-1, interleukin-6).
- The extent of oxidation and the inflammatory response are under genetic control, and primary or genetic lipoprotein disorders have been classified into six categories commonly used for the phenotypical description of hyperlipidemia (Table 8–1). Secondary forms of hyperlipidemia also exist, and several drug classes may elevate lipid levels (e.g., progestins, β blockers, thiazide diuretics, corticosteroids).
- The primary defect in familial hypercholesterolemia is the inability to bind LDL to the LDL receptor (LDL-R) or, rarely, a defect of internalizing the LDL-R complex into the cell after normal binding. This leads to lack of LDL degradation by cells and unregulated biosynthesis of cholesterol, with total cholesterol and LDL-C being inversely proportional to the deficit in LDL receptors.

TABLE 8–1. Fredrickson–Levy–Lees Classification of Hyperlipoproteinemia

Type	Lipoprotein Elevation	Approximate Mean Lipid Elevation: *Cholesterol (mg/dL)*	*Triglycerides (mg/dL)*
I	Chylomicrons	324	3316
IIa	LDL[a]	368	148
IIb	LDL + VLDL	354	135
III	IDL (LDL_1)	441	694
IV	VLDL	251	438
V	VLDL + chylomicrons	373	2071

[a]Heterozygotes for familial hypercholesterolemia.

Adapted from Schafer EJ, Levy RI. Pathogenesis and management of lipoprotein disorders. *N Engl J Med* 1985; 312:1302.

▶ CLINICAL PRESENTATION

- Familial hypercholesterolemia is characterized by a selective elevation in plasma LDL and deposition of LDL-derived cholesterol in tendons (xanthomas) and arteries (atheromas).
- Familial lipoprotein lipase deficiency is characterized by a massive accumulation of chylomicrons and a corresponding increase in plasma triglycerides or a type I lipoprotein pattern. Presenting manifestations include repeated attacks of pancreatitis and abdominal pain, eruptive cutaneous xanthomatosis, and hepatosplenomegaly beginning in childhood. Symptom severity is proportional to dietary fat intake, and consequently to the elevation of chylomicrons. Accelerated atherosclerosis is not associated with this disease.
- Patients with familial type III hyperlipoproteinemia develop the following clinical features after age 20: xanthoma striata palmaris (yellow discolorations of the palmar and digital creases); tuberous or tuberoeruptive xanthomas (bulbous cutaneous xanthomas); and severe atherosclerosis involving the coronary arteries, internal carotids, and abdominal aorta.
- Type IV hyperlipoproteinemia is common and occurs primarily in adult patients who are obese, diabetic, and hyperuricemic and do not have xanthomas. It may be secondary to alcohol ingestion and can be aggravated by stress, progestins, oral contraceptives, thiazides, or β blockers.
- Type V (VLDL + chylomicrons) is characterized by abdominal pain, pancreatitis, eruptive xanthomas, and peripheral polyneuropathy. These patients are commonly obese, hyperuricemic, and diabetic; alcohol intake, exogenous estrogens, and renal insufficiency tend to be exacer-

bating factors. The risk of atherosclerosis is increased with this disorder.

▶ DIAGNOSIS

- Total cholesterol and HDL should be measured in all adults 20 years of age or older at least once every 5 years.
- Once hyperlipidemia is suspected, two major components of the evaluation are the history (including age, gender, and, if female, menstrual and estrogen replacement status) and physical examination and laboratory investigations.
- A complete history and physical exam should assess the following: (1) presence or absence of cardiovascular risk factors or definite cardiovascular disease in the individual; (2) family history of premature cardiovascular disease or lipid disorders; (3) presence or absence of secondary causes of hyperlipidemia, including concurrent medications; and (4) presence or absence of xanthomas, abdominal pain, or history of pancreatitis, renal or liver disease, peripheral vascular disease, or cerebral vascular disease (carotid bruits, stroke, or transient ischemic attack).
- Measurement of plasma cholesterol (which is about 3% lower than serum determinations), triglyceride, and HDL-C levels after a 12-hour or longer fast is important, because triglycerides may be elevated in nonfasted individuals; total cholesterol is only modestly affected by fasting.
- Two determinations, 1–8 weeks apart, with the patient on a stable diet and weight, and in the absence of acute illness, are recommended to minimize variability and to obtain a reliable baseline. If the total cholesterol is greater than 200 mg/dL, a second determination is recommended and, if the values are more than 30 mg/dL apart, the average of three values should be used.
- If the physical examination and history are insufficient to diagnose a familial disorder, then agarose-gel lipoprotein electrophoresis is useful to determine which class of lipoproteins is affected. If the triglyceride levels are below 400 mg/dL and neither type III hyperlipidemia nor chylomicrons are detected by electrophoresis, then one can calculate VLDL-C and LDL-C concentrations: VLDL-C = triglyceride/5; LDL-C = total cholesterol − (VLDL-C + HDL-C). Initial testing uses total cholesterol for case finding but subsequent management decisions should be based on LDL-C.
- Because total cholesterol is comprised of cholesterol derived from LDL, VLDL, and HDL, determination of HDL-C is useful when total plasma cholesterol is elevated. HDL-C may be elevated by moderate alcohol ingestion (less than 2 drinks per day), physical exercise, smoking cessation, weight loss, oral contraceptives, phenytoin, and terbutaline. HDL may be lowered by smoking, obesity, a sedentary lifestyle, and drugs such as β blockers.

- Diagnosis of lipoprotein lipase deficiency is based on low or absent enzyme activity with normal human plasma or apolipoprotein C-II, a cofactor of the enzyme. II

▶ DESIRED OUTCOME

- The goals of treatment are to reduce total and LDL cholesterol in order to prevent the development of new atherosclerotic plaques in coronary arteries, to halt progression of established lesions, and to induce the regression of existing lesions. Data from secondary and primary intervention trials also provide evidence that CHD morbidity and mortality as well as total mortality can be reduced with diet and drug therapy.

▶ TREATMENT

GENERAL GUIDELINES

- The Adult Treatment Panel II of the National Cholesterol Education Panel (NCEP) has recommended that total cholesterol determinations and risk factor assessment be used in the initial classification of adults (Table 8–2).
- If the total cholesterol is below 200 mg/dL and the HDL is higher than 35 mg/dL, no further follow-up is recommended for patients without known CHD and less than two risk factors (Table 8–3).
- In patients with borderline high blood cholesterol, assessment of risk factors is needed to more clearly define disease risk.
- When the serum total cholesterol is 200 mg/dL or higher, or when the HDL cholesterol is less than 35 mg/dL or at borderline high levels with two or more risk factors, a lipoprotein analysis (two measurements 1–8 weeks apart) to measure total and HDL cholesterol and triglycerides is recommended so that LDL-C may be estimated.
- Decisions regarding management are based on the LDL-C levels. The goals of therapy expressed as LDL-C levels and the level of initiation of diet and drug therapy are provided in Table 8–4. The extent of lipid

TABLE 8–2. Initial Classification of Cholesterol and Triglycerides

Classification	Total Cholesterol (mg/dL)	LDL Cholesterol (mg/dL)	HDL Cholesterol (mg/dL)	Triglycerides (mg/dL)
Desirable/normal	< 200	< 130	—	< 200
Borderline-high	200–239	130–159	—	200–400
High	≥ 240	> 160	> 60	400–1000
Very high	—	—	—	> 1000
Low	—	—	< 35	—

TABLE 8–3. Risk Status Based on Presence of CHD Risk Factors Other Than LDL Cholesterol[a]

Positive Risk Factors

Age

- Men: ≥ 45 years
- Women: ≥ 55 years or premature menopause without estrogen replacement therapy

Family history of premature CHD (definite myocardial infarction or sudden death before 55 years of age in father or other male first-degree relative, or before 65 years of age in mother or other female first-degree relative)

Current cigarette smoking

Hypertension (≥ 140/90 mm Hg or on antihypertensive medication)

Low HDL cholesterol (< 35 mg/dL)

Diabetes mellitus

Negative Risk Factor[b]

- High HDL cholesterol (≥ 60 mg/dL)

[a]High risk is defined as a net of two or more CHD risk factors or the presence of coronary or peripheral atherosclerosis.
[b]If the HDL cholesterol level is ≥ 60 mg/dL, subtract one risk factor, because high HDL cholesterol levels decrease CHD risk.

TABLE 8–4. Treatment Decisions Based on LDL Cholesterol

	Initiation Level (mg/dL)	LDL Goal (mg/dL)
Dietary Therapy		
Without CHD and < 2 risk factors	≥ 160	< 160
Without CHD and ≥ 2 risk factors	≥ 130	< 130
With CHD	> 100	≤ 100
	Consideration Level (mg/dL)	**LDL Goal (mg/dL)**
Drug Treatment		
Without CHD and < 2 risk factors	≥ 190[a]	< 160
Without CHD and ≥ 2 risk factors	≥ 160	< 130
With CHD	≥ 130[b]	≤ 100

[a]In men less than 35 years old and premenopausal women with LDL cholesterol levels of 190 to 219 mg/dL, drug therapy should be delayed except in high-risk patients such as those with diabetes.
[b]In patients with CHD and LDL cholesterol levels of 100 to 129 mg/dL, the clinician should excercise clinical judgment in deciding whether to initiate drug treatment.

reduction is related to CHD risk reduction, and the goals outlined in the tables should be considered as *minimal* goals. If possible, dietary means should be used to attain even lower LDL-C to achieve further reductions in CHD risk.

- Secondary forms of hyperlipidemia should be managed initially by correcting the underlying abnormality, including modification of drug therapy when appropriate.

DIETARY THERAPY

- The objectives of dietary therapy are to decrease progressively the intake of total fat, saturated fatty acids (i.e., saturated fat), and cholesterol and to achieve a desirable body weight.
- Dietary modification, weight control, and increased physical activity are essential first steps in the treatment of most lipid disorders. The recommended dietary approach is outlined in Table 8–5.
- The basic rationale for reducing dietary cholesterol, saturated fat, and excessive calories is based on the overproduction of VLDL and, subsequently, LDL. Excessive dietary intake of cholesterol and saturated fatty acids leads to decreased hepatic clearance of LDL and deposition of LDL and oxidized LDL in peripheral tissues.
- The predicted reduction in total serum cholesterol following institution of the step I diet is 3–14%, with average reductions of about 5–7% in men consuming 13–14% of their calories as saturated fat. Progressing

TABLE 8–5. Dietary Therapy of High Blood Cholesterol

Nutrient[a]	Step I Diet	Recommended Intake	Step II Diet
Total fat		≤ 30% of total calories	
Saturated fatty acids	8–10% of total calories		< 7% of total calories
Polyunsaturated fatty acids		Up to 10% of total calories	
Monounsaturated fatty acids		Up to 15% of total calories	
Carbohydrates		≥ 55% of total calories	
Cholesterol	< 300 mg/d		< 200 mg/d
Total calories		To achieve and maintain desirable body weight	

[a]Calories from alcohol not included.

to step II diet therapy should provide an additional reduction of about 3–7%.

- Each phase of the diet should be maintained for a minimum of 4–6 weeks for the minimal goal; however, the optimal response may not be seen for 3–6 months or more. In general, drug therapy should not be instituted until the trial of diet has continued for 6 months in primary prevention except in patients with severe forms of hyperlipidemia, those with two or more risk factors, or definite CHD.
- Reduction of cholesterol and saturated fat intake provides a reduction of CHD risk regardless of the time of intervention (primary versus secondary). Diet modification works adjunctively with other risk factor interventions, such as cessation of smoking and treating hypertension. Continuation of diet therapy is imperative if drug therapy is to be optimal.
- Increased intake of soluble fiber in the form of oat bran, pectins, certain gums, and psyllium products can result in useful adjunctive reductions in total and LDL cholesterol (5–20%), but these dietary alterations or supplements should not be substituted for more active forms of treatment. They have little or no effect on HDL-C or triglyceride concentrations. These products may also be useful in managing constipation associated with the bile acid sequestrants.
- Fish oil supplementation has a fairly large effect in reducing triglycerides and VLDL-C, but it either has no effect on total and LDL cholesterol or may cause elevations in these fractions.

PHARMACOLOGIC THERAPY

- The effect of drug therapy on lipids and lipoproteins is shown in Table 8–6.
- Recommended drugs of choice for each lipoprotein phenotype and alternate agents are given in Table 8–7.
- Available products and their doses are provided in Table 8–8.

Bile Acid Sequestrants (Cholestyramine and Colestipol)

- The primary action of both agents is to bind bile acids in the intestinal lumen, with a concurrent interruption of enterohepatic circulation of bile acids, which decreases the bile acid pool size and stimulates hepatic synthesis of bile acids from cholesterol. Depletion of the hepatic pool of cholesterol results in an increase in cholesterol biosynthesis and an increase in the number of LDL-R on the hepatocyte membrane, which stimulates an enhanced rate of catabolism from plasma and lowers LDL levels. The increase in hepatic cholesterol biosynthesis may be paralleled by increased hepatic VLDL production and, consequently, bile acid resins may aggravate hypertriglyceridemia in patients with combined hyperlipidemia.
- Bile acid sequestrants are useful in treating primary hypercholesterolemia (familial hypercholesterolemia, familial combined hyperlipidemia, type IIa hyperlipoproteinemia).

II

TABLE 8–6. Effects of Drug Therapy on Lipids and Lipoproteins

Drug	Mechanism of Action	Effects on Lipids	Effects on Lipoproteins
Cholestyramine and colestipol	↑ LDL catabolism, ↓ cholesterol absorption	↓ Cholesterol	↓ LDL, ↑ VLDL
Niacin	↓ LDL and VLDL synthesis	↓ Triglyceride and cholesterol	↓ VLDL, ↓ LDL, ↑ HDL
Fibric acids			
Clofibrate	↑ VLDL clearance,	↓ Triglyceride and cholesterol	↓ VLDL and LDL, ↑ HDL
Gemfibrozil Fenofibrate	↓ VLDL synthesis	↓ Triglyceride and cholesterol	↓ VLDL, ↑ ↓ LDL, ↑ HDL
Lovastatin, pravastatin, simvastatin, fluvastatin, atorvastatin, cerivastatin	↑ LDL catabolism, inhibit LDL synthesis	↓ Cholesterol	↓ LDL

TABLE 8–7. Lipoprotein Phenotype and Recommended Drug Treatment

Lipoprotein Type	Drug of Choice	Combination Therapy
I	Not indicated	—
IIa	HMG Co-ARI (statins)	Niacin or BAR
	Cholestyramine or colestipol	Statins or niacin
	Niacin	Statins or BAR
		ERT/HRT[a]
IIb	Statins	BAR, fibric acid, or niacin
	Fibric acids	Statins, niacin, or BAR[b]
	Niacin	Statins or fibric acid
III	Fibric acids	Statins or niacin
	Niacin	Statins or fibric acid
IV	Fibric acids	Niacin
	Niacin	Fibric acid
V	Fibric acids	Niacin
	Niacin	Fish oils

HMG Co-ARI, hydroxymethylglutaryl coenzyme-A reductase inhibitor; BAR, bile acid resin; ERT/HRT, estrogen replacement therapy or hormone replacement therapy.

[a]In selected women, ERT may be first-line therapy and may be adequate to reach LDL-C and HDL-C targets. ERT/HRT may also be combined with statins, BAR, or fibric acids.

[b]BAR is not used as first-line therapy if triglycerides are elevated at baseline, because hypertriglyceridemia may be worsened with BAR alone.

TABLE 8–8. Comparison of Drugs Used in the Treatment of Hyperlipidemia

Generic Name	Brand Name	Dosage Forms	Usual Daily Dose	Maximum Daily Dose
Cholestyramine	Questran Questran Light Prevalite	Bulk powder/4-g packets	8 g tid	32 g
Colestipol HCl	Colestid	Bulk powder/5-g packets 1-g tablets	10 g bid 8 g bid	30 g 16 g
Niacin	(Various)	50-, 100-, 250-, and 500-mg tablets; 125-, 250-, and 500-mg capsules	2 g tid	9 g
Fenofibrate	Tricor	67 mg capsules	201 mg	201 mg
Clofibrate	Atromid-S	500-mg capsules	1 g bid	2 g
Gemfibrozil	Lopid	300- and 600-mg capsules	600 mg bid	1.2 g
Lovastatin	Mevacor	10-, 20-, and 40-mg tablets	20–40 mg	80 mg
Pravastatin	Pravachol	10-, 20-, and 40-mg tablets	10–20 mg	40 mg
Simvastatin	Zocor	5-, 10-, 20-, 40- and 80-mg tablets	10–20 mg	80 mg
Fluvastatin	Lescol	20- and 40-mg capsules	20–40 mg	80 mg
Atorvastatin	Lipitor	10-, 20-, and 40-mg tablets	10 mg	80 mg
Cerivastatin	Baycol	0.2-, 0.3- and 0.4-mg tablets	0.4 mg[a]	0.4 mg

[a]In moderate to severe renal insufficiencies the initial dose should be 0.2 or 0.3 mg/d

- Gastrointestinal complaints of constipation, bloating, epigastric fullness, nausea, and flatulence are most commonly reported. These adverse effects can be managed by increasing the fluid intake, modifying the diet to increase bulk, and by use of stool softeners.
- The gritty texture and bulk may be minimized by mixing the powder with orange drink or juice. Colestipol may have better palatability because it is odorless and tasteless. Tablet forms of bile acid sequestrants should help in improving compliance with this form of therapy.
- Other potential adverse effects include impaired absorption of fat-soluble vitamins A, D, E, and K with high doses; hypernatremia and hyperchloremia; gastrointestinal obstruction; and reduced bioavailability of acidic drugs such as coumarin anticoagulants, digitoxin, nicotinic acid, thyroxine, acetaminophen, hydrocortisone, hydrochlorothiazide, loperamide, and possibly iron. Drug interactions may be avoided by alternating administration times with an interval of 6 hours or greater between the bile acid resin and other drugs.

Niacin

- Niacin (nicotinic acid) reduces the hepatic synthesis of VLDL, which in turn leads to a reduction in the synthesis of LDL. Niacin also increases HDL by reducing its catabolism.

- The principal use of niacin is for mixed hyperlipemia or as a second-line agent in combination therapy for hypercholesterolemia. It is also considered to be the first-line agent or an alternative for the treatment of hypertriglyceridemia.
- Niacin has many common adverse drug reactions; fortunately, most of the symptoms and biochemical abnormalities seen do not require discontinuation of therapy.
- Cutaneous flushing and itching appear to be prostaglandin mediated and can be reduced by aspirin 325 mg given shortly before niacin ingestion. Taking the dose with meals and slowly titrating the dose upward may minimize these effects. Concomitant alcohol and hot drinks may magnify flushing and pruritus with niacin, and they should be avoided at the time of ingestion. Gastrointestinal intolerance is also a common problem.
- Potentially important laboratory abnormalities occurring with niacin therapy include elevated liver function tests, hyperuricemia, and hyperglycemia. Niacin-associated hepatitis is more common with sustained-release preparations, and their use should be restricted to patients intolerant of regular-release products. Niacin is contraindicated in patients with active liver disease, and it may exacerbate preexisting gout and diabetes.
- **Nicotinamide** should *not* be used in the treatment of hyperlipidemia, because it does not effectively lower cholesterol or triglyceride levels.

HMG-CoA Reductase Inhibitors (Atorvastatin, Cerivastatin, Fluvastatin, Lovastatin, Pravastatin, Simvastatin)

- Reductase inhibitors interrupt the conversion of HMG-CoA to mevalonate, the rate-limiting step in *de novo* cholesterol biosynthesis, by inhibiting HMG-CoA reductase. Reduced synthesis of LDL-C and enhanced catabolism of LDL mediated through LDL receptors appear to be the principal mechanisms for lipid-lowering effects.
- When used as monotherapy, the HMG-CoA reductase inhibitors are the most potent total and LDL cholesterol lowering agents and among the best tolerated.
- Total and LDL cholesterol are reduced in a dose-related fashion by 30% or more on average when added to dietary therapy, with the effects being more pronounced in nonfamilial hypercholesterolemia than in the familial form. Atorvastatin is the most potent drug for lowering total cholesterol and LDL-C, with LDL-C reductions of 38–54% at doses ranging from 10 to 80 mg.
- Combination therapy with bile acid sequestrants and statins is rational as LDL receptor numbers are increased, leading to greater degradation of LDL-C; intracellular synthesis of cholesterol is inhibited; and enterohepatic recycling of bile acids is interrupted.
- Constipation occurs in less than 10% of patients taking reductase inhibitors. Other adverse effects include elevated serum transaminase

levels (primarily alanine aminotransferase), elevated creatine kinase levels, and myopathy.

Gemfibrozil

- Gemfibrozil, a fibric acid derivative of clofibrate, reduces the synthesis of VLDL and, to a lesser extent, apolipoprotein B with a concurrent increase in the rate of removal of triglyceride-rich lipoproteins from plasma.
- As a single agent, it is effective in reducing VLDL but a reciprocal rise in LDL may occur, and total cholesterol values may remain relatively unchanged. Plasma HDL concentrations may rise 10–15% or more with gemfibrozil.
- Gastrointestinal complaints occur in 3–5% of patients, rash in 2%, dizziness in 2.4%, and transient elevations in transaminase levels and alkaline phosphatase in 4.5% and 1.3%, respectively.
- Similar to clofibrate, gemfibrozil may enhance the formation of gallstones associated with an increase in the lithogenic index; however, the rate is low (0.6%) and similar to that seen with placebo in the Helsinki Heart Study.
- Gemfibrozil may potentiate the effects of oral anticoagulants as seen with clofibrate, but this is not well documented.

Clofibrate

- Clofibrate increases the activity of lipoprotein lipase and reduces to a lesser extent the synthesis or secretion of VLDL from the liver into the plasma. Clofibrate is less effective than gemfibrozil or niacin in reducing VLDL production.
- Although clofibrate has been suggested as the drug of choice for type III hyperlipoproteinemia, it has not been shown to reduce cardiovascular mortality and it has numerous well-documented and serious adverse effects, relegating it to third-line therapy after niacin or gemfibrozil.
- Clofibrate may induce gallstones (4.7%, clofibrate; 0.54%, placebo), promote ventricular ectopy, and potentially cause gastrointestinal malignancy causing a greater overall mortality than placebo alone.
- A myositis syndrome of myalgia, weakness, stiffness, malaise, and elevations in creatine kinase and aspartate aminotransferase may occur and seems to be more common in patients with renal insufficiency.
- Enhanced hypoprothrombinemic and hypoglycemic effects are reported to occur when clofibrate is given to patients on coumarin anticoagulants and sulfonylurea compounds, but the mechanisms for these interactions are not well understood.

Neomycin and Dextrothyroxine

- Although these drugs have been used as alternative drugs for primary hypercholesterolemia, the advent of more potent and safer agents such as the reductase inhibitors has further reduced their potential role in therapy.

Fish Oil Supplementation

- Diets high in omega-3 polyunsaturated fatty acids (from fish oil), most commonly eicosapentaenoic acid (EPA), reduce cholesterol, triglycerides, LDL-C, VLDL-C, and may elevate HDL-C.
- Fish oil supplementation may be most useful in patients with hypertriglyceridemia, but its role in treatment is not well defined.
- Complications of fish oil supplementation such as thrombocytopenia and bleeding disorders have been noted, especially with high doses (EPA, 15–30 g/d).

TREATMENT RECOMMENDATIONS

- Treatment of type I hyperlipoproteinemia is directed toward reduction of chylomicrons derived from dietary fat with the subsequent reduction in plasma triglycerides. Total daily fat intake should be no more than 10–25 g/d, or approximately 15% of total calories. Secondary causes of hypertriglyceridemia should be excluded or, if present, the underlying disorder should be treated appropriately.
- Primary hypercholesterolemia (familial hypercholesterolemia, familial combined hyperlipidemia, type IIa hyperlipoproteinemia) is treated with the bile acid sequestrants (cholestyramine and colestipol), HMG-CoA reductase inhibitors, or niacin.
- Combined hyperlipoproteinemia (type IIb) may be treated with reductase inhibitors, niacin, or gemfibrozil to lower LDL cholesterol without elevating VLDL and triglycerides. Niacin is the most effective agent and may be combined with a bile acid sequestrant. Cholestyramine or colestipol alone in this disorder may elevate VLDL and triglycerides and their use as single agents for treating combined hyperlipoproteinemia should be avoided.
- Type III hyperlipoproteinemia may be treated with niacin, gemfibrozil, fenofibrate, or (rarely) clofibrate. Fish oil supplementation may be an alternative therapy.
- Type V hyperlipoproteinemia requires a stringent restriction of the fat component of dietary intake. In addition, drug therapy is indicated, as outlined in Table 8–7, if the response to diet alone is inadequate. Medium-chain triglycerides, which are absorbed without chylomicron formation, may be used as a dietary supplement for caloric intake if needed for both types I and V.

Combination Drug Therapy

- Combination therapy may be considered after adequate trials of monotherapy and in patients documented as being compliant to the prescribed regimen. Two to three monthly lipoprotein determinations should confirm lack of response prior to initiation of combination therapy.
- Contraindications to and drug interactions with combined therapy should be screened carefully, as well as consideration of the extra cost of drug product and monitoring that may be required.

- An HMG-CoA reductase inhibitor and a bile acid sequestrant or niacin with a bile acid sequestrant provide the greatest reduction in total and LDL cholesterol.
- Regimens intended to increase HDL levels should include either gemfibrozil or niacin, and it should be remembered that reductase inhibitors combined with either of these drugs may result in a greater incidence of hepatotoxicity or myositis.
- Familial combined hyperlipidemia may respond better to a fibric acid and a reductase inhibitor than to a fibric acid and a bile acid sequestrant.

TREATMENT OF HYPERTRIGLYCERIDEMIA

- Lipoprotein pattern types I, III, IV, and V are associated with hypertriglyceridemia, and these primary lipoprotein disorders should be excluded prior to implementing therapy.
- A positive family history of CHD is important in identifying patients at risk for premature atherosclerosis. If a patient with CHD has elevated triglycerides, the associated abnormality is probably a contributing factor to CHD and should be treated.
- The goal of therapy is to lower triglycerides and VLDL particles that may be atherogenic, increase HDL, and reduce LDL. Success in treatment is defined as a reduction in triglycerides below 500 mg/dL.
- High serum triglycerides (Table 8–2) should be treated by achieving desirable body weight, consumption of a low saturated and cholesterol diet, regular exercise, smoking cessation, and restriction of alcohol (in selected patients).
- Drug therapy with niacin should be considered in patients with borderline-high triglycerides accompanied by established CHD, family history of premature CHD, concomitant high LDL-C or low HDL-C, and genetic forms of hypertriglyceridemia associated with CHD.
- Niacin should not be used in diabetics because of the risk of worsening glycemic control. Alternative therapies include gemfibrozil, reductase inhibitors, and fish oil.

► EVALUATION OF THERAPEUTIC OUTCOMES

- Short-term evaluation of therapy for hyperlipidemia is based on response to diet and drug treatment as measured in the clinical laboratory by total cholesterol, LDL-C, HDL-C, and triglycerides.
- Patients treated for primary prevention may have no symptoms or clinical manifestations of a genetic lipid disorder (e.g., xanthomas), so monitoring is solely laboratory based. The goals for LDL and HDL cholesterol are provided in Table 8–4.
- In patients treated for secondary intervention, symptoms of atherosclerotic cardiovascular disease, such as angina or intermittent claudication, may improve over months to years. Xanthomas or other external manifestations of hyperlipidemia should regress with therapy.

- Lipid measurements should be obtained in the fasted state to minimize interference from chylomicrons and, once the patient is stable, monitoring is needed at intervals of 6 months to 1 year.
- Patients with multiple risk factors and established CHD should also be monitored and evaluated for progress in managing their other risk factors such as hypertension, smoking cessation, exercise and weight control, and glycemic control (if diabetic).
- Evaluation of dietary therapy with diet diaries and recall survey instruments allows information about diet to be collected in a systemic fashion and may improve patient adherence to dietary recommendations.

See Chapter 19, Hyperlipidemia, authored by Robert L. Talbert, PharmD, FCCP, BCPS, for a more detailed discussion of this topic.

Chapter 9

▶ HYPERTENSION

▶ DEFINITION

- Based on the impact on risk for cardiovascular morbidity and mortality, the Sixth Joint National Committee on the Detection, Evaluation, and Treatment of High Blood Pressure (JNC-VI) classifies adult blood pressure as shown in Table 9–1.
- If the diastolic blood pressure (DBP) is less than 90 mm Hg and the systolic blood pressure (SBP) is 140 mm Hg or higher, then the term *isolated systolic hypertension* is applicable. Isolated systolic hypertension is believed to result from the pathophysiology of aging and portends an increased risk of cardiovascular morbidity and mortality.
- A marked or sharp increase in DBP is considered a hypertensive crisis, which may represent either a hypertensive emergency—an elevation of diastolic blood pressure accompanied by acute target organ injury—or a hypertensive urgency—severe hypertension without signs or symptoms of acute target organ complications.

▶ PATHOPHYSIOLOGY

- Hypertension is a heterogeneous disorder that may result either from a specific cause (secondary hypertension) or from some underlying pathophysiologic mechanism stemming from an unknown etiology (primary or essential hypertension). Secondary hypertension accounts for fewer than 5% of cases, and most of these are caused by chronic renal disease or renovascular disease. Other conditions causing secondary hypertension include pheochromocytoma, Cushing's syndrome, primary aldosteronism, coarctation of the aorta, and exogenous substances such as estrogens, glucocorticoids, licorice, sympathomimetic amines, nonsteroidal anti-inflammatory drugs (NSAIDs), chronic alcohol use, and tyramine-containing foods in combination with monoamine oxidase (MAO) inhibitors.
- Multiple factors may contribute to the development of primary hypertension. Postulated mechanisms include:
  - A pathologic disturbance in the central nervous system (CNS), autonomic nerve fibers, adrenergic receptors, or baroreceptors.
  - Abnormalities in either the renal or tissue autoregulatory processes for sodium excretion, plasma volume, and arteriolar constriction.
  - Humoral abnormalities involving the renin–angiotensin–aldosterone system (RAS), natriuretic hormone, or hyperinsulinemia.
  - A deficiency in the local synthesis of vasodilating substances in the vascular endothelium, such as prostacyclin, bradykinin, and nitric oxide, or an increase in the production of vasoconstricting substances such as angiotensin II and endothelin I.

TABLE 9–1. Adult Blood Pressure Classification

Category	Systolic (mm Hg)	Diastolic (mm Hg)
Optimal	<120	<80
Normal	<130	<85
High normal	130–139	85–89
Hypertension		
Stage 1	140–159	90–99
Stage 2	160–179	100–109
Stage 3	≥180	≥110

- Increased sodium intake together with an inherited defect in the kidney's ability to excrete sodium, leading to an increase in circulating natriuretic hormone, which inhibits intracellular sodium transport resulting in increased vascular reactivity.
- Increased intracellular concentration of calcium, leading to altered vascular smooth muscle function and increased peripheral vascular resistance.

- Early in the course of primary hypertension, the blood pressure may fluctuate between abnormal and normal levels. As the disease progresses, peripheral vascular resistance increases and patients develop a sustained increase in blood pressure. In most cases the DBP does not exceed 115 mm Hg. Individuals with secondary hypertension are more likely to experience severe elevations in blood pressure. Only a small proportion of patients suffering from primary hypertension develops accelerated or severe hypertension.
- The target organ damage secondary to chronic hypertension principally involves the brain, the eye, the heart, and the kidney. The main causes of death in hypertensive subjects are cerebrovascular accidents, cardiovascular events, and renal failure. The probability of premature death from any of these causes increases with increasing SBP or DBP.

▶ CLINICAL PRESENTATION

- Patients with uncomplicated primary hypertension are usually asymptomatic initially. As the hypertension progresses, however, symptoms characteristic of cardiovascular, cerebrovascular, or renal disease may occur as the patient develops target organ damage.
- Patients with secondary hypertension usually complain of symptoms suggestive of the underlying disorder. For example, patients with pheochromocytoma may have a history of paroxysmal headaches, sweating, tachycardia, palpitations, orthostatic dizziness, or syncope. In primary aldosteronism, hypokalemic symptoms of muscle cramps and

weakness may be present. Patients with hypertension secondary to Cushing's syndrome may complain of weight gain, polyuria, edema, menstrual irregularities, recurrent acne, or muscular weakness.

▶ DIAGNOSIS

- Frequently, the only sign of primary hypertension on physical examination is an elevated blood pressure. As the disease progresses, signs of end-organ damage begin to appear, chiefly related to pathologic changes in the eye, brain, heart, kidneys, and peripheral blood vessels.
- The funduscopic exam may reveal arteriolar narrowing, arteriovenous nicking, retinal hemorrhages, and infarcts. Papilledema suggests a malignant stage of high blood pressure requiring rapid treatment.
- Auscultation of the heart may identify an accentuated second heart sound (S_2), a systolic ejection murmur, an S_4 gallop, or an S_3 gallop sound associated with heart failure.
- The physical examination may provide clues for diagnosing secondary hypertension. For example, patients with renal artery stenosis may have an abdominal systolic–diastolic bruit; patients with Cushing's syndrome may have the classic physical features of moon face, buffalo hump, hirsutism, and abdominal striae.
- A low serum potassium before antihypertensive therapy is begun may suggest mineralocorticoid-induced hypertension. The presence of protein, blood cells, and casts in the urine may indicate an underlying parenchymal kidney disease as the cause of hypertension.
- Routine laboratory tests that should be obtained in all patients prior to initiating drug therapy include hemoglobin and hematocrit, urinalysis, serum potassium and creatinine, liver function tests, and electrocardiogram (ECG). Total and high density lipoprotein (HDL) cholesterol, plasma glucose, and serum uric acid are indicated to assess other risk factors and to develop baseline data for monitoring drug-induced metabolic changes.
- More specific laboratory tests are used to diagnose secondary hypertension. These include plasma norepinephrine and urinary metanephrine for pheochromocytoma, plasma and urinary aldosterone levels for primary aldosteronism, and plasma renin activity, captopril stimulation test, renal vein renins, and renal artery angiography for renovascular disease.
- A single reading of blood pressure elevation does not constitute a diagnosis of hypertension. If the blood pressure taken on two or more subsequent days is 140/90 mm Hg or higher, then a diagnosis of hypertension is confirmed.

▶ DESIRED OUTCOME

The long-term goal for the treatment of hypertension is to reduce blood pressure to the desired goal with minimal adverse effects in order to reduce target organ damage and prevent the development of the cerebrovascular, cardiovascular, ophthalmic, and renal complications of the disease.

▶ TREATMENT

GENERAL PRINCIPLES

- The treatment plan for hypertension should include measures to minimize contributing factors and to reduce or prevent other known risk factors. Obesity, hyperlipidemia, glucose intolerance, excessive salt intake, cigarette smoking, and alcohol consumption are important risk factors that should be addressed. The JNC-VI treatment algorithm is presented in Figure 9–1.
- Initial treatment steps should include lifestyle modifications, including: (1) a sensible dietary program designed for gradual weight reduction, if appropriate, and for reducing the saturated fat and salt content of the diet; (2) restriction of alcohol intake, which may worsen hypertension; (3) cessation of smoking; and (4) regular aerobic exercise, if medically feasible.
- Pharmacologic therapy should be individualized based on a patient's age, race, known pathophysiologic variables, and concurrent conditions. Treatment should be designed not only to lower blood pressure safely and effectively, but also to avoid or reverse hyperlipidemia, glucose intolerance, and left ventricular hypertrophy.
- Individual drug selection should also be based on safety, efficacy, cost, and the presence of concomitant diseases and other risk factors. Table 9–2 provides a list of agents currently available for the treatment of hypertension in the United States.

DIURETICS

- Thiazides are generally the diuretics of choice for the treatment of hypertension, and all are equally effective in lowering blood pressure. In patients with adequate renal function [i.e., glomerular filtration rate (GFR) >30 mL/min], thiazides are more effective hypotensive agents than loop diuretics. As renal function declines, however, sodium and fluid accumulate, and the use of a more potent diuretic is necessary to counter the effects that volume and sodium expansion have on arterial blood pressure.
- The potassium-sparing diuretics are weak antihypertensive agents when used alone but provide an additive hypotensive effect when used in combination with thiazide or loop diuretics. Moreover, they counteract the potassium- and magnesium-losing properties of other diuretic agents.
- Acutely, diuretics lower blood pressure by causing a diuresis. The reduction in plasma volume and stroke volume associated with a diuresis decreases cardiac output and, consequently, blood pressure. The initial drop in cardiac output produced by the diuresis causes a compen-

II

Begin or continue life-style modifications
Not at goal blood pressure (< 140/90 mm Hg) Lower goals for patients with diabetes or renal disease
Initial drug choices*
Uncomplicated hypertension†
Diuretics
β-blockers
Specific indications for the following drugs
ACE inhibitors
Angiotensin II receptor blockers
α-blockers
α-β-blockers
β-blockers
Calcium antagonists
Diuretics
Compelling indications†
Diabetes mellitus (type 1) with proteinuria
• ACE inhibitors
Heart failure
• ACE inhibitors
• Diuretics
Isolated systolic hypertension (older persons)
• Diuretics preferred
• Long-acting dihydropyridine calcium antagonists
Myocardial infarction
• β-blockers (non-ISA)
• ACE inhibitors (with systolic) dysfunction)
• Start with a low dose of a long-acting once-daily drug, and titrate dose.
• Low-dose combinations may be appropriate.
Not at goal blood pressure
No response or troublesome side effects
Inadequate response but well tolerated
Substitute another drug from a different class.
Add a second agent from a different class (diuretic if not already used).
Not at goal blood pressure
Continue adding agents from other classes. Consider referral to a hypertension specialist.

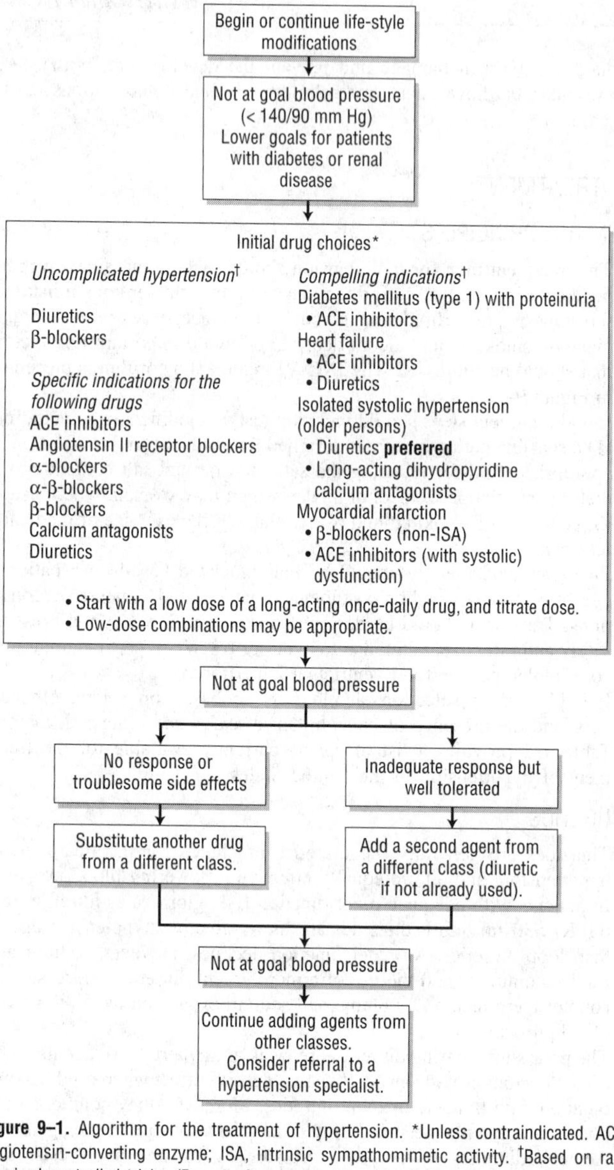

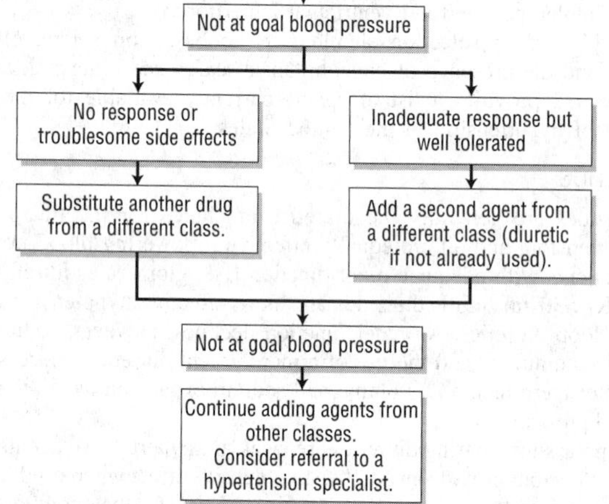

Figure 9–1. Algorithm for the treatment of hypertension. *Unless contraindicated. ACE, angiotensin-converting enzyme; ISA, intrinsic sympathomimetic activity. †Based on randomized controlled trials. *(From the Sixth Report of the Joint National Committee on Prevention, Detection, Evaluation, and Treatment of High Blood Pressure. Arch Intern Med 1997;157:2413–2446.)*

satory increase in peripheral vascular resistance. With continuing diuretic therapy, the extracellular fluid volume and plasma volume return almost to pretreatment levels, and peripheral vascular resistance falls below its pretreatment baseline. The reduction in peripheral vascular resistance is responsible for the long-term hypotensive effectiveness. It has been postulated that thiazides lower blood pressure by mobilizing sodium and water from arteriolar walls. II

- When diuretics are used in combination with other antihypertensive agents, an additive hypotensive effect is usually observed because of independent mechanisms of action. Furthermore, many nondiuretic antihypertensive agents induce salt and water retention, which is counteracted by concurrent use of a diuretic.
- Side effects of thiazides include hypokalemia, hypomagnesemia, hypercalcemia, hyperuricemia, hyperglycemia, hyperlipidemia, and sexual dysfunction. Loop diuretics cause a lesser effect on serum lipids and glucose, but hypocalcemia may occur. Short-term studies indicate that indapamide does not adversely affect lipids or glucose tolerance or cause sexual dysfunction.
- The hypokalemia and hypomagnesemia caused by thiazide and loop diuretics may lead to cardiac arrhythmias, especially in patients receiving digitalis therapy, patients with left ventricular hypertrophy, and patients with ischemic heart disease. Hypokalemia may be prevented by using low daily doses (e.g., 12.5–25 mg of **hydrochlorothiazide** or 25 mg of **chlorthalidone**) and reducing sodium and increasing potassium in the diet.
- Potassium-sparing diuretics may cause hyperkalemia, especially in patients with renal insufficiency or diabetes, and in patients receiving concurrent treatment with an ACE inhibitor, NSAIDs, or potassium supplements. **Spironolactone** may cause gynecomastia.

CENTRAL α_2-RECEPTOR AGONISTS

- **Clonidine, guanabenz, guanfacine,** and **methyldopa** all lower blood pressure primarily by stimulating α_2-adrenergic receptors in the brain, which reduces sympathetic outflow from the vasomotor center in the brain and increases vagal tone. Stimulation of presynaptic α_2 receptors peripherally may contribute to the reduction in sympathetic tone. Consequently, heart rate is decreased, cardiac output decreases slightly, total peripheral resistance is lowered, plasma renin activity is reduced, and baroreceptor reflexes are blunted.
- Chronic use results in sodium and fluid retention, which appear to be most prominent with methyldopa. Low doses of either clonidine, guanfacine, or guanabenz can be used to treat mild hypertension without the addition of a diuretic.
- Sedation and dry mouth are common side effects of these antihypertensive agents. These symptoms may diminish or completely abate with chronic use of low doses. As with other centrally acting antihypertensive drugs, these agents may cause depression.

TABLE 9–2. The Antihypertensive Agents

Drug	Dose Range (mg/d)	
	Initial	*Maximum*
Diuretics		
Thiazides and related sulfonamide diuretics		
Bendroflumethiazide	2.5	5
Benzthiazide	25	50
Chlorothiazide sodium	250	500
Chlorthalidone	12.5	50
Cyclothiazide	1	2
Hydrochlorothiazide	12.5	50
Hydroflumethiazide	25	50
Indapamide	1.25	5
Methyclothiazide	2.5	5
Metolazone	2.5	5
Polythiazide	2	4
Quinethazone	50	100
Trichlormethiazide	2	4
Loop diuretics		
Bumetanide	0.5	10
Ethacrynic acid	25	200
Furosemide	40	240
Potassium-sparing agents		
Amiloride hydrochloride	5	10
Spironolactone	25	100
Triamterene	25	100
Adrenergic Inhibitors		
β-Adrenergic blockers		
Acebutolol	200	800
Atenolol	25	100
Betaxolol	5	40
Bisoprolol	2.5	20
Carteolol	2.5	10
Metoprolol tartrate	50	300
Nadolol	20	320
Oxprenolol hydrochloride	160	480
Penbutolol	10	80
Pindolol	10	60
Propranolol hydrochloride	40	480
Propranolol, long-acting (LA)	80	480
Timolol maleate	20	60
Centrally-acting adrenergic inhibitors		
Clonidine hydrochloride	0.2	1.2

continued

II

TABLE 9–2. continued

Drug	Dose Range (mg/d)	
	Initial	*Maximum*
Centrally-acting adrenergic inhibitors (cont.)		
Guanabenz acetate	8	32
Guanfacine	1	3
Methyldopa	500	2000
Peripherally-acting adrenergic antagonists		
Guanadrel sulfate	10	150
Guanethidine monosulfate		
Reserpine	0.05	0.25
α_1-Adrenergic blockers		
Doxazosin	1	16
Prazosin hydrochloride	2	20
Terazosin	1	5
Combined α- and β-adrenergic blockers		
Carvedilol	12.5	50
Labetolol	200	1200
Vasodilators		
Hydralazine hydrochloride	50	300
Minoxidil	5	100
Angiotensin-converting Enzyme Inhibitors		
Benazepril	5	40
Captopril	25	150
Enalapril maleate	5	40
Fosinopril	10	80
Lisinopril	5	80
Moexipril	7.5	30
Quinapril	5	80
Ramipril	1.25	20
Trandolapril	1	4
Angiotensin II Receptor Agonists		
Candesartan	16	32
Irbesartan	150	300
Losartan	50	100
Valsartan	80	320
Telmisartan	20	80
Eposartan	300	600
Tasosartan	25	100
Calcium Channel Antagonists		
Amlodipine	2.5	10
Diltiazem hydrochloride	120	360
Felodipine	2.5	20
Isradipine	5	20
Nicardipine	60	120
Nifedipine	30	180
Nisoldipine	20	60
Verapamil hydrochloride	120	480

- Rebound hypertension may rarely occur when a central α-receptor agonist is stopped. This is thought to occur secondary to a compensatory increase in norepinephrine release that follows discontinuation of presynaptic α-receptor stimulation.
- Methyldopa rarely may cause hepatitis or hemolytic anemia. A transient elevation in liver function tests is occasionally associated with methyldopa therapy and is clinically unimportant. A persistent increase in serum transaminases or alkaline phosphatase may herald the onset of fulminant hepatitis, which can be fatal. A Coombs'-positive hemolytic anemia occurs in less than 1% of patients receiving methyldopa, although 20% exhibit a positive direct Coombs' test without anemia.
- The transdermal delivery system for clonidine is applied to the skin and left in place 1 week before being replaced. It reduces blood pressure while facilitating compliance and avoiding the high peak serum drug concentrations that are thought to contribute to adverse effects. The disadvantages of this system are its cost, a 20% incidence of local skin rash or irritation, and a 2- or 3-day delay in onset of effect.

PERIPHERAL α_1-RECEPTOR BLOCKERS

- **Prazosin, terazosin,** and **doxazosin** are selective α_1-receptor blockers that do not alter α_2-receptor activity and therefore do not usually cause reflex tachycardia.
- At low doses, selective α blockers may be used as monotherapy in the treatment of mild hypertension. At higher doses, fluid and sodium accumulation necessitate concurrent diuretic therapy to maintain hypotensive efficacy.
- CNS side effects include lassitude, vivid dreams, and depression. The so-called "first-dose phenomenon" is characterized by orthostatic hypotension, transient dizziness or faintness, palpitations, and even syncope occurring within 1–3 hours of the first dose, or subsequently after the first increased dose. These episodes can be obviated by having the patient take the first dose, and first increased dose, at bedtime. Occasionally, orthostatic dizziness persists with chronic administration.

β-Adrenergic Blockers

- The exact hypotensive mechanism of β-adrenergic blockers (β blockers) is not known. Postulated mechanisms include reduction in cardiac output through negative chronotropic and inotropic effects on the heart, a central action on β receptors in the brain, reduction in renin release from the kidney, and possibly blockade of peripheral β receptors on the surface of presynaptic sympathetic neuronal endings.
- Even though there are important pharmacodynamic and pharmacokinetic differences among the various β blockers (Table 9–3), there is no difference in their clinical antihypertensive efficacy.
- At low doses, **bisoprolol, metoprolol, atenolol,** and **acebutolol** are cardioselective and bind more avidly to β_1 receptors than to β_2

TABLE 9–3. Pharmacodynamic and Pharmacokinetic Properties of the β-Adrenergic Blocking Agents

	α-Blockade	β_1-Selectivity	MSA	ISA	Lipid Solubility	Bioavailability (%)	Half-life (h)
Acebutolol	0	+	+	+	Low	20–60	3–4
Atenolol	0	+	0	0	Low	50	6–9
Betaxolol	0	+	±	0	Low	100	14–24
Bisoprolol	0	++	0	0	Low	80	9–12
Carteolol	0	0	0	+	Low	50	6
Carvedilol	+	0	0	0	High	25–35	7–10
Labetalol	+	0	+	0	Moderate	40	3–5
Metoprolol	0	+	0	0	Moderate	50	3–4
Nadolol	0	0	0	0	Low	30	14–24
Penbutolol	0	0	0	+	High	100	5
Pindolol	0	0	+	+++	Moderate	100	3–4
Propranolol	0	0	+	0	High	35	4–6
Timolol	0	0	0	0	Low	75	3–4

MSA = membrane stabilizing activity; ISA = intrinsic sympathomimetic activity.

receptors. As a result, they are less likely to provoke bronchospasm and vasoconstriction and may be safer than nonselective β blockers in patients with asthma, chronic obstructive pulmonary disease (COPD), diabetes, and peripheral vascular disease. Cardioselectivity is a dose-dependent phenomenon, and the effect is lost at higher doses.

- **Pindolol, penbutolol, carteolol,** and **acebutolol** possess intrinsic sympathomimetic activity (ISA) or partial β-receptor agonist activity and are therefore capable of maintaining normal basal sympathetic tone while blocking the effects of excessive adrenergic stimulation. When sympathetic tone is low, as it is during resting states, β receptors are partially stimulated, so resting heart rate, cardiac output, and peripheral blood flow are not reduced when receptors are blocked. Theoretically, these drugs may be less hazardous in patients with borderline heart failure, sinus bradycardia, or perhaps even peripheral vascular disease.
- All β blockers are capable of exerting a membrane-stabilizing action on cardiac cells if large enough doses are given, but the dose required usually greatly exceeds that used in treating hypertension or cardiac arrhythmias.
- Pharmacokinetic differences among β blockers can be found in first-pass metabolism, serum half-lives, degree of lipophilicity, and route of elimination. Propranolol and metoprolol undergo extensive first-pass metabolism. Atenolol and nadolol, which have relatively long half-lives, are excreted renally, and the dosage of each may need to be

adjusted in patients with renal insufficiency. Even though the half-lives of the other β blockers are much shorter, once-daily administration may still be effective. β Blockers vary in terms of their lipophilic properties and CNS penetration.

- Side effects from β blockade in the myocardium include bradycardia, atrioventricular conduction abnormalities, and heart failure. Pulmonary β blockade may lead to acute exacerbations of bronchospasm in patients with asthma or COPD. Blocking β_2 receptors in arteriolar smooth muscle may aggravate intermittent claudication or Raynaud's phenomenon and may cause cold extremities as a result of decreased peripheral blood flow.
- Abrupt cessation of β-blocker therapy may produce unstable angina, myocardial infarction, or even death in patients predisposed to ischemic myocardial events. In patients without coronary artery disease, abrupt discontinuation of β-blocker therapy may be associated with sinus tachycardia, increased sweating, and generalized malaise. For these reasons, it is always prudent to taper the dose gradually over 14 days before discontinuation.
- Adverse effects on serum lipids and glucose tolerance may offset some of the beneficial effects on cardiovascular morbidity and mortality. β Blockers increase serum triglyceride levels and decrease HDL cholesterol levels. β Blockers with α-blocking properties produce no appreciable change in serum lipid concentration. Also, β blockers with ISA do not affect serum lipids adversely and may even increase HDL cholesterol.
- β Blockers may induce glucose intolerance by inhibiting insulin secretion and by generating insulin resistance. These adverse effects are not usually associated with the use of β blockers that possess ISA or α-receptor blocking properties.

ANGIOTENSIN-CONVERTING ENZYME (ACE) INHIBITORS

- ACE is widely distributed in many tissues. It is present in several different cell types, but its principal location is in endothelial cells. Because the vascular endothelium covers a large surface area, the major site for angiotensin II production in the body is the blood vessels, not the kidney. ACE inhibitors block the conversion of angiotensin I to angiotensin II, a potent vasoconstrictor and stimulator of aldosterone secretion. Blockade of angiotensin II also increases the compliance of large arteries, which may effectively prevent or reverse left ventricular hypertrophy. ACE inhibitors also block the degradation of bradykinin and stimulate the synthesis of other vasodilating substances including prostaglandin E_2 and prostacyclin. The observation that ACE inhibitors lower blood pressure in patients with normal plasma renin and ACE activity clearly indicates the importance of tissue production of ACE as a cause of increased vascular resistance.
- **Captopril** has a relatively short half-life and is usually administered two to three times daily. Recent studies indicate that once-daily admin-

istration of captopril may be adequate for the treatment of hypertension in salt-restricted patients. The remaining ACE inhibitors have long half-lives and are given once or twice daily in the treatment of hypertension. II
The absorption of captopril is reduced 30–40% by the presence of food in the stomach.

- The most serious adverse effects of the ACE inhibitors are neutropenia and agranulocytosis, proteinuria, glomerulonephritis, and angioedema; these effects occur in less than 1% of patients. Patients with preexisting renal or connective tissue diseases appear to be most vulnerable to the renal and hematologic side effects. Patients with bilateral renal artery stenosis or unilateral stenosis of a solitary functioning kidney and patients dependent on the vasoconstrictive effect of angiotensin II on the efferent arteriole are particularly susceptible to developing acute renal failure on ACE inhibitors.
- Approximately 10% of patients who receive captopril develop a skin rash, which is usually transient and disappears despite continued treatment. A reversible loss of taste or taste disturbance (dysgeusia) has been reported in about 6% of patients receiving captopril. The higher incidence of skin rash, dysgeusia, and proteinuria with captopril has been attributed to its sulfhydryl group, which is not present on enalapril or lisinopril. Approximately 10–20% of patients develop a persistent cough; these patients may be switched to an angiotensin II receptor antagonist.
- Acute hypotension may occur at the onset of ACE inhibitor therapy, especially in patients who are severely sodium or volume depleted. It may be necessary to discontinue diuretics and reduce the dosage of other antihypertensive agents before initiating therapy. Initiating therapy at the lowest dose possible and administering the first dose at bedtime may also minimize acute hypotension.
- ACE inhibitors are absolutely contraindicated in pregnancy because serious neonatal problems, including renal failure and death, have been reported when mothers took these agents during the second and third trimesters of pregnancy.
- Hyperkalemia is seen primarily in patients with renal disease or diabetes mellitus (especially with type IV renal tubular acidosis) or patients on concomitant NSAIDs, potassium supplements, or potassium-sparing diuretics.

ANGIOTENSIN II RECEPTOR ANTAGONISTS

- **Losartan, valsartan, candesartan,** and **irbesartan** are angiotensin analogues that inhibit the renin system by competing directly with angiotensin II for tissue binding sites. Therefore, they block the effects of angiotensin II generated by either ACE or the enzyme chymase.
- These drugs appear to have effects on blood pressure and systemic and renal hemodynamics that are comparable to the ACE inhibitors. They are less likely than ACE inhibitors to cause a nonproductive cough or hyperkalemia.

VASODILATORS

II • **Hydralazine** and **minoxidil** cause direct arteriolar smooth muscle relaxation through mechanisms that increase the intracellular concentration of cyclic guanosine monophosphate (GMP).

- A compensatory activation of the baroreceptor reflexes results in an increase in sympathetic outflow from the vasomotor center, producing an increase in heart rate, cardiac output, and renin release. Consequently, the hypotensive effectiveness of direct vasodilators diminishes in time unless the patient is also taking a sympathetic inhibitor and a diuretic. In older patients, baroreceptor mechanisms may be blunted enough that blood pressure may be lowered with vasodilatory therapy without causing sympathetic overactivity.
- Direct vasodilator use can precipitate angina in patients with underlying coronary artery disease unless the baroreceptor reflex mechanism is completely blocked with a sympathetic inhibitor; the β-adrenergic blocking agents are most effective.
- Hydralazine may cause a dose-related, reversible lupus-like syndrome, which is more common in slow acetylators of the drug. Lupus-like reactions can usually be avoided by using total daily doses of less than 200 mg. Other hydralazine side effects include dermatitis, drug fever, peripheral neuropathy, hepatitis, and vascular headaches.
- Minoxidil causes a reversible hypertrichosis on the face, arms, back, and chest. Other side effects include pericardial effusion and a nonspecific T-wave change on the ECG.

CALCIUM CHANNEL ANTAGONISTS

- Calcium channel antagonists cause relaxation of cardiac and smooth muscle by blocking voltage-sensitive calcium channels, thereby reducing the entry of extracellular calcium into the cells. Vascular smooth muscle relaxation leads to vasodilation and a corresponding reduction in blood pressure.
- **Verapamil** decreases heart rate, slows atrioventricular (AV) nodal conduction, and produces a negative inotropic effect that may precipitate heart failure in subjects with borderline cardiac reserve. **Diltiazem** decreases atrioventricular conduction and heart rate to a lesser extent than verapamil.
- Diltiazem and verapamil rarely cause cardiac conduction abnormalities such as bradycardia, AV block, and heart failure. Both can cause anorexia, nausea, peripheral edema, and hypotension. Verapamil causes constipation in about 7% of patients.
- **Nifedipine** is a dihydropyridine derivative that has potent peripheral vasodilating effects, causing a baroreceptor-mediated reflex increase in heart rate. It does not usually alter conduction through the AV node. Nifedipine rarely may cause an increase in the frequency, intensity, and duration of angina in association with acute hypotension. However, this effect may be obviated by using sustained-

released formulations. Other side effects of nifedipine include dizziness, flushing, headache, peripheral edema, mood changes, and various gastrointestinal complaints. Other dihydropyridine derivatives include **amlodipine, felodipine, isradipine, nicardipine,** and **nisoldipine.**

POSTGANGLIONIC SYMPATHETIC INHIBITORS

- **Guanethidine** and **guanadrel** deplete norepinephrine from postganglionic sympathetic nerve terminals and inhibit the release of norepinephrine in response to sympathetic nerve stimulation. This results in a reduction in cardiac output and peripheral vascular resistance.
- Postural hypotension is common because reflex-mediated vasoconstriction is blocked by these drugs. Other undesired side effects include impotence, diarrhea (due to unopposed parasympathetic activity), and weight gain. These drugs are usually reserved for patients with refractory hypertension because of their side effect profiles.

RESERPINE

- **Reserpine** depletes norepinephrine from sympathetic nerve endings and blocks the transport of norepinephrine into its storage granules. When the nerve is stimulated, less than the usual amount of norepinephrine is released into the synapse. This reduces sympathetic tone, decreasing peripheral vascular resistance and blood pressure.
- Its use is associated with significant sodium and fluid retention, and it should be administered in combination with a diuretic.
- Reserpine's strong inhibition of sympathetic activity allows increased parasympathetic activity to occur, which is responsible for side effects of nasal stuffiness, increased gastric acid secretion, diarrhea, and bradycardia.
- The most important side effect is a dose-related mental depression, which is a consequence of CNS depletion of catecholamines and serotonin. The problem can be minimized by not exceeding 0.25 mg daily.

DIFFERENTIAL APPROACH TO THE MANAGEMENT OF HYPERTENSION

- Hypertension is a heterogeneous disorder that poses special therapeutic problems in several specific clinical situations, as shown in Table 9–4.

Hypertension in Childhood

- In most cases, the factors associated with hypertension in children are identical to those in adults. However, secondary hypertension is much more common in children than in adults.
- Renal disease (e.g., pyelonephritis, glomerulonephritis, renal artery stenosis, renal cysts) is the most common cause of secondary hypertension in children. Medical or surgical management of the underlying renal disorder usually restores normal blood pressure.

TABLE 9–4. Differential Antihypertensive Therapy in Specific Clinical Situations

	Advantageous	Disadvantageous
Heart failure	ACE inhibitor, diuretic	β Blockers (in some cases), Ca channel antagonists (except amlodipine)
Angina	β Blocker, Ca channel antagonist	Hydralazine, minoxidil
Elderly	Diuretic, α-agonist, Ca channel antagonist	
Black	Diuretic, Ca channel antagonist	β Blocker as initial agent
Young	β Blocker, α-agonist, ACE inhibitor	Diuretic
Diabetes	ACE inhibitor, α-Agonist, Ca channel antagonist	β Blocker, diuretic
Bronchospasm	Ca channel antagonist	β Blocker, ACE inhibitor
Pregnancy	Methyldopa, hydralazine, labetolol	Diuretic, β blocker
Renal insufficiency	α-Agonist, Ca channel antagonist, minoxidil, hydralazine, loop diuretic	Thiazide diuretic, potassium-sparing agents
Tachycardia	β Blocker, α-agonist, verapamil, diltiazem	Nifedipine, hydralazine, minoxidil
Hyperlipidemia	α Blocker, ACE inhibitor, Ca channel antagonist	Diuretic, β blocker
Gout/hyperuricemia	α-Agonist, α-blocker, Ca channel antagonist, ACE inhibitor	Diuretic, ACE inhibitor[a]

ACE, angiotensin-converting enzyme; Ca, calcium; COPD, chronic obstructive pulmonary disease.
[a]ACE inhibitors may increase urinary clearance of uric acid thereby reducing hyperuricemia but increasing the risk of uric acid deposition in the urine or kidneys.

- In many young people, primary hypertension is associated with an increased cardiac output and a normal plasma volume and total peripheral vascular resistance. This hyperdynamic or hyperkinetic circulatory state might best be treated with a β blocker. Alternative agents include clonidine, guanfacine, or guanabenz, which lower serum norepinephrine levels and reduce hyperadrenergic activity.

Hypertension in Pregnancy

- Preeclampsia can lead rapidly to life-threatening complications for both the mother and fetus; it usually presents after 20 weeks' gestation in primigravid women. The diagnosis is based on the appearance of hypertension or a significant increase in blood pressure with proteinuria, edema, or both.
- Definitive treatment of preeclampsia is delivery or abortion, and this is clearly indicated if pending or frank eclampsia (preeclampsia plus convulsions) is present. Otherwise, measures such as restriction of activity, bed rest, and close monitoring are in order. If drug treatment of hyper-

tension is indicated (DBP >100 mm Hg), methyldopa (or perhaps another α-agonist) is the recommended drug of choice.

- β blockers appear safe and effective in simple hypertension of pregnancy even though there is some concern about effects on fetal heart rate, glucose intolerance, and growth retardation. II

Hypertension in Elderly Patients

- Elderly patients may present with either isolated systolic hypertension or an elevation in both systolic and diastolic blood pressure. In the double-blind placebo-controlled trial called the Systolic Hypertension in the Elderly Program (SHEP), active treatment of isolated systolic hypertension resulted in a 36% reduction in the incidence of total stroke and a 27% reduction in the total number of cardiovascular events.
- The JNC-VI recommends a reduction in the SBP to less than 160 mm Hg for patients with a SBP greater than 180 mm Hg and a reduction in blood pressure by 20 mm Hg for those with SBP between 160 and 179 mm Hg.
- Elderly patients are usually more sensitive to volume depletion and sympathetic inhibition, and treatment generally should be initiated with a small dose of a diuretic (e.g., 12.5 mg of hydrochlorothiazide) and increased gradually. If diuretic therapy alone does not achieve the desired reduction in SBP, a sympathetic inhibitor can be added at low doses with gradual increases. Calcium channel blockers or β blockers should be considered in elderly patients with hypertension and angina, and ACE inhibitors might be preferred for hypertensive patients with heart failure. The pharmacologic management of diastolic hypertension in the elderly is similar to that outlined for isolated systolic hypertension.

Hypertension in African Americans

- Hypertension is more common and more severe in black persons than other races. Differences in electrolyte homeostasis, glomerular filtration rate, sodium excretion and transport mechanisms, plasma renin activity, and blood pressure response to plasma volume expansion have been noted.
- Supplemental potassium and calcium have both been shown to cause a modest reduction in blood pressure in some studies.
- The lower plasma renin activity and increased blood pressure response to sodium and fluid loading observed suggest a more sodium- and volume-dependent hypertension. Black individuals are hyperresponsive to diuretic therapy; therefore, diuretics are usually recommended as initial treatment.
- If diuretic therapy alone does not provide adequate control, addition of a sympathetic inhibitor is appropriate. Diuretic therapy combined with β blockers or ACE inhibitors is equally effective in hypertensive blacks and whites.
- Calcium channel antagonists are as effective as diuretics for initial treatment and provide an alternative that may be preferable under certain conditions.

Hypertension with Diabetes Mellitus

- The blood pressure treatment goal in diabetic patients with hypertension is 130/85 mm Hg or less, if tolerated.
- Diuretics and β blockers generally should be avoided in diabetic hypertensive patients because they cause insulin resistance and glucose intolerance. β blockers also mask most of the signs and symptoms of hypoglycemia (tremor, tachycardia, palpitations), delay recovery from hypoglycemia, and may produce elevations in blood pressure due to vasoconstriction caused by unopposed α-receptor stimulation during the hypoglycemic recovery phase.
- The α_1 antagonists may increase the risk of orthostatic hypotension, and the α_2 agonists may cause a paradoxical increase in blood pressure. These effects appear to be due to a more sensitive autonomic nervous system in patients with diabetic neuropathy.
- ACE inhibitors may increase insulin sensitivity and provide renal protective effects. Thus, these agents may be considered the preferred pharmacologic treatment of hypertension in the diabetic subject. However, hyperkalemia may occur in diabetic patients with type 4 renal tubular acidosis or in any diabetic on potassium supplements or potassium-sparing diuretics.

Hypertension with Hyperlipidemia

- Because hyperlipidemia compounds the risk of coronary artery disease, it should be effectively managed or prevented in hypertensive patients.
- Thiazide diuretics and β blockers without ISA or α-blocking properties may affect serum lipids adversely, although it is controversial whether the effect persists over time.
- α-adrenergic agonists decrease LDL cholesterol and increase HDL cholesterol levels, giving them some advantage over other agents.
- ACE inhibitors and calcium channel antagonists have no effect on serum lipids.

Hypertension and Coronary Artery Disease

- For hypertensive patients with ischemic heart disease, β blockers and calcium channel antagonists lower blood pressure and reduce myocardial oxygen demand. The cardiac stimulation that may occur with nifedipine or β blockers with ISA, however, may make these agents less desirable in this clinical setting.
- Reducing the DBP excessively may compromise coronary perfusion, especially in patients with fixed coronary artery stenosis, and lead to myocardial infarction (MI).
- For secondary prevention of infarction in hypertensive patients, calcium channel blockers do not afford the same degree of benefit as β blockers. Diltiazem has been shown to reduce reinfarction in patients with non–Q-wave infarcts and may reduce cardiac events in post-MI patients who do not have heart failure.

Hypertension and Heart Failure

- In patients with heart failure, captopril, enalapril, and ramipril have been shown to improve symptomatology and reduce mortality. Because of the high renin and angiotensin II status of patients with heart failure, therapy should be initiated at low doses to avoid a profound drop in blood pressure.
- A β blocker or nondihydropyridine calcium channel antagonist may improve left ventricular filling and cardiac output in patients with reduced cardiac output due to diastolic dysfunction. However, these agents may worsen heart failure in patients with systolic decompensation.

HYPERTENSIVE URGENCIES AND EMERGENCIES

- Hypertensive urgencies may be treated effectively with oral loading using:
    - clonidine, with 0.2 mg given initially followed by 0.2 mg hourly until the DBP falls below 110 mm Hg or a total of 0.7 mg has been administered; a single dose may be sufficient.
    - captopril, with oral doses of 25–50 mg given at 1- to 2-hour intervals.
- Hypertensive emergencies must be treated aggressively immediately to salvage viable tissue. DBP should not be lowered below 100–110 mm Hg over several minutes to several hours depending on the clinical situation. Precipitous drops in blood pressure to the normotensive range or lower may lead to end-organ ischemia or infarction. After the goal DBP is reached, treatment should be designed to hold that level of pressure for several days to allow physiologic adjustments in autoregulatory function. Then the blood pressure can be further reduced to normotensive levels.
    - **Nitroprusside** is the agent of choice for minute-to-minute control in most cases. It is usually given as a continuous IV infusion at a rate of 0.5–8.0 μg/kg/min. Its onset of hypotensive action is immediate and its effect disappears within 2–5 minutes of discontinuation of the infusion. When the infusion must be continued longer than 72 hours, serum thiocyanate levels should be measured, and the infusion should be discontinued if the level exceeds 12 mg/dL. The risk of thiocyanate toxicity is increased in patients with impaired renal function. Other side effects of nitroprusside include fatigue, nausea, anorexia, disorientation, psychotic behavior, muscle spasms, and, rarely, hypothyroidism. Nitroprusside administration requires constant intra-arterial pressure monitoring.
    - **IV nitroglycerin** may be given at a rate of 5–100 μg/min. As with oral nitrates, IV nitroglycerin is associated with tolerance over 24–48 hours.
    - **Diazoxide** given in small IV bolus doses (50–100 mg every 5–10 minutes) or by slow IV infusion over 15–30 minutes avoids the precipitous fall in pressure that occurs when given as a 300-mg rapid IV bolus. Because diazoxide increases plasma volume, it is common practice to give a diuretic concurrently unless the patient is

volume depleted. Diazoxide has quick onset and a duration of action ranging from 4–12 hours. It occasionally causes overshoot hypotension, which can be reversed by pressor agents. Other side effects include nausea, vomiting, tachycardia, hyperglycemia, and hyperuricemia.

- **Trimethaphan camsylate** is a ganglionic blocking agent that is particularly useful for treating hypertension in patients with acute aortic dissection. It is administered by continuous IV infusion with constant or frequent intra-arterial pressure monitoring at an initial infusion rate of 1 mg/min; the dose can be adjusted up to 10 mg/min. Its onset of action is immediate and its effects disappear within 10 minutes of discontinuation. Trimethaphan may cause profound orthostatic hypotension, ileus, urinary retention, dry mouth, and visual impairment. Respiratory arrest has been reported at infusion rates greater than 5 mg/min.
- **Labetolol** may be given at an initial dose of 20 mg by slow IV injection over a 2-minute period, followed by repeated injections of 40–80 mg at 10-minute intervals, up to a total dose of 300 mg. It can also be administered by continuous infusion at an initial rate of 2 mg/min and adjusted according to blood pressure response. Because of its α-blocking effects, labetolol can cause orthostatic hypotension. Other side effects include nausea, vomiting, paresthesias, sweating, dizziness, flushing, and headaches.
- **Hydralazine** may be given intravenously by diluting 10–20 mg in 20 mL of 5% dextrose in water (D_5W) and administering it at a rate of 0.5–1.0 mL/min. Its onset of action ranges from 10–30 minutes and its effects last 2–4 hours. Because the hypotensive response is less predictable than with other parenteral agents, its major role is in the treatment of eclampsia or hypertensive encephalopathy associated with renal insufficiency.
- **Nicardipine IV** may be administered for short-term treatment of hypertension using doses of 5–15 mg/h, which is adjusted by 1–2.5 mg/h after 15 minutes. Headaches, nausea, and vomiting are common side effects, and the use of the agent increases heart rate by 8–18 beats per minute.

► EVALUATION OF THERAPEUTIC OUTCOMES

- The goal of antihypertensive treatment is to maintain arterial blood pressure below 140/90 mm Hg to prevent cardiovascular morbidity and mortality. If feasible, attempts to lower blood pressure to <120/80 may be pursued.
- Either self-recorded measurements or automatic ambulatory blood pressure monitoring should be performed to establish effective 24-hour control. Readings should be taken after 2–4 weeks of initiating or making changes in therapy. Once the goal level is achieved, readings need to be evaluated only every 3–6 months in asymptomatic patients.

- Patients receiving treatment should be questioned periodically about changes in their general health perception, energy level, physical functioning, and overall satisfaction with treatment.
- A careful history should be taken for chest pain, palpitations, dizziness, dyspnea, orthopnea, slurred speech, and loss of balance to assess the likelihood of cardiovascular and cerebrovascular hypertensive complications.
- Other parameters used to assess therapeutic efficacy include changes in funduscopic findings, left ventricular hypertrophy regression on ECG or echocardiogram, resolution of proteinuria, and improvement in renal function.
- Patients should be monitored routinely for adverse drug effects, as discussed previously in this chapter.

See Chapter 10, Hypertension, authored by David W. Hawkins, PharmD, Henry I. Bussey, PharmD, and L. Michael Prisant, MD, for a more detailed discussion of this topic.

Chapter 10

▶ ISCHEMIC HEART DISEASE

▶ DEFINITION

Ischemic heart disease (IHD) is defined as a lack of oxygen and decreased or no blood flow in the myocardium. The disease results from coronary artery narrowing or obstruction and is manifested as the clinical syndrome of angina pectoris. IHD has many clinical expressions including stable exertional angina; unstable (rest, preinfarction, crescendo) angina; silent myocardial ischemia; acute coronary insufficiency; coronary vasomotion or vasospasm associated with atypical, variant, or Prinzmetal's angina; and myocardial infarction (MI).

▶ PATHOPHYSIOLOGY

- The major determinants of myocardial oxygen demand (MVo_2) are heart rate, contractility, and intramyocardial wall tension. Wall tension is thought to be the most important factor. Because the consequences of IHD usually result from increased demand in the face of a fixed oxygen supply, alterations in MVo_2 are important as a cause of ischemia and for interventions intended to alleviate it.
- A clinically useful indirect estimate of MVo_2 is the double product (DP), which is heart rate (HR) multiplied by systolic blood pressure (SBP) ($DP = HR \times SBP$). The DP does not consider changes in contractility (an independent variable), and because only changes in pressure are considered, volume loading of the left ventricle and increased MVo_2 related to ventricular dilation are underestimated.
- MVo_2 and the caliber of the resistance vessels delivering blood to the myocardium are the prime determinants in the occurrence of ischemia.
- The normal coronary system consists of large epicardial or surface vessels (R_1) that offer little resistance to myocardial flow and intramyocardial arteries and arterioles (R_2), which branch into a dense capillary network to supply basal blood flow. Under normal circumstances, the resistance in R_2 is much greater than that in R_1. Myocardial blood flow is inversely related to arteriolar resistance and directly related to the coronary driving pressure.
- Atherosclerotic lesions occluding R_1 increase arteriolar resistance, and R_2 can vasodilate to maintain coronary blood flow. With greater degrees of obstruction, this response is inadequate, and the coronary flow reserve afforded by R_2 vasodilation is insufficient to meet oxygen demand. Relatively severe stenosis (80–85%) may provoke ischemia and symptoms at rest while less severe stenosis may allow a reserve of coronary blood flow for exertion.
- The diameter and length of obstructing lesions and the influence of pressure drop across an area of stenosis affect coronary blood flow

and function of the collateral circulation. Dynamic coronary obstruction can occur in normal vessels and vessels with stenosis in which vasomotion or spasm may be superimposed on a fixed stenosis. Persisting ischemia may promote growth of developed collateral blood flow. II

- Critical stenosis occurs when the obstructing lesion encroaches on the luminal diameter and exceeds 70–80%. Lesions creating obstruction of 50–70% may reduce blood flow, but these obstructions are not consistent, and vasospasm and thrombosis superimposed on a "noncritical" lesion may lead to clinical events such as MI. If the lesion enlarges from 80% to 90%, resistance in that vessel is tripled. Coronary reserve is diminished at about 85% obstruction due to vasoconstriction.
- Abnormalities of ventricular contraction can occur, and regional loss of contractility may impose a burden on the remaining myocardial tissue, resulting in heart failure, increased MVO_2, and rapid depletion of oxygen stores. Zones of tissue with marginal blood flow may develop that are at risk for more severe damage if the ischemic episode persists or becomes more severe. Nonischemic areas of myocardium may compensate for the severely ischemic and border zones of ischemia by developing more tension than usual in an attempt to maintain cardiac output. Changes at the cellular level may impair the association of actin and myosin. The left or right ventricular dysfunction that ensues may be associated with clinical findings of an S_3, dyspnea, orthopnea, tachycardia, fluctuating blood pressure, transient murmurs, and mitral or tricuspid regurgitation.

► CLINICAL PRESENTATION

- The classic symptoms associated with typical chest pain and angina due to IHD appear in Table 10–1. For some patients, the presenting symptoms due to ischemia differ from the classical symptoms, and these are referred to as anginal equivalents.
- Patients suffering from variant or Prinzmetal's angina secondary to coronary spasm are more likely to experience pain at rest and in the early morning hours. Pain is not usually brought on by exertion or emotional stress nor relieved by rest; the electrocardiogram (ECG) pattern is that of current injury with ST elevation rather than depression.
- Unstable angina is generally defined as the presence of one or more of the following: (1) new onset (<2 months) exertional angina resulting in marked limitations of ordinary physical activity; (2) recent (<2 months) acceleration of angina as reflected by an increase in severity; or (3) pain at rest which lasts for >20 minutes.
- Ischemia may also be painless or "silent" in many patients due to a higher threshold and tolerance for pain.

TABLE 10–1. Characteristics of Angina Pectoris

Quality
Sensation of pressure or heavy weight on the chest
Burning sensation
Feeling of tightness
Shortness of breath with feeling of constriction about the larynx or upper trachea
Visceral quality (deep, heavy, squeezing, aching)
Gradual increase in intensity followed by gradual fading away
Location
Over the sternum or very near to it
Anywhere between epigastrium and pharynx
Occasionally limited to left shoulder and left arm
Rarely limited to right arm
Limited to lower jaw
Lower cervical or upper thoracic spine
Left interscapular or suprascapular area
Duration
0.5–30 min
Precipitating factors
Relationship to exercise
Effort that involves use of arms above the head
Cold environment
Walking against the wind
Walking after a large meal
Emotional factors involved with physical exercise
Fright, anger
Coitus
Nitroglycerin relief
Relief of pain occurring within 45 sec to 5 min of taking nitroglycerin
Radiation
Medial aspect of left arm
Left shoulder
Jaw
Occasionally right arm

From Helfant RH, Banka VS. A Clinical and Angiographic Approach to Coronary Heart Disease. *Philadelphia, FA Davis, 1978, p 47, with permission.*

► DIAGNOSIS

- Important aspects of the clinical history include the nature or quality of the chest pain, precipitating factors, duration, pain radiation, and the response to nitroglycerin or rest. There appears to be little relationship between the historical features of angina and the severity or extent of coronary artery vessel involvement. Ischemic chest pain may resemble pain arising from a variety of noncardiac sources, and the differential diagnosis of anginal pain from other etiologies may be difficult based on history alone.

II

- The patient should be asked about major risk factors for coronary disease, including smoking and a family history of coronary artery disease (CAD), familial lipid disorders, and diabetes mellitus.
- There are few signs on physical examination to indicate the presence of CAD. Findings on the cardiac examination may include abnormal precordial systolic bulge, decreased intensity of S_1, paradoxical splitting of S_2, S_3 (ventricular gallop), S_4 (atrial gallop), apical systolic murmur, and diastolic murmur. Elevated heart rate or blood pressure can yield an increased DP and may be associated with angina. Other noncardiac physical findings suggesting that significant cardiovascular disease may be present include abdominal aortic aneurysms or peripheral vascular disease.
- Other than risk-factor screening (lipid profiling, fasting glucose to exclude diabetes), there are no specific laboratory tests that are useful in diagnosing CAD. Cardiac enzymes should be normal in the angina patient.
- The ECG is normal in about one-half of patients with angina who are not experiencing an acute attack. Typical ST-T wave changes include depression, T-wave inversion, and ST-segment elevation. Variant angina is associated with ST-segment elevation, whereas silent ischemia may produce elevation or depression. Significant ischemia is associated with ST-segment depression of >2 mm, exertional hypotension, and reduced exercise tolerance.
- Exercise tolerance (stress) testing (ETT) is useful for a history of chest pain that is equivocal, for risk stratification, implementation of medical versus surgical therapy, and to assess the efficacy of treatment. Ischemic ST depression that occurs during ETT is an independent risk factor for cardiac events and cardiovascular mortality. Thallium (^{201}Tl) myocardial perfusion scintigraphy may be used in conjunction with ETT to detect reversible and irreversible defects in blood flow to the myocardium.
- Radionuclide angiocardiography (performed with technetium-99*m*, a radioisotope) is used to measure ejection fraction (EF), regional ventricular performance, cardiac output, ventricular volumes, valvular regurgitation, asynchrony or wall motion abnormalities, and intracardiac shunts.
- Echocardiography is useful for direct visualization of lesions in the left main coronary artery and in detecting the presence of ventricular aneurysms, assessing EF, and detecting regional or global left ventricular (LV) function abnormalities that occur during ischemia episodes.
- Ambulatory ECG (Holter) monitoring is useful in detecting ischemia during symptomatic and asymptomatic episodes and provides information for an extended period of time.

- Cardiac catheterization and angiography in patients with suspected CAD are used diagnostically to document the presence and severity of disease as well as for prognostic purposes.

▶ DESIRED OUTCOME

The goals of treatment are to relieve the patient's symptoms, maintain functional capacity, minimize adverse effects of treatment, and prevent progression to MI.

▶ TREATMENT

MODIFICATION OF RISK FACTORS

- Primary prevention through the identification and modification of risk factors should result in a significant impact on the prevalence of IHD. Secondary intervention is effective in reducing subsequent morbidity and mortality.
- Risk factors are additive and can be classified as alterable or unalterable. Unalterable risk factors include gender, age, family history or genetic composition, environmental influences, and, to some extent, diabetes mellitus. Risk factors that can be altered include smoking, hypertension, hyperlipidemia, obesity, sedentary lifestyle, hyperuricemia, psychosocial factors such as stress and type A behavior patterns, and the use of certain drugs that may be detrimental including progestins, corticosteroids, cyclosporine, thiazide diuretics, and β blockers. Although thiazide diuretics and β blockers (nonselective without intrinsic sympathomimetic activity) may elevate both cholesterol and triglycerides by 10–20%, and these effects may be detrimental, no objective evidence exists from prospective well-controlled studies to support avoiding these drugs.
- Alcohol ingestion in small to moderate amounts (<40 g/d of pure ethanol) reduces the risk of CAD; however, consumption of large amounts (>50 g/d) or binge drinking of alcohol are associated with increased mortality from stroke, malignant neoplasms, and cirrhosis.

PHARMACOLOGIC THERAPY

β-Adrenergic Blocking Agents

- Decreased heart rate, decreased contractility, and a slight to moderate decrease in blood pressure with β-adrenergic receptor antagonism reduce MVO_2. The overall effect in patients with effort-induced angina is a reduction in oxygen demand. β blockers do not improve oxygen supply and, in certain instances, unopposed α-adrenergic stimulation may lead to coronary vasoconstriction.
- β blockers improve symptoms in about 80% of patients with chronic exertional stable angina, and objective measures of efficacy demonstrate improved exercise duration and delay in the time at which ST-

segment changes and initial or limiting symptoms occur. β blockade may allow angina patients previously limited by symptoms to perform more exercise and ultimately improve overall cardiovascular performance through a training effect. II

- Postacute MI patients with angina are particularly good candidates for β blockade because of a reduced risk of reinfarction. A beneficial effect on mortality has been demonstrated with timolol, propranolol, and metoprolol. Patients with preexisting LV dysfunction may receive digitalis glycosides to maintain cardiac output if β blockade is necessary for IHD.
- β blockade is effective in chronic exertional angina as monotherapy and in combination with nitrates and/or calcium channel antagonists. β blockers are the first-line drugs in chronic angina requiring daily maintenance therapy because they are more effective in reducing episodes of silent ischemia, reducing early morning peak of ischemic activity, and improving mortality after Q-wave MI than nitrates or calcium channel blockers. If β blockers are ineffective or not tolerated, then monotherapy with a calcium channel blocker or combination therapy may be instituted. Reflex tachycardia from nitrates can be blunted with β blocker therapy, making this a useful combination. Patients with severe angina, rest angina, or variant angina may be better treated with calcium channel antagonists.
- Initial doses of β blockers should be at the lower end of the usual dosing range and titrated to response. General guidelines include the objective of lowering resting heart rate to 50–60 beats per minute and limiting maximal exercise heart rate to about 100 beats per minute or less. Heart rate with modest exercise should be no more than about 20 beats per minute above resting heart rate (or a 10% increment over resting heart rate).
- There is little evidence to suggest superiority of any particular β blocker. Those with longer half-lives may be dosed less frequently, but even propranolol may be dosed twice a day in most patients with angina. The ancillary property of intrinsic sympathomimetic activity appears to be detrimental in patients with rest or severe angina because the reduction in heart rate would be minimized, therefore limiting a reduction in MVO_2. Cardioselective β blockers may be used in some patients to minimize adverse effects such as bronchospasm. Combined nonselective β and α blockade with labetolol may be useful in some patients with marginal LV reserve.
- Adverse effects associated with β blockade include hypotension, heart failure, bradycardia and heart block, bronchospasm, peripheral vasoconstriction and intermittent claudication, and altered glucose metabolism. Central nervous system adverse effects include fatigue, malaise, and depression. Abrupt withdrawal of therapy in patients with angina has been associated with increased severity and number of pain episodes and MI. Tapering of therapy over the course of 2 days should minimize the risk of withdrawal reactions if therapy is to be discontinued.

Nitrates

- The major mechanism of action of nitrates appears to be mediated indirectly through a reduction of myocardial oxygen demand secondary to venodilation and arterial–arteriolar dilation, leading to a reduction in wall stress from reduced ventricular volume and pressure. Direct actions on the coronary circulation include dilation of large and small intramural coronary arteries, collateral dilation, coronary artery stenosis dilation, abolition of normal tone in narrowed vessels, and relief of spasm.
- Nitrate therapy may be used to terminate an acute anginal attack, prevent effort- or stress-induced attacks, or for long-term prophylaxis. Sublingual, buccal, or spray **nitroglycerin** products are the treatment of choice for the alleviation of anginal attacks because of rapid absorption (Table 10–2). Prevention of symptoms may be accomplished by the prophylactic use of oral or transdermal products, but the development of tolerance may be problematic.
- **Sublingual nitroglycerin** 0.3–0.4 mg relieves pain in about 75% of patients within 3 minutes, with another 15% becoming pain free in 5–15 minutes. Pain persisting beyond about 20–30 minutes after the use of two or three nitroglycerin tablets is suggestive of evolving MI or unstable angina, and the patient should be instructed to seek emergency aid.
- Chewable, oral, and transdermal products are acceptable for the long-term prophylaxis of angina; dosing of the longer acting preparations should be adjusted to provide a hemodynamic response. This may require doses of oral **isosorbide dinatrate** (ISDN) ranging from 10–60 mg as often as every 3–4 hours due to tolerance or first-pass metabolism. Intermittent (10–12 hours on, 12–14 hours off) transdermal nitroglycerin therapy has been shown to produce modest but significant

TABLE 10–2. Nitrate Products

Product	Onset (min)	Duration	Initial Dose
Nitroglycerin			
IV	1–2	3–5 min	5 μg/kg/min
SL/lingual	1–3	30–60 min	0.3 mg
PO	40	3–6 h	2.5–9 mg tid
Ointment	20–60	2–8 h	½–1 inch
Patch	40–60	> 8 h	1 patch
Erythritol tetranitrate	5–30	4–6 h	5–10 mg tid
Pentaerythritol tetranitrate	30	4–8 h	10–20 mg tid
Isosorbide dinitrate			
SL/chewable	2–5	1–2 h	2.5–5 mg tid
PO	20–40	4–6 h	5–20 mg tid
Isosorbide mononitrate	30–60	6–8 h	20 mg qd, bid[a]

[a]Product dependent.

improvement in exercise time in chronic stable angina. Because nitrates work primarily through a reduction in MVO_2, the DP can be used to optimize the dose of sublingual and oral nitrate products. II

- Nitrates may be combined with other drugs with complementary mechanisms of action for chronic prophylactic therapy. Combination therapy is generally used in patients with more frequent symptoms or symptoms that do not respond to β blockers alone (nitrates plus β blockers or calcium channel blockers), in patients intolerant of β blockers or calcium channel blockers, and in patients having an element of vasospasm leading to decreased supply (nitrates plus calcium channel blockers).
- Pharmacokinetic characteristics common to nitrates include a large first-pass effect of hepatic metabolism, short to very short half-lives (except for isosorbide mononitrate [ISMN]), large volumes of distribution, high clearance rates, and large interindividual variations in plasma or blood concentrations. The half-life of nitroglycerin is 1–5 minutes regardless of route, hence the potential advantage of sustained-release and transdermal products. ISDN is metabolized to isosorbide 2 mono- and 5-mononitrate (ISMN). ISMN has a half-life of about 5 hours and may be given once or twice daily depending on the product chosen.
- Patients should be instructed to keep nitroglycerin in the original, tightly closed glass container and to avoid mixing with other medication. Patients should also be aware that enhanced venous pooling in the sitting or standing positions may improve the effect as well as the symptoms of postural hypotension.
- Adverse reactions include postural hypotension, reflex tachycardia, headaches and flushing, and occasional nausea. Excessive hypotension may result in MI or stroke. Noncardiovascular adverse effects include rash (especially with transdermal nitroglycerin) and methemoglobinemia with high doses given for extended periods.
- Because both the onset and offset of tolerance to nitrates occurs quickly, one dosing strategy to circumvent it is to provide a daily nitrate-free interval of 8 to 12 hours. ISDN, for example, should not be used more often than three times per day if tolerance is to be avoided.

Calcium Channel Antagonists

- Direct actions of the calcium antagonists include vasodilation of systemic arterioles and coronary arteries, leading to a reduction of arterial pressure and coronary vascular resistance as well as depression of the myocardial contractility and conduction velocity of the SA and AV nodes. Reflex β-adrenergic stimulation overcomes much of the negative inotropic effect, and depression of contractility becomes clinically apparent only in the presence of LV dysfunction and when other negative inotropic drugs are used concurrently.
- **Verapamil** and **diltiazem** cause less peripheral vasodilation than **nifedipine** and, consequently, the risk of myocardial depression is

greater with these two agents. Conduction through the AV node is predictably depressed with verapamil and to some extent with diltiazem, and they must be used with caution in patients with preexisting conduction abnormalities or in the presence of other drugs with negative chronotropic properties.

- MV_{O_2} is reduced with use of all the calcium channel antagonists primarily because of reduced wall tension secondary to reduced arterial pressure. Overall, the benefit provided by calcium channel antagonists is related to reduced MV_{O_2} rather than improved oxygen supply.
- In contrast to the β blockers, calcium channel antagonists have the potential to improve coronary blood flow through areas of fixed coronary obstruction by inhibiting coronary artery vasomotion and vasospasm.
- Good candidates for calcium channel antagonists in angina include patients with contraindications or intolerance to β blockers, coexisting conduction system disease (excluding the use of verapamil and possibly diltiazem), Prinzmetal's angina, concurrent hypertension, and severe ventricular dysfunction. **Amlodipine** is probably the drug of choice in severe ventricular dysfunction, and the other drugs in this class should be used with caution if the EF is <40%.

MANAGEMENT OF STABLE EXERTIONAL ANGINA PECTORIS (FIGURE 10–1)

- After assessing and manipulating alterable risk factors, a regular exercise program should be undertaken in a graduated fashion and with adequate supervision to improve cardiovascular and muscular fitness.
- Nitrate therapy should be the first step in managing acute attacks for patients with chronic stable angina if the attacks are infrequent (i.e., a few times per month) or for prophylaxis of symptoms when undertaking activities known to precipitate attacks. If angina occurs no more often than once every few days, then sublingual nitroglycerin or the spray or buccal products may be sufficient.
- For episodes of "first-effort" angina occurring in a predictable fashion, nitroglycerin may be used in a prophylactic manner with the patient taking 0.3–0.4 mg sublingually about 5 minutes prior to the anticipated time of activity. Nitroglycerin spray may be useful when inadequate saliva is produced to rapidly dissolve sublingual nitroglycerin or if a patient has difficulty opening the container. The response usually lasts about 30 minutes.
- When angina occurs more frequently than once a day, chronic prophylactic therapy should be instituted. β-adrenergic blocking agents may be preferable because of less frequent dosing and other desirable pharmacologic properties (e.g., potential cardioprotective effects, antiarrhythmic effects, lack of tolerance, antihypertensive efficacy). The appropriate dose should be determined by the goals outlined for heart rate and DP. An agent should be selected that is well tolerated by individual patients at a reasonable cost. Patients most likely to respond well to β blockade are those with a high resting heart rate and those

with a relatively fixed anginal threshold (i.e., their symptoms appear at the same level of exercise or workload on a consistent basis).

- Calcium channel antagonists have the potential advantage of improving coronary blood flow through coronary artery vasodilation as well as decreasing MVo_2 and may be used instead of β blockers for chronic prophylactic therapy. They are as effective as β blockers and are most useful in patients who have a variable threshold for exertional angina. Calcium antagonists may provide better skeletal muscle oxygenation, resulting in decreased fatigue and better exercise tolerance. They can be used safely in many patients with contraindications to β-blocker therapy. The available drugs have similar efficacy in the management of chronic stable angina. Patients with conduction abnormalities and moderate to severe LV dysfunction (EF <35%) should be treated cautiously with verapamil. Diltiazem has significant effects on the AV node and can produce heart block in patients with preexisting conduction disease or when other drugs with effects on conduction (e.g., digoxin, β blockers) are used concurrently. Nifedipine may cause excessive heart rate elevation, especially if the patient is not receiving a β blocker, and this may offset its beneficial effect on MVo_2. The combination of calcium channel blockers and β blockers may increase exercise duration and decrease ECG evidence of ischemia; this combination may be more useful than adding nitrates to β-blocker therapy. Because both β blockers and calcium antagonists have the potential for depressing contractility, this combination should be used with care in patients with poor ventricular function.
- When angina occurs more than once a day, chronic prophylactic therapy with long-acting forms of nitroglycerin (oral or transdermal), ISDN, ISMN, and pentaerythritol trinitrate may also be effective. Monotherapy with nitrates should not be first-line therapy unless β blockers and calcium channel blockers are contraindicated or not tolerated. A nitrate-free interval of 8 hours per day or longer should be provided to maintain efficacy. Dose titration should be based on changes in the DP. The choice among nitrate products should be based on familiarity with the preparation, cost, and patient acceptance.

MANAGEMENT OF UNSTABLE ANGINA PECTORIS (Figure 10–2)

- Precipitation of the acute ischemic syndromes of unstable angina and MI are thought to be due to progression of atherosclerosis, acute coronary thrombosis, coronary artery spasm, and platelet aggregation. Patients at high risk of death or nonfatal MI are those presenting with prolonged ongoing (>20 minutes) rest pain, pulmonary edema related to ischemia, angina at rest with dynamic ST changes of ≥1 mm, angina with new or worsening mitral regurgitation, S_3 or rales, and angina with hypotension. Unstable angina differs from stable angina in that the primary event is thought to be a reduction in coronary blood flow rather than an increase in MVo_2.
- Initial patient management should include history, physical examination, ECG (within 20 minutes), bed rest with continuous monitoring for

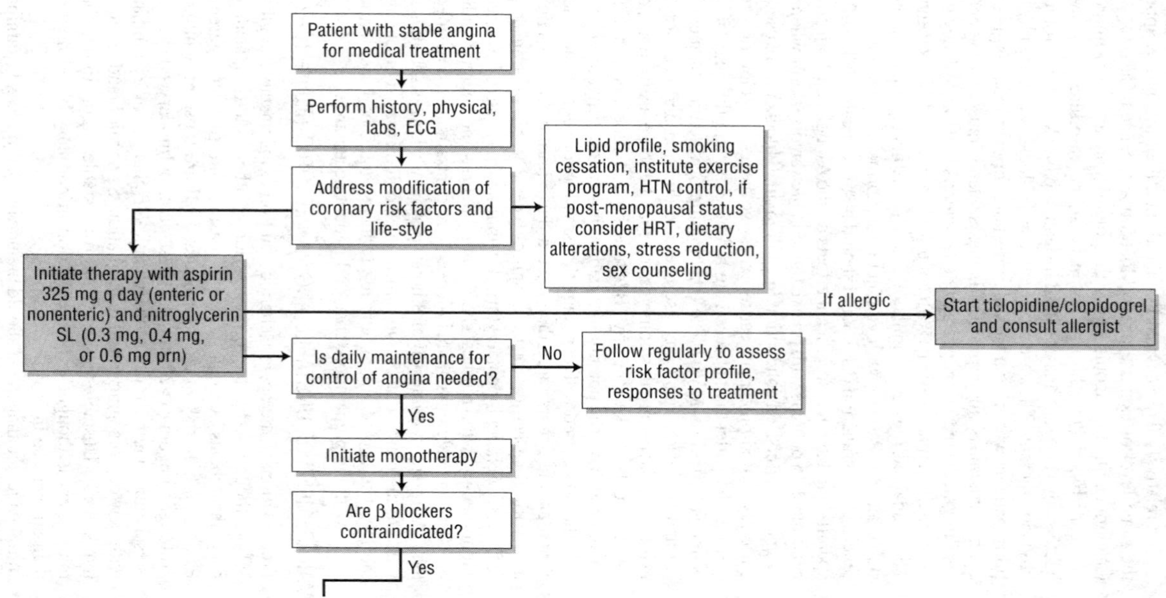
Patient with stable angina for medical treatment
Perform history, physical, labs, ECG
Address modification of coronary risk factors and life-style
Lipid profile, smoking cessation, institute exercise program, HTN control, if post-menopausal status consider HRT, dietary alterations, stress reduction, sex counseling
Initiate therapy with aspirin 325 mg q day (enteric or nonenteric) and nitroglycerin SL (0.3 mg, 0.4 mg, or 0.6 mg prn)
If allergic
Start ticlopidine/clopidogrel and consult allergist
Is daily maintenance for control of angina needed?
No
Follow regularly to assess risk factor profile, responses to treatment
Yes
Initiate monotherapy
Are β blockers contraindicated?
Yes

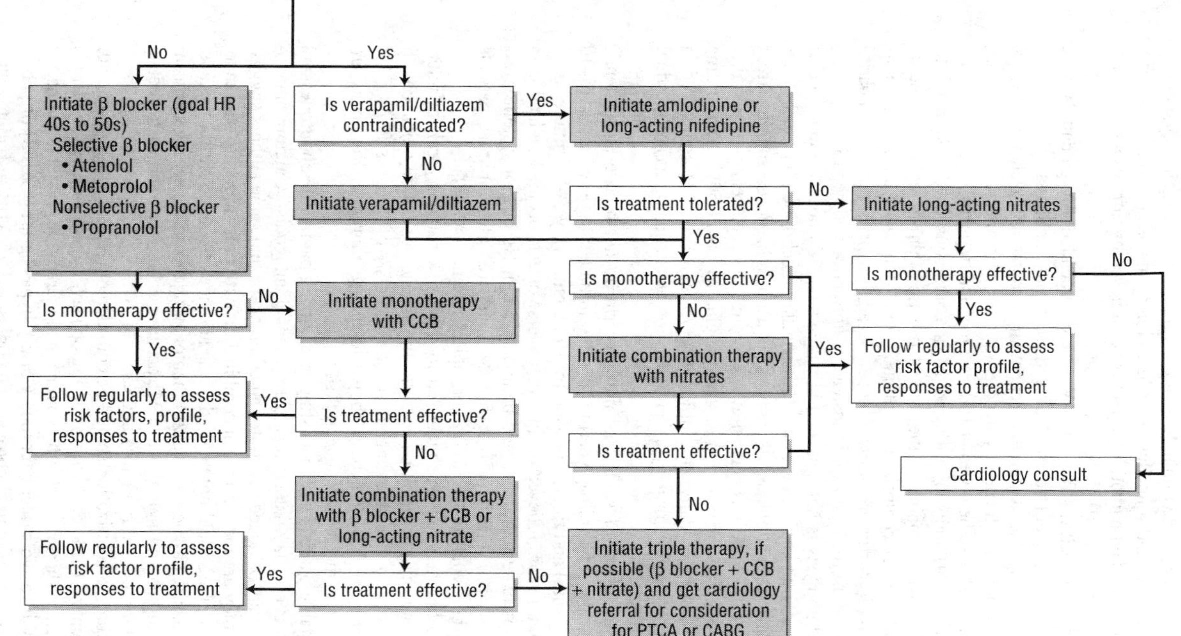

Figure 10–1. Algorithm for chronic stable angina. HR, heart rate; HTN, hypertension; HRT, hormone replacement therapy; CCB, calcium channel blocker; PTCA, percutaneous transluminal coronary angioplasty; CABG, coronary artery bypass grafting.

ischemia and arrhythmia detection, supplemental oxygen if cyanotic or hypoxemic, and immediate consideration of the use of aspirin, heparin, β blockers, and narcotics (if pain is not relieved by nitrates and β blockers) (see Figure 10–2).

- **Morphine sulfate** 2–5 mg IV is recommended for patients whose symptoms are not relieved after three serial sublingual nitroglycerin tablets or whose symptoms recur with adequate anti-ischemia therapy (unless contraindicated by hypotension or intolerance).
- **Aspirin** should be dosed at 160–325 mg, and **heparin** is given as an IV bolus of 80 units/kg followed by a continuous IV infusion of 18 units/kg/h to maintain the activated partial thromboplastin time at 1.5–2.5 times control and continued for 2–5 days or until revascularization is performed. Low-molecular-weight heparin (e.g., enoxaparin) may be useful with aspirin instead of unfractionated heparin.
- Thrombolysis is not indicated in patients who do not have evidence of acute ST-segment elevation or left bundle branch block on ECG.
- Long-term antiplatelet therapy with aspirin in doses ranging from 324–1300 mg/d has been shown to reduce the occurrence of mortality and nonfatal infarction in unstable angina by about 50%. **Ticlopidine** (250 mg twice daily) or **clopidogrel** (75 mg/d) may be considered in patients with aspirin hypersensitivity or recent major gastrointestinal bleeding.
- If three doses of sublingual nitroglycerin do not relieve the patient's pain, then IV nitroglycerin may be initiated at low doses (5–10 μg/kg/min) and titrated upward by 10 μg/min every 5–10 minutes until symptoms are relieved or limiting adverse effects occur. A reduction in SBP is expected and should be about 15 mm Hg or to a systolic pressure of 100–110 mm Hg. After 24 hours free of symptoms, patients may be switched over to oral or topical nitrates.
- IV β blockers are recommended for high-risk patients (oral for intermediate- and low-risk patients) in the absence of contraindications. β blockers in unstable angina reduce the risk of progression to MI slightly but have not been shown to reduce mortality. Regimens are similar to those used in acute MI.
- Unstable patients with persisting or recurring pain while on nitrates and β blockers may receive a calcium channel antagonist. Calcium antagonists may be added to nitrates and β blockers, and some authors suggest that they are most useful in combination with pretreatment β blockade. Nifedipine should not be used in the absence of concurrent β blockade. Diltiazem may be more useful than other agents in the setting of unstable angina and non–Q-wave MI because it has been shown to reduce reinfarction and refractory angina.
- Cardiac catheterization should be considered in the following groups of patients: (1) patients with prior angioplasty, bypass surgery, or MI; (2) patients who fail to stabilize on medical therapy; (3) patients opting for early invasive strategy (coronary artery bypass graft [CABG] or percutaneous transluminal coronary angioplasty [PTCA]); (4) patients with

Patient entry

Likelihood of CAD assessment

Initial evaluation; history, physical exam, ECG

Patient with known CAD

Simultaneous interactive evaluation

Risk assessment

Does patient meet likelihood of CAD or risk criteria for ischemia?

No → Alternate diagnosis/not ischemic heart disease; exit from this guideline

Yes

Does patient meet criteria for unstable angina?

No → Stable angina: exit from this guideline

Yes

Does patient meet criteria for thrombolytic therapy?

Yes → Reperfusion-eligible myocardial infarction: exit from this guideline

High-risk and intermediate-risk patients

Relieve pain and reduce ischemia

1. IV NTG
2. Morphine
3. β blockers IV/PO
4. Aspirin
5. CCB if uncontrolled with NTG and β blockers
6. UF heparin or LMWH

Yes

Pain persists?

Yes → Catheterization and revascularization

No

Patient counseling and assessment of patient preferences regarding early revascularization strategy

Patient chooses early invasive management

Yes → Catheterization and revascularization

No → Continue medical therapy

Pain persists?

Yes → Catheterization and revascularization

No → Nonintensive management

Figure 10–2. Algorithm for unstable angina. CAD, coronary artery disease; CCB, calcium channel blocker; NTG, nitroglycerin, UF, unfractionated; LMWH, low molecular weight heparin.

high-risk clinical findings or noninvasive test results; or (5) patients with significant heart failure or LV dysfunction.

- CABG is recommended for patients found to have ≥50% occlusion of the left main artery or ≥70% three-vessel disease with depressed LV function (EF <0.50). Patients with two-vessel disease with proximal LAD stenosis ≥95% and depressed LV function should be referred promptly for CABG or PTCA. Patients with significant CAD who fail to stabilize on medical therapy or have symptoms with low levels of exertion or have ischemia accompanied by heart failure should have prompt revascularization.
- If cardiac catheterization is not indicated, noninvasive exercise or pharmacologic stress testing should be performed in low- and intermediate-risk patients who have been free of angina and heart failure for 48 hours.
- In the event of prolonged chest pain and ischemic ECG changes unrelieved by nitrate therapy or calcium channel antagonists, one may assume total occlusion of a coronary vessel and steps should be taken to restore blood flow (e.g., thrombolytic therapy either alone or preceding PTCA).

CORONARY ARTERY SPASM AND VARIANT ANGINA PECTORIS

- All patients should be treated for acute attacks and maintained on prophylactic treatment for 6–12 months after the initial episode. Aggravating factors such as alcohol or cocaine use and cigarette smoking should be eliminated.
- Nitrates are the mainstay of therapy, and most patients respond rapidly to sublingual nitroglycerin or ISDN. IV and intracoronary nitroglycerin may be very useful for patients not responding to sublingual preparations.
- Because calcium channel antagonists may be more effective, have few serious adverse effects in effective doses, and can be given less frequently than nitrates, some consider them the agents of choice for variant angina. Nifedipine, verapamil, and diltiazem are all equally effective as single agents for the initial management of variant angina and coronary artery spasm. In patients unresponsive to calcium channel antagonists alone, nitrates may be added. Combination therapy with nifedipine plus diltiazem or nifedipine plus verapamil has been reported to be useful in patients unresponsive to single-drug regimens.
- β blockers have little or no role in the management of variant angina as they may induce coronary vasoconstriction and prolong ischemia, as documented by continuous ECG monitoring.
- The effects of aspirin in variant angina have not been as successful as in unstable angina, perhaps reflecting differences in the underlying pathophysiology.

► EVALUATION OF THERAPEUTIC OUTCOMES

- Subjective measures of drug response include the number of painful episodes, amount of rapid-acting nitroglycerin consumed, and patient-reported alterations in activities of daily living (e.g., time to walk two blocks, number of stairs climbed without pain).

- Objective clinical measures of response include HR, blood pressure, and the DP as a measure of MVO_2. Nitrates may increase HR but lower SBP, whereas calcium channel blockers and β blockers reduce the DP. II
- Objective assessment also includes the resolution of ECG changes at rest, during exercise, or with ambulatory ECG monitoring.
- Monitoring for major adverse effects includes headache and dizziness with nitrates; fatigue and lassitude with β blockers; and peripheral edema, constipation, and dizziness with calcium channel blockers.
- The ECG is very useful, particularly if the patient is experiencing chest pain or other symptoms thought to be of ischemic origin. ST-segment deviations are very important, and the extent of their deviation is related to the severity of ischemia.
- ETT may also be used to evaluate the response to therapy, but the expense and time needed to perform this test preclude its routine use.
- Cardiac catheterization, radionuclide scans, and echocardiography are used primarily for risk stratification and selecting patients for more invasive procedures rather than for monitoring therapy.
- A comprehensive plan includes ancillary monitoring of lipid profiles, fasting plasma glucose, thyroid function tests, hemoglobin/hematocrit, and electrolytes.
- For variant angina, reduction in symptoms and nitroglycerin consumption as documented by a patient diary can assist the interpretation of objective data obtained from ambulatory ECG recordings. Evidence of efficacy includes the reduction of ischemic events, both ST-segment depression and elevation. Additional evidence is a reduced number of attacks of angina requiring hospitalization, and the absence of MI and sudden death.

See Chapter 12, Ischemic Heart Disease, authored by Robert L. Talbert, PharmD, FCCP, BCPS, for a more detailed discussion of this topic.

Chapter 11

▶ MYOCARDIAL INFARCTION

▶ DEFINITION

Myocardial infarction (MI) results from a sudden interruption of blood supply to an area of myocardium resulting from complete, or near complete, occlusion of a coronary artery. The occlusion persists long enough that myocardial function is compromised and myocardium becomes necrotic (nonviable).

▶ PATHOPHYSIOLOGY

- Coronary artery disease (CAD) is the primary underlying process that leads to MI. Fatty streaks are deposited on coronary artery endothelium and may progress to form atherosclerotic plaques, depending on the absence or presence of specific risk factors (hypertension, diabetes mellitus, smoking, and hyperlipidemia).
- If progression occurs, plaques develop, proliferate, and eventually disrupt the integrity and function of the endothelium. Myocardial ischemia may occur owing to the narrowing of one or more coronary arteries. However, thrombus formation, not coronary artery narrowing, is believed to be the cause of >85% of acute MIs. The precipitating event is disruption of a coronary plaque, which initiates a thrombotic process.
- Infarction is characterized by a "wavefront" of ischemia that progresses from the endocardium to the epicardium. If coronary blood flow is not restored, myocardium dies within approximately 3 hours, based on animal models. Despite this rapid time course, a significant percentage of myocardium is salvageable after as long as 12–24 hours of ischemia, perhaps because of the presence of collateral blood flow within the infarcted area.
- Anterior wall MI (AWMI) involves the anterior wall of the left ventricle and most often represents occlusion of the left anterior descending (LAD) artery (Figure 11–1). AWMI involves a much larger area of myocardium than inferior wall MI (IWMI) and, consequently, there is a risk of a greater loss of myocardium and myocardial function.
- Although isolated right ventricular infarction accounts for <3% of all acute MIs, infarction of the right ventricle occurs in nearly 50% of patients with IWMI. In many patients, the right coronary artery (RCA) is a large, dominant vessel that not only supplies the right ventricle but also supplies a significant portion of inferior wall of the left ventricle. Therefore, occlusion of the RCA may result in an IWMI or the combination of an IWMI and right ventricular MI, depending on where the occlusion in the RCA occurs.

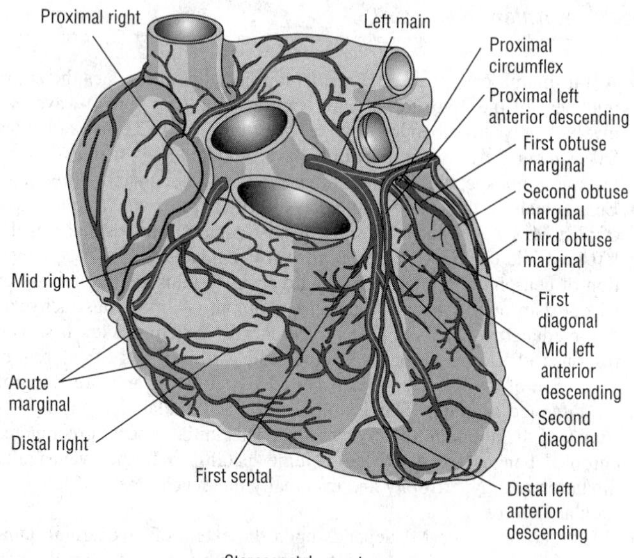

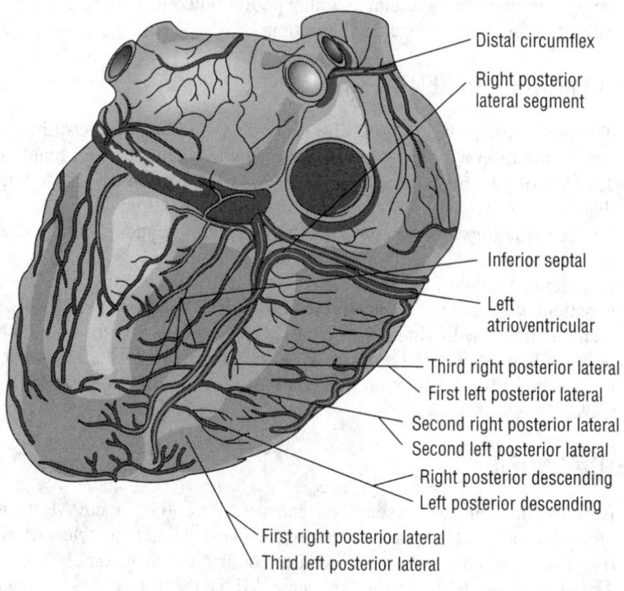

Figure 11–1. Coronary artery anatomy with sternocostal and diaphragmatic views.

- A transmural, or Q-wave, MI results in injury that penetrates the entire thickness of the myocardial wall. Nontransmural, or non–Q-wave, MI involves only the subendocardial myocardium; the ECG may not show ST-segment elevation but may only have subtle findings such as T wave inversion, nonspecific ST-T–wave changes, or ST-segment depression.
- Enlargement of the left ventricle plays a critical role in the development of post-MI heart failure and subsequent mortality. The response of the left ventricle to injury (called *ventricular remodeling*) involves activation of neurohumoral and renin–angiotensin systems and the release of vasopressin once a decrease in cardiac output occurs. Sinus tachycardia, mediated by activation of the adrenergic system, occurs first as a response to a drop in cardiac output and, within hours of infarction, expansion of the infarcted area occurs due to thinning and stretching of the infarcted segment. This is followed by acute dilatation and hypertrophy of the noninfarcted myocardium. This initial process precipitates chronic changes in ventricular volume leading to further ventricular dilatation and hypertrophy and eventually the development of left ventricular failure.
- Outcome after acute MI depends upon the extent of myocardial damage, left ventricular function, infarct location, the presence or absence of heart failure, and patient age. Anterior wall infarction tends to be larger and therefore associated with a poorer outcome than inferior wall infarction or right ventricular infarction.

▶ CLINICAL PRESENTATION

- The predominant symptom is chest pain that is frequently described as chest pressure or a squeezing sensation rather than pain. As many as 15–25% of patients with acute MI have no pain, particularly those with diabetes mellitus who may have autonomic dysfunction.
- Physical findings may include diaphoresis, nausea and vomiting, arm tingling/numbness, and shortness of breath.
- Hypotension, clear lung fields, and elevated jugular venous pressure in a patient with an IWMI are indications of right ventricular involvement. Patients with right ventricular MI may present with or quickly develop hemodynamic compromise or cardiogenic shock. Because of right ventricular dysfunction, there is inadequate filling of the left ventricle.

▶ DIAGNOSIS

- Because the clinical presentation cannot differentiate acute MI from other cardiac and noncardiac causes of chest pain, objective criteria (ECG, cardiac enzymes) are needed to confirm the diagnosis.
- The diagnostic ECG feature of acute MI is the Q wave associated with a pattern of ST-segment changes. The earliest change in the ECG is associated with the T wave; it may be prolonged, peaked, or

inverted. T wave alterations are soon followed by ST-segment elevation. A Q wave may or may not be present on the initial ECG or may appear hours or sometimes days after MI.

- Serial blood samples for the determination of cardiac enzyme concentrations should be obtained every 6–8 hours for 24 hours if MI is suspected. Creatine kinase (CK) concentration peaks within 24 hours after acute MI, followed by a decline and return to baseline by the third or fourth day. There must be an elevation of the total CK with at least a 4% CK-MB isoenzyme fraction to confirm the diagnosis of Q wave MI. The higher the total CK and percent MB, the larger the infarct. Peak lactate dehydrogenase (LDH) concentrations usually occur between 3 and 4 days after MI and return to normal by day 14. The utility of serial LDH determinations is limited; if the patient presents late (beyond 24 hours) from the onset of symptoms, determination of serial LDH concentrations may be useful in confirming the diagnosis. Peak concentrations should be at least two times above normal with an increase in the LDH-1 fraction that ultimately exceeds the concentration of the LDH-2 fraction (referred to as the LDH "flip").
- The diagnosis of Q wave acute MI is made if the following criteria are met: the presence of ischemic chest pain for at least 30 minutes and/or ST-segment elevation on the ECG with the subsequent development of pathological Q waves. The diagnosis is then confirmed by a rise in cardiac enzymes as described above.

▶ DESIRED OUTCOME

The primary goals of therapy for patients with acute MI are to relieve pain and anxiety, minimize infarct size, salvage ischemic myocardium, prevent or minimize complications, and reduce mortality and improve quality of life.

▶ TREATMENT

GENERAL PRINCIPLES

- Admission to an intensive care or coronary care unit is mandatory for close observation and acute care.
- Close monitoring of vital signs, symptoms, and the ECG is recommended for the first 48–72 hours after MI in uncomplicated patients. Continued intensive monitoring is recommended beyond 72 hours if the patient is hemodynamically unstable and has persistent ischemia and/or hemodynamically significant cardiac arrhythmias.
- Activity should be restricted for the first 2–3 days and gradually increased as tolerated by the patient.
- The diet should include use of multiple small meals, sodium restriction, and reduced content of saturated fats and cholesterol.

- A stool softener, either docusate sodium 100 mg or docusate calcium 240 mg once or twice a day, is recommended to avoid the stress associated with defecation.
- If possible, patients with presumed acute MI should have three large-bore (18-gauge) peripheral intravenous (IV) lines placed upon admission to the emergency department to permit prompt drug therapy and facilitate collection of blood for diagnostic tests.
- Pertinent laboratory tests on admission should include CBC with platelet count, activated partial thromboplastin time (aPTT), prothrombin time (PT) and international normalized ratio (INR). If the patient receives thrombolytic therapy, regular assessment of hemoglobin, hematocrit, and platelets should be obtained.
- For the first 2–3 hours of acute MI, supplemental oxygen (2–4 L/min by nasal cannula) should be administered because even uncomplicated patients may be moderately hypoxic.

PHARMACOLOGIC THERAPY

Analgesics

- IV **morphine sulfate** is the drug of choice for acute pain associated with MI. It results in peripheral arteriolar dilation, which decreases systemic vascular resistance and reduces myocardial oxygen demand (MVo_2). It also reduces afterload and decreases circulating concentrations of catecholamines, which may reduce the likelihood of ventricular arrhythmias.
- IV morphine should be administered slowly in small doses of 2–5 mg every 5–15 minutes, as needed. Some patients with persistent pain may require maintenance doses of 4–8 mg every 4–6 hours.
- Therapy should be continued until pain relief is achieved or an unacceptable end point, such as hypotension (systolic blood pressure <90 mm Hg), is reached. Patients should be monitored closely for hypotension, respiratory depression, and allergic reactions.

Nitroglycerin

- The purpose of **nitroglycerin** (NTG) therapy is to relieve myocardial ischemia via coronary vasodilation. Data from the ISIS-4 trial suggest that nitrate therapy may reduce the risk of early death in MI patients. Therefore IV nitroglycerin is used to manage ischemia for the first 24–48 hours, especially in MI patients with heart failure, large or AWMI, persistent ischemia, or hypertension. Use beyond 48 hours should be reserved for patients with persistent chest pain, heart failure, or hypertension.
- Sublingual (SL) NTG (0.4 mg) is frequently used to determine whether chest pain is due to MI or ischemia. Typically, 0.4 mg SL NTG is administered, and chest pain intensity and the ECG are assessed. This dose may be repeated three times, once every 5 minutes, as long as heart rate and blood pressure are stable. If the ECG changes persist despite relief of chest pain, the diagnosis is MI.

- IV NTG is preferred in the management of MI because it is easily titrated. Therapy may be initiated with an infusion of 5–10 µg/min via an infusion pump. The infusion may be increased every 5–10 minutes by 5–10 µg/min increments for chest pain relief, resolution of ECG abnormalities, or until the systolic blood pressure is between 90 and 100 mm Hg. The duration of therapy for an uncomplicated MI should not exceed 48 hours.
- Heart rate and blood pressure must be monitored during IV NTG administration. If hypotension develops, the rate of infusion should be reduced or gradually discontinued. IV fluids should be administered if the patient remains hypotensive upon discontinuation. If the patient becomes either symptomatically tachycardic or bradycardic, the NTG infusion rate should be decreased. The ECG should also be closely monitored for reemergence of ischemia, even if the patient does not have recurrent chest pain.
- Headache is common with NTG (>50%); decreasing the infusion rate and use of acetaminophen may be effective and should be given consideration prior to discontinuation of the NTG infusion.

Lidocaine

- Although ventricular tachycardia (VT) and ventricular fibrillation (VF) are the most common consequences of MI, prophylactic **lidocaine** is not recommended because it has not been shown to reduce mortality and is associated with potentially serious risks.
- Lidocaine has no role in the early management (within 48 hours) of MI unless the patient experiences VF and/or unsustained VT. Refer to Chapter 5 for details regarding the use of lidocaine and other antiarrhythmics in the management of VT/VF.

Early Administration of β-Adrenergic Blockers

- Administration of β blockers within 12 hours of the onset of chest pain reduces the incidence of ventricular arrhythmias, recurrent ischemia, and reinfarction, and, most important, mortality in patients with acute MI.
- If there are no contraindications, β-blocker therapy is recommended within 12 hours of symptom onset for MI patients whether or not they receive thrombolytic therapy.
- The choice of agent does not appear to be an issue except that those with intrinsic sympathomimetic activity (ISA) should be avoided since they have not been shown to be of benefit. Examples of IV dosing regimens include:
  - **Propranolol** 0.1 mg/kg in two to three divided doses every 10 minutes
  - **Metoprolol** 15 mg in three divided doses every 5 minutes
  - **Atenolol** 5–10 mg in two divided doses every 5–10 minutes
- An oral regimen can be initiated 6–12 hours after the last IV dose depending on the β blocker used. An algorithm outlining the decision-

making process for acute β-blocker therapy with metoprolol is outlined in Figure 11–2.

II

Late Administration of β-Adrenergic Blockers

- The goal of late (at least 24 hours after MI) oral administration of β-blocker therapy is prevention of recurrent infarction and death. Studies have demonstrated an improvement in survival and a reduction in reinfarction when therapy is initiated as early as 24 hours and as late as 28 days after MI. Patients with mild heart failure appear to benefit at least as much as patients with normal LV function. Long-term β-blocker therapy is recommended in all but low-risk patients and those with a contraindication to β-blocker therapy.
- Examples of dosing regimens include:
  - Propranolol 180–240 mg/d in four divided doses
  - Metoprolol 100 mg twice daily
  - Atenolol 100 mg once daily
  - Timolol 10 mg twice daily

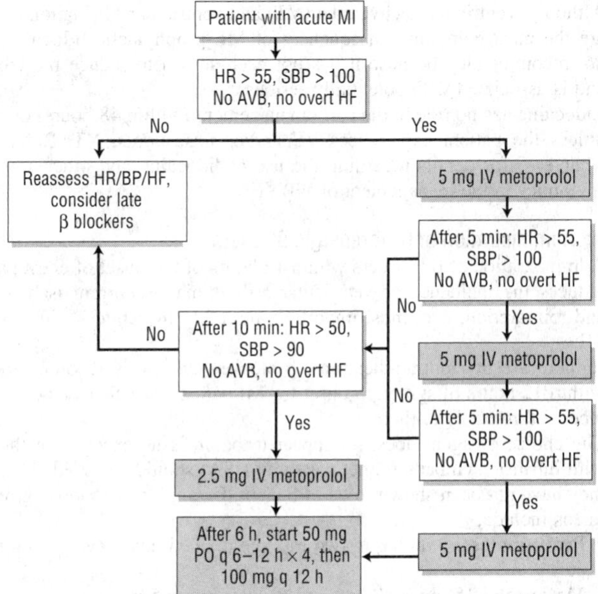

Figure 11–2. Algorithm for the administration of early IV metoprolol to patients with acute myocardial infarction. HR, heart rate; SBP, systolic blood pressure; AVB, atrioventricular block; HF, heart failure.

- Whenever possible, the dose should be maximized unless this is intolerable to the patient.
- For secondary prevention, β-blocker therapy should be continued indefinitely.

Calcium Channel Antagonists

- There is no evidence that calcium channel antagonists confer a mortality benefit in the setting of acute MI. In the acute phase, only **diltiazem** or **verapamil** may be used when there is a clear indication such as persistent angina or hypertension that is unresponsive to β blockers, or when β blockers are contraindicated in either of these two situations.
- Diltiazem and verapamil may also be appropriate for patients with a rapid ventricular rate associated with ventricular fibrillation as long as there is no evidence of heart failure, LV dysfunction, or AV block.
- Diltiazem is recommended for patients with non–Q-wave MI for the prevention of post-MI angina and reinfarction. Calcium channel antagonists are not routinely recommended in patients with Q-wave MI.
- In patients with non–Q-wave MI who have no contraindications, diltiazem 90 mg every 6 hours should be initiated between 24 and 72 hours after the onset of MI and continued for 1 year.
- Heart rate, blood pressure, and the frequency of anginal episodes should be monitored closely. Other side effects of diltiazem include constipation, nausea, and dizziness.
- Because of equivocal results from clinical trials, calcium channel blockers are not recommended for routine use for secondary prevention of acute MI.

Thrombolytic Therapy

- Agents approved for use by the FDA in patients with acute MI in the United States include:
  - **Alteplase** (recombinant tissue-type plasminogen activator [Activase])
  - **Anistreplase** (anisoylated plasminogen streptokinase activator complex or APSAC [Eminase])
  - **Reteplase** (recombinant plasminogen activator [Retavase])
  - **Streptokinase** (Streptase/Kabikinase)
- These agents improve myocardial oxygen supply by dissolving the thrombus associated with acute MI, reestablishing blood flow to ischemic myocardium. Consequently, the extent of myocardial necrosis and infarct size are limited and the likelihood of survival is significantly improved if thrombolysis is achieved in a timely fashion.
- Patients who present within the first 12 hours after onset of chest pain should be evaluated as candidates for thrombolytic therapy. Patients who present between 12 and 24 hours may be considered if they have signs and symptoms of ongoing ischemia such as persistent ST-segment elevation and chest pain. Patients who present after 24 hours should not be considered eligible.

- Absolute and relative contraindications to thrombolytic therapy are outlined in Table 11–1. The presence of more than one relative contraindication is considered an *absolute* contraindication to therapy. Age is neither an absolute nor relative contraindication.
- Although there may be a slight mortality benefit in favor of alteplase, it is more expensive than streptokinase. The choice of thrombolytic agent is less important than ensuring that a thrombolytic drug is given in a timely manner to eligible patients.
- Current recommendations call for the administration of thrombolytic therapy to patients with ECG evidence of Q-wave MI who present within 12 hours of the onset of chest pain without contraindications to therapy. Eligible patients should be treated as soon as possible, but preferably within 70 minutes from the time they present to the emergency department, with one of the following regimens:
    - Alteplase: 15 mg IV bolus followed by 0.75 mg/kg infusion (not to exceed 50 mg) over 30 minutes followed by 0.5 mg/kg infusion (not to exceed 35 mg) over the next 60 minutes
    - Anistreplase: 30 units IV over 2 minutes
    - Reteplase: 10 units IV over 2 minutes followed by a second 10 units over 2 minutes 30 minutes later
    - Streptokinase: 1.5 million units in 50 mL of normal saline or D_5W IV over 60 minutes
- A lytic state characterized by a fall in fibrinogen concentration, an increase in fibrin degradation products, and prolongation of the aPTT

TABLE 11–1. Relative and Absolute Contraindications to Thrombolytic Therapy in Patients with Acute Myocardial Infarction

Absolute Contraindications
History of hemorrhagic stroke at any time; other strokes or cerebrovascular events within 1 year
Possible aortic dissection
Acute pericarditis
Active internal bleeding (does not include menses)
Known intracranial neoplasm
Relative Contraindications/Cautions
Severe uncontrolled hypertension (BP >180/110 mm Hg) or history of chronic severe hypertension
Recent trauma or surgery (i.e., within 2 to 4 wk)
History of cerebrovascular accident > 1 year ago
Active peptic ulcer
Current use of anticoagulation therapy (INR ≥ 2 to 3)
Known bleeding diathesis
Previous allergic reaction to streptokinase or anistreplase; use alteplase
Significant liver dysfunction
Pregnancy
Recent internal bleeding
Prolonged CPR (>10 min)
Noncompressible vascular punctures

increases the risk of bleeding. Hemorrhagic stroke is the most serious adverse effect; others include hypotension and allergic reactions (primarily with streptokinase).

- Successful reperfusion with thrombolytic therapy can be assessed by normalization of the ECG, relief of chest pain, and onset of reperfusion arrhythmias, which are usually ventricular in nature.
- Patients in whom symptoms of MI persist beyond 1 to 2 hours from the start of thrombolytic therapy may benefit from rescue percutaneous transluminal coronary angioplasty (PTCA).

Antithrombotic Therapy

Aspirin

- **Aspirin** is a potent inhibitor of platelet cyclooxygenase with a rapid onset, usually before aspirin concentrations are detectable in the systemic circulation.
- Aspirin 160–325 mg should be chewed and swallowed as soon as possible after the onset of symptoms or immediately after presentation to the emergency department whether or not the patient is considered a candidate for thrombolytic therapy. Exceptions include aspirin allergy or GI intolerance. Patients with a history of aspirin allergy may receive **ticlopidine, clopidogrel,** or **dipyridamole.**
- For secondary prevention, aspirin has been shown to reduce the risk of recurrent cardiovascular events when started within days or even years of acute MI. A single loading dose of 300–325 mg followed by long-term therapy with 75 or 80 mg/d may be started in patients not already receiving aspirin as part of their acute MI care. Enteric-coated aspirin reduces the incidence of GI side effects (stomach pain, heartburn, nausea).
- Patients should be evaluated regularly for signs and symptoms of recurrent ischemia, as up to 30–40% of patients experience recurrent ischemia or reinfarction despite aspirin therapy.

Heparin

- When combined with thrombolytic therapy, IV **heparin** may have a beneficial effect on maintaining artery patency, but this comes at the expense of an increased risk of bleeding. Ongoing trials are evaluating use of a weight-based dosing regimen and established guidelines for the adjustment of heparin based on the aPTT. Until more information is acquired, the current recommendations for concomitant heparin therapy are as follows:
  - Alteplase and reteplase: Heparin 70 U/kg bolus followed by a continuous infusion of 15 U/kg/h at the time the thrombolytic therapy is initiated.
  - Streptokinase or anistreplase: Initiation of a continuous heparin infusion of 15 U/kg/h without a bolus dose starting 4 hours after the thrombolytic or when the aPTT returns to <2 times control. With these two agents, IV heparin is recommended only for patients at high risk for systemic embolization (e.g., patients with a large MI or

AWMI, atrial fibrillation, history of previous thromboembolic event, or visualized LV thrombus).

- In the absence of a thrombolytic agent, IV heparin may be used in MI patients who are at high risk for thromboembolism (i.e., large MI or AWMI, atrial fibrillation, history of embolus, or known LV thrombus).
- In patients with AWMI, use of full-dose IV heparin should continue for 48 hours to prevent LV thrombus formation. Heparin should be followed by warfarin therapy titrated to prolong the INR to 2.0 to 3.0 for 1 to 3 months.
- When used for prevention of thromboembolic complications of MI, subcutaneous heparin (7500 units twice daily) is recommended to begin within 12–18 hours after the onset of chest pain. This should be continued until the patient is ambulatory; follow-up therapy with warfarin is not necessary.

Warfarin

- **Warfarin** is currently recommended for secondary prevention in MI patients who are intolerant or allergic to aspirin. In these patients, the warfarin dose should be titrated to an INR of 2.0–3.0 and continued for up to 2 years.
- Patients with persistent or paroxysmal atrial fibrillation, extensive LV wall motion abnormalities, and severe LV dysfunction (LVEF <35%) may also benefit from warfarin prophylaxis.
- The combination of aspirin and warfarin is not recommended for secondary prevention.

Angiotensin-Converting Enzyme (ACE) Inhibitors

- Use of an ACE inhibitor within the first 24 hours of an MI is recommended if there is no significant hypotension and there are no other contraindication to ACE inhibitor use.
- In patients with clinical evidence of heart failure or in asymptomatic patients with an ejection fraction ≤40%, therapy should be continued indefinitely. For those without evidence of LV dysfunction, therapy can be discontinued after 4–6 weeks of therapy.
- ACE inhibitors should be withheld until thrombolytic therapy has been completed and the patient's blood pressure has stabilized (i.e., systolic blood pressure >100 mm Hg).
- Initial doses should not exceed **lisinopril** 5 mg, **captopril** 6.25 mg, or **trandolapril** 1 mg. The goal doses are those used in the clinical trials (lisinopril 10 mg/d, captopril 50 mg 2 or 3 times/d, and trandolapril 4 mg once daily).

NONPHARMACOLOGIC THERAPY

Primary PTCA

- Recent randomized trials have shown primary PTCA to produce superior reductions in mortality rate and recurrent MI compared with thrombolysis. However, few hospitals in the United States are capable of providing an emergency PTCA service. The delay in transferring patients to one of these facilities may offset any benefit associated with use of the procedure.

- Because of these practical limitations, primary PTCA is considered to be most beneficial as an alternative to thrombolysis for patients with cardiogenic shock, severe left ventricular dysfunction, and perhaps those at high risk of bleeding. To retain its potential benefits, the procedure must be performed in a timely manner by skilled individuals at high-volume centers.

▶ EVALUATION OF THERAPEUTIC OUTCOMES

- At the time of or near the time of hospital discharge, patients should be carefully evaluated to ensure the appropriate plan for rehabilitation.
- Patients should understand important aspects of their medications, particularly secondary prevention; modification of risk factors such as smoking, high cholesterol, and hypertension; exercise program; and diet.
- An objective assessment of a patient's prognosis and stratification for risk of recurrent cardiovascular events should be made, usually by exercise tolerance testing (ETT) and determination of left ventricular function. ETT with continuous ECG and blood pressure monitoring will determine the overall exercise capacity of the patient, blood pressure response to exercise, and if angina occurs, at what point during exercise it occurs, as well as if activity precipitates arrhythmias. Submaximal exercise testing can usually be performed just prior to hospital discharge and can then be followed by a full exercise test 1 month after infarction.
- High-risk patients are easily identified by their low exercise capability, failure of the systolic blood pressure to rise above the resting value during exercise (frequently referred to as an inadequate blood pressure response to exercise), and chest pain associated with ischemic changes on the ECG.
- Current guidelines recommend that post-MI patients undergo exercise testing annually following acute MI.
- Left ventricular function may be evaluated by echocardiography, coronary angiography, or radionuclear ventriculograms.

See Chapter 13, Myocardial Infarction, authored by Kathleen A. Stringer, PharmD, FCCP, and Larry M. Lopez, PharmD, FCCP, for a more detailed discussion of this topic.

Chapter 12

▶ SHOCK

▶ DEFINITION

Shock refers to conditions manifested by hemodynamic alterations (e.g., hypotension, tachycardia, low cardiac output [CO], and oliguria) caused by intravascular volume deficit (hypovolemic shock), myocardial pump failure (cardiogenic shock), or peripheral vasodilation (septic, anaphylactic, or neurogenic shock). The underlying problem in these situations is inadequate tissue perfusion resulting from circulatory failure.

▶ PATHOPHYSIOLOGY

- Shock results in failure of the circulatory system to deliver sufficient oxygen (O_2) to body tissues despite normal or reduced O_2 consumption. General pathophysiologic mechanisms of different forms of shock are similar, except for initiating events.
- Hypovolemic shock is characterized by acute intravascular volume deficiency owing to external losses or internal redistribution of extracellular water. This type of shock can be precipitated by hemorrhage, burns, trauma, intestinal obstruction, and dehydration from considerable insensible fluid loss, over-aggressive loop-diuretic administration, and severe vomiting or diarrhea. Relative hypovolemia leading to hypovolemic shock occurs during significant vasodilation, which accompanies anaphylaxis, sepsis, and neurogenic shock.
- Regardless of the etiology, fall in blood pressure (BP) is compensated by an increase in sympathetic outflow, activation of the renin–angiotensin system, and other humoral factors that stimulate peripheral vasoconstriction. Compensatory vasoconstriction redistributes blood away from extremities and kidneys toward vital organs (e.g., heart, brain) in an attempt to maintain oxygenation, nutrition, and organ function.
- Severe metabolic lactic acidosis often develops secondary to tissue ischemia and causes localized vasodilation, which further exacerbates the impaired cardiovascular state.

▶ CLINICAL PRESENTATION

- Shock presents with a diversity of signs and symptoms. Hypotension, tachycardia, tachypnea, confusion, and oliguria are common symptoms. Myocardial and cerebral ischemia, pulmonary edema (cardiogenic shock), and multisystem organ failure often follow.
- Significant hypotension (sytolic blood pressure [SBP] <90 mm Hg) with reflex sinus tachycardia (>120 beats/min) is often observed in the hypovolemic patient. Clinically, the patient presents with extremities cool to

the touch and a "thready" pulse. If coronary hypoxia persists, cardiac arrhythmias may occur, which eventually lead to irreversible myocardial pump failure, pulmonary edema, and cardiovascular collapse. II

- In the patient with extensive myocardial damage, chest auscultation may reveal heart sounds consistent with valvular heart disease (regurgitation, outflow obstruction) or significant ventricular dysfunction (S_3). Chest roentgenogram may detect dissecting ascending aortic aneurysm (widened mediastinum) or cardiomegaly (large heart shadow).
- Altered sensorium (confusion or combativeness) may be one of the first symptoms of shock.
- Respiratory alkalosis secondary to hyperventilation is usually observed secondary to CNS stimulation of ventilatory centers as a result of trauma, sepsis, or shock. Lung auscultation may reveal rales (pulmonary edema) or absence of breath sounds (pneumothorax, hemothorax). Chest roentgenogram can confirm early suspicions or disclose an undetected abnormality such as pneumonia (pulmonary infiltrates). Continued insult to the lungs may result in adult respiratory distress syndrome (ARDS).
- Kidneys are exquisitely sensitive to changes in perfusion pressures. Moderate alterations can lead to significant changes in glomerular filtration rate (GFR). Oliguria, progressing to anuria, occurs because of vasoconstriction of afferent arterioles.
- Skin is often cool, pale, or cyanotic (bluish) due to hypoxemia. Sweating results in a moist, clammy feel. Digits will have severely slowed capillary refill.
- Redistribution of blood flow away from the gastrointestinal (GI) tract may cause stress gastritis, gut ischemia, and in some cases, infarction, resulting in GI bleeding.
- Reduced hepatic blood flow, especially in vasodilatory forms of shock, can alter metabolism of endogenous compounds and drugs. Progressive liver damage (shock liver) manifests as elevated serum hepatic transaminases and unconjugated bilirubin. Impaired synthesis of clotting factors may increase prothrombin time (PT), international normalized ratio (INR), and activated partial thromboplastin time (aPTT).

▶ DIAGNOSIS AND MONITORING

- Information from noninvasive and invasive monitoring (Table 12–1) and evaluation of past medical history, clinical presentation, and laboratory findings are key components in establishing the diagnosis as well as in assessing general mechanisms responsible for shock. Regardless of the etiology, consistent findings include hypotension (SBP <90 mm Hg), depressed cardiac index (CI <2.2 L/min/m^2), tachycardia (heart rate [HR] >100 beats/min), and low urine output (<20 mL/h).
- Noninvasive assessment of BP using the sphygmomanometer and stethoscope may be inaccurate in the shock state.

TABLE 12–1. Hemodynamic and Oxygen Transport Monitoring Parameters

Parameter	Normal Value
Blood pressure (systolic/diastolic)	100–130/70–85 mm Hg
Mean arterial pressure (MAP)	80–100 mm Hg
Pulmonary artery pressure (PAP)	25/10 mm Hg
Mean pulmonary artery pressure (MPAP)	12–15 mm Hg
Central venous pressure (CVP)	2–6 mm Hg
Pulmonary capillary wedge pressure (PCWP)	8–12 (normal), 15–18 (ICU) mm Hg
Heart rate (HR)	60–80 beats/min
Cardiac output (CO)	4–7 L/min
Cardiac index (CI)	2.8–3.6 L/min/m^2
Stroke volume index (SVI)	30–50 mL/m^2
Systemic vascular resistance index (SVRI)	1300–2100 dyne•sec/m^2cm^5
Pulmonary vascular resistance index (PVRI)	45–225 dyne•sec/m^2cm^5
Arterial oxygen saturation (Sao_2)	97% (range, 95%–100%)
Mixed venous oxygen saturation (Svo_2)	75% (range, 60%–80%)
Arterial oxygen content (Cao_2)	20.1 vol % (range, 19–21)
Venous oxygen content (Cvo_2)	15.5 vol % (range, 11.5–16.5)
Oxygen content difference ($C(a\text{-}v)o_2$)	5 vol % (range, 4–6)
Oxygen consumption index (Vo_2)	131 mL/min/m^2 (range, 100–180)
Oxygen delivery index (Do_2)	578 mL/min/m^2 (range, 370–730)
Oxygen extraction ratio (O_2 ER)	25% (range, 22%–30%)
Mucosal pH (pHi)	7.40 (range, 7.35–7.45)
Index	Parameter indexed to body surface area

- Pulmonary artery catheterization using the Swan–Ganz catheter is frequently performed for invasive monitoring of central cardiovascular pressures. This flow-directed balloon-tipped catheter is inserted via the subclavian or internal jugular vein through the superior vena cava, right atrium, and ventricle, into the pulmonary artery. Depending on the location of its tip, a Swan–Ganz catheter can be used to determine central venous pressure (CVP), which is essentially the same as right atrial pressure (RAP) and therefore an estimate of intravascular volume and right ventricular preload; pulmonary artery systolic and diastolic pressures (PAS and PAD); and pulmonary capillary wedge pressure (PCWP), which affords an estimate of the left ventricular end diastolic volume and a major determinant of left ventricular preload.
- Cardiac output (2.5–3 L/min) and Svo_2 (70–75%) may be very low in the patient with extensive myocardial damage. These values are determined by Swan–Ganz catheterization.

- Respiratory alkalosis is associated with low partial pressure of O_2 (Pao_2) (25–35 mm Hg) and alkaline pH, but normal bicarbonate. The first two values are measured by arterial blood gas, which also yields partial pressure of carbon dioxide ($Paco_2$) and Sao_2. Circulating Sao_2 can also be measured by an oximeter, which is a noninvasive method that is fairly accurate and useful at the patient's bedside.
- Renal function can be grossly assessed by hourly measurements of urine output, but estimation of creatinine clearance based on isolated serum creatinine values in critically ill patients may yield erroneous results. Decreased renal perfusion and aldosterone release result in sodium retention, and thus, low urinary sodium (U_{Na} <30 mEq/L).
- In normal individuals, oxygen consumption (Vo_2) is dependent on oxygen delivery (Do_2) up to a certain critical level (Vo_2 flow dependency). At this point, tissue oxygen requirements have apparently been satisfied and further increases in Do_2 will not alter Vo_2 (flow independency). However, studies in critically ill patients show a continuous, pathologic dependence relationship of Vo_2 on Do_2. These indexed parameters are calculated as: $Do_2 = CI \times Cao_2$ and $Vo_2 = CI \times (Cao_2 - Cvo_2)$, where CI = cardiac index, Cao_2 = arterial oxygen content, and Cvo_2 = mixed-venous oxygen content. Currently available data do not support the concept that patient outcome or survival is altered by treatment measures directed to achieve supranormal levels of Do_2 and Vo_2.
- The Vo_2 to Do_2 ratio (oxygen extraction ratio or o_2ER) can be used to assess adequacy of perfusion and metabolic response. Patients who are able to increase Vo_2 when Do_2 is increased show improved survival. However, low Vo_2 and o_2ER values are indicative of poor oxygen utilization and lead to greater mortality.
- Serum lactate concentrations may be used as another measure of tissue oxygenation and may show better correlation with outcome than oxygen transport parameters in some patients.
- Gastric tonometry measures gut luminal Pco_2 at equilibrium by placing a saline-filled gas-permeable balloon in the gastric lumen. Increases in mucosal Pco_2 and calculated decreases in intramucosal pH (pHi) are associated with mucosal hypoperfusion and perhaps increased mortality. However, the presence of acid–base disorders, systemic bicarbonate administration, arterial blood gas measurement errors, enteral feeding solutions, or stool in the gut may confound pHi determinations. Some clinicians believe that gastric mucosal Pco_2 may be more accurate than pHi.

▶ DESIRED OUTCOME

The initial goal is to support oxygen delivery through the circulatory system by assuring effective intravascular plasma volume, optimal oxygen-carrying capacity, and adequate BP while definitive diagnostic and therapeutic strategies are being determined. The ultimate goals are to prevent further progression of the disease with subsequent organ damage and, if possible, to reverse organ dysfunction that has already occurred.

▶ TREATMENT

GENERAL PRINCIPLES

- Figure 12–1 contains an algorithm summarizing one approach to the adult patient presenting with hypovolemic shock. It presumes that initial rehydration attempts have been unsuccessful in restoring circulation.
- Supplemental oxygen should be initiated at the earliest signs of shock, beginning with 4–6 L/min via nasal cannula or 6–10 L/min by face mask.
- Fluid resuscitation is essential. Different therapeutic options are discussed below.
- If fluid challenge does not achieve desired end points, pharmacologic support is necessary with inotropic and vasoactive drugs.

FLUID RESUSCITATION FOR HYPOVOLEMIC SHOCK

- Initial fluid resuscitation consists of isotonic crystalloid (0.9% sodium chloride or lactated Ringer's solution), colloid (5% plasmanate or albumin, 6% hetastarch), or whole blood. Choice of solution is based on oxygen-carrying capacity (e.g., hemoglobin, hematocrit), cause of hypovolemic shock, accompanying disease states, degree of fluid loss, and required speed of fluid delivery.
- Most clinicians agree that crystalloids should be the initial therapy of circulatory insufficiency. Crystalloids are preferred over colloids as initial therapy for burn patients because they are less likely to cause interstitial fluid accumulation. If volume resuscitation is suboptimal following several liters of crystalloid, colloids should be considered. Some patients may require blood products to assure maintenance of oxygen-carrying capacity, as well as clotting factors and platelets for blood hemostasis.

Crystalloids

- Crystalloids consist of electrolytes (e.g., Na^+, Cl^-, K^+) in water solutions, with or without dextrose. **Lactated Ringer's** solution may be preferred because it is unlikely to cause the hyperchloremic metabolic acidosis seen with infusion of large amounts of normal saline.
- Crystalloids are administered at a rate of 500–2000 mL/h, depending on the severity of the deficit, degree of ongoing fluid loss, and tolerance to infusion volume. Usually 2–4 L of crystalloid normalizes intravascular volume.
- Advantages of crystalloids include rapidity and ease of administration, compatibility with most drugs, absence of serum sickness, and low cost.

- The primary disadvantage is the large volume necessary to replace or augment intravascular volume. Approximately 4 L of normal saline must be infused to replace 1 L of blood loss. In addition, dilution of II colloid oncotic pressure leading to pulmonary edema is more likely to follow crystalloid than colloid resuscitation.

Colloids

- Colloids are larger molecular-weight solutions (>30,000 daltons) that have been recommended for use in conjunction with or as replacements for crystalloid solutions. Albumin is a monodisperse colloid because all of its molecules are of the same molecular weight, whereas hetastarch and dextran solutions are polydisperse compounds with molecules of varying molecular weight. Colloids are useful because their increased molecular weight corresponds to an increased intravascular retention time (in the absence of increased capillary permeability). However, even with intact capillary permeability, the colloid molecular will eventually leak through capillary membranes.
- **Albumin 5% and 25%** concentrations are available. It takes approximately 3 to 4 times as much lactated Ringer's or normal saline solution to yield the same volume expansion as 5% albumin solution. However, albumin is much more costly than crystalloid solutions. The 5% albumin solution is relatively iso-oncotic, whereas 25% albumin is hyperoncotic and tends to pull fluid into the compartment containing the albumin molecules. In general, 5% albumin is used for hypovolemic states. The 25% solution should probably not be used for acute circulatory insufficiency unless diluted with other fluids or unless it is being used in patients with excess total body water but intravascular depletion, as a means of pulling fluid into the intravascular space.
- **Hetastarch 6%** has comparable plasma expansion to 5% albumin solution but is usually less expensive, which accounts for much of its use. Hetastarch should be avoided in patients with severe bleeding conditions such as subarachnoid hemorrhage, since it may aggravate bleeding due to mechanisms such as decreased factor VIII activity. Microamylase formation may cause elevations in serum amylase concentration that may lead to an inaccurate diagnosis of pancreatitis.
- **Dextran 40, dextran 70,** and **dextran 75** are available for use as plasma expanders (the number indicates the average molecular weight × 1000). These solutions are not used as often as albumin or hetastarch for plasma expansion, possibly due to concerns related to aggravation of bleeding (i.e., anticoagulant action resulting from inhibiting stasis of microcirculation) and anaphylaxis that is more likely to occur with the higher molecular weight solutions.
- The theoretical advantage of colloids is their prolonged intravascular retention time compared to crystalloid solutions. In contrast to isotonic crystalloid solutions that have substantial interstitial distribution within minutes of intravenous administration, colloids remain in the intravas-

II

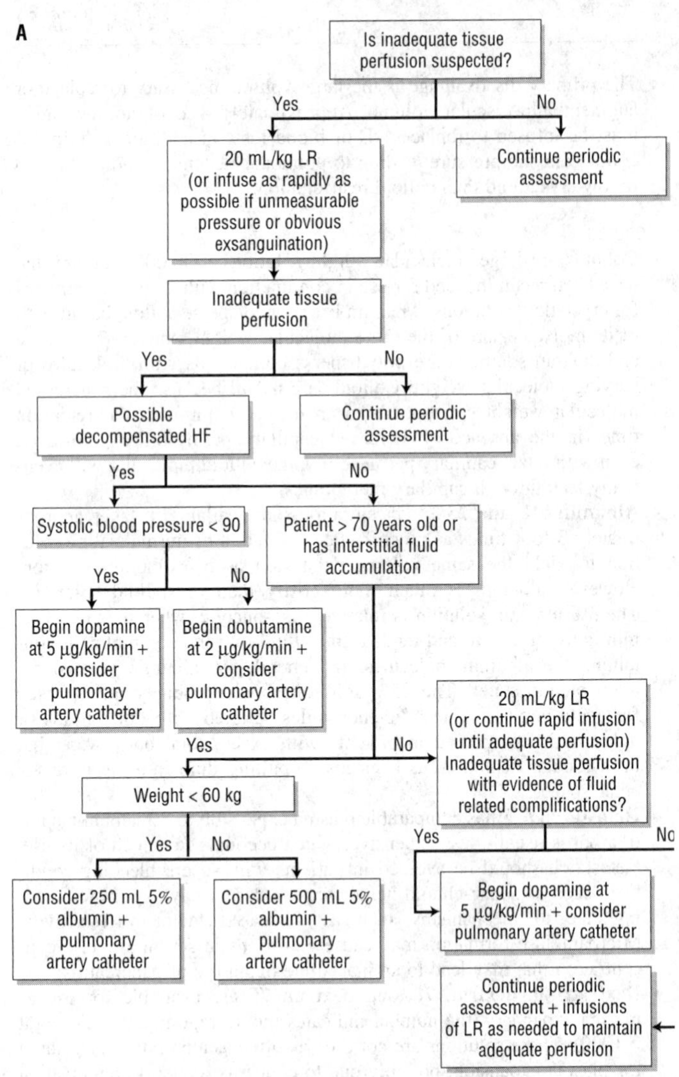

Figure 12–1. Hypovolemia protocol for adults. This protocol is not intended to replace or delay therapies such as surgical intervention or blood products for restoring oxygen-carrying capacity or hemostasis. If available, some measurements may be used in addition to those listed in the algorithm, such as mean arterial pressure or pulmonary artery catheter recordings. The latter may be used to assist in medication choices (agents with primary pressor effects may be desirable in patients with normal cardiac outputs, whereas dopamine or dobutamine may be indicated in patients with suboptimal cardiac outputs).

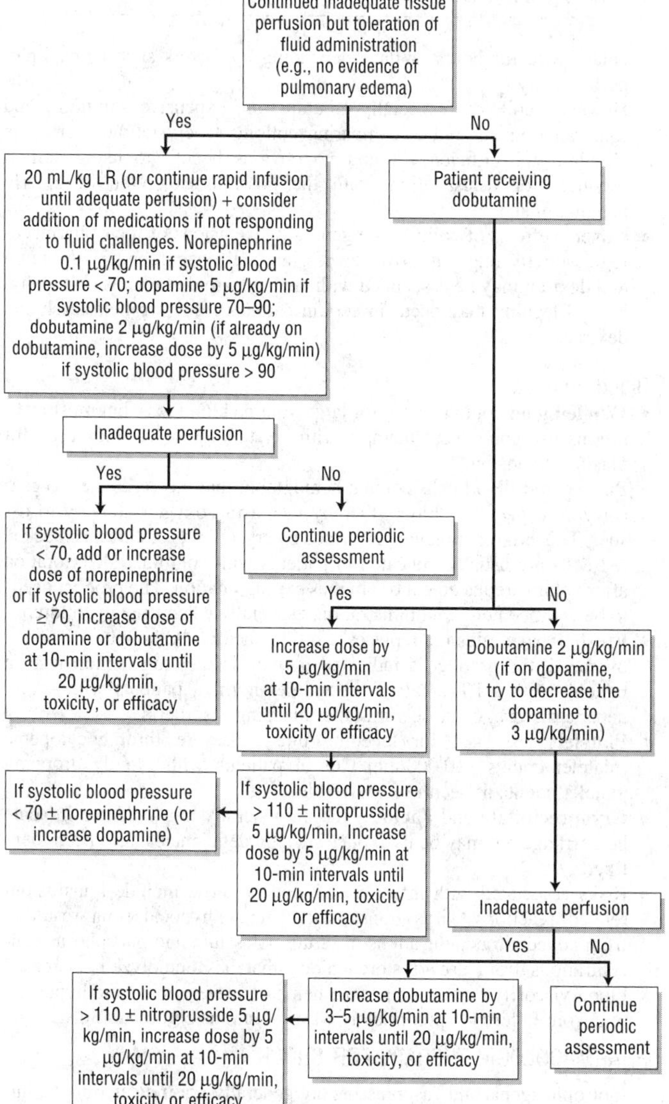

Figure 12–1 (continued). Lower maximal doses of the medications in this algorithm should be considered when pulmonary artery catheterization is not available. LR, lactated Ringer's solution; HF, heart failure. Colloids that may be substituted for albumin are hetastarch 6% and dextran 40.

cular space for hours or days depending on factors such as capillary permeability.
- However, colloids (especially albumin) are expensive solutions, and four randomized studies comparing colloids to crystalloids for acute circulatory insufficiency found no obvious benefit to using colloid products for resuscitation, with the possible exception of elderly patients in shock.
- Adverse effects of colloids are generally extensions of their pharmacologic activity (e.g., fluid overload, dilutional coagulopathy). Albumin and dextran may be associated with anaphylactoid reactions or anaphylaxis. Bleeding may occur in certain patients receiving hetastarch and dextrans.

Blood Products

- **Whole blood** could be used for large volume blood loss, but most institutions use component therapy, with crystalloids or colloids used for plasma expansion.
- **Packed red blood cells** contain hemoglobin that increases the oxygen-carrying capacity of blood, thereby increasing oxygen delivery to tissues. This is a function not performed by crystalloids or colloids. Packed red cells are usually indicated in patients with continued deterioration after volume replacement or obvious exsanguination. The product needs to be warmed before administration, especially when used in children.
- **Fresh frozen plasma** replaces clotting factors. Although it is often overused, the product is indicated if there is ongoing hemorrhage in patients with a PT or aPTT >1.5 times normal, patients with severe hepatic disease, or those with other bleeding disorders.
- **Platelets** are used for bleeding due to severe thrombocytopenia (platelet counts <10,000/mm^3) or in patients with rapidly dropping platelet counts as seen in massive bleeding.
- **Cryoprecipitate** and **Factor VIII** are generally not indicated in acute hemorrhage but may be used once specific deficiencies have been identified.
- Risks associated with infusion of blood products include transfusion-related reactions, virus transmission (rare), hypocalcemia resulting from added citrate, elevations in serum potassium and phosphorus concentrations from use of stored blood that has hemolyzed, increased blood viscosity from supranormal hematocrit elevations, and hypothermia from failure to appropriately warm solutions before administration.

PHARMACOLOGIC THERAPY FOR SHOCK

- Inotropic agents and vasopressors are generally not indicated in the initial treatment of hypovolemic shock (assuming that fluid therapy is adequate), as the body's normal response is to increase cardiac output and constrict blood vessels to maintain blood pressure. However, once the cause of circulatory insufficiency has been stopped or treated and fluids have been optimized, medications may be needed in patients who continue to have signs and symptoms of inadequate tissue perfusion. Pressor agents such as norepinephrine and high-dose dopamine should be avoided if at all possible, since they may increase blood pressure at the expense of peripheral tissue ischemia. In patients with unstable blood pressure despite massive fluid replacement and increasing interstitial fluid accumulation, inotropic agents such as dobutamine are preferred if blood pressure is adequate (SBP ≥90 mm Hg) because they should not aggravate the existing vasoconstriction. When pressure cannot be maintained with inotropes, or when inotropes with vasodilatory properties cannot be used due to concerns about inadequate blood pressure, pressors may be required as a last resort.

- The choice of vasopressor or inotropic agent in septic shock should be made according to the needs of the patient. An algorithm for the use of these agents in septic shock is shown in Figure 12–2. The traditional approach is to start with dopamine, then norepinephrine; dobutamine is added for low cardiac output states, and occasionally epinephrine and phenylephrine are used when necessary.
- The receptor selectivity of vasopressors and inotropes are listed in Table 12–2. In general, these drugs are rapid acting with short durations of action and are given as continuous infusions. Potent vasoconstrictors such as norepinephrine and phenylephrine should be given through central veins due to the possibility of extravasation and necrosis with peripheral administration. Careful monitoring and calculation of infusion rates is advised, because dosing adjustments are made frequently and varying admixture concentrations are used in volume-restricted patients.
- **Dopamine** is often the initial vasopressor used in septic shock because it increases BP by increasing myocardial contractility and vasoconstriction. Although dopamine has been reported to have dose-related receptor activity at dopamine (DA_1), β_1, and α_1 receptors, this dose–response relationship has not been confirmed in critically ill patients. In patients with septic shock, there is overlap of hemodynamic effects with doses as low as 3 μg/kg/min. Doses of 5–10 μg/kg/min are initiated to improve mean arterial pressure (MAP). In septic shock, these doses increase CI by improving ventricular contractility, heart rate, arterial pressure, and systemic vascular resistance. The clinical utility of dopamine in septic shock is limited, because large doses are frequently necessary to maintain CO and BP. At doses above 20 μg/kg/min, there is limited further improvement in cardiac performance and regional hemodynamics. Its use is also hampered frequently by tachycardia and tachydysrhythmias. Other adverse effects limiting its use include increases in PCWP, pulmonary shunt, and decreases in PaO_2. Dopamine should be used with caution in patients with elevated preload, as it may worsen pulmonary edema. Low doses of dopamine (1–3 μg/kg/min) are clinically useful in critically ill patients with septic shock with vasopressors or in oliguric patients. The goal in both situations is to preserve or increase urine output by way of dopamine's

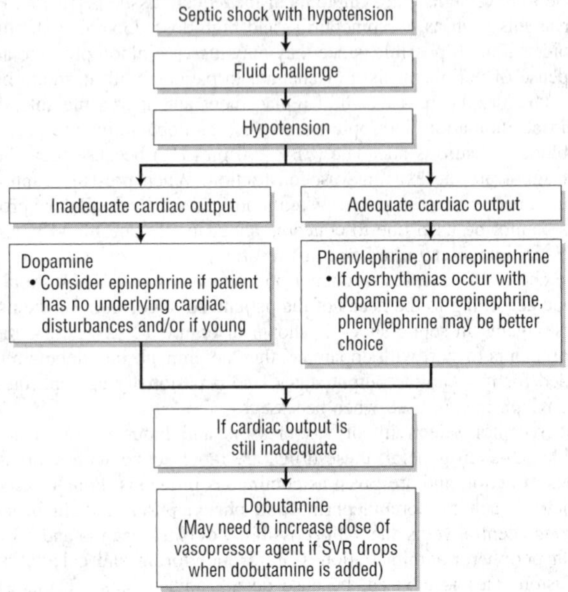

Figure 12–2. Algorithmic approach to the use of vasopressors and inotropes in septic shock. Approach is intended to be used in conjunction with clinical judgment, hemodynamic monitoring parameters, and therapeutic end points. *(Modified from Society of Critical Care Med (SCCM). Practice parameters on adult hemodynamic support of sepsis.* Crit Care Med *[in press].)*

dopaminergic (DA_1 agonist) activity at low doses. When other vasopressors or inotropes are used, low doses of dopamine may be started concurrently. Dopamine is commonly found to be ineffective or not tolerated when used in pressor doses and another agent is added. The dopamine dose is then titrated down to improve mesenteric and renal blood flow. In the setting of oliguria (either with or without bacteremia/septic shock), low-dose dopamine is initiated in an attempt to convert oliguric renal failure to nonoliguric renal failure.

- **Dobutamine** is primarily a selective β_1 agonist with mild β_2 and vascular α_1 activity, resulting in strong positive inotropic activity with vasodilatory properties. Dobutamine produces a larger increase in CO and is less dysrhythmogenic than dopamine. Clinically, the increased myocardial contractility and subsequent reflex reduction in sympathetic tone lead to a decrease in systemic vascular resistance (SVR). Even though dobutamine is optimally used for low CO states with high filling pressures or in cardiogenic shock, vasopressors may be needed to counteract arterial vasodilation. The addition of dobutamine to epi-

TABLE 12–2. Receptor Pharmacology of Selected Inotropic and Vasopressor Agents Used in Septic Shock[a]

Agent	α_1	α_2	β_1	β_2	DA[b]
Dobutamine (500 mg/250 mL D_5W or NS)					
2–10 μg/kg/min	+	0	++++	++	0
>10–20 μg/kg/min	++	0	++++	+++	0
Dopamine (800 mg/250 mL D_5W or NS)					
1–3 μg/kg/min	0	0	+	0	++++
3–10 μg/kg/min	0/+	0	++++	++	++++
>10–20 μg/kg/min	+++	0	++++	+	0
Dopexamine (investigational)					
0.5–4.0 μg/kg/min	0	0	++[c]	+++	++++
Epinephrine (2 mg/250 mL D_5W or NS)					
0.01–0.05 μg/kg/min	++	++	++++	+++	0
>0.05 μg/kg/min	++++	++++	+++	+	
Norepinephrine (4 mg/250 mL D_5W or NS)					
0.02–3.0 μg/kg/min (2–20 μg/min)	+++	+++	+++	+/++	0
Phenylephrine (50 μg/250 mL D_5W or NS)					
0.5–9 μg/kg/min	+++	+	?	0	0

[a]Activity ranges from no activity (0) to maximal (++++) activity or ? when activity is not known.
[b]DA, dopaminergic.
[c]Dopexamine inhibits neuronal reuptake of norepinephrine.

nephrine-treated patients can improve mucosal perfusion as measured by improvements in pHi and arterial lactate concentrations. Dobutamine should be started with doses ranging from 2.5–5.0 μg/kg/min. Doses above 5.0 μg/kg/min may provide limited beneficial effects on oxygen transport values and hemodynamics and may increase adverse cardiac effects. Infusion rates should be guided by clinical end points. Decreases in PaO_2 and increases in PvO_2, as well as myocardial adverse effects such as tachycardia, ischemic changes on ECG, tachydysrhythmias, and hypotension are seen.

- **Norepinephrine** is a combined α and β agonist, but it primarily produces vasoconstriction, thereby increasing SVR. It generally produces either no change or a slight decrease in CO. Norepinephrine is frequently initiated after vasopressor doses of dopamine (4–20 μg/kg/min) and/or combined use with dobutamine (2–40 μg/kg/min) fail to achieve desired goals. Doses of dopamine and dobutamine are kept constant, stopped altogether, or in some instances, dopamine is kept at low doses for purported renal protection. Norepinephrine 0.02–2.0 μg/kg/min reliably and predictably improves hemodynamic parameters to normal or supranormal values in the majority of patients with septic shock.
- **Phenylephrine** is a pure α agonist and is thought to increase blood pressure through vasoconstriction. It may also increase contractility and

CO. Phenylephrine may be beneficial in septic shock because of its selective α agonism, primary vascular effects, rapid onset, and short duration. Phenylephrine should be used when a pure vasoconstrictor is desired in patients who may not require or do not tolerate the β effects of dopamine with or without dobutamine. It is generally initiated at dosages of 0.5 μg/kg/min and may be titrated quickly to the desired effect. Adverse effects such as tachydysrhythmias are infrequent when it is used as a single agent or with higher doses.

- **Epinephrine** has combined α and β agonist effects and has traditionally been reserved as the vasopressor of last resort because of reports of peripheral vasoconstriction, particularly in the splanchnic and renal beds. At the high infusion rates used in septic shock, α-adrenergic effects are predominantly seen, and SVR and MAP are increased. It may be an acceptable single agent in septic shock due to its combined vasoconstrictor and inotropic effects. Epinephrine may be particularly useful when used earlier in the course of septic shock in young patients and those without known cardiac abnormalities. Infusion rates of 0.04–1.0 μg/kg/min alone increase hemodynamic and oxygen transport variables to supranormal levels without adverse effects in patients without coronary heart disease. Large doses (0.05–1.0 μg/kg/min) are required when epinephrine is added to other agents. Smaller doses (0.1–0.5 μg/kg/min) are effective if dobutamine and dopamine infusions are kept constant. Although Do_2 increases mainly as a function of consistent increases in CI (and a more variable increase in SVR), Vo_2 may not increase and o_2ER may fall. Lactate concentrations may rise during the first few hours of epinephrine therapy but normalize over the ensuing 24 hours in survivors. Caution must be used before considering epinephrine for managing hypoperfusion in patients with coronary artery disease to avoid ischemia, chest pain, and myocardial infarction.
- **Dopexamine** is an investigational catecholamine with marked intrinsic agonist activity at β_2 receptors with less activity at dopaminergic DA_1 and DA_2 receptors. Stimulation of cardiac β_2 receptors may result in a reflex baroreceptor stimulation and mild inotropic activity. It has no clinically significant β_1–agonist activity and no α effects. It is used in low cardiac output states with coexisting elevated systemic or pulmonary vascular resistance. It has been used in acute heart failure, impaired left ventricular function after surgery, and in septic shock. As with dobutamine in septic shock, dopexamine is most frequently used in combination with a pressor agent such as norepinephrine or dopamine, due to coexisting refractory hypotension.

▶ EVALUATION OF THERAPEUTIC OUTCOMES

- The initial monitoring of a patient with suspected volume depletion should include vital signs, urine output, mental status, and physical examination.

- Placement of a central venous pressure (CVP) line provides a useful (although indirect and insensitive) estimate of the relationship between increased right atrial pressure and cardiac output.
- The indications for pulmonary artery catheterization are controversial. Because there is a lack of well-defined outcome data associated with this procedure, its use is presently best reserved for complicated cases of shock not responding to conventional fluids and vasopressor therapy. Complications related to pulmonary artery catheterization insertion, maintenance, and removal include damage to vessels and organs during insertion, arrhythmias, infections, and thromboembolic damage.
- Laboratory tests indicated for the ongoing monitoring of shock include electrolytes and renal function tests (BUN, serum creatinine); complete blood count to assess possible infection, oxygen-carrying capacity of the blood, and ongoing bleeding; prothrombin time and activated partial thromboplastin time to assess clotting ability; and lactate concentration and base deficit to detect inadequate tissue perfusion.
- Cardiovascular and respiratory parameters should be monitored continuously (Table 12–1). Trends, rather than specific CVP or PCWP numbers, should be attempted because of interpatient variability in response.
- Successful fluid resuscitation should increase SBP (>90 mm Hg), CI (>2.2 L/min/m^2), and urine output (0.5–1 mL/kg/h) while decreasing SVR to the normal range (900–1200 dynes-s/cm^5). MAP of >60 mm Hg should be achieved to ensure adequate cerebral and coronary perfusion pressure.
- Intravascular volume overload is characterized by high filling pressures (CVP > 12–15 mm Hg, PCWP > 20–24 mm Hg) and decreased CO (<3.5 L/min). If volume overload occurs, furosemide 20–40 mg should be administered by slow IV push to produce rapid diuresis of intravascular volume and "unload" the heart through venous dilation.
- Coagulation problems are primarily associated with low levels of clotting factors in stored blood as well as dilution of endogenous clotting factors and platelets following administration of the blood. As a result, a coagulation panel (PT, INR, aPTT) should be checked in patients undergoing replacement of 50–100% or more of blood volume in 12–24 hours.

See Chapter 21, Use of Vasopressors and Inotropes in the Pharmacotherapy of Shock, authored by Maria I. Rudis, PharmD, ABAT, BCPS, Bertil Wagner, PharmD, FCCM, and Joseph F. Dasta, MS, FCCM; and Chapter 22, Hypovolemic Shock, authored by Brian L. Erstad, PharmD, for a more detailed discussion of this topic.

Chapter 13

▶ STROKE

▶ DEFINITION

Stroke is the syndrome caused by disruption in blood flow to the brain resulting in sudden onset of a focal neurologic deficit that persists for at least 24 hours. Stroke is a major manifestation of cerebrovascular disease, which in turn refers to any type of pathophysiologic vascular disease of the brain.

▶ PATHOPHYSIOLOGY

- Vascular pathology leading to stroke can include any abnormality of the vessel, blood flow, or blood quality. Vessel abnormalities include many processes such as developmental defects, arteritis, aneurysm, hypertensive disease, vasoconstriction, and atherosclerosis. Blood flow can be affected by vessel disease and also by thrombotic or embolic processes. Decreased blood flow in the brain (i.e., ischemia) or cerebral bleeding can produce these abnormalities.
- When a stroke occurs, the resulting neurologic manifestations depend upon the location of the insult in the brain and the extent of ischemia, infarct, or hemorrhage.
- Infarction accounts for 85% of all strokes; of these, 80% are caused by cerebrovascular disease, 15% by cardiogenic embolism, and 5% by other unusual causes. Hemorrhage into the brain tissue and subarachnoid hemorrhages account for about 15% of all strokes.

TREATABLE RISK FACTORS

- Hypertension is the major predisposing treatable risk factor for stroke and is strongly related to atherothrombotic brain infarction as well as cerebral hemorrhage.
- Individuals with cardiac diseases (e.g., coronary heart disease, heart failure, left ventricular hypertrophy, and arrhythmias [i.e., atrial fibrillation]) have more than twice the stroke risk compared with those with normal cardiac function.
- Transient ischemic attacks (TIAs) are focal ischemic neurologic deficits lasting <24 hours. TIAs precede an ischemic stroke in about 60% of cases; 35% of untreated patients develop a stroke within 5 years of a TIA.
- Multiple factors identified in the Framingham study [i.e., elevated systolic blood pressure, elevated serum cholesterol, glucose intolerance, cigarette smoking, and left ventricular hypertrophy by electrocardiogram (ECG)] can be used to identify the 10% of the population who will have one-third of the strokes.

CEREBROVASCULAR DISEASE

Atherothrombotic Disease

- Atherosclerosis of brain arteries is a process similar to that found in extracranial vessels. Atherosclerosis and subsequent plaque formation result in arterial narrowing or occlusion and constitute the most common cause of aortacranial stenosis. Thrombosis is most likely to occur where plaque causes the most vessel narrowing. Embolism can produce a stroke when a clot, plaque, or platelet aggregate breaks off into the circulation and blocks an artery. Platelets contribute to thrombosis. Platelet activation, whether by plaque formation or trauma, initiates a series of events including release of adenine diphosphate (ADP) from platelets, which enhances platelet aggregation. Aggregation is consolidated by coagulation factors, red and white blood cells, and formation of a fibrin network. Thromboxane A_2 promotes platelet aggregation and vasoconstriction, which is balanced by prostacyclin (PGI_2), a vasodilator and inhibitor of platelet aggregation. The atherosclerotic process is variable; resultant ischemic consequences depend on adequacy of blood flow and collateral circulation and embolism.

Cerebral Ischemia

- Cerebral ischemia can be global or focal. Global ischemia is associated with lack of collateral blood flow, and irreversible brain damage occurs in 4–8 minutes. In focal ischemia, collateral circulation may allow for survival of brain cells and reversal of neuronal damage after ischemia.
- Cell function can be preserved for up to 4 hours provided reductions in cerebral blood flow (CBF) are between ranges associated with electrical (i.e., 15–18 mL/100 g/min) and ionic failure (10 mL/100 g/min).
- When CBF is 10 mL/100 g/min, metabolic derangements [e.g., accumulation of lactic acid, adenosine triphosphate (ATP) depletion, and increased intracellular calcium] ultimately decrease cell integrity, increase membrane permeability, perpetuate intracellular acidosis, and impair cell function.
- Swelling is one of the primary responses of brain tissue to acute injury. Movement of plasma into the extracellular space results in increased intracranial pressure, which can result in brain herniation.

Lacunar Infarcts

- Lacuna refers to the small cavity left after necrotic tissue has been removed. Occlusion of small arterial branches of the circle of Willis and of anterior, middle, and posterior cerebral and basilar arteries can result in infarcts deep in the cerebral hemispheres and brain stem. The associated pathophysiology is somewhat different compared with that of infarcts located closer to the brain surface. The pathophysiology has been described as being a degenerative process in the media of the artery (lipohyalinosis), leading to vessel occlusion.

II

Transient Ischemic Attacks

- TIA pathophysiology involves the atherosclerotic process of thrombus formation in cerebrovascular arteries and low CBF. Small microemboli break off from the cerebral thrombus and lodge in distal areas, producing temporary focal cerebral dysfunction.

CEREBRAL EMBOLISM

- Any region of the brain can be affected by embolism; however, the middle cerebral artery is commonly involved.
- Cerebral embolism secondary to thrombotic disease usually has a rapid onset and is not preceded by a TIA. Because there is less time for collateral circulation to develop than in cerebral thrombosis, embolic strokes are often functionally devastating.
- Chronic atrial fibrillation is the most common cause of cardiogenic embolism and is the most common sustained arrhythmia (see Chapter 5).
- Factors that increase the risk of embolism in patients with valvular heart disease include mitral stenosis with or without incompetence (versus mitral incompetence alone), atrial fibrillation, increased left atrial size, increased age, and previous embolic event.
- Thrombus formation on prosthetic cardiac valves is related to valve-induced turbulence in blood flow and thrombogenic potential of valve material. The early Starr–Edwards valve and original Bjork–Shiley valve have higher embolic rates than newer valves. Bioprosthetic valves (e.g., Hancock, Carpentier–Edwards, Lonescu–Shiley) have a central flow design, which produces less turbulence, and a biologic material (i.e., porcine valve), which is less thrombogenic.
- The highest frequency of emboli induced by infective endocarditis is associated with infections on the left side of the heart that produce large, mobile vegetations from *Haemophilus parainfluenzae,* or slow-growing, fastidious, gram-negative bacilli, fungi *(Aspergillus* spp.), and *Streptococcus viridans.*

INTRACRANIAL HEMORRHAGE

- Frequent causes of hemorrhagic stroke are hypertensive intracerebral hemorrhage, ruptured saccular aneurysms, hemorrhage associated with bleeding disorders, and arteriovenous malformations. Bleeding from a ruptured artery allows for an extravasation of blood into brain tissue and mass formation. Brain tissue is pushed, displaced, and compressed; brain functions may be impaired.

► CLINICAL PRESENTATION

- Neurologic manifestations differ depending on stroke type; location of insult; and extent of ischemia, infarct, or hemorrhage. Stroke may show varied manifestations, which are reversible or irreversible and which range from hemiplegia to sensory deficits. Hemiplegia may or may not be accompanied by other manifestations.

- Thrombosis of cerebral vessels produces variable clinical manifestations compared with embolic disease or intracranial hemorrhage. Stroke is preceded by TIA(s) in >50% of cases. If thrombosis involves internal carotid and middle cerebral arteries, focal symptoms may include mono- or hemiplegia, mono- or hemiparesthesia, blindness in one eye, and speech disturbance. If the vertebrobasilar system is involved, symptoms may include dizziness, diplopia, numbness, impaired vision, and dysarthria. Usually these attacks are short lived and resolve in <10 minutes. Stroke itself most often develops suddenly as a single attack. Stroke in evolution or progressing stroke evolves over hours, days, or weeks. Most cerebral thrombotic strokes occur at rest while sleeping or after arising. Headache may precede other symptoms, but it is often absent.
- Clinical presentation of lacunar infarcts varies depending on their location. The most frequently occurring lacunar syndrome is pure motor hemiparesis (e.g., hemiparesis or hemiplegia of arm, leg, face, and trunk) due to infarction in the posterior portion of the internal capsule. Mild dysarthria occurs without sensory or consciousness alterations or visual field defects. Affected body parts display the same degree of weakness. In contrast, stroke in the cortical region usually leads to unequal distribution of weakness.
- Most TIAs last 5–10 minutes; those lasting ≥1 hour may result from embolism. Symptoms are determined by lesion location.
- Onset of cerebral embolism is characteristically abrupt, often occurring in an awake patient. Cardiogenic embolism is associated with multifocal neurologic findings.
- Clinical manifestations of intracranial hemorrhage have an abrupt onset; changes generally occur over minutes to hours (up to 24 hours). Most patients lose consciousness, which is often preceded by head pain and dizziness. Headache is more likely to occur at the onset than with thromboembolism (50% versus <25% of cases). Neck rigidity, convulsions, and vomiting are common. Hypertension-related external capsule (putaminal) hemorrhage is manifested by rapid onset of hemiplegia, loss of consciousness, and conjugate deviation of eyes to the contralateral side. As the lesion enlarges, compression of the upper brain stem produces deepening coma, dilated and fixed pupils, Babinski signs, bilateral motor hypertonus, and irregular respirations. Internal capsule (thalamic) hemorrhage is also characterized by rapid onset; however, loss of vision occurs on the same side as optic nerve involvement in the internal capsule. Gaze disturbances include defective vertical and lateral gaze, fixed downward deviation of eyes, and unequal pupils.

▶ DIAGNOSIS

- It is challenging to diagnose accurately a particular lesion because of variations in presentation; however, good clinical examination can help to locate a lesion and to delineate between ischemic and hemorrhagic stroke. Imaging studies [e.g, computed tomography (CT) scan and magnetic resonance imaging (MRI)] are important diagnostic tools. CT scan results must be known before initiating therapy of stroke with anticoagulants or platelet antiaggregating agents.
- Diagnosis of atherothrombotic stroke requires evaluation of clinical presentation and laboratory findings. Tests may include cerebral arteriography, CT and MRI scans, radioactive brain scan study (e.g., technetium scan), head x-rays, electroencephalogram (EEG), ECG, transcranial Doppler studies, and lumbar puncture (LP). Arteriogram is the definitive test for arterial occlusion or narrowing; however, because of associated neurologic risk, arteriogram should be reserved for unclear diagnosis or pending vascular surgery. Hydration may reduce the risks of arteriogram. Because of these risks, brain imaging is most important. CT scan is often normal during the first 48 hours after thrombotic infarct. In contrast, MRI can adequately detect small infarcts in the cortical surface and elsewhere usually within 1 hour of occurrence. Promising new techniques include digital subtraction angiography, transesophageal echocardiography, xenon blood flow, and positron emission tomography (PET) scan.
- CT or MRI scan can provide evidence of lacunar infarction if performed within 7–10 days; however, infarcts <2 mm may be missed.
- Diagnosis of TIA is confounded by short duration, which necessitates reliance on the patient's recollection of symptoms. Laboratory studies are performed to rule out blood or other disorders that may decrease CBF. Embolism of cardiac origin should be considered by performing ECG, chest x-ray, and echocardiography, especially with the two-dimensional technique.
- Cardiogenic embolism should be considered when the following are present: patient older than age 60, sudden onset of maximal neurologic deficit, prior cortical infarct, history of valvular heart disease or left ventricular myocardial infarct, and atrial fibrillation or heart failure. Two-dimensional, M-mode, and transesophageal echocardiography are all useful for demonstrating thrombi, valve dysfunction, and cardiac dysfunction. ECG may indicate arrhythmia (e.g., atrial fibrillation). MRI and CT are being evaluated for their ability to detect cardiogenic emboli.
- In hypertensive intracerebral hemorrhage, important diagnostic clues are sudden onset and quick evolution of physical findings, and history of hypertension. Ocular signs are helpful in localizing hemorrhages of putaminal and thalamic origin; funduscopic examination may reveal periarteriolar hemorrhages and decreased arteriolar size. CT is the diagnostic procedure of choice because it can detect small amounts of blood and distinguish between hemorrhage and infarction.

▶ DESIRED OUTCOME

The desired outcome depends on the etiology of stroke. The major treatment goals for ischemic stroke are to: (1) remove or limit the obstruction to flow in the vessel; and (2) protect brain cells distal to the obstruction or blockage from suffering hypoxic changes. II

▶ TREATMENT

GENERAL PRINCIPLES

- A comprehensive approach to cerebrovascular disease consists of general prophylaxis against stroke and vascular disease, supportive and medical management during the acute phase of stroke, mitigation of the pathologic or atherothrombotic process, and appropriate rehabilitative and physical therapy programs during the poststroke period.
- Control of hypertension, hyperlipidemia, obesity, tobacco use, and other risk factors is essential to overall care of the patient with cerebrovascular disease.

ISCHEMIC CEREBROVASCULAR DISEASE

Anticoagulants

- Anticoagulation should not be used routinely for TIAs and should not be used at all for completed stroke. Anticoagulation is still controversial for progressing stroke; however, individual judgment must be used when intracerebral hemorrhage has been ruled out by CT scan.
- If indicated, **heparin** should be administered acutely by continuous IV infusion to a target activated partial thromboplastin time (aPTT) of 1.5 times control value.
- If indicated, **warfarin** should overlap with heparin for approximately 5 days. The target international normalized ratio (INR) is 2.0–3.0.

Antiplatelet Agents

- **Aspirin** 325 mg/d is recommended for prophylaxis of thromboembolism in patients with completed stroke, because prior stroke is a risk for another stroke. Aspirin 325–1300 mg/d is recommended in preventing TIAs and stroke. Enteric-coated products may be better tolerated by some individuals and may be used if needed.
- **Ticlopidine** 250 mg twice daily can be used for secondary prevention of stroke as an alternative in patients who cannot tolerate aspirin or in whom aspirin has not been effective. However, it has a significant side effect profile and is costly. Side effects include gastrointestinal complaints, bone marrow suppression, rash, diarrhea, and elevation of serum cholesterol. Reversible neutropenia occurs in up to 2% of patients; it is recommended that patients have CBCs with differential performed every 2 weeks for 3 months after therapy initiation.

- **Clopidogrel** 75 mg/d has similar efficacy to ticlopidine but does not require monitoring for neutropenia. It can be used in place of ticlopidine but not as a substitute for aspirin.

Thrombolytic Agents

- **Alteplase** carries FDA approval for use in acute ischemic stroke, but several other thrombolytics have also been investigated.
- Alteplase must be initiated within 3 hours of onset, and diagnosis of ischemic stroke (including CT scan) must be made by a physician with expertise in verifying stroke. Alteplase is not recommended when the time of stroke onset cannot be ascertained reliably (e.g., strokes recognized on awakening).
- The recommended dose of alteplase is 0.9 mg/kg (maximum 90 mg) infused over 60 minutes, with 10% of the total dose administered as an initial IV bolus over 1 minute.
- Hemorrhage is the most common and potentially severe complication of thrombolytic therapy for acute ischemic stroke. Treatment should only be administered if bleeding complications can be managed promptly. Patients should not receive any antiplatelet agents or anticoagulants for 24 hours after the use of alteplase.

Surgical Therapy

- Surgery is performed to prevent cerebral infarctions and TIAs by removing the source of occlusion and/or embolus, which should increase CBF to an ischemic area. Carotid endarterectomy is the most common surgical procedure for occlusive cerebrovascular disease. Indications are TIAs and mild completed stroke in the presence of ulcerated or highly stenotic (>75%) plaque. Carotid endarterectomy was superior to medical treatment alone in symptomatic patients with stenosis of ≥70%, but it was not beneficial in patients with <70% stenosis.

CEREBRAL EMBOLISM OF CARDIAC ORIGIN

- Immediate anticoagulation with heparin should be considered to reduce the risk of recurrent embolic events if CT scan documents absence of hemorrhagic transformation. Heparin is usually given 24 hours after stroke onset without a loading dose; aPTT should be maintained no greater than 1.5 times control. Warfarin (INR 2.0–3.0) should follow heparin therapy.
- Patients at high risk of embolic events because of atrial fibrillation should receive prophylactic chronic anticoagulation with warfarin. Because of the potential for intracerebral hemorrhage in elderly patients and the probability of lifetime treatment, subgroups with high and low rates of stroke have been identified.
  - Younger low-risk patients (<75 years) and patients with lone atrial fibrillation can be treated with aspirin 325 mg/d.
  - High-risk patients in whom anticoagulation is judged to be safe can be treated with warfarin to an INR of 2.0–3.0.

- High-risk patients >75 years may be treated with lower intensity warfarin at an INR of 1.5–2.5. Aspirin is the alternative.
- Anticoagulation is necessary for most patients with atrial fibrillation who have had an ischemic stroke.

- Patients who have had prosthetic cardiac valve replacement should begin anticoagulation immediately after surgery to reduce risk of thromboembolism. The regimen depends on valve type.
  - Mechanical prosthetic cardiac valve: Six hours after implantation, therapy should begin with IV heparin to maintain aPTT at 1.5–2 times control, followed by subcutaneous heparin 10,000 U every 12 hours after chest tube removal until discharge. Warfarin should be started as soon as possible after the operation and dosed to maintain INR of 2.5–3.5. **Aspirin** 80–160 mg/d or **dipyridamole** 5–6 mg/kg/d may be added to warfarin for additional protection. For patients who cannot take oral anticoagulants, **dipyridamole plus sulfinpyrazone** 800 mg/d may be tried empirically.
  - Bioprosthetic cardiac valve: Initial heparin therapy is similar to that given to patients with a mechanical prosthetic cardiac valve. For mitral valve, warfarin therapy should be initiated soon after operation and continued for 3 months at a less intense INR of 2.0–3.0. Warfarin (INR of 2.0–3.0) should be continued indefinitely in patients who have atrial fibrillation, enlarged left atrium, or previous thromboembolism. For aortic valve and sinus rhythm, anticoagulation is optional; aspirin 325 mg/d can be used empirically.

INTRACRANIAL HEMORRHAGE

- Surgery can be performed in the acute or early stage to remove the clot by aspiration or evacuation in patients whose hemorrhage is near the brain surface and who are not comatose.
- To reduce edema around the hemorrhage, **mannitol** 0.25–2 g/kg can be administered intravenously every 4–8 hours until the serum osmolality is raised between 300 and 310 mOsm/L. This regimen is also suitable for ischemic stroke; however, cerebral edema is rarely present unless there is a large infarction in the middle cerebral artery. Corticosteroids (e.g., dexamethasone) are no longer recommended.
- Cerebral vasospasm in subarachnoid hemorrhage can be severe; reserpine, kanamycin, isoproterenol, aminophylline, and nitroprusside have all failed. Dopamine, 3–6 μg/kg/min, has been used, but there is a risk of rebleeding. Barbiturate coma has been used to reduce intracranial pressure when dopamine or mannitol has not been successful.

▶ EVALUATION OF THERAPEUTIC OUTCOMES

- Treatable single risk factors should be vigorously addressed. When risk factors occur in combination, therapy is initiated aggressively, with particular emphasis on hypertension and lifestyle changes. Blood pressure is monitored to ensure effective management of hypertension; drug-induced hypotension must be avoided. Lipid profiles, body weight, tobacco use, and other risk factors should also be monitored.

- Patients receiving anticoagulant therapy are carefully monitored for maintenance of appropriate coagulation parameters and for minor and major bleeding.
- Patients receiving aspirin are monitored for gastrointestinal bleeding because risk of bleeding is slightly increased.
- Patients receiving ticlopidine are monitored for side effects and potential drug interactions. Complete blood count with differential should be performed every 2 weeks for 3 months to detect the occurrence of reversible neutropenia.

See Chapter 18, Stroke, authored by J. Chris Bradberry, PharmD, for a more detailed discussion of this topic.

Chapter 14

▶ THROMBOEMBOLIC DISORDERS

▶ DEFINITION

Venous thromboembolism includes both venous thrombosis and pulmonary embolism. A deep vein thrombosis (DVT) is a thrombus composed of cellular material (red and white blood cells, platelets) bound together with fibrin strands, which form in the venous portion of the vasculature. A pulmonary embolism (PE) is a thrombus or foreign substance that arises from the systemic circulation and lodges in the pulmonary artery or one of its branches, causing complete or partial obstruction of pulmonary blood flow.

▶ PATHOPHYSIOLOGY

- Three primary components—venous stasis, vascular injury, and hypercoagulability (Virchow's triad)—play a role in the development of a thrombus.
- Venous stasis is characterized by altered or decreased blood flow in the deep veins of the lower limbs resulting from immobility, prolonged bed rest, massive obesity, venous obstruction, heart failure, hypovolemia, varicose veins, late-stage pregnancy, shock, or severe myocardial infarction.
- Vascular wall injury or endothelial damage occurs from mechanical (e.g., venipuncture, fractures) or chemical (e.g., potassium, hypertonic glucose) trauma that evokes an inflammatory response (phlebitis), in addition to locally activating the coagulation cascade to form an intraluminal thrombus.
- Hypercoagulability and excessive activation of the coagulation cascade can occur in activated protein C resistance; deficiencies of protein C, protein S, or antithrombin III; and certain types of malignancy.
- The coagulation cascade can be triggered through either the intrinsic or extrinsic pathways (Figure 14–1). The intrinsic pathway is activated by the contact of factor XII with exposed collagen from damaged subendothelial vessels. The extrinsic pathway is activated by the exposure of blood to tissue thromboplastin, a tissue factor released after vascular wall damage.
- Most venous thrombi involve the veins of the lower extremities where they develop behind venous valve cusps or at bifurcations in the intramuscular veins of the calf. Consequences of DVT include the postphlebitic syndrome, compromise of venous blood flow to the lower extremity, chronic venous insufficiency, and embolization of the thrombus to the lungs or elsewhere.

II

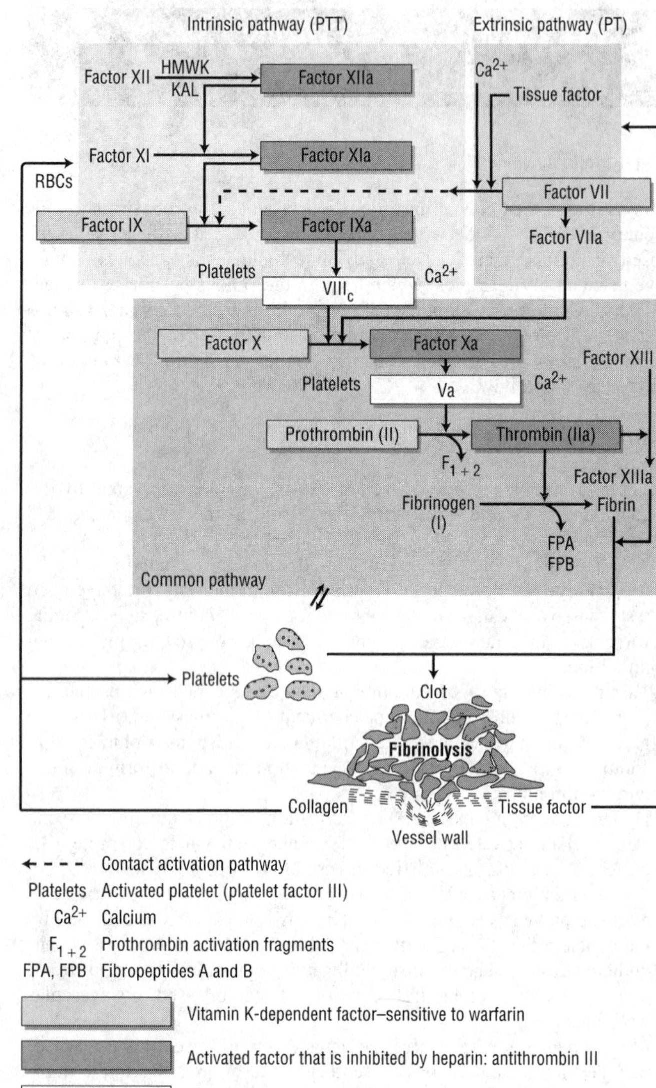

Intrinsic pathway (PTT)
Extrinsic pathway (PT)
Factor XII
HMWK
KAL
Factor XIIa
Ca2+
Tissue factor
Factor XI
Factor XIa
RBCs
Factor VII
Factor IX
Factor IXa
Factor VIIa
Platelets
VIIIc
Ca2+
Factor X
Factor Xa
Factor XIII
Platelets
Va
Ca2+
Prothrombin (II)
Thrombin (IIa)
F1 + 2
Factor XIIIa
Fibrinogen (I)
Fibrin
FPA
FPB
Common pathway
Platelets
Clot
Fibrinolysis
Collagen
Tissue factor
Vessel wall
Contact activation pathway
Platelets Activated platelet (platelet factor III)
Ca2+ Calcium
F1 + 2 Prothrombin activation fragments
FPA, FPB Fibropeptides A and B
Vitamin K-dependent factor–sensitive to warfarin
Activated factor that is inhibited by heparin: antithrombin III
Cofactors VIIIa and Va–inhibited by protein C

- In most patients, venous thrombi and PE are broken up by the endogenous lytic system, with complete clot resolution occurring over several weeks.
- The pulmonary effects of a PE may include the formation of an alveolar dead space, pneumoconstriction, arterial hypoxemia, loss of pulmonary surfactant (which occurs after 24 hours) leading to atelectasis and transudation of alveolar fluid into alveolar spaces, and pulmonary infarction (<10%).
- Hemodynamically, a PE increases pulmonary vascular resistance and subsequently right ventricular afterload. If these changes become marked, they may lead to tricuspid regurgitation, pulmonary hypertension, right ventricular failure, and low cardiac output.

▶ CLINICAL PRESENTATION

- Venous thrombi frequently are clinically silent. The most common clinical symptoms include pain, tenderness, swelling, and discoloration. The pain and tenderness are usually localized to the calf in patients with calf vein thrombosis and tend to be more diffuse and intense in patients with proximal vein thrombosis.
- Edema secondary to proximal vein obstruction or vascular inflammation is most often responsible for the swelling and ranges in severity. The swelling typically is localized or unilateral and can occur with or without pain. Patients with DVT may exhibit a discolored lower extremity from cyanosis because of a large venous obstruction; it may also be pale secondary to reflex arterial vasospasm or reddish from perivascular inflammation.
- Physical signs that may be present include a palpable cord and a positive Homan's sign (a nonspecific and insensitive test).
- Symptoms of postphlebitic syndrome may range from chronic pain and swelling in the lower extremities to the formation of stasis ulcers and the development of infection.
- Although many PE are clinically silent, signs and symptoms may include a sudden onset of unexplained dyspnea, cough, tachypnea,

◄

Figure 14–1. Scheme of the hemostatic system, showing interaction of vessel wall, platelets, coagulation pathways, and fibrinolytic system. Important features of the coagulation pathways include the contact activation phase, vitamin K-dependent factors (affected by warfarin), the activated serine proteases that are inhibited by heparin: antithrombin III, and the role of platelets and calcium. Factors VIIIc and Va are nonenzymatic cofactors that are inactivated by protein C. The protime (PT) measures the function of the extrinsic and common pathways; the partial thromboplastin time (PTT or APTT) measures the function of the intrinsic and common pathways. HMWK, high-molecular-weight kininogen; KAL, kallikrein; RBCs, red blood cells. *(Adapted from Stead RB: Regulation of hemostasis, in Goldhaber SZ (Ed):* Pulmonary Embolism and Deep Vein Thrombosis. *Philadelphia, W.B. Saunders, 1985, p 28, with permission.)*

tachycardia, pleuritic chest pain, and anxiety or a feeling of impending doom. Diaphoresis, substernal chest pain, and hemoptysis (which may indicate pulmonary infarction or congestive atelectasis) are sometimes seen.

- Patients with massive PE often present with signs of circulatory collapse, such as syncope or shock due to a reduced cardiac output, or with evidence of acute cor pulmonale or right ventricular failure.

▶ DIAGNOSIS

- The diagnosis of DVT or PE should be suspected in any patient with suggestive clinical signs and symptoms. Because none are specific, objective testing methods are necessary.
- A medical history, medication history, and thorough physical examination are important in identifying underlying risk factors that may have led to the development of the thrombus.

DIAGNOSTIC TECHNIQUES FOR DVT

- Diagnostic techniques may visualize the thrombus (contrast venography, ultrasound, magnetic resonance imaging); measure obstructions to venous outflow (impedance plethysmography, Doppler ultrasound); or detect the incorporation of radiolabeled proteins into the developing thrombus (^{125}I-fibrinogen scan, monoclonal antibodies).
- When venous thrombosis is suspected clinically, a noninvasive test (impedance plethysmography, Doppler ultrasound, or real-time ultrasound) should be performed initially. If the test is positive (in the absence of conditions known to produce a false-positive result), anticoagulant therapy should be initiated. If the test is negative, repeat serial exams are obtained between days 5–7 and again between days 10–14. Serial testing is necessary because these tests are insensitive to calf vein thrombosis, which is clinically important only when it extends into the proximal veins. If the test becomes positive during serial testing, the patient is diagnosed with DVT and anticoagulant therapy is initiated. Positive tests occurring in the presence of conditions known to produce false-positives (e.g., heart failure) should be confirmed by venography.

DIAGNOSTIC TECHNIQUES FOR PE

- An electrocardiogram (ECG), chest roentgenogram, and arterial blood gas should be obtained in any patient with suspected PE. ECG patterns may include nonspecific ST-segment elevations or depression, T wave inversion, right axis deviation, new incomplete right bundle-branch block, or evidence of right ventricular hypertrophy. The radiographic patterns may include effusions, infiltrates, enlargement of right descending pulmonary artery, Westermark's sign (avascular lung zones), and elevation of the diaphragm.

- An arterial blood gas may be useful in assessing the degree of ventilation; however, approximately 10–20% of patients with PE have Po_2 values of >80 mm Hg.
- A ventilation–perfusion (V/Q) radionuclide scan estimates the probability of PE based on the anatomic patterns of injected and inhaled radioactive materials. Pulmonary perfusion defects are nonspecific, so assessment of ventilation is necessary. Because an embolus obstructs arterial blood flow in one of the pulmonary arteries but does not affect ventilation, this scan can detect areas that are being ventilated but not perfused (a V/Q mismatch). If results are inconclusive, further objective testing is necessary to confirm the diagnosis of PE.
- Pulmonary angiography may be indicated when there is a nondiagnostic V/Q scan with or without a normal IPG in a patient with a picture suggestive of PE; disagreement between V/Q scan interpretation and clinical impression; a contraindication to anticoagulation; and anticipation of thrombolytic therapy, inferior vena cava interruption, or embolectomy.
- New plasma markers, such as D-dimer, are currently being investigated as negative predictors of DVT and PE. Normal D-dimer concentrations (<500 ng/mL) have been shown to be strongly predictive of a normal pulmonary angiogram. However, current data are insufficient to allow complete reliance on this test as a diagnostic tool for PE.

► DESIRED OUTCOME

The main objectives of treating venous thrombosis are to prevent the development of pulmonary embolism and the postphlebitic syndrome, to reduce morbidity from the acute event, and to achieve these objectives with a minimum of adverse effects and cost. Successful treatment of DVT should prevent extension of the thrombus, prevent embolism to the lungs, and restore patency to the venous circulation while maintaining normal venous valve function.

► TREATMENT

GENERAL PRINCIPLES

- In any patient suspected of having a DVT or PE, empiric therapy (e.g., heparin) is started to decrease the risk of further embolic events while waiting for the results of diagnostic tests.
- General management of DVT includes bed rest, with the heels elevated above the heart to enhance venous return, and administration of nonaspirin analgesics for pain.
- For PE, oxygen should be given and, if necessary, patients should be mechanically ventilated.
- Coagulation tests (APTT, PT, INR) should be performed prior to the initiation of therapy to establish the patient's baseline values, which assists in determining the end point for heparin therapy and guides later oral anticoagulation with warfarin.

UNFRACTIONATED HEPARIN

- **Unfractionated heparin** is a heterogeneous mixture of polymers ranging from 3000 to 30,000 daltons with varying antithrombotic activity. Apparently, only a small and distinct fraction of the heparin molecule is responsible for most of the anticoagulant effect.
- The anticoagulant function of heparin is thought to depend on its ability to bind to and catalyze antithrombin III (ATIII) or heparin cofactor, a circulating anticoagulant that neutralizes the proteolytic activities of several clotting factors that have a serine residue at their enzymatically active site (XII, XI, X, and IX, kallikrein, and thrombin).
- Heparin halts further growth and propagation of the thrombus, allowing the endogenous thrombolytic system to eradicate the existing clot. In addition, heparin may also promote thrombus resolution.
- Heparin is indicated in patients with a thrombus extending above the popliteal vein because of the high risk of PE and postphlebitic syndrome in these patients. Patients with symptomatic calf vein thrombosis should also receive heparin. Patients with superficial thrombophlebitis should not receive anticoagulation. Heparin is clearly indicated for patients with documented PE and is also used for the prevention of venous thromboembolism.
- Contraindications include hypersensitivity to the drug, active bleeding, hemophilia, thrombocytopenia, intracranial hemorrhage, bacterial endocarditis, active tuberculosis, ulcerative lesions of the GI tract, severe hypertension, threatened abortion, or visceral carcinoma.
- Figure 14–2 is an algorithm for the acute management of DVT or PE with heparin therapy and management of excessive anticoagulation. Doses should be based on total body weight with a loading dose of 70–100 U/kg followed by an initial IV infusion rate of 15–25 U/kg/h. One popular regimen is an initial dose of 80 U/kg followed by 18 U/kg/h. Continuous intravenous (IV) infusion is the recommended method of administration because it produces a more consistent degree of anticoagulation and may be associated with lower risk for bleeding than intermittent bolus dosing.
  - The activated partial thromboplastin time (APTT) should be checked no sooner than 6 hours after beginning the heparin infusion or after any dosage change (target APTT: 1.5–2.0 times control).
  - Once the target APTT is achieved, daily monitoring is indicated for minor dosing adjustments.
  - In uncomplicated patients or less extensive disease, a short course of heparin therapy may be appropriate (4–5 days of continuous IV heparin with warfarin started on day 1). Patients with massive pulmonary embolism or ileofemoral thrombosis may require a more traditional duration of heparin therapy (i.e., 10 days), with warfarin being started on day 5 to ensure an overlap period of 4–5 days.
- If continuous infusion is not feasible, intermittent IV injections may be given every 4 hours in most patients, with APTT performed 3.5–4 hours after the heparin injection.

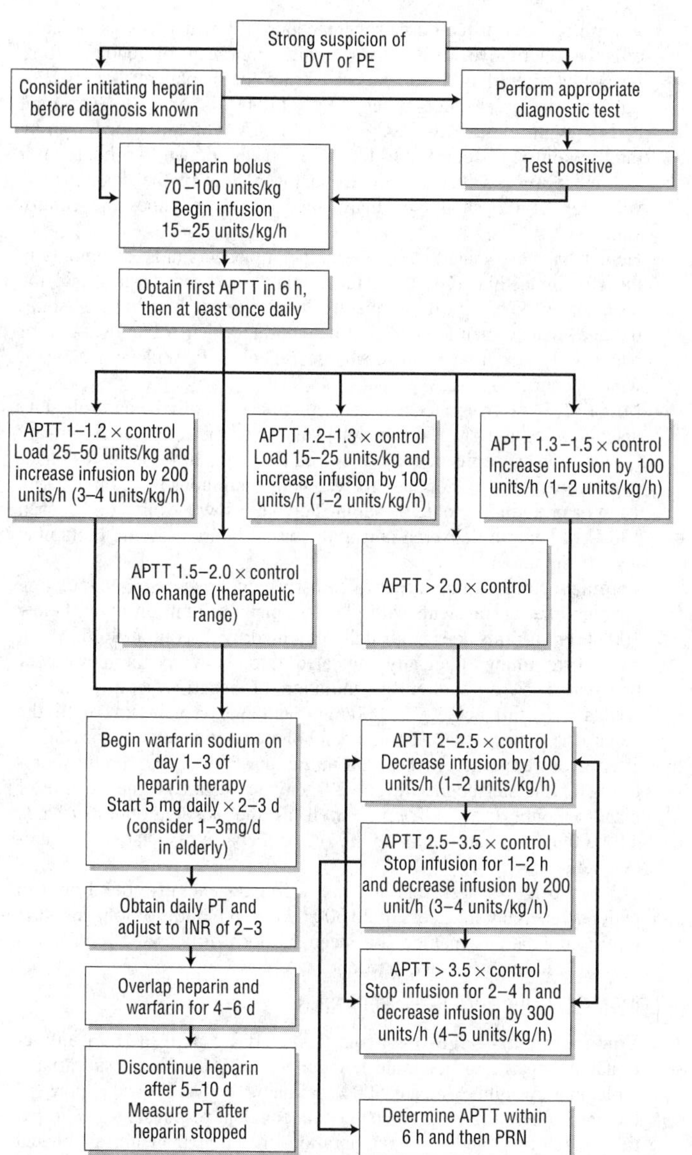

Figure 14–2. Algorithm for the acute management of DVT or PE with heparin. *(Adapted from Carter BL. Therapy of acute thromboembolism with heparin and warfarin.* Clin Pharm *1991;10:503–518.)*

- Intermittent, adjusted-dose subcutaneous (SC) heparin is a safe, effective alternative method for the initial treatment of venous thrombosis that simplifies treatment and allows for outpatient therapy. Initial heparin doses should be 15,000–17,500 U or 250 U/kg total body weight administered SC every 12 hours. The initial dose can be rapidly adjusted according to the APTT value drawn 4–6 hours after the first dose and then once daily at the middle of the dosing interval. The APTT should be maintained above 1.5 times the control value.
- Hemorrhage associated with heparin therapy occurs most commonly in the gastrointestinal (GI) tract, the urinary tract, soft tissues, and the oropharynx. The most frequently encountered bleeding episodes include melena, hematomas, and hematuria, which occur in 2–3% of patients. Less common are ecchymosis, epistaxis, and hematemesis, which occur in 0.5–1.2% of patients.
- Minor bleeding from an excess of heparin can usually be controlled by discontinuing the drug. For major bleeding or the threat of significant hemorrhage, specific therapy is warranted (e.g., blood transfusion or **protamine sulfate**). For patients receiving continuous infusion heparin, 1 mg of protamine should be administered by slow IV infusion for each 100 U of heparin delivered during the past 4 hours (≤50 mg protamine over 10 minutes).
- Thrombocytopenia may occur as an early, slight decrease in circulating platelets that is transient, with platelet counts seldom dropping below 100,000/mm^3; this does not usually require drug discontinuation. A rare but severe immunologically mediated thrombocytopenia may occur between 5–14 days after the initiation of heparin therapy. Platelet counts may fall below 100,000/mm^3 and will remain low until the heparin is discontinued. Thromboembolic complications may occur in arteries or veins (i.e., myocardial infarction, DVT, PE). Careful monitoring of platelet counts (every 2–3 days) to evaluate the decline of platelet count (i.e., >30%) as well as the absolute number (i.e., <100,000/mm^3) can minimize the risk of heparin-associated thrombocytopenia.
- Osteoporosis has been reported rarely and is generally found only in patients receiving in excess of 20,000 U/d for 6 months or longer. Other rare complications include skin necrosis, local urticaria, hypoaldosteronism, and hypersensitivity reactions.

LOW-MOLECULAR-WEIGHT HEPARINS

- **Low-molecular-weight heparins** (LMWH) are derived from unfractionated heparin to elaborate compounds with smaller, less variable molecular weights (mean 5000 daltons). LMWH have improved bioavailability, a more predictable anticoagulant response, less interpatient variability, and a longer duration of action than unfractionated heparin.

- Although LMWH have a preferential effect on activated factor X with fewer effects on thrombin and platelets, this has not been conclusively proven to result in a lower incidence of bleeding complications than with unfractionated heparin. The LMWH are associated with a lower risk of heparin-induced thrombocytopenia and its associated thrombotic effects than unfractionated heparin. II
- The APTT is not altered during LMWH therapy, but plasma anti-Xa activity may be measured to monitor the anticoagulant effect. No routine monitoring is required when LMWH are used for the prevention of DVT. When used for treating established venous thromboembolism (not presently an FDA-approved indication), anti-Xa levels should be measured at least once at the beginning of therapy to assure that an adequate level of anticoagulation is achieved and to assess the risk of hemorrhage.
- LMWH have been used for the treatment of established DVT and PE because the predictable dose–response relationship permits standard once or twice daily dosing, there is no need for routine laboratory monitoring, they are well-absorbed and can be self-administered on an outpatient basis, and their use reduces the number of inpatient hospital days.
- Overall, clinical trials have shown LMWH to be at least as safe and effective as unfractionated heparin for the initial treatment of DVT or nonmassive PE and as safe and effective as adjusted-dose warfarin for the prevention of recurrent venous thromboembolism. However, further large-scale studies are needed to more clearly define the role of individual LMWH for these clinical indications. Unfractionated heparin and warfarin currently remain the drugs of choice.

WARFARIN

- **Warfarin** prevents formation of γ-carboxyglutamic acid residues (by blocking the carboxylation system) and release of certain proteins that are deficient in γ-carboxyglutamic acid. Six vitamin K-dependent proteins are involved in the coagulation system (factors II, VII, IX, X, and proteins C and S), whose synthesis is inhibited by warfarin.
- Warfarin is indicated after the initial course of heparin therapy to prevent recurrent thromboembolic complications that may occur particularly in the first 3 months after DVT or PE.
- Although inhibition of coagulation factors occurs 12–24 hours after oral administration, the antithrombotic effects may not occur until 2–7 days after the initiation of therapy.
- Warfarin is indicated for at least 3 months after an initial episode of DVT and indefinitely for long-term anticoagulation in patients with recurrent venous thromboembolism.
- All of the contraindications listed for heparin also apply to warfarin. Relative contraindications for warfarin include severe hepatic or renal disease, vitamin K deficiency, chronic alcoholism, a requirement for

intensive salicylate or NSAID therapy, and the inability of the patient to comply with the regimen.

- Warfarin can be initiated at any time during heparin treatment and should be initiated as soon as it becomes apparent that oral anticoagulation will be used. Initiation of warfarin should occur before IV heparin is discontinued to prevent a break in the level of anticoagulation. The overlapping period of heparin and warfarin should be 4–5 days because of the delayed onset of the effect of warfarin and the hypercoagulable state occurring after heparin is discontinued. Heparin can usually be discontinued once the INR is within the desired range for 2 consecutive days.
- Warfarin should be initiated with small doses (approximately 5 mg/d for 2–4 days); elderly patients (i.e., age >65 years) may need even lower initial doses (i.e., 1–3 mg/d).
- Warfarin therapy is monitored by the INR (target: 2.0–3.0 for DVT or PE) every 24–48 hours after therapy is initiated and until the INR results have stabilized (i.e., INRs that are similar for 2 or 3 consecutive days with the same warfarin dosage) or until a maintenance dose is determined.
- The frequency of fatal, major, and major plus minor bleeding during warfarin therapy has been estimated to be 0.6, 3.0, and 9.6%, respectively. Table 14–1 outlines guidelines for reversing the anticoagulant effect of warfarin according to the INR and the clinical situation (i.e., presence of bleeding). **Vitamin K** given orally, SC, or by slow IV infusion will usually reverse the effects of warfarin in 6–12 hours. Patients who will be resumed on warfarin therapy should receive lower doses of vitamin K (e.g., <1 mg) to avoid full normalization of the INR and subsequent warfarin resistance.
- Warfarin-induced skin necrosis and purple toe syndrome are rare non-dose-related side effects of warfarin.
- Warfarin should be avoided in pregnant women because it crosses the placenta and causes fetal malformation at *any* time during pregnancy. Heparin is currently the anticoagulant of choice in pregnancy because it does not cross the placenta and does not cause fetal complications. During lactation, heparin is not secreted in breast milk and can be safely administered to nursing mothers.
- Because of the large number of food–drug and drug–drug interactions with warfarin, close monitoring and additional INR determinations may be indicated whenever other medications are initiated or discontinued or an alteration in consumption of vitamin K–containing foods is noted.

THROMBOLYTIC THERAPY

- Thrombolytic agents are not generally accepted as a standard form of therapy for DVT or PE because of potential bleeding complications, lack of mortality differences and adequate long-term follow-up among studies performed, the amount of patient monitoring required once therapy is initiated, and the substantial cost of these agents.

TABLE 14–1. Reversing the Anticoagulant Effect of Warfarin

Clinical Situation	Recommended Treatment Action
INR >3 but <6, patient is not bleeding, and rapid reversal is not indicated for reasons of surgical intervention	Omit the next few warfarin doses and resume warfarin therapy at a lower dose when the INR is between 2 and 3
INR ≥ 6 but <10 and the patient is not bleeding, or more rapid reversal is required because the patient requires elective surgery	Administer vitamin K 0.5–1 mg, oral or SC; reduction in INR will occur within 8 h; INR may be in the range of 2–3 in 24 h. If the INR at 24 h is still high, a second dose of vitamin K 0.5 mg SC can be given. Warfarin can then be restarted at a lower dose
INR ≥ 10 but <20 and the patient is not bleeding	Vitamin K 3–5 mg, oral or SC, should be given with the INR reduced substantially at 6 h. The INR should be checked every 6–12 h, and vitamin K can be repeated as necessary
Major warfarin overdose (e.g., INR >20) or a rapid reversal of an anticoagulant effect is required because of serious bleeding	Vitamin K 10 mg slow IV infusion (e.g., over 20–30 min) and the INR checked every 6 h. Vitamin K may be repeated every 12 h and supplemented with plasma transfusion or factor concentrate depending on the urgency of the situation
Life-threatening bleeding or serious warfarin overdose	Replacement with factor concentrates as indicated supplemented with vitamin K 10 mg slow IV infusion (e.g., over 20–30 min). Vitamin K may be repeated as necessary depending on the INR

Adapted from Hirsh J, Poller L. The international normalized ratio: a guide to understanding and correcting its problems. Arch Intern Med *1994;154:282–288, with permission.*

- All thrombolytics are plasminogen activators and act either directly (urokinase, alteplase) or indirectly (streptokinase). Plasminogen, an inactive proteolytic enzyme, is converted to plasmin, which has the ability to lyse fibrin, as well as to hydrolyze fibrinogen and other coagulation factors, leading to a systemic lytic state.
- Proposed indications for thrombolytic therapy of thromboembolic disease include massive/submassive PE with hemodynamic compromise, massive PE without hemodynamic compromise, submassive PE in patients who cannot tolerate further cardiopulmonary compromise, heparin treatment failures, and extensive proximal DVT. Thrombolytic agents offer the greatest benefit to PE patients with acute decompensation (hypotension and low cardiac output); their role in patients with less severe episodes remains to be defined.
- Patients receiving thrombolytics should have a documented diagnosis of thromboembolism and evidence that the thrombus is of recent origin (within the last 7 days).

- Three thrombolytic agents and regimens are available for treatment of DVT and PE:
  - **Streptokinase:** Loading dose of 250,000 units in normal saline or 5% dextrose in water IV over 30 minutes followed by a continuous IV infusion of 100,000 U/h for 24 (PE) to 72 (DVT) hours.
  - **Urokinase:** Loading dose of 4400 U/kg in normal saline or 5% dextrose in water IV over 10 minutes followed by 4400 U/kg/h IV for a total of 12 hours (PE).
  - **Alteplase:** 100 mg by IV infusion over 2 hours (PE).
- Laboratory monitoring is used to determine whether some degree of systemic fibrinolysis has been achieved. The thrombin time or APTT should be performed prior to the administration of thrombolytic therapy and 3–4 hours after the initiation of treatment. As long as test values during the thrombolytic infusion are prolonged beyond the control value, it can be assumed that a lytic state has been established.
- Once thrombolytic therapy is discontinued and the thrombin time or APTT has fallen to less than twice the normal values (usually in 2–4 hours), continuous IV heparin should be given followed by warfarin therapy.
- Thrombolytic therapy is associated with a 6–30% frequency of major bleeding complications in patients treated for DVT and approximately 20% for patients being treated for PE. Minor bleeding or oozing at cutaneous puncture sites can be controlled locally with pressure dressings. In cases of serious bleeding, thrombolytic therapy should be discontinued quickly. If blood replacement is indicated, whole blood or blood products (packed red blood cells, fresh-frozen plasma, or cryoprecipitate) may be given. In situations where bleeding unresponsive to blood replacement therapy must be rapidly corrected, **ε-aminocaproic acid** (EACA) may be given in 5-g doses.
- Allergic or hypersensitivity reactions associated with streptokinase include urticaria, itching, flushing, nausea, headache, and transient elevation or decrease of systolic blood pressure. Anaphylaxis (1.3–2.5%) has ranged in severity from minor breathing difficulties to bronchospasm, periorbital swelling, or angioneurotic edema. Mild allergic reactions have been reported with urokinase and alteplase.
- Fever is more common with streptokinase therapy but can also occur with urokinase and alteplase. Allergic and febrile reactions may be treated with antihistamines, and acetaminophen is effective for fever. Corticosteroids have also been used for the prophylaxis of these adverse reactions.
- Hypotension can occur with rapid infusions of streptokinase and has also been reported with urokinase and alteplase. The hypotension can often be prevented by slowing the rate of administration.

SURGICAL THERAPY

- Thrombectomy for DVT is reserved for patients with severe limb ischemia.

- Pulmonary embolectomy and venous interruption are the most common procedures considered for PE. The placement of percutaneous transvenous filters (i.e., Greenfield filter) and umbrellas (Mobin–Uddin) may prevent recurrence of thromboembolism from the lower extremities. Pulmonary embolectomy may be considered in life-threatening situations, but it is associated with a high mortality rate.

PREVENTION OF VENOUS THROMBOEMBOLISM

- General guidelines for identifying patients at risk for thromboembolism are contained in Table 14–2.
- Nonpharmacologic prophylactic techniques include early ambulation, leg elevation, leg exercises, elastic compression or thromboembolic deterrent (TED) stockings, intermittent calf compression, electrical stimulation of calf muscles during surgery, and inferior vena cava interruption.
- Low-dose unfractionated heparin therapy involves the administration of 5000 U SC every 8–12 hours. Dosing every 8 hours (15,000 U/d) is no more effective (except in very high risk general surgery patients) and may be associated with a slightly higher rate of bleeding episodes. In surgery patients, heparin should be started 2 hours before the surgical procedure and then given every 8 to 12 hours thereafter.
- Adjusted-dose infractionated heparin (given subcutaneously every 12 hours) has also been used in high-risk patients in whom low-dose heparin is not effective or has limited effectiveness (i.e., hip surgery patients). The APTT is drawn 4–6 hours after the first dose and at the midpoint of the dosing interval thereafter to slightly prolong the APTT (1.1–1.2 times control). The average daily dose is 15,000 to 18,000 units.
- Warfarin has been used in high-risk patients in either a fixed low dose (1–2 mg daily) or a dose adjusted to prolong the INR to 2.0–3.0. Because of the risk of bleeding and the need for repeated laboratory monitoring, warfarin should be reserved for high-risk patients (e.g., major orthopedic procedures or history of recurrent venous thrombosis).
- LMWH are effective for prophylaxis of venous thromboembolism; current FDA-approved indications and dosage regimens are included in Table 14–3.
- **Danaparoid sodium** (Orgaron) is an LMW glycosaminoglycan (mean molecular weight 6000 daltons) that has had heparin and heparin-like fragments removed during the extraction process, yielding a mixture of heparan sulfate (84%), dermatan sulfate (12%), and chondroitin sulfate (4%). This structural difference results in a low degree of cross-reactivity (0–20%) between danaparoid and heparin or LWMH, making it an alternative agent in patients with heparin-induced thrombocytopenia. It is currently indicated for prophylaxis of venous thromboembolism in patients undergoing elective hip replacement surgery. The dose is 750 anti-Xa units SC twice daily. The first dose

TABLE 14–2. Guidelines for Prophylaxis of Thromboembolism

Type of Surgery/Indication	Recommended Prophylaxis
General Surgery	
Low risk (minor surgery, < 40 y old, no risk factors)	Early ambulation
Moderate risk (major surgery, > 40 y old, no additional risk factors)	GCS, LDUH (every 12 h), or IPC[a]
High risk (major surgery, > 40 y old, with additional risk factors)	LDUH (every 8 h) or LMWH
Above but prone to wound complications (hematoma)	IPC
Very high risk (above with multiple risk factors)	LDUH (every 8 h), LMWH, or dextran **with** IPC[b]
	Warfarin (INR 2.0–3.0) may be used in select patients
Total hip replacement	LMWH, low-intensity warfarin (INR 2.0–3.0), or ADUH; GCS or IPC may be additive[c]
Hip fracture surgery	LMWH or low-intensity warfarin (INR 2.0–3.0); IPC may be additive[d]
Total knee replacement	LMWH or IPC[e]
Multiple trauma patients (especially patients with hip and lower extremity fractures)	IPC, warfarin, or LMWH
High-risk orthopedic and multiple-trauma patients, other prophylaxis contraindicated	IVC filter
Neurosurgery-intracranial	IPC and/or GCS; LDUH (alternative); LDUH and IPC may be additive in high-risk patients
Acute spinal cord injury with paralysis[f]	ADUH or LMWH; warfarin (alternative) GCS or IPC may be additive
Myocardial infarction	LDUH or full-dose heparin; IPC and/or GCS useful if heparin contraindicated
Ischemic stroke with lower extremity paralysis	LDUH or LMWH; IPC and GCS also effective
General medicine patients with VTE risk factors	LDUH or LMWH
Long-term indwelling central venous catheters	Warfarin 1 mg daily

[a]LDUH should be started 2 h preoperatively and given every 12 h postoperatively. GCS and IPC should be applied during surgery, if possible, and throughout the postoperative period.

[b]LDUH and LMWH should be started preoperatively; dextran should be started intraoperatively; IPC should be applied intraoperatively.

[c]LMWH should begin postoperatively; warfarin should be started preoperatively or immediately postoperatively; ADUH should be started postoperatively. Duration of prophylaxis is **at least** 7–10 d postoperatively regardless of the duration of hospital stay; risk may be as long as 2 mo.

[d]LMWH should be started preoperatively.

[e]LMWH should be started postoperatively; IPC should be started intraoperatively or immediately postoperatively and should be worn continuously except during ambulation.

[f]Greatest risk is during the first 2 wk after injury; prophylaxis should be continued for a minimum of 3 mo in patients unable to ambulate.

GCS, graduated compression stockings; LDUH, low-dose unfractionated heparin at a dose of 5000 units; IPC, intermittent pneumatic compression; LMWH, low-molecular-weight heparin; ADUH, adjusted-dose unfractionated heparin; IVC, inferior vena cava; VTE, venous thromboembolism.

TABLE 14–3. LMWH for Prophylaxis of Venous Thromboembolism in Patients at Risk for Thromboembolic Complications

Generic Name (Brand Name)	Indications	Dose	Administration Schedule
Enoxaparin (Lovenox)	Patients undergoing hip or knee replacement surgery	30 mg SC bid	First dose given within 12–24 h postoperatively
	Patients undergoing abdominal surgery	40 mg SC qd	First dose given 2 h prior to surgery Continue until the risk of DVT is diminished; usual duration is 7–10 days
Dalteparin (Fragmin)	Patients undergoing abdominal surgery	2500 anti-Xa units SC qd (5000 anti-Xa units in high-risk patients)	First dose given 1–2 h preoperatively, then qd for 5–10 days postoperatively
Ardeparin (Normiflo)	Patients undergoing knee replacement surgery	50 anti-Xa units/kg actual weight SC bid	First dose given on the evening of the day of surgery or the following morning; continue for up to 14 days or until the patient is fully ambulatory.

should be administered 1–4 hours preoperatively with subsequent doses beginning at least 2 hours postoperatively for 7–10 days or until the risk is diminished.

▶ EVALUATION OF THERAPEUTIC OUTCOMES

- Patients should be monitored for the resolution of symptoms, the development of recurrent thrombosis, and symptoms of the postphlebitic syndrome, as well as for adverse effects from treatment.
- Patients treated for DVT should be initially monitored twice daily and then daily for changes in pain, limb circumference, swelling, and tenderness.
- Patients treated for DVT or PE should be monitored for signs and symptoms of PE every shift for 1–2 days, followed by daily monitoring for the incidence or changes in dyspnea, apprehension, cough, pleuritic chest pain, and hemoptysis.
- Repeat arterial blood gases and/or V/Q studies may be indicated to assess progress of antithrombotic therapy in patients being treated for PE.
- Patients should be examined twice daily during hospitalization for signs of bleeding including IV catheter sites, hematomas, and ecchy-

mosis. Intramuscular injections should be avoided in patients receiving therapeutic heparin doses.

- A platelet count should be obtained prior to heparinization, every 2 or 3 days during therapy, and after the discontinuation of therapy to monitor for heparin-associated thrombocytopenia.
- Hemoglobin and hematocrit are indicated prior to heparinization and every 1–2 days during therapy to identify the presence of bleeding. The stool should be examined daily for the presence of blood.
- Alterations in warfarin dosage should be made in small increments to prevent excessive changes in the INR.
- Careful follow-up and weekly monitoring of the INR is required during the first 4 weeks of therapy after discharge from the hospital. Changes in diet, exercise, clinical state, social habits, and compliance frequently alter maintenance dose requirements. Once a stable therapeutic warfarin dose has been attained, the INR can be monitored less frequently (i.e., once monthly).

See Chapter 17, Thromboembolic Disorders, authored by Sharon M. Erdman, PharmD, Susan K. Chuck, PharmD, and Keith A. Rodvold, PharmD, FCCP, BCPS, for a more detailed discussion of this topic.

Dermatologic Disorders

Edited by Barbara G. Wells, PharmD, FASHP, FCCP, BCPP

Chapter 15

▶ ACNE

▶ DEFINITION

- Acne is a common, self-limiting, multifactorial disease involving inflammation of the sebaceous follicles of the face and upper trunk.

▶ PATHOPHYSIOLOGY

- Acne pathogenesis is depicted in Figure 15–1. Major pathophysiologic features of acne are shown in Table 15–1.
- A widening of the follicular canal with an increase in cell production occurs. Sebaceous glands atrophy, and sebum mixes with excess loose cells in the follicular canal to form a keratinous plug. This appears as a "blackhead," or open comedo. Trauma or inflammation may lead to formation of a "whitehead," or closed comedo.
- Increased androgen activity at puberty triggers growth of sebaceous glands and enhances sebum production. Sebum consists of glycerides, wax esters, squalene, and cholesterol. Glyceride is converted to free fatty acids and glycerol by lipases which are products of *Propionibacterium acnes* (*P. acnes*). Free fatty acids may irritate the follicular wall and cause increased cell turnover and inflammation. *P. acnes* is antigenic and can increase antibody formation leading to an inflammatory response, and immune-complex-mediated complement activation may lead to vascular leakage, mast cell degranulation, and leukocyte chemotaxis. Hydrolytic enzymes released by complement activation may damage the follicle wall. *P. acnes* may also evoke a cell-mediated immune response.
- The primary change in acne is an alteration in the pattern of keratinization within the follicle. Increased production of loosely adherent keratin cells has been correlated with obstruction of the follicles seen in comedo formation.

▶ CLINICAL PRESENTATION

- The clinical presentation of acne can range from a mild comedonal form to severe inflammatory necrotic acne of the face, chest, and back.
- Fibrosis associated with healing may lead to permanent scarring.

III

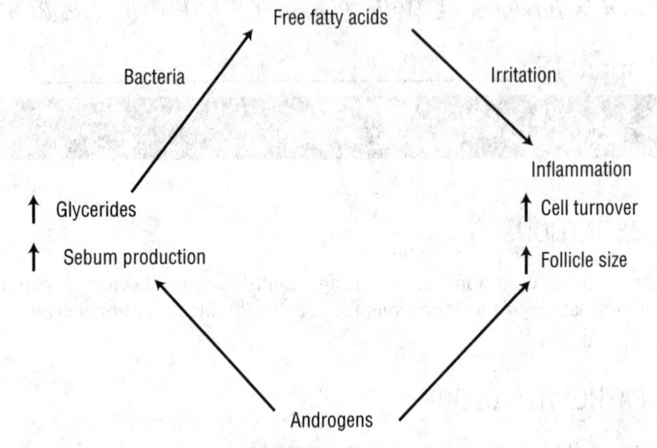

Figure 15–1. Acne pathogenesis.

TABLE 15–1. Major Pathophysiologic Features of Acne and Responsive Pharmacotherapeutic Agents

Feature	Systemic Drug	Topical Drug
Sebum production/secretion	Estrogens Antiandrogens Spironolactone Isotretinoin	None established
Abnormal desquamation of follicular epithelium	Isotretinoin Antibiotics	Tretinoin Salicylic acid Adapalene Tazarotene
P. acnes proliferation	Tetracycline Minocycline Doxycycline Erythromycin Clindamycin Cotrimoxazole Isotretinoin	Erythromycin Clindamycin Benzoyl peroxide Azelaic acid
Inflammation	Corticosteroids Isotretinoin Nonsteroidal anti-inflammatory agents	Metronidazole Intralesional corticosteroids Sulfur Adapalene Azelaic acid

▶ DIAGNOSIS

- Diagnosis is established by a mixture of lesions of acne (comedones, pustules, papules, nodules, cysts) on the face, back, or chest. The presence of 5 to 10 comedones is usually considered diagnostic.

▶ DESIRED OUTCOME

The goal of treatment is to heal lesions and to prevent or minimize scarring.

▶ TREATMENT

- Topical and oral treatment guidelines are shown in Tables 15–2 and 15–3.

TOPICAL PHARMACOLOGIC THERAPY

Benzoyl Peroxide

- **Benzoyl peroxide** is an effective treatment for mild and moderately severe acne. It increases sloughing rate of epithelial cells and loosens the follicular plug. Further studies are required to assess the tumorigenic potential of benzoyl peroxide.
- Benzoyl peroxide is decomposed on the skin by cysteine, liberating free oxygen radicals that oxidize bacterial proteins. Daily application of 10% benzoyl peroxide for 2 weeks can reduce free fatty acid levels by 50% and *P. acnes* levels by 98%.
- Side effects include dryness, irritation, and contact dermatitis. To limit irritation, therapy may be initiated with a low potency product (2.5%), and then the strength may be increased (5–10%) or application frequency slowly increased (every other day, then each day, then twice daily).
- Gel formulations are usually most potent, whereas the lotion, creams, and soaps are weaker potency. The alcohol-based preparations generally cause more dryness and irritation. Fair or moist skin is more sensitive, thus patients should be advised to apply medication to dry skin at least 30 minutes after washing.

Sulfur, Resorcinol, and Salicylic Acid

- **Sulfur, resorcinol,** and **salicylic acid** are keratolytic and mildly antibacterial. Keratolytic refers to the effect of solubilization of the intracellular cement of keratin cells in the stratum corneum.
- Combinations of these agents are often considered synergistic.
- They are not considered to be effective comedolytic agents as are benzoyl peroxide and tretinoin.
- Disadvantages include odor created by a hydrogen sulfide reaction of sulfur with the skin, the brown scale from resorcinol, and salicylism from long-term use of high concentrations of salicylic acid on permeable skin.

TABLE 15–2. Topical Acne Treatment Guidelines

Active Ingredient	Formulation	Strength (%)	Regimen	Potential Side Effects
Benzoyl peroxide	Soaps, lotions, creams, gels	2.5–10	Initially every other day, or daily, then twice daily	Irritation based on form/strength Bleaching/staining of clothing
Tretinoin	Creams, gels, solution, microsphere gel, liquid polymer	0.025–0.05	Initially every other day or daily	Moderate erythema, burning, stinging, pruritus Concomitant use of other irritants increases likelihood of undue irritation
Sulfur/resorcinol/salicylic acid	Creams, lotions, gels, soaps	0.5–10 in various combinations	Daily	
Clindamycin	Solution, gel, lotion	1	Twice daily	Drying, gastrointestinal effects (*P. colitis*)
Tetracycline	Solution	2.2	Twice daily	Burning and stinging following application, skin discoloration
Erythromycin	Solution, powder, gel	1.5–2	Twice daily	Drying, erythema
Adapalene	Gel, lotion	0.03–0.1	Daily	Moderate erythema, drying, stinging, burning, pruritus
Azelaic acid	Cream	20	Twice daily	Mild, transient, local erythema, burning, pruritus
Tazarotene	Gel	0.1	Daily or twice daily	Moderate erythema, burning, stinging, pruritus

TABLE 15–3. Oral Acne Treatment Guidelines

Active Ingredient	Formulation	Strength (mg)	Regimen	Potential Side Effects
Tetracycline	Tablets, capsules	250–500	1 g/d initial; if no response in 2–3 weeks or severe acne, 2–3 g/d. Maintenance 125–500 mg/d	Gastrointestinal upset, photoreactivity, drug and food interactions
Minocycline	Tablets, capsules, suspension	50–100	100 mg twice daily	CNS effects (dizziness, drowsiness), discoloration of skin
Doxycycline	Tablets, capsules, suspension, syrup	50–100	50–100 mg twice daily	Discoloration, gastrointestinal upset (esophagitis), photoreactivity
Erythromycin	Tablets as various salts	250–500	1 g/d as base; if no response in 2–3 weeks or severe acne, 2–3 g/d. Maintenance 250–500 mg/d	Gastrointestinal upset, cutaneous reactions, drug interations
Clindamycin	Capsules	75, 150, 300	300–450 mg/d	Diarrhea, pseudomembranous colitis
Isotretinoin	Capsules	10, 20, 40	0.5–1 mg/kg/d two divided doses Maximum of 2 mg/kg/d	Cheilitis, erythema, dryness, gastrointestinal effects, teratogenicity

Topical Antibacterial Products

- Inhibition of *P. acnes* is most effectively accomplished by **clindamycin,** but this does not necessarily correlate with clinical response.
- A topical preparation of **erythromycin** plus **zinc** is reported to be significantly better than 500 mg/d oral **tetracycline** in reducing overall acne severity and papule lesion counts.
- Disadvantages of topical antibiotic agents include occasional irritation and stinging. On the skin, tetracycline photooxidizes to produce a visible yellow tinting. Diarrhea and pseudomembranous colitis may occur with the use of topical clindamycin.

Azelaic Acid

- Topical **azelaic acid** apparently interferes with DNA synthesis in some of the bacteria associated with acne vulgaris. It significantly reduced inflamed lesions after 1 month and noninflamed lesions after 2 months.
- Topical 20% azelaic acid cream is a twice daily, cost-effective, product effective for mild to moderate acne.

Tretinoin

- **Tretinoin** (topical vitamin A acid) increases cell turnover in the follicular wall and decreases cohesiveness of cells, leading to extrusion of comedones and inhibition of the formation of new comedones. It also decreases the number of cell layers in the stratum corneum from 14 to 5. A "flare" of acne may suddenly appear after 3–6 weeks of treatment, followed by clinical clearing in 8–12 weeks.
- Side effects include irritation, erythema, peeling, allergic contact dermatitis, and increased sensitivity to sun exposure, wind, cold, and other irritants.
- Irritation may be managed by titrating strength and frequency of application. Treatment can be initiated with 0.025% cream for mild acne in people with sensitive and nonoily skin, 0.01% gel for moderate acne in easily irritated skin with oily complexions, and 0.025% gel for moderate acne with nonsensitive and oily skin.
- **Retin-A Micro** (microsphere vehicle of porous beads) and **Avita** (liquid polymer vehicle) are new formulations that are less irritating than products with standard vehicles.
- Concomitant use of an antibacterial agent with tretinoin can decrease keratinization, inhibit *P. acnes,* and decrease inflammation. A combination of benzoyl peroxide each morning and tretinoin at bedtime may enhance efficacy and be less irritating than either agent used alone.

Adapalene

- **Adapalene** is a retinoid with potent anti-inflammatory and comedolytic properties. The 0.1% gel can be used as an alternative to tretinoin 0.025% gel in patients with mild to moderate acne, with better patient tolerability.
- Exposure to sunlight should be limited. It is not recommended during pregnancy or lactation.

Tazarotene

- **Tazarotene** is a synthetic acetylenic retinoid that is converted to tazarotenic acid following topical application. It binds to retinoic acid receptors and can alter expression of genes involved in cell proliferation, differentiation, and inflammation.
- The 0.1% gel is slightly more effective than the 0.05% gel. III
- Side effects include erythema, pruritus, stinging, and burning.

SYSTEMIC THERAPY

Oral Antibacterial Agents

- Oral antibiotics are effective and relatively safe for inflammatory types of acne.
- **Tetracycline** (and derivatives), **erythromycin, clindamycin,** and **trimethoprim–sulfamethoxazole** decrease the percentage of free fatty acids in skin surface lipids and also decrease numbers of *P. acnes.* Tetracycline also reduces the amount of keratin in sebaceous follicles and inhibits chemotaxis, phagocytosis, complement activation, and cell-mediated immunity. **Minocycline** and **doxycycline** have enhanced penetration into tissue and sebaceous follicles compared to tetracycline.
- Drawbacks to use of tetracycline include drug-food interactions with dairy products, photosensitivity, gastrointestinal disturbances, and predisposition to superinfections (e.g., vaginal candidiasis). Disadvantages of minocycline include vestibular toxicity, drug-induced lupus, and discoloration of skin and teeth.
- Side effects of clindamycin include diarrhea and risk for pseudomembranous colitis.
- Trimethoprim–sulfamethoxazole should perhaps be reserved for refractory cases to minimize the risk of resistance.
- **Ampicillin** and tetracycline apparently decrease the intestinal flora needed to hydrolyze conjugated ethinyl estradiol excreted into bile, thus enterohepatic recirculation is interrupted and the amount of active estrogen is reduced. Women taking oral contraceptives given ampicillin or tetracycline should be informed of the potential for contraceptive failure.

Oral Contraceptives

- The combination of **norgestimate** and **ethinyl estradiol** has been shown to increase sex hormone-binding globulin (SHBG), causing a decrease in unbound, biologically active androgens.
- **Ortho Tri-Cyclen** is approved for antiacne therapy. Oral contraceptives containing 0.035 mg of ethinyl estradiol along with a triphasic dose of norgestimate can be an effective treatment alternative for moderate acne in women.

Isotretinoin

- **Isotretinoin** is indicated for patients with severe recalcitrant comedonal acne unresponsive to conventional therapies. A recent survey found that most dermatologists recommend that oral isotretinoin be considered for patients with moderate or mild acne who respond with less than 50% improvement after 6 months of conventional therapies.

- It decreases sebum production, changes sebum composition, inhibits *P. acnes,* inhibits inflammation, and alters patterns of keratinization within follicles.
- After 16 weeks of therapy, it produced a >70% success rate and a remission of >20 months.
- Adverse effects are often dose-related and include dry lips (90% of patients), dryness and desquamation of the face (30%), hypertriglyceridemia (25%), conjunctivitis and eye irritation, muscle and joint pain, skeletal hyperostosis, increased creatinine phosphokinase, increased blood glucose, photosensitivity, pseudotumor cerebri, excess granulation tissue, and a high incidence of teratogenicity.
- Dosing guidelines range from 0.5 to 1.0 mg/kg/d, while the cumulative dose taken by patients during a treatment course may be the major factor influencing long-term outcome. Best results are usually attained with cumulative doses of 120 to 150 mg/kg.

▶ EVALUATION OF THERAPEUTIC OUTCOMES

- Information regarding pathogenic factors and the importance of medication compliance should be conveyed to patients.
- Patients should understand that effectiveness of any therapeutic regimen may require 6–8 weeks and that they may also notice an exacerbation of acne after initial therapy.

See Chapter 88, Acne and Psoriasis, authored by Nina H. Han, PharmD, Phillip A. Nowakowski, PharmD, and Dennis P. West, PhD, FCCP, for a more detailed discussion of this topic.

Chapter 16

▶ PSORIASIS

▶ DEFINITION

Psoriasis is a common chronic disease characterized by recurrent exacerbations and remissions of thickened, erythematous, and scaling lesions.

▶ PATHOPHYSIOLOGY

- The cause of psoriasis is unknown. Possible etiologies are shown in Table 16–1.
- Psoriatic epidermal cells proliferate at a rate sevenfold faster than normal epidermal cells. Duration of the cell cycle is 37.5 hours, versus 300 hours in normal skin.
- Psoriatic skin shows evidence of increased metabolic activity and increased cGMP, DNA, RNA, IgG, and C3. Arachidonic acid levels are 30 times normal, and prostaglandin E_2 levels are 50% higher than normal.
- Climate, stress, infection, trauma, and drugs may aggravate psoriasis. Warm seasons and sunlight improved psoriasis in 80% of patients, whereas 90% of patients worsen in cold weather. Infection (e.g., streptococcal, upper respiratory) may be a precipitating factor. Injury (e.g., rubbing, venipuncture, bites, surgery) to normal appearing skin may precipitate psoriasis (Koebner response). Lithium carbonate and β-adrenergic blocking agents exacerbate psoriasis.

▶ CLINICAL PRESENTATION

- Lesions are characterized by sharply demarcated, erythematous papules and plaques often covered with silver-white fine scales. Lesions start small and enlarge over time.
- Scalp psoriasis ranges from diffuse scaling on an erythematous scalp to thickened plaques with exudation, microabscesses, and fissures. Trunk, back, arm, and leg lesions may be generalized, scattered, discrete, drop-like lesions or large plaques. Palms, soles, face, and genitalia may be involved, as well. Usually pustular psoriasis affects the palms and soles symmetrically. Affected nails are often pitted and associated with subungual keratotic material.
- Psoriatic arthritis is a distinct clinical entity in which both psoriatic lesions and inflammatory arthritis occur.

▶ DIAGNOSIS

- The diagnosis is made based on history and physical exam, which reveals characteristic lesions as described previously. Patients assessment is summarized in Table 16–2.

TABLE 16–1. Possible Etiologic Factors of Psoriasis

Possible Etiologic Factors of Psoriasis
Defects in epidermal cell cycle
Disruption in arachidonic acid metabolism
Genetics
III Exogenous trigger factors
Climate
Stress
Infection
Trauma
Drugs
Immunologic mechanisms

▶ DESIRED OUTCOME

The goal of therapy is to achieve complete clearing of lesions, but partial clearing using regimens with decreased toxicity and increased patient acceptability is acceptable in some cases.

▶ TREATMENT

- Drug treatments are listed in Table 16–3, and treatment guidelines are shown in Tables 16–4 and 16–5.

TOPICAL PHARMACOLOGIC THERAPY

Emollients and Keratolytics

- Emollients hydrate the stratum corneum and minimize water evaporation. They may enhance desquamation, eliminate scaling, and decrease itching.
- Moisturizers often need to be applied three times daily.
- Side effects of moisturizers include folliculitis and allergic contact dermatitis.

TABLE 16–2. Psoriatic Patient Assessment

Psoriatic Patient Assessment
Onset and duration of psoriasis
Family history
Exacerbating factors
Previous history of antipsoriasis agents with efficacy and side effect data
All current and recent topical and systemic medications
Environmental and occupational exposure to chemicals and toxins
Allergies (food, drug, environmental)

TABLE 16–3. Examples of Drug Treatments for Psoriasis

Topical	Systemic
Emollients and keratolytics	Ultraviolet-A and oral psoralens (systemic PUVA)
Coal tar	Methotrexate
Anthralin	Retinoids
Calcipotriene	Sulfasalazine
Acitretin	Cyclosporine
Tazarotene	Tacrolimus
Mycophenolate mofetil	
Methotrexate	
UVA and topical psoralens (topical PUVA)	

- Keratolytics are used to remove scales and decrease hyperkeratosis. **Salicylic acid** is the most frequently used agent, usually used in 2–10% strengths. Lower concentrations have a keratin-dispersing effect, whereas concentrations of 5% or higher have a corneolytic (exfoliative) action.
- Side effects of salicylic acid include local irritation and salicylism with nausea, vomiting, tinnitus, or hyperventilation.

Coal Tar

- **Coal tar** contains multiple hydrocarbon compounds formed by distillation of bituminous coal.
- Ultraviolet B (UVB) light-activated coal tar photoadducts with epidermal DNA, and inhibits DNA synthesis, leading to reduction in plaque elevation.
- Disadvantages include unpleasant odor, staining of skin and clothing, ability to reversibly darken or alter light hair colors, and ability to tarnish silver jewelry.
- It may be applied directly to skin and may also be used in bath water and as a shampoo.
- Although many of its polynuclear aromatic hydrocarbons are known carcinogens, no increase in cancer risk has been identified. However, there are cases indicating a higher rate of cutaneous carcinoma in patients exposed to coal tar and UV light.

Topical Corticosteroids

- They halt synthesis and mitosis of DNA in epidermal cells and appear to inhibit phospholipase A, lowering the amounts of arachidonic acid, prostaglandins, and leukotrienes in the skin and reducing erythema and pruritus. As antipsoriatic agents, they are best used adjunctively with a product that specifically functions to normalize epidermal hyperproliferation.
- Low-potency products have a modest anti-inflammatory effect and are safest for long-term application, for application on the face and inter-

TABLE 16–4. Topical Psoriasis Treatment Guidelines

Active Ingredient	Formulation	Strength	Regimen	Potential Side Effects
Emollients	Lotions, creams, ointments	N/A	Three to four times daily	Folliculitis, contact dermatitis
Salicylic acid (keratolytic)	Gels, lotions	2–10%	Two to three times daily	Can be irritating Has resulted in salicylism
Coal tar	Creams, gels, lotions, ointments, solutions	1–48.5%	Apply in evening, allowing to remain through the night	Messy and burdensome Can be irritating Photoreactions
Anthralin	Creams, ointments	0.1–1%	Usually in the evening, allowing to remain through the night. Short contact regimens have also been used	Stains skin and clothing Can be irritating
Calcipotriene	Ointment, solution, cream	0.005%	Apply twice daily, no more than 100 g/wk, for up to 8 days	Burning and stinging in 10% of patients
Corticosteroids	Creams, lotions, ointments, solutions	Variable potency	Two to four times daily for maintenance; may use occlusion at night	Local tissue atrophy, striae, epidermal thinning, glucocorticoid systemic effects
Methoxsalen	Lotion	1%	Apply to area prior to UVA therapy	Photoreaction, exaggerated burning

TABLE 16–5. Oral Psoriasis Treatment Guidelines

Active Ingredient	Formulation	Strength	Regimen	Potential Side Effects
Sulfasalazine	Suspension, tablets	250 mg/5 mL, 500 mg	3–4 g/d	Gastrointestinal upset
Methoxsalen	Capsules	10 mg	Dosed on body weight 2 hours before UVA exposure	Burns, erythema, gastrointestinal upset, CNS effects, ocular damage
Methotrexate	Tablets, injection	2.5 mg; 20–25 mg/mL	2.5–5 mg every 12 hours for three doses every week	Anemia, leukopenia, thrombocytopenia, gastrointestinal upset
Acitretin	Capsules	10 mg, 25 mg	25–50 mg daily	Dry mouth and lips, eye irritation, arthralgia, monitor liver function tests
Cyclosporine	Capsules, solution	25 mg, 100 mg; 100 mg/mL	3–4 mg/kg/d in two divided doses; may increase to 5 mg/kg/d in one month if no response	Nephrotoxicity, gastrointestinal upset, hypertension, tremor, monitor liver function tests
Tacrolimus	Capsules	1 mg, 5 mg	0.15 mg/kg twice daily; titrate based on side effects	Nephrotoxicity, gastrointestinal upset

triginous areas, for use with occlusion, and in infants and young children.

- Medium-potency products are used in moderate inflammatory dermatoses (e.g., chronic eczematous dermatoses).
- High-potency preparations are used for more severe inflammatory der-
III matoses. They may be used for an intermediate duration, or for longer periods on thickened skin. They may also be used on the face and intertriginous areas, but only for a short treatment duration.
- Very high potency products are used for short durations and on small surface areas. Occlusive dressings should not be used with these products. There is a high likelihood of skin atrophy with the use of very high potency preparations.
- Ointments are considered the most clinically effective preparation for psoriasis. They are not suited for use in areas such as the axilla, groin, or other intertriginous areas where maceration and folliculitis may develop secondary to the occlusive effect. Creams are often preferred by patients and may be used in intertriginous areas.
- For severe acute forms of psoriasis, a patient may be instructed to apply a high-potency topical steroid every 2 hours for 24–48 hours, followed by application three to four times daily. For maintenance application two to four times daily is adequate.
- Adverse effects include tissue atrophy, degeneration, and striae. If detected early, these effects may be reversible with discontinuation. Thinning of epidermis and purpura may occur. Acneform eruptions and masking of symptoms of bacterial or fungal skin infections have been reported. Systemic side effects include risk of suppression of the hypothalamic–pituitary–adrenal axis, hyperglycemia, and development of cushinoid features. Tachyphylaxis and rebound psoriasis after abrupt cessation of topical corticosteroid therapy can also occur.

Anthralin

- **Anthralin** appears to inhibit DNA synthesis by intercalation between DNA strands. It may also decrease epidermal proliferation by mitochondrial inhibition.
- Irritation, inflammation, and staining of skin and clothing are common.
- Application for 20 minutes has been found effective with decreased side effects. Titrating the strength of anthralin slowly from 0.1–0.25% to a concentration of 0.5–1% may minimize irritation. It should be applied only to affected areas of skin.

Calcipotriene

- **Calcipotriene** is a synthetic vitamin D analogue. It inhibits cell proliferation and induction of cell differentiation.
- Improvement usually requires 2 weeks of treatment, and approximately 70% of patients demonstrate marked improvement after 8 weeks. Maintenance therapy may be required.
- Side effects include burning, stinging, dry skin, peeling, rash, and worsening of psoriasis. Hypercalcemia is rare.

Tazarotene

- **Tazarotene** is a synthetic retinoid that is hydrolyzed to its active metabolite, tazarotenic acid, which has affinity for retinoic acid receptors.
- It affects abnormal differentiation, hyperproliferation of the keratinocyte, and inflammation.
- The 0.05% and 0.1% gels applied once daily are effective for mild to moderate plaque-type psoriasis. Application of the gel to eczematous skin or to more than 20% of body surface area is not recommended. The 0.1% gel is somewhat more efficacious, but the 0.05% gel causes less irritation.
- Adverse effects are dose- and frequency-related and include pruritus, burning, stinging, and erythema.

SYSTEMIC PHARMACOLOGIC THERAPY

Acitretin

- **Acitretin** is an aromatic retinoid. Acitretin plus UVB combination treatment is a possible therapeutic regimen in severe psoriasis.
- The initial recommended dose is 25 or 50 mg; therapy is continued until lesions have resolved.
- Side effects include dry lips, mouth, eyes, and nose; dry skin; pruritus; scaling; hair loss; hepatotoxicity; skeletal changes; hypercholesterolemia; and hypertriglyceridemia.
- It is a teratogen and contraindicated in females who are pregnant or who plan pregnancy within 3 years following drug discontinuation.

Cyclosporine

- **Cyclosporine** inhibits an early step in T-cell activation, and also has anti-inflammatory activity.
- Adverse effects are renal dysfunction, hypertension, paresthesias, hypertrichosis, gingival hyperplasia, and gastrointestinal disorders.
- Intralesional cyclosporine has been clinically effective; a topical preparation can serve as monotherapy or as a dose-sparing modality in conjunction with systemically administered cyclosporine.

Tacrolimus

- **Tacrolimus,** an immunosuppressant, has been found effective in treatment of recalcitrant plaque-type psoriasis.
- Doses of 0.05 mg/kg/d (increased up to 0.15 mg/kg/d as needed) are efficacious.
- Adverse effects include diarrhea, paresthesias, insomnia, and renal insufficiency.

Sulfasalazine

- Oral **sulfasalazine** (3–4 g/d for 8 weeks) has been reported to be effective for plaque-type psoriasis in some patients. When used alone, it is not as effective as **methotrexate, psoralens** plus ultraviolet A (UVA) light, or **etretinate,** but it has a lowered incidence of severe side effects.

COMBINATION THERAPY

Systemic Therapy-Photochemotherapy: Oral and Topical Psoralen and Long-wave Ultraviolet A Light

- Use of **psoralens** with UVA **(PUVA)** controls psoriasis in nearly 90% of patients.
- Psoralens react with nucleic acids and intercalate between base pairs. When DNA is irradiated with long-wave ultraviolet light (320–400 nm, UVA) the psoralens covalently bind to pyrimidine bases, forming a cross-link.
- Candidates for PUVA therapy usually have severe incapacitating psoriasis unresponsive to topical therapies without history of photosensitivity, skin cancers, cataracts, or x-ray of the skin. **Methoxsalen (8-methoxypsoralen or 8-MOP)** is usually dosed at 0.6–0.8 mg/kg and is given 2 hours before exposure to UVA. Dosing of UVA is determined by skin type and history of previous response to UV radiation.
- **Trioxsalen** baths and UV light are also beneficial for psoriasis.

▶ EVALUATION OF THERAPEUTIC OUTCOMES

- Monitoring for disease resolution and side effects is critical to successful therapy. Positive response to therapy is noted as normalization of involved areas of skin as measured by reduced erythema and scaling as well as flattening of plaques.
- Patients should understand the general concepts of therapy, and the importance of compliance should be emphasized.
- Achievement of efficacy by any therapeutic regimen requires days to weeks. Initial dramatic response may be achieved with some agents such as corticosteroids; however, sustained benefit with pharmacologically specific antipsoriatic therapy usually requires about 2–4 weeks for noticeable response.

See Chapter 88, Acne and Psoriasis, authored by Nina H. Han, PharmD, Phillip A. Nowakowski, PharmD, and Dennis P. West, PhD, FCCP, for a more detailed discussion of this topic.

Endocrinologic Disorders

Edited by Terry L. Schwinghammer, PharmD, FCCP, BCPS

Chapter 17

▶ DIABETES MELLITUS

▶ DEFINITION

The term diabetes mellitus describes a series of complex and chronic metabolic disorders characterized by symptomatic glucose intolerance. All diabetics eventually show abnormalities of insulin secretion and complications of the disease, such as vascular and neurologic abnormalities; most manifest some degree of cellular resistance to insulin in type 2 diabetes mellitus.

▶ PATHOPHYSIOLOGY

DIABETES CLASSIFICATION

- In 1997, the American Diabetes Association Expert Committee on the Diagnosis and Classification of Diabetes Mellitus recommended use of the terms type 1 and type 2 to simply the labels for the primary forms of diabetes.
  - Type 1 diabetes (previously termed insulin dependent or juvenile-onset diabetes) is primarily due to pancreatic islet β-cell destruction, usually leading to absolute insulin deficiency. These patients are prone to developing diabetic ketoacidosis (DKA) if insulin is withheld. This form results from an autoimmune process, but environmental factors such as infectious, chemical, and dietary agents may be contributing factors in the expression of the disease.
  - Type 2 diabetes (previously termed non-insulin dependent or adult-onset diabtetes) is the more prevalent form and results from insulin resistance with a relative (rather than absolute) defect in the secretion of insulin.
- Smaller etiologic categories include secondary diabetes, impaired glucose tolerance (IGT), impaired fasting glucose (IFG), and gestational diabetes mellitus (GDM).

CARBOHYDRATE METABOLISM

- Carbohydrates are metabolized in the body to glucose, which is absorbed from the gastrointestinal (GI) tract into the bloodstream and oxidized in skeletal muscle to produce energy. Glucose is also stored in the liver in the form of glycogen and is converted in adipose tissue to fats and triglycerides.
- Insulin is produced and stored in the ß cells of the pancreas; its release increases uptake of glucose by the tissues, increases liver glycogen lev-

els, decreases glycogen breakdown (glycogenolysis) by the liver, increases synthesis of fatty acids, decreases breakdown of fatty acids into ketone bodies, and promotes incorporation of amino acids into proteins.

- Glucose can diffuse into the brain without the aid of insulin, but muscle and fat require the presence of insulin to receive glucose for energy. If glucose is not available or cannot enter muscle and adipose tissue, these tissues convert amino acids and fatty acids to carbohydrates (gluconeogenesis). If deprivation continues, the tissue will eventually metabolize stored fats, resulting in the production of free fatty acids that are eventually oxidized to ketone bodies.
- Plasma glucose concentrations are usually maintained between 40 and 160 mg/dL. Symptoms of hypoglycemia are usually present at concentrations <40 mg/dL. Plasma concentrations in excess of 180 mg/dL usually exceed the renal tubular maximal threshold for reabsorption, and glucose spills into the urine.
- Counterregulatory hormones that increase blood glucose levels include glucagon, growth hormone, epinephrine, glucocorticoids, and thyroid hormone; somatostatin reduces blood glucose levels because it suppresses glucagon secretion and inhibits absorption of glucose from the GI tract.
- Macrovascular complications of diabetes include coronary heart disease, stroke, and peripheral vascular disease. Microvascular complications include nephropathy, retinopathy, and neuropathy.

▶ CLINICAL PRESENTATION

TYPE 1 DIABETES

- The classic symptoms of diabetes include polyuria, polydipsia, and polyphagia (increased appetite with increased calorie intake).
- Osmotic diuresis from urinary glucose produces polyuria, which can lead to dehydration with accompanying polydipsia.
- Because glucose cannot be adequately transported into cells, the hunger sensation is triggered, resulting in polyphagia.
- Other common symptoms in type 1 patients include weight loss, weakness, and dry skin. The onset of these symptoms is rapid, and secondary ketoacidosis is common.

TYPE 2 DIABETES

- Type 2 diabetes presents gradually and may be present without symptoms.
- Because obesity is common, weight changes and/or polyphagia may be absent or go unnoticed.
- Polyuria and fatigue may be presenting complaints, but most type 2 diabetics are discovered because of an abnormal blood or urine glucose on routine physical examination or screening.

DIABETIC KETOACIDOSIS (DKA)

- Patients in DKA often present with:
  - Lethargy (from hyperglycemia, hyperosmolality, ketonemia, and acidosis).
  - Hyperventilation with possible Kussmaul's respirations (from compensatory respiratory alkalosis).
  - Fruity odor to the breath (from acetonemia).
  - Changes in mental status (from hyperosmolality).
  - Nausea and vomiting (from metabolic acidosis). IV
  - Abdominal pain (from gastric distention).
  - Thirst and polyuria (from osmotic diuresis) or decreased urine output [from progressive DKA causing decreased glomerular filtration rate (GFR)].
  - Dry mucous membranes and poor skin turgor (from dehydration).
  - Tachycardia.

► DIAGNOSIS

- All persons over the age of 45 should be tested for diabetes with subsequent screening every 3 years if blood glucose is normal. Persons at risk for developing diabetes (e.g., those with a diabetic family member) should be tested at younger ages.
- Pregnant women do not need to be screened for gestational diabetes if they meet the following criteria: <25 years old, normal body weight, no family history of diabetes, *and* not a member of an ethnic group with a high incidence of diabetes.
- The 1997 revised diagnostic criteria for diabetes mellitus are contained in Table 17–1.
- Impaired fasting glucose (IFG) is defined as FPG ≥110 mg/dL but <126 mg/dL.

TABLE 17–1. Criteria for the Diagnosis of Diabetes Mellitus

Diabetes can be diagnosed by any of three ways, confirmed on a different day by any one of the following three methods:

1. Symptoms of diabetes plus a casual plasma glucose concentration ≥160 mg/dL. Casual is defined as any time of day without regard to time since last meal. The classic symptoms of diabetes include polyuria, polydipsia, and unexplained weight loss.
2. Fasting plasma glucose (FPG) ≥126 mg/dL. Fasting is defined as no caloric intake for at least 8 hours.
3. Oral glucose tolerance test (OGTT) with the two-hour postload value ≥200 mg/dL. The test should be performed as described by the World Health Organization, using a glucose load containing the equivalent of 75-g anhydrous glucose dissolved in water.

The FPG is the preferred test because it is simple, convenient, widely available, acceptable to patients, and inexpensive compared to the OGTT.

- Impaired glucose tolerance (IGT) is diagnosed when the 2-hour post-load sample of the oral glucose tolerance test (OGTT) is ≥140 mg/dL but <200 mg/dL.
- Diagnosis of DKA is established by testing for the presence of signs and symptoms and one or more of the following: (1) urine ketones, (2) serum ketones, (3) lowered serum bicarbonate level, and (4) lowered arterial pH. Patients usually have an increased anion gap. More than three-fourths of patients exhibit an increased serum amylase, but its cause and significance are unclear.

▶ DESIRED OUTCOME

The goals of diabetes treatment are to maintain the blood glucose level in an acceptable range throughout the day to prevent symptoms of hyperglycemia, prevent the long-term microvascular and neurologic complications of the disease, and minimize the likelihood of hypoglycemia. Desirable plasma glucose and glycosylated hemoglobin (HbA_{1c}) levels are listed in Table 17–2.

▶ TREATMENT

GENERAL PRINCIPLES

- Patient education about the causes, symptoms, complications, and treatment of diabetes is essential for proper management.
- A diet plan for type 1 patients should be based on healthy daily nutrition to allow flexibility in insulin therapy and home monitoring. Dietary therapy for type 2 patients should be directed toward achieving blood glucose, lipid, and blood pressure goals and weight loss, if appropriate. About 10–20% of total daily calories should come from protein, which is the same recommendation as for the general population. Less than 10% of the total daily caloric intake should come from saturated fats, and up to 10% from polyunsaturated fats, leaving 60–70% of the total calories from carbohydrates and monounsaturated fats.
- Appropriate physical activity should be recommended (unless contraindicated) to improve insulin sensitivity and possibly improve glu-

TABLE 17–2. Goals of Therapy

Parameter	Normal	Acceptable	Fair	Poor
Fasting plasma glucose (mg/dL)	< 110	< 140	< 200	> 200
Postprandial plasma glucose (mg/dL)	< 140	< 175	< 235	> 235
Glycosylated hemoglobin[a] (%)	< 6	< 8	8–9.5	> 10

[a]Increase limits 10% for elderly patients.

cose tolerance. Exercise can also help promote weight loss and maintain ideal body weight when combined with restricted caloric intake.

ORAL AGENTS

- Oral agents are indicated for type 2 diabetics who have failed to control blood glucose adequately despite weight loss, proper diet, and exercise. A treatment algorithm for implementing therapy of type 2 diabetes is shown in Figure 17–1.

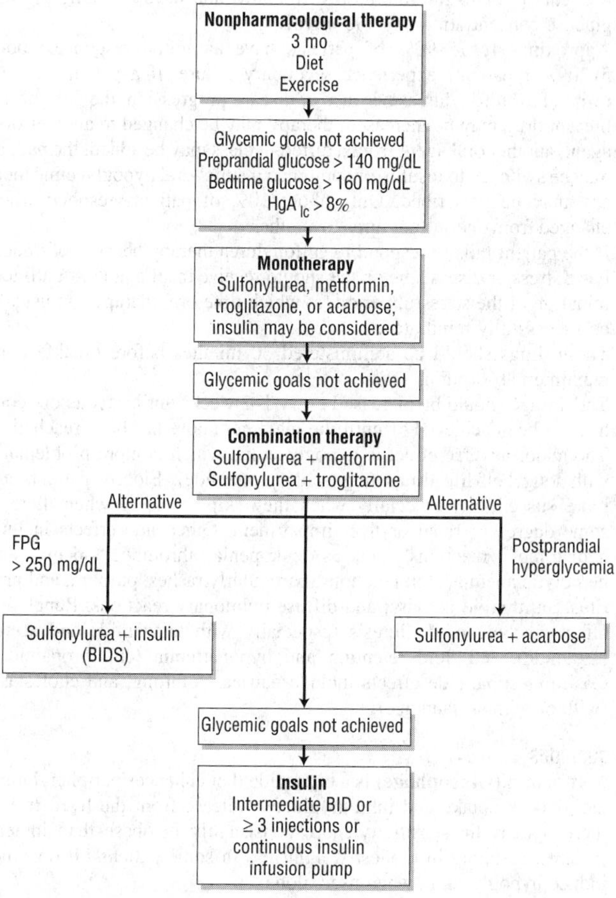

IV 

Nonpharmacological therapy
3 mo
Diet
Exercise

↓

Glycemic goals not achieved
Preprandial glucose > 140 mg/dL
Bedtime glucose > 160 mg/dL
HgA$_{1c}$ > 8%

↓

Monotherapy
Sulfonylurea, metformin, troglitazone, or acarbose; insulin may be considered

↓

Glycemic goals not achieved

↓

Combination therapy
Sulfonylurea + metformin
Sulfonylurea + troglitazone

Alternative: FPG > 250 mg/dL → Sulfonylurea + insulin (BIDS)

Alternative: Postprandial hyperglycemia → Sulfonylurea + acarbose

↓

Glycemic goals not achieved

↓

Insulin
Intermediate BID or
≥ 3 injections or
continuous insulin infusion pump

Figure 17–1. Treatment algorithm for type 2 diabetes mellitus.

Sulfonylureas (Table 17–3)

- Sulfonylureas initially increase ß-cell insulin secretion; later extrapancreatic effects may include reducing the rate of hepatic glucose production, increasing insulin receptor sensitivity and/or number, and potentiation of postreceptor insulin effects.
- There are few therapeutic differences among these agents; except for hypoglycemia, the second-generation oral hypoglycemics appear to produce fewer side effects than do the older drugs.
- The best candidates for sulfonylurea therapy are patients who are at least 40 years of age at the onset of the disease, have been diabetic for <5 years prior to the initiation of therapy, and have a fasting plasma glucose concentration of <300 mg/dL.
- Approximately 75–90% of patients have an initial response; about 5–20% of patients experience secondary failure. If a patient fails to respond to sulfonylureas because of disease progression, the dose of the present drug may be increased, therapy may be changed to another oral agent, another oral agent from a different class may be added, the patient may be switched to insulin, or combined insulin–oral hypoglycemic therapy may be prescribed. Only about 10% of patients respond when changed from one sulfonylurea to another.
- If the patient fails to respond to sulfonylurea therapy because of underlying stress or disease, he or she should receive insulin at least until termination of the stressful period, at which time oral therapy can usually be successfully reinitiated.
- These drugs should be administered 30 minutes before breakfast for maximum absorption.
- The dosage should be increased every 1–2 weeks until satisfactory control has been achieved or until the maximum dose has been reached.
- The major adverse effect is hypoglycemia, which is more problematic with long half-life drugs (e.g., chlorpropamide). Elderly patients are more susceptible, especially when they skip meals or when there is some degree of renal or liver impairment. Other side effects include hematologic reactions such as leukopenia, thrombocytopenia, and hemolytic anemia; skin reactions, particularly rashes, purpura, and pruritus; antithyroid activity; and diffuse pulmonary reactions. Renal side effects include mild diuresis (especially with tolazamide and acetohexamide), and fluid retention and hyponatremia (chlorpropamide). Gastrointestinal side effects include nausea, vomiting, and cholestasis (with or without jaundice).

Biguanides

- **Metformin (Glucophage)** is a biguanide that enhances peripheral muscle glucose uptake and inhibits glucose release from the liver. It also increases insulin sensitivity more consistently in obese than in lean patients, resulting in modest weight loss in some patients. It does not induce hypoglycemia when used alone.

- Metformin is as effective as a sulfonylurea in controlling blood glucose levels.
- The most frequent side effects are gastrointestinal (diarrhea up to 30%). Lactic acidosis occurs rarely, and is more likely in patients with renal disease (SCr >1.5 mg/dL for males, >1.4 mg/dL for females), liver disease, history of alcohol abuse, acute/chronic metabolic acidosis, and patients with conditions that predispose them to renal insufficiency or hypoxia.
- Patients undergoing radiographic dye studies are advised to stop metformin for 2 days prior to the study since hyperosmolar contrast dyes cause dehydration and predispose patients to metformin accumulation secondary to renal insufficiency.

α-Glucosidase Inhibitors

- **Acarbose (Precose)** inhibits the enzyme α-glucosidase in the brush border of the intestine that facilitates absorption of starch and disaccharides such as sucrose. This decreases the absorption rate of carbohydrate, slowing or lowering the peak postprandial blood glucose concentration without causing hypoglycemia.
- Studies have demonstrated a decrease in postprandial blood glucose with some improvement of HbA_{1c} but less than that observed with sulfonylureas or metformin.
- Acarbose is indicated for monotherapy or in combination with insulin, a sulfonylurea, or metformin.
- The usual recommended dose is 50–100 mg with each large meal; the dose should be gradually increased to minimize side effects.
- The most common side effects are flatulence, diarrhea, and abdominal cramps. When used in combination with a hypoglycemic agent (sulfonylurea or insulin), patients must be taught the importance of treating hypoglycemia with glucose- (dextrose-) based products because acarbose will block absorption of more complex disaccharide sugars (e.g., sucrose).
- **Miglitol (Glyset)** is another agent in this class. The recommended starting dose is 25 mg with the first bite of each main meal.

Thiazolidinediones

- **Troglitazone (Rezulin)** decreases gluconeogenesis, increases glucose uptake and utilization in skeletal muscle, and increases glucose uptake and decreases fatty acid output in adipose tissue. It decreases insulin resistance and lowers fasting plasma glucose and HbA_{1c} concentrations. It does not affect insulin secretion.
- The drug is FDA-approved for use in type 2 patients currently taking insulin but inadequately controlled (HbA_{1c} >8.5% and insulin >30 units/d in multiple injections). It is also indicated for use as monotherapy or in combination with a sulfonylurea.
- The initial dose is 200 mg once daily with a meal; the dose may be increased to 400 mg once daily after 2–4 weeks.

TABLE 17–3. Oral Agents for Diabetes

Generic (Trade)	Onset (h)	Half-Life (h)	Duration (h)	Recommended Starting Dose		Maximum Dose per Day	Metabolism/ Elimination
				Nonelderly	Elderly		
Sulfonylureas							
Tolbutamide (Orinase)	1	5.6	6–12	1–2 g/d	500 mg/d to 500 mg twice daily	2–3 g	Metabolized in liver to inactive metabolites that are excreted renally
Acetohexamide (Dymelor)	1	5	10–14	250 mg–1.5 g/d	125–250 mg/d	1.5 g	Metabolized in liver; metabolite's potency is equal to or greater than that of parent compound; renally eliminated
Tolazamide (Tolinase)	4–6	7	10–14	100–250 mg/d	100 mg/d	750 mg–1 g	Metabolized in liver; metabolite less active than parent compound; renally eliminated
Chlorpropamide (Diabinese)	1	35	72	250 mg/d	100 mg/d	500 mg	Metabolized in liver; also excreted unchanged in the urine
Glyburide (DiaBeta, Micronase)	1.5	2–4	18–24	2.5 mg/d	1.25–2.5 mg/d	20 mg	Metabolized in liver; 50% of metabolites eliminated in urine, 50% in feces

TABLE 17–3. continued

Generic (Trade) Name	Onset (h)	Half-Life (h)	Duration (h)	Recommended Starting Dose		Maximum Dose per Day	Metabolism/ Elimination
				Nonelderly	Elderly		
Glyburide, micronized (Glynase)	1.5	2–4	18–24	1.5 mg	1.5–3 mg	12 mg	Metabolized in liver; 50% metabolites eliminated urine, 50% in feces
Glipizide (Glucotrol, Glucotrol XL)	1	3–7	10–24	5 mg/d	2.5–5 mg/d	40 mg	Metabolized in liver to inactive metabolites; renally eliminated
Glimepiride (Amaryl)	2	4–6	18–28	1–2 mg/d	0.5–1 mg/d	8 mg	Metabolized in liver to inactive metabolities
Biguanides Metformin (Glucophage)	1.5	1.5–4.9	16–20	500 mg	500–1000 mg	2550 mg	Urinary excretion
α-Glucosidase Inhibitors Acarbose (Precose)	0.5	1–2	4	25 mg/d	25 mg/d	300 mg/d	Nonabsorbed, excreted in feces
Thiazolidinediones Troglitazone (Rezulin)	1–2	4–6	16–24	200 mg with food	200 mg with food	600 mg	Metabolized in liver

- For patients not responding to the usual dose of 400 mg after 1 month, the dose may be increased to 600 mg. If patients do not respond adequately to 600 mg after 1 month, the drug should be discontinued and alternative treatment options pursued.
- Hepatic dysfunction, characterized as idiosyncratic hepatocellular damage, has been reported rarely with troglitazone. The reaction is more common in the first year of therapy. Liver function tests (alanine aminotransferase, ALT) should be performed before therapy and monthly for the first 8 months of therapy, every 2 months for the remainder of the first year, and periodically thereafter. Therapy should not be started in patients with ALT levels >1.5 times the upper limit of normal. Treatment should be stopped if the ALT rises above 3 times the upper limit of normal.
- Troglitazone does not induce hypoglycemia when used alone.
- The drug is substantially more expensive than sulfonylureas.

Meglitinides

- **Repaglinide (Prandin)** is a nonsulfonylurea moiety of glyburide. It closes ATP-dependent potassium channels in the β-cell membrane and increases intracellular calcium, resulting in increased insulin secretion. It is indicated as monotherapy or as combination therapy with metformin.
- It has a short duration of action and must be taken immediately (usually within 15 minutes) before eating. Patients who skip or add a meal should skip (or add) a dose for that meal. The starting dose is 0.5 mg prior to each meal for patients not previously treated with blood glucose-lowering agents or whose HbA_{1c} is <8%. For patients previously treated and whose HbA_{1c} is ≥8%, the initial dose is 1 or 2 mg before each meal.
- The response should be assessed (usually by fasting blood glucose) after at least 1 week of therapy, and the preprandial dose may be doubled at weekly intervals up to 4 mg until satisfactory response is achieved. The maximum daily dose is 16 mg. The drug has an adverse effect profile that is generally comparable to that of sulfonylurea drugs.

Oral Hypoglycemic Combinations

- The combination of a sulfonylurea and metformin, troglitazone, or acarbose may lower blood glucose by a greater amount than one of the agents alone.
- Oral agents and insulin have also been used in combination. When a sulfonylurea is combined with insulin, the insulin is initially given at bedtime and the sulfonylurea in the mornings (BIDS—bedtime insulin, daytime sulfonylurea). The sulfonylurea increases insulin secretion while the bedtime insulin suppresses hepatic glucose production. Patients poorly controlled on this regimen may require multiple insulin injections throughout the day.

INSULINS

- Table 17–4 compares the onset, peak, and duration of various insulin preparations. **Lispro** is an insulin analog that has more rapid absorption and can be administered immediately before meals, thereby allowing more flexibility in dosing. It may also cause fewer severe hypoglycemic episodes than unmodified regular insulin.
- **Regular insulin** is a solution and can be administered by the intravenous (IV), intramuscular (IM), or subcutaneous (SC) route. Insulin lispro is a solution intended for SC administration. All other types of insulin are suspensions and can be administered subcutaneously only. IV
- **NPH** and **Lente insulins** differ in their ability to be mixed with other types of insulin. NPH and regular insulins can be combined in the same syringe and refrigerated for up to 21 days without changes in potency. Lente insulin has an excess of zinc that binds with regular insulin and delays its absorption. The interaction also produces more Lente insulin, possibly causing hypoglycemia when the absorption of Lente reaches its peak. Because the interaction occurs within 15 minutes after mixing and lasts for 24 hours, patients should be instructed either to inject the mixture immediately or to consistently wait 24 hours before administration.

TABLE 17–4. Onset, Peak, and Duration of Various Insulin Preparations by Species

Type of Insulin	Onset (h)	Peak (h)	Effective Duration (h)
Animal			
Short acting			
Regular	0.5–2	3–4	6–8
Intermediate acting			
NPH	4–6	8–14	16–20
Lente	4–6	8–14	16–20
Long acting			
Ultralente	8–14	Minimal	24–36
Human			
Rapid acting			
Lispro	0.25	0.5–1.5	2–4
Short acting			
Regular	0.5–1	2–3	4–6
Intermediate acting			
NPH	2–4	4–10	10–16
Lente	3–4	4–12	12–18
Long acting			
Ultralente	6–10	Minimal	20–24

- NPH insulin should not be combined with Lente insulins. Human NPH and human regular preparations can be mixed with no adverse consequences.
- Type 2 patients can be started on a single injection of 15–20 U/d of an intermediate-acting (NPH or Lente) insulin with dosage adjustments made according to plasma glucose levels. Patients receiving insulin for the first time should be started on human insulin.
- Since many type 1 and type 2 patients do not exhibit 24-hour control on a single daily injection, twice daily injections of NPH and regular insulin are often used. The first injection contains two-thirds of the total daily dose (NPH-to-regular ratio of 2:1) and is given 30 minutes before breakfast. The second injection (NPH-to-regular ratio of 1:1) is given 30 minutes before the evening meal. Premixed NPH/regular insulins are available in a ratio of 70:30.
- If regular insulin only is used, the patient's total daily insulin requirement is divided into four equal doses, each given 30 minutes before meals and at bedtime (given with a snack).
- Continuous subcutaneous insulin infusion (CSII) by pump is administered continuously and as bolus doses before meals. Because of a high incidence of complications, pump use should be restricted to patients who are knowledgeable, stable, and well motivated.
- Guidelines for dose adjustments based on clinical response are given in Table 17–5.

TREATMENT OF HYPOGLYCEMIA

- In a conscious patient, immediate treatment involves the administration of food, preferably sugar. Eight Lifesavers, 4–6 ounces of a sugar-containing soft drink, a piece of fruit, one-half cup fruit juice, 2–3 glucose tablets (5 g each), a tube of glucose gel, or 1 cup skim milk usually reverses the symptoms in 10–20 minutes.
- In an unconscious patient, 1 mg of **glucagon** injected subcutaneously should provide relief within 10–15 minutes. Patients who weigh less than 20 kg should receive 0.5 mg. Common side effects are nausea and vomiting. Once the patient regains consciousness, oral liquids containing sugar should be administered. In a hospitalized hypoglycemic patient, 50 mL of $D_{50}W$ provides rapid reversal of symptoms.

TREATMENT OF DKA

- Therapy should be targeted toward correcting dehydration, reducing the plasma glucose concentration to normal, reversing the acidosis and ketosis, replenishing electrolyte and volume losses, and identifying the underlying cause.
- Normal saline should be administered at a rate of 1 L/h for 2–3 hours. After the patient's heart rate, rhythm, and blood pressure have normalized, IV fluids can be changed to 0.45% sodium chloride.

TABLE 17–5. Adjusting Insulin Dosages Based on Clinical Response

Problem	Time Problem Experienced	Possible Solutions
Hyperglycemia	Fasting	If the patient is receiving a single dose of an intermediate-acting insulin, split into 2 doses: ⅔ of total dose before breakfast, ⅓ of dose before supper. If the patient is receiving split-dose intermediate insulin, increase presupper dose or move present dose to a later time in the evening.
	Midmorning	Add regular insulin to morning dose.
	Midafternoon	Increase morning NPH or Lente dose, **OR** add regular insulin at lunch time.
	Bedtime	Add regular insulin with presupper dose if not currently receiving, **OR** increase regular insulin at presupper dose.
	Early morning (2:00–3:00 AM)	Consider pronounced dawn effect. Give the presupper dose later in the evening.
Hypoglycemia	Fasting	Decrease evening insulin dose, but first check timing of AM test and dose.
	Midmorning	Decrease or omit prebreakfast dose of regular insulin.
	Midafternoon	Decrease morning NPH or Lente dose. Be sure patient is withdrawing correct dosage into syringe in the correct order if he or she is receiving more than one type of insulin.
	Bedtime	Instruct patient to eat a bedtime snack and/or check dose of afternoon NPH/Lente dose. Decrease presupper dose of regular insulin. Decrease presupper dose of intermediate-acting insulin if it is being administered earlier in the afternoon.
	Early morning (2:00–3:00 AM)	Consider Somogyi effect. Decrease the evening dose of intermediate-acting insulin.

If more than one monitoring time throughout the day is abnormal, try to adjust only one insulin dose at a time. Adequately titrating more than one dose adjustment and gauging the effects is quite difficult and often creates more adjustment problems.

IV

- Low-dose IV regular insulin may be initiated with a bolus of 0.1 U/kg before starting a continuous infusion (e.g., dilute 100 units of regular insulin in 100 mL of 0.9% sodium chloride and infuse at an initial rate of 0.1 U/kg/h.) Plasma glucose determinations should be made hourly. If there has been less than a 10% drop in 2 hours, then the insulin drip rate should be doubled.

- When the plasma glucose concentration declines to approximately 250 mg/dL, the primary IV fluid should be changed from 0.45% sodium chloride to 5% dextrose in 0.45% sodium chloride and the insulin infusion rate should be cut in half to avoid hyperchloremic acidosis and to prevent hypoglycemia.
- The end point of insulin therapy is not euglycemia but correction of acidosis and ketonemia. The insulin infusion should be continued until the acidosis has been corrected (arterial pH >7.30, plasma glucose concentration <250 mg/dL, anion gap 13–17, serum bicarbonate >15 mEq/L, no ketonemia).

- Electrolytes depleted from osmotic diuresis and acidosis should be replaced as quickly as possible. Sodium is generally replaced by administering 2–4 L of normal saline during the initial management of DKA. Potassium can be replaced by adding 40–60 mEq to each liter of IV fluid and administering it at a rate of 10–20 mEq/h.
- Phosphate replacement should be instituted if the serum level approaches the lower end of the normal range.
- Bicarbonate is generally administered only to patients whose arterial pH is below 7.0 or when the serum bicarbonate is very low (<5 mEq/L). When indicated, bicarbonate should be administered via infusion of 50 mEq (or 1 mEq/kg) over 1 hour. The goal of therapy is to raise the arterial pH to 7.10–7.15.

TREATMENT OF NEUROPATHY

- Symptoms may begin as tingling, or burning sensations, particularly in the distal tissues with a definite loss in vibratory sensation. The patient may eventually lose all sensation in a particular area, becoming unable to detect hot, cold, or pain. Circulation is usually impaired to these areas because of diabetes-related vascular changes.
- Narcotic analgesics and nonsteroidal anti-inflammatory drugs (NSAIDs) may provide some relief for painful neuropathy.
- Anticonvulsants (phenytoin and carbamazepine) should be reserved for severe cases that have been resistant to other treatments.
- Psychotropic drugs, such as tricyclic antidepressants, trazodone, fluoxetine, and phenothiazines, have mixed favorable responses but seem to provide greater pain relief than anticonvulsants. Doses for the treatment of painful neuropathies should be low initially and titrated to effect.
- Neurogenic bladder, with loss of autonomic mediated urinary continence, may benefit from treatment with bethanechol and/or anticholinergics.
- Symptoms of gastroparesis (nausea, vomiting, abdominal distension) may be reduced with prokinetic agents (metoclopramide or cisapride).
- Treatment for diabetic diarrhea has included anticholinergic agents, dietary change, antibiotics, bulk and bile salt resins, kaolin/pectin, and diphenoxylate/atropine. Octreotide has shown some promise in this disorder.

TREATMENT OF RETINOPATHY

- Nonproliferative retinopathy can be treated with laser photocoagulation therapy that may help to arrest progression and decrease the loss of vision associated with macular edema.
- Because hypertension and smoking lead to more rapid progression of ocular damage, it is very important to halt or to eliminate these risk factors.
- Aldose reductase inhibitors are investigational agents that have not yet been proven to be beneficial in progressive retinopathy. IV

TREATMENT OF NEPHROPATHY

- Microalbuminuria (urinary albumin excretion of 30–300 mg/d) is a harbinger of diabetic nephropathy; aggressive management of hypertension and microalbuminuria delays progression of nephropathy. Patients should be screened yearly for microalbuminuria, and ACE inhibitor therapy should be initiated if it is present. ACE inhibitors should be given to all type 1 diabetics with microalbuminuria even if normotensive. Many clinicians would also use ACE inhibitors in normotensive type 2 diabetics, although there is less evidence of a positive effect. Preliminary studies suggest that angiotensin-receptor antagonists may be beneficial in patients unable to tolerate ACE inhibitors.
- ACE inhibitors are most useful during the early stages of diabetic nephropathy. When an ACE inhibitor is started, the patient may have a transient rise in serum creatinine, which usually returns to baseline within a few days. Caution must be advised, however, when using these agents in severe renal disease, since ACE inhibitors can worsen or cause renal impairment.

▶ EVALUATION OF THERAPEUTIC OUTCOMES

- Blood glucose determination is the standard for diabetes monitoring. Most patients use whole-blood glucose determinations as a means of monitoring diabetic control in the ambulatory setting. In the laboratory, serum or plasma is utilized. Chemically impregnated strips or hand-held electronic glucose monitoring machines that use strips are available that can monitor whole-blood glucose from several drops of blood obtained by a fingerstick. The goals of therapy are included in Table 17–2.
- The HbA_{1c} is useful for monitoring long-term control of diabetes (see Table 17–2). Bringing the blood glucose under control for 4–6 weeks will result in a fall in the percentage of HbA_{1c}. However, a patient must have experienced hyperglycemia for 1–4 weeks before the HbA_{1c} concentration rises substantially.
- Urine glucose testing is the least expensive monitoring device but has several limitations. Urine testing may lack correlation between urine and blood glucose values. The tests are technique dependent, and the

patient must read the results at the appropriate time. Urine ketone determination (e.g., Ketostix) is commonly recommended to patients with type 1 diabetes or who are ketosis prone.

- For monitoring therapy of DKA, plasma or whole-blood glucose concentrations should be monitored hourly until they have stabilized below 250 mg/dL. Electrolytes, especially potassium, should be monitored every hour until stabilized within the normal range, then every 2–4 hours until the acidosis has been corrected. Heart rhythm should be monitored, especially in comatose patients.

IV

See Chapter 70, Diabetes Mellitus, authored by Condit F. Steil, PharmD, CDE, for a more detailed discussion of this topic.

Chapter 18

▶ THYROID DISORDERS

▶ DEFINITION

Thyroid disorders encompass a variety of disease states affecting thyroid hormone production or secretion that result in alterations in metabolic stability. Hyperthyroidism and hypothyroidism are defined as the clinical and biochemical syndromes resulting from increased and decreased thyroid hormone production, respectively.

▶ THYROID HORMONE PHYSIOLOGY

- The thyroid hormones thyroxine (T_4) and triiodothyronine (T_3) are formed on thyroglobulin, a large glycoprotein synthesized within the thyroid cell. Inorganic iodide enters the thyroid follicular cell and is oxidized by thyroid peroxidase and is covalently bound (organified) to tyrosine residues of thyroglobulin.
- The iodinated tyrosine residues monoiodotyrosine (MIT) and diiodotyrosine (DIT) combine (couple) to form iodothyronines in reactions catalyzed by thyroid peroxidase. Thus, DIT and DIT combine to form T_4, while MIT and DIT form T_3.
- Thyroid hormone is liberated into the bloodstream by the process of proteolysis within thyroid cells. T_4 and T_3 are transported in the bloodstream by three proteins: thyroid-binding globulin (TBG), thyroid-binding prealbumin (TBPA), and albumin. Only the unbound (free) thyroid hormone is able to diffuse into the cell, elicit a biologic effect, and regulate thyroid-stimulating hormone (TSH) secretion from the pituitary.
- T_4 is secreted solely from the thyroid gland, but <20% of T_3 is produced there; the majority of T_3 is formed from the breakdown of T_4 catalyzed by the enzyme 5′-monodeiodinase found in peripheral tissues. T_3 is about five times more active than T_4.
- T_4 may also be acted on by the enzyme 5′-monodeiodinase to form reverse T_3, which has no significant biologic activity.
- Thyroid hormone production is regulated by TSH secreted by the anterior pituitary, which in turn is under negative feedback control by the level of free thyroid hormone and the positive influence of hypothalamic thyrotropin-releasing hormone (TRH). Thyroid hormone production is also regulated by extrathyroidal deiodination of T_4 to T_3, which can be affected by nutrition, nonthyroidal hormones, drugs, and illness.

▶ THYROTOXICOSIS (HYPERTHYROIDISM)

PATHOPHYSIOLOGY

- Thyrotoxicosis results when tissues are exposed to excessive levels of T_4, T_3, or both. In Graves' disease, hyperthyroidism results from the action of thyroid-stimulating antibodies (TSAb) directed against the thyrotropin receptor on the surface of the thyroid cell. These immunoglobulin G (IgG) antibodies bind to the receptor and activate the enzyme adenylate cyclase in the same manner as TSH.

CLINICAL PRESENTATION

- Symptoms include nervousness, emotional lability, easy fatigability, heat intolerance, loss of weight concurrent with an increased appetite, increased frequency of bowel movements, palpitations, proximal muscle weakness (noted on climbing stairs or arising from a sitting position), and scanty or irregular menses in women.
- Physical signs may include warm, smooth, moist skin and unusually fine hair; separation of the end of the fingernails from the nail beds (onycholysis); retraction of the eyelids and lagging of the upper lid behind the globe upon downward gaze (lid lag); tachycardia at rest, a widened pulse pressure, and a systolic ejection murmur; occasional gynecomastia in men; a fine tremor of the protruded tongue and outstretched hands; and hyperactive deep tendon reflexes.
- Graves' disease is manifested by hyperthyroidism, diffuse thyroid enlargement, and the extrathyroidal findings of exophthalmos, pretibial myxedema, and thyroid acropachy. The thyroid gland is usually diffusely enlarged, with a smooth surface and consistency varying from soft to firm. In severe disease, a thrill may be felt and a systolic bruit may be heard over the gland.
- In painful subacute (viral, or DeQuervain's) thyroiditis, patients complain of severe pain in the thyroid region, which often extends to the ear on the affected side. Low-grade fever is common, and systemic signs and symptoms of thyrotoxicosis are present. The thyroid gland is firm and exquisitely tender on physical examination.
- Painless (silent, lymphocytic, postpartum) thyroiditis has a triphasic course that mimics that of painful thyroiditis. Most patients present with mild thyrotoxic symptoms; lid retraction and lid lag are present but exophthalmos is absent. The thyroid gland may be diffusely enlarged but thyroid tenderness is absent.
- Thyroid storm is a life-threatening medical emergency characterized by severe thyrotoxicosis, high fever (often >103°F), tachycardia, tachypnea, dehydration, delirium, coma, nausea, vomiting, and diarrhea. Precipitating factors include infection, trauma, surgery, radioactive iodine treatment, and withdrawal from antithyroid drugs.

DIAGNOSIS

- An elevated 24-hour radioactive iodine uptake (RAIU) indicates *true hyperthyroidism,* i.e., the patient's thyroid gland is actively overproducing T_4, T_3, or both (normal RAIU 10–30%).
  - TSH-induced hyperthyroidism is diagnosed by evidence of peripheral hypermetabolism, diffuse thyroid gland enlargement, elevated

  free thyroid hormone levels, and elevated serum immunoreactive TSH concentrations. Because the pituitary gland is extremely sensitive to even minimal elevations of free T_4, a detectable TSH level in any thyrotoxic patient indicates the inappropriate production of TSH.
  - TSH-secreting pituitary adenomas are diagnosed by demonstrating lack of response to TRH stimulation, elevated TSH α-subunit levels, and radiologic imaging.
  - An autonomous thyroid nodule (toxic adenoma) usually occurs with larger nodules (i.e., those more than 4 cm in diameter). If the T_4 level is normal, a T_3 level is measured to rule out T_3 toxicosis. Once a radioiodine scan has demonstrated that the toxic thyroid adenoma would collect more radioiodine than the surrounding tissue, independent function is documented by a failure of the autonomous nodule to decrease its iodine uptake during exogenous T_3 administration.
  - In multinodular goiters, a thyroid scan will show patchy areas of autonomously functioning thyroid tissue.
- A low RAIU indicates the excess thyroid hormone is not a consequence of thyroid gland hyperfunction. This may be seen in subacute thyroiditis, painless thyroiditis, struma ovarii, follicular cancer, and factitious ingestion of exogenous thyroid hormone.
- In thyrotoxic Graves' disease, there is an increase in the overall hormone production rate with a disproportionate increase in T_3 relative to T_4 (Table 18–1). Saturation of TBG is increased owing to the elevated levels of serum T_4 and T_3, which is reflected in an elevated T_3 resin uptake. As a result, the concentrations of free T_4, free T_3, and the free T_4 and T_3 indices are increased to an even greater extent than are the measured serum total T_4 and T_3 concentrations. The TSH level is undetectable owing to negative feedback by elevated levels of thyroid hormone at the pituitary. The diagnosis of thyrotoxicosis is confirmed by measurement of the serum T_4 concentration, T_3 resin uptake (or free T_4), and TSH. An increased 24-hour RAIU (obtained in nonpregnant

TABLE 18–1. Thyroid Function Test Results in Different Thyroid Conditions

	Total T_4	Free T_4	Total T_3	T_3 Resin Uptake	Free Thyroxine Index	TSH
Normal	4.5–12.5 μg/dL	0.8–1.5 ng/dL	80–220 ng/dL	22–34%	1.0–4.3 U	0.2–4.8 μIU/mL
Hyperthyroid	↑↑	↑↑	↑↑↑	↑	↑↑↑	↓↓
Hypothyroid	↓↓	↓↓	↓	↓↓	↓↓↓	↑↑
Increased TBG	↑	Normal	↑	↓	Normal	Normal

TSH, thyroid-stimulating hormone; TBG, thyroid-binding globulin.

individuals) documents that the thyroid gland is inappropriately utilizing the iodine to produce more thyroid hormone at a time when the patient is thyrotoxic.

- In subacute thyroiditis, thyroid function tests typically run a triphasic course in this self-limited disease. Initially, serum thyroxine levels are elevated due to release of preformed thyroid hormone from disrupted follicles. The 24-hour RAIU during this time is <2% owing to thyroid inflammation and TSH suppression by the elevated thyroxine level. As the disease progresses, intrathyroidal hormone stores are depleted, and the patient may become mildly hypothyroid with an appropriately elevated TSH level. During the recovery phase, thyroid hormone stores are replenished and serum TSH elevation gradually returns to normal.

DESIRED OUTCOME

The therapeutic objectives for hyperthyroidism are to normalize the production of thyroid hormone; minimize the symptoms and long-term consequences of the disorder; and provide individualized therapy based on the type and severity of disease, patient age and gender, existence of nonthyroidal conditions, and response to previous therapy.

TREATMENT

Antithyroid Medications (Table 18–2)

Thiourea Drugs

- The thioureas **propylthiouracil (PTU)** and **methimazole** block thyroid hormone synthesis by inhibiting the peroxidase enzyme system of the thyroid gland, thus preventing oxidation of trapped iodide and subsequent incorporation into iodotyrosines and ultimately iodothyronine ("organification"), and by inhibiting coupling of monoiodotyrosine and diiodotyrosine to form T_4 and T_3. PTU (but not methimazole) also inhibits the peripheral conversion of T_4 to T_3.
- The thioureas are the preferred treatment for children and pregnant women. The increased risk of hypothyroidism following RAI or surgery makes thioureas a reasonable treatment alternative in young adults.
- Usual initial doses include PTU 300–600 mg daily (usually in 4 divided doses) or methimazole 30–60 mg/d (usually in 3 divided doses). Some evidence suggest single daily doses of either drug may be effective.
- Improvement in symptoms and laboratory abnormalities should ensue within 4–8 weeks, at which time a tapering regimen to maintenance doses can be started. Dosage changes should be made on a monthly basis, since the endogenously produced T_4 will reach a new steady-state concentration in this interval. Typical daily maintenance doses are PTU 50–300 mg and methimazole 5–30 mg.
- If clinical improvement is not observed, consider noncompliance, insufficient dosage to block hormone synthesis, and inadequate dosing interval if a single daily dose has been used.

TABLE 18–2. Management of Hyperthyroidism

Modality	Maintenance Dose (mg/d)	Maximum Dose (mg/d)	Indications
Thiourea drugs			First-line therapy for Graves' hyperthyroidism, short-term therapy before ^{131}I or surgery
Propylthiouracil (PTU), 50-mg tablets	200–600	1200	
Methimazole (Tapazole), 5- and 10-mg tablets	10–60	120	
β-Adrenergic antagonists[a]			Adjunctive therapy; often required for thyroiditis
Propranolol	80–160	480	
Nadolol	80–160	320	
Iodine-containing compounds			Preparation for surgery; thyrotoxic crisis
Lugol's solution	750	750	
Potassium iodide (SSKI)	10–300	400	
Miscellaneous			
Potassium perchlorate	NA	NA	No routine indications
Lithium carbonate	NA	NA	No routine indications
Glucocorticoids			Severe subacute thyroiditis; thyrotoxic crisis
Radioactive iodine (RAI, ^{131}I)	NA	5–29 mCi	First-line therapy for Graves' hyperthyroidism; treatment of choice for recurrent thyrotoxicosis; young adults to elderly; contraindicated in pregnancy, children, and active ophthalmopathy
Surgery	NA	NA	Patients should be euthyroid prior to surgery; caution in elderly; cold iodine given prior to surgery

SSKI, saturated solution of potassium iodide; NA, not applicable.
[a]Not approved in the United States by the FDA for the treatment of thyrotoxicosis.

IV

- Antithyroid drug therapy should continue for 12–24 months to induce a long-term remission. The presence of TSAb is predictive for relapse.
- Patients should be monitored every 6–12 months after remission. If a relapse occurs, alternate therapy with RAI is preferred to a second course of antithyroid drugs, as subsequent courses of therapy are less likely to induce remission.
- Minor adverse reactions include pruritic maculopapular rashes, arthralgias, fever, and a benign transient leukopenia (WBC <4000/mm^3). The alternate thiourea may be tried in these situations, but cross-sensitivity occurs in about 50% of patients.

- Major adverse effects include agranulocytosis (with fever, malaise, gingivitis, oropharyngeal infection, and a granulocyte count <250/mm^3), aplastic anemia, a lupus-like syndrome, polymyositis, gastrointestinal intolerance, hepatotoxicity, and hypoprothrombinemia. Agranulocytosis, if it occurs, almost always develops in the first 3 months of therapy; routine monitoring is not recommended because of its sudden onset. Patients who have experienced a *major* adverse reaction to one thiourea drug should not be converted to the alternate drug because of cross-sensitivity.

Iodides

- Iodide acutely blocks thyroid hormone release, inhibits thyroid hormone biosynthesis by interfering with intrathyroidal iodide utilization, and decreases the size and vascularity of the gland.
- Symptom improvement occurs within 2–7 days of initiating therapy, and serum T_4 and T_3 concentrations may be reduced for a few weeks.
- Iodides are often used as adjunctive therapy to prepare a patient with Graves' disease for surgery, to acutely inhibit thyroid hormone release and quickly attain the euthyroid state in severely thyrotoxic patients with cardiac decompensation, or to inhibit thyroid hormone release following radioactive iodine therapy.
- **Potassium iodide** is available as a saturated solution (**SSKI,** 38 mg iodide per drop), or as **Lugol's solution,** containing 6.3 mg of iodide per drop (Table 18–2).
- The typical starting dose of SSKI is 3–10 drops daily (120–400 mg) in water or juice. When used to prepare a patient for surgery, it should be administered 7–14 days preoperatively.
- As an adjunct to radioactive iodine (RAI), SSKI should not be used before, but rather 3–7 days after RAI treatment so that the radioactive iodide can concentrate in the thyroid.
- Adverse effects include hypersensitivity reactions (skin rashes, drug fever, rhinitis, conjunctivitis); salivary gland swelling; "iodism" (metallic taste, burning mouth and throat, sore teeth and gums, symptoms of a head cold, and sometimes stomach upset and diarrhea); and gynecomastia.

Adrenergic Blockers

- β blockers (especially **propranolol**) have been used widely to ameliorate thyrotoxic symptoms such as palpitations, anxiety, tremor, and heat intolerance. They have no effect on peripheral thyrotoxicosis and protein metabolism and do not reduce TSAb or prevent thyroid storm. Propranolol and **nadolol** partially block the conversion of T_4 to T_3 but this contribution to the overall therapeutic effect is small.
- β blockers are usually used as adjunctive therapy with antithyroid drugs, RAI, or iodides when treating Graves' disease or toxic nodules; in preparation for surgery; or in thyroid storm. β blockers are primary therapy only for thyroiditis and iodine-induced hyperthyroidism.

- Propranolol doses required to relieve adrenergic symptoms are variable but an initial dose of 20–40 mg four times daily is effective (heart rate <90 beats/min) for most patients.
- β blockers are contraindicated in patients with heart failure unless it is due solely to tachycardia (high output) and in patients who have developed cardiomyopathy and heart failure. Other side effects include nausea, vomiting, anxiety, insomnia, lightheadedness, bradycardia, and hematologic disturbances.
- Centrally acting sympatholytics (e.g., **clonidine**) and calcium channel antagonists (e.g., **diltiazem**) may be useful for symptom control when contraindications to β blockade exist. IV

Radioactive Iodine (RAI)

- **Sodium iodide 131 (^{131}I)** is an oral liquid that concentrates in the thyroid and initially disrupts hormone synthesis by incorporating into thyroid hormones and thyroglobulin. Over a period of weeks, follicles that have taken up RAI and surrounding follicles develop evidence of cellular necrosis and fibrosis of the interstitial tissue.
- RAI is the agent of choice for Graves' disease, toxic autonomous nodules, and toxic multinodular goiters. It is also the preferred treatment for debilitated, cardiac, and elderly patients and patients who have had a failure or toxic reaction on drug therapy. RAI is also used in patients who relapse after surgery. Pregnancy is an absolute contraindication to the use of RAI.
- β blockers are the primary adjunctive therapy to RAI, since they may be given anytime without compromising RAI therapy.
- In patients whose symptoms are not controlled with β blockers alone, symptomatic control with adjunctive thioureas to attain a euthyroid state up until 1 week prior to RAI is warranted because of the slow onset of effect with RAI. Patients with cardiac disease and elderly patients are often treated with thioureas prior to RAI ablation because thyroid hormone levels will transiently increase following RAI treatment, owing to release of performed thyroid hormone.
- Thioureas should not routinely be administered after RAI, because their use is associated with a higher incidence of early post-treatment recurrence or persistence of hyperthyroidism.
- If iodides are administered, they should be given 3–7 days *after* RAI to prevent interference with the uptake of RAI in the thyroid gland.
- The goal of therapy is to destroy overactive thyroid cells, and a single dose of 4000–8000 rads results in a euthyroid state in 60% of patients at 6 months or less. A second dose of RAI should be given 6 months after the first RAI treatment if the patient remains hyperthyroid.
- Hypothyroidism commonly occurs months to years following RAI. The acute, short-term side effects include mild thyroidal tenderness and dysphagia. Long-term follow-up has not revealed an increased risk for development of thyroid carcinoma, leukemia, or congenital defects.

Surgery

- Surgical removal of the thyroid gland is the treatment of choice for coexisting cold nodules, extremely large goiters (over 80 g), and patients with contraindications to thioureas (i.e., allergy or adverse effects) and RAI (i.e., pregnancy).
- If thyroidectomy is planned, PTU or methimazole is usually given until the patient is biochemically euthyroid (usually 6–8 weeks), followed by the addition of iodides (500 mg/d) for 10–14 days before surgery to decrease the vascularity of the gland. Levothyroxine may be added to maintain the euthyroid state while the thioureas are continued.
- Propranolol has been used for several weeks preoperatively and 7–10 days after surgery to maintain a heart rate <90 beats/min. Combined pretreatment with propranolol and 10–14 days of potassium iodide also has been advocated.
- Complications of surgery include persistent or recurrent hyperthyroidism (up to 18%), hypothyroidism (up to about 49%), hypoparathyroidism (up to 4%), and vocal cord abnormalities (up to 5%). The frequent occurrence of hypothyroidism requires periodic follow-up for identification and treatment.

Treatment of Thyroid Storm

- The following therapeutic measures should be instituted promptly: suppression of thyroid hormone formation and secretion, antiadrenergic therapy, administration of corticosteroids, and treatment of associated complications or coexisting factors that may have precipitated the storm (Table 18–3).

TABLE 18–3. Drug Dosages Used in the Management of Thyroid Storm

Drug	Regimen
Propylthiouracil	900–1200 mg/d PO in four or six divided doses
Methimazole	90–120 mg/d PO in four or six divided doses
Sodium iodide	Up to 2 g/d IV in single or divided doses
Lugol's solution	5–10 drops PO tid in water or juice
Saturated solution of potassium iodide	1–2 drops PO tid in water or juice
Esmolol	50–150 μg/kg/min IV
Propranolol	40–80 mg PO every 6 h
Dexamethasone	5–20 mg/d PO or IV in divided doses
Prednisone	25–100 mg/d PO in divided doses
Methylprednisolone	20–80 mg/d IV in divided doses
Hydrocortisone	100–400 mg/d IV in divided doses

- PTU in large doses is the preferred thiourea because it interferes with the production of thyroid hormones and blocks the peripheral conversion of T_4 to T_3.
- Iodides, which rapidly block the release of preformed thyroid hormone, should be administered *after* PTU is initiated to inhibit iodide use by the overactive gland.
- General supportive measures, including acetaminophen as an antipyretic (aspirin or other nonsteroidal anti-inflammatory drugs [NSAIDs] may displace bound thyroid hormone), fluid and electrolyte replacement, sedatives, digitalis, antiarrhythmics, insulin, and antibiotics should be given as indicated. Plasmapheresis and peritoneal dialysis have been used to remove excess hormone when the patient has not responded to more conservative measures.

EVALUATION OF THERAPEUTIC OUTCOMES

- After therapy (thioureas, RAI, or surgery) for hyperthyroidism has been initiated, patients should be evaluated on a monthly basis until they reach a euthyroid condition.
- Clinical signs of continuing thyrotoxicosis or the development of hypothyroidism should be noted.
- If hypothyroidism develops after RAI treatment or surgery, thyroxine replacement may be given. The goal is to maintain both the free thyroxine level and the TSH concentration in the normal range. Once a stable dose of thyroxine is identified, the patient may be followed every 6–12 months.

▶ HYPOTHYROIDISM

PATHOPHYSIOLOGY

- The vast majority of hypothyroid patients have thyroid gland failure (primary hypothyroidism). Causes include chronic autoimmune thyroiditis (Hashimoto's disease), iatrogenic hypothyroidism, iodine deficiency, enzyme defects, thyroid hypoplasia, and goitrogens.
- Pituitary failure (secondary hypothyroidism) is an uncommon cause resulting from pituitary tumors, surgical therapy, external pituitary radiation, postpartum pituitary necrosis, metastatic tumors, tuberculosis, histiocytosis, and autoimmune mechanisms.

CLINICAL PRESENTATION

- Adult manifestations of hypothyroidism include dry skin, cold intolerance, weight gain, constipation, weakness, lethargy, fatigue, loss of ambition or energy, depression, and slowed and hoarse speech. In children, thyroid hormone deficiency may manifest as growth retardation.
- Physical signs include coarse skin and hair, cold skin, periorbital puffiness, bradycardia, muscle cramps, myalgia, and stiffness. Reversible

neurologic syndromes such as carpal tunnel syndrome, polyneuropathy, and cerebellar dysfunction may also occur. Objective weakness (with proximal muscles being affected more than distal muscles) and slow relaxation of deep tendon reflexes are common.
- Most patients with pituitary failure (secondary hypothyroidism) have clinical signs of generalized pituitary insufficiency such as abnormal menses and decreased libido, or evidence of a pituitary adenoma such as visual field defects, galactorrhea, or acromegaloid features.

- Myxedema coma is the end stage of long-standing uncorrected hypothyroidism and is manifested by hypothermia, advanced stages of hypothyroid symptoms, and altered sensorium ranging from delirium to coma. Untreated disease is associated with a high mortality rate.

DIAGNOSIS

- A rise in the TSH level is the first evidence of primary hypothyroidism. Many patients have a T_4 level within the normal range (compensated hypothyroidism) and few, if any, symptoms of hypothyroidism. As the disease progresses, the T_4 concentration drops below the normal level. The T_3 concentration is often maintained in the normal range despite a low T_4. The RAIU is not a useful test in the evaluation of a hypothyroid patient.
- Pituitary failure (secondary hypothyroidism) should be suspected in a patient with decreased levels of thyroxine and inappropriately normal or low TSH levels.

DESIRED OUTCOME

The treatment goals for hypothyroidism are to normalize thyroid hormone concentrations in tissue, provide symptomatic relief, prevent neurologic deficits in newborns and children, and reverse the biochemical abnormalities of hypothyroidism.

TREATMENT OF HYPOTHYROIDISM

- **Levothyroxine** (L-thyroxine) is the drug of choice for thyroid hormone replacement and suppressive therapy, because it is chemically stable, relatively inexpensive, free of antigenicity, and has uniform potency; however, any of the commercially available thyroid preparations can be used (Table 18–4).
- Although T_3 (and not T_4) is the biologically active form, levothyroxine administration results in a pool of thyroid hormone that is readily and consistently converted to T_3.
- Cholestyramine, sucralfate, aluminum hydroxide, ferrous sulfate, soybean formula, and dietary fiber supplements may impair the absorption of levothyroxine from the gastrointestinal tract. Drugs that increase nondeiodinative T_4 clearance include rifampin, carbamazepine, and possibly phenytoin. Amiodarone may block the conversion of T_4 to T_3.

TABLE 18–4. Thyroid Preparations Used in the Treatment of Hypothyroidism

Drug/Dosage Form	Content	Relative Dose
Thyroid, USP Armour Thyroid, ¼-, ½-, 1-, 1½-, 2-, 3-, 4-, and 5-grain tablets	Desiccated beef or pork thyroid gland	1 grain (equivalent to 60 μg of T_4)
Thyroglobulin Proloid, ½-, 1-,1½-, 2-, and 3-grain tablets	Partially purified pork thyroglobulin	1 grain
Levothyroxine Synthroid, Levothroid, 25-, 50-, 75-, 88-, 100-, 112-, 125-, 137-,150-, 175-, 200-, and 300-μg tablets; 200 and 500 μg/vial injection	Synthetic T_4	50–60 μg
Liothyronine Cytomel, 5-, 25-, and 50-μg tablets	Synthetic T_3	15–37.5 μg
Liotrix Euthyroid, Thyrolar, ¼-, ½-, 1-, 2-, and 3-strength tablets	Synthetic T_4:T_3 in 4:1 ratio	50–60 μg T_4 and 12.5–15 μg T_3

IV

- Substitution of generic levothyroxine preparations should be undertaken with caution, as products may not be bioequivalent.
- The average maintenance dose for most adults is about 110–120 μg/d, but there is a wide range of replacement doses, necessitating individualized therapy and appropriate monitoring to determine an appropriate dose.
- Young patients with long-standing disease and patients over age 45 without known cardiac disease can be started on 50 μg daily of levothyroxine and increased to 100 μg daily after 1 month.
- The recommended initial daily dose for older patients or those with known cardiac disease is 25 μg/d titrated upward in increments of 25 μg at monthly intervals to prevent stress on the cardiovascular system.
- Patients with subclinical hypothyroidism and marked elevations in TSH (>10 μIU/mL) and high titers of TSAb or prior treatment with ^{131}I may benefit from treatment with levothyroxine of 50–75 μg per day.
- Serum TSH concentration is the most sensitive and specific monitoring parameter for adjustment of levothyroxine dose. Concentrations begin to fall within hours and are usually normalized within 2 to 6 weeks. An elevated TSH level indicates insufficient replacement.
- TSH and T_4 concentrations should both be checked monthly until a euthyroid state is achieved. Serum T_4 concentrations can be useful in detecting noncompliance, malabsorption, or changes in levothyroxine product bioequivalence. TSH may also be used to check for noncompliance.

- In patients with hypothyroidism caused by hypothalamic or pituitary failure, alleviation of the clinical syndrome and restoration of serum T_4 to the normal range are the only criteria available for estimating the appropriate replacement dose of levothyroxine.
- TSH suppressive levothyroxine therapy may also be given to patients with nodular thyroid disease and diffuse goiter, to patients with a history of thyroid irradiation, and to patients with thyroid cancer.
- **Thyroid USP** (or desiccated thyroid) has unpredictable hormonal stability. Inexpensive generic brands may not be bioequivalent.

- **Thyroglobulin** is standardized biologically to give a T_4:T_3 ratio of 2.5:1. It is more expensive than thyroid extract and has no clinical advantages.
- **Liothyronine** (synthetic T_3) has uniform potency but has a higher incidence of cardiac adverse effects, higher cost, and difficulty in monitoring with conventional laboratory tests. Response is monitored with TSH assays.
- **Liotrix** (T_4:T_3 in a 4:1 ratio) is chemically stable, pure, and has a predictable potency but is expensive. It lacks therapeutic rationale because about 35% of T_4 is converted to T_3 peripherally.
- Excessive doses of thyroid hormone may lead to heart failure, angina pectoris, and myocardial infarction. Allergic or idiosyncratic reactions can occur with the natural animal-derived products such as desiccated thyroid and thyroglobulin but they are extremely rare with the synthetic products used today. Excess exogenous thyroid hormone may reduce bone density and increase the risk of fracture.

TREATMENT OF MYXEDEMA COMA

- Immediate and aggressive therapy with IV bolus thyroxine 300–500 μg is needed to prevent mortality.
- Glucocorticoid therapy with IV hydrocortisone 100 mg every 8 hours should be given until coexisting adrenal suppression is ruled out.
- Consciousness, lowered TSH concentrations, and normal vital signs are expected within 24 hours.
- Maintenance doses of thyroxine are typically 75–100 μg IV until the patient stabilizes and oral therapy is begun.
- Supportive therapy must be instituted to maintain adequate ventilation, euglycemia, blood pressure, and body temperature. Underlying disorders such as sepsis and myocardial infarction must be diagnosed and treated.

EVALUATION OF THERAPEUTIC OUTCOMES

- Patients with uncomplicated hypothyroidism receiving typical doses of levothyroxine will have an increase in metabolic activity and be out of the myxedematous zone within 1 week of initiating therapy.
- An impressive diuresis usually occurs within 2–3 days, with an improvement in the puffy facial appearance and with weight loss.

Speech, skin temperature, mental alertness, and physical activity show improvement within 72 hours.

- Levothyroxine is the drug of choice in pregnant women, and the objective of treatment is to decrease TSH to <6 μIU/mL and to maintain T_4 concentrations in the range of ~2–4 μg/dL.
- In children with hypothyroidism developing beyond 2–3 years of age, normal CNS and physiologic development are expected with thyroid replacement therapy.

See Chapter 71, Thyroid Disorders, authored by Charles A. Reasner, II, MD, FACE, and Robert L. Talbert, PharmD, FCCP, BCPS, for a more detailed discussion of this topic.

Chapter 19

PORTAL HYPERTENSION AND CIRRHOSIS

DEFINITIONS

- Alcoholic liver disease (ALD) is defined as chronic insufficiency of the liver as a result of alcohol abuse.
- Cirrhosis is defined as a chronic inflammatory and degenerative disease of the liver characterized by progressive loss of liver mass, reduced function, and increased resistance to blood flow through the liver.
- Portal hypertension is defined as increased pressure of the portal circulation resulting in venous congestion and varices.

PATHOPHYSIOLOGY

- Alcohol is one of the most common causes of liver disease worldwide.
  - Up to 90% of deaths due to cirrhosis may be prevented by elimination of alcohol use.
  - ALD is associated with chronic ingestion of 60–80 g of ethanol daily for long periods of time (e.g., >10 years).
- ALD can be viewed as a progressive, chronic condition with four basic stages.
  - The initial lesion, steatosis, or fatty metamorphosis, may begin as early as the first drink.
  - If the pattern of heavy alcohol use is continued, these lesions become necrotic, inducing a mild inflammatory reaction called alcoholic hepatitis or steatonecrosis. Lysis and necrosis of the fat-filled hepatocytes provoke an immune response. Alcohol may lead to cell necrosis by increasing the metabolic rate of cells that are already relatively hypoxic.
  - In some cases, these lesions lead to a third stage involving fibrotic changes of cirrhosis. The fibrosis that occurs in alcoholic hepatitis often obliterates the central veins, leading to portal vein hypertension even before the patient has progressed to cirrhosis.
  - The end point of the disease is hepatic failure and death. Cirrhosis leading to hepatic failure and its complications is the terminal event in ALD. The fibrosis may compress the hepatic veins, decreasing hepatic outflow, and thus lead to portal hypertension.

▶ CLINICAL PRESENTATION AND DIAGNOSIS

- Patients with ALD typically present with scleral icterus, spider angiomata (star-shaped vascular defects observed on the skin) generally observed on the trunk, and palmar erythema.
- Icterus, also called jaundice, is characterized by a yellow tinge to the skin or eyes that is noticeable when total bilirubin levels exceed 3–5 mg %.
- The liver is usually distended. Typically, the spleen is palpable because of increased pressures from the portal hypertension.
- Gynecomastia is common in males because of the testicular atrophy induced by alcohol.

LABORATORY

- With advancing liver disease, less bilirubin (a breakdown product of hemoglobin) is conjugated by the liver, leading to increases in indirect bilirubin (insoluble form which is bound to plasma proteins) in blood. Liver cell death leads to release of conjugated bilirubin (or direct bilirubin) from the liver into the systemic circulation. Excess bilirubin may be filtered by the kidneys, giving urine the characteristic "cola" color and leads to accumulation in the epidermis and sclera.
- Alkaline phosphatase, an enzyme made in the cells lining the biliary tract and in bone tissue, increases in the blood with processes that disrupt bile flow.
- With alcoholic hepatitis, values of alanine aminotransferase (ALT) and aspartate aminotransferase (AST) may reach into the hundreds (normal range for these is generally 5–40 IU/dL). As liver disease progresses into cirrhosis, the transaminases may actually fall, despite decreasing liver function.
- With ALD, a disproportionate increase in γ-glutamyltranspeptidase (GGTP, a biliary excretory enzyme that is more specific for liver disease) can be expected and is a useful diagnostic clue.
- As liver damage progresses, protein synthesis decreases. Prolongation of clotting tests such as prothrombin time and activated partial thromboplastin time can be expected. The serum albumin may fall as low as 2 g/dL (normal 4.5–5.5 g/dL).
- The Child–Pugh classification is frequently used to stratify patients into categories for selection of various therapies (Table 19–1).

PORTAL HYPERTENSION

- Portal hypertension in cirrhosis is the direct result of increased mechanical resistance to blood flow through the liver. Thus, the manifestations of portal hypertension are primarily the result of low-pressure vessels handling high-pressure loads. Esophageal and abdominal varices often develop; these can rupture and sometimes lead to life-threatening hemorrhage.
- Another significant complication of portal hypertension is ascites.

TABLE 19–1. Child–Pugh Grading of Liver Disease

Clinical and Biochemical Measurements	Points Scored for Increasing Abnormality		
	1	2	3
Encephalopathy (grade)	None	1 and 2	3 and 4
Ascites	Absent	Slight	Moderate
Bilirubin (mg/dL)	1–2	2–3	>3
Albumin (g/dL)	3.5	2.8–3.5	<2.8
Prothrombin time (increased sec)	1–4	4–6	>6

Total score for five factors is determined. Score ≤ 6 indicates highly survivable disease. Score 7–9 indicates moderate disease and score ≥ 10 indicates end-stage disease.

DECREASED LIVER FUNCTION

- With cirrhosis, there is a progressive loss of parenchymal mass and basic hepatocyte function that results in a decrease in protein synthesis and utilization of available substrates.
- A loss of enzymes leads to a decrease in the ability of the liver to metabolize both drugs and endogenous toxins, which then begin to accumulate.
- A decrease in serum albumin leads to a decrease in the protein binding of certain drugs and a decrease in the serum oncotic pressure.
- Vitamin K-dependent coagulation factors (II, VII, IX, X) synthesized by the liver slowly diminish, resulting in an increased frequency of bleeding problems.
- The ability of the hepatic transaminases to detoxify ammonia is decreased. Ammonia, octopamine, mercaptans, phenols, methanethiols, and other by-products of metabolism begin to accumulate. Along with this decrease in transamination, there is an apparent increase in ammonia production in the gut.
- There is some evidence that benzodiazepine-receptor reactivity is increased and that an endogenous benzodiazepine-receptor ligand accumulates in liver disease.
- There is an increase in aromatic amino acids (AAAs) at a rate 24 times the production of branched-chain amino acids (BCAAs).

HEPATIC ENCEPHALOPATHY

- Hepatic encephalopathy (HE) is a syndrome of altered mental status associated with liver impairment and is characterized by impaired cognitive skills, worsened motor abilities, and steadily depressed levels of consciousness, beginning with somnolence and ending with coma.
- The spectrum of impairment is broad and may be classified in stages as the syndrome progresses (Table 19–2).
- The cause of HE is not known; several factors, such as increased blood levels of ammonia and aromatic amino acids, have been associated with the development of HE (Table 19–3).

TABLE 19–2. Scale for Assessing the Depth of Hepatic Encephalopathy

Grade	Cognitive/Motor	Behavior
1	Mild tremor, altered handwriting	Anxiety, insomnia, mild confusion
2	Dysarthria, ataxia asterixis	Lethargy, disorientation
3	Seizures, muscle twitching	Delirium, bizarre behavior
4	Posturing	Coma

From Barber JR, Teasley KM. Clin Pharm *1984;3:245–253, with permission.*

- There are a variety of precipitating causes for hepatic encephalopathy including infection, constipation, metabolic alkalosis, excess dietary protein, gastrointestinal bleeding, azotemia, and some drugs (e.g., sedative/hypnotics, opiates).
- There is also a tremendous increase in the relative levels of aromatic amino acids in the encephalopathic patient. The abnormal ratio of BCAAs to AAAs in liver disease allows for enhanced CNS entry of tryptophan, tyrosine, and phenylalanine.

PHARMACOKINETIC/PHARMACODYNAMIC CHANGES ASSOCIATED WITH LIVER FAILURE

- There is currently no mathematical approach useful for adjusting drug doses in patients with liver failure.
- The most important parameter when adjusting drug doses for liver impairment is the clinical response.

Some pharmacokinetic/pharmacodynamic changes with liver disease include:

- Highly extracted drugs tend to be affected more by changes in hepatic blood flow than by changes in metabolism. The opposite is true of low-extraction ratio drugs. Cirrhosis, which reduces liver blood flow, would

TABLE 19–3. Theories for the Development of Hepatic Encephalopathy

Toxin	Description
Ammonia	Direct neurotoxin
Multiple synergistic neurotoxins	Mercaptans (produced by dietary methionine), elevated free fatty acids
False neurotransmitters	Elevated aromatic amino acids lead to increased serotonin, octopamine, and phenylethylamine (depressants) while decreasing dopamine and noradrenaline (stimulants)
γ-Aminobutyric acid neurotransmission	Endogenous and/or exogenous benzodiazepine-like compounds

have a greater effect on high extraction drugs (such as lidocaine, labetalol, and propranolol).

- Highly protein-bound drugs have increased unbound (or free) fractions owing to reduced protein (e.g., albumin concentrations).
- An increased free fraction also means that there is more drug available to be metabolized by the still-functioning hepatic enzymes. Thus, until these enzymes become saturated, the clearance of a highly protein-bound drug during liver impairment can increase and the half-life can shorten.
- Drugs that are excreted through the bile may accumulate in these patients.
- Dramatic shifts in fluid can be expected in ALD, thus increasing the distribution volume of drugs with low protein binding.
- The clinical components of liver disease also can change the dose–response relationships of drugs. Encephalopathic patients will be much more sensitive to central nervous system (CNS) depressants.
- Bleeding varices may increase the absorption of drugs that would normally exhibit poor absorption.
- Diarrhea associated with hepatitis will decrease the absorption of many drugs.

► DESIRED OUTCOME

GENERAL PRINCIPLES

The ideal goal for treatment of ALD is that the patient stops drinking alcohol before irreversible hepatic damage has occurred. This would reduce long-term complications. When there is chronic liver dysfunction, the goals are restoration of liver function or at least prevention of further damage, and avoidance of life-threatening complications. With chronic liver dysfunction, reduction in disease symptoms is important as is restoration of nutritional status.

► TREATMENT

GENERAL PRINCIPLES

- The most important treatment for ALD is the discontinuance of alcohol exposure. With discontinuation of alcohol exposure, many patients improve dramatically.
- After the discontinuation of alcohol, the therapy for ALD is primarily symptomatic.

ALCOHOLIC HEPATITIS

- A treatment algorithm for alcoholic hepatitis is shown in Figure 19–1.
- In alcoholic hepatitis, glucocorticoids are sometimes used during the acute phase to decrease the inflammatory response to the alcoholic hyaline and other antigenic substances present. Dramatic improvement in

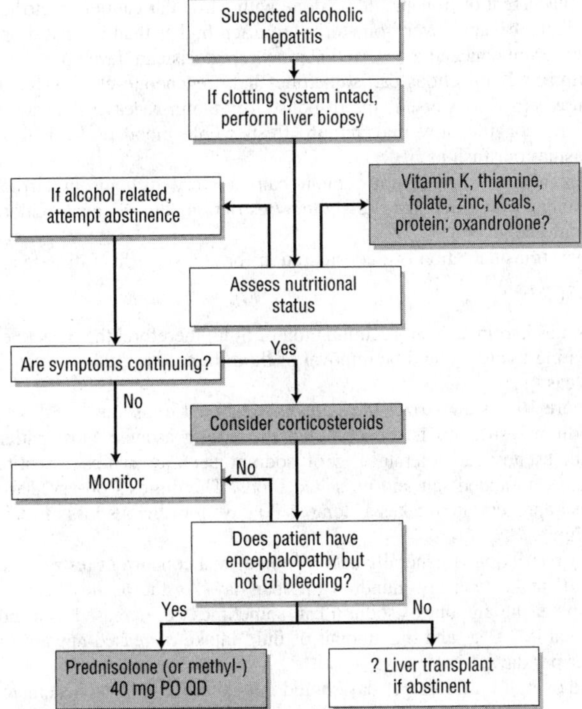

Figure 19–1. Treatment algorithm for a patient with alcoholic hepatitis.

V

short-term mortality has been demonstrated with **methylprednisolone** in very sick patients.

- Encephalopathy was a predictor for success of corticosteroids. The presence of GI bleeding can reverse the positive effects of glucocorticoids.
- Generally, **prednisolone** or methylprednisolone are the preferred steroids since they do not require liver metabolism to an active compound as prednisone does.

CIRRHOSIS

- The treatment of cirrhosis is also symptomatic, directed at the manifestations in the particular patient.
- If the patient shows signs of nutritional deficiency, it should be corrected. Deficiencies in folate, thiamine, and vitamin C are very common and often severe. In addition, potassium, phosphorus, magnesium, and iron can be quite low in these patients.

- Replacement of iron should be done with particular caution in cirrhotic patients, because liver iron stores are often higher than normal despite low serum concentrations, and hemochromatosis can develop.
- **Vitamin K** injections can sometimes help regenerate clotting factors, but as cirrhosis worsens the response to vitamin K lessens. Treatment of the coagulopathy may require fresh whole blood or fresh frozen plasma transfusions.
- Replenishment of serum protein can be very difficult in cirrhotic patients who often require protein restriction, but adequate calories should be given.
- Liver transplantation is a consideration for end-stage liver disease.

ASCITES

- Ascites is primarily an accumulation of fluid; therefore, the objective in treating ascites should be removal of fluid. In practice, this is often not an easy task.
- Figure 19–2 summarizes the stepwise treatment of ascites.
- Sodium restriction is the first step in treating ascites. Most patients with ascites can tolerate 1 g of sodium per day, which essentially means no added salt and no salted foods. The diuresis observed from this approach, often takes as long as 30 days for obvious loss of ascites volume.
- Salt restriction is generally accompanied by a concurrent restriction of fluid intake to a few hundred mL per day. As the ascites begins to resolve, the amount of sodium can sometimes be increased to a more tolerable 2–3 g, and the amount of fluid intake increased upward to a liter per day.
- The overall fluid loss per day should not exceed 1–2 L. Nonedematous patients should not be diuresed beyond a weight loss of about 0.5 kg/d. Diuresis that is too brisk can lead to problems of relative dehydration and a potentially fatal hepatorenal syndrome.
- Paracentesis or diuretic therapy can be used to deplete the volume of ascites when sodium and fluid restriction fail to produce adequate diuresis.
- Many patients who continue to develop ascites, and those who do not respond to diuretics or paracentesis, may be eligible to receive a LeVeen or peritoneovenous shunt.
- Diuretic therapy for ascites is effective in most patients; however, the process is slow (35–40 days of continuous therapy may be required before the ascites resolves).
- The diuretic most frequently used is **spironolactone,** because of its ability to inhibit the action of aldosterone in the kidney tubule. The dose of spironolactone required ranges from 100–800 mg/d and is usually not effective without concurrent sodium and water restriction.
- The onset of the diuretic effect with spironolactone is slow, 3–5 days in some cases, and **furosemide** or **amiloride** are sometimes added to increase the rate of weight loss.

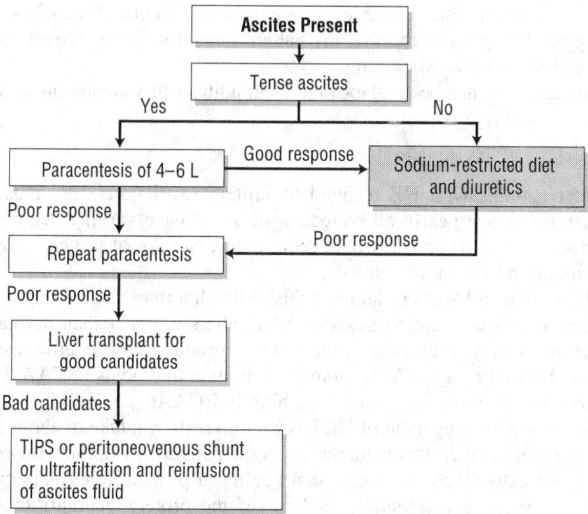

Figure 19–2. Treatment algorithm for the management of ascites.

PORTAL HYPERTENSION

- The therapy for portal hypertension is directed at reducing flow to the portal bed. Operative procedures such as splenectomy or portacaval shunts attempt to do this mechanically.
- Drug therapy with **propranolol** is also used with some success at a dose sufficient to decrease the blood pressure by 25 mm Hg or to reduce the heart rate by 20–25%.
- Propranolol reduces the incidence of first rebleeding and lowers the mortality rate relative to placebo. However, it produces desirable (decreased portal vein pressure) and undesirable effects (decreased liver blood flow) precipitating encephalopathy.
- Selective β blocker **(metoprolol)** reduces portal hypertension without reducing hepatic blood flow.
- Sclerotherapy is the direct injection of a chemical with necroinflammatory or thrombotic properties **(ethanolamine, sodium tetradecyl sulfate,** and **sodium morrhuate)** into the varix to manage the acute bleeding episode or to prevent relapse. There is no consensus regarding the sclerosant of choice.
- An intravenous infusion of **vasopressin** at 0.2–0.6 unit per minute can be used to treat acutely bleeding varices.
- Coronary and venous thrombosis can occur along with arrhythmias secondary to ischemia as a result of the use of vasopressin. Increases in

blood pressure are possible as are severe vascular headaches and angina. It is prudent to have any patient treated with vasopressin monitored by electrocardiogram.

- Nitroglycerin has been advocated as an adjunct to vasopressin to limit the coronary vasospasm.

HEPATIC ENCEPHALOPATHY

- Most patients with HE respond to protein restriction. Care must be exercised since nearly all patients with ALD have varying degrees of protein malnutrition and would require at least 60 g of protein daily to maintain positive nitrogen balance.
- The source and types of amino acids in the diet may also be important, because aromatic amino acids (AAAs), already higher than normal in cirrhotics, can be utilized in the CNS to produce false neurotransmitters. This ratio of AAAs to branched-chain amino acids (BCAAs) can be reversed by the use of feedings high in BCAAs.
- The classic management of HE has been to restrict intake to about 20 g of protein per day; this is increased as the patient's symptoms improve. An alternative theory suggests that quality of protein rather than quantity is important, especially in light of the protein malnutrition and anorexia present in this population.
- In latent (i.e., subclinical) HE, oral BCAA improves psychomotor disturbances and automobile-driving capacity compared to placebo.
- The status of BCAA in acute HE is uncertain. In contrast, oral BCAA has improved some measures in chronic HE including liver function tests (increased serum albumin), nutritional measures (amino-acid profile, nitrogen balance), and mortality, in some studies. To prevent negative nitrogen balance, stable cirrhotic patients may require 0.5–1 g/kg of protein. However, catabolic states such as alcoholic hepatitis require intakes of 1.0 g/kg of protein.
- Therapies that reduce the blood ammonia level appear to be effective in the management of HE that does not respond to protein restriction alone (Figure 19–3).
- **Lactulose** decreases the rate of urea breakdown and thus decreases the ammonia in the blood derived from the gut. Optimally, the lactulose dose should be titrated to produce two to three stools per day. Lactulose should be started at 50 mL every hour until catharsis occurs.
- **Neomycin** given orally is also used to change colonic flora and decrease blood ammonia. The optimal dosing regimen is not known; however, a starting dose of 0.5 g four times daily may be used up to 4–6 g/d.
- The benzodiazepine antagonist **flumazenil** is an alternative when conventional treatment of HE has failed. Rapid and startling clinical response has been reported with doses of 0.2–15 mg IV in uncontrolled studies. Studies show improvement in 40–70% of patients treated with flumazenil and no response to placebo.

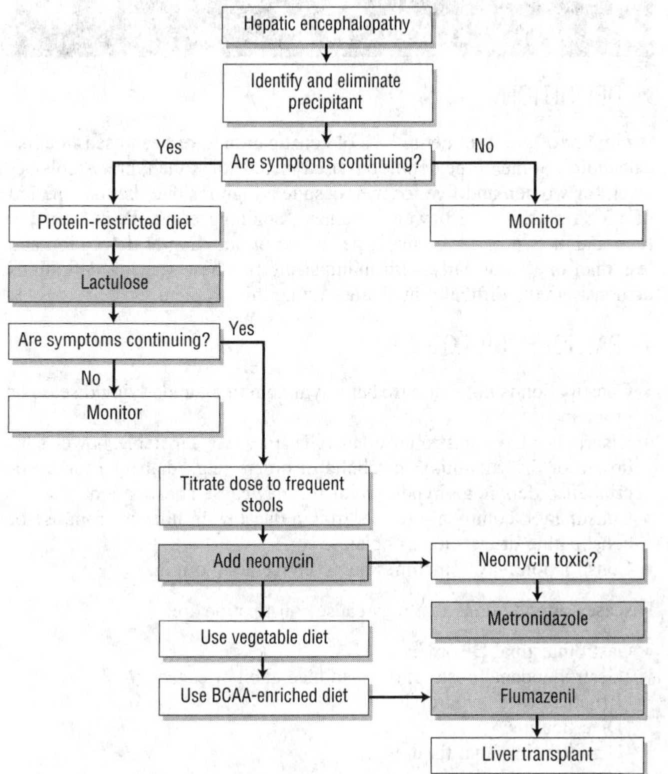

Figure 19–3. Treatment algorithm for the management of hepatic encephalopathy.

► EVALUATION OF THERAPEUTIC OUTCOMES

- A careful drug history on initial evaluation is important to avoid hepatotoxins and to identify drugs that may require dosage adjustment.
- The status for vaccination against hepatitis B should be determined.
- A thorough nutritional assessment should be performed along with determination of nutritional parameters.
- Periodic liver biopsies can be used to track disease progress.
- Mental status exams are useful to assess encephalopathy.

See Chapter 35, Portal Hypertension and Cirrhosis, authored by Mark A. Gill, PharmD, and William R. Kirchain, PharmD, CDE, for a more detailed discussion of this topic.

Chapter 20

▶ CONSTIPATION

▶ DEFINITION

A number of different definitions of constipation have been used in clinical studies. Some of the definitions used include: less than three stools per week for women and five for men despite a high residue diet or a period of >3 days without a bowel movement; straining at stool >25% of the time and/or two or fewer stools per week; or straining at defecation and less than one stool daily with minimal effort. These varying definitions demonstrate the difficulty in characterizing this problem.

▶ PATHOPHYSIOLOGY

- Constipation is not a disease but a symptom of an underlying disease or problem.
- Disorders of the gastrointestinal (GI) tract (e.g., irritable bowel syndrome or diverticulitis), metabolic disorders (e.g., diabetes), or endocrine disorders (e.g., hypothyroidism) may cause constipation.
- Constipation commonly results from a diet low in fiber or from use of constipating drugs such as opiates.
- Constipation may sometimes be psychogenic in origin.

Diseases or conditions that may cause constipation are:

- Gastrointestinal Disorders
  - Gastroduodenal obstruction from ulceration or cancer
  - Irritable bowel syndrome
  - Diverticulitis
  - Hemorrhoids, anal fissures
  - Ulcerative proctitis
  - Tumors
- Metabolic and Endocrine Disorders
  - Diabetes mellitus
  - Hypothyroidism
  - Panhypopituitarism
  - Pheochromocytoma
  - Hypercalcemia
- Pregnancy
- Neurogenic Constipation
  - Head trauma
  - Central nervous system tumors
  - Stroke
  - Parkinson's disease
- Psychogenic Constipation
  - Psychiatric disorders
  - Inappropriate bowel habits

- Drug-Induced Constipation
  - Analgesics
  - Inhibitors of prostaglandin synthesis
  - Opiates
  - Anticholinergics
  - Antihistamines
  - Antiparkinsonian agents (e.g., benztropine or trihexyphenidyl)
  - Phenothiazines
  - Tricyclic antidepressants
  - Antacids containing calcium carbonate or aluminum hydroxide
  - Barium sulfate
  - Clonidine
  - Diuretics (nonpotassium sparing)
  - Ganglionic blockers
  - Iron preparations
  - Muscle blockers (d-tubocurarine, succinylcholine)
  - Polystyrene sodium sulfonate
- All opiate derivatives are associated with constipation, but the degree of intestinal inhibitory effects seems to differ between agents. Orally administered opiates appear to have greater inhibitory effect than parenterally administered agents; oral codeine is well known as a potent antimotility agent.
- Agents with anticholinergic properties inhibit bowel function by parasympatholytic actions on innervation to many regions of the GI tract, particularly the colon and rectum. Many types of drugs possess anticholinergic action, and these agents are used commonly in hospitalized and nonhospitalized patients.

▶ CLINICAL PRESENTATION

- The patient presenting with constipation usually complains of abdominal discomfort and distention. They may also complain of straining at stool, lumpy or hard stools, or a feeling of incomplete evacuation.
- Constipation may vary in implication from a minor discomfort in the otherwise healthy adult to a symptom of colon cancer or other serious diseases.
- A basis for evaluation and treatment should be a thorough history including questions about the nature of the constipation.
- It is important to ascertain whether the patient perceives the problem as infrequent bowel movements, stools of insufficient size, a feeling of fullness, or difficulty and pain on passing stool.
- The patient should be asked about the frequency of bowel movements and the chronicity of constipation. The patient also should be carefully questioned about usual diet and laxative regimens. Does the patient have a diet consistently deficient in high-fiber items and containing mainly highly refined foods? What laxatives or cathartics has the patient used to attempt relief of constipation?

- The patient should be questioned about other concurrent medications, with interest toward agents that might cause constipation.
- The laxative abuser may present with contradictory findings, sometimes diarrhea or weight loss. Laxative abusers may also have vomiting, abdominal pain, lassitude, thirst, edema, and bone pain (due to osteomalacia). With prolonged abuse, patients may have fluid and electrolyte imbalances (most commonly hypokalemia), protein losing gastroenteropathy with hypoalbuminemia, and syndromes resembling colitis. Laxative abusers frequently deny laxative use.

▶ DESIRED OUTCOME

A major goal for treatment of constipation is prevention of constipation by alteration of lifestyle (particularly diet). For acute constipation, the goal is to relieve symptoms and restore normal bowel function.

▶ TREATMENT

GENERAL APPROACH TO TREATMENT

- General measures believed to be beneficial in managing constipation include dietary modification to increase the amount of fiber consumed daily, exercise, adjustment of bowel habits so that a regular and adequate time is made to respond to the urge to defecate, and increasing fluid intake.
- If an underlying disease is recognized as the cause of constipation, attempts should be made to correct it. GI malignancies may be removed through a surgical resection. Endocrine and metabolic derangements are corrected by the appropriate methods.
- Potential drug causes of constipation should be identified. For some medications (e.g., antacids), nonconstipating alternatives exist. If no reasonable alternatives exist to the medication thought to be responsible for constipation, consideration should be given to lowering the dose. If a patient must remain on constipating medications, then more attention must be paid to general measures for prevention of constipation, as discussed next.

DIETARY MODIFICATION AND BULK-FORMING AGENTS

- The most important aspect of the therapy for constipation for the majority of patients is dietary modification to increase the amount of fiber consumed. Patients should be advised to include at least 14 g of crude fiber in their daily diets.
- Fruits, vegetables, and cereals have the highest fiber content.
- A trial of dietary modification with high-fiber content should be continued for at least 1 month before effects on bowel function are determined.

- The patient should be cautioned that abdominal distention and flatus may be particularly troublesome in the first few weeks, particularly with high bran consumption.

▶ SURGERY

- In a small percentage of patients presenting with complaints of constipation, surgical procedures (such as intestinal resection) are necessary. Surgery is usually necessary with most colonic malignancies and with GI obstruction from a number of causes.

PHARMACOLOGIC THERAPY

- The various types of laxatives are discussed in this section. The agents are divided into three general classifications: (1) those causing softening of feces in 1–3 days (bulk-forming laxatives, docusates, and lactulose); (2) those that result in soft or semifluid stool in 6–12 hours (diphenylmethane derivatives and anthraquinone derivatives); and (3) those causing water evacuation in 1–6 hours (saline cathartics, castor oil, and polyethylene glycol-electrolyte lavage solution).
- Dosage recommendations for laxatives and cathartics are provided in Table 20–1.

Recommendations

- The basis for treatment and prevention of constipation should consist of bulk-forming agents in addition to dietary modifications that increase dietary fiber.
- For most nonhospitalized persons with acute constipation, the infrequent use (less than every few weeks) of most laxative products is acceptable; however, before more potent laxative/cathartics are used, relatively simple measures may be tried. For example, acute constipation may be relieved by the use of a tap-water enema or a glycerin suppository; if neither is effective, the use of low doses of diphenylmethane or anthraquinone derivatives or saline laxatives (e.g., milk of magnesia) may provide relief.
- If laxative treatment is required for longer than 1 week, the person should be advised to consult a physician to determine if there is an underlying cause of constipation that requires treatment with agents other than laxatives.
- For some bedridden or geriatric patients, or others with chronic constipation, bulk-forming laxatives remain the first line of treatment, but the use of more potent laxatives may be required relatively frequently. Agents that may be used in these situations include diphenylmethane and anthraquinone derivatives, milk of magnesia, and lactulose.
- In the hospitalized patient without GI disease, constipation may be related to the use of general anesthesia and/or opiate substances. Most orally or rectally administered laxatives may be used. For prompt initi-

TABLE 20–1. Dosage Recommendations for Laxatives and Cathartics

Agent	Recommended Dose
Agents that Cause Softening of Feces in 1–3 d	
Bulk-forming agents	
Methylcellulose	4–6 g/d
Polycarbophil	4–6 g/d
Psyllium	Varies with product
Emollients	
Docusate sodium	50–360 mg/d
Docusate calcium	50–360 mg/d
Docusate potassium	100–300 mg/d
Lactulose	15–30 mL orally
Sorbitol	30–50 g/d orally
Mineral oil	15–30 mL orally
Agents that Result in Soft or Semifluid Stool in 6–12 h	
Bisacodyl (oral)	5–15 mg orally
Phenolphthalein	30–270 mg orally
Cascara sagrada	Dose varies with formulation
Senna	Dose varies with formulation
Magnesium sulfate (low dose)	<10 g orally
Agents that Cause Watery Evacuation in 1–6 h	
Magnesium citrate	18 g in 300 mL water
Magnesium hydroxide	2.4–4.8 g orally
Magnesium sulfate (high dose)	10–30 g orally
Sodium phosphates	Varies with salt used
Bisacodyl	10 mg rectally
Polyethylene glycol–electrolyte preparations	4 L

ation of a bowel movement, a tap-water enema or glycerin suppository is recommended, or milk of magnesia.

- The approach to the treatment of constipation in young persons should consider neurologic, metabolic, or anatomic abnormalities when constipation is a persistent problem. When not related to an underlying disease, the approach to constipation is similar to that in an adult.
- Prokinetic agents (such as cisapride) may be used in patients with neurologic disorders such as Parkinson's disease or chronic idiopathic constipation.
- Patients with chronic, intractable constipation are commonly found to have slow GI transit, pelvic floor dysfunction, both of the above, or irri-

table bowel syndrome. With failure of medical management, surgery may be indicated in patients with slow transit. Behavioral treatments such as biofeedback are successful in about 70% of patients with pelvic floor dysfunction.

Emollient Laxatives (Docusates)

- These surfactant agents, **docusate** in its various salts, work by facilitating the mixing of aqueous and fatty materials within the intestinal tract. They may increase water and electrolyte secretion in the small and large bowel.
- These products result in a softening of stools within 1–3 days.
- Emollient laxatives are not effective in treating constipation but are used mainly to prevent constipation. They may be helpful in situations where straining at stool should be avoided, such as after recovery from myocardial infarction, with acute perianal disease, or after rectal surgery.
- It is unlikely that these agents are very effective in preventing constipation if major causative factors (e.g., heavy opiate use, uncorrected pathology, inadequate dietary fiber) are not concurrently addressed.

V

Lubricants

- **Mineral oil** is the only lubricant laxative in routine use and acts by coating stool and allowing easier passage. It inhibits colonic absorption of water, thereby increasing stool weight and decreasing stool transit time.
- Generally, the effect on bowel function is noted after 2 or 3 days of use.
- Mineral oil is helpful in situations similar to those suggested for docusates: to maintain a soft stool and avoid straining for relatively short periods of time (a few days to 2 weeks).
- Mineral oil may be absorbed systemically and cause a foreign-body reaction in lymphoid tissue. Also, in debilitated or recumbent patients, mineral oil may be aspirated causing lipoid pneumonia.

Lactulose and Sorbitol

- **Lactulose** is a disaccharide that causes an osmotic effect retained in the colon.
- Lactulose is generally not recommended as a first-line agent for the treatment of constipation because it is costly and not necessarily more effective than agents such as milk of magnesia. It may be justified as an alternative for acute constipation and has been found to be particularly useful in elderly patients.
- Occasionally, the use of lactulose may result in flatulence, cramps, diarrhea, and electrolyte imbalances.
- **Sorbitol,** a monosaccharide, is occasionally used as a laxative, exerting its effect by osmotic action. It is as effective as lactulose and much less expensive.

Diphenylmethane Derivatives

- The two commonly used agents in this class are **bisacodyl** and **phenolphthalein.**

- Bisacodyl stimulates the mucosal nerve plexus of the colon; the mechanism of action of phenolphthalein is poorly understood.
- The dose of these agents for effective use in various individuals appears to vary greatly. A dose that causes no effects in one patient may result in excessive cramping and fluid evacuation in another.
- Their use is acceptable intermittently (every few weeks) to treat constipation or as a bowel preparation before diagnostic procedures in which cleansing of the colon is necessary.
- The patient taking phenolphthalein-containing laxatives should be cautioned that it may turn urine pink.

Anthraquinone Derivatives

- The agents in this class are **cascara sagrada, sennosides,** and **casanthrol.**
- Effects are limited to the colon, and stimulation of Auerbach's plexus may be involved.
- Recommendations for the use of these agents are similar to those for the diphenylmethane derivatives. In most cases, intermittent use is acceptable; daily use should be strongly discouraged.

Saline Cathartics

- Saline cathartics are composed of relatively poorly absorbed ions such as magnesium, sulfate, phosphate, and citrate, which produce their effects primarily by osmotic action to retain fluid in the GI tract.
- These agents may be given orally or rectally.
- A bowel movement may result within a few hours after oral doses and in 1 hour or less after rectal administration.
- These agents should be used primarily for acute evacuation of the bowel, which may be necessary before diagnostic examinations, after poisonings, and in conjunction with some anthelmintics to eliminate parasites.
- Agents such as **milk of magnesia** (an 8% suspension of magnesium hydroxide) may be used occasionally (every few weeks) to treat constipation in otherwise healthy adults.
- Saline cathartics should not be used on a routine basis to treat constipation. With fecal impactions, the enema formulations of these agents may be helpful.

Castor Oil

- **Castor oil** is metabolized in the GI tract to an active compound, ricinoleic acid, which stimulates secretory processes, decreases glucose absorption, and promotes intestinal motility, primarily in the small intestine.
- Castor oil usually results in a bowel movement within 1–3 hours of administration.
- Because the agent has such a strong purgative action, it should not be used for the routine treatment of constipation.

Glycerin

- This agent is usually administered as a 3-g suppository and exerts its effect by osmotic action in the rectum.
- As with most agents given as suppositories, the onset of action is usually less than 30 minutes.
- **Glycerin** is considered a very safe laxative, although it may occasionally cause rectal irritation. Its use is acceptable on an intermittent basis for constipation, particularly in children.

Polyethylene Glycol-Electrolyte Lavage Solution

- Whole-bowel irrigation with **polyethylene glycol-electrolyte lavage solution (PEG-ELS)** has become popular for colon cleansing before diagnostic procedures or colorectal operations.
- Four liters of this solution is administered over 3 hours to obtain complete evacuation of the GI tract.
- The solution is not recommended for the routine treatment of constipation and its use should be avoided in patients with intestinal obstruction.

Other Agents

- Tap-water enemas may be used to treat simple constipation. The administration of 200 mL of water by enema to an adult often results in a bowel movement within one-half hour. Soapsuds are no longer recommended for use in enemas because their use may result in proctitis or colitis.
- **Cisapride** is a GI prokinetic agent that is used in GI motility disorders. It has been demonstrated to be effective in relieving acute constipation in both adults and children. The agent is considerably more expensive than most alternatives.

See Chapter 34, Diarrhea and Constipation, authored by R. Leon Longe, PharmD, and Joseph T. DiPiro, PharmD, FCCP, for a more detailed discussion of this topic.

Chapter 21

▶ DIARRHEA

▶ DEFINITION

Diarrhea is the abnormal frequency and liquidity of fecal discharge compared with the normal stools. Frequency and consistency are variable within and between individuals. For example, some individuals defecate as many as three times per day, while others defecate only two or three times per week.

▶ PATHOPHYSIOLOGY

- Diarrhea is an imbalance in absorption and secretion of water and electrolytes. If absorption of water in the small bowel and colon decreases or secretion increases beyond normal, diarrhea results. Normally, the absorption of water and electrolytes exceeds secretory fluxes.
- Four general pathophysiologic mechanisms disrupt water and electrolyte balance, leading to diarrhea. These four mechanisms are the basis of diagnosis and therapy. They are (1) a change in active ion transport by either decreased sodium absorption or increased chloride secretion; (2) a change in intestinal motility; (3) an increase in luminal osmolarity; and (4) an increase in tissue hydrostatic pressure.

These mechanisms have been related to four broad clinical diarrheal groups: secretory, osmotic, exudative, and altered intestinal transit.

- Secretory diarrhea occurs when a structurally similar substance (e.g., vasoactive intestinal peptide or bacterial toxin) increases secretion or decreases absorption of large amounts of water and electrolytes.
- Poorly absorbed substances retain intestinal fluids, making osmotic diarrhea.
- Inflammatory gut diseases can cause exudative diarrhea by discharge of mucus, proteins, or blood into the gut.
- Intestinal motility can be altered by reduced contact time in the small intestine, premature emptying of the colon, and by bacterial overgrowth.

▶ CLINICAL PRESENTATION

- Diarrhea is divided into acute and chronic disorders. Usually, acute diarrheal episodes subside within 72 hours of onset. Chronic diarrhea involves frequent attacks during 2–3 extended periods.
- With acute diarrhea, the patient complains of abrupt onset of frequent watery, loose stools, flatulence, malaise, and abdominal pain. Intermittent periumbilical or lower right quadrant pain with cramps and audible bowel sounds is characteristic of small intestinal disease. When pain is

TABLE 21–1. Drug-Induced Diarrhea

- Laxatives
- Antacids (magnesium-containing)
- Antibiotics
  - Clindamycin
  - Tetracyclines
  - Sulfonamides
  - Any broad-spectrum antibiotic
- Antihypertensives
  - Reserpine
  - Guanethidine
  - Methyldopa
  - Guanabenz
  - Guanadrel
- Cholinergics
  - Bethanechol
  - Metoclopramide
  - Neostigmine
- Cardiac agents
  - Quinidine
  - Digitalis
  - Digoxin

present in large intestinal diarrhea, it is a gripping, aching sensation with tenesmus (straining ineffective and painful stooling). In chronic diarrhea, previous bouts, weight loss, anorexia, and chronic weakness are important findings.

- Americans traveling abroad may experience traveler's or parasitic diarrhea. Recent ingestion of bacteria-contaminated foods identifies "food poisoning" as a possible etiology. An attentive dietary history identifies offending foods (e.g., dairy products with lactose intolerance). With AIDS patients, opportunistic pathogens may cause diarrheal illness.
- Many agents, including antibiotics and other drugs, cause diarrhea (Table 21–1). Laxative abuse for weight loss may also result in diarrhea.
- With diarrhea, physical examination of the abdomen may detect hyperperistalsis with borborygmi (growling stomach sounds) and generalized or local tenderness. A rectal examination detects masses or possibly fecal impaction, a common cause of diarrhea in the elderly.
- For unexplained diarrhea, especially in chronic situations, special tests are used, including stool examination for parasites and ova, blood, mucus, or fat. Stool osmolality, pH, and electrolytes may also be assessed. Direct endoscopic visualization and biopsy can be used to diagnose conditions such as colitis. Radiographic studies are helpful in diagnosing neoplastic and inflammatory conditions.

▶ DESIRED OUTCOME

The therapeutic goals of diarrhea treatment are to prevent excessive water, electrolyte, and acid–base disturbances, provide symptomatic relief, treat curable causes of diarrhea, and manage secondary disorders causing diarrhea. Clinicians must clearly understand that diarrhea, like a cough, may be a body defense mechanism for ridding itself of harmful substances or pathogens. The correct therapeutic response is not necessarily to stop diarrhea at all costs!

▶ TREATMENT

GENERAL PRINCIPLES

- Management of the diet is a first priority for treatment of diarrhea (Figures 21–1 and 21–2). Most clinicians recommend stopping solid foods for 24 hours and avoiding dairy products.

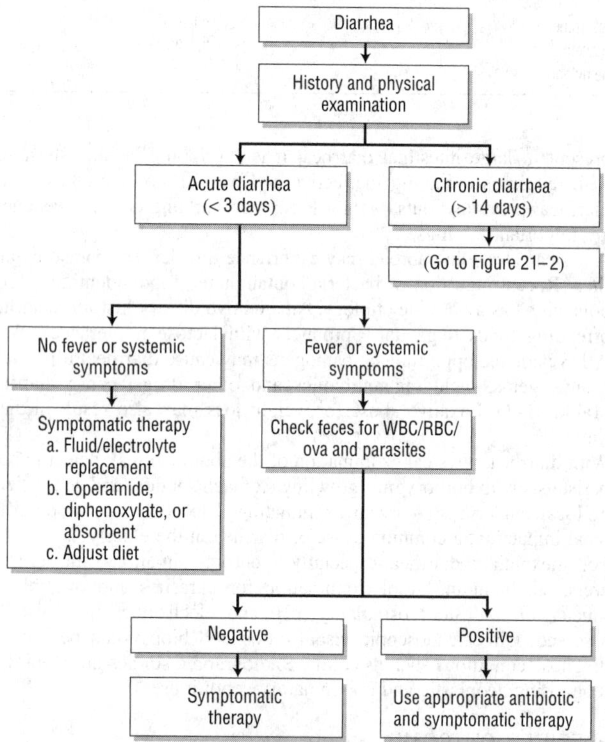

Figure 21–1. Recommendations for treating acute diarrhea. Follow these steps: (1) Perform a complete history and physical examination. (2) Is the diarrhea acute or chronic? If acute diarrhea, check for fever and/or systemic signs and symptoms (i.e., toxic patient). If systemic illness (fever, anorexia, volume depletion), check for infectious source. If positive for infectious diarrhea, use appropriate antibiotic/anthelminthic drug, and symptomatic therapy. If negative for infectious cause, use only symptomatic treatment. (3) If no systemic findings, then use symptomatic therapy, based on severity of volume depletion, oral or parenteral fluid/electrolytes, antidiarrheal agents (see Table 21–3), and diet.

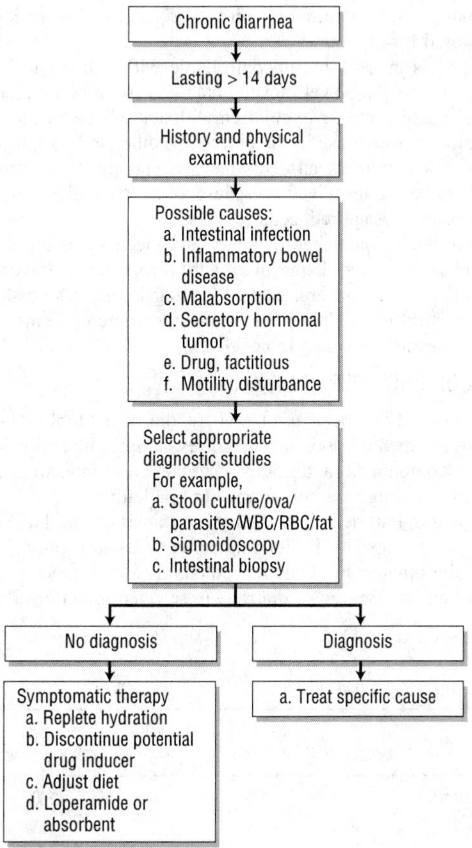

V

Figure 21–2. Recommendations for treating chronic diarrhea. Follow these steps: (1) Perform a careful history and physical examination. (2) The possible causes of chronic diarrhea are many. These can be classified into intestinal infections (bacterial, protozoal), inflammatory (Crohn's disease, ulcerative colitis), malabsorption (lactose intolerance), secretory hormonal tumor (intestinal carcinoid tumor, VIPoma), drug (antacid), factitious (laxative abuse), or motility disturbance (diabetes mellitus, irritable bowel syndrome, hyperthyroidism). (3) If the diagnosis is uncertain, selected appropriate diagnostic studies should be ordered. (4) Once diagnosed, treatment is planned for the underlying cause with symptomatic antidiarrheal therapy. (5) If no specific cause can be identified, symptomatic therapy is prescribed.

- When nausea or vomiting is mild, a digestible low-residue diet is administered for 24 hours.
- If vomiting is present and uncontrollable with antiemetics, nothing is taken by mouth. As bowel movements decrease, a bland diet is begun. Feeding should continue in children with acute bacterial diarrhea.
- Overzealous laxative use in the elderly, whether self- or physician-prescribed, is a common cause of diarrhea and must be identified and stopped. Other drugs that may cause or worsen diarrhea should be stopped or the dosage reduced.
- Repletion and maintenance of water and electrolytes are the primary treatment measures until the diarrheal episode ends. If vomiting and dehydration are not severe, enteral feeding is the less costly and preferred method. In the United States, many commercial oral rehydration preparations are available (Table 21–2).

PHARMACOLOGIC THERAPY

- Various drugs have been used to treat diarrhea (Table 21–3). These drugs are grouped into several categories: antimotility, adsorbents, antisecretory compounds, antibiotics, enzymes, and intestinal microflora. Usually, these drugs are not curative but palliative.
- Opiates and opioid derivatives delay the transit of intraluminal content or increase gut capacity, prolonging contact and absorption. The limitations of the opiates are addiction potential (a real concern with long-term use) and worsening of diarrhea in selected infectious diarrheas.

TABLE 21–2. Oral Rehydration Solutions

	WHO–ORS[a]	Pedialyte (Ross)	Rehydralyte (Ross)	Infalyte (Mead Johnson)	Resol[b] (Wyeth)
Osmolality (mOsm/L)	333	249	304	200	269
Carbohydrates (g/L)[b]	20	25	25	30[c]	20
Calories (cal/L) 77	85	100	100	126	80
Electrolytes (mEq/L)					
Sodium	90	45	75	50	50
Potassium	20	20	20	25	20
Chloride	80	35	65	45	50
Citrate	—	30	30	34	34
Bicarbonate	30	—	—	—	—
Calcium	—	—	—	—	4
Magnesium	—	—	—	—	4
Sulfate	—	—	—	—	—
Phosphate	—	—	—	—	5

[a]World Health Organization Oral Rehydration Solution.
[b]Carbohydrate is glucose.
[c]Rice syrup solids are carbohydrate source.

TABLE 21–3. Selected Antidiarrheal Preparations

	Dose Form	Adult Dose
Antimotility		
Diphenoxylate	2.5 mg/tablet 2.5 mg/5 mL	5 mg qid; do not exceed 20 mg/day
Loperamide	2 mg/capsule	Initially 4 mg, then 2 mg after each loose stool; do not exceed 16 mg/day
Paregoric	1 mg/5 mL, 2 mg/5 mL (morphine)	5–10 mL 1–4 times daily
Opium tincture	5 mg/mL (morphine)	0.6 mL qid
Difenoxin	1 mg/tablet	Two tablets, then one tablet after each loose stool; up to 8 tablets per day
Adsorbents		
Kaolin–pectin mixture	5.7 g kaolin + 130.2 mg per 30 mL	30–120 mL after each loose stool
Polycarbophil	500 mg/tablet	Chew 2 tablets qid or after each loose stool; do not exceed 12 tablets per day
Attapulgite	750 mg/15 mL, 300 mg/7.5 mL, 750 mg/tablet, 600 mg/tablet, 300 mg/tablet	1200–1500 mg after each loose bowel movement or every 2 hours; up to 9000 mg per day
Antisecretory		
Bismuth subsalicylate	1050 mg/30 mL, 262 mg/15 mL, 524 mg/15 mL, 262 mg/tablet	Two tablets or 30 mL every 30 minutes to 1 hour as needed up to 8 doses per day
Enzymes (lactase)	1250 neutral lactase units per 4 drops 3300 FCC lactase units per tablet	3–4 drops taken with milk or dairy product, 1 or 2 tablets as above
Bacterial replacement (*Lactobacillus acidophilus*, *L. bulgaricus*)		2 tablets or 1 granule packet 3 to 4 times daily; give with milk, juice, or water
Octreotide	0.05 mg/mL, 0.1 mg/mL, 0.5 mg/mL	Initial: 50 μg subcutaneously 1–2 times per day and titrate dose based on indication up to 600 μg/day in 2–4 divided doses

V

- Adsorbents are used for symptomatic relief (Table 21–3). Adsorbents are nonspecific in their action; they adsorb nutrients, toxins, drugs, and digestive juices. Coadministration with other drugs reduces their bioavailability.
- **Lactobacillus preparation** is a controversial treatment that is intended to replace colonic microflora. This supposedly restores intestinal functions and suppresses the growth of pathogenic microorganisms. However, a dairy-product diet containing 200–400 g of lactose or dextrin is equally effective in recolonization.
- Anticholinergic drugs, such as atropine, block vagal tone and prolong gut transit time. Their value in controlling diarrhea is questionable and limited by side effects.
- V **Bismuth subsalicylate** blocks copious fluid flow in secretory diarrheas. It is effective and safe in treatment and prevention of traveler's diarrhea.
- The role of antibiotics for treatment of diarrhea is controversial. Antibiotics are curative if the causative organism is susceptible, but most infectious diarrheas are self-limiting and treated with supportive therapy.
- **Octreotide,** a synthetic octapeptide analogue of endogenous somatostatin, is prescribed for the symptomatic treatment of carcinoid tumors and vasoactive intestinal peptide-secreting tumors (VIPomas). Octreotide is used in selected patients with carcinoid syndrome. Octreotide blocks the release of serotonin and other active peptides and is effective in controlling diarrhea and flushing. Dosage range for managing diarrhea associated with carcinoid tumors is 100–600 mg/d in two to four divided doses subcutaneously.

▶ EVALUATION OF THERAPEUTIC OUTCOMES

- Therapeutic outcomes are directed to key symptoms, signs, and laboratory studies. The constitutional symptoms usually improve within 24–72 hours.
- One should check the frequency and character of bowel movements each day along with the vital signs and improving appetite.
- The clinician also needs to monitor body weight, serum osmolality, serum electrolytes, complete blood cell count, urinalysis, and cultures (if appropriate). With the urgency/emergency situation, evaluation of the volume status of the patient is the most important outcome.
- Toxic patients (those with fever, dehydration, hematochezia, hypotensive) require hospitalization; they need intravenous electrolyte solutions and empiric antibiotics while awaiting cultures. With quick management, they usually recover within a few days.

See Chapter 34, Diarrhea and Constipation, authored by R. Leon Longe, PharmD and Joseph T. DiPiro, PharmD, FCCP, for a more detailed discussion of this topic.

Chapter 22

▶ GASTROESOPHAGEAL REFLUX DISEASE

▶ DEFINITION

Gastroesophageal reflux refers to the retrograde movement of gastric contents from the stomach into the esophagus. Gastroesophageal reflux disease (GERD) refers to any symptomatic clinical condition or histologic alteration that results from episodes of gastroesophageal reflux. When the esophagus is repeatedly exposed to refluxed material for prolonged periods of time, inflammation of the esophagus (i.e., reflux esophagitis) can occur. Gastroesophageal reflux must precede the development of GERD or reflux esophagitis.

▶ PATHOPHYSIOLOGY

- In many patients with GERD, the problem is not that they produce too much acid, but that the acid produced spends too much time in contact with the esophageal mucosa.
- A primary factor influencing the occurrence of esophageal reflux is the lower esophageal sphincter pressure (Table 22–1). Patients may have decreased gastroesophageal sphincter pressures related to spontaneous transient lower esophageal sphincter relaxations, transient increases in intra-abdominal pressure, or an atonic lower esophageal sphincter.
  - Problems with other normal mucosal defense mechanisms may also contribute to the development of GERD. These factors include decreased esophageal clearance, delayed gastric emptying, and reduced mucosal resistance.
  - Aggressive factors that may promote esophageal damage upon reflux into the esophagus include gastric acid, pepsin, bile acids, and pancreatic enzymes. The composition and volume of the refluxate are the most important aggressive factors in determining the consequences of gastroesophageal reflux.

▶ CLINICAL PRESENTATION

- The hallmark symptom of gastroesophageal reflux and esophagitis is heartburn or pyrosis. It is classically described as a substernal sensation of warmth or burning that may radiate to the neck. It is waxing and waning in character and is often aggravated by activities that potentiate gastroesophageal reflux (e.g., supine position, bending over).
- Other symptoms that may occur in patients with GERD include regurgitation, water brash (hypersalivation), dysphagia (difficulty swallowing), odynophagia (pain on swallowing), and hemorrhage.

TABLE 22–1. Factors That Affect Lower Esophageal Sphincter Pressure[a]

Decrease Pressure	Increase Pressure
Foods	
Carminatives (peppermint, spearmint)	Protein meal
Chocolate	
Fatty meal	
Coffee, cola, tea, citrus juices	
Tomato juice	
Onions, garlic	
Drugs	
Anticholinergics	Prokinetic agents (bethanechol cisapride, metoclopramide)
Barbiturates	
Benzodiazepines (diazepam)	Edrophonium
Caffeine	Methacholine
Calcium channel blockers	Norepinephrine
Dopamine	Pentagastrin
Estrogen	Phenylephrine
Ethanol	
Isoproterenol	
Narcotics (meperidine, morphine)	
Nicotine (smoking)	
Nitrates	
Phentolamine	
Progesterone	
Theophylline	
Hormones/Physiologic Factors	
Cholecystokinin	Gastric alkalinization
Estrogen	Gastrin
Gastric acidification	Prostaglandin F_2
Glucagon	
Progesterone	
Prostaglandins (E_1, E_2, A_2)	
Secretin	
Vasoactive intestinal peptide (VIP)	

[a] *Adapted from Weinberg DS, Kadish SL. The diagnosis and management of gastroesophageal reflux disease.* Medical Clinics of North America *1996;80(2):411–429.*

- Symptoms that are more atypical of GERD include nonallergic asthma, chronic cough, hoarseness, pharyngitis, and chest pain that mimics angina.
- The severity of the symptoms of gastroesophageal reflux does not usually correlate with the degree of esophagitis, but it does correlate with the duration of reflux.
- Gastroesophageal reflux may lead to many severe complications, including esophageal ulceration, stricture formation, esophageal perfo-

ration, pharyngeal/oral disturbances, hemorrhage, and Barrett's esophagus.

▶ DIAGNOSIS

- The most useful tool in the diagnosis of gastroesophageal reflux is the clinical history, including both presenting symptoms and associated risk factors.
- Endoscopy allows visualization and biopsy of the esophageal mucosa to assess the severity of esophageal injury. Histologic changes can only be diagnosed by endoscopy with biopsy. Endoscopy can also detect esophageal stricture and hiatal hernia, although it is less sensitive than the barium esophagogram.
- The barium esophagogram is less expensive than endoscopy but lacks the sensitivity and specificity needed to accurately determine the presence of mucosal injury. However, the barium esophagogram is the most sensitive test for detecting esophageal strictures or obstruction in patients presenting with dysphagia. It can also detect the presence of hiatal hernia and assess esophageal motor function.
- Provocative tests such as the acid perfusion (Bernstein) test, gastrointestinal scintiscanning, and maneuvers to induce reflux during the barium esophagogram are used to establish a causal relationship between the patient's symptoms and abnormal acid exposure, especially when esophagitis is not present. In general, these tests have limited utility in the diagnosis of routine GERD.
- Twenty-four hour ambulatory pH monitoring is useful in patients who continue to have symptoms without evidence of esophageal damage, patients who are refractory to standard treatment, and patients who present with atypical symptoms (e.g., chest pain or pulmonary symptoms). Ambulatory pH monitoring documents the percentage of time the intraesophageal pH is low. It is very effective in determining the frequency and severity of reflux.
- Esophageal manometry is useful in excluding motility disorders and should be performed in any patient who is a candidate for antireflux surgery.
- Patients who present with atypical chest pain often require both cardiac and esophageal evaluations. The diagnosis is complicated because esophageal pain may cause electrocardiographic disorders, and both esophageal and cardiac disorders may occur simultaneously.

▶ DESIRED OUTCOME

The multifold goals of treatments are to alleviate/eliminate the patient's symptoms, decrease the frequency and duration of gastroesophageal reflux, promote healing of the injured mucosa, and prevent the development of complications.

▶ TREATMENT

GENERAL PRINCIPLES

- Therapeutic modalities utilized in the treatment of gastroesophageal reflux are targeted at reversing the various pathophysiologic abnormalities.
- Specifically, therapy is directed at increasing lower esophageal sphincter pressure, enhancing esophageal acid clearance, improving gastric emptying, protecting the esophageal mucosa, decreasing the acidity of the refluxate and the gastric volume available to be refluxed. (Figure 22–1).
- Treatment is categorized into the following modalities: lifestyle changes, pharmacologic interventions, and surgical interventions.
- The initial therapeutic modality used is, in part, dependent on the condition of the patient (degree of esophagitis, presence of complications, etc.). However, historically, a stepwise approach has been used, starting with noninvasive lifestyle modifications (Tables 22–2 and 22–3).

ANTACIDS AND ANTACID–ALGINIC ACID PRODUCTS

- **Antacids** are commonly used in the treatment of gastroesophageal reflux because of their acid-neutralizing ability. Antacids are generally used to provide symptomatic relief in patients who have mild to moderate intermittent symptoms. Documentation of their efficacy for treatment of reflux and esophagitis in placebo-controlled clinical trials is lacking.

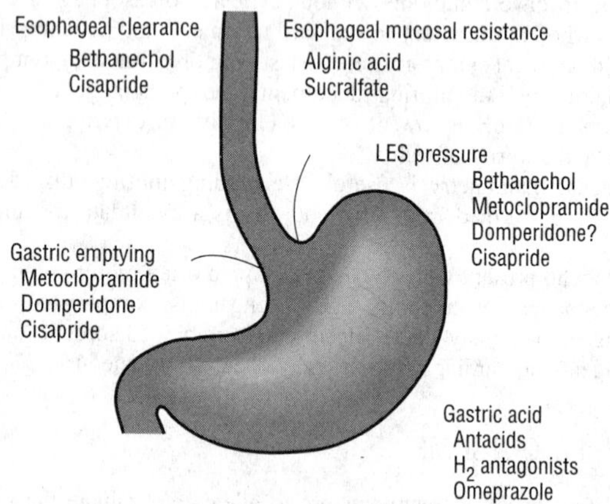

Figure 22–1. Therapeutic interventions in the management of gastroesophageal reflux disease. Pharmacologic interventions are targeted at improving defense mechanisms or decreasing aggressive factors. LES = lower esophageal sphincter.

TABLE 22–2. Therapeutic Approach to Gastroesophageal Reflux Disease

Patient Presentation	Recommended Treatment Regimen	Comments
Phase I		
Intermittent, mild heartburn	Lifestyle changes and antacids (Maalox TC 1–2 tsp 20 min to 1 h pc and hs; Gaviscon 2 tabs (pc and hs); calcium carbonate 0.5–1 g as needed) **and/or** Low-dose, OTC H_2-receptor antagonists (each taken up to bid) Climetidine 200 mg[a] Famotidine 10 mg[a] Nizatidine 75 mg Ranitidine 75 mg	Lifestyle changes should be started initially and continued throughout the course of treatment. If symptoms are unrelieved with Phase I therapy, then begin Phase IIa therapy.
Phase IIa		
Mild to moderate, typical symptoms not relieved by Phase I therapy **or** Atypical symptoms with nonerosive GERD (per endoscopy)	Lifestyle modifications **plus** Standard doses of H_2-receptor antagonists for 6–12 weeks Climetidine 400 mg bid Famotidine[b] 20 mg bid Nizatidine[c] 150 mg bid Ranitidine[c] 150 mg bid **or** Prokinetic agent[d] cisapride 10 mg qid or 20 mg bid (up to 20 mg qid)	For typical symptoms, treat empirically with Phase IIa therapy. If symptoms are relieved, treat recurrences on "as needed" basis. If symptoms recur frequently, consider maintenance therapy (MT) with lowest effective dose of ranitidine[e], cisapride, or a proton pump inhibitor[f] (PPI). Note: Most patients will require standard doses for MT. For atypical symptoms, obtain endoscopy (if possible) to evaluate mucosa. If nonerosive GERD present, give a trial of H_2-receptor antagonist therapy. If symptoms are relieved, consider MT. (May require a PPI for MT.) For patients with typical or atypical symptoms resistant to Phase IIa therapy, or for patients with erosive disease per endoscopy, begin Phase IIb therapy.

V

TABLE 22–2. continued

Patient Presentation	Recommended Treatment Regimen	Comments
Phase IIb		
Moderate to severe symptoms not relieved by Phase I or IIa therapy **or** "Erosive disease," or other complication such as strictures or Barrett's esophagus, noted on endoscopy	Titrate to higher, more frequent dose of H_2-receptor antagonist for 8–12 weeks Climetidine[g] 400 mg qid OR 800 mg bid Famotidine[g] 40 mg bid Nizatidine 150 mg qid Ranitidine[g] 150 mg qid **or** Omeprazole[h] 20 mg qd (up bid) for 8 weeks Lansoprazole[i] 30 mg qd (up to bid) for 8 weeks	If symptoms relieved with Phase IIb therapy, consider MT with the lowest effective dose. APPI is the drug of choice for both treatment and MT in patients with "erosive disease" or in patients with other complications. PPIs are also preferred for patients with atypical symptoms not responding to standard doses of H_2-receptor antagonists. Patients not responding to Phase IIb therapy, including those with persistent atypical symptoms, should be evaluated via ambulatory 24-h pH monitoring to confirm diagnosis of GERD (if possible). If GERD is present, consider Phase III therapy.
Phase III		
Surgery		Manometry should be performed in anyone who is a candidate for surgery.

[a]FDA labeled indication: heartburn, acid indigestion, and sour stomach (OTC).
[b]FDA labeled indication: GERD (for up to 6 weeks).
[c]FDA labeled indication: GERD.
[d]Concurrent use of an H_2-receptor antagonist and a prokinetic agent may be useful in patients with GERD and motor dysfunction. Review contraindications before using cisapride.
[e]FDA labeled indication: Maintenance of healing erosive esophagitis (150 mg bid).
[f]FDA labeled indication: To maintain healing of erosive esophagitis (omeprazole 20 mg daily, lansoprazole 15 mg daily).
[g]FDA labeled indication: Erosive esophagitis up to 12 weeks.
[h]FDA labeled indication: Erosive esophagitis (up to 8 weeks) and poorly responsive symptomatic GERD.
[i]FDA labeled indication: Erosive esophagitis (up to 8 weeks).

TABLE 22–3. Nonpharmacologic Treatment With Lifestyle Modifications

- Elevate the head of the bed (increases esophageal clearance)
  - Use 6 to 8 inch blocks under the head of the bed
  - Sleep on a foam wedge
- Dietary changes
  - Avoid foods that may decrease lower esophageal sphincter pressure (fats, chocolate, alcohol, peppermint, and spearmint)
  - Avoid foods that have a direct irritant effect on the esophageal mucosa (spicy foods, orange juice, tomato juice, and coffee)
  - Include protein-rich meals in diet (augments lower esophageal sphincter pressure)
  - Eat small meals and avoid eating immediately prior to sleeping (within 3 h if possible) (decreases gastric volume)
  - Weight reduction (reduces symptoms) V
- Stop smoking (decreases spontaneous esophageal sphincter relaxation)
- Avoid alcohol (increases amplitude of the lower esophageal sphincter, peristaltic waves, and frequency of contraction)
- Avoid tight-fitting clothes
- Discontinue, if possible, drugs that may promote reflux (calcium channel blockers, β blockers, nitrates, theophylline)
- Take drugs that have a direct irritant effect on the esophageal mucosa with plenty of liquid if they cannot be avoided (tetracyclines, quinidine, KCl, iron salts, aspirin, nonsteroidal anti-inflammatory drugs)

- The antacid product combined with **alginic acid (Gaviscon)** is not a potent neutralizing agent but it does form a highly viscous solution that floats on the surface of the gastric contents. This may mechanically impair reflux or coat the esophagus, thereby preventing mucosal contact of the irritants in the refluxate. Studies have shown that the product usually relieves symptoms of reflux, but data indicating endoscopic healing are lacking.
- Antacids have a short duration, which necessitates frequent administration throughout the day to provide continuous acid neutralization. Typical doses are two tablets four times daily after meals and at bedtime. Night-time acid suppression cannot be maintained with bedtime doses of antacids.

H_2 ANTAGONISTS: CIMETIDINE, RANITIDINE, FAMOTIDINE, AND NIZATIDINE

- The H_2 antagonists have historically been the mainstay in the treatment of GERD. These agents decrease gastric acid secretion which results in a less irritating refluxant. In addition, inhibition of gastric acid secretion results in a lower volume of gastric fluid available to be refluxed.
- Clinical trials clearly indicate that the efficacy of H_2 antagonists in the management of GERD is extremely variable and is frequently lower than desired.

- Response to the H_2 antagonists appears to be dependent on the severity of disease, duration of therapy, and dosage regimen used. The more severe the esophageal damage, the poorer the response to H_2 antagonists.
- Prolonged therapy with H_2 antagonists (8 weeks or more) is frequently used when treating patients with GERD.
- In general, standard-dose H_2 antagonists provide symptomatic improvement in about 60% of patients. Because of the somewhat disappointing endoscopic healing rates observed with standard dosages (about 48%), many recent studies have evaluated the efficacy of higher doses. For nonerosive disease, H_2 antagonists are given in standard doses (**cimetidine** 400 mg four times a day or 800 mg twice daily, **ranitidine** 150 mg twice daily, **famotidine** 20 mg twice daily, or **nizatidine** 150 mg twice daily).
- Patients not responding to standard regimens and those with erosive disease may obtain greater acid suppression and endoscopic healing rates with higher doses and/or four times daily dosing (cimetidine 800 mg twice daily, famotidine 40 mg twice daily, nizatidine 150 mg four times daily, ranitidine 150 mg four times daily).
- Relatively low, nonprescription doses have been shown to be effective in providing symptomatic relief of intermittent heartburn and in preventing meal-provoked heartburn in patients with mild disease.
- In general, H_2 antagonists are well tolerated. The most common adverse effects are headache, somnolence, fatigue, dizziness, and either constipation or diarrhea.
- Since all of the H_2 antagonists are efficacious, selection of the specific agent to be used in the management of GERD should be based on other factors such as differences in pharmacokinetics and safety profiles, as well as cost.

PROTON PUMP INHIBITORS: OMEPRAZOLE AND LANSOPRAZOLE

- **Omeprazole** and **lansoprazole** inhibit gastric acid secretion by inhibiting gastric H^+/K^+-adenosine triphosphatase.
- Proton pump inhibitors are the drugs of choice in patients with moderate to severe erosive esophagitis, patients with GERD not responding to H_2 antagonist therapy, and patients with complicated symptoms (Barrett's esophagus, strictures). Relapse is common in these patients, and long-term maintenance therapy is generally indicated.
- Clinical trials clearly indicate that proton pump inhibitors are superior to H_2 antagonists in controlling symptoms and healing esophagitis in patients with severe GERD. They are also more cost-effective in patients with severe disease.
- Omeprazole treatment for 4–8 weeks provides symptomatic relief in 71–96% of patients and healing rates of 62–94%. Healing rates after 8 weeks of treatment with lansoprazole 30 mg daily are similar to those achieved after 8 weeks of omeprazole 20 mg daily.

- Patients should be instructed to take the proton pump inhibitor in the morning before breakfast to maximize efficacy. Because these drugs degrade in acidic environments, they are formulated in delayed-release capsules containing enteric-coated granules. The contents of the capsule can be mixed in applesauce for patients who are unable to swallow the capsules. In patients with nasogastric tubes, the contents should be mixed in an acidic fruit juice such as apple or orange juice. In patients with feeding tubes placed directly into the duodenum, the contents should be mixed in a basic solution such as sodium bicarbonate.
- Proton pump inhibitors are usually well tolerated. Potential adverse effects include headache, dizziness, somnolence, diarrhea, constipation, and nausea.

PROKINETIC AGENTS: BETHANECHOL, METOCLOPRAMIDE, AND CISAPRIDE

- **Bethanechol, metoclopramide,** and **cisapride** have been shown to increase lower esophageal sphincter pressure and thereby may minimize the number of reflux episodes. Bethanechol and cisapride have also been shown to improve esophageal clearance.
- Metoclopramide and cisapride promote gastric emptying and thus may be of benefit in patients with GERD, many of whom have delayed gastric emptying. Bethanechol does not improve gastric emptying.
- Although bethanechol has been shown to increase lower esophageal sphincter pressure and improve esophageal clearance, its side-effect profile severely limits its use. Oral bethanechol may cause abdominal cramps, urinary frequency, malaise, blurred vision, and diarrhea. It may also increase gastric acid secretion.
- Cisapride is thought to increase lower esophageal sphincter pressure and accelerate gastric emptying through the facilitation of acetylcholine release at the myenteric plexus. The efficacy of cisapride 10 mg four times daily is similar to that of the H_2 antagonists (e.g., cimetidine 400 mg four times daily or ranitidine 150 mg twice daily) in mild esophagitis. However, it is more expensive and offers no real advantage in patients with normal gastrointestinal motility. Unlike **metoclopramide,** it is devoid of antidopaminergic effects and, therefore, does not cause extrapyramidal side effects or prolactin secretion.
- The most common adverse effects include transient abdominal cramping, borborygmi, diarrhea, and loose stools. Cisapride should be avoided in patients taking other drugs that inhibit the cytochrome P450 3A4 isoenzyme, as potentially life-threatening interactions have been reported. Cisapride should generally be reserved for patients who do not respond adequately to lifestyle modifications, antacids, and acid-reducing agents because of cardiac events and deaths associated with its use. An ECG should be performed before initiating cisapride therapy.

- Metoclopramide, a dopamine antagonist, increases lower esophageal sphincter pressure in a dose-related manner and accelerates gastric emptying in gastroesophageal reflux.
- Metoclopramide may provide symptomatic improvement for some patients with GERD, but endoscopic healing has not been demonstrated.
- A limiting factor with metoclopramide therapy is the high incidence of adverse effects. Most commonly reported adverse reactions were somnolence, nervousness, fatigue, dizziness, weakness, depression, diarrhea, and rash. Other possible adverse reactions include anxiety, insomnia, and extrapyramidal reactions, and increased prolactin levels.

MUCOSAL PROTECTANTS: SUCRALFATE

- **Sucralfate** is a nonabsorbable aluminum salt of sucrose octasulfate that has very limited value in the treatment of GERD.
- In general, sucralfate appears effective in some patients and may therefore be a suitable alternative to standard-dose H_2 antagonists or antacid–alginic acid therapy for treating mild esophagitis.
- Sucralfate is generally well tolerated. Side effects include constipation, dry mouth, nausea, and abdominal discomfort. Aluminum may accumulate in patients with renal dysfunction. Sucralfate may also lead to hypophosphatemia, presumably due to phosphate binding in the gut. Sucralfate may also reduce the absorption of several other medications.

COMBINATION THERAPY

- Combination therapy should be reserved for those patients failing to respond to high-dose proton pump inhibitor therapy or for those patients who obviously have multifactorial problems contributing to their disease (e.g., esophagitis + motor dysfunction). The most frequently used combinations include H_2 antagonists with prokinetic agents.

MAINTENANCE THERAPY

- Although healing and/or symptomatic improvement may be achieved via many different therapeutic modalities, 70–90% of patients relapse within 1 year of discontinuation of therapy.
- Long-term maintenance therapy should be considered to prevent complications and worsening of esophageal function in patients who have symptomatic relapse after discontinuation of therapy or dosage reduction, including patients with complications such as Barrett s esophagus, strictures, or hemorrhage.
- H_2 antagonists in standard doses (e.g., ranitidine 150 mg twice daily) and cisapride may be effective maintenance therapy for patients with mild disease. However, proton pump inhibitors (omeprazole 20 mg or lansoprazole 30 mg daily) are the drugs of choice for maintenance treatment of moderate to severe esophagitis. Lower doses (e.g., omeprazole 10 mg daily) or alternate-day regimens may be beneficial in patients with mild disease.

SURGERY

- Surgical intervention (Nissen, Belsey Mark IV, or Hill operations) is indicated when the patient fails to respond to conservative and pharmacologic treatment modalities, strictures are present, major bleeding occurs, and pulmonary complications exist.

▶ EVALUATION OF THERAPEUTIC OUTCOMES

- The short-term goals are to relieve symptoms such as heartburn and regurgitation so that they do not impair the patient's quality of life.
- The frequency and severity of symptoms should be monitored and patients should be counseled on symptoms that may suggest the presence of complications requiring immediate medical attention, such as dysphagia or odynophagia.
- Patients should also be monitored for the presence of atypical symptoms such as cough, nonallergic asthma, or chest pain. These symptoms require further diagnostic evaluation.

See Chapter 30, Gastroesophageal Reflux Disease, authored by Dianne B. Williams, PharmD for a more detailed discussion of this topic.

Chapter 23

▶ HEPATITIS, VIRAL

▶ DEFINITION

Viral hepatitis refers to the clinically important hepatotrophic viruses responsible for hepatitis A (HAV), hepatitis B (HBV), delta hepatitis (HDV), hepatitis C (HCV), and hepatitis E (HEV). Those viruses that cause hepatitis as part of a generalized illness, such as Epstein-Barr virus, herpes simplex virus, measles virus, and cytomegalovirus, are not discussed in this chapter. Viral hepatitis has several clinical forms (acute, fulminant, chronic), defined by duration or severity of infection.

Acute viral hepatitis is a systemic viral infection of up to but not exceeding 6 months in duration that produces inflammatory necrosis of the liver. Chronic viral hepatitis describes prolongation or continuation of the hepatic necroinflammatory process 6 months or more beyond the onset of the acute illness.

▶ PATHOPHYSIOLOGY

ACUTE VIRAL HEPATITIS

- Once virions gain access to the circulation (usually by oral or parenteral innoculation or through sexual contact), they accumulate in hepatic sinusoids and are internalized by the hepatocytes.
- The internalized viral particles replicate within the hepatocyte. Infective viral particles are then shed into blood, bile, and other body secretions.
- The duration of the incubation stage is virus specific and varies (Table 23–1). The host is essentially asymptomatic during the incubation stage of the infection.
- The hepatotrophic viruses cause hepatic injury either because of the host immune response or from direct viral damage to hepatocytes. Cellular and humoral immune response is directed against viral antigens found on the host hepatocyte membranes and/or circulating within the vascular compartment.
- Clinical symptoms are accompanied by moderate to marked elevations of the serum bilirubin, gamma globulin, and hepatic transaminases (4–10 times normal).
- Viral serologic markers and host antibodies are detectable during this stage of the illness.
- HBV is not cytopathic.
- The liver injury (like HAV infection) is immune related and T lymphocytes are important for both the host cellular and humoral responses.

CHRONIC VIRAL HEPATITIS

- A weak cell-mediated immune response has been demonstrated in patients with persistent HBV infection. In healthy carriers, an absent or poor cell-mediated response results in persistent viral replication but only minimal liver dam-

TABLE 23–1. Important Features of Hepatitis Viruses

	Hepatitis A	Hepatitis B	Hepatitis C	Hepatitis D	Hepatitis E	Hepatitis G
Virus	HAV	HBV	HCV	HDV	HEV	HGBV or HGV[a]
Family	Picornavirus	Hepadnavirus	Flavivirus	Satellite	Calcivirus	Flavivirus
Size (nm)	27	42	30–60	40	32	?
Genome	ssRNA	dsDNA	ssRNA	ssRNA	ssRNA	ssRNA
Incubation (d)	14–45	40–180	35–84	40–180 coinfection 14–45 superinfection	14–60	? ?
Transmission	Fecal–oral	Parenteral Sexual Perinatal Mucous membrane	Parenteral Sexual Perinatal (?) Mucous membrane	Parenteral Sexual (?) Perinatal	Fecal–oral	Parenteral
Serologic markers						
Antigens	HAVAg	HBsAg HBcAg HBeAg	HCVAg	HDVAg	Not available	?
Antibodies	Anti-HAV	Anti-HBs Anti-HBc Anti-HBe	Anti-HCV	Anti-HDV	Not available	?
Viral markers	HAV RNA	HBV DNA DNA polymerase	HCV RNA	HDV RNA	Not available	HGBV-C RNA
Clinical illness						
Children	Anicteric	Anicteric 70%	Anicteric 75%	Not known	High % anicteric	Not determined if associated with clinical illness
Adults	Icteric	Icteric 30%	Most Icteric	Icteric 25%	Not known	
Acute mortality (%)	0.3	0.2–1	0.2	2–20	10 (pregnancy)	?
Chronicity (%)	No	2–7 Neonates 90	70–80	2–70	No	?
Hepatocellular carcinoma	No	Yes	Yes	Yes	No	?

[a]Comprised of several RNA viruses: HGBV-A, HGBV-B, HGBV-C.

V

age. Patients with chronic HBV infection are deficient in producing, or responding to, interferon (IFN), which results in incomplete direction of the lymphocyte to the target infected cell.

- If persistent viral replication and subsequent hepatocyte inflammatory destruction continue unabated, the number of functioning hepatocytes gradually decreases over time, and fibrosis resulting from cellular repair mechanisms distorts the basic cellular architecture. Hepatic nodules are thus formed.
- When widespread, the hepatic fibrosis with nodule formation is termed cirrhosis.
- The consequences of cirrhosis do not differ with regard to initial etiologies and can produce portal hypertension and ascites.

▶ CLINICAL PRESENTATION

- The natural history of the infection is divided into three stages based on viral serologic markers: incubation, acute hepatitis, and convalescence.
- Clinical severity of illness varies widely from asymptomatic, anicteric hepatitis to fulminant hepatitis, a rapidly fatal disease.
- Most patients with acute viral hepatitis develop only a few, mild symptoms and minimal hepatocyte damage. This mild disease is called acute anicteric hepatitis.
- The minimal degree of liver cell damage is reflected by mild elevations of serum bilirubin, gamma globulin, and hepatic transaminases (ALT, AST) values to about twice normal.
- A subset of patients experiences enough hepatocyte destruction to produce significant liver function derangement characterized by interruption of bilirubin metabolism and flow, resulting in jaundice.
- The preicteric phase is frequently associated with nonspecific influenza-like symptoms consisting of anorexia, nausea, fatigue, and malaise. The icteric phase is generally accompanied by fever, right upper quadrant abdominal pain, nausea, vomiting, dark urine, acholic stools, and worsening of systemic symptoms.
- Clinical symptoms are accompanied by moderate to marked elevations of serum bilirubin, gamma globulin, and hepatic transaminase (4–10 times normal).
- Viral serologic markers and host antibodies are detectable during this stage of the illness.
- Most patients with either acute anicteric or icteric hepatitis go through the convalescence stage to complete recovery without developing complications or chronic sequelae.
- The duration of disease stages and the risk for developing chronic sequelae are virus-specific phenomena (Table 23–1).

HEPATITIS A

- HAV infection usually produces a mild, self-limited illness, lasting <2 months, and rarely results in fulminant hepatitis or death.

- Clinical symptoms are age dependent, with children less than 6 years old generally displaying a mild, influenza-like illness without clinical jaundice.
- In contrast, infected adults display the characteristic clinical syndrome of acute hepatitis with elevated hepatic transaminase levels and jaundice. Pruritus may be the primary complaint of this latter patient group.
- No cases of a chronic carrier state or chronic hepatitis have been reported. However, up to 20% of patients relapse with acute hepatitis 2–8 weeks after the initial illness.
- The diagnosis of acute HAV infection depends on clinical suspicion, characteristic symptoms (if present), elevated aminotransferases and bilirubin, and a positive anti-HAV IgM.

HEPATITIS B

- In the typical case of acute HBV infection, the incubation period is followed by a symptomatic prodromal phase consisting of malaise, fatigue, weakness, anorexia, myalgias, and arthralgias.
- Clinical manifestations of HBV infection are age dependent. Newborns infected with HBV are generally asymptomatic, while about one-third of adult patients with acute HBV infection have symptoms.
- Of the approximately 65% of adults with subclinical infection, most recover completely.
- Twenty-five percent have symptomatic illness with jaundice and 1% develop fulminant hepatic failure during the acute illness. Jaundice may persist for several weeks.
- Approximately 10% of adult patients develop chronic or persistent infection. Chronicity is more likely to occur in patients with mild, anicteric forms of acute hepatitis, and is much more likely to occur when the infection is acquired as a newborn or infant.
- Over a period of years, about 25% of adults with chronic HBV infection develop chronic active hepatitis (CAH), and a smaller percentage progress to cirrhosis.
- Extrahepatic manifestations such as neuropathies, glomerulonephritis, pancreatitis, and hematopoietic stem cell suppression (aplastic anemia, thrombocytopenia) are occasionally seen.
- HBV has four gene regions that produces viral proteins that can be detected: the nucleocapsid region (HBcAg and HBeAg), the envelope region (HBsAg), the P region (DNA polymerase), and the poorly understood X region. In typical acute HBV infection, antibody markers to HBV antigens proceed in sequence from the development of HBsAg followed by HBeAg (30–60 days prior to onset of clinical symptoms) through to the appearance of anti-HBs in late convalescence.

HEPATITIS C

- Acute hepatitis C is clinically indistinguishable from other types of viral hepatitis.

- The clinical course is generally mild with <25% of patients developing jaundice. Major complaints are frequently limited to fatigue and malaise.
- Similar to other types of viral hepatitis, the hepatic transaminase values in HCV hepatitis vary from mildly to markedly elevated.
- Extrahepatic manifestations occcassionally occur including polyarteritis nodosa, erythema multiforme, thrombocytopenia, serum sickness, rash, and blood dyscrasias.
- Unlike the other types, HCV infections characteristically demonstrate a pattern of widely fluctuating enzyme values over the course of the infection.
- An important feature of this form of hepatitis is that up to 90% of cases progress to chronic infection.
- Within 5 years, 30–35% develop CAH and 20–33% progress to cirrhosis. Others who eventually develop cirrhosis and hepatic failure do so after up to 20 years of indolent, asymptomatic infection. Chronic HCV infection-related cirrhosis is an etiologic factor in the development of hepatocellular carcinoma.
- Seroconversion to anti-HCV appears from 4–8 weeks following initial exposure. HCV RNA is detectable by PCR as early as 1 week after infection.
- To assess chronic HCV, liver biopsy is the only reliable indicator of disease progression.

DELTA HEPATITIS VIRUS

- Coinfection with HIV and HBV occurs commonly. Superinfection of HDV in patients with HBV infection may also occur.
- In coinfection, the acute delta hepatitis is almost always self-limited and follows the usual course of HBV infection. A biphasic rise in liver transaminase levels may be seen, the first peak attributable to HBV and the second to HDV.
- In HDV superinfection, delta viral replication occurs rapidly due to the persistent HBV infection, providing a ready supply of HBsAg. Liver injury and clinical symptoms appear quickly and may be severe, leading to a fulminant course. Many of these patients develop chronic liver disease and some develop HCC.
- In acute superinfection of a chronic HBV carrier, markers for acute HBV are negative. HBsAg, HDVAg, and anti-HDV IgM are usually present. In acute coinfection, HDVAg, anti-HDV IgM, and markers for acute HBV are usually present. Anti-HDV IgG follows. Currently, only a test for total anti-HDV is commercially available.

HEPATITIS E VIRUS

- Infection with HEV follows a benign course, except in pregnant women; women who contract HEV during the third trimester are at considerable risk for developing fulminant hepatitis. The diagnosis is made on clinical grounds in conjunction with exclusion of other viruses.

HEPATITIS G VIRUS

- HGV can cause persistent infection and viremia.
- It is not clear if HGV causes clinical illness.

FULMINANT HEPATITIS

- Liver injury that results in fulminant hepatic necrosis and hepatic failure is relatively rare. When it occurs, death results in a few days or weeks in nearly 80% of cases.
- In the United States, fulminant hepatitis is mainly due to HBV, and occasionally, HCV.
- Manifestations of hepatic failure include metabolic encephalopathy, coma, coagulation defects, ascites, and edema. In fulminant liver failure, complications include gastrointestinal hemorrhage, sepsis, cerebral edema, renal failure, lactic acidosis, and disseminated coagulopathy, with death resulting from bleeding, cerebral edema, hypoglycemia, infection, and/or multisystem organ failure.

CHRONIC HEPATITIS

- The clinical findings, course, and histologic features are similar in all patients with chronic hepatitis regardless of the etiologic agent. Sixty to 80% of all cases are related to HBV or HCV infection.
- In either chronic HBV or chronic HCV, if the patient is symptomatic, fatigue, malaise, anorexia, and weight loss are common. Many patients have a history of jaundice.
- On physical examination, hepatomegaly is usually present, but the stigmata of chronic liver disease (spider nevi, splenomegaly, palmar erythema, testicular atrophy, caput medusa, female escutcheon) are generally absent until late in the disease course.
- Mild but persistent elevations of the serum aminotransferases, bilirubin, and gamma globulin levels are most commonly seen.
- In chronic hepatitis C, the patient is often asymptomatic, yet liver biopsy demonstrates ongoing liver injury and progressive histologic changes. Serum enzymes can be normal or only mildly elevated; unfortunately, the patient is on an insidious course that progresses to complications after a period of 15–20 years.
- Complications of chronic hepatitis include cirrhosis, hepatic failure, and HCC.
- Unlike acute hepatitis, physical symptoms do not correlate well with the severity of liver injury. Many patients are asymptomatic and therefore are diagnosed only after elevated serum liver transaminases and/or HBsAg are found in patients' serum upon routine testing.

▶ DESIRED OUTCOME

- For acute hepatitis, the desired outcomes are resolution of symtoms, prevention of disease spread, and avoidance of hepatotoxic substances.
- For chronic hepatitis, the goals are to prevent progression to end-stage liver disease and to prevent infected patients from serving as reservoirs of infection.
- Since no known therapy can consistently eradicate HBV, end points of therapy include normalization of serum aminotransferase levels, disappearance of HBV DNA, and improvement of liver histology.

▶ TREATMENT

ACUTE HEPATITIS

- Management of acute viral hepatitis is primarily supportive. General measures include a healthy diet, rest, maintaining fluid balance, and avoidance of hepatotoxic drugs and alcohol.
- The patient should avoid becoming fatigued; bed rest may be required during the acute phase of the illness.
- Management includes monitoring for development of chronic liver disease and preventing disease spread.
- Treatments that offer no benefit include special diets, corticosteroids, and antiemetics. **Vitamin K** is recommended only if the patient has a prolonged prothrombin time. Hospitalization is necessary only for those who have prolonged vomiting, coagulation defects, or fulminant hepatitis.
- Preliminary trials and case reports of the use of **IFN-alpha** and **IFN-beta** as therapy in acute HBV and HCV infections are promising. Because not all studies have demonstrated IFN to be useful, further studies are ongoing to define the role of IFN in acute hepatitis treatment.
- The role of antiviral agents is undefined.

FULMINANT HEPATITIS

- There is no specific treatment for fulminant hepatic failure. Management of fulminant hepatitis focuses on recognition, prevention of complications, and aggressive treatment of complications.
- Measures that improve survival of patients include intensive supportive care plus early referral for liver transplantation. Specific measures include:
  - Fresh frozen plasma administered for bleeding.
  - H_2 blocker therapy given to prevent gastrointestinal (GI) bleeding.
  - Aggressive antibiotic therapy used for infections.
  - Management of cerebral edema including intracranial-pressure monitoring and administration of **mannitol** (0.3–0.4 g/kg body weight as a 20% solution).

- Urgent liver transplantation is the therapy of choice for patients with fulminant hepatic failure.
- Patients do not benefit from administration of corticosteroids, heparin, insulin, or glucagon.
- The role of antiviral therapy is not clear, however, **foscarnet** and the combination of **interferon** and **cyclosporin** have been beneficial.

CHRONIC VIRAL HEPATITIS

- General therapeutic measures in patients with compensated chronic hepatitis include exercise as tolerated, avoidance of potentially hepatotoxic drugs and chemicals (e.g., alcohol), and a healthy diet.
- Sexual partners and children of patients with chronic HBV should be vaccinated against hepatitis B. V
- Effective treatment of chronic viral hepatitis should decrease morbidity and mortality and prevent infected patients from serving as reservoirs of infection.
- The decision to treat patients with chronic hepatitis should not be made based on the presence or absence of symptoms or the degree of abnormality of biochemical tests. The activity and extent of the liver disease do not correlate with the level of serum aminotransferases or the patient's symptoms.

Interferons

- **IFN** is now the treatment of choice for patients with chronic HBV, HCV, and HDV infection. Unfortunately, only a proportion of patients respond favorably; considerably fewer have lasting response; very few are cured.
- Patients who should be treated with INF are those with persistent elevations in serum aminotransferases, detectable viral and antibody markers in serum, chronic hepatitis on liver biopsy, and compensated liver disease.
- Recombinant IFNs **(alfa-2A, Roferon A,** Hoffmann-LaRoche; **alpha-2B, Intron A,** Schering) and lymphoblastoid IFN **(alpha-n1, Wellferon,** Burroughs Wellcome) are effective in relieving symptoms and halting progression of chronic hepatitis B in one-third to one-half of immunocompetent patients from Western countries. Remissions are marked by loss of HBV DNA, HBeAg, normalization of serum aminotransferases, and improvement in liver histology.
- Effective dosing regimens of IFN in clinically stable adult patients with chronic HBV are 5 million units (MU) daily or 10 MU subcutaneously three times weekly for 4–6 months. One specific regimen (FDA-approved) for IFN-alpha-2b is 5 MU 5 days per week or 10 MU every other day for 16 weeks.
- Laboratory monitoring parameters during INF treatment include the serum aminotransferases, HBeAg, and HBV DNA. Clinical vigilance for decompensation is essential.

- Use of IFN in patients with cirrhosis is controversial. These patients appear to respond to IFN at rates similar to those with less advanced disease; however, IFN side effects are more common and severe, even life-threatening.
- Patients with HBV in whom IFN should not be used include those whose liver disease has progressed to end stage (very low serum albumin, prolonged prothrombin time, elevated bilirubin, leukopenia, thrombocytopenia, bleeding esophageal varices, ascites, encephalopathy, and/or progressive jaundice), those with liver disease of other causes, patients on immunosuppressive therapy, patients actively abusing drugs, those with significant psychiatric illness, and those with significant other medical illnesses such as cardiac, renal, or thyroid disease that are not successfully treated.
- IFN therapy may lead to complete eradication of HCV infection in long-term responders. IFN-alpha-2b at a dose of 3 MU three times weekly for 6–12 months is approved for treatment of chronic hepatitis C. One-third to one-half of treated patients improve, but approximately 50% of responders relapse within 6 months when therapy is discontinued. Patients who respond should be continued for at least 12 months.
- INF therapy for chronic HCV should be offered to those with disabling disease, histologically advanced disease, patients with rapidly progressive disease, those with markedly elevated aminotransferase levels, and those with serum HCV RNA levels.
- In chronic delta hepatitis, high-dose IFN-alpha treatment (5 MU daily or 9 MU three times weekly for at least 12 months) produces disease improvement in about 50% of patients. Unfortunately, relapse is common when therapy is stopped, and these patients have a high rate of drug-related adverse effects necessitating dosage reduction or termination of therapy. Prolonged IFN therapy may be necessary to achieve a sustained response.
- The side effects of IFN are frequent enough that the patient should be informed about them before treatment begins. Early side effects include fatigue, malaise, muscle aches, headaches, changes in appetite, fever, chills, nausea, and sleep disturbance. Late adverse reactions include those previously mentioned plus mild myelosuppression, bacterial infection, weight loss, loss of libido, thyroiditis, alopecia, IFN-induced autoimmune hepatitis (very rarely), exacerbation of other autoimmune phenomena, development of a variety of autoantibodies (e.g., antinuclear antibody, smooth muscle antibody, or antibody to thyroid microsomal antigen), irritability, anxiety, depression, attention span deficits, seizures, psychosis, delirium, and, most commonly, fatigue.

Monitoring of IFN Therapy

- Pre- and posttherapy monitoring for INF efficacy includes liver biopsy, and serum measurement of anti-HCV antibodies, RNA for HCV, HbcAg, HbsAg, HBV DNA, and anti-HBs for HBV.

- Ongoing monitoring of IFN toxicity includes complete blood counts weekly during the first 2 weeks of therapy and monthly thereafter. Other laboratory monitoring includes serum aminotransferases, prothrobin time, alkaline phophatase, albumin, and bilirubin concentrations before therapy, monthly for the first 3 months, then every 2 months.
- Patients should be asked about level of performance, mood changes, and symptoms.
- The dose of IFN should be decreased by 50% if any of the following develop: fatigue that interferes with the daily routine, daily nausea with occasional vomiting, granulocytopenia (less than 750/mm^3), and/or thrombocytopenia (less than 50,000/mm^3).
- IFN should be immediately discontinued if any of the following develop: fatigue that requires bed rest, vomiting more than twice daily, profound granulocytopenia (less than 500/mm^3), or thrombocytopenia (less than 30,000/mm^3).

Nucleoside Analogs in Chronic HBV

- **Lamuvidine** inhibits HBV replication in chronically HBV infected immunocompetent patients coinfected with HIV and HBV.
- Lamuvidine oral dose is 100–300 mg per day (300–600/d for those infected with both HIV and HBV) for 3–12 months.
- Side effects for lamuvidine include anemia, nausea, neuropathy, elevated serum lipases, and liver enzymes.

Corticosteroids

- Corticosteroids lead to reduced hepatic inflammation, but also result in dramatic increases in viral replication. In addition, withdrawal of the steroids causes a flare in hepatitis disease activity. Thus, corticosteroids can cause further decompensation and death in patients with clinically unstable disease.
- Patients with mild disease and low levels of HBV DNA can be tried on a 4- to 8-week tapering course of **prednisone** (e.g., decreasing daily doses of 60, 40, and 20 mg, each for 2 weeks) followed by IFN-alpha 3 to 5 MU daily for 16 weeks.
- Combination of corticosteroids with IFN have not demonstrated added benefit for HBV.

Liver Transplantation

- Liver transplantation is an option for patients with end-stage chronic liver disease secondary to viral infection. Recurrent viral hepatitis B infection in the transplanted liver almost always occurs.
- The primary strategy to protect the graft from reinfection is to transplant HBV DNA negative patients and then treat them for life with HBIG.

PREVENTION OF VIRAL HEPATITIS

- The mainstays of hepatitis prevention are risk reduction, education, passive immunization with immune globulins, and, for hepatitis B, active immunization through vaccination programs.

TABLE 23–2. Recommended Dosing of Havrix and Vaqta

Vaccine	Vaccine Recipient's age (years)	Dose	Volume (mL)	Number of Doses	Schedule (months)[b]
Havrix	2–18	720 ELISA units[a]	0.5	2	0, 6–12
	> 18	1440 ELISA units	1.0	2	0, 6–12
Vaqta	2–17	25 units	0.5	2	0, 6–18
	> 17	50 units	1.0	2	0, 6

[a]Havrix is also available as 360 ELISA units per dose, three-dose schedule for persons 2 to 18 years of age. The 720 ELISA units per dose, two-dose schedule is preferred.

[b]0 months represents the timing of the initial dose; subsequent numbers represent months after the initial dose.

- HBV and HCV spread are reduced, but not eliminated, through screening of blood donors and testing for HBsAg and anti-HCV.

HEPATITIS A PREVENTION

- The spread of HAV can be controlled by cautious handling of fomites contaminated with feces coupled with good handwashing techniques. Universal precautions are used to prevent hepatitis spread within the hospital setting.
- Prevention of HAV has traditionally focused on avoiding exposure as well as preexposure and postexposure prophylaxis with **immune globulin (IG).**
- A single dose of IG of 0.02 mL/kg intramuscularly (IM) is recommended for travelers to high-risk areas if travel is for <3 months. For lengthy stays, 0.06 mL/kg IM should be given every 3–5 months. Dosing is the same for adults and children.
- HAV vaccines given preexposure substantially lower the risk of infection. A protective efficacy of 94% has been demonstrated. Immunization is indicated for individuals 2 years of age or greater who are at increased risk of hepatitis A infection. Approved dosing recommendations are shown in Table 23–2. The initial dose ahould be given at least 2 weeks prior to expected exposure.
- The postexposure prophylactic benefit from IG is greatest early in the incubation period and is of no benefit more than 2 weeks after exposure. A single IG dose of 0.02 mL/kg IM is used for postexposure prophylaxis of hepatitis A.
- Groups recommended for active immunization against hepatitis A are given in Table 23–3.
- Vaccine side effects include injection site reactions, malaise, fever, fatigue, and GI upset.

TABLE 23–3. Groups Recommended for Active Immunization Against Hepatitis A

Persons at increased risk for HAV infection or its consequences
Travelers to countries that have high or intermediate endemicity of infection[a]
Injection drug users
Men who have sex with men
Persons who have occupational risk for infection, e.g., persons working with nonhuman primates
Persons who have chronic liver disease
Persons with clotting factor disorders
Children living in communities that have high rates of hepatitis A (help prevent recurrent epidemics)
Children and young adults in communities that have intermediate rates of hepatitis A (help control ongoing and prevent future epidemics)
Contacts of case-patients

[a]Africa, Asia (except Japan), the Mediterranean basin, Eastern Europe, the Middle East, Central and South America, Mexico, Greenland, and parts of the Caribbean. Essentially all countries other than Australia, Canada, Japan, New Zealand, countries in Western Europe, and Scandinavia.

TABLE 23–4. Recommendations for Hepatitis B Prophylaxis Following Percutaneous or Permucosal Exposure

Vaccination Status of Exposed Person	Treatment According to HBsAg Status of Source		
	HBsAg-Positive	*HBsAg-Negative*	*Source Not Tested or Unknown*
Unvaccinated	HBIG $\times$ 1[a] and initiate vaccine[b]	Initiate vaccine[b]	Initiate vaccine[b]
Previously vaccinated, known responder	Test exposed person for anti-HBs level If adequate,[c] no treatment If inadequate or titer unknown, 1 vaccine booster dose	No treatment	No treatment
Previously vaccinated, known nonresponder	HBIG $\times$ 2 (1 month apart) or HBIG $\times$ 1, plus 1 dose of vaccine	No treatment	If known high-risk source, may treat as if source were HBsAg-positive
Previously vaccinated, response unknown	Test exposed person for anti-HBs level If inadequate,[c] HBIG $\times$ 1, plus 1 vaccine booster dose If adequate, no treatment If titer unknown, 1 vaccine booster dose	No treatment	Test exposed person for anti-HBs level If inadequate,[c] vaccine booster dose If adequate, no treatment

[a]HBIG dose 0.06 mL/kg IM.
[b]HB vaccine dose; see Table 23–5.
[c]Adequate anti-HBs is $\geq$10 mIU/mL by radioimmunoassay or enzyme immunoassay.

HEPATITIS B PREVENTION

- Two products are available for prevention of hepatitis B infection: **hepatitis B vaccine,** which provides active immunity, and **HBIG,** which provides temporary passive immunity.
- The goals of immunization against viral hepatitis include prevention of the short-term viremia that can lead to transmission of infection, clinical disease, and chronic HBV infection.

Hepatitis B Immune Globulin (HBIG)

- Postexposure prophylaxis for HBV is recommended for perinatal exposure of infants of HBV-carrier mothers, sexual exposure to HBsAg-positive persons, accidental percutaneous or permucosal exposure to HBsAg-positive blood, and exposure of an infant to a caregiver who has acute hepatitis B.
- HBIG is used only in postexposure prophylaxis. The recommended dose is 0.06 mL/kg administered intramuscularly. Guidelines for use are listed in Tables 23–4 and 23–5.

Hepatitis B Vaccine

- **Hepatitis B vaccines** contain 5–40 g HBsAg protein per mL adsorbed onto aluminum per mL of vaccine, with thimerosal added as preserva-

TABLE 23–5. Recommended Doses and Schedules of Currently Licensed HB Vaccines

	Vaccine	
Group	*Recombivax HB[a] dose, µg (mL)*	*Engerix-B[a,b] dose, µg (mL)*
Infants of HBsAg-positive mothers	Adult formulation: 5 (0.5) Pediatric formulation: 5 (1)[c]	10 (0.5)
Other infants and children <11 years	Adult formulation: 2.5 (0.25) Pediatric formulation: 2.5 (0.5)[c]	10 (0.5)
Children and adolescents 11–19 years	5 (0.5)	10 (0.5)
Adults age 20 years and greater	10 (1.0)	20 (1.0)
Dialysis patients and other immunocompromised persons	40 (1.0)[d]	40 (2.0)[e,f]

[a]Usual schedules:

Infants: Three doses given at birth, at 1–2 months, and at 6–18 months or, for infants, with other routine immunizations at 1–2 months of age, 4 months, and 6–18 months.

Older children and adults: Three doses given at 0, 2, and 6 months or, at 0, 2, and 4 months. Higher titers of HBsAb are achieved with the last two doses of vaccine being spaced at least 4 months apart.

[b]Alternative approved schedule: Four doses, one given at 0, 1, 2, and 12 months.

[c]A special pediatric formulation of Recombivax HB is available that contains 5 µg/mL.

[d]Special formulation for dialysis patients.

[e]Two 1.0-mL doses given at different sites.

[f]Four-dose schedule recommended at 0, 1, 2, and 6 months.

tive. Side effects of the vaccine are soreness at the injection site, headache, fatigue, and fever.

- The dose of HBsAg to induce the desired antibody response/protective effect varies between the two available vaccines (Table 23–5).
- HBV vaccine is given as a series of three IM doses into the deltoid (anterolateral thigh in infants), given over a period of months. An adequate anti-HBs response is seen in more than 90% of healthy adults and 95% of infants and children.
- Dosing guidelines for infants are listed in Table 23–6. All infants (>2000 g) born to HbsAg-positive women should be vaccinated within 12 hours of birth with HBV vaccine and one dose of HBIG.
- Hepatitis B vaccines are inactivated and can be simultaneously administered with other vaccines.
- Postvaccination testing for immunity is only important for persons at risk of poor antibody response and for those at very high risk of exposure.
- Nonresponders and inadequate responders should be immediately revaccinated with one or two injections of vaccine and then every year or two thereafter.

TABLE 23–6. Recommended Schedule of Immunoprophylaxis to Prevent Perinatal or Sexual Transmission of HBV Infection

Vaccine Recipient	Immunoprophylaxis	Timing
Infant born to HBsAg-positive mother	Vaccine dose 1	Within 12 hours of birth
	HBIG[a]	Within 12 hours of birth
	Vaccine doses 2 and 3[b]	Usual schedule
Infant born to mother not screened for HBsAg	Vaccine dose 1	Within 12 hours of birth
	HBIG	If mother is found to be HBsAg-positive, administer dose to infant as soon as possible, but no later than 1 week after birth
	Vaccine doses 2 and 3[b]	Usual schedule
Sexual exposure	HBIG[d]	Single dose within 14 days of sexual contact
	Vaccine dose 1	At time of HBIG treatment[e]

[a] 0.5 mL intramuscularly, at a site different from that used for the vaccine.

[b] The four-dose schedule for Engerix-B can also be used.

[c] The first dose of vaccine is the same as that for the infant of an HBsAg-positive mother. If the mother is found to be HBsAg-positive, that dose is continued. If the mother is found to be HBsAg-negative, the remaining vaccine doses are those appropriate for other infants and children.

[d] 0.06 mL/kg intramuscularly.

[e] The first dose can be given at the same time as the HBIG dose but in a different site; subsequent doses should be given as recommended in Table 23–5.

- Hemodialysis patients have decreased seroconversion rates, decreased antibody titers to surface antigens, and a faster rate of loss of antibody after HBV vaccination. These patients require higher vaccine doses or an increased number of doses. A special formulation of **Recombivax HB** (40 mg/mL) is available for these patients. A more rapid rise in antibody concentration is observed with a 0-, 1-, 2-, and 6-month vaccination schedule in these patients, although overall conversion rate is similar whether the final (fourth) dose is given 6 or 12 months after the series begins.

Groups Recommended for Preexposure Vaccination

- The primary eradication strategy for hepatitis B is routine infant vaccination, which, over several decades, could eliminate transmission of the virus.
- The groups currently recommended for preexposure vaccination are listed in Table 23–7.

Postexposure Prophylaxis for Hepatitis B

- HBIG and HBV vaccine are recommended in combination for postexposure prophylaxis. The antibody response to the vaccine is not attenuated by administration of HBIG.

TABLE 23–7. High-Risk Groups Recommended for Preexposure Hepatitis B Vaccination

High-Risk Groups
All 11- to 12-year-old children who have not previously received hepatitis B vaccine
All unvaccinated children ages < 11 years who are Pacific Islanders or who reside in households of first-generation immigrants from countries where HBV is of high or intermediate endemicity
Health care and public safety workers who have occupational exposure to blood
Injection-drug users
Heterosexual individuals who have had more than one sexual partner in the previous 6 months and/or those with a recent episode of a sexually transmitted disease
Sexually active homosexual or bisexual males
Hemodialysis patients
Recipients of certain blood products (i.e., patients with hemophilia and other clotting disorders)
Clients and staff of institutions for the developmentally disabled
Household and sexual contacts of HBsAg positive persons
Household contacts of adoptees from countries where HBV is highly endemic
Populations where HBV is highly endemic (e.g., Alaskan Eskimos)
Inmates of long-term correctional facilities
International travelers to highly endemic HBV regions for >6 months and who have close contact with the local population; also short-term travelers who have contact with blood, or sexual contact with residents in high- or intermediate-risk areas
Unvaccinated infants under 12 months exposed to acute HBV infection through primary caregiver
Household contacts with blood exposure to a patient with acute HBV infection

[a]The CDC recommends that all newborns be vaccinated against hepatitis B.

- Hepatitis B vaccination is recommended for any person not previously vaccinated who is exposed to blood potentially containing HBsAg. The source should be tested for HBsAg. If positive, the exposed person should receive HBIG (Tables 23–4 and 23–5).
- Current recommendations also include administration of both HBIG and HBV vaccine to neonates with HBV exposure, although vaccination without HBIG may be effective.
- Hepatitis C prevention.
- No HCV vaccine is currently available.
- Progress that focuses on reducing HIV transmission should decrease HCV transmission in high-risk groups.

See Chapter 38, Viral Hepatitis, authored by Marsha A. Raebel, PharmD, FCCP, BCPS, and Shirley M. Palmer, PharmD, for a more detailed discussion of this topic.

Chapter 24

▶ INFLAMMATORY BOWEL DISEASE

▶ DEFINITION

There are two forms of idiopathic inflammatory bowel disease (IBD): ulcerative colitis, a mucosal inflammatory condition confined to the rectum and colon, and Crohn's disease, a transmural inflammation of gastrointestinal (GI) mucosa that may occur in any part of the GI tract. The etiologies of both conditions are unknown, but they may have a common pathogenetic mechanism.

▶ PATHOPHYSIOLOGY

- The major theories of the cause of IBD involve infectious or immunologic causes. The infectious theory assumes that the body is reacting normally to an unrecognized pathogen, whereas the immunologic theory assumes that the immune system is acting inappropriately to antigens to which most people are exposed, leading to an autoimmune reaction (Table 24–1).
- Ulcerative colitis and Crohn's disease differ in two general respects: anatomic sites and depth of involvement within the bowel wall. There is, however, overlap between the two conditions, with a small fraction of patients showing features of both diseases (Table 24–2).

ULCERATIVE COLITIS

- Ulcerative colitis is confined to the colon and rectum, and affects primarily the mucosa and the submucosa. The primary lesion occurs in the crypts of the mucosa (crypts of Lieberkuhn) in the form of a crypt abscess.

CROHN'S DISEASE

- Crohn's disease is a transmural inflammatory process. The terminal ileum is the most common site of the disorder (14–30%), but it may occur in any part of the GI tract.
- About two-thirds of patients have some colonic involvement, and 15–25% of patients have only colonic disease.
- Patients often have normal bowel separating segments of diseased bowel; that is, the disease is often discontinuous.
- Complications of Crohn's disease may involve the intestinal tract or organs unrelated to it. Small-bowel stricture and subsequent obstruction is a complication that may require surgery. Fistula formation is common and occurs much more frequently than with ulcerative colitis.

TABLE 24–1. Proposed Etiologies for Inflammatory Bowel Disease

Infectious Agents
- Viruses
- L-forms of bacteria
- Mycobacteria
- Chlamydia

Genetics
- Metabolic defects
- Connective tissue disorders

Environmental Factors
- Diet
- Smoking (Crohn's disease)

Immune Defects
- Altered host susceptibility
- Immune-mediated mucosal damage

Psychologic Factors
- Stress
- Emotional or physical trauma
- Occupation

TABLE 24–2. Comparison of the Clinical and Pathologic Features of Crohn's Disease and Ulcerative Colitis

Feature	Crohn's Disease	Ulcerative Colitis
Intestinal		
Malaise, fever	Common	Uncommon
Rectal bleeding	Intermittent about 50%	Common
Abdominal tenderness	Common	May be present
Abdominal mass	Very common (especially with ileocolitis)	Not present
Abdominal pain	Very common	Unusual
Abdominal wall and internal fistulas	Very common	Rare
Endoscopic		
Rectal disease	About 20%	Almost 100%
Diffuse, continuous symmetric involvement	Uncommon	Very common
Aphthous or linear ulcers	Common	Rare
Pathologic		
Continuous disease	Rare	Very common
Rectal involvement	Rare	Common
Ileal involvement	Very common	Rare
Asymmetry	Very common	Rare
Strictures	Common	Rare
Fistulas	Very common	Rare
Discontinuity	Common	Rare
Transmural involvement	Common	Rare
Crypt abscesses	Rare	Very common
Granulomas	Common	Rare

- Systemic complications of Crohn's disease are common, and similar to those found with ulcerative colitis. Arthritis, iritis, skin lesions, and liver disease often accompany Crohn's disease.

▶ CLINICAL PRESENTATION

ULCERATIVE COLITIS

- There is a very wide range of ulcerative colitis presentation. Symptoms may range from mild abdominal cramping with frequent small-volume bowel movements to profuse diarrhea.
- Most patients with ulcerative colitis experience intermittent bouts of illness after varying intervals with no symptoms.
- Mild disease has been defined as less than four stools daily without anemia, tachycardia, weight loss, or hypoalbuminemia, and severe disease as greater than six stools daily with the signs just listed.
- Patients with moderate disease have more prominent abdominal discomfort and usually present with diarrhea and bleeding as the major complaint. They may be noted to have a low-grade fever.
- With severe disease, the patient is usually found to be in acute distress, has profuse bloody diarrhea, and often has a high fever with leukocytosis and hypoalbuminemia. Often the patient is dehydrated and therefore may be tachycardic and hypotensive.

CROHN'S DISEASE

- As with ulcerative colitis, the presentation of Crohn's disease is highly variable. A single episode may not be followed by further episodes, or the patient may experience continuous, unremitting disease. Commonly, a patient may first present with a perirectal or perianal lesion.
- The course of Crohn's disease is characterized by periods of remission and exacerbation. Some patients may be free of symptoms for years, while others experience chronic problems in spite of medical therapy.

Complications

- Local complications (involving the colon) occur in the majority of ulcerative colitis patients. Relatively minor complications include hemorrhoids, anal fissures, or perirectal abscesses.
- A major complication is toxic megacolon, a severe condition that occurs in 1–3% of patients with ulcerative colitis or Crohn's disease.
- The risk of colonic carcinoma is much greater in patients with ulcerative colitis as compared with the general population.
- Approximately 11% of patients with ulcerative colitis have hepatobiliary complications including fatty liver, pericholangitis, chronic active hepatitis, cirrhosis, cholangiocarcinoma, and gallstones.
- Arthritis is found to be present in about 5% of patients. Arthritis is typically migratory and involves one or a few joints. The joints most often affected, in decreasing frequency, are the knees, hips, ankles, wrists, and elbows.

- Ocular complications, including iritis, uveitis, episcleritis, or conjunctivitis, occur in about 10% of patients with IBDs. The most commonly reported symptoms include blurred vision, headaches, eye pain, and photophobia.
- Skin and mucosal lesions are associated with IBDs, including erythema nodosum, pyoderma gangrenosum, and aphthalous ulceration. Most studies report 5–10% of IBD patients experience dermatologic or mucosal complications.

► DESIRED OUTCOME

Goals of treatment may vary considerably among patients and include
V resolution of acute inflammatory processes and attendant complications (e.g., fistulas, abscesses), alleviation of systemic manifestations (e.g., arthritis), maintenance of remission from acute inflammation, or surgical palliation or cure. The approach to the therapeutic regimen differs considerably with varying goals as well as with the two diseases, ulcerative colitis and Crohn's disease.

► TREATMENT

GENERAL APPROACH

- Treatment of IBD centers on agents used to lessen the inflammatory process. Aminosalicylates, corticosteroids, antimicrobials, and immunosuppressive agents such as azathioprine and 6-mercaptopurine are commonly used to treat active disease and, for some agents, to lengthen remission from disease.
- In addition to the use of drugs, surgical procedures are sometimes performed when active disease is not adequately controlled or when the required drug dosages pose an unacceptable risk of adverse effects.

NONPHARMACOLOGIC TREATMENT

Nutritional Support

- Proper nutritional support is an important aspect of the treatment of patients with IBD because patients with moderate to severe disease are often malnourished.
- Many patients with IBD, although not the majority, have lactase deficiency and therefore, diarrhea may be associated with milk intake. In these patients, avoidance of milk or supplementation with lactase generally improves their symptoms.
- The nutritional needs of the majority of patients can be adequately addressed with enteral supplementation. Patients who have severe disease may require a course of parenteral nutrition.

Surgery

- For ulcerative colitis, colectomy may be performed when the patient has disease uncontrolled by maximum medical therapy or when there are complications of the disease such as colonic perforation, toxic dilatation (megacolon), uncontrolled colonic hemorrhage, or colonic strictures.

- Although surgery (proctocolectomy) is curative for ulcerative colitis, this is not the case for Crohn's disease.
- The indications for surgery with Crohn's disease are not as well established as they are for ulcerative colitis, and surgery is usually reserved for the complications of the disease.

PHARMACOLOGIC THERAPY

- Drug therapy plays an integral part in the overall treatment of IBD. None of the drugs used for IBD is curative; at best they serve to control the disease process. V
- The major types of drug therapy used in IBD include aminosalicylates, corticosteroids, immunosuppressives **(azathioprine, 6-mercaptopurine, cyclosporin),** antimicrobials **(metronidazole),** and other agents used investigationally, such as immune enhancers (e.g., **levamisole** or **bacillus Calmette-Guerin, BCG**), mast cell stabilizers **(cromolyn sodium),** and antibodies against tumor necosis factor alpha.
- **Sulfasalazine,** an agent that combines a sulfonamide (sulfapyridine) antibiotic and 5-aminosalicylic acid (5-ASA, mesalamine) in the same molecule, has been used for many years to treat IBD. The active component of sulfasalazine is 5-ASA (mesalamine), which has a local anti-inflammatory effect on the lumen of the intestine; however, other mechanisms are still considered (Table 24–3).

TABLE 24–3. Mesalamine Derivatives for Treatment of Inflammatory Bowel Disease

Product	Trade Name(s)	Formulation	Dose/Day (g)	Site of Action
Sulfasalazine	Azulfidine	Tablet	4–6	Colon
Mesalamine	Rowasa, Salofalk, Claversal, Pentasa	Enema	1–4	Rectum, terminal, colon
	Rowasa	Suppository	1	Rectum
	Asacol	Mesalamine coated with Eudragit-S (delayed release acrylic resin)	2.4–4.8	Distal ileum and colon
	Pentasa	Mesalamine encapsulated in ethylcellulose microgranules (oral tablet)	2–4	Small bowel and colon
Olsalazine	Dipentum	Dimer of 5-ASA oral capsule	1.5–3	Colon
Balsalazide	Colazide	Capsule	2–6	Colon

- Corticosteroids and **adrenocorticotropic hormone (ACTH)** have been widely used for the treatment of ulcerative colitis and Crohn's disease and are used in moderate to severe disease.
- Immunosuppressive agents such as **azathioprine** and **6-mercaptopurine** (a metabolite of azathioprine) are sometimes used for the treatment of IBDs. These agents are generally reserved for cases that are refractory to steroids and may be associated with serious adverse effects such as lymphomas, pancreatitis, or nephrotoxicity.
- Antimicrobial agents, particularly **metronidazole,** are frequently used in attempts to control Crohn's disease. Metronidazole has been demonstrated to be of value in some patients with active Crohn's disease, particularly when it involves the perineal area or fistulas.

Ulcerative Colitis

Mild to Moderate Disease

- The first line of drug therapy for the patient with mild to moderate colitis is oral sulfasalazine or an oral mesalamine derivative.
- For proctitis or distal colitis the preferred therapy is rectally administered steroids or mesalamine.
- Sulfasalazine therapy should be instituted at 500 mg/d orally and increased every few days up to 4 g or the maximum tolerated (up to 8 g/d).
- Oral mesalamine derivatives (such as those listed in Table 24–3) are reasonable alternatives to sulfasalazine for treatment of ulcerative colitis (Figure 24–1).
- Steroids have a place in the treatment of moderate to severe ulcerative colitis. **Prednisone** dosages in the range of 40–60 mg/d have been superior to regimens of 20 mg/d in producing remission.
- Overall, steroids and sulfasalazine appear to be equally efficacious; however, the response to steroids may be evident sooner.
- **Transdermal nicotine** has been shown to improve symptoms of patients with active ulcerative colitis (when given along with mesalamine).

Severe or Intractable Disease

- Patients with uncontrolled severe colitis or incapacitating symptoms require hospitalization for effective management. Under these conditions, patients generally receive nothing by mouth to put the bowel at rest; however, the benefit of enteral nutrition in these patients has been demonstrated. Most medication is given by the parenteral route.
- With severe colitis, there is a much greater reliance on parenteral steroids and surgical procedures. Sulfasalazine or mesalamine derivatives have not been proven beneficial for treatment of severe colitis.
- Steroids have been valuable in the treatment of severe disease because the use of these agents may allow some patients to avoid colectomy. A trial of prednisone or parenteral equivalent of 1 mg/kg/d (up to 60 mg) is warranted in most patients before proceeding to colectomy, unless the condition is grave or rapidly deteriorating.

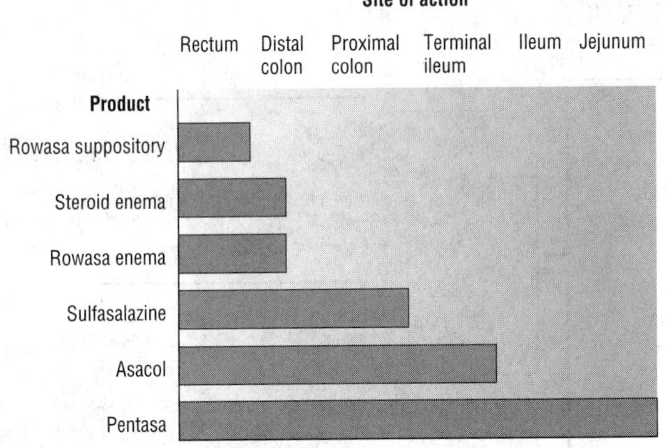

Figure 24–1. Site of activity of various agents to treat inflammatory bowel disease.

- Continuous intravenous infusion of cyclosporine (4 mg/kg/d) is recommended for patients with severe ulcerative colitis refractory to steroids.

Maintenance of Remission

- Once remission from active disease has been achieved, the goal of therapy is to maintain remission.
- The major agents used for maintenance of remission are sulfasalazine and the mesalamine derivatives.
- Steroids do not have a role in the maintenance of remission with ulcerative colitis because they have been demonstrated to be ineffective. Steroids should be gradually withdrawn after remission is induced (over 3–4 weeks). If they are continued, the patient will be exposed to steroid side effects without likelihood of benefits.
- Azathioprine has been demonstrated effective in preventing relapse of ulcerative colitis for periods of up to 2 years. However, 3–6 months may be required for beneficial effect.

Crohn's Disease (Figure 24–2)

Active Crohn's Disease

- The goal of treatment for active Crohn's disease is to achieve remission; however, in many patients, reduction of symptoms so that the patient may carry out normal activities or reduction of the steroid dose required for control is a significant accomplishment.
- In the majority of patients, active Crohn's disease is treated with **sulfasalazine**, **mesalamine** derivatives, or **steroids**, although **azathioprine**, **6-mercaptopurine**, or **metronidazole** are frequently used.

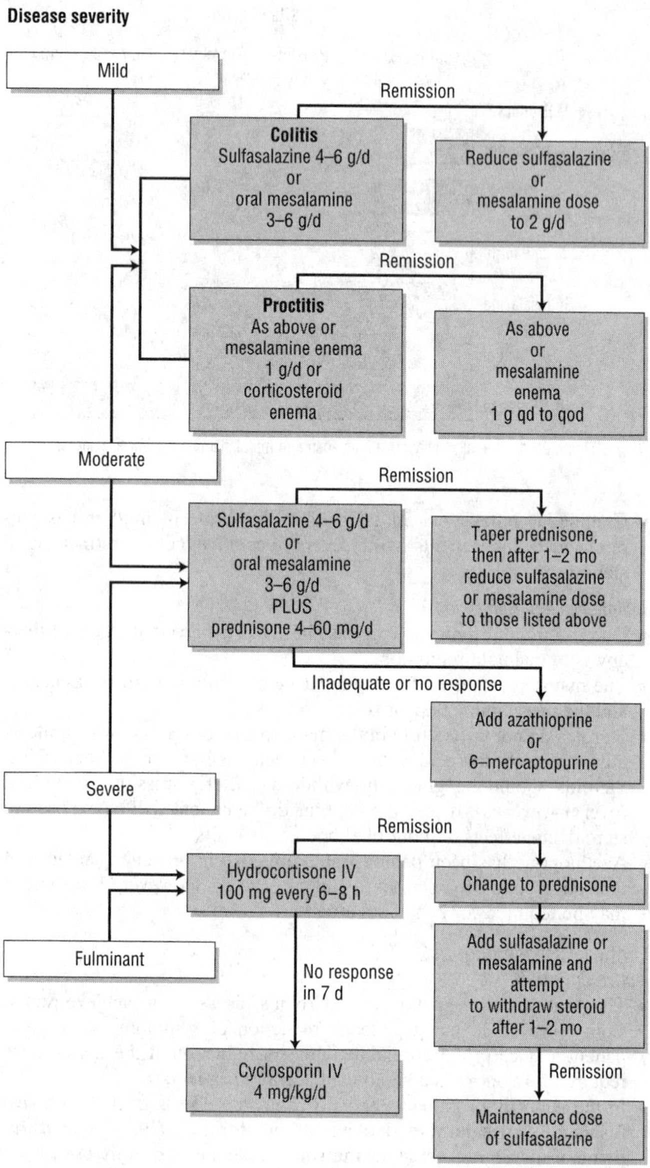

Disease severity

Mild

Remission

Colitis
Sulfasalazine 4–6 g/d
or
oral mesalamine
3–6 g/d

Reduce sulfasalazine
or
mesalamine dose
to 2 g/d

Remission

Proctitis
As above or
mesalamine enema
1 g/d or
corticosteroid
enema

As above
or
mesalamine
enema
1 g qd to qod

V

Moderate

Remission

Sulfasalazine 4–6 g/d
or
oral mesalamine
3–6 g/d
PLUS
prednisone 4–60 mg/d

Taper prednisone,
then after 1–2 mo
reduce sulfasalazine
or mesalamine dose
to those listed above

Inadequate or no response

Add azathioprine
or
6–mercaptopurine

Severe

Remission

Hydrocortisone IV
100 mg every 6–8 h

Change to prednisone

Add sulfasalazine or
mesalamine and
attempt
to withdraw steroid
after 1–2 mo

Fulminant

No response
in 7 d

Cyclosporin IV
4 mg/kg/d

Remission

Maintenance dose
of sulfasalazine

Figure 24–2. Treatment approaches for ulcerative colitis.

- Sulfasalazine is more effective when Crohn's disease involves the colon and in patients who have not undergone surgery for their disease.
- Other mesalamine derivatives (such as **Pentasa** or **Asacol**) that release mesalamine in the small bowel may be more effective than sulfasalazine for ileal involvement.
- Steroids are frequently used for the treatment of active Crohn's disease, particularly with more severe presentations. Steroids are preferred for treatment of severe Crohn's disease, mainly because these agents can be given parenterally and response to therapy may occur sooner.
- Once remission is achieved, however, it may prove difficult to reduce steroid dosage without reintroduction of active disease.
- Metronidazole may be useful in some patients with Crohn's disease, particularly in patients with colonic involvement or those with perineal disease.
- The immunosuppressive agents (azathioprine and 6-mercaptopurine) are generally limited to use in patients not achieving adequate response to standard medical therapy, or to reduce steroid doses when toxic doses are required. The usual dose of azathioprine is 2–2.5 mg/kg/d and 1–1.5 mg/kg/d for 6-mercaptopurine.
- Cyclosporine has also demonstrated benefit in active Crohn's disease. It appears that the dose of cyclosporine is important in determining efficacy. An oral dose of 5 mg/kg/d was not effective, whereas 7.9 mg/kg/d was effective. However, toxic effects limit application of the higher dosage.

Maintenance of Remission

- Prevention of recurrence of disease is clearly more difficult with Crohn's disease than with ulcerative colitis. Sulfasalazine and oral mesalamine derivatives are effective in preventing acute recurrences in quiescent Crohn's disease.
- Steroids also have no place in the prevention of recurrence of Crohn's disease; these agents do not appear to alter the long-term course of the disease.
- Although the published data are not consistent, there is evidence to suggest that azathioprine and 6-mercaptopurine are effective in maintaining remission in Crohn's disease.

SELECTED COMPLICATIONS

Toxic Megacolon

- The treatment required for toxic megacolon includes general supportive measures to maintain vital functions, consideration for early surgical intervention, and drugs (steroids and antimicrobials).
- Aggressive fluid and electrolyte management is required for dehydration.
- When the patient has lost significant amounts of blood (through the rectum), blood replacement is also necessary.

- Steroids in high dosages should be administered intravenously to reduce acute inflammation. Doses as high as 2 mg/kg/d of **prednisone** equivalent have been recommended (generally administered as **hydrocortisone**).
- Antimicrobial regimens that are effective against enteric aerobes and anaerobes (e.g., **aminoglycoside** with **clindamycin** or metronidazole, **imipenem,** or **extended-spectrum penicillin with a β-lactamase inhibitor**) should be administered from the time of diagnosis and continued until patient improvement is assured.

Systemic Manifestations

- The common systemic manifestations of IBD include arthritis, anemia, skin manifestations such as erythema nodosum and pyoderma gangrenosum, uveitis, and liver disease.
- Anemia may be a common problem where there is significant blood loss from the GI tract. When the patient can consume oral medication, **ferrous sulfate** should be administered.
- For arthritis associated with IBD, **aspirin** or other **NSAIDs** may be beneficial, as well as steroids.

► SPECIAL CONSIDERATIONS

PREGNANCY

- Drug therapy for IBD is not a contraindication for pregnancy, and most pregnancies are well managed in patients with these diseases. The indications for medical and surgical treatment are similar to those in the nonpregnant patient. If a patient has an initial bout of IBD during pregnancy, a standard approach to treatment should be initiated.

ADVERSE DRUG REACTIONS TO AGENTS USED FOR TREATMENT OF IBD

- Sulfasalazine is often associated with either dose related or idiosyncratic adverse drug effects. Dose-related side effects usually include GI disturbances such as nausea, vomiting, diarrhea, or anorexia, but may also include headache and arthralgia.
- Patients receiving sulfasalazine should receive oral **folic acid** supplementation since sulfasalazine inhibits folic acid absorption.
- Non–dose-related adverse effects of sulfasalazine include rash, fever, or hepatotoxicity most commonly, as well as relatively uncommon but serious reactions such as pancreatitis and hepatitis.
- Oral mesalamine derivatives may impose a lower frequency of adverse effects compared with sulfasalazine. Many patients who are intolerant to sulfasalazine will tolerate oral mesalamine derivatives.
- The well-appreciated adverse effects of corticosteroids include hyperglycemia, hypertension, osteoporosis, fluid retention and electrolyte disturbances, myopathies, psychosis, and reduced resistance to infec-

tion. In addition, corticosteroid use may cause adrenocortical suppression. Specific regimens for withdrawal of corticosteroid therapy have been suggested.

- Immunosuppressants such as azathioprine and 6-mercaptopurine have a significant potential for adverse reactions including bone marrow suppression and have been associated with lymphomas (in renal transplant patients) and pancreatitis.

▶ EVALUATION OF THERAPEUTIC OUTCOMES

- The success of therapeutic regimens to treat IBDs can be measured by patient-reported complaints, signs and symptoms, direct physician examination (including endoscopy), history and physical examination, selected laboratory tests, and quality of life measures.
- To create more objective measures, disease-rating scales or indices have been created. The Crohn's Disease Activity Index (CDAI) is a commonly used scale, particularly for evaluation of patients during clinical trials. The scale incorporates eight elements: (1) number of stools in the past 7 days; (2) sum of abdominal pain ratings from the past 7 days; (3) rating of general well-being in the past 7 days; (4) use of antidiarrheals; (5) body weight; (6) hematocrit; (7) finding of abdominal mass; and (8) a sum of symptoms present in the past week. Elements of this index provide a guide for those measures that may be useful in assessing the effectiveness of treatment regimens.
- Standardized assessment tools have also been constructed for ulcerative colitis. Elements in these scales include (1) stool frequency; (2) presence of blood in the stool; (3) mucosal appearance (from endoscopy); and (4) physician's global assessment based on physical examination, endoscopy, and laboratory data.

See Chapter 32, Inflammatory Bowel Disease, authored by Joseph T. DiPiro, PharmD, FCCP, and Robert Schade, MD, for a more detailed discussion of this topic.

Chapter 25

▶ NAUSEA AND VOMITING

▶ DEFINITION

Nausea is usually defined as the inclination to vomit or as a feeling in the throat or epigastric region alerting an individual that vomiting is imminent. Vomiting is defined as the ejection or expulsion of gastric contents through the mouth, often requiring a forceful event.

▶ PATHOPHYSIOLOGY

- Specific etiologies associated with nausea and vomiting are presented in Table 25–1.
- Table 25–2 presents specific cytotoxic agents categorized by their emetogenic potential. Although some agents may have greater emetogenic potential than others, combinations of agents, high doses, clinical settings, psychologic conditions, prior treatment experiences, and unusual stimuli to sight, smell, or taste may alter a patient's response to a drug treatment.
- A variety of other common etiologies have been proposed for the development of nausea and vomiting in cancer patients. These are presented in Table 25–3.
- The three consecutive phases of emesis include nausea, retching, and vomiting. Nausea, the imminent need to vomit, is associated with gastric stasis. Retching is the labored movement of abdominal and thoracic muscles before vomiting. The final phase of emesis is vomiting, the forceful expulsion of gastric contents due to gastrointestinal (GI) retroperistalsis.
- Vomiting is triggered by afferent impulses to the vomiting center, a nucleus of cells in the medulla. Impulses are received from sensory centers, such as the chemoreceptor trigger zone (CTZ), cerebral cortex, and visceral afferents from the pharynx and GI tract. When excited, afferent impulses are integrated by the vomiting center, resulting in efferent impulses to the salivation center, respiratory center, and the pharyngeal, GI, and abdominal muscles, leading to vomiting.
- The CTZ, located in the area postrema of the fourth ventricle of the brain, is a major chemosensory organ for emesis and is usually associated with chemically induced vomiting.
- Numerous neurotransmitter receptors are located in the vomiting center, CTZ, and GI tract. Examples of such receptors include cholinergic and histaminic, dopaminergic, opiate, serotonin, and benzodiazepine receptors. It is theorized that chemotherapeutic agents, their metabolites, or other emetic compounds trigger the process of emesis through stimulation of one or more of these receptors.

TABLE 25–1. Specific Etiologies of Nausea and Vomiting

Gastrointestinal
- Gastric outlet obstruction
- Motility disorders
- Intra-abdominal emergencies
  - Intestinal obstruction
  - Acute pancreatitis
  - Acute pyelonephritis
  - Acute cholecystitis
  - Acute cholangitis
  - Acute viral hepatitis
- Acute gastroenteritis

Cardiovascular Diseases
- Acute myocardial infarction
- Congestive heart failure
- Shock and circulatory collapse

Neurologic Processes
- Midline cerebellar hemorrhage
- Increased intracranial pressure
- Migraine headache
- Vestibular disorders
- Head trauma

Metabolic Disorders
- Diabetes mellitus (diabetic ketoacidosis)
- Addison's disease
- Renal disease (uremia)

Psychogenic Causes
- Self-induced
- Anticipatory

Therapy-Induced Causes
- Cytotoxic chemotherapy
- Radiation therapy
- Theophylline preparations (intolerance, toxic)
- Anticonvulsant preparations (toxic)
- Digitalis preparations (toxic)
- Opiates
- Amphotericin
- Antibiotics

Drug Withdrawal
- Opiates
- Benzodiazepines

Miscellaneous Causes
- Pregnancy
- Any swallowed irritant (foods, drugs)
- Noxious odors
- Operative procedures

TABLE 25–2. Emetogenic Potential of Cytotoxic Chemotherapy

Most Emetogenic	Moderate	Least Emetogenic
Amsacrine	Azacytidine	Asparaginase
Cisplatin	Etoposide	Bleomycin
Cyclophosphamide	Mitomycin C	Busulfan
Dacarbazine	Procarbazine	Chlorambucil
Dactinomycin	Thiotepa	Cytarabine
Daunorubicin		Diaziquone
Doxorubicin		Estramustine
Hexamethylmethamine		Floxuridine
Mechlorethamine		Fluorouracil
Mitoxantrone		Hydroxyurea
Nitrosoureas		Melphalan
Streptozocin		Mercaptopurine
		Methotrexate
		Teniposide
		Thioguanine
		Vinca alkaloids

TABLE 25–3. Nonchemotherapy Etiologies of Nausea and Vomiting in Cancer Patients

Fluid and electrolyte abnormalities	Peritonitis
Hypercalcemia	Metastases
Volume depletion	Brain
Water intoxication	Meninges
Adrenocortical insufficiency	Hepatic
Drug induced	Uremia
Opiates	Infections (septicemia, local)
Antibiotics	Radiation therapy
Gastrointestinal obstruction	
Increased intracranial pressure	

Adapted from Frytak S, Moertel CG. Management of nausea and vomiting in the cancer patient. JAMA *1981; 245:393–396, with permission. Copyright 1981, American Medical Association.*

- Anticipatory nausea and vomiting may be elicited either by specific stimuli associated with the administration of noxious, often cytotoxic, agents or by the anxiety associated with such treatments.

► CLINICAL PRESENTATION

- Nausea and vomiting may be classified as either simple or complex. The term simple applies to those episodes of nausea and/or vomiting described by one of the following criteria: (1) occur occasionally and are self-limiting or relieved by the minimal use of antiemetic methods or medications; (2) account for little patient deterioration such as fluid–electrolyte imbalances, pain, or noncompliance with prescribed therapies; or (3) are not related to the administration of or exposure to noxious agents.
- The term complex is used when describing a patient's clinical course as including symptoms that are not adequately or readily relieved by the administration of a single antiemetic method or medication; lead to progressive patient deterioration secondary to fluid–electrolyte imbalances, pain, or noncompliance with prescribed therapies; or are caused by noxious agents or psychogenic events.
- Nausea and vomiting occur frequently after operative procedures; those of the abdomen, eye, ear, nose, and throat are generally associated with higher incidences of nausea and vomiting than other procedures. Women experience a three-fold higher incidence of nausea and vomiting as compared to men, independent of the type of operation or anesthetic. Children are about twice as susceptible as adults.
- Other risk factors that may be associated with an increase in postoperative symptoms include patient variables such as obesity, increased age, a history of motion sickness or prior postoperative emesis, as well as

drug therapy variables such as the choice of premedication or general anesthetic agent.

- Many women experience nausea and vomiting during pregnancy; however, the etiology of hyperemesis gravidarum is not well understood.

▶ DESIRED OUTCOME

- The overall goal of antiemetic therapy is to prevent or eliminate nausea and vomiting without adverse effects.

▶ TREATMENT

GENERAL PRINCIPLES

- Most cases of nausea and vomiting are self-limiting, resolve spontaneously, and require only symptomatic therapy.
- Antiemetic therapy is indicated in patients with electrolyte disturbances secondary to vomiting, severe anorexia or weight loss, or progression of disease either owing to refusal of continued therapy or poor nutritional status.

NONPHARMACOLOGIC MANAGEMENT

- For patients with simple complaints, perhaps related to food or beverage consumption, a change in diet may be appropriate.
- Symptoms related to labyrinthe changes produced by motion may benefit by assuming a stable position.
- Psychogenic vomiting may benefit from psychological interventions, hypnosis, behavioral modifications, and guided mental imagery.

PHARMACOLOGIC MANAGEMENT

- Antiemetic drugs [over-the-counter (OTC) and prescription] are most often recommended to treat nausea and vomiting. Provided that a patient can and will adhere to oral dosing, a suitable and effective agent can often be selected; however, for certain other patients, oral medications may be inappropriate because of their inability to retain any appreciable oral ingestion. In these patients, the rectal or injectable route of administration might be preferred.
- Information concerning commonly available antiemetic preparations is compiled in Table 25–4.
- For most conditions, a single-agent antiemetic is preferred; however, for those patients not responding to such therapy and those receiving highly emetogenic chemotherapy, multiple-agent regimens are usually recommended.

TABLE 25–4. Common Antiemetic Preparations and Adult Dosage Regimens

Drug (Brand name)	Adult Dosage Regimen	Dosage Form/Route	Availability
Antacids			
Antacids (various)	15–30 mL every 2–4 h prn	Liquid	OTC
Histamine H_2 Antagonists			
Cimetidine (Tagament HB)	200 mg bid prn	Tab	OTC
Famotidine (Pepcid AC)	10 mg bid prn	Tab	OTC
Nizatidine (Axid AR)	75 mg bid prn	Tab	OTC
Ranitidine (Zantac 75)	75 mg bid prn	Tab	OTC
Antihistaminic–Anticholinergic Agents			
Benzquinamide (Emete-Con)	25–50 mg every 3–4 h prn	IM, IV	Rx
Buclizine (Bucladin-S)	50 mg twice daily	Tab	Rx
Cyclizine (Marezine)	50 mg every 4–6 h prn	Tab, IM	Rx/OTC
Dimenhydrinate (Dramamine)	50–100 mg every 4–6 h prn	Tab, chew tab, cap, liquid, IM, IV	Rx/OTC
Diphenhydramine (Benadryl)	10–50 mg every 4–6 h prn	Tab, cap, liquid, IM, IV	Rx/OTC
Hydroxyzine (Vistril, Atarax)	25–100 mg every 6 h prn	Tab, cap, liquid, IM	Rx
Meclizine (Bonine, Antivert)	25–50 mg every 24 h prn	Tab, chew tab, cap	Rx/OTC
Promethazine (Phenergan)	12.5–25 mg every 4–6 h prn	Tab, liquid, IM, IV, supp	Rx
Pyrilamine (Nisaval)	25–50 mg three to four times daily	Tab	Rx/OTC
Scopolamine (Transderm Scop)	0.5 mg every 72 h prn	Transdermal patch	Rx
Trimethobenzamide (Tigan)	200–250 mg three to four times daily prn	Cap, IM, supp	Rx
Phenothiazines			
Chlorpromazine (Thorazine)	10–25 mg every 4–6 h prn	SR, cap, tab, liquid, IM, IV	Rx
	50–100 mg every 6–8 h prn	Supp	Rx
Fluphenazine (Prolixin)	1.25–2.5 mg every 6–8 h prn	Tab, liquid, IM	Rx
Perphenazine (Trilafon)	8–30 mg/d divided prn	Tab, liquid, IM, IV	Rx
Prochlorperazine (Compazine)	5–10 mg three to four times daily prn	SR, cap, tab, liquid IM, IV	Rx
	25 mg twice daily prn	Supp	Rx

Promazine (Sparine)	25–50 mg every 4–6 h prn	Tab, IM	Rx
Thiethylperazine (Torecan)	10 mg 3 times daily	Tab, IM, supp	Rx
Cannabinoids			
Dronabinol (Marinol)	5–7.5 mg/m^2 every 2–4 h prn	Cap	Rx (C-II)
Nabilone (Cesamet)	1–2 mg two to three times daily prn	Cap	Rx (C-II)
Butyrophenones			
Haloperidol (Haldol)	1–5 mg every 12 h prn	Tab, liquid, IM, IV	Rx
Droperidol (Inapsine)	2.5–5.0 mg every 4–6 h prn	IM, IV	Rx
Corticosteroids			
Dexamethasone (Decadron)	10 mg prior to chemotherapy, repeat with 4–8 mg every 6 h for total of four doses	IV	Rx
Methylprednisolone (Solu-Medrol)	125–500 mg every 6 h for total of four doses	IV	Rx
Benzodiazepines			
Lorazepam (Ativan)	0.5–4.0 mg prior to chemotherapy	IV	Rx (C-IV)
Diazepam (Valium)	2–5 mg every 3 h	Tab	Rx (C-IV)
Selective Serotonin Antagonists			
Dolasetron (Anzemet), for CINV	1.8 mg/kg 30 min prior to chemotherapy (undiluted, up to 100 mg over 30 sec, or diluted, over 30 min	IV	Rx
	or		
	100 mg within 1 h before chemotherapy	Tab	Rx
Dolasetron (Anzemet), for PONV undiluted as single injection	12.5 mg 15 min before the cessation of anesthesia	IV	Rx
	or		
	100 mg within 2 h before surgery	Tab	Rx
Granisetron (Kytril), for CINV	10 μg/kg prior to chemotherapy (diluted, infuse, over 5 min, or undiluted over 30 sec)	IV	Rx

continued

TABLE 25–4. continued

Drug (Brand name)	Adult Dosage Regimen	Dosage Form/Route	Availability
Granisetron (Kytril) for PONV	20–40 μg/kg 30 min before end of anesthesia	IV	Rx
Ondansetron (Zofran), for CINV	32 mg prior to chemotherapy as a single dose (diluted, give over 15 min), or 0.15 mg/kg prior to chemotherapy, repeat at 4 and 8 h	IV	Rx
	or		
	8 mg 30 min prior to chemotherapy, repeat at 4 and 8 h and every 12 h for 1–2 days after chemotherapy completion	Tab	Rx
Ondansetron (Zofran), for PONV	4 mg prior to induction of anesthesia or postoperatively (undiluted, give over 2–5 min)	IV	Rx
	or		
	16 mg given 1 h before anesthesia	Tab	Rx
Miscellaneous Agents			
Metoclopramide (Reglan), for CINV	1–2 mg/kg every 2 h × 2, then every 3 h × 3	IV	Rx
Metoclopramide (Reglan), for PONV	10–20 mg about 10 min prior to anesthesia	IV	Rx
Metoclopramide (Reglan), for delayed CINV	0.5 mg/kg or 20 mg every 6 h prn, days 2 to 4	Tab	Rx
Dextrose, fructose, phosphoric acid (Emetrol)	15–30 mL every 1–3 h prn	Liquid	OTC
Diphenidol (Vontrol)	25–50 mg every 4 h prn	Tab	Rx

Rx, prescription; OTC, over the counter; cap, capsule; chew tab, chewable tablet; IM, intramuscular; IV, intravenous; liquid, oral syrup, concentrate, suspension; SR cap, sustained-release capsule; supp, rectal suppository; tab, tablet; CINV, chemotherapy-induced nausea and vomiting; PONV, postoperative nausea and vomiting.

- The treatment of simple nausea and vomiting usually requires minimal therapy. Both OTC and prescription drugs useful in the treatment of simple nausea and vomiting are usually effective in small, infrequently administered doses.
- The management of complex nausea and vomiting may require aggressive drug therapy, possibly with more than one antiemetic agent.
- For patients receiving highly emetogenic chemotherapy, antiemetic regimens may include one or more of the following agents: **prochlorperazine, metoclopramide, ondansetron, granisetron, dexamethasone,** or **lorazepam** (see the section "Chemotherapy-induced Nausea and Vomiting" [CINV]).

DRUG CLASS INFORMATION

Antacids

- Single or combination OTC antacid products, especially those containing magnesium hydroxide, aluminum hydroxide, and/or calcium carbonate, may provide sufficient relief of simple nausea/vomiting, primarily through gastric acid neutralization.
- Common antacid dosage regimens for the relief of nausea and vomiting include one or more small doses of single- or multiple-agent products.

Antihistamines, Anticholinergics

- Antiemetic drugs from the antihistaminic–anticholinergic category may be appropriate in the treatment of simple symptomology. However, when used alone, each provides little efficacy in patients with more complex complaints such as those caused by cytotoxic chemotherapy.
- Adverse reactions that may be apparent with the use of the antihistaminic–anticholinergic agents primarily include drowsiness or confusion, blurred vision, dry mouth, urinary retention, and possibly tachycardia, particularly in elderly patients.

Phenothiazines

- Phenothiazines are most useful in patients with simple nausea and vomiting or in those receiving mildly emetogenic doses of chemotherapy.
- Rectal administration is most preferred when parenteral administration is impractical or oral medications cannot be retained and are therefore ineffective.
- In many patients, low doses of phenothiazine drugs may not be effective, while larger doses may produce unacceptable risks.
- Problems associated with these drugs include troublesome and potentially dangerous side effects, including extrapyramidal reactions, hypersensitivity reactions with possible liver dysfunction, marrow aplasia, and excessive sedation.

Butyrophenone (Haloperidol and Droperidol)

- Preoperative doses may range from 2.5 to 10 mg, while dosage regimens during cytotoxic chemotherapy have been documented as low as

0.5–2.5 mg by intermittent injection to as great as 1.0–1.5 mg/h by IV infusion.
- Adverse reactions resulting from the use of the butyrophenone compounds primarily include sedation and the possibility of dystonic reactions.

Corticosteroids

- Corticosteroids have been used successfully in the management of CINV with few problems.
- Reported adverse effects have included mood changes ranging from anxiety to euphoria as well as headache, a metallic taste in the mouth, abdominal discomfort, hyperglycemia, and itchy throat.

Metoclopramide

- **Metoclopramide** increases lower esophageal sphincter tone, aids gastric emptying, and accelerates transit through the small bowel, possibly through the release of acetylcholine.
- Because the adverse reactions to metoclopramide include extrapyramidal effects, IV **diphenhydramine** 25–50 mg should be prophylactically administered or provided on-call for its anticipated need.

Serotonin Antagonists (Ondansetron, Granisetron, Dolasetron)

- 5-HT_3 selective serotonin antagonists act by blocking serotonin receptors located in the area postrema and possibly vagal afferent fibers in the upper GI tract.
- Although potentially important agents for cancer patients, 5-HT_3 serotonin receptor antagonists have provided no beneficial effects in reducing motion sickness when compared with placebo.

Other Agents

- Phosphorated carbohydrate solutions (mixtures of fructose, dextrose, and phosphoric acid) are available OTC and may be administered in 15- to 30-mL doses as often as every 3 hours or as needed. This combination is safe and effective in patients with morning sickness.

CHEMOTHERAPY-INDUCED NAUSEA AND VOMITING

Droperidol

- **Droperidol,** usually given intravenously, has been documented as safe and effective, even in ambulatory cancer patients.
- Although the optimal antiemetic dose of droperidol for patients receiving chemotherapy is not well established, many patients benefit from small doses, particularly when combined with other antiemetic drugs.

Corticosteroids

- During therapy with mildly to moderately emetogenic agents, **dexamethasone** appears to be comparable to **metoclopramide** and superior to **prochlorperazine** when each is used alone; however, metoclopramide has shown greater efficacy with highly emetogenic regimens, especially those including cisplatin.

- Dexamethasone has often been administered parenterally as a single dose of 8–20 mg prior to chemotherapy, followed by oral doses of 4–12 mg up to 24 hours after completion of chemotherapy. Usually, **methylprednisolone** has been administered prior to chemotherapy in a dose of 250 mg. After chemotherapy, up to four subsequent doses have been given.

Metoclopramide

- **Metoclopramide** is commonly prescribed in multiagent combination protocols for the prevention and treatment of complex nausea and vomiting in response to chemotherapy administration, particularly cisplatin.
- Metoclopramide is given in high doses (1–2 mg/kg intravenously), with one dose administered approximately 30 minutes prior to chemotherapy. Up to four subsequent doses are given at 2-hour intervals after chemotherapy.

5-HT_3 Serotonin Antagonists (Ondansetron, Granisetron, Dolasetron)

- Several selective 5-HT_3 serotonin antagonists, are safe and effective in the treatment of nausea and vomiting associated with cytotoxic chemotherapy and radiation therapy.
- **Ondansetron** is usually administered intravenously 30 minutes prior to chemotherapy at a dose of 0.15 mg/kg over 15 minutes. Similar subsequent doses are given 4 and 8 hours after the first dose.
- In adults and children at least 2 years of age, **granisetron** should be intravenously infused in a dose of 10 mg/kg over 5 minutes, beginning within 30 minutes before the initiation of chemotherapy, only on the day(s) chemotherapy is given. Oral doses of 1 mg may be used in adults.
- Some patients have experienced a reduction of efficacy with multiple-day chemotherapy or after several cycles of chemotherapy. In this situation, some clinicians recommend the addition of a corticosteroid to the regimen to increase the response rate.

Dronabinol and Nabilone

- The cannabinoids **dronabinol** and **nabilone** are effective antiemetic agents, even when other regimens have failed. Dronabinol, D-9-tetrahydrocannabinol (THC), is the major psychoactive substance present in marijuana.
- Cannabinoids are only indicated for nausea and vomiting associated with cancer chemotherapy.
- There is a strong correlation between a subjective "high" and antiemetic efficacy. Nabilone has been associated with less euphoric effects than dronabinol.

- Administration of the cannabinoids should be initiated the night before chemotherapy because failure to achieve adequate blood concentrations will likely result in vomiting.

Benzodiazepines

- Benzodiazepines (particularly **lorazepam**) represent the best of the therapeutic alternatives in the treatment of anticipatory nausea and vomiting. Dosage regimens include one dose before and multiple doses after each treatment with cytotoxic chemotherapy.

POSTOPERATIVE NAUSEA AND VOMITING

- A variety of pharmacologic approaches are available and may be prescribed as single or combination therapy for nausea and vomiting following an operative procedure including **promethazine, prochlorperazine, scopolamine, diphenhydramine, lorazepam,** and **ephedrine.**
- With or without antiemetic therapy, nonpharmacologic methods (including assisting patients with movement and providing particularly close attention to adequate hydration and pain management) may be effective in reducing the potential for emesis and should be universally applied.
- Metoclopramide has been of inconsistent value for postoperative nausea and vomiting.
- Selective serotonin antagonists are very effective in the prevention of postoperative nausea and vomiting but are much more expensive than alternative agents.

DISORDERS OF BALANCE

- Beneficial therapy for patients with nausea and vomiting associated with disorders of balance can reliably be found among the antihistaminic–anticholinergic agents, particularly scopolamine.
- Neither the antihistaminic nor the anticholinergic potency appears to correlate well with the ability of these agents to prevent or treat the nausea and vomiting associated with motion sickness.

COMBINATION ANTIEMETIC PROTOCOLS

- The management of complex nausea and vomiting may require various combinations of from two to five antiemetic drugs.
- The primary goal of combination antiemetic regimens is to select beneficial agents that have different pharmacologic mechanisms as well as toxic effects that are not considered additive or synergistic. Combinations often include **metoclopramide, diphenhydramine,** and **dexamethasone**.
- Other agents that may be added to the regimen include droperidol, diazepam, **thiethylperazine, secobarbital, pentobarbital, chlorpromazine,** or **prochlorperazine**.
- Dexamethasone may be combined with **ondansetron** or **granisetron**.

- The ideal multiagent antiemetic protocol has not been well defined. Protocols utilizing injectable metoclopramide or a serotonin antagonist appear to have a high degree of efficacy in preventing nausea and vomiting, even in patients receiving cisplatin.

ANTIEMETIC USE DURING PREGNANCY

- Agents that have commonly been prescribed during pregnancy include phenothiazines (**prochlorperazine** and **promethazine**), the antihistaminic–anticholinergic agents (**dimenhydrinate, diphenhydramine, meclizine,** and **scopolamine**), **metoclopramide,** and **pyridoxine.**
- The efficacy of antiemetics has been questioned while the importance of other management plans (including emphasis on fluid and electrolyte management, vitamin supplements, and efforts aimed at reducing psychosomatic complaints) has been addressed.
- Presently, **cyclizine** and **meclizine** are considered the drugs of choice for the treatment of nausea and vomiting during pregnancy.
- Teratogenicity is a major consideration for the use of antiemetic drugs during pregnancy and is the primary factor that dictates the drug of choice. Of the agents commonly used, those that have demonstrated teratogenicity in animals include diphenhydramine, meclizine, prochlorperazine, and thiethylperazine; however, in humans meclizine has not been shown to have these same effects.
- Most authors currently do not recommend metoclopramide because its use during pregnancy requires further study. In addition, serotonin antagonists cannot be recommended in this setting, even though animal studies to date have revealed no harm.

► EVALUATION OF THERAPEUTIC OUTCOMES

- The etiology of a patient's nausea and vomiting determines the expected outcome of antiemetic therapy. Depending on their ability to tolerate antiemetics, symptomatic relief is often unattainable until definitive therapy can be instituted (i.e., delivery of fetus, GI surgery, correction of metabolic disorders, or removal of emetogenic agents).
- If nausea and vomiting persist despite maximal and frequent dosing of an antiemetic agent, an agent with a different mechanism of action is administered. In addition, the patient should be examined closely to elicit any signs of volume contraction and assess the need for aggressive fluid replacement.
- Individualized therapy is recommended through drug selection and dosage adjustment.
- Monitoring criteria for drug therapy includes the subjective assessment of the severity of nausea as well as objective parameters such as the number of vomiting episodes each day, the volume of vomitus lost, and evaluation of fluid, acid–base balance, and electrolyte status, with particular attention to serum sodium, potassium, and

chloride concentrations. In addition, evaluation of renal function may become important, particularly in patients with volume contraction and progressive electrolyte disturbances. Specific parameters include daily urine volume, urine specific gravity, and urine electrolyte concentrations.

- Physical assessment of patients should include evaluation of mucous membranes and skin turgor, since dryness of these tissues may be indicative of significant volume loss.

See Chapter 33, Nausea and Vomiting, authored by A. Thomas Taylor, PharmD for a more detailed discussion of this topic.

Chapter 26

▶ PANCREATITIS

▶ DEFINITION

Acute pancreatitis (AP) is an inflammatory disorder of the pancreas resulting from premature activation of proteolytic enzymes within the pancreas. It is characterized by a discrete episode of symptoms, with restoration of normal exocrine and endocrine function when the cause is removed.

Chronic pancreatitis (CP) results in functional and structural damage to the pancreas that persists after the causative factor is eliminated. The disease is often progressive and loss of pancreatic function is irreversible.

▶ PATHOPHYSIOLOGY

- The etiologic factors associated with AP are presented in Table 26–1. Ethanol abuse (30%) and gallstone-associated biliary tract disease (30–70%) account for most cases in the United States. A cause cannot be identified in 10–15% of cases.
- A number of medications have been implicated in AP, but a causal association is difficult to confirm because ethical and practical considerations prevent rechallenge with the suspected agent.
- Table 26–2 lists drugs according to their certainty to cause AP. A definite association is based on the temporal relationship of drug administration to abdominal pain and hyperamylasemia or on a positive response to rechallenge with the offending agent. Suggestive evidence exists for drugs with a probable association, whereas evidence is inadequate or contradictory for drugs having a possible association.

ACUTE PANCREATITIS

- The pathophysiology of AP is related to autodigestion of the pancreas.
- Several mechanisms may initiate enzymatic activation within the pancreas, including reflux of duodenal contents containing enterokinase, activated pancreatic enzymes, and bile salts into the pancreatic duct; disruption of the pancreatic ducts and extravasation of juice as a result of gallstone-induced ductal hypertension; and intracellular activation of proteases by lysosomal enzymes.
- After initial acinar cell injury, pancreatic enzymes leak into the interstitium and cause edema and inflammation. Lipase damages fat cells, producing substances that cause further pancreatic and peripancreatic injury.
- Injured acinar cells liberate chemoattractants that attract neutrophils, macrophages, and other cells to the area of inflammation. Leukocyte stimulation results in the release of a wide variety of destructive mediators, such as elastase, platelet activating factor, reactive oxygen

TABLE 26–1. Etiology of Acute Pancreatitis

Structural: gallstones, pancreatic tumors, sphincter of Oddi dysfunction
Toxins: ethanol consumption, scorpion venom, organophosphorous insecticides
Infectious: bacterial, viral, parasitic
Metabolic: hyperlipidemia, hypercalcemia
Medications: (see Table 26–2 for specific drugs)
Trauma: accidental pancreatic trauma, postoperative pancreatitis, ERCP[a]
Vascular: vasculitis, atherosclerosis, coronary bypass surgery
Miscellaneous: congenital, idiopathic, cystic fibrosis, Crohn's disease

[a] ERCP, endoscopic retrograde cholangiopancreatography.

TABLE 26–2. Medications Associated With Acute Pancreatitis

Definite Association	Probable Association	Possible Association	
5-Aminosalicylic acid	Ampicillin	Acetaminophen	Interleukin-2
Asparaginase	Bumetamide	Amiodarone	Isoniazid
Azathioprine	Calcium	Amoxapine	Isotretinoin
Didanosine	Cimetidine	Carbamazepine	Ketoprofen
Estrogens	Chlorthalidone	Cholestyramine	Lipid emulsion
Furosemide	Cisplatin	Clarithromycin	Mefenamic acid
Pentamidine	Clozapine	Clonidine	Metolazone
6-Mercaptopurine	Corticosteroids	Cyclosporine	Nitrofunantoin
Methyldopa	Cytarbine	Cyproheptadine	Octreotide
Metronidazole	Enalapril	Danazol	Ondansetron
Sulfonamides	Ethacrynic acid	Diazoxide	Opiates
Sulindac	Ifosfamide	Diphenoxylate	Oxyphenbutazone
Tetracycline	Lisinopril	Ergotamine	Paclitaxel
Thiazide diuretics	Meglumine antimoniate	Erythromycin	Phenolphthalein
Valproic acid	Phenformin	Famciclovir	Propoxyphene
	Piroxicam	Granisetron	Rifampicin
	Procainamide	Gold therapy	Ranitidine
	Salicylates	Ibuprofen	Tryptophan
	Sodium stibogluconate	Indomethacin	Warfarin
	Zalcitabine	Interferon-α	

species, and cytokines. Prostaglandins, histamine, and kinins are released from the inflamed pancreas into the circulation causing vascular permeability, vasodilation, and tissue edema.

- When digestive enzymes and toxic products of leukocyte secretion enter the circulation, they combine to produce widespread injury of extra-abdominal organs.
- Local complications include acute fluid collection, pancreatic necrosis, abscess, pseudocyst formation, and pancreatic ascites. Systemic complications include pulmonary, cardiovascular, hematologic, renal, metabolic, and central nervous system abnormalities.

CHRONIC PANCREATITIS

- Chronic pancreatitis results in functional and structural damage to the pancreas that persists after the causative factor is eliminated. In contrast to ethanol-induced CP, structural and functional changes may improve in obstructive CP when the obstruction is removed.
- In most individuals, CP is progressive and loss of pancreatic function is irreversible. Permanent destruction of pancreatic tissue usually leads to exocrine and endocrine insufficiency.
- Cystic fibrosis is a cause of pancreatic exocrine insufficiency in children.
- Prolonged ethanol consumption is the main cause of CP in the United States, accounting for approximately 70% of all cases, while half of the remaining 30% of nonethanol cases are idiopathic.
- Infrequent causes of CP include hyperparathyroidism (and other chronic hypercalcemic states), protein-calorie malnutrition, heredity, trauma, pancreatic divisum, and obstruction of the main pancreatic duct by tumors, scars, stenosis, and pseudocysts. Although cholelithiasis may coexist with CP, gallstones rarely lead to chronic disease.
- In ethanol-induced CP, changes in the composition of pancreatic secretion lead to the precipitation of protein within the pancreatic ducts. The precipitates form protein plugs that occlude the secondary pancreatic ducts, causing duct dilation and increased intraductal pressure, inflammation, acinar cell atrophy, fibrosis, scarring, and eventual calcification.
- A minority of patients develop complications including pancreatic pseudocyst, abscess, and ascites or common bile duct obstruction leading to cholangitis or secondary biliary cirrhosis.

► CLINICAL PRESENTATION

ACUTE PANCREATITIS

- The spectrum of acute pancreatitis varies from mild, which is usually self-limiting, to severe, in which the severity of the attack correlates with the degree of the pancreatic involvement and complications.
- Typical signs and symptoms and their incidence include abdominal pain (95%), radiation of pain to back (50%), abdominal distention

(75%), nausea and vomiting (80%), low-grade fever (75%), hypotension (30%), mental aberrations (25%), and jaundice (20%).
- The initial presentation ranges from mild abdominal discomfort to excruciating pain, shock, and respiratory distress. Abdominal pain, the major symptom of nearly all patients, is usually epigastric, often radiating to either of the upper quadrants or the back. The onset is usually sudden and the intensity is often described as "knifelike" or "boring." Generally, the pain of AP tends to be steady and usually persists for several days.
- The majority of patients with AP recover uneventfully. Mortality rates appear to be influenced by the etiology of the disease and whether the acute attack is an initial or recurrent episode.

CHRONIC PANCREATITIS

- The main features of CP are abdominal pain, malabsorption, weight loss, and diabetes. Prolonged jaundice occurs in about 10% of patients.
- Abdominal pain is the most prominent clinical feature and is classically described as dull, constant, epigastric, and radiating to the back.
- Steatorrhea (excessive loss of fat in the feces) and azotorrhea (excessive loss of protein in the feces) are seen in the majority of patients once significant pancreatic destruction occurs.
- Diarrhea may occur secondary to fat malabsorption.
- Nausea, vomiting, anorexia, and weight loss are often seen.
- Pancreatic diabetes is usually a late manifestation commonly associated with pancreatic calcification.
- Patients with alcoholic CP usually present with an initial acute attack followed by successive attacks that are slower to resolve. Continued ethanol use leads to chronic abdominal pain and progressive exocrine and endocrine insufficiency.
- In 50% of patients, the pain diminishes in about 5–10 years after the onset of symptoms.
- Steatorrhea, calcification, and diabetes usually develop after 10–20 years of heavy ethanol ingestion. Most patients present with varying degrees of pain, malnutrition, and glucose intolerance.

► DIAGNOSIS

ACUTE PANCREATITIS

- The gold standard for diagnosis of AP is surgical examination of the pancreas or pancreatic histology. In the absence of these procedures, the diagnosis depends on the recognition of an etiologic factor, the clinical signs and symptoms, abnormal laboratory tests, and imaging techniques that predict the severity and course of the disease.
- Acute pancreatitis and its complications may be associated with leukocytosis, hyperglycemia, hypoalbuminemia, and mild hyperbilirubinemia. Elevations in serum alkaline phosphatase and liver transaminases are common.

- Dehydration may lead to hemoconcentration with elevated hemoglobin, hematocrit, blood urea nitrogen (BUN), and serum creatinine concentration.
- Marked hypocalcemia is an indication of severe necrosis.
- Some patients with severe pancreatitis develop thrombocytopenia and a prolongation in the prothrombin time.
- The serum amylase concentration usually rises within 24 hours of the onset of symptoms and returns to normal over the next 3–5 days. Serum amylase elevations do not correlate with either the etiology or severity of the disease.
- Serum lipase is specific to the pancreas and concentrations are usually elevated in AP. Serum lipase persists longer than serum amylase elevations and can be detected in the serum after the amylase has returned to normal.

- Urine amylase is increased in AP and may be elevated for 7–10 days after serum values have returned to normal.
- A plain radiographic film of the abdomen may suggest AP. Abdominal ultrasonography is indicated in patients with suspected biliary involvement. A computed tomography (CT) scan is extremely useful in most patients with AP. Contrast-enhanced CT distinguishes interstitial from necrotizing pancreatitis but does not distinguish between fat necrosis and acute fluid collection. Endoscopic retrograde cholangiopancreatography (ERCP) is used to visualize and remove bile duct stones in patients with gallstone pancreatitis.

CHRONIC PANCREATITIS

- The classic triad of calcification, steatorrhea, and diabetes usually confirms the diagnosis of CP.
- Serum amylase and lipase concentrations usually remain normal unless the pancreatic duct is blocked or a pseudocyst is present.
- The white blood cell count, fluid balance, and electrolyte concentrations usually remain normal unless fluids and electrolytes are lost due to vomiting and diarrhea.
- Malabsorption of fat can be detected by Sudan staining of the feces or a 72-hour quantitative measurement of fecal fat.
- Imaging techniques are helpful in detecting calcification of the pancreas, other causes of pain (ductal obstruction secondary to stones, strictures, or pseudocysts), and in differentiating CP from pancreatic cancer.
- ERCP may assist in the diagnosis and permits the identification of surgically correctable lesions.

► DESIRED OUTCOME

- The primary goal of treatment of acute pancreatitis is resolution of the inflammatory process such that patient symptoms are relieved and irreversible pancreatic damage does not occur.

- The goal of treatment of uncomplicated CP is directed at the control of chronic pain and the correction of malabsorption and glucose intolerance.

► TREATMENT

ACUTE PANCREATITIS (FIGURE 26–1)

- Initial treatment is aimed at relieving pain, replacing fluids, minimizing complications, and preventing pancreatic necrosis and infection.
- Discontinue medications listed in Table 26–2 whenever possible.
- In the early phase of the attack, most patients are treated by withholding food or liquids in order to minimize exocrine stimulation of the pancreas.
- Nasogastric (NG) aspiration is beneficial in patients with profound pain, severe disease, paralytic ileus, and intractable vomiting.
- IV fluids may be required to maintain intravascular volume and blood pressure in severe pancreatitis.
- Intravenous **potassium, calcium,** and **magnesium** should be used to correct deficiency states.
- **Insulin** may be needed to treat hyperglycemia.
- Total parenteral nutrition is a useful adjunct in restoring and maintaining the nutritional status.
- Secondary infections require the use of antibiotics and surgical intervention.
- Analgesics should be administered to reduce the severity of abdominal pain. Begin therapy with parenteral **meperidine** (50–100 mg) at regular intervals (e.g., every 4 hours). Theoretically it causes less spasm of the sphincter of Oddi than other narcotic medications.
- In patients with mild to moderate AP, the inhibition of gastric acid secretion by antisecretory drugs does not appear to be more effective than NG suction or withholding food when these modalities are used to diminish the pain associated with pancreatic exocrine secretion.
- **Octreotide** should be considered in patients with severe AP. Preliminary reports indicate that octreotide 0.1 mg subcutaneously every 8 hours may decrease sepsis, the length of hospital stay, and perhaps mortality.
- The use of prophylactic antibiotics does not offer any therapeutic advantage in patients with mild ethanol-induced AP who do not have necrosis. Prophylaxis is not routinely recommended for all patients with severe AP because of conflicting mortality data and concerns regarding antibiotic resistance. Antibiotic prophylaxis may be considered for patients with severe necrotic AP or disruption of the pancreatic ductal system.

CHRONIC PANCREATITIS

- In patients with ethanol-induced CP, abstinence is the most important factor in the prevention of chronic pain in the early stages of the disease.
- Small and frequent meals (six meals per day) and a diet restricted in fat

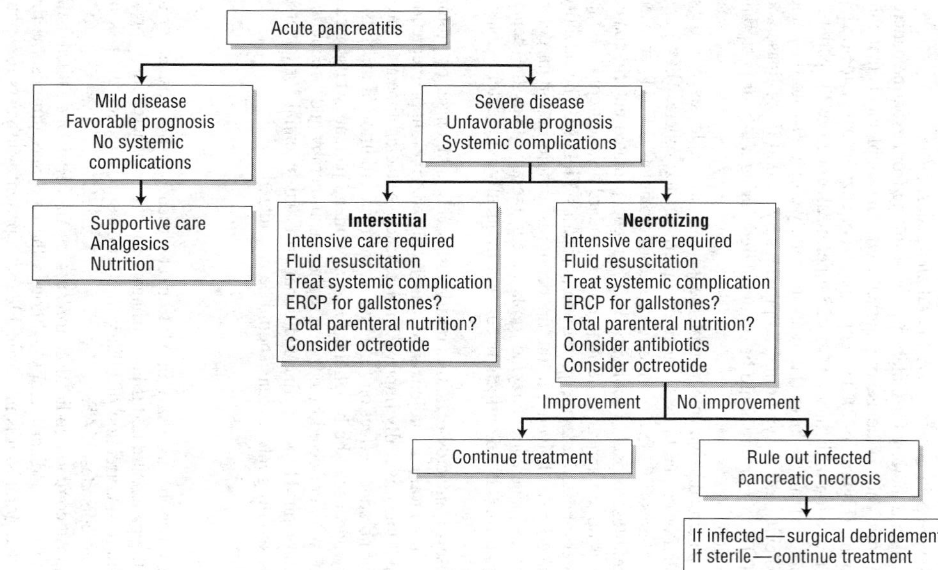
Acute pancreatitis
Mild disease
Favorable prognosis
No systemic complications
Severe disease
Unfavorable prognosis
Systemic complications
Supportive care
Analgesics
Nutrition
Interstitial
Intensive care required
Fluid resuscitation
Treat systemic complication
ERCP for gallstones?
Total parenteral nutrition?
Consider octreotide
Necrotizing
Intensive care required
Fluid resuscitation
Treat systemic complication
ERCP for gallstones?
Total parenteral nutrition?
Consider antibiotics
Consider octreotide
Improvement
No improvement
Continue treatment
Rule out infected pancreatic necrosis
If infected—surgical debridement
If sterile—continue treatment

Figure 26–1. Algorithm for evaluation and treatment of acute pancreatitis.

(50–75 g/d) is recommended to minimize postprandial pancreatic secretion and resulting pain.

- Pain management should begin with simple analgesics such as **aspirin** or **acetaminophen**. If pain persists, the response to exogenous pancreatic enzymes is evaluated in patients with mild to moderate nonalcoholic pancreatitis. Parenteral narcotics are reserved for those patients with severe pain unresponsive to oral analgesics.
- The standard therapy for malabsorption resulting from exocrine pancreatic insufficiency is the use of pancreatic enzyme supplements that contain lipase (Figure 26–2). The combination of enzyme supplementation and a reduction in dietary fat (to <25 g per meal) enhances the patient's nutritional status, reduces (but does not totally correct) steatorrhea, and may alleviate other symptoms. Approximately 30,000 IU of lipase and 10,000 IU of trypsin should be administered during a 4-hour postprandial period.
- Oral pancreatic enzyme supplements are available as powders, uncoated or coated tablets, capsules, enteric-coated spheres (ECS) and microspheres (ECMS), or enteric-coated microtablets (ECMT) encased in a cellulose capsule (Table 26–3). Microencapsulated enteric-coated products do not appear to be superior to standard doses of conventional nonenteric-coated enzyme preparations such as **Viokase.** The quantity of active lipase delivered to the duodenum is a more important determinant in pancreatic enzyme replacement therapy than the actual dosage form. GI side effects occur less frequently with enteric-coated products.
- The use of antacids or antisecretory drugs (H_2 antagonists or proton pump inhibitors) as adjuncts to pancreatic enzyme supplementation does not unequivocally improve their efficacy. Antacids appear to have little or no added effect on reducing steatorrhea. Addition of an antisecretory agent may be beneficial for symptomatic patients whose steatorrhea is not corrected by enzyme replacement therapy and a reduction in dietary fat. However, the additional cost and potential for adverse effects and drug interactions should be considered.

SURGERY

- Surgery may be necessary in AP to treat a pseudocyst or abscess or to drain the pancreatic bed if hemorrhagic or necrotic pancreatitis is present. Surgical correction of biliary tract disease may reduce the risk of recurrent episodes of AP.
- The most common indication for surgery in CP is abdominal pain refractory to medical therapy. Although the pain may diminish as the gland deteriorates, it is unreasonable that a patient wait years for spontaneous relief.
- Surgical procedures that alleviate pain include a subtotal pancreatectomy, decompression of the pancreatic duct, or interruption of the splanchnic nerves.

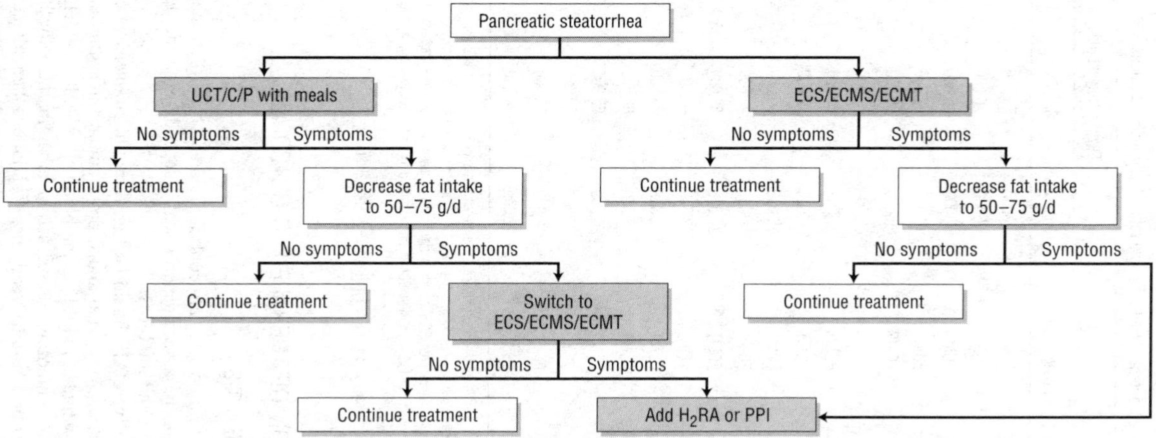

Pancreatic steatorrhea

UCT/C/P with meals

No symptoms → Continue treatment

Symptoms → Decrease fat intake to 50–75 g/d

No symptoms → Continue treatment

Symptoms → Switch to ECS/ECMS/ECMT

No symptoms → Continue treatment

Symptoms → Add H_2RA or PPI

ECS/ECMS/ECMT

No symptoms → Continue treatment

Symptoms → Decrease fat intake to 50–75 g/d

No symptoms → Continue treatment

Symptoms → Add H_2RA or PPI

Figure 26–2. Algorithm for treatment of pancreatic steatorrhea. UCT, uncoated tablet; C, capsule; P, powder; ECS, enteric-coated sphere; ECMS, enteric-coated microsphere; ECMT, enteric-coated microtablet; H_2RA, H_2-receptor antagonist; PPI, proton pump inhibitor.

TABLE 26–3. Enzyme Content of Selected Pancreatic Enzyme Preparations

Product	Dosage Form[b]	Enzyme Content (units)[a]		
		Lipase	*Amylase*	*Protease*
Cotazym	C	8000	30,000	30,000
Cotazym-S	ECS	5000	20,000	20,000
Creon-5	ECMS	5000	16,600	18,750
Creon-10	ECMS	10,000	33,200	37,500
Creon-20	ECMS	20,000	66,400	75,000
Ku-Zyme HP	C	8000	30,000	30,000
Pancrease	ECMS	4500	20,000	25,000
Pancrease MT-4	ECMT	4500	12,000	12,000
Pancrease MT-10	ECMT	10,000	30,000	30,000
Pancrease MT-16	ECMT	16,000	48,000	48,000
Pancrease MT-20	ECMT	20,000	56,000	44,000
Pancrezyme 4X[c]	UCT	12,000	60,000	60,000
Ultrase MT-12	ECMT	12,000	39,000	39,000
Ultrase MT-18	ECMT	18,000	58,500	58,500
Ultrase MT-20	ECMT	20,000	65,000	65,000
Viokase	UCT	8000	30,000	30,000
Viokase[d]	P	16,800	70,000	70,000
Zymase	ECS	12,000	24,000	24,000

[a] All listed products contain pancrealipase. Pancrealipase contains not less than 24 USP units of lipase activity, not less than 100 USP units of amylase activity, and not less than 100 USP units of protease activity per mg.
[b] C, powder encased in a cellulose capsule; ECS, enteric-coated sphere encased in a cellulose capsule; ECMS, enteric-coated microspheres encased in a cellulose capsule; ECMT, enteric-coated microtablets encased in a cellulose capsule; UCT, uncoated tablet; P, powder.
[c] Vegetable origin (suitable for vegetarians or those with allergies to beef and pork).
[d] Units of 0.7 g of powder.

▶ EVALUATION OF THERAPEUTIC OUTCOMES

ACUTE PANCREATITIS

- In patients with mild AP, pain control, fluid and electrolyte status, and nutrition should be assessed periodically depending on the degree of abdominal pain and fluid loss.
- Patients with severe AP should be transferred to an intensive care unit for close monitoring of vital signs, prothrombin time, fluid and electrolyte status, white blood cell count, blood glucose, lactate dehydrogenase, aspartate aminotransferase, serum albumin, hematocrit, blood urea nitrogen, and serum creatinine. Continuous hemodynamic and arterial blood gas monitoring is essential. Serum lipase, amylase, and bilirubin require less frequent monitoring. The patient should also be

monitored for signs of infection, relief of abdominal pain, and adequate nutritional status.

CHRONIC PANCREATITIS

- The severity and frequency of abdominal pain should be assessed periodically to determine the efficacy of the analgesic regimen.
- The effectiveness of pancreatic enzyme supplementation is measured by improvement in body weight and stool consistency or frequency. The 72-hour stool test for fecal fat may be used when the adequacy of treatment is in question.
- Serum uric acid and folic acid concentrations should be monitored yearly in patients prone to hyperuricemia or folic acid deficiency.
- Blood glucose must be monitored carefully in diabetic patients.

See Chapter 37, Pancreatitis, authored by Rosemary R. Berardi, PharmD, FASHP, and Patricia A. Montgomery, PharmD, for a more detailed discussion of this topic.

Chapter 27

▶ PEPTIC ULCER DISEASE

▶ DEFINITION

Peptic ulcer disease (PUD) refers to a group of ulcerative disorders of the upper gastrointestinal (GI) tract that require acid and pepsin for their formation. Ulcers differ from superficial mucosal erosions in that they extend deeper into the muscularis mucosa.

▶ PATHOPHYSIOLOGY

- The pathogenesis of duodenal (DU) and gastric ulcer (GU) is multifactorial and most likely reflects a combination of pathophysiologic abnormalities, environmental, and genetic factors.
- Most peptic ulcers occur in the presence of acid and pepsin when *Helicobacter pylori* (HP), NSAIDs, or other possible factors disrupt normal mucosal defense and healing mechanisms. About 30–50% of patients with DU are hypersecretors of gastric acid. Factors responsible for acid hypersecretion include increased parietal cell mass, increased basal secretory drive [high basal acid output/maximal acid output (BAO/MAO) ratio], and increased postprandial secretory drive.
- A strong association exists between HP (formerly *Campylobacter pylori*) and PUD. Most patients with DU and GU who are not taking NSAIDs have evidence of HP infection and antral gastritis.
- HP may cause ulcer by impairing mucosal defense by elaboration of toxins and enzymes, or increasing antral gastrin release which leads to increased acidity.
- There is overwhelming evidence linking chronic NSAID (including aspirin) use and hemorrhagic gastric erosions, gastric ulcers, and (less commonly) duodenal ulcers. Chronic NSAID therapy produces gastroduodenal injury by two mechanisms: a direct irritant action on the mucosa and a systemic effect whereby endogenous prostaglandin synthesis is inhibited.
- The association between corticosteroids alone and PUD remains controversial. However, patients receiving concurrent corticosteroids and NSAIDs are at increased risk of developing NSAID-induced ulcers.
- Cigarette smoking increases the risk for the development and recurrence of DU and GU, and the risk appears to be proportional to the amount smoked. Smoking also impairs ulcer healing and promotes recurrence.
- Although clinical observation supports the belief that ulcer patients are adversely affected by stressful life events, controlled studies have failed to document a cause-and-effect relationship.
- The causal association between specific dietary substances and PUD has not been substantiated. Ethanol may cause acute gastric mucosal damage, but is not clearly the cause of ulcers.

▶ CLINICAL PRESENTATION

- Epigastric pain is the classic and most frequent symptoms of peptic ulcer disease. The pain is often described as burning but can present as a vague discomfort, abdominal fullness, or cramping (Table 27–1). Many patients with DU describe a typical nocturnal pain that awakens them at night.
- Patients with PUD often present with dyspeptic symptoms such as heartburn, belching, and bloating. Nausea, vomiting, anorexia, and weight loss are more common in GU.
- The severity of symptoms varies from patient to patient and, in some patients, symptoms may be seasonal, occurring more frequently in the spring or fall.
- Patients consuming NSAIDs and the elderly are often symptom free prior to bleeding or perforation.
- Complications of HP- and NSAID-induced ulcers include GI bleeding, perforation into the peritoneal cavity, penetration into an adjacent structure (e.g., pancreas, biliary tract, or liver), and gastric outlet obstruction. Bleeding may be insidious or present as melena or hematemesis. Perforation is association with sudden, sharp, severe pain, beginning first in the epigastrium but quickly spreading over the entire abdomen.

TABLE 27–1. Clinical Features of Duodenal Ulcer (DU), Gastric Ulcer (GU), and Nonulcer Dyspepsia (NUD)

Feature	DU	GU	NUD
Pain	++++	++++	++++
Primary pain is epigastric pain	++++	+++	+++
Frequently severe	+++	+++	++
Occurs in clusters (episodic)	+++	+	++
Occurs at night (nocturnal)	++++	++	++
Radiates to back	++	++	++
Relieved by antacids	++++	++++	+++
Increased by food	++	+	++
Relieved by food	+++	++	++
Heartburn	+++	+	++
Bloating	+++	+++	+++
Belching	+++	+++	+++
Nausea	++	+++	++
Vomiting	++	+++	+
Anorexia	+	++	+
Weight loss	++	++	+

Frequencies represent estimates and are categorized as being consistent (++++), frequent (+++), infrequent (++), or rare (+). None of the features are always present or always absent.

Symptoms of gastric outlet obstruction typically occur over several months and include early satiety, bloating, anorexia, nausea, vomiting, and weight loss.
- The natural history of PUD is characterized by periods of exacerbations and remissions. Most ulcers will eventually heal on their own, but the healing process is accelerated with treatment.

▶ DIAGNOSIS

- The physical examination usually reveals epigastric tenderness which occurs between the umbilicus and the xiphoid process and less commonly radiates to the back.
- Routine laboratory tests are not helpful in establishing a diagnosis of uncomplicated PUD.
- The hematocrit, hemoglobin, and stool hemoccult tests are used to detect bleeding.
- The diagnosis of HP can be made using invasive or noninvasive tests. The invasive methods require upper GI endoscopy with a mucosal biopsy taken for histology, culture, or detection of urease activity. The ^{13}C and ^{14}C urea breath tests are noninvasive methods that require that patients ingest radiolabeled urea, which, in the presence of urease, forms ammonia and radiolabeled bicarbonate. Serologic tests are useful to detect antibodies directed against HP but are not useful to assess HP eradication, as antibody titers to HP may take 6 months to 2 years or longer to return to the uninfected range.
- Serologic tests are the initial screening test of choice because they are quick, inexpensive, and reliable; urea breath testing may be used if there is concern about a positive serologic test. When endoscopy is indicated, the primary diagnosis should be established using the rapid urease test. Culturing for antibiotic sensitivity is not practical at this time.
- The diagnosis of PUD depends on visualizing the ulcer crater, either by upper GI radiography or endoscopy. DU should be distinguished from other acid-peptic diseases, and benign GU must be distinguished from those that are malignant. Therefore, the diagnosis depends on radiologic or endoscopic findings. Fiber optic endoscopy detects more than 90% of peptic ulcers.

▶ DESIRED OUTCOME

The ultimate goals of PUD treatment are relief of ulcer pain, acceleration of ulcer healing, prevention of ulcer recurrence, and reduction of ulcer-related complications.

▶ TREATMENT

- An algorithm for the treatment of chronic PUD is presented in Figure 27–1.

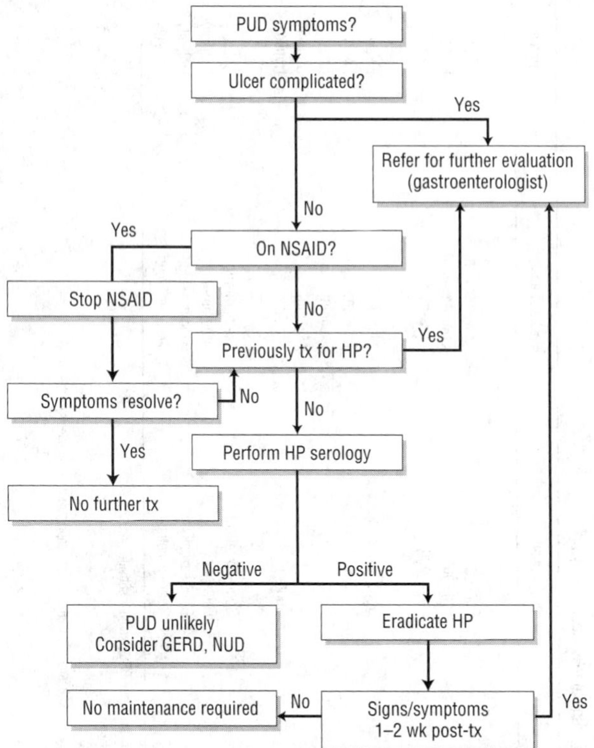

Figure 27–1. Algorithm for the evaluation and treatment (tx) of chronic peptic ulcer disease (PUD). HP, *Helicobacter pylori*; NSAID, nonsteroidal anti-inflammatory drug; GERD, gastroesophageal reflux disease NUD, nonulcer dyspepsia.

V

- Patients with PUD should eliminate or reduce psychological stress, cigarette smoking, and the use of NSAIDs (including aspirin). If NSAIDs cannot be discontinued, use of lower doses, less damaging agents, and coadministration with food or antacids should be encouraged.
- Although there is no need for a special diet, patients should avoid foods and beverages (e.g., spicy foods, caffeine, alcohol) that cause dyspepsia or exacerbate ulcer symptoms.
- **Antacids** may be used in conjunction with other antiulcer medications to relieve occasional ulcer symptoms.
- Eradication is recommended for all HP-infected patients with an active ulcer, a history of ulcer-related complications, or who require maintenance therapy. Testing for HP is only recommended if eradication ther-

V

TABLE 27–2. Comparison of Therapeutic Strategies Used to Eradicate *Helicobacter pylori*

Strategy	Efficacy[a]	Adverse Effects[b]	Compliance[c]
Two-Drug Regimens			
Amoxicillin + PPI	Poor–fair	Low–medium	Likely
Clarithromycin + PPI	Fair–good	Low–medium	Likely
Clarithromycin + RBC	Fair–good	Low–medium	Likely
Three-Drug Regimens			
Clarithromycin + metronidazole + PPI	Good–excellent	Medium	Likely
Clarithromycin + amoxicillin + PPI	Good–excellent	Low–medium	Likely
Amoxicillin + metronidazole + PPI	Good	Medium	Likely
Clarithromycin + metronidazole + RBC	Good	Medium	Unlikely
Tetracycline + metronidazole + sucralfate	Good	Medium	Unlikely
Four-Drug Regimens			
BSS + metronidazole + tetracycline + H_2RA[d]	Good–excellent	Medium–high	Unlikely
BSS + metronidazole + amoxicillin + H_2RA[d]	Fair–good	Medium–high	Unlikely
BSS + metronidazole + tetracycline + PPI	Good–excellent	Medium–high	Unlikely
BSS + metronidazole + clarithromycin + PPI	Good–excellent	Medium–high	Unlikely

PPI, proton pump inhibitor; H_2RA, H_2-receptor antagonist; RBC, ranitidine bismuth citrate; BSS, bismuth subsalicylate.

[a]Efficacy (eradication rate) = Excellent (>90%); Good (>80%–90%); Fair (>70%–80%); Poor (<70%).

[b]Safety (frequency of clinically important adverse effects) = High; Medium; Low.

[c]Complicance (estimate based on total number of tablets or capsules, frequency of administration, and clinically important adverse effects) = Likely; Unlikely.

[d]H_2RA indicated when used in patients with an active ulcer.

apy is planned. An individualized regimen should be selected based on efficacy, tolerability, drug interaction potential, antibiotic resistance, cost, and the likelihood of patient adherence (Tables 27–2 and 27–3). Most patients should receive a **proton pump inhibitor** (PPI) based three-drug regimen, as they are superior to two-drug regimens. **Bismuth-based** four-drug regimens are effective but involve complicated dosing schedules and are associated with a higher incidence of adverse effects. Patients with an active ulcer should receive cotherapy with an antisecretory drug [PPI or **H_2 receptor antagonist** (H_2RA)] for relief of ulcer symptoms. If a second course of therapy is required, the regimen should contain different antibiotics.

- Treatment with a conventional antiulcer drug alone (an H_2RA or **sucralfate** for 6–8 weeks or a PPI for 4 weeks) may be an alternative to HP eradication (Table 27–4) but is discouraged because of the high rate of ulcer recurrence and ulcer-related complications. Combination therapy with these agents does not enhance efficacy and increases costs.
- Maintenance therapy with a low-dose H_2RA or PPI (Table 27–4) should be limited to high-risk patients who fail HP eradication, patients with severe complications, or those with HP-negative ulcers.
- Most uncomplicated NSAID-induced ulcers heal with standard regimens of an H_2RA, PPI, or sucralfate if the NSAID is discontinued. If the NSAID must be continued or if the ulcer is large, PPIs are the drugs of choice because they accelerate ulcer healing. A higher PPI dose (e.g., **omeprazole** 40 mg/d) should be used, as these ulcers tend to heal at a slower rate. If HP is present, treatment should be initiated with an eradication regimen that contains a PPI. Patients at risk of developing serious ulcer-related complications while on NSAIDs should receive prophylactic cotherapy. H_2RAs and PPIs may be useful in relieving dyspeptic symptoms and may prevent ulcers, but cotherapy with **misoprostol** remains the treatment of choice for preventing NSAID-induced GU and DU.
- Emergency surgery is required in some patients for bleeding, perforation, or obstruction. Surgical procedures usually include vagotomy with pyloroplasty or vagotomy with antrectomy.

▶ EVALUATION OF THERAPEUTIC OUTCOMES

- Patients should be monitored for symptomatic relief of ulcer pain as well as potential adverse effects and drug interactions related to drug therapy.
- Ulcer pain typically resolves in a few days when NSAIDs are the cause of the symptoms and within 7 days upon initiation of antiulcer therapy. Most patients with uncomplicated PUD will be rendered symptom free with any one of the recommended antiulcer regimens.
- The persistence or recurrence of symptoms after 14 days of treatment suggests failure of ulcer healing or an alternative diagnosis such as cancer.

TABLE 27–3. Drug Treatment Regimens Used to Eradicate *Helicobacter pylori*

Drug	Dose	Frequency	Duration
1. Clarithromycin[a]	500 mg	tid	14d
Omeprazole[b,c]	40 mg	qd	14d
2. Amoxicillin[d]	1 g	tid	14d
Lansoprazole[b,c]	30 mg	tid	14d
3. Amoxicillin	1 g	bid–tid	14d
Omeprazole[b,c]	20 g	bid	14d
4. Clarithromycin[a]	500 mg	tid	14d
Ranitidine bismuth citrate	400 mg	bid	28d
5. Clarithromycin[a]	500 mg	bid	10–14d
Amoxicillin	1 g	bid	10–14d
Lansoprazole[b,c]	30 mg	bid	10–14d
6. Clarithromycin	500 mg	bid	10–14d
Metronidazole	500 mg	bid	10–14d
Omeprazole[b,c]	20 mg	bid	10–14d
7. Clarithromycin	500 mg	bid	14d
Metronidazole	500 mg	bid	14d
Ranitidine bismuth citrate	400 mg	bid	14–28d
8. Bismuth subsalicylate[a]	525 mg	qid	14d
Metronidazole	250 mg	qid	14d
Tetracycline	500 mg	qid	14d
H_2RA[e]	As directed using conventional ulcer-healing dosage regimen		28d
9. Bismuth subsalicylate	525 mg	qid	14d
Metronidazole	250 mg	qid	14d
Amoxicillin	500 mg	qid	14d
H_2RA[e]	As directed using conventional ulcer-healing dosage regimen		28d
10. Bismuth subsalicylate	525 mg	qid	7–10d
Metronidazole	500 mg	qid	7–10d
Tetracycline	500 mg	qid	7–10d
Omeprazole[b,c]	20 mg	bid	7–10d
11. Bismuth subsalicylate	525 mg	qid	7–10d
Metronidazole	500 mg	qid	7–10d
Clarithromycin	500 mg	bid	7–10d
Omeprazole[b,c]	20 mg	bid	7–10d
12. Tetracycline	500 mg	qid	14d
Metronidazole	500 mg	qid	14d
Sucralfate	1 g	qid	14–28d

[a]Approved by the Food and Drug Administration (FDA).
[b]When eradicating *Helicobacter pylori,* only proton pump inhibitor may be used in its recommended eradication dosage.
[c]In patients with an ulcer at the time of initiation of therapy, the proton pump inhibitor may be extended to 28 days using conventional anti-ulcer dosages.
[d]Approved by the FDA for patients unable to tolerate clarithromycin.
[e]When treating an ulcer, any H_2-receptor antagonist (H_2RA) may be used in its conventional ulcer healing dosage regimen.

TABLE 27–4. Oral Drug Treatment Regimens Used to Heal Ulcers or Maintain Ulcer Healing

Drug	Ulcer Healing		Maintenance of Ulcer Healing	
	Duodenal Ulcer	*Gastric Ulcer*	*Duodenal Ulcer*	*Gastric Ulcer*
H_2-Receptor Antagonists				
Cimetidine	300 mg qid[a]	300 mg qid[a]	400 mg hs[a]	400–800 mg hs
	400 mg bid[a]	800 mg hs[a]	—	—
	800 mg hs[a]	—	—	—
Famotidine	20 mg bid[a]	20 mg bid	20 mg hs[a]	20 mg hs
	40 mg hs[a]	40 mg hs[a]	—	—
Nizatidine	150 mg bid[a]	150 mg bid[a]	150 mg hs[a]	150–300 mg hs
	300 mg hs[a]	300 mg hs[a]	—	—
Ranitidine	150 mg bid[a]	150 mg bid[a]	150 mg hs[a]	150[a]–300 mg hs
	300 mg hs[a]	300 mg hs	—	—
Proton Pump Inhibitors				
Omeprazole	20 mg qd[a]	40 mg qd[a]	20 mg qd	20–40 mg qd
Lansoprazole	15 mg qd[a]	30 mg qd[a]	15[a] mg qd	15–30 mg qd
Mucosal Defense				
Sucralfate	1 g qid[a]	1 g qid	1 g qd/bid	1 g qid
	2 g bid	2 g bid	—	—

[a]Approved by the Food and Drug Administration (FDA).

- The majority of patients with uncomplicated HP-positive ulcers do not require confirmation of ulcer healing or HP eradication. Exceptions include patients with a complicated ulcer, gastric mucosa-associated lymphoid tissue (MALT) lymphoma, or gastric cancer. When endoscopy is not indicated, the urea breath test is the best noninvasive method to verify eradication after treatment. The test should be delayed for at least 4 weeks after the completion of HP eradication therapy to avoid confusing bacterial suppression with eradication.
- Ulcer patients, especially the elderly or other high-risk patients on NSAIDs, should be closely monitored for signs and symptoms of bleeding, obstruction, penetration, and perforation.
- Follow-up endoscopy to determine if ulcers or HP are present is justified in patients with frequent symptomatic recurrence, refractory disease, complications, or suspected hypersecretory states.

See Chapter 31, Peptic Ulcer Disease, authored by Rosemary R. Berardi, PharmD, FASHP, for a more detailed discussion of this topic.

Gynecologic and Obstetric Disorders

Edited by Barbara G. Wells, PharmD, FASHP, FCCP, BCPP

Chapter 28

▶ CONTRACEPTION

▶ EFFECTIVENESS

- Failure inherent in the proper use of the contraceptive alone is called a "method failure" or "perfect use failure." "User failure" or "typical use failure" takes into account inaccuracies in the user's abilities to follow directions, such as skipping an oral contraceptive pill (Table 28–1).

▶ HORMONAL METHODS OF CONTRACEPTION

COMPOSITION AND FORMULATIONS

- **Estrogens** and/or **progestins** inhibit ovulation and alter cervical mucus and the endometrium by suppressing the production of follicle-stimulating hormone (FSH) and the luteinizing hormone (LH) surge.
- The progestin-only **"minipill"** (28 days of active hormone/cycle) is generally used for women who have contraindications or intolerance to estrogens, smokers, older than 35 years of age, and women who are breast feeding, as it is less effective than the combination pill and is associated with irregular bleeding and increased frequency of functional ovarian cysts.
- **Mestranol,** which is converted to **ethinyl estradiol (EE)** in the liver, is 50% less potent than EE.
- Progestins vary in progestational, estrogenic, antiestrogenic, and androgenic activity.
- Third-generation oral contraceptives (OCs) contain newer progestins (e.g., **norgestimate, desogestrel, gestodene**) that appear to have no estrogenic effects and are less androgenic than **levonorgestrel.**
- The composition and activity of OCs are shown in Table 28–2.

CONSIDERATIONS WITH ORAL CONTRACEPTIVE USE

- Absolute and relative contraindications to the use of OCs are shown in Table 28–3. Guidelines for use of OCs in selected medical disorders are shown in Table 28–4.
- Generally, OCs are an acceptable form of birth control for nonsmoking women up to the age of menopause. Women over 40 years old use the lowest dose estrogen products.

TABLE 28–1. Comparison of Reversible Methods of Contraception

Method	Absolute Contraindications	Advantages	Disadvantages	Percent of Women with Pregnancy (%)[a]	
				Lowest Expected	*Typical Use*
Episodic Contraceptive Methods					
Spermicides alone	Allergy to spermicide	Inexpensive No office visit required Some protection against STDs	High user failure rate Must be reapplied before each act of intercourse May cause local irritation in either partner May enhance HIV transmission (?)	3.0	21.0
Condoms, male	Allergy to latex or rubber	Inexpensive Readily available No office visit required STD protection, including HIV (latex only)	Poor acceptance Possibility of breakage Efficacy decreased by oil-based lubricants Latex can cause allergic reactions in either partner	2.0	12.0
Condoms, female (Reality)	Allergy to polyurethane History of toxic shock syndrome	Can be inserted just before intercourse or ahead of time; provides protection for 48 hours STD protection, including HIV	Dislike ring hanging outside vagina Cumbersome	5	21
Diaphragm with spermicide	Allergy to latex rubber or spermicide Recurrent UTIs History of toxic shock syndrome Abnormal gynecologic anatomy	Low cost Decreased incidence of cervical neoplasia STD protection, including HIV Can be inserted for up to 6 hours before intercourse	Office visit required Decreased efficacy with increased frequency of intercourse Must be refitted after significant change in weight (± 10 pounds) Increased incidence of vaginal yeast and UTI infections Increased incidence of toxic shock syndrome Efficacy affected by oil-based lubricants Cervical irritation	6.0	18.0

Cervical cap (Prentif)	Allergy to rubber or spermicide History of toxic shock syndrome Abnormal gynecologic anatomy Abnormal Pap smear	Low cost STD protection, including HIV Can be inserted just before or ahead of time; provides protection for 48 hours	Office visit required May be difficult for patient to use correctly Decreased efficacy with parity Not possible to fit all patients	6.0	18.0
Hormonal Methods					
OCs	Hepatic adenomas Thromboembolic disorders or history thereof Cerebrovascular or coronary artery disease Known or suspected breast cancer Undiagnosed abnormal gynecologic bleeding Cardiovascular risk factors (relative contraindication) Jaundice with pregnancy or previous pill use	Decreased risk of pelvic inflammatory disease, ovarian and endometrial cancer Improvement in endometriosis (probably) Fewer functional ovarian cysts (possibly) Less salpingitis; ectopic pregnancy Prevention of benign breast disease (fibroadenoma and fibrocystic changes) Less rheumatoid arthritis (possibly) Increased bone density (possibly) Improvement in acne and hirsutism *Significant improvement in menstrually related problems:* fewer cramps; less flow for fewer days; less iron-deficiency anemia; more predictable menses; elimination of mittelschmerz: less dysmenorrhea and premenstrual tension syndrome	Increased risk of benign hepatocellular adenomas Mild increased risk of thromboembolism and stroke May elevate blood pressure No protection against most STDs Estrogenic side effects (nausea, breast tenderness, fluid retention) Progestogen side effects (acne, increased appetite, depression) Increased risk of myocardial infarction in older smokers, nausea, headache	0.1	3.0

continued

TABLE 28–1. continued

Method	Absolute Contraindications	Advantages	Disadvantages	Percent of Women with Pregnancy (%)[a]	
				Lowest Expected	*Typical Use*
Progestin-only OCs	Undiagnosed abnormal gynecologic bleeding	May be used by lactating women and women with cardiovascular risk Allows avoidance of estrogen-related side effects Protection against PID, iron deficiency anemia, and dysmenorrhea	Frequent spotting and/or amenorrhea Increased risk of ectopic pregnancy Must take every day at the same time	0.5	3.0
Progestin Implants *Norplant and Norplant II (Levonorgestrel)* *Capronor (Levonorgestrel)* *Implanon (3-Ketodesogestrel)* *Uniplant (nomegestrol acetate)*	Undiagnosed abnormal gynecologic bleeding Acute liver disease Benign or malignant liver tumors Known or suspected breast cancer Active thrombophlebitis or thromboembolic disease	Passive contraception Duration of efficacy varies; effective up to 5 years with Norplant in women < 154 pounds Effects are quickly reversible Less menstrual cramping and mittelschmerz No suppression of lactation No metabolic disturbances Can be considered for use in women who have diabetes, hypertension, gall bladder disease, history of cardiovascular or thromboembolic disease, SLE, or sickle cell disease; in women who are smokers or lactating	Requires outpatient surgical procedure Irregular menstrual bleeding, headaches, weight gain (?), acne Progestin side effects Local infection or bruising on insertion; removal may be difficult Expensive initially High discontinuation rate Unacceptable in patients using some anticonvulsants	0.2	0.2

Depo-Provera	Pregnancy Undiagnosed abnormal gynecologic bleeding Known or suspected breast cancer Liver disease (relative contraindication) Severe depression (relative contraindication) Severe cardiovascular disease (relative contraindication)	No suppression of lactation No increased risk of thromboembolism Passive contraception No drug interactions May decrease seizures Effective for 3 months Can be considered for use in women who have seizure disorders, diabetes, hypertension, gall bladder disease, history of cardiovascular or thromboembolic disease, SLE, or sickle cell disease; in women who are smokers or lactating	Irregular menstrual bleeding, headache, weight gain, acne Delayed return of fertility Possible increased risk of breast cancer in younger users Decreased HDL Progestin side effects Decreased bone density in long-term users Office visit required	0.3	0.3
Intrauterine Devices (Hormonal and nonhormonal)					
Copper-T 380A (Paragard)	Multiple sexual partners/partner with multiple partners (high risk for STDs) History of PID or ectopic pregnancy, acute pelvic infection Abnormal uterine cavity/pelvic surgery/undiagnosed vaginal bleeding Uterine or cervical cancer	Passive contraception Long-term contraception (can remain in place up to 10 years) Less expensive per year and easier for some patients No delay in return of fertility after removal	Increased heavy bleeding Spotting between periods Increased cramping and dysmenorrhea Increased risk of ectopic pregnancy Office visit required Rarely uterine perforation	0.8	<1.0

continued

TABLE 28–1. continued

Method	Absolute Contraindications	Advantages	Disadvantages	Percent of Women with Pregnancy (%)[a]	
				Lowest Expected	*Typical Use*
Progesterone T (Progestasert)	Postpartum endometritis or infected abortion in previous 3 months Acute cervicitis or vaginitis, (including BV) until infection controlled	Remains in place for 1 year Decreased cramping and dysmenorrhea Decrease in menstrual blood loss No delay in return of fertility after removal	Office visit required Must be changed each year Increased risk of ectopic pregnancy Rarely uterine perforation	2.0	<2.0
Levonorgestrel IUD	Conditions associated with increased susceptibility to infections, including leukemia, AIDS, IV drug abuse, and corticosteroid use Valvular heart disease (±) Nulliparity (±) Genital actinomyces Wilson's disease[b] Allergy to copper[b]	Constant rate of hormone release for 5 years Possibly, the single most effective reversible contraceptive method over 5-year period Decreased cramping and dysmenorrhea Reduced incidence of PID and menorrhagia Combines benefits of Norplant and Copper-T	Office visit required Irregular menstrual bleeding (?) Rarely uterine perforation	Not available	

[a]Failure rates during first year of use, United States.
[b]Contraindication for copper IUD only.
STD, sexually transmitted disease; UTI, urinary tract infection; PID, pelvic inflammatory disease; SLE, systemic lupus erythematosus; HDI, high-density lipoprotein cholestesterol; BV, bacterial vaginosis.

- **Combination OCs** can cause small increases in blood pressure.
- When an OC is prescribed for a patient with history of glucose intolerance, a product containing one of the new progestins (i.e., desogestrel or norgestimate) or a low dose of a **norethindrone-type progestin** is recommended.
- Generally, synthetic progestins decrease high-density lipoprotein (HDL) and increase low-density lipoprotein (LDL). Estrogens have the opposite effect and may increase triglycerides. Most low-dose combination OCs do not significantly impact HDL, LDL, triglycerides, or total cholesterol.
- Estrogens play a dose-related role in development of venous thrombosis and pulmonary embolism (PE), especially in smokers or those with conditions that predispose to coagulation abnormalities.
- The increased risk of venous thromboembolism (VTE) appears to be limited to current OC users, and the 20-μg EE products do not appear to have an effect on clotting parameters, even in smokers.
- Some progestins also appear to have a procoagulant effect. The third-generation OCs containing gestodene or desogestrel had a two-fold greater risk of nonfatal VTE than the older low-dose combination OCs.
- Thrombotic and hemorrhagic stroke have been associated with OC use, but the increased risk is extremely low with the low-dose OCs.
- Diabetes, hypertension, obesity, and especially smoking appear to act synergistically with OCs to increase the risk of cardiovascular disease.
- The risk for ovarian and endometrial cancer decreases with OC use.
- Women taking or within 10 years of stopping OCs have a small increase in the risk of breast cancer. The impact of the low-dose OCs on breast cancer risk is unknown.

SELECTING AN ORAL CONTRACEPTIVE

- Most clinicians routinely prescribe a combination OC that possesses hormonal activity equivalent to 50 μg or less of EE.
- Women with a history of migraine, heavy menstrual cramps, or severe nausea during pregnancy may be estrogen-sensitive and may benefit from an OC containing a very low dose of estrogen. However, they should be cautioned that spotting may occur and that missed pills could result in breakthrough ovulation.
- Women with a history of weight gain, fatigue, varicose veins, or toxemia during pregnancy may be progestin-sensitive and may benefit from an OC with low progestational activity.
- Women with a history of irregular heavy menses, oily skin, hirsutism, and acne may be androgen-sensitive and may benefit from a pill with high progestational and low androgenic activity.
- In women taking anticonvulsants, an OC containing greater estrogenic activity may be more effective; however, other forms of contraception are strongly recommended.

TABLE 28–2. Composition of Commonly Prescribed Oral Contraceptives[a]

Product	Composition				Spotting and BTB[b] (%)
	Estrogen	*μg*	*Progestin*	*mg*	
50 μg Estrogen					
Ovral	E. estradiol	50	Norgestrel	0.5	4.5
Norlestrin 2.5/50	E. estradiol	50	Nor. acetate	2.5	5.1
Genora/Norethin/Norinyl/ Ortho-Novum 1/50	Mestranol	50	Norethindrone	1.0	10.6
Ovcon 50	E. estradiol	50	Norethindrone	1.0	11.9
Demulen 50	E. estradiol	50	Ethy. diacetate	1.0	13.9
Norlestrin 1/50	E. estradiol	50	Nor. acetate	1.0	13.6
Sub 50 μg Estrogen Monophasic					
Lo-Ovral	E. estradiol	30	Norgestrel	0.3	9.6
Desogen/Ortho-Cept	E. estradiol	30	Desogestrel	0.15	9.9
Ovcon 35	E. estradiol	35	Norethindrone	0.4	11.0
Levlen/Nordette/Min-Ovral[c]	E. estradiol	30	Levonorgestrel	0.15	14.0
Ortho-Cyclen	E. estradiol	35	Norgestimate	0.25	14.3
Brevicon/Modicon/Nelova 0.5/35	E. estradiol	35	Norethindrone	0.5	14.6
Brevicon/Ortho 0.5/35[c]					
Genora/Nelova/Norethin/Norinyl/ Ortho-Novum 1/35 Ortho 1/35[c]	E. estradiol	35	Norethindrone	1.0	14.7
Loestrin 1.5/30	E. estradiol	30	Nor. acetate	1.5	25.2
Loestrin/Minestrin[c] 1/20	E. estradiol	20	Nor. acetate	1.0	29.7
Aleese	E. estradiol	20	Levonorgestrel	0.1	
Demulen 1/35	E. estradiol	35	Ethy. diacetate	1.0	37.4

Sub 50 μg Estrogen Multiphasic[d]					
Ortho Novum 7/7/7	E. estradiol	35 (7)	Norethindrone	0.5 (7)	12.2
	E. estradiol	35 (7)	Norethindrone	0.75 (7)	
	E. estradiol	35 (7)	Norethindrone	1.0 (7)	
Jenest	E. estradiol	35 (7)	Norethindrone	0.5 (7)	14.1
	E. estradiol	35 (14)	Norethindrone	1.0 (14)	
Tri-Levlen/TriPhasil	E. estradiol	30 (6)	Levonorgestrel	0.05 (6)	15.1
Triquilar[c]	E. estradiol	40 (5)	Levonorgestrel	0.075 (5)	
	E. estradiol	30 (10)	Levonorgestrel	0.125 (10)	
Tri-Norinyl	E. estradiol	35 (7)	Norethindrone	0.5 (7)	14.7
Synphasic[c]	E. estradiol	35 (7)	Norethindrone	1.0 (9)	
	E. estradiol	35 (7)	Norethindrone	0.5 (5)	
Estrostep 21	E. estradiol	20 (5)▲	Nor. acetate	1.0	18 (first cycle)
Estrostep FE	E. estradiol	30 (7)■			
	E. estradiol	35 (9)●			
Tri-Cyclen	E. estradiol	35 (7)	Norgestimate	0.180 (7)	17.5
	E. estradiol	35 (7)	Norgestimate	0.215 (7)	
	E. estradiol	35 (7)	Norgestimate	0.250 (7)	
Ortho Novum 10-11	E. estradiol	35 (10)	Norethindrone	0.5 (10)	19.6
	E. estradiol	35 (11)	Norethindrone	1.0 (11)	
Progestin Only					
Ovrette	None	—	Norgestrel	0.075	34.9
Micronor/Nor Q.D.	None	—	Norethindrone	0.35	42.3

[a]Oral contraceptives containing greater than 50 μg of estrogen are not included in this chart. These products are generally not necessary to prevent conception and are associated with an increase in serious complications. Women who may need to use the higher strength estrogen include women who have had a contraceptive failure while *properly* taking a product containing 50 μg of estrogen, women who are concomitantly taking a medication which decreases the efficacy of the estrogen or women who have severe acne. The higher dose estrogen products are also used to treat other conditions such as ovarian cysts, endometriosis, and dysfunctional uterine bleeding.

[b]Reported prevalence of breakthrough bleeding (BTB) and spotting in the third cycle of use. Information was submitted to the FDA by the manufacturer. These rates are derived from individual studies conducted by various investigators, and therefore information should not be precisely compared.

[c]Canadian trade name.

[d]Number in parentheses indicates number of tablets (days) in each phase.

E. estradiol, ethinyl estradiol; Ethy. diacetate, ethynodiol diacetate; Nor. acetate, norethindrone acetate; BTB, breakthrough bleeding. ▲, ■, ● = tablet shapes.

TABLE 28–3. Absolute and Relative Contraindications to the Use of Oral Contraception

Absolute Contraindications

1. Thrombophlebitis, thromboembolic disorders, cerebral vascular disease, coronary occlusion, or a past history of these conditions, or conditions predisposing to these problems.
2. Markedly impaired liver function. Steroid hormones are contraindicated in patients with hepatitis until liver function tests return to normal.
3. Known or suspected breast cancer.
4. Undiagnosed abnormal vaginal bleeding.
5. Known or suspected pregnancy.
6. Smokers over the age of 35.

Relative Contraindications Requiring Clinical Judgment and Informed Consent

1. **Migraine headaches:** In retrospective studies of high-dose formulations, migraine headaches have been associated with an increased risk of stroke, however, some women report an improvement in their headaches.
2. **Hypertension:** A woman under 35 who is otherwise healthy and whose blood pressure is controlled by medication can elect to use OCs. If an OC-related increase in blood pressure occurs, discontinuing the OC usually results in a return to pretreatment blood pressure values within 3–6 months.
3. **Uterine leiomyoma:** This is no longer a contraindication with the low-dose formulations. There is evidence that the risk of leiomyomas is decreased by 31% in women who used higher dose oral contraception for 10 years. However, a case-control study with lower dose OCs found neither a decrease nor an increase in risk. The administration of low-dose oral contraceptives to women with leiomyomata does not stimulate fibroid growth, and is associated with a reduction in menstrual bleeding.
4. **Gestational diabetes:** Low-dose formulations do not produce a diabetic glucose tolerance response in women with previous gestational diabetes, and there is no evidence that oral contraception increases the incidence of overt diabetes mellitus. Women with previous gestational diabetes can use oral contraception with annual assessment of the fasting glucose level.
5. **Elective surgery:** The recommendation that oral contraception should be discontinued 4 weeks before elective surgery to avoid an increased risk of postoperative thrombosis is based on data derived from high-dose products. If possible, it is safer to follow this recommendation, but it is probably less critical with low-dose OCs. It is more prudent to maintain contraception right up to the performance of a sterilization procedure, and this short, outpatient operation probably carries very minimal risk.
6. **Epilepsy:** Oral contraceptives do not exacerbate epilepsy, and in some women, improvement in seizure control has occurred. Antiepileptic drugs, however, may decrease the effectiveness of oral contraception.
7. **Obstructive jaundice in pregnancy:** Not all patients with this history will develop jaundice on OCs, especially with the low-dose formulations.
8. **Sickle cell disease or sickle C disease:** Patients with sickle cell trait can use oral contraception. The risk of thrombosis in women with sickle cell disease or sickle C diseases is theoretical (and medical-legal). Effective protection against pregnancy in these patients warrants the use of low-dose oral contraception.
9. **Diabetes mellitus:** Effective prevention of pregnancy outweighs the small risk of complicating vascular disease in diabetic women who are under age 35 and otherwise healthy.
10. **Gallbladder disease:** Oral contraceptives do not cause gallstones, but may accelerate the emergence of symptoms when gallstones are already present.

TABLE 28–4. OC Use and Medical Problems

Coagulation disorders: Estrogens increase the risk of thrombotic events, including MI, in a dose-related manner. The use of estrogen containing OCs in women who are predisposed to coagulation disorders is contraindicated. However, the use of OCs in women with coagulation disorders *who have been properly anticoagulated* may be considered, because OCs lower the risk of fetal exposure to warfarin, bleeding corpus luteum cysts, and excessive blood loss during menses.

Gestational diabetes: There is no contraindication to OC use following gestational diabetes.

Diabetes mellitus: Oral contraception can be used by diabetic women less than 35 years old, who do not smoke and are otherwise healthy (especially in an absence of diabetic vascular complications).

Hypertension: Low-dose oral contraception can be used in women less than 35 years old with hypertension controlled by medication, and who are otherwise healthy and do not smoke.

Pregnancy-induced hypertension: Women with pregnancy-induced hypertension can use OCs as soon as the blood pressure is normal in the postpartum period.

Hemorrhagic disorders: Women with hemorrhagic disorder and women taking anticoagulants can use OCs. Inhibition of ovulation can avoid the problem of hemorrhagic corpus luteum in these patients. A reduction in menstrual blood loss is another important benefit.

Gallbladder disease: Oral contraception use may precipitate a symptomatic attack in women known to have stones or a positive history for gallbladder disease, and therefore, should either be used very cautiously or not at all.

Obesity: An obese woman who is otherwise healthy can use low-dose OCs.

Hepatic disease: Oral contraception can be utilized when liver function tests return to normal. Follow-up liver function tests should be obtained after 2–3 months of use.

Seizure disorders: There is no impact of OCs on pattern or frequency of seizures; anticonvulsant drugs can decrease efficacy of OCs and Norplant, increasing the risk of contraceptive failure. Some clinicians advocate the use of higher dose (50 µg estrogen) products or Depo-Provera.

Mitral valve prolapse: Oral contraception use is limited to nonsmoking patients who are asymptomatic (no evidence of regurgitation). Patients with atrial fibrillation, migraine headaches, or clotting factor abnormalities should consider progestin-only methods or the IUD (prophylactic antibiotics should cover IUD insertion in mitral regurgitation if present).

Systemic lupus erythematosus: Oral contraceptive use can exacerbate systemic lupus erythematosus, and the vascular disease associated with lupus represents a contraindication to estrogen-containing OCs. The progestin-only methods can be considered.

Migraine headaches: Low-dose OCs (the lowest estrogen formulations) can be tried with careful surveillance in women with common migraine headaches. Daily administration can prevent menstrual migraine headaches. Oral contraception is best avoided in women with classic migraine headaches associated with neurologic symptoms.

Sickle cell disease: Patients with sickle cell trait can use OCs. The risk of thrombosis in women with sickle cell disease or sickle C is theoretical (and medical-legal). Effective protection against pregnancy in these patients warrants the use of low-dose OCs.

Benign breast disease: Benign breast disease is not a contraindication for oral contraception; with 2 years of use, the condition may improve.

Congenital heart disease or valvular heart disease: Oral contraception is contraindicated only if there is marginal cardiac reserve or a condition that predisposes to thrombosis.

continued

TABLE 28–4. continued

Hyperlipidemia: Because low-dose OCs have negligible impact on the lipoprotein profile, hyperlipidemia is not an absolute contraindication, with the exception of very high levels of triglycerides (which can be made worse by estrogen). If vascular disease is already present, OCs should be avoided. If other risk factors are present, especially smoking, OCs are not recommended. Dyslipidemic patients who begin OCs should have their lipoportein profiles monitored monthly for a few visits to ensure no adverse impact. If the lipid abnormality cannot be held in control, an alternative method of contraception should be used. OCs containing desogestrel, norgestimate, or gestodene can increase HDL levels, but it is not known if this change is clinically significant.

Depression: Low-dose oral contraceptives have minimal, if any, impact on mood.

Smoking: Oral contraception is absolutely contraindicated in smokers over the age of 35. In patients 35 years old and less, heavy smoking (15 or more cigarettes per day) is a relative contraindication. The relative risk of cardiovascular events is increased for women of all ages who smoke and use OCs; however, because the actual incidence of cardiovascular events is so low at a young age, the real risk is very low for young women, although it increases with age. An ex-smoker (for at least one year) should be regarded as a nonsmoker. Risk is only linked to active smoking.

Pituitary prolactin-secreting adenomas: Low-dose OCs can be used in the presence of microadenomas.

Infectious mononucleosis: Oral contraception can be used as long as liver function tests are normal.

Ulcerative colitis: There is no association between oral contraception and ulcerative colitis; women with this problem can use OCs. Oral contraceptives are absorbed mainly in the small bowel.

DRUG INTERACTIONS

- Table 28–5 shows a summary of clinically significant drug interactions.

PATIENT INSTRUCTIONS

- Written information in the patient package insert should be supplemented with verbal information on how the medication works and recognition of common and serious side effects [e.g., breast tenderness, bloating, breakthrough bleeding (BTB), spotting, nausea]. Patients should be aware of the danger signals that require immediate medical attention (Table 28–6).
- Instructions for when to start taking the medication should be provided (either Sunday start or on the first day of the next menses).
- If the patient forgets to take one pill, she should take it as soon as she remembers. If she does not remember to take the pill until the next scheduled pill, she may take two pills at once. If she misses two pills in a row, she may take two pills for the next 2 days. If she misses more than two pills, she should call her physician. If she misses one or more pills in a cycle, barrier method should be used for the rest of that cycle.
- An additional method of contraception is recommended during use of the initial pack of pills and during any time that she has severe diarrhea or vomiting for several days.

TABLE 28–5. Pill Interactions with Other Drugs

Interacting Drugs	Adverse Effects (Probable Mechanism)	Comments and Recommendations
Acetaminophen (Tylenol and others)	Possible decreased pain-relieving effect (increased metabolism)	Monitor pain-relieving response
Alcohol	Possible increased effect of alcohol	Use with caution
Ampicillin	Decreased contraceptive effect	Low but unpredictable incidence; use back-up method of contraception
Anticoagulants (oral)	Decreased anticoagulant effect	Use with caution and monitor INR
Antidepressants (Elavil, Norpramin, Tofranil, and others)	Possible increased antidepressant pharmacologic effect	Monitor for adverse effects
Barbiturates (phenobarbital and others)	Decreased contraceptive effect	Avoid simultaneous use; use alternative contraceptive for patients with epilepsy (i.e., DMPA)
Benzodiazepine tranquilizers (Ativan, Librium, Serax, Tranxene, Valium, Xanax, and others)	Possible increased or decreased tranquilizer effects including psychomotor impairment	Use with caution; greatest impairment during drug-free week in oral contraceptive dosage
Beta blockers (Corgard, Inderal, Lopressor, Tenormin)	Possible increased ß blocker pharmacologic effect	Monitor cardiovascular status
Carbamazepine (Tegretol)	Possible decreased contraceptive effect	Avoid simultaneous use; use alternative contraceptive for patients with epilepsy (i.e., DMPA)
Corticosteroids (cortisone)	Possible increased corticosteroid toxicity	Clinical significance not established
Griseofulvin (Fulvicin, Grifulvin V, and others)	Decreased contraceptive effect	Use back-up method of contraception
Hypoglycemics (Tolbutamide, Diabinese, Orinase, Tolinase)	Possible decreased hypoglycemic effect	Monitor blood glucose
Methyldopa (Aldoclor, Aldomet, and others)	Possible decreased antihypertensive effect, especially with high dose OCs	Monitor blood pressure
Phenytoin (Dilantin)	Decreased contraceptive effect, possible increased phenytoin effect	Use alternative contraceptive (i.e., DMPA); monitor phenytoin concentration
Primidone (Mysoline)	Decreased contraceptive effect	Use alternative contraceptive (i.e., DMPA)
Rifampin	Decreased contraceptive effect	Use back-up method of contraception; use alternate method if planned concomitant use is long term
Tetracycline	Decreased contraceptive effect	Use back-up contraception
Theophylline (Bronkotabs, Marax, Primatene, Quibron Tedral, Theor-Dur, and others)	Decreased contraceptive effect; increased theophylline effect	Monitor theophylline concentration
Troglitazone (Rezulin)	Decreased contraceptive effect	Use alternative contraceptive
Troleandomycin (TAO)	Jaundice (additive)	Avoid simultaneous use
Vitamin C	Increased serum concentration and possible increased adverse effects of estrogens with 1 g or more per day of vitamin C	Avoid high dose of vitamin C

INR, International Normalized Ratio; DMPA, depomedroxyprogesterone acetate.

TABLE 28–6. Symptoms of a Serious or Potentially Serious Nature

Symptom	Possible Cause
Serious: OCs Should Be Stopped Immediately	
Loss of vision, proptosis, diplopia, papilledema	Retinal artery thrombosis
Unilateral numbness, weakness, or tingling	Hemorrhagic or thrombotic stroke
Severe pains in chest, left arm, or neck	Myocardial infarction
Hemoptysis	Pulmonary embolism
Severe pains, tenderness or swelling, warmth, or palpable cord in legs	Thrombophlebitis
Slurring of speech	Hemorrhagic or thrombotic stroke
Hepatic mass or tenderness	Liver neoplasm
Potentially Serious: OCs May Be Continued with Caution While Patient Is Being Evaluated	
Absence of menses	Pregnancy
Spotting or breakthrough bleeding	Cervical, endometrial, or vaginal cancer
Breast mass, pain, or swelling	Breast cancer
Right upper-quadrant pain	Cholecystitis, cholelithiasis, or liver neoplasm
Midepigastric pain	Thrombosis of abdominal artery or vein, myocardial infarction, or pulmonary embolism
Migraine (vascular or throbbing) headache	Vascular spasm which may precede thrombosis
Severe nonvascular headache	Hypertension, vascular spasm
Galactorrhea	Pituitary adenoma
Jaundice, pruritus	Cholestatic jaundice
Depression	Vitamin B_6 deficiency
Uterine size increase	Leiomyomata, adenomyosis, pregnancy

From Dickey R P. Managing Contraceptive Pill Patients, *7th ed. Durant, OK: Essential Medical Information Systems, 1993:148–149.*

- If she received an antibiotic, she may need to use an additional method of contraception for the course of antibiotics and the rest of that cycle. Patients taking minipills should be advised to use a backup method for 48 hours if they are 3 or more hours late in taking their daily progestin dose.

POSTCOITAL "MORNING-AFTER" PILLS

- To prevent pregnancy after unprotected intercourse, a dose of one of the following 6 brands can be taken within 72 hours of unprotected intercourse with a follow up dose 12 hours after the first: **Ovral** (2 tablets/dose); **Nordette, Lo/Ovral, Triphasil, Levlen,** or **TriLevlin** (4 tablets/dose).

LONG-ACTING INJECTABLE OR IMPLANTABLE PROGESTINS

- **Sustained progestin** exposure blocks the LH surge, thus preventing ovulation. Should ovulation occur, progestins reduce ovum motility in the fallopian tubes, thin the endometrium, and thicken cervical mucus.

Medroxyprogesterone Acetate

- **Depomedroxyprogesterone acetate (DMPA)**, 150 mg administered by deep intramuscular (IM) injection in the gluteal or deltoid muscle within 5 days after the onset of menstrual bleeding, inhibits ovulation. The dose should be repeated every 3 months.
- Compared to the 100 mg/mL strength, the 400 mg/mL strength has inconsistent bioavailability, may be less effective, is more painful, and is not approved for contraception.
- DMPA can be used in lactating women and in women with sickle cell disease. It does not alter blood pressure or increase the risk of thromboembolic disorders. It may be used in women with seizure disorders and may even decrease the frequency of seizures.
- The median time to conception from the first omitted dose is 6 months.
- The incidence of irregular bleeding decreases from 30% in the first year to 10% thereafter. After 2 years of therapy, 68% of women report amenorrhea. Because estrogen concentrations may be lower than normal, women can lose bone density. Other side effects are breast tenderness, weight gain, and depression. Minor elevations in serum total triglycerides and decreases in serum HDL have occurred.
- DMPA may enhance the growth of already existing tumors.

Progestin Subdermal Implants

- **Norplant** is a set of six implantable, nonbiodegradable, soft, silicone rubber capsules, each filled with 36 mg of crystalline levonorgestrel. These capsules are inserted under the skin to provide continuous contraception for up to 5 years.
- Failure rates may be unacceptable during the fourth and fifth year in women weighing >154 pounds, and replacement after three years in heavier women is recommended.
- **Norplant II,** a two-rod, 150-mg implant system providing 3 years of contraception, may prove easier to insert and remove.
- Most women return to baseline ovulatory patterns within 1 month of removal of Norplant.
- Drugs that significantly increase hepatic enzymes, including most anticonvulsants and rifampin, lower efficacy.

▶ BARRIER TECHNIQUES AND SPERMICIDES

- These methods include the diaphragm, cervical cap, sponge (no longer available in the United States), condom, and **spermicide.**
- They can reduce the rate of transmission of sexually transmitted diseases.
- The diaphragm may be inserted as long as 6 hours before intercourse and must be left in place for at least 6 hours after intercourse. If intercourse occurs more than once within 6 hours, more spermicide must be inserted.

- Diaphragm users appear to have a lower incidence of cervical neoplasia, but an increased incidence of urinary tract infections.
- The **Prentif cervical cap** is a soft rubber cup that fits over the cervix like a thimble. It is used with a spermicide. It is less messy to use than a diaphragm and remains effective for more than one episode of intercourse (up to 48 hours) without adding more spermicide. Women should not wear the cap for more than 48 hours.
- Most condoms made in the United States are made of latex rubber and are impermeable to viruses; however condoms made of lamb intestine are not.
- When used with any other barrier method, the effectiveness of condoms theoretically approaches 95%. Water-soluble lubricants are preferable, as mineral oil-based medications or lubricants (e.g., **Cleocin vaginal cream, Premarin vaginal cream, Vagistat 1, Femstat, Monistat vaginal suppositories**) can decrease the strength of the latex.

- The condom for women **(Reality)** appears to be as effective as the diaphragm. It may be more effective than the male condom in preventing transmission of herpes.
- Most spermicides contain **nonoxynol-9,** a surfactant that destroys sperm cell walls and offers some protection against sexually transmitted diseases and cervical cancer.
- Additional spermicides must be used each time intercourse is repeated.

▶ PHARMACOECONOMIC CONSIDERATIONS

- The copper intrauterine device, vasectomy, Norplant, and **Depo-Provera** are the most cost-effective methods. OCs are more cost-effective than barrier methods, spermicides, withdrawal, and periodic abstinence.

▶ EVALUATION OF THERAPEUTIC OUTCOMES

- Initial OC use should be reevaluated during the first 3–6 months of therapy to determine if the patient is experiencing any adverse effects and if she wishes to continue.
- All users of OCs should have blood pressure monitored regularly.
- Glucose tolerance should be periodically monitored when an OC is prescribed for a patient with a history of glucose intolerance.
- OC users should receive at least annual cytology screening for cervical cancer.

See Chapter 76, Contraception, authored by Kathryn K. Bucci, PharmD, BCPS, and Deborah Stier Carson, PharmD, BCPS, for a more detailed discussion of this topic.

Chapter 29

▶ HORMONE REPLACEMENT THERAPY

▶ DEFINITION

Menopause is the loss of ovarian function leading to a state of permanent amenorrhea. The climacteric spans several years and includes a series of physiologic and psychologic changes. A period of amenorrhea lasting 1 year is used clinically to define the onset of menopause.

▶ PHYSIOLOGY

- The major circulating estrogen during the reproductive years is 17β-estradiol (E_2) produced primarily by the ovaries. Estrone has approximately one-third the estrogenic potency of estradiol. In the postmenopausal period, virtually all circulating estradiol is derived from conversion of estrone in adipose tissue. Estrone concentrations exceed estradiol by about four-fold afer menopause.

GONADOTROPINS

- Postmenopausal decline in estradiol production causes diminished negative-feedback on the anterior pituitary, resulting in a compensatory increase in secretion of the gonadotropins, follicle-stimulating hormone (FSH) and luteinizing hormone (LH). This results in the level of FSH exceeding LH (opposite of the premenopausal period).
- Peak levels of FSH and LH are reached 2–3 years after menopause and remain stable or decline slightly over the remaining years of life.

▶ CLINICAL PRESENTATION

GENITOURINARY ATROPHY

- With diminished estrogen concentrations, the vagina, vulva, urethra, and trigone of the bladder atrophies, and this continues over many years. There is also thinning of hair of the mons, and shrinkage of the labia minora.
- Vaginal epithelium becomes pale and thin, and there is reduced secretion. The vaginal pH becomes alkaline. Atrophic vaginitis characterized by itching, bleeding, or dyspareunia may occur.
- Postmenopausal women are more prone to the urethral syndrome (e.g., a recurrent, nonbacterial urethritis) and to bacteriuria.

VASOMOTOR INSTABILITY

- Hot flushes (or flashes) are experienced by 75–85% of women following natural menopause and 37–50% of premenopausal women who undergo bilateral oophorectomy. They are most common 12–24 months after the last menstrual period and gradually subside thereafter.

- Symptoms of the hot flash may include increased skin temperature, increased heart rate, nausea, dizziness, headache, palpitations, and diaphoresis.
- **Estrogen** is the traditional treatment for hot flashes, but **medroxyprogesterone** in relatively high doses and some **ergot alkaloids** are also effective.

OSTEOPOROSIS

- Bone loss is associated with declining estrogen levels in the perimenopausal and menopausal periods.
- Vertebral crush fractures are most common, but hip fractures have the most serious sequelae. Twelve to 20% of patients who suffer a hip fracture die from complications within 6 months.

- The greatest risk of postmenopausal osteoporosis occurs in slender, sedentary females of Caucasian or Asian descent. Other risk factors include smoking, chronic alcohol use, low calcium intake, malignancy, rheumatoid arthritis, endocrine disorders, and chronic use of certain drugs (e.g., corticosteroids).

CARDIOVASCULAR DISEASE

- After natural or surgical menopause, the incidence of coronary artery disease increases.

OTHER SYMPTOMS

- Other symptoms include insomnia, fatigue, irritability, depression, crying spells, anxiety, and impaired memory. Most women experience some change in sexual function in the years immediately before and after menopause.

▶ DIAGNOSIS

- The diagnosis of menopause should involve a comprehensive medical history and physical examination with complete blood count and measurement of serum FSH. In the absence of other disease processes, a serum FSH of ≥30 pg/mL indicates that the woman is menopausal.
- Altered thyroid function and pregnancy must be excluded.

▶ DESIRED OUTCOME

- The goal of hormone replacement therapy (HRT) is relief of vasomotor, genitourinary, and associated symptoms, and the prevention of osteoporosis and cardiovascular disease.

▶ TREATMENT

NONHORMONAL TREATMENT

- Nonpharmacologic measures are generally not very helpful, but aerobic exercise and resistance training may help with cardiovascular disease, obesity, muscle weakness, and osteoporosis. Behavioral symptoms may respond to counseling.
- For treatment and prevention of osteoporosis, see Chapter 3.
- For vaginal dryness and dyspareunia, a mucoadherent lubricant, **polycarbophil,** is available without a prescription. It is long-acting and lowers pH.
- Exercise and diet, along with smoking cessation, stress reduction, and moderation in alcohol consumption are the foundation of prevention of cardiovascular disease.

ESTROGEN REPLACEMENT THERAPY

- Indications for estrogen replacement therapy (ERT) include relief from vasomotor symptoms, genitourinary dysfunction, and some psychologic changes, as well as prevention or treatment of osteoporosis. It also reduces cardiovascular morbidity and mortality.

Pharmacology

- **Estrogens** attach to receptors in the cytoplasm of target organs including ovaries, uterus, fallopian tubes, vagina, bladder, urethra, breast, skin, adrenals, cardiovascular system, gastrointestinal (GI) tract, and the central nervous system (CNS). The estrogen–protein complex diffuses through the nuclear membrane and binds within the cell nucleus. Synthesis of DNA, RNA, and other proteins increases, altering response tissue.
- Exogenous estrogen products are shown in Table 29–1. Injectable estrogens are not generally used for menopausal symptoms because of poor patient acceptance and fluctuating plasma concentrations.
- **Conjugated equine estrogens** are a mixture of estrogen compounds, mostly sulfates and glucuronides, some of which are not found in humans.
- Oral absorption of **estradiol** is more reliable with micronized formulations, but estradiol is metabolized significantly on first pass through the liver to less active metabolites.
- Estrogen in **vaginal creams** is a feasible treatment for urogenital and other menopausal symptoms. Estradiol is metabolized very little as it is absorbed from the vagina, resulting in increased plasma concentrations. Unfortunately, these concentrations return to baseline in approximately 6 hours; they are not widely used.
- The **transdermal patch** is applied to the skin, usually on the lower trunk. This offers convenience with little metabolism of estradiol and precise dosing.

TABLE 29–1. Estrogen Products

Agent	Dosage Form	Dose	Indications
Estrone aqueous suspension	Injection	0.1–5 mg IM 2–3 times/week	A,B
Estrogenic substance or estrogen aqueous suspension (primarily estrone) injection	Injection	0.1–1.0 mg IM 2–3 times/week	A,B
Estradiol cypionate (in oil)	Injection	1–5 mg IM weekly for 3–4 weeks	C
Estradiol valerate (in oil)	Injection	10–20 mg every 4 weeks	A,B,C
Conjugated estrogens	Oral	0.03–1.25 mg/d[a]	A,B,C,D
Conjugated estrogens/medroxyprogesterone acetate	Oral	0.625 mg/2.5 mg per day[b]	C,D
Conjugated estrogens/medroxyprogesterone acetate	Oral	0.625 mg/d for 14 days,[b] then 0.625 mg/5 mg per day for 14 days[b]	C,D
Estradiol, micronized	Oral	0.5–2 mg/d[a]	A,B,C,D
Esterified estrogens (75–85% estrone sulfate and 6–15% sodium equilin)	Oral	0.3–1.25 mg/d[a]	A,B,C,D
Estropipate (piperazine estrone sulfate)	Oral	0.75–6 mg/d[a]	A,B,C
Ethinyl estradiol	Oral	0.02–1.5 mg/d[a]	A,C
Quinestrol	Oral	0.1 mg/d for 7 days, then 0.1 mg once weekly	A,B,C
Chlorotrianisene	Oral	12–25 mg/d for 21 days	A,B,C
Estropipate vaginal cream	Topical	3–6 mg daily for 3 weeks	B
Estradiol micronized vaginal cream	Topical	Daily[c]	B
Conjugated estrogens vaginal cream	Topical	1.25–2.5 mg/d for 3 weeks	B
Dienestrol vaginal cream	Topical	Once or twice daily[c]	B
Estrone vaginal cream	Topical	2–4 mg/d	B
Estradiol transdermal	Transdermal	0.05–0.1 mg system twice weekly	A,B,C,D

[a]May administer continuously or cyclically with 3 weeks of daily estrogen followed by 1 week off.
[b]Blister pack dosage cards used for single prescription convenience in continuous or cyclic combination regimens.
[c]Typical regimen: Initial therapy one dose daily for 2 weeks, followed by 2 additional weeks of daily therapy at one-half dose, followed by maintenance therapy of one dose 1–3 times/week for three weeks.
Check drug information references for specific regimens.
A, replacement therapy of estrogen deficiency-associated conditions (e.g., female hypogonadism); B, senile vaginitis and Kraurosis vulvae; C, moderate to severe vasomotor symptoms associated with menopause; D, osteoporosis.

- Transdermal administration of estrogens results in estradiol levels equivalent to those in the early to mid-follicular phase and an estrone-to-estradiol ratio of approximately 1 to 1, which closely resembles the premenopausal state. Unlike oral ERT, transdermal estrogen has no significant effect on the production of certain hepatic proteins, renin substrate, sex-hormone-binding globulin, thyroxine-binding globulin, and cortisol-binding globulin. Although controversial, the effects of transdermal ERT on the lipid profile appear to be less favorable than with orally administered estrogens.
- Administration of **transdermal estrogen** may be either continuous, or in 3-week cycles with 1 week estrogen free. The addition of a **progestin** is recommended for the last 10–13 days of the cycle in women receiving cyclic therapy who have an intact uterus.

Clinical Use

- The presence of any estrogen-dependent cancer should be ruled out before the initiation of ERT. If not recently done, mammography should be performed.
- Figure 29–1 shows a decision analysis model to determine which patients would achieve at least 6 months of additional life expectancy from HRT. The authors of this study estimated that 99% of healthy postmenopausal women would benefit from HRT.

Vasomotor Instability

- Symptoms of vasomotor instability respond to ERT.
- The addition of a progestin (e.g., **medroxyprogesterone acetate, norethindrone, norgestrel,** or **micronized oral progesterone**) is standard therapy in women with an intact uterus to counter the increased risk of endometrial cancer.
- For women in whom cyclical bleeding is unacceptable, an alternative involves continuous administration of estrogens with the addition of a progestin for 10–12 days each month. Some clinicians advocate continuous administration of estrogens and lower dose progestins (2.5–5 mg daily of medroxyprogesterone acetate) as an effective alternative to cyclic therapy, which also avoids withdrawal bleeding.

Urogenital Atrophy

- Therapy is generally initiated with the smallest dose to restore the vaginal epithelium, usually 2–4 g of **estradiol cream** given once daily for 1–2 weeks initially, then half-doses for an additional 2 weeks. Maintenance therapy can be continued with 1 g given one to three times weekly in the usual cyclic manner. Alternatives to estradiol cream include **dienestrol, conjugated estrogens,** or **estropipate cream** given in the same cyclic manner.
- Oral, transdermal, or vaginal ERT often relieves urogenital symptoms in the same doses discussed for vasomotor instability.

VI

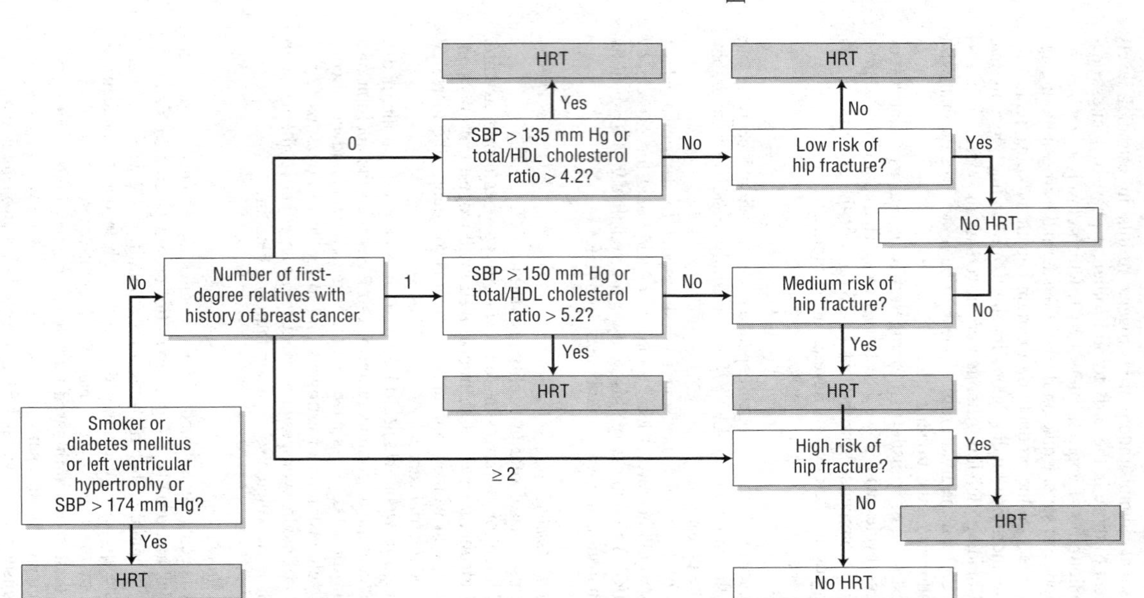

Figure 29–1. Decision analysis model to determine patients who would achieve at least 6 months of additional life expectancy from HRT. HDL, high-density lipoprotein; SBP, systolic blood pressure.

Osteoporosis

- The response of bone to ERT is a reduced rate of resorption with normal mineralization of the remodeling unit. Estrogens alone do not restore bone that has been lost.
- HRT should be begun soon after menopause (preferable within 3 years). If HRT is discontinued, bone loss begins immediately. At least 7 years of HRT is necessary to achieve persistent bone density; this benefit extends to women of age 75 years. Protective effects against hip fracture also wane, but are not eliminated, with age. Thus some clinicians recommend starting HRT at menopause and never stopping.
- The dose of conjugated estrogen required to prevent bone loss is 0.625 mg/d. Lower doses (e.g., 0.312 mg/d) may prevent bone loss if used with high daily doses of **elemental calcium** (1500 mg/d). Alternative regimens are esterified estrogens (0.625 mg/d), oral ethinyl estradiol (0.02 mg/d), micronized 17β-estradiol (1 mg/d), and transdermal estrogen patches (delivering estradiol 0.05–0.10 mg administered as one patch twice weekly). VI
- Adequate intake of calcium and regular weight-bearing exercise are also important adjunctive treatments.

Cardiovascular Disease

- Estrogens lower low-density lipoprotein (LDL) cholesterol and increase high-density lipoprotein (HDL) cholesterol. Other mechanisms such as platelet effects and direct effects on vessel wall physiology may also be cardioprotective. While triglycerides may be higher in estrogen users, blood pressure and fasting blood glucose levels are unchanged or lower.
- Estrogen therapy has shown a ≥50% reduction in cardiovascular morbidity and mortality.
- Progestins may attenuate the benefits on HDL. However, cardiovascular benefits of combined treatment on HDL have been confirmed.

PROGESTIN THERAPY

- Progestins alone are as effective as estrogens for relief of vasomotor symptoms and are also useful in treatment and prevention of osteoporosis.
- Administration of a progestin for 12 days each month with ERT decreases risk of estrogen-induced irregular bleeding, endometrial hyperplasia, and carcinoma; protects against breast carcinoma; and enhances estrogen prophylaxis of osteoporosis.
- The 17-hydroxyprogesterone derivatives are used primarily in HRT but are associated with depression and anxiety symptoms. Medroxyprogesterone acetate is the progestin generally used.

Clinical Use

- The usual dose of medroxyprogesterone acetate is 2.5–5 mg/d with ERT to prevent endometrial hyperplasia.

- Medroxyprogesterone acetate (20 mg/d) orally has been used alone to treat vasomotor instability. Alternatively, depot medroxyprogesterone acetate 50–100 mg intramuscularly given every 2–3 months is as effective as conjugated estrogens.
- When estrogen is contraindicated, medroxyprogesterone acetate, 5–10 mg/d, or the depot injection, 100–200 mg every 2–3 months, may be an alternative for treatment of osteoporosis.

Adverse Effects

- When used alone or with ERT, a premenstrual tension-like syndrome (physical and behavioral symptoms) may occur along with weight gain, headache, and drowsiness. Dosage reduction or switching progestins may help.
- Progestins cause a dose-related decrease in HDL and an increase in LDL. When given with ERT, they should be used at the minimum dosage required for endometrial protection.

PHARMACOECONOMIC CONSIDERATIONS

- The cost per quality adjusted life-year (QALY) saved ranged from $5600 in symptomatic women with no increased breast cancer risk and no HRT side effects treated for 10 years to $139,000 in women with increased risk of breast cancer, who had no menopausal symptoms, but did suffer HRT adverse effects.

▶ EVALUATION OF THERAPEUTIC OUTCOMES

- In women taking HRT, routine visits with regular breast examinations, PAP smears, and monitoring of the cardiovascular system (blood pressure, lipid profile, symptoms) and skeleton are indicated. All women receiving ERT should practice regular breast self-examination along with annual physician breast examinations and routine mammography.
- Periodic endometrial biopsy to screen for endometrial hyperplasia should be done in women receiving unopposed estrogen.

▶ RISKS AND BENEFITS

- Overall, HRT use was associated with a 37% decrease in mortality from any cause, but the apparent benefit declined after 10 or more years to a 20% decrease in mortality due to increase in incidence of breast cancer. There may be a 30% decrease in mortality risk from cancers overall.
- Estrogen users have a four- to eight-fold increase in risk of endometrial cancer. The addition of progestin to ERT confers protection against endometrial hyperplasia.
- A history of thromboembolism is a relative contraindication to estrogen therapy. Despite producing increased amounts of clotting factors, estrogens do not produce a hypercoagulable state. Clinical trials have shown

no increase in risk of thromboembolism in postmenopausal women receiving ERT.

- There is a significant benefit of HRT on risk of cardiovascular disease. This is attributed to their effects on lipids and lipoproteins. Synthetic progestins have an effect on lipoproteins that is opposite that of estrogens.
- Progestins produce a dose-related increase in blood pressure by causing sodium and water retention.
- There may also be a benefit of ERT in prevention of Alzheimer's disease.

See Chapter 78, Hormone Replacement Therapy, authored by Mark C. Pugh, PharmD, and Patricia Moynahan Mullins, PharmD, for a more detailed discussion of this topic.

Chapter 30

▶ PREGNANCY AND LACTATION: THERAPEUTIC CONSIDERATIONS

▶ DIAGNOSIS OF PREGNANCY

- Pregnancy may be confirmed by the presence of human chorionic gonadotropin (HCG). Serum tests such as radioimmunoassay (RIA) and enzyme-linked immunosorbent assay (ELISA) can detect concentrations as low as 5 mIU/mL (present about 6–10 days after implantation). Urine tests using monoclonal antibodies can usually detect concentrations of HCG in the 20–40 mIU/mL range (1–2 weeks after fertilization).
- Quantitative serum assays for HCG should be used in the diagnosis of ectopic pregnancies or suspected pregnancy loss.
- Home pregnancy tests using monoclonal antibodies are sensitive and specific, but false negatives occur 25% of the time usually due to errors in performing the test. False positives occur <3% of the time. Home tests fail to detect 50% of ectopic pregnancies.

▶ NORMAL COURSE OF PREGNANCY

- The normal gestation period is 267 days from conception or 280 days from the first day of the last menstrual period. The average weight gain is 24 pounds, 3 pounds during the first trimester and 1 pound per week during the last 16 weeks.
- During pregnancy it is common to give a **multivitamin.** Many pregnant patients may require supplemental **iron,** and most prescription prenatal vitamins contain at least 60 mg elemental iron. Pregnant women should ingest at least 1.2 grams of elemental **calcium** daily, either from diet or through supplementation.
- All women of childbearing age capable of becoming pregnant should take at least 0.4 mg of **folic acid** daily to reduce the incidence of neural tube defects. Patients should never take more than 0.8 mg of folic acid daily without physician supervision.

▶ DRUG EFFECTS ON THE FETUS

- Major structural abnormalities occur in 2–4% of births in the United States. If minor malformations, such as ear tags or extra digits are included, this increases to 10%. About 25% of abnormalities are probably due to genetic predisposition, while 2–3% are drug-induced. All drugs should be avoided during pregnancy unless absolutely necessary, and the lowest effective dose should be used for the shortest duration possible.

- The Food and Drug Administration (FDA) requires that all drugs marketed after 1983 be assigned a pregnancy risk category (Table 30–1).
- Factors that influence the teratogenicity of a drug include the genotype of the mother and fetus, embryonic stage at exposure, the dose, specificity of the agent, and the simultaneous exposure to other agents.
- Teratogens may cause spontaneous abortion, congenital abnormalities, intrauterine growth retardation, mental retardation, carcinogenesis, and mutagenesis.
- Drug exposure around the time of conception and implantation may kill the fetus. If exposure occurs in the first 12–15 days after conception, when the cells are still totipotential (i.e., if one cell is damaged or killed, another can assume its function), the fetus may not be damaged. The first 3 months are the most critical in terms of malformations. Functional and behavior defects have been associated with drug exposure later in gestation.
- Effects of medication on labor and delivery should be considered. **Salicylate** use late in gestation can cause increased bleeding at delivery and delay the onset of labor.

PLACENTAL TRANSPORT

- Drugs with molecular weights <400, highly unionized, and lipophilic drugs cross the placenta more readily. Most drugs have molecular weights between 250 and 400 and cross the placenta by simple diffusion. Other factors influencing placental transfer are degree of protein binding, maternal and fetal blood flow, the area available for exchange, and the amount of placental metabolism.
- Many drugs reach concentrations in the fetus at 50% to over 100% of maternal blood levels. The fetus may have higher free drug concentrations than the mother, as the concentration of blood proteins is lower in the fetus. Fetal drug clearance may be slower than in healthy adults.

TABLE 30–1. FDA Categories for Drug Use in Pregnancy

Category A: Controlled studies in women fail to demonstrate a risk to the fetus in the first trimester, and the possibility of fetal harm appears remote.

Category B: Either animal studies do not indicate a risk to the fetus and there are no controlled studies in pregnant women, or animal studies have indicated fetal risk, but controlled studies in pregnant women failed to demonstrate a risk.

Category C: Either animal studies indicate a fetal risk and there are no controlled studies in women or there are no available studies in women or animals.

Category D: There is positive evidence of fetal risk, but there may be certain situations where the benefit might outweigh the risk (life-threatening or serious diseases where other drugs are ineffective or carry a greater risk).

Category X: There is definite fetal risk based on studies in animals or humans or based on human experience, and the risk clearly outweighs any benefit in pregnant women.

From Content format for labeling of human prescription drugs. Fed Reg *1979;44: 37434–37467.*

TABLE 30–2. Medications Known to Be Teratogens

Alcohol	Isotretinoin
Androgens	Lithium
Anticonvulsants	Live vaccines
Antineoplastics	Methimazole
Cocaine	Penicillamine
Diethylstilbestrol	Tetracyclines
Etretinate	Warfarin
Iodides (including radioactive iodine)	

SPECIFIC AGENTS

VI The following is not a complete list of drugs affecting the fetus, and the reader is referred to the primary literature. Drugs with known, suspected, and no known teratogenic effects are listed in Tables 30–2, 30–3, and 30–4, and nonteratogenic adverse effects are shown in Table 30–5.

Benzodiazepines

- **Diazepam** has been associated with facial clefts.
- The floppy infant syndrome, neonatal central nervous system (CNS) depression, and withdrawal symptoms may occur following chronic benzodiazepine use during the last trimester and when large doses are administered shortly before delivery.

Lithium

- Infants exposed to **lithium** during the first trimester have an increased risk of developing abnormalities, 75% of which are cardiovascular (e.g., Epstein's anomaly).
- When administered late in pregnancy, manifestations of neonatal toxicity include cyanosis, hypotonia, bradycardia, and electrocardiographic abnormalities.

Sex Hormones

- **Progestogens** and **androgens,** including **danazol,** are associated with masculinization of the female fetus.
- Progestogens, primarily those present in oral contraceptives, may produce the VACTERL syndrome: vertebral, anal, cardiovascular, tracheal,

TABLE 30–3. Medications Suspected to Be Teratogens

ACE inhibitors	Oral hypoglycemic agents
Benzodiazepines	Progestogens
Estrogens	Quinolones

TABLE 30–4. Medications With No Known Teratogenic Effects[a]

Acetaminophen	Narcotic analgesics
Cephalosporins	Penicillins
Corticosteroids	Phenothiazines
Docusate sodium	Thyroid hormones
Erythromycin	Tricyclic antidepressants
Multiple vitamins	

[a]No drug is absolutely without risk during pregnancy. These drugs appear to have a minimal risk when used judiciously in usual doses under clinical supervision.

esophageal, renal, and limb defects. This is a rare event, and a more likely problem resulting from progestin exposure is abnormal sex organ development.

- **Diethylstilbestrol (DES)** causes a number of reproductive tract abnormalities in both female and male offspring exposed in utero, the most common being vaginal clear cell adenocarcinoma in daughters of mothers taking DES.
- **Estrogens** and progestogens are contraindicated during pregnancy.

Isotretinoin

- **Isotretinoin,** a vitamin A isomer, is a potent teratogen (e.g., craniofacial, CNS, and cardiac defects). Women of child-bearing age should have a negative pregnancy test before initiating treatment and must use at least two reliable methods of contraception during therapy and for 1 month after the last dose.

Antineoplastic Agents

- All antineoplastic agents except **cyclosporin A** have teratogenic potential in animals.

TABLE 30–5. Medications With Nonteratogenic Adverse Effects in Pregnancy

Antithyroid drugs	Diuretics
Aminoglycosides	Isoniazid
Aspirin	Narcotic analgesics (chronic use)
Barbiturates (chronic use)	Nicotine
Benzodiazepines	Nonsteroidal anti-inflammatory agents
β blockers	Oral hypoglycemic agents
Caffeine	Propylthiouracil
Chloramphenicol	Sulfonamides
Cocaine	

Antibiotics

- All **tetracyclines** have been reported to cause congenital abnormalities, particularly staining of the teeth and retardation of the developing skeletal system.
- In animal studies, **fluoroquinolones** were shown to cause erosion of the cartilage and other arthropathies in fetuses. These drugs should not be used in pregnancy.

▶ TREATMENT OF CONDITIONS CAUSED OR EXACERBATED BY PREGNANCY

NAUSEA AND VOMITING

- Half of all pregnant patients experience some degree of nausea and vomiting during the first trimester, especially upon arising. For some women, nausea lasts throughout the day and throughout pregnancy. Hyperemesis gravidarum, nausea that cannot be controlled and results in dehydration and malnutrition, can be life-threatening and requires immediate therapy, usually with intravenous fluids, electrolytes, and antiemetics. Total parenteral nutrition and enteral feeding have been effective.
- Medication must be considered for patients whose nausea persists despite dietary alterations. Medications used most often include **phenothiazines, meclizine, cyclizine, dimenhydrinate, doxylamine,** and **pyridoxine.** Recently **ondansetron,** a category B drug, has been used effectively.

HEARTBURN

- Heartburn during pregnancy may result from relaxation of the cardiac sphincter and increased pressure in the stomach caused by the enlarging uterus. Recommendations include smaller, more frequent meals, avoiding food and liquids other than water for at least 3 hours before bedtime, and elevating the head of the bed with blocks.
- **Magnesium** and/or **aluminum hydroxides** are usually effective, and duration of action is several hours. **Sucralfate** is poorly absorbed, and no adverse effects to the fetus have been reported.

CONSTIPATION

- Constipation is common, and pregnant women should be encouraged to add fiber to their diet, increase their fluid intake (eight 8-oz glasses of water daily), and exercise moderately (e.g., walking).
- **Surfactants** and **bulk laxatives** are the agents of choice. **Mineral oil** should be avoided.

HEMORRHOIDS

- Correction of constipation and use of stool softeners and sitz baths are usually helpful in reducing discomfort.

- External medications are preferred over those inserted into the rectum because many drugs are absorbed rectally. **Topical anesthetics** and **steroids** are usually avoided.

COAGULATION DISORDERS

- Anticoagulation is necessary if there is a history of deep vein thrombosis, a prosthetic heart valve, deficiencies of certain clotting factors, or antiphospholipid antibodies.
- **Warfarin** should be avoided.
- **Subcutaneous (SC) heparin** and **low molecular weight heparin (LMWH)** are the anticoagulants of choice for chronic use during pregnancy. Heparin does not cross the placenta, and heparin's effects can be reversed by **protamine sulfate.** There are no reports of congenital malformations caused by heparin or LMWH.
- Conversion from oral anticoagulants to subcutaneous heparin or LMWH should be considered for those wishing to become pregnant. Advantages of LMWH over SC heparin include less risk for thrombocytopenia and osteoporosis, once daily dosing, and simplified monitoring.

▶ TREATMENT OF PREGNANCY-SPECIFIC CONDITIONS

PREGNANCY-INDUCED HYPERTENSION

- Pregnancy-induced hypertension can be life-threatening. Gestational hypertension is diagnosed when the blood pressure exceeds 140/90 mm Hg in the absence of proteinuria or pathologic edema.
- Mild preeclampsia is hypertension accompanied by proteinuria (≥300 mg/24 h or 100 mg/dL in two random samples 6 hours apart) and/or pathologic edema.
- Preeclampsia is severe when proteinuria exceeds 4 g/24 h or persistent dipstick values of 2+, blood pressure is 160/110 mm Hg or severe headache, visual disturbances, or epigastric pain are noted.
- Eclampsia is the development of generalized tonic–clonic seizures in a patient with pregnancy-induced hypertension.
- Pregnancy-aggravated hypertension is defined as preexisting essential hypertension with a 15 mm Hg increase in diastolic or 30 mm Hg increase in systolic blood pressure after the 24th week of gestation.
- Eight-five percent of patients with preeclampsia are primiparas, particularly those who are very young or at the upper end of the reproductive age range. Other risk factors include essential hypertension, family history of preeclampsia, multiple fetuses, and molar pregnancies.
- Prevention of preeclampsia with low-dose **aspirin** has been suggested for patients at high risk for developing the disorder. The recommended dose is 60 mg/d and is usually initiated at the 24th to 28th week and continued until the onset of labor. Low-dose aspirin has not been shown to be useful in the treatment of existing preeclampsia or eclampsia.

- Treatment for preeclampsia is delivery if the pregnancy is at term. If not at term, treatment is bed rest with frequent monitoring of blood pressure, urine protein, serum chemistries, and platelets. Antihypertensive medications have not been shown to prolonging gestation. Severely preeclamptic women must be hospitalized, begun on parenteral **magnesium sulfate** to prevent seizures, and delivered. IV administration may be preferred, as magnesium carries a risk of toxicity, and an IV infusion may be quickly discontinued. IV administration is initiated with a loading dose of 4 grams and followed by an infusion of 1–3 g/h using a controlled infusion pump. Another regimen begins with a 4-grams IV load with simultaneous intramuscular injection of 10 grams (5 grams in each buttock) followed by 5 grams IM every 4 hours. The large volume IM injections are painful, and **lidocaine** may be used to minimize discomfort.
- Close monitoring of patients receiving magnesium sulfate is essential. The optimum serum concentration for prevention of seizures is 4–7 mEq/L. Reflexes should be checked every hour. Urine output should be >25 mL/h, and respirations should be >10/min. IV administration of 1 gram of **calcium gluconate** (10 mL of 10% solution) usually reverses mild magnesium toxicity. Magnesium levels should be determined in "floppy" neonates exposed to magnesium prior to delivery.
- Seizures not controlled by magnesium may respond to IV **diazepam** or **phenytoin.**
- A systolic reading of ≥160–180 mm Hg or a diastolic reading of ≥110 mm Hg should be treated with an IV antihypertensive. **Hydralazine,** 5–10 mg IV, is given initially, followed by 10 mg every 20 minutes as needed to decrease diastolic blood pressure to below 100 mm Hg. An infusion may also be necessary. **Propranolol** may be useful in opposing the cardiac side effects of hydralazine (tachycardia, palpitations, flushing), but it should not be used alone to control blood pressure. IV **labetalol,** an α- and β-adrenergic blocker, may be an alternative to hydralazine as it has a faster onset of effectiveness with less reflex tachycardia. Hydralazine tends to be more effective.
- Neither **diazoxide, nitroprusside,** nor diuretics are recommended in these patients. Calcium channel blockers may be useful for acute hypertensive episodes in pregnancy, but further study is required.

PRETERM LABOR

- Uterine contractions with cervical changes prior to the 37th week of gestation are termed preterm labor. Inhibition of labor is not usually attempted before the 20th week.
- Drug therapy is most successful when the cervix is dilated <4 cm and membranes are intact. Premature rupture of membranes is usually considered a contraindication to inhibition of labor, but it may be advantageous to administer pharmacologic agents to delay delivery 24–48 hours to allow glucocorticoids to enhance fetal lung maturity.

- Although the efficacy of tocolytics has been questioned, most clinicians choose to treat preterm labor.

β-Agonists

- **Ritodrine** is the only β-adrenergic drug approved in the United States for premature labor, but **terbutaline** is also used. Terbutaline is as effective and less expensive than ritodrine and is available IV, subcutaneously, and orally.
- Side effects of both drugs include hypotension, tachycardia, hypokalemia (with parenteral therapy), palpitations, tremor, anxiety, angina, and headache. The fluid of choice is 5% dextrose in water (less incidence of pulmonary edema than with isotonic saline). Limiting the fluid intake to 2500 mL/24 h may also decease the likelihood of pulmonary edema.
- IV infusion of ritodrine or terbutaline is usually continued for 12 hours after contractions cease. Oral medication is initiated 30 minutes before the infusion is stopped. Terbutaline has also been given by subcutaneous pump for maintenance.

Magnesium Sulfate

- **Magnesium sulfate** is also effective in inhibiting preterm labor at serum levels of 6–8 mEq/L. In addition to monitoring the patellar reflex, urine output, and respirations, some protocols require serial magnesium levels every 6 hours. It may be the agent of choice for diabetic patients.
- Serious neonatal effects are uncommon unless the treatment fails and the delivery occurs during the infusion. Respiratory depression in the mother can be reversed by administration of 10 mL of 10% **calcium gluconate.**

Others

- Oral and rectal **indomethacin** are effective for preterm labor, but potential side effects to the fetus include premature closure of the ductus arteriosus, poor cardiopulmonary adaptation after delivery, necrotizing enterocolitis, intracranial hemorrhage, and renal dysfunction. Therefore, use of indomethacin is limited to 72 hours.
- **Nifedipine** has been used as a tocolytic agent.

INDUCTION OF LABOR

- Indications include severe maternal infection; uterine bleeding; preeclampsia, eclampsia, or chronic hypertension; diabetes mellitus; macrosomia; maternal renal insufficiency; premature rupture of membranes after the 36th week; polyhydramnios; evidence of placental insufficiency; isoimmunization; and postdate pregnancy.
- The ergot alkaloids are not used to induce labor at term or in late pregnancy.

- The prostaglandin **dinoprostone** is available as a gel and vaginal insert, both of which are approved for labor induction. The suppository is approved only for termination in early pregnancy. The gel or insert is used with electronic fetal and uterine monitoring. **Oxytocin** is usually administered several hours later.
- **Misoprostol** has been used for labor induction by both vaginal and oral routes. It is less expensive than dinoprostone.
- Hyperstimulation with any of the above agents can be reversed with β-adrenergic tocolytic agents.
- Oxytocin is the drug used most often to induce labor, augment inadequate labor, and decrease postpartum bleeding. Some clinicians begin with 2 mU/min, increasing by 1 mU/min every 20–30 minutes; others use as much as 6 mU/min increasing by 6 mU every 20–30 minutes. The maximum dose of 20 mU/min should generally not be exceeded, unless internal monitoring of the magnitude of uterine contractions is being used. The goal is contractions that last 45 to 60 seconds at intervals of 2–3 minutes. Fetal monitoring is also required.
- Side effects of oxytocin include uterine rupture (infrequent), fetal hypoxia (reduced uteroplacental blood flow), maternal hypotension, hypoglycemia, and fluid retention.
- Contraindications include abnormal fetal positions or presentations, cephalopelvic disproportion, previous classical cesarean section, some other previous uterine surgeries, and a firm, closed, uneffaced, posterior cervix. Patients with functional class III or IV heart disease are not good candidates for oxytocin use.

▶ TREATMENT OF CHRONIC MEDICAL DISORDERS IN PREGNANCY

DIABETES

- Patients should be normoglycemic before conception and during the first trimester as congenital malformations associated with diabetes seem to be related to poor control during the first 8 weeks. Patients with highest risk of complications include those with vasculopathy, poor glucose control, a previous stillbirth, and noncompliance.
- Complications of diabetic pregnancies include fetal macrosomia, polyhydramnios, malformations, and respiratory distress syndrome. During pregnancy, diabetic patients have an increased risk of hypoglycemia and ketoacidosis.
- Glucose tests using whole blood are preferred over urine tests. Glucose should be monitored fasting, before meals, and at bedtime daily. Monitoring 1 hour after a meal once weekly may also be useful. Evaluation of glycosylated hemoglobin once each trimester is also recommended. Most women should be able to maintain glucose levels between 60–120 mg/dL.

- Only intermediate-acting and fast-acting insulins should be used. **NPH** or **lente insulin,** combined with **regular insulin,** should be given subcutaneously in two divided doses daily. About 70% of pregnant patients have increased insulin requirements after the 24th week, and requirements will usually double by the end of pregnancy.
- Oral hypoglycemic agents should be discontinued before conception and are contraindicated during pregnancy, as they can cause fetal and neonatal hypoglycemia and have teratogenic effects.
- Gestational diabetes (glucose intolerance of pregnancy) develops during the second half of pregnancy in about 2–3% of patients. If a diabetic diet does not control glucose, insulin should be started.
- Tight glucose control should be maintained during labor and delivery. An IV infusion of 1 liter of 5% dextrose with 10 units of regular insulin given at a rate of 100 mL/h may be given. Additional glucose or insulin may be given to maintain glucose at approximately 100 mg/dL. Alternatively, IV administration of 50 grams of glucose every 6 hours, with regular insulin given subcutaneously as needed can be used. Blood glucose should be checked every 1–2 hours.
- Immediately after delivery of the placenta, insulin requirements drop and remain lower for 24–72 hours, and hypoglycemic shock is common during this period.
- Breastfeeding is encouraged; lower insulin requirements during lactation are expected.

THYROID DISEASE

- Preeclampsia, maternal heart failure, and stillbirths are more common in hyperthyroid pregnancies than normal pregnancies or adequately treated hyperthyroid pregnancies.
- **Methimazole** and **propylthiouracil (PTU)** are equally effective. PTU is generally preferred. The dose must be individualized.
- Hypothyroidism in pregnancy should be treated with **thyroxine** replacement.

CHRONIC HYPERTENSION

- Chronic hypertension in pregnancy is described as hypertension present at conception or developing before the 20th week of gestation. Up to one-third of hypertensive patients have superimposed preeclampsia.
- Blood pressure should be controlled. It is common for blood pressure to decrease in the second trimester. Mild hypertension should be treated with bed rest (at least 1 hour at lunch, 1 hour in the afternoon, and 10 hours at night).
- Patients not responding may be treated with **methyldopa. Propranolol, labetalol,** and **hydralazine** are second-line drugs. If propranolol is used, it should be discontinued 1–2 weeks before delivery, and the neonate observed for adverse effects. Oral hydralazine may be less effective than propranolol, but may be useful near delivery.

- **Diuretics, reserpine,** and **angiotensin-converting enzyme (ACE) inhibitors** should not be used during pregnancy. Until more data are available, calcium channel blockers should be avoided as well.

EPILEPSY

- During pregnancy, about 25% of epileptics experience an exacerbation of disease, 25% have fewer seizures, and 50% have no change.
- Although it is difficult to separate the effects of medication from the effects of the disease, most evidence supports a role of antiepileptic drugs (AEDs) in causing congenital problems (e.g., orofacial clefts, skeletal anomalies, CNS malformations, cardiac abnormalities, and mental retardation). The risk of maternal seizures is considered more harmful to the fetus than teratogenicity.
- Patients who have been seizure-free for several years should undergo a trial of medication withdrawal before becoming pregnant. Patients with recurrent epilepsy who are on AEDs should be advised that they have a 90% chance of having a normal child, but that the risk of congenital abnormalities and mental retardation is twice that of the normal population.
- Treatment with one AED is preferred, but if monotherapy fails, a second drug should be initiated and the first drug gradually withdrawn during the course of 7 days. A trial using a third drug may be tried, but if monotherapy with the third drug does not succeed, a trial with two AEDs is indicated.
- Serum concentrations of most AEDs are lower during pregnancy, but seizure frequency may not increase because free concentrations of the drug do not decline proportionally with total concentrations. Serum concentrations should be evaluated at least bimonthly and the dose adjusted according to concentration, seizure frequency, and side effects.
- In a large percentage of neonates exposed to AEDs, coagulopathy occurs within 24 hours after delivery due to a deficiency of the vitamin K-dependent clotting factors. All babies exposed to AEDs should receive 2 mg of **vitamin K** at birth, and cord blood should be sent for clotting studies. Some clinicians give pregnant patients receiving AEDs prophylactic oral vitamin K, 20 mg daily, the last 1–3 weeks before delivery. Folate deficiency also occurs in patients on AEDs, and prophylaxis is recommended to prevent megaloblastic anemia.
- The American Academy of Obstetrics and Gynecology recommends **phenobarbital** as the AED of choice during pregnancy, but it can be teratogenic, and some studies have suggested behavioral abnormalities and impaired intellect in babies exposed in utero. Higher doses are usually required during pregnancy to maintain serum concentrations. Coagulopathy and folate deficiency can occur, and neonates may experience CNS depression and withdrawal at delivery. Neonatal withdrawal symptoms do not usually begin for 4–7 days after delivery and may last 2–6 months. Withdrawal is characterized by neuromuscular

excitability, hyperactivity, sleep disturbances, excessive crying, tremulousness, vomiting, or diarrhea.

- **Phenytoin** is probably more teratogenic than phenobarbital, and it also causes coagulopathy, and vitamin deficiencies, but neonatal CNS depression and withdrawal do not occur. About 10% of infants exposed to phenytoin will manifest the full syndrome of fetal hydantoin syndrome, and 30% will have some features. The syndrome includes craniofacial abnormalities, growth retardation, limb defects, cardiac lesions, hernias, and distal digital and nail hypoplasias.
- **Carbamazepine** is teratogenic, and defects include spina bifida, craniofacial defects, nail hypoplasia, and developmental delays.
- **Valproic acid** should be avoided in women of child-bearing age, as it causes malformations including cleft palate, renal defects, and neural tube defects.
- **Trimethadione,** the most potent teratogen of the AEDs, is contraindicated in pregnancy.

ASTHMA

- During pregnancy, one-third of asthmatics experience improvement of their disease, and one-third worsen. Severe asthma may have an adverse effect on pregnancy outcome.
- Of the antiasthmatic drugs, only the iodides are absolutely contraindicated in pregnancy.
- When steroids are required, **prednisone** and **prednisolone** are suggested because fetal serum concentrations of these are lower than other steroids. Severe attacks and status asthmaticus are managed as in the nonpregnant patient.
- Prostaglandins for cervical ripening or induction of labor should be avoided in asthmatic patients as they can precipitate acute attacks. For postpartum hemorrhage, **prostaglandin E_2** is preferred over **prostaglandin $F_{2\alpha}$** because it is less likely to cause bronchospasm.

HIV

- All seropositive pregnant women should be offered **zidovudine,** as it decreases the perinatal transmission of HIV-1 (by 67.5% in one study). It is given to the mother as early as 14 weeks or as late as 34 weeks, is given IV during labor, and orally to the infant for 6 weeks after delivery. Seropositive mothers should not breastfeed.

▶ LACTATION

- Drugs that decrease milk production include **sympathomimetics, nicotine, levodopa, bromocriptine, ergot alkaloids, pyridoxine, monoamine oxidase inhibitors,** and **androgens.** Drugs that may increase milk production and may cause galactorrhea include antipsychotics, **cimetidine, metoclopramide, reserpine, amoxapine,** and **methyldopa.**

- Drugs contraindicated by nursing mothers include **amphetamines, bromocriptine, cocaine, ergotamine, lithium, nicotine,** most antineoplastic drugs, and drugs of abuse.

USE OF SELECTED AGENTS DURING LACTATION

- Ingestion of large quantities or chronic use of **alcohol** may cause CNS depression, weakness, and abnormal growth.
- **Caffeine** can cause irritability and sleeplessness in breast-fed infants. Moderate use (1–2 cups/d) of coffee is considered acceptable if tolerated by the infant.
- **Nicotine** should be avoided by lactating women, as it is excreted in breast milk and can cause decreased milk production. Nausea, vomiting, diarrhea, tachycardia, and restlessness may occur in nursing infants exposed to nicotine.
- Most analgesics are excreted in breast milk in low concentrations that should not be harmful to the baby; large doses or chronic use should be considered with caution.

- All antibiotics cross into breast milk. There is potential to cause candidiasis, diarrhea, and thrush in the nursing infant. **Penicillins, cephalosporins,** and **erythromycin** are usually considered permissible for nursing mothers. **Sulfonamides** are permitted if the nursing infant is healthy and full-term. **Chloramphenicol, tetracycline,** and **isoniazid** should be avoided. If **metronidazole** is required, a single 2-gram dose should be used, and the breasts should be pumped for 24–48 hours before nursing is resumed.
- AEDs are generally considered permissible during breastfeeding, but the infant should be observed for sedation and poor feeding.
- All laxatives, with the exception of bulk-forming products, potentially cross into breast milk, but occasional use is not likely to be harmful.
- Diabetic mothers using insulin may breast-feed as it is not excreted into breast milk.

See Chapter 74, Pregnancy and Lactation: Therapeutic Considerations, authored by Janet McCombs, PharmD, and Margaret K. Cramer, MD, FACOG, for a more detailed discussion of this topic.

Hematologic Disorders

Edited by Cindy W. Hamilton, PharmD

Chapter 31

▶ ANEMIAS

▶ DEFINITION

Anemias are a group of diseases characterized by a decrease in either hemoglobin or red blood cells (RBCs), resulting in a decrease in the oxygen-carrying capacity of blood.

▶ PATHOPHYSIOLOGY

- Anemias can be classified on the basis of RBC morphology, etiology, or pathophysiology (Table 31–1). The most common anemias are included in this chapter.
- Morphologic classifications are based on cell size. Megaloblasts are large nucleated precursors that typically are associated with deficiencies of folate or vitamin B_{12}. Microcytes are small cells that typically are associated with iron deficiency; corresponding iron concentrations may be normal (normochromic) or decreased (hypochromic).
- Iron-deficiency anemia accounts for 25% of anemias and is usually caused by inadequate dietary intake, inadequate gastrointestinal absorption, increased iron demands (e.g., pregnancy), blood loss, and chronic diseases.
- Vitamin B_{12}- and folate-deficiency anemias are caused by inadequate intake, decreased absorption, and inadequate utilization. Deficiency of intrinsic factor may cause decreased absorption of vitamin B_{12} (i.e., pernicious anemia). Celiac disease is the most common cause of folate malabsorption. Folate-deficiency anemia also may be caused by hyperutilization due to pregnancy, hemolytic anemia, myelofibrosis, malignancy, chronic inflammatory disorder, long-term dialysis, or growth spurt. Drugs may cause megaloblastosis by reducing absorption of vitamin B_{12} or folate (e.g., phenytoin, phenobarbital, primidone), or by interfering with corresponding metabolic pathways (e.g., methotrexate).
- Anemia of chronic disease is a hypoproliferative anemia associated with infectious, inflammatory, or neoplastic diseases that last >1–2 months. Anemia of renal failure is addressed separately in this chapter and in Chapter 78. Although the cause of anemia of chronic disease is uncertain, the etiology may involve blocked iron release from marrow reticuloendothelial cells, which may be mediated by cytokines that inhibit the production or action of erythropoietin or that inhibit RBC production.

TABLE 31–1. Classification Systems for Anemias

I. Morphology
- Macrocytic
  - Megaloblastic anemias
    - Vitamin B_{12} deficiency
    - Folic acid deficiency anemia
- Hypochromic, microcytic
  - Iron deficiency anemia
  - Genetic anomaly
    - Sickle cell anemia
    - Thalassemia
    - Other hemoglobinopathies (abnormal hemoglobins)
- Normocytic anemias
  - Recent blood loss
  - Hemolysis
  - Bone marrow failure
  - Anemias of chronic disease
  - Renal failure
  - Endocrine disorders
  - Myeloplastic anemias

II. Etiology
- Deficiency
  - Iron
    - Vitamin B_{12}
    - Folic acid
    - Pyridoxine
- Central—caused by impaired bone marrow function
  - Anemia of chronic disease
  - Anemia of the elderly
  - Malignant bone marrow disorders
- Peripheral
  - Bleeding (hemorrhage)
  - Hemolysis (hemolytic anemias)

III. Pathophysiology
- Excessive blood loss
  - Recent hemorrhage
    - Trauma
    - Peptic ulcer
    - Gastritis
    - Hemorrhoids
  - Chronic hemorrhage
    - Vaginal bleeding
    - Peptic ulcer
    - Intestinal parasites
    - Nonsteroidal anti-inflammatory agents
- Excessive red cell destruction
  - Extracorpuscular (i.e., outside the cell) factors
    - RBC antibodies
    - Drugs
    - Physical trauma to RBC (artificial valves)
    - Excessive sequestration in the spleen
  - Intracorpuscular factors
    - Heredity
    - Disorders of hemoglobin synthesis
- Inadequate production of mature RBCs
  - Deficiency of nutrients (B_{12}, folic acid, iron, protein)
  - Deficiency of erythroblasts
    - Aplastic anemia
    - Isolated (often transient) erythroblastopenia
    - Folic acid antagonists
    - Antibodies
  - Conditions with infiltration of bone marrow
    - Lymphoma
    - Leukemia
    - Myelofibrosis
    - Carcinoma
  - Endocrine abnormalities
    - Hypothyroid
    - Adrenal insufficiency
    - Pituitary insufficiency
  - Chronic renal disease
  - Chronic inflammatory disease
    - Granulomatous diseases
    - Collagen-vascular diseases
  - Hepatic disease

- The etiology of anemia of chronic renal failure is multifactorial. Decreased renal production of erythropoietin is the primary mechanism. Other factors include decreased RBC life span caused by uremia, increased folate demand plus depleted body stores, and dialysis-induced blood and iron loss.
- Anemia is one of the most common clinical problems in the elderly. Age-related reductions in bone marrow reserve may render the elderly patient more susceptible to anemia that is caused by multiple minor and often unrecognized diseases (e.g., nutritional deficiencies) that negatively affect erythropoiesis.
- Hemolytic anemia, one of the least common anemias, occurs when the RBC life span is shorter than its normal length of 120 days. Of the many potential etiologies, the most common are RBC membrane defects (e.g., hereditary spherocytosis), altered hemoglobin solubility or stability (e.g., sickle cell anemia and thallasemias), and changes in intracellular metabolism (e.g., glucose-6-phosphate dehydrogenase [G6PD] deficiency). Hemolysis results from the action of the spleen and reticuloendothelial system on damaged RBCs. Depending on the mechanism, hemolytic anemia can be mild, chronic, compensated, and lifelong, or it may be acute, severe, and life threatening. Sickle cell anemia is discussed in Chapter 32.

► CLINICAL PRESENTATION

- Signs and symptoms of anemia depend on the onset and cause of the anemia. Anemia of recent onset usually is manifested by cardiorespiratory symptoms such as tachycardia, light-headedness, and breathlessness. Chronic anemia is manifested by fatigue, headache, vertigo, faintness, sensitivity to cold, pallor, and loss of skin tone.
- Iron-deficiency anemia is manifested by spooning of the nails (koilonychia), angular stomatitis and glossitis, and craving for substances low in iron (pica); however, symptoms do not appear until hemoglobin concentrations fall below 8 or 9 g/dL.
- Vitamin B_{12}- and folate-deficiency anemias are manifested by cardiorespiratory symptoms. Vitamin B_{12} anemia is distinguished by neuropsychiatric abnormalities, especially paresthesias and ataxia, which are absent in patients with folate-deficiency anemia.

► DIAGNOSIS

- Evaluation of anemia involves a complete blood count including RBC indices, reticulocyte index, examination of the peripheral blood smear, and stool for occult blood (Table 31–2).
- The earliest laboratory change associated with iron-deficiency anemia is decreased serum ferritin (<10–12 ng/mL), which is followed by decreased transferrin saturation (<15%), decreased serum iron con-

TABLE 31–2. Normal Hematologic Values

Test	Reference Range (yr)			
	2–6	*6–12*	*12–18*	*18–49*
Hemoglobin (g/dL)	11.5–13.0	11.5–15.5	M 13.0–16.0 F 12.0–16.0	M 13.5–17.5 F 12.0–16.0
Hematocrit (%)	34.0–40.0	35.0–45.0	M 37.0–49.0 F 36.0–46.0	M 41.0–53.0 F 36.0–46.0
MCV (fL)	75–87	77–95	M 78–98 F 78–102	80–100
MCHC (%)	—	31–37	31–37	31–37
MCH (pg/cell)	24–30	25–33	25–35	26–34
RBC (million/mm^3)	3.9–5.3	4.0–5.2	M 4.5–5.3	M 4.5–5.9
Reticulocyte count, absolute (%)				0.5–1.5
Serum iron (μg/dL)		50–120	50–120	M 50–160 F 40–150
TIBC (μg/dL)	250–400	250–400	250–400	250–400
RDW (%)				11–16
Ferritin (ng/mL)	7–140	7–140	7–140	M 15–200 F 12–150
Folate (ng/mL)				1.8–16[a]
Vitamin B_{12} (pg/mL)				100–900[a]
Erythropoietin (U/mL)				0.01–0.03

[a]Varies by assay method.

MCV, mean corpuscular volume; MCHC, mean corpuscular hemoglobin concentration; MCH, mean corpuscular hemoglobin; RBC, red blood cell; RDW, RBC distribution width; TIBC, total iron-binding capacity.

VII

centrations, and increased total iron-binding concentration (TIBC >400 μg/dL). Hemoglobin, hematocrit, and RBC indices usually remain normal until later stages of iron-deficiency anemia.

- Macrocytic anemias, such as vitamin B_{12}- and folate-deficiency anemias, are characterized by mean corpuscular volume (MCV) of >100 μm^3. One of the earliest and most specific indications of macrocytic anemia is hypersegmented polymorphonuclear leukocytes on the peripheral blood smear.
- Vitamin B_{12} and folate concentrations can be measured to differentiate between the corresponding deficiency anemias. A vitamin B_{12} value of <150 pg/mL, together with appropriate peripheral smear and clinical symptoms, is diagnostic of vitamin B_{12}-deficiency anemia. The Schilling test, which is usually abnormal in patients with pernicious anemia, should be performed if the vitamin B_{12} value is <200 pg/mL. The vitamin B_{12} determination should be repeated in 1–3 months, if the value is 200–300

pg/mL. With folate-deficiency anemia, RBC folate concentrations are more predictive of tissue concentrations than serum folate concentrations.

- Diagnosis of anemia of chronic disease is usually one of exclusion, with consideration of iron-deficiency anemia as the primary or coexisting anemia. Serum iron is usually decreased, but, unlike iron-deficiency anemia, serum ferritin is normal or increased and TIBC is increased. The bone marrow reveals an abundance of iron; the peripheral smear reveals normocytic anemia. The hematocrit may be as low as 25% in 20% of patients.

▶ DESIRED OUTCOME

The ultimate goals of treatment in the anemic patient are to (1) alleviate signs and symptoms, (2) correct the underlying etiology (e.g., restore depleted stores of iron or other elements required for RBC production), and (3) prevent recurrence of anemia.

▶ TREATMENT

IRON-DEFICIENCY ANEMIA

- Treatment of iron-deficiency anemia consists of dietary supplementation and administration of therapeutic iron preparations. **Oral iron** therapy with soluble ferrous iron salts that are not enteric coated and not slow- or sustained-release is recommended at a daily dosage of 200 mg elemental iron in two or three divided doses (Table 31–3). Food also plays a significant role because iron is poorly absorbed from vegetables, grain products, dairy products, and eggs; iron is best absorbed from meat, fish, and poultry.
- Patients with iron-deficiency anemia may require **parenteral iron** therapy if there is iron malabsorption, intolerance of oral iron therapy, or noncompliance. Iron dextran may be given intramuscularly by Z-tract administration, or intravenously by multiple slow injections of the undiluted solution or by infusion of the diluted solution. Dosage is determined by the etiology of the anemia (Table 31–4). After an initial

TABLE 31–3. Iron Products

Salt	Elemental Iron (%)
Ferrous sulfate	20
Ferrous sulfate, exsiccated	30
Ferrous gluconate	12
Ferrous fumarate	33
Ferric pyrophosphate	12
Ferrous carbonate	48

TABLE 31–4. Equations for Calculating Doses of Iron Dextran

In patients with iron deficiency anemia:
mg of iron = W × (100 – %Hb) × 0.3
where *W* is the patient's weight in pounds and %Hb is the patient's observed hemoglobin expressed as a percentage of the normal hemoglobin concentration (assuming 14.8 g of hemoglobin per 100 mL is equivalent to 100% concentration).
If the patient weighs 13.6 kg (30 lb) or less, the dose is 80% of the calculated amount.
In patients with anemia secondary to blood loss (hemorrhagic diathesis or long-term dialysis):
mg of iron = blood loss × hematocrit
where blood loss is in milliliters and hematocrit is expressed as a decimal fraction.

test dose of 25 mg intramuscularly or intravenously (or 5–10 minutes of the diluted intravenous infusion solution), patients should be monitored for 1 hour for adverse reactions such as allergic reactions, including anaphylaxis.

VII

VITAMIN B_{12}-DEFICIENCY ANEMIA

- Vitamin B_{12}-deficiency anemia is treated with replacement therapy. **Cyanocobalamin** or **hydroxycobalamin** 800–1000 μg is injected daily for 1–2 weeks until symptoms subside, followed by 100–1000 μg once weekly until hemoglobin and hematocrit values return to normal. Thereafter, 100–1000 μg is injected monthly for life. Oral vitamin B_{12} is rarely indicated unless the individual has a nutritional deficiency.

FOLATE-DEFICIENCY ANEMIA

- Treatment of folate-deficiency anemia is initiated with **oral folate** 1–5 mg daily for approximately 4 months; 1 mg daily is usually sufficient. Long-term therapy may be required if the etiology is a chronic condition that cannot be corrected.

ANEMIA OF CHRONIC DISEASE AND RENAL FAILURE

- Treatment of anemia of chronic disease is less specific than that of other anemias. This type of anemia usually subsides when the inflammation subsides. Iron therapy is not effective when the inflammation is present. RBC transfusions are effective but should be limited to episodes of inadequate oxygen transport. Erythropoietin may be indicated because erythropoietin concentrations are low relative to the severity of anemia; however, studies yielded mixed results, except in patients with rheumatoid arthritis.
- Recombinant human erythropoietin or **epoetin alfa** reverses the anemia of chronic renal failure in essentially all patients, circumvents the inherent risks of RBC transfusions, and therefore has become the mainstay of treatment. Epoetin alfa should be initiated at a dosage of 50–100

U/kg three times weekly until the hematocrit approaches 36%; the dosage should be titrated to maintain a hematocrit of 30–36%. Although epoetin alfa may be administered intravenously or subcutaneously, the latter method may be preferred because it provides more sustained concentrations. The agent of choice for preventing concomitant iron deficiency is oral ferrous sulfate, 325 mg once daily at bedtime.

HEMOLYTIC ANEMIA

- Treatment of hemolytic anemia is determined by etiology. The treatment of choice for hereditary spherocytosis is splenectomy. Because there is no specific therapy to compensate for G6PD deficiency, treatment consists of avoiding oxidant medications and chemicals.

► EVALUATION OF THERAPEUTIC OUTCOMES

- In patients with iron-deficiency anemia, therapeutic doses of iron should raise hemoglobin by 1–2 g/dL per week. The patient should be reevaluated if hemoglobin does not increase by 2 g/dL in the course of 3 weeks or if reticulocytosis does not occur within 7–10 days. Iron therapy is continued until iron stores are restored to normal, which usually requires at least 3–6 months. VII
- Signs and symptoms of megaloblastic anemia usually subside soon after starting vitamin B_{12} or folate therapy. The patient should be reevaluated if reticulocytosis does not occur after 2–3 days, hemoglobin does not rise after 1 or 2 weeks, or leukocyte and platelet counts do not normalize after 1 week.
- In patients with anemia of chronic failure, the goal of epoetin alfa therapy is to maintain a hematocrit of 30–36%. Iron depletion is a major reason for failure to respond to epoetin therapy; iron therapy is considered if the transferrin saturation is at least 20% and the serum ferritin is <100 ng/mL. Blood pressure is monitored because approximately 30–47% of patients receiving epoetin alfa experience elevated diastolic blood pressure; antihypertensive therapy may need to be adjusted.

See Chapter 91, Anemias, authored by Thomas T. Sproat, PharmD, BCPS, PA-C, for a more detailed discussion of this topic.

Chapter 32

▶ SICKLE CELL ANEMIA

▶ DEFINITION

Sickle cell disease is a group of hemolytic anemias caused by genetic defects in hemoglobin, which result in sickle-shaped red blood cells (RBCs).

▶ PATHOPHYSIOLOGY

- The biochemical defect causing development of sickle cell disease involves an amino acid in the β polypeptide chain of the hemoglobin molecule; the α chain is normal.
- The most common abnormal hemoglobin in the United States is hemoglobin S, where sickle cell trait occurs in 8% of the black population and sickle cell anemia occurs in 0.3%. Hemoglobin C can be detected in 3% of the corresponding population. Other abnormal hemoglobins are E, which is found in the Far East, and D, which is found in India, Pakistan, Afghanistan, and Iran.
- Two genes for hemoglobin S result in a homozygote with sickle cell anemia, while only one results in a heterozygote with sickle cell trait. It should be noted, however, that the heterozygotes may experience pathology, especially if they are double heterozygotes with hemoglobin S and either hemoglobin C or thalassemia.
- Clinical manifestations of sickle cell disease are attributable to impaired circulation, RBC destruction, and stasis of blood flow.
- When RBCs contain hemoglobin S, their membranes become damaged, which cause cells to lose potassium and water. This dehydrated state enhances the formation of sickle-shaped RBCs. With repeated episodes, these RBCs retain calcium, become more rigid, and eventually assume irreversible sickle shapes.
- The presence of sickle-shaped RBCs increases blood viscosity and encourages sludging in the capillaries and small vessels. Such obstructive events lead to local tissue hypoxia, which accentuates the pathologic process.
- Not all clinical manifestations are readily attributable to sickling of RBCs. For example, reticuloendothelial function may be impaired because of functional asplenia, which in turn increases the risk of bacterial infection and of disseminated intravascular coagulation (DIC).

▶ CLINICAL PRESENTATION

- Sickle cell disease is associated with many clinical manifestations (Table 32–1). Symptoms do not appear until after 4–6 months of age because of the oxygen-carrying capability of fetal hemoglobin and because hemoglobin F is less likely to sickle.

TABLE 32–1. Manifestations of Sickle Cell Disease: Crises and Complications

Crisis	**Characteristic**
Vaso-occlusive	Infarction/pain
Hemolytic	Massive hemolysis
Splenic sequestration	Sequestration of red blood cells
Aplastic	Bone marrow failure
Organ system	**Complication**
Pulmonary	Acute chest syndrome
Neurologic	Various, including cerebrovascular accident
Dermatologic	Chronic ulcers
Cardiovascular	Hypertrophy
Genitourinary	Priapism, hematuria, hyposthenuria
Skeletal	Aseptic necrosis, osteomyelitis
Ocular	Retinal problems
Hepatic	Cholelithiasis

- Common initial findings are pneumonia or pain and swelling of the hands and feet (e.g., hand-and-foot syndrome or dactylitis). Splenomegaly is also common in children.
- Usual clinical signs and symptoms of sickle cell disease are chronic anemia, fever and pallor, arthralgia, scleral icterus, abdominal pain, weakness, anorexia, fatigue, and hematuria.
- Children experience delayed growth and sexual maturation. Additional physical findings are protuberant abdomen and exaggerated lumbar lordosis, asthenic appearance with long extremities and tapered fingers, and barrel-shaped chest.
- Sickle cell crisis may be precipitated by fever, infection, dehydration, hypoxia, acidosis, sudden temperature change, or a combination of factors. The most common type of crisis is vasoocclusive or infarctive, which is manifested by pain over the involved areas without changes in hemoglobin or other laboratory values. This type of crisis may affect hands and feet, joints and extremities, abdomen, liver, and lungs. Less common types of crises are aplastic, hemolytic, and splenic sequestration (see Table 32–1).
- Complications of sickle cell disease include acute chest syndrome, neurologic abnormalities due to cerebrovascular occlusion, chronic ulcers of the inner aspect of the lower leg, cholelithiasis, cardiovascular abnormalities, priapism, destructive bone and joint problems, ocular complications, and renal complications. Acute chest syndrome is characterized by cough, dyspnea, chest pain, fever, pulmonary infiltration, and equivocal response to antibiotic therapy; the etiology may or may not be pulmonary infarction.
- Patients with sickle cell trait are usually asymptomatic, except for impaired renal function and dilute urine, increased risk of dehydration, and hematuria.

▶ DIAGNOSIS

- The diagnosis should be considered in any black patient with hemolytic anemia, especially if there is a history of painful crises, arthropathies, ankle ulcers, or other clinical manifestations.
- Evaluation of a blood sample from a patient with sickle cell anemia will reveal reduced hemoglobin, increased reticulocyte count, usually increased platelet and leukocyte counts, and sickle forms on the peripheral smear.
- The screening test for hemoglobin disorders is electrophoresis on cellulose acetate, followed by solubility testing for sickling.
- The presence of abnormal hemoglobin is confirmed by citrate agar electrophoresis, quantifying of hemoglobin fractions, alkali denaturation, and family studies.

▶ DESIRED OUTCOME

The goal of treatment is to decrease the number of sickle cell crises, prevent complications, and improve the quality of life.

▶ TREATMENT

GENERAL PRINCIPLES

- Treatment is primarily supportive.
- Patients with sickle cell disease should receive pneumococcal and hemophilus b conjugate vaccines at appropriate ages.

SICKLE CELL CRISIS

- Hydration and analgesics are the core interventions for sickle cell crisis, but there is no consensus on specific guidelines.
- Daily hydration of 3–4 L is recommended, which may be administered intravenously or, if feasible, orally.
- **Morphine** is replacing **meperidine** as the narcotic analgesic of choice because morphine has a longer duration of action and avoids problems resulting from accumulation of metabolites that may be toxic, especially in patients with sickle cell disease.
- Opioids should be administered on a scheduled basis because as-needed dosing does not provide effective pain control. Patient-controlled analgesia (PCA) combines the advantages of providing steady analgesic blood concentrations with the ability to administer additional bolus doses.
- Because crises may be precipitated by infection, an infectious etiology should be considered. *Streptococcus pneumoniae, Haemophilus influenzae, and Salmonella* are the most likely pathogens.
- Mild cases may be treated on an outpatient basis with rest, hydration, warmth, and oral analgesics. Oral analgesic options include **non-**

steroidal anti-inflammatory drugs (NSAIDs) or **acetaminophen,** generally in combination with **codeine** or a codeine derivative.

- Splenic sequestration crisis is a major cause of mortality in young patients. Treatment includes whole-blood transfusion to correct hypovolemia, and broad-spectrum antibiotic therapy including coverage for *S. pneumoniae and H. influenzae.* Although controversial, splenectomy is probably merited after a life-threatening crisis or after repetitive episodes.
- Treatment of aplastic crisis is primarily supportive. Blood transfusion may be indicated for severe anemia. Antibiotic therapy is generally not warranted because an infectious etiology is probably viral rather than bacterial.
- There is no specific treatment for hemolytic crises. Treatment is primarily supportive and may include blood transfusions.

TRANSFUSION AND OTHER ACUTE INTERVENTIONS

- Transfusion therapy may be beneficial in carefully selected patients. It has been used to treat life-threatening complications of sickle cell disease, such as central nervous system infarction or multiorgan failure associated with sickle cell crisis. Transfusion has also been used before childbirth and before surgery. After a stroke, chronic transfusion may reduce the risk of subsequent stroke and halt clinical progression. VII
- The risks of transfusion therapy include iron overload, acquired viral infection, and sensitization to transfusion products. The conventional dosage of the iron chelator, **deferoxamine,** is 1–2 g by subcutaneous infusion over 10–12 hours. A higher dosage, such as 6 g/day intravenously at a rate of 15 mg/kg/h, may be required for large iron stores or noncompliance.
- Conventional therapeutic approaches to priapism are often ineffective in patients with sickle cell disease. Acute intervention may consist of vasoconstrictors (e.g., **phenylephrine, epinephrine**) or vasodilators (e.g., β agonists **[terbutaline], hydralazine**). More invasive approaches, such as aspiration of the corpora cavernosa or surgery, may be required. Preventative measures that have occasionally been successful include **stilbestrol** and gonadotropin-releasing hormone analogue.
- In patients with idiopathic unilateral renal hematuria, high fluid intake is indicated to prevent clotting and urethral colic. Iron therapy and possibly transfusions should be used as needed for blood loss. Nephrectomy may be required for massive hemorrhaging.

► LONG-TERM AND NEW STRATEGIES

- Current therapeutic interventions do not necessarily prevent complications. **Folic acid,** 1 mg daily, is given empirically because of increased demand caused by accelerated erythropoiesis; however, there are no controlled clinical trials indicating that supplementation is essential.

- Prophylactic **penicillin** prevents pneumococcal septicemia and meningitis, but this approach has been criticized because of the risk of promoting development of drug-resistant strains, compliance problems, and uncertainty about the duration of therapy.
- New strategies that are being considered to decrease gelation of sickle cells include **hydroxyurea, butyrate,** and **clotrimazole.** Of these, hydroxy-urea is the most appealing, but the ideal regimen is unknown.
- Studies of **pentoxifylline** yielded mixed results regarding the ability of this agent to decrease the number and severity of sickle cell crises.
- Bone marrow transplantation produces dramatic results in patients with sickle cell disease. The procedure involves marrow ablation followed by transplantation of marrow harvested from a matched sibling donor. This procedure is limited by the shortage of suitable donors and by substantial toxicity.

▶ EVALUATION OF THERAPEUTIC OUTCOME

- Patients receiving hydration for sickle cell crisis should be monitored to prevent overhydration.

VII
- Folate levels and mean corpuscular volume (MCV) should be monitored to detect possible folate deficiency and megaloblastic anemia.
- The number, severity, and duration of sickle cell crises should be monitored to evaluate the effectiveness of long-term interventions such as gelation inhibitor therapy.
- Patients receiving hydroxyurea should be monitored for myelotoxicity; slight neutropenia may contribute to the drug's efficacy.
- The effectiveness of analgesic therapy is evaluated by subjective assessments by patients and health care practitioners.
- Patients should be monitored for bacterial infections, especially infections caused by *S. pneumoniae, H. influenzae,* and *Salmonella.* When infections occur, appropriate antibiotic therapy should be initiated.

See Chapter 93, Sickle Cell Anemia, authored by Clarence E. Curry, Jr., PharmD, and Eula D. Beasley, PharmD, for a more detailed discussion of this topic.

Infectious Diseases

Edited by Joseph T. DiPiro, PharmD, FCCP

Chapter 33

▶ ANTIMICROBIAL REGIMEN SELECTION

A generally accepted systematic approach to the selection and evaluation of an antimicrobial regimen is shown in (Table 33–1). "Empiric" antimicrobial regimen is begun before the offending organism is identified while "definitive" therapy is instituted when the causative organism is known.

▶ CONFIRMING THE PRESENCE OF INFECTION

FEVER

- Fever is defined as a controlled elevation of body temperature above the normal range of 36–37.8°C. Fever is a manifestation of many disease states other than infection.
- Many drugs have been identified as causes of fever. Drug-induced fever is defined as persistent fever in the absence of infection or other underlying condition. The fever must coincide temporally with the administration of the offending agent and disappear promptly upon its withdrawal, after which it remains normal.
- Fever patterns (e.g., high-spiking or low-grade sustained) are believed by some to be helpful in establishing the etiology of the increased temperature. Overall, characterization of the fever pattern probably offers little in the general assessment of the patient.

SIGNS AND SYMPTOMS

White Blood Cell Count

- Most infections result in elevated white blood cell (WBC) counts (leukocytosis) because of the mobilization of granulocytes and/or lymphocytes to ingest and destroy invading microbes. The generally accepted range of normal values for WBC counts is between 4000 and 10,000/mm^3.
- Classically, bacterial infections are associated with elevated granulocyte counts (neutrophils, basophils), often with immature forms (band neutrophils) seen in peripheral blood smears (left-shift). With infection, peripheral leukocyte counts may be very high, but are rarely higher than 30,000–40,000/mm^3. Low leukocyte counts after the onset of infection indicate an abnormal response and are generally associated with a poor prognosis for bacterial infection.
- Relative lymphocytosis, even with normal or slightly elevated total WBC counts, is generally associated with viral or fungal infections.

TABLE 33–1. Systematic Approach for Selection of Antimicrobials

A. Confirm the presence of infection
  1. Fever
  2. Signs and symptoms
  3. Predisposing factors

B. Identification of the pathogen
  1. Collection of infected material
  2. Stains
  3. Serologies
  4. Culture

C. Selection of presumptive therapy
  1. Host factors
  2. Drug factors

D. Monitor therapeutic response
  1. Clinical assessment
  2. Laboratory tests
  3. Assessment of therapeutic failure

- Many types of infections, however, may be accompanied by a completely normal WBC count and differential.

Pain and Inflammation

- The classic signs of pain and inflammation may accompany infection and are manifested by swelling, erythema, tenderness, and purulent drainage. Unfortunately, these are visibly apparent only if the infection is superficial or in a bone or joint.
- The manifestations of inflammation in deep-seated infections such as meningitis, pneumonia, endocarditis, and urinary tract infection must be ascertained by examining tissues or fluids. For example, the presence of polymorphonuclear leukocytes (neutrophils) in spinal fluid, lung secretions (sputum), and urine is highly suggestive of bacterial infection.

Other Factors

- Table 33–2 lists factors that predispose patients to infection. Generally, immunosuppressive disease states lead to a wide variety of infections (e.g., AIDS), while other diseases may predispose the patient to a certain type of infectious disease (e.g., recurrent meningococcal infection with complement deficiency). Information from the patient's history regarding underlying disease is vitally important, since the presence of an underlying condition may not only predispose patients to infection, but also may modify the likely offending pathogen.
- Many factors predisposing to infection are related to disruption of the host's integumentary barriers. For example, trauma, burns, and iatrogenic wounds induced in surgery may lead to a substantial risk of infection depending on the severity and location of the injury or disruption.

TABLE 33–2. Factors Predisposing to Infection

Alterations in normal flora of the host	Immunosuppression secondary to
Disruption of natural barriers	Malnutrition
Skin and mucous membranes	Underlying disease (hereditary or acquired)
Cilia of respiratory tract	Hormones (e.g., pregnancy, corticosteroids)
pH and motility of bowel	Drugs (e.g., cytotoxic agents)
Age	

► IDENTIFICATION OF THE PATHOGEN

- Infected body materials must be sampled, if at all possible or practical, before the institution of antimicrobial therapy, for two reasons. First, Gram stain of the material may rapidly reveal bacteria, or acid-fast stain may detect mycobacteria or actinomycetes. Second, a delay in obtaining infected fluids or tissues until after therapy is started may result in false-negative culture results or alterations in the cellular and chemical composition of infected fluids.
- Blood cultures should nearly always be performed in the acutely ill, febrile patient. Less accessible fluids or tissues must be obtained based on localized signs or symptoms (e.g., spinal fluid in meningitis, joint fluid in arthritis). Abscesses and cellulitic areas should also be aspirated.
- Once positive Gram stain and/or culture results are obtained, the clinician must be cautious in determining whether the organism recovered is a true pathogen, a contaminant, or is part of the normally expected flora from the site of specimen collection.
- Caution must be taken in the evaluation of positive culture results from normally sterile sites (e.g., blood, cerebrospinal fluid, joint fluid). The recovery of bacteria normally found on the skin in large quantities (e.g., coagulase-negative staphylococci, diphtheroids) from one of these sites may be a result of contamination of the specimen rather than a true infection.

► SELECTION OF PRESUMPTIVE THERAPY

- To select rational antimicrobial therapy for a given infection, a variety of factors must be considered. These include the severity and acuity of the disease, host factors, factors related to the drugs used, and the necessity for use of multiple agents.
- There are generally accepted drugs of choice for the treatment of most pathogens (Table 33–3). The drugs of choice are compiled from a variety of sources and are intended as guidelines rather than specific rules for antimicrobial use.

TABLE 33–3. Drugs of Choice, First choice, *Alternative(s)*

Gram-Positive Cocci

Streptococcus (groups A, B, C, G, and *S. bovis*)

Penicillin-sensitive

Erythromycin, FGC,[c,d] azithromycin, clarithromycin,[e] vancomycin

Streptococcus pneumoniae[f]

Penicillin-sensitive

Erythromycin, FGC,[c,d] cefotaxime or ceftriaxone,[d,g] chloramphenicol[h]

Penicillin-resistant (MIC ≥ 2.0 μg/mL)

Vancomycin (check sensitivities for TGC,[d,o] cefepime,[d] imipenem,[r] grepafloxacin,[i] levofloxacin,[i] sparfloxacin,[i] trovafloxacin[i])

***Streptococcus, viridans* group**

Penicillin G ± gentamicin[i]

Vancomycin ± gentamicin, FGC[c,d]

Enterococcus faecalis (generally not as resistant to antibiotics as *E. faecium*)

Serious infection (endocarditis, meningitis, pyelonephritis with bacteremia)

Ampicillin (or penicillin G) + gentamicin or streptomycin

Vancomycin with gentamicin or streptomycin

Urinary Tract Infection (UTI)

Ampicillin, amoxicillin, doxycycline,[j] ciprofloxacin,[j] levofloxacin[j]

Enterococcus faecium (generally more resistant to antibiotics than *E. faecalis*); no regimen proven efficacious for vancomycin-resistant *E. faecium;* recommend consultation with infectious disease physician

Staphylococcus aureus

Methicillin (oxacillin)-sensitive

PRP[k]

FGC,[c,d] trimethoprim–sulfamethoxazole, clindamycin,[l] vancomycin, BLIC,[m] imipenem

Methicillin (oxacillin)-resistant

Vancomycin ± rifampin or gentamicin

VIII *Trimethoprim–sulfamethoxazole, doxycycline,[j] either ± rifampin*

Teicoplanin (investigational Hoechst Marion Roussel)

Gram-Negative Cocci

Moraxella (Branhamella) catarrhalis

Amoxicillin/clavulanate

Trimethoprim–sulfamethoxazole, erythromycin, azithromycin, clarithromycin,[e] doxycycline,[j] SGC,[d,n] TGC,[d,o] TGCpo[d,p]

***Neisseria gonorrhoeae* (also give concomitant treatment for *Chlamydia trachomatis*)**

Uncomplicated infection

Ceftriaxone,[d] cefixime,[d] cefpodoxime[d]

APPG,[q] ciprofloxacin,[j] ofloxacin,[j] cefotaxime,[d] spectinomycin

Disseminated gonnococcal infection

Ceftriaxone[d] + doxycycline[j]

TGC[d,o]

Neisseria meningitidis

Penicillin G

TGC,[d,o] chloramphenicol[h]

Gram-Positive Bacilli

Clostridium perfringens

Penicillin G ± clindamycin

Clindamycin, metronidazole, doxycycline,[j] cefazolin,[d] imipenem,[r] chloramphenicol[h]

Clostridium difficile

Oral metronidazole

Oral vancomycin, oral bacitracin

Gram-Negative Bacilli

Acinetobacter spp.

Imipenem or meropenem either plus amikacin

ESP,[s] fluoroquinolone,[j,t] trimethoprim–sulfamethoxazole, ampicillin/sulbactam

TABLE 33–3. continued

Gram-Negative Bacilli continued

Bacteroides fragilis (and others)

Metronidazole

BLIC,[u] clindamycin, cephamycin,[d,v] ESP,[s] imipenem[r]

Enterobacter spp.

Fluoroquinolone,[j,w] imipenem, meropenem, or cefepime any plus AMG[x]

ESP,[s] trimethoprim–sulfamethoxazole, or TGC[d,o] any plus AMG[x] or TGCpo[d,p]

Escherichia coli

FGC[c,d]

AMG,[x] SGC,[d,n] TGC,[d,o] TGCpo,[d,p] ampicillin, fluoroquinolone[j,y]

Gardnerella vaginalis

Metronidazole

Clindamycin

Haemophilus influenzae

BLIC,[u] azithromycin, or ampicillin/amoxicillin if β-lactamase negative

TGC,[d,o,r] trimethoprim–sulfamethoxazole, SGC,[d,n] chloramphenicol,[h] erythromycin, clarithromycin,[e] ciprofloxacin,[j,r] imipenem,[r] meropenem,[r] TGCpo[d,p]

Klebsiella pneumoniae

TGC,[d,o] (for UTI: AMG[x])

Trimethoprim–sulfamethoxazole, FGC,[c,d] SGC,[d,n] fluoroquinolone,[j,z] BLIC,[u] ESP,[s] imipenem[r]

Legionella spp.

Erythromycin ± rifampin

Trimethoprim–sulfamethoxazole, ciprofloxacin,[j] ofloxacin,[j] clarithromycin,[e] azithromycin

Pasteurella multocida

Penicillin G

Doxycycline,[j] BLIC,[u] trimethoprim–sulfamethoxazole, ceftriaxone[d,r]

Proteus mirabilis

Ampicillin

Trimethoprim–sulfamethoxazole, most antibiotics except PRP[k]

***Proteus* (indole-positive) (including *Providencia rettgeri, Morganella morganii, Proteus vulgaris*)**

TGC,[d,p] fluoroquinolone[j,y]

Trimethoprim–sulfamethoxazole, BLIC,[u] ESP,[s] aztreonam,[aa] imipenem[r]

Providencia stuartii

TGC,[d,o] fluoroquinolone[j,t]

Trimethoprim–sulfamethoxazole, ESP,[s] aztreonam,[aa] imipenem[r]

Pseudomonas aeruginosa

ESP[s] or ceftazidime either plus AMG[x]

UTI only: AMG[x]

Ciprofloxacin,[j] aztreonam,[aa] imipenem,[r] meropenem[r] any plus AMG[x]

Salmonella typhi

Ciprofloxacin[j] or TGC[d,o]

Trimethoprim–sulfamethoxazole, ampicillin/amoxicillin, chloramphenicol[h]

Salmonella **(non-*typhi*)**

Ceftriaxone,[bb]

Trimethoprim–sulfamethoxazole, ampicillin/amoxicillin, ciprofloxacin,[j] chloramphenicol[h]

Serratia marcescens

TGC[d,o] ± Gentamicin

Trimethoprim–sulfamethoxazole, ciprofloxacin,[j] ESP,[s] BLIC,[u] aztreonam,[aa] imipenem,[r] meropenem[r]

Stentrophomonas (Xanthomonas) maltophilia

Trimethoprim–sulfamethoxazole

Ciprofloxacin,[j] ofloxacin,[j] ceftazidime

Miscellaneous Microorganisms

Nocardia

Trimethoprim–sulfamethoxazole (high dose)

continued

TABLE 33–3. continued

Sulfonamide,[cc] doxycycline,[j] (imipenem,[r] ceftriaxone[d]/cefuroxime[d] either plus amikacin), cycloserine[h]

Chlamydia pneumoniae

Doxycycline[j] or erythromycin

Azithromycin, clarithromycin[e]

Chlamydia trachomatis

Doxycycline[j] or azithromycin

Mycoplasma pneumoniae

Erythromycin, azithromycin, clarithromycin[e]

Doxycycline[j]

Spirochetes

Treponema pallidum

Penicillin G

Doxycycline,[j] ceftriaxone[d]

Borrelia burgdorferii

(choice depends on stage of disease)

Doxycycline[j] or amoxicillin

High-dose penicillin, ceftriaxone,[d] cefotaxime,[d] cefuroxime axetil,[d] azithromycin, clarithromycin[e]

---

[a]Either aqueous penicillin G or benzathine penicillin G (pharyngitis only).

[b]Only for soft-tissue infections or upper respiratory infections (pharyngitis, otitis media).

[c]First-generation cephalosporins. Intravenous: cefazolin; oral: cephalexin, cephradine, or cefadroxil.

[d]Some penicillin-allergic patients may react to cephalosporins.

[e]Do not use in pregnant patients.

[f]*S. pneumoniae* susceptibility to penicillin is expressed as the following: sensitive (MIC < 0.1 μg/mL), intermediate (MIC 0.1 to 1.0 μg/mL), and resistant (MIC ≥ 2.0 μg/mL). For intermediate strains, cefotaxime or ceftriaxone may be used for meningitis and either high-dose penicillin (≥ 12 MU/day) or cefuroxime may be used for pneumonia. For resistant strains, sensitivites should be used to guide therapy for meningitis and pneumonia. Resistance has been reported to erythromycin, clindamycin, trimethoprom–sulfamethoxazole, clarithromycin, azithromycin, and chloramphenicol. Quinupristin/dalfopristin (an investigational agent available from Rhone Poulenc Rorer (610-454-3071) has been sensitive to all strains tested.

VIII

[g]For the treatment of meningitis.

[h]Reserve for serious infection when less toxic drugs are not effective.

[i]Gentamicin should be added if tolerance or moderately susceptible (MIC^3 0.1 g/mL) organisms are encountered; streptomycin is used but may be more toxic.

[j]Not for use in pregnant patients or children less than 18 years old.

[k]Penicillinase-resistant penicillin: nafcillin or oxacillin.

[l]Not reliably bactericidal, so should not be used for endocarditis.

[m]β-lactamase inhibitor combination. IV: ampicillin/sulbactam; oral: amoxicillin/clavulanate.

[n]Second-generation cephalosporins. IV: cefuroxime; oral: cefuroxime aextil, cefaclor, cefprozil.

[o]Third-generation cephalosporins. IV: cefotaxime, ceftizoxime, ceftriaxone.

[p]Third-generation cephalosporins. Oral: cefixime, cefpodoxime, ceftibutin.

[q]Aqueous procaine penicillin G.

[r]Should only be used in serious infection.

[s]Extended-spectrum penicillin: ticarcillin, mezlocillin, or piperacillin.

[t]Ciprofloxacin. IV/PO: ofloxacin; IV/PO, norfloxacin.

[u]β-lactamase inhibitor combination: ampicillin/sulbactam, ticarcillin/clavulanate, piperacillin/tazobactam.

[v]Cefoxitin, cefotetan, cefmetazole.

[w]Ciprofloxacin. IV/PO, levofloxacin; IV/PO, ofloxacin; IV/PO, lomefloxacin, norfloxacin, sparfloxacin.

[x]Aminoglycosides: gentamicin, tobramycin, amikacin—use per sensitivities.

[y]Ciprofloxacin. IV/PO, levofloxacin; IV/PO, ofloxacin; IV/PO, lomefloxacin, norfloxacin.

[z]Ciprofloxacin. IV/PO, levofloxacin; IV/PO, ofloxacin; IV/PO, lomefloxacin, sparfloxacin.

[aa]Generally reserved for patients with hypersensitivity reactions to penicillin.

[bb]Antibiotics should not be given for gastroenteritis, because the carrier state may be prolonged without significant clinical benefit.

[cc]Sulfisoxazole, sulfadiazine (preferred for central nervous system [CNS] disease), trisulfapyrimidines.

- Local susceptibility data should be considered whenever possible rather than information published by other institutions or national compilations when selecting antimicrobial regimens.
- Empiric therapies are directed at organisms that are frequently known to cause the infection in question. The severity and/or acuity of the infectious process dictates the necessity for use of empiric antimicrobial therapy.

HOST FACTORS

- In evaluating a patient for initial or empiric therapy, the factors listed in Table 33–4 should be considered.
- Patients with diminished renal and/or hepatic function will accumulate certain drugs unless dosage is adjusted. Any concomitant therapy the patient is receiving may influence both the selection of drug therapy, the dosage, and monitoring.
- A list of selected drug interactions involving antimicrobials and antimicrobial interference with laboratory tests is provided in Table 33–5.

DRUG FACTORS

- In selecting an antimicrobial agent for empiric therapy, the kinetic disposition of the agent is an important consideration. This is partly because of cost considerations (less frequent dosing is less costly) and also because drugs should be selected that are best suited for the organ elimination capacity of the patient. VIII
- The relevance of tissue concentrations of antimicrobials has long been disputed. The central nervous system (CNS) is one body site where antimicrobial penetration is relatively well defined and correlations with clinical outcomes are established. Drugs that do not reach significant concentrations in cerebrospinal fluid (CSF) should be avoided in treating meningitis.
- Apart from the bloodstream, other body fluids where drug concentration data are clinically relevant include urine, synovial fluid, and peritoneal fluid.

TABLE 33–4. Host Factors in Selection of Antimicrobial Therapy

Allergy or history of adverse drug reactions
Age of patient
Pregnancy
Genetic or metabolic abnormalities
Renal and hepatic function
Site of the infection
Concomitant drug therapy
Underlying disease state(s)

TABLE 33–5. Antimicrobial Interactions

Antimicrobial	Other Agent(s)	Results of Interaction
Aminoglycosides	Neuromuscular blocking drugs	Increased neuromuscular blockade
	Other nephrotoxins or ototoxins (e.g., cisplatin amphotericin B, ethacrynic acid, vancomycin, cyclosporine)	Increased nephrotoxicity or ototoxicty
	Penicillins	Inactivation of both drugs (a particular problem in renal failure and when obtaining drug levels)
Sulfonamides	Sufonylureas	Hypoglycemia
	Phenytoin	Increased serum concentration of phenytoin leading to toxicity
	Oral anticoagulants (warfarin derivatives)	Enhanced hypoprothrombinemia
Chloramphenicol	Phenytoin, tolbutamide, ethanol	Increased serum concentration of other agents and enhanced pharmacologic effect or increased toxicity
Metronidazole (also cefamandole, moxalactam, cefoperazone)	Ethanol (including ethanol-containing medications)	Disulfiram-like reaction
Macrolides, azalides	Theophylline	Increased serum theophylline concentration
Fluconazole	Terfenadine, astemizole, cisapride	Cardiac arrhythmias
	Terfenadine, cisapride	Cardiac arrhythmias
	Phenytoin, warfarin	Inhibits metabolism of these drugs
	Rifampin	Enhances metabolism of fluconazole
Itraconazole	Astemizole, terfenadine, cisapride	Cardiac arrhythmias
	Phenytoin, warfarin	Inhibits metabolism of these drugs
	Rifampin	Enhances metabolism of itraconazole
Quinolones (norfloxacin, ciprofloxacin, ofloxacin, lomefloxacin, enoxacin grepafloxacin, levofloxacin, sparfloxacin, trovafloxacin)	Multivalent cations (antacids, iron, sucralfate, zinc)	Decreased absorption of quinolone
	Theophylline	Inhibits metabolism of theophylline (ciprofloxacin, grepafloxacin, and enoxacin)
	Antiarrhythmics	Increased Q/T interval (grepafloxacin and sparfloxacin)
Rifampin	Coumarin anticoagulants	Decreased anticoagulant effect (increased metabolsim of drug)
	Quinidine	Decreased effect of quinidine
	Digoxin	Decreased effect of digoxin
	Methadone	Narcotic withdrawl
	Propranolol	Decreased effect of propranolol
	Oral contraceptives	Decreased effect (pregnancy)
	Fluconazole; ketoconazole	Decreased antifungal effect
Tetracyclines	Antacids, iron, calcium	Inhibit intestinal absorption of tetracycline
Penicillins and cephalosporins	Uricosuric agents (probenecid, high-dose asprin, etc.)	Block excretion of β-lactams, causing higher serum levels
	Copper reduction test for glycosuria (Clinitest tablets)	False-positive test for glycosuria (not seen with glucose oxidase method)
Isoniazid	Phenytoin	Increased serum concentrations of both

TABLE 33–6. Total Economic Impact of Antimicrobial Therapy

Drug acquisition cost
Storage and inventory cost
Preparation by pharmacy and nursing staff, distribution, administration
Monitoring
Adverse effects
Impact on length of stay
Cost of control systems

- Certain basic pharmacokinetic parameters such as area under the concentration-vs-time curve (AUC) and maximal plasma concentration (C_{max}) can be predictive of treatment outcome when specific ratios of AUC or C_{max} to the minimum inhibitory concentration (MIC) are achieved. This is relevant for those antimicrobials that produce concentration-dependent bactericidal effects, for example, aminoglycosides and fluoroquinolones.
- When such concentration-dependent killing is coupled with a prolonged postantibiotic effect (PAE) (a prolonged lag period of growth following a brief exposure to an antimicrobial), it is possible to modify dosage regimens to take advantage of these effects (e.g., larger, less frequent doses for aminoglycosides). VIII
- Antimicrobials that affect cell wall synthesis (e.g., β-lactams) do not produce concentration-dependent killing and they do not produce prolonged PAE, but rather have time-dependent bactericidal effects. Therefore, the most important pharmacodynamic relationship for these antimicrobials is the duration that drug concentrations exceed the MIC.
- If one has the choice of two drugs that are equally efficacious yet one is less toxic, the less toxic drug, even if more costly, should be selected.
- The costs of drug therapy are increasing dramatically, especially as new products derived from biotechnology are introduced. The total cost of antimicrobial therapy includes much more than just the acquisition cost of the drugs. The total economic impact of antimicrobial therapy is detailed in Table 33–6.

► COMBINATION ANTIMICROBIAL THERAPY

- Combinations of antimicrobials are generally used to broaden the spectrum of coverage for empiric therapy, achieve synergistic activity against the infecting organism, and prevent the emergence of resistance.

BROADENING THE SPECTRUM OF COVERAGE

- Increasing the coverage of antimicrobial therapy is generally necessary in mixed infections where multiple organisms are likely to be present. This is the case in intra-abdominal and female pelvic infections in which a variety of aerobic and anaerobic bacteria may produce disease.

- The other clinical situation in which increased spectrum of activity is desirable is in nosocomial infection. Hospital-acquired infections, except as previously noted, are generally caused by only one organism, but many different organisms may be possible.

SYNERGISM

- The achievement of synergistic antimicrobial activity is advantageous for infections caused by gram-negative bacilli in immunosuppressed patients.
- Traditionally, combinations of aminoglycosides and β-lactams have been used since these drugs together generally act synergistically against a wide variety of bacteria. However, the data supporting superior efficacy of synergistic over nonsynergistic combinations is weak.
- Synergistic combinations may produce better results in infections caused by *Pseudomonas aeruginosa,* in certain infections caused by *Enterococcus* sp. and, perhaps, in patients with profound, persistent neutropenia.

PREVENTING RESISTANCE

- The use of combinations to prevent the emergence of resistance is widely applied but not often realized. The only circumstance where this has been clearly effective is in the treatment of tuberculosis.

DISADVANTAGES OF COMBINATION THERAPY

- Although there are potentially beneficial effects from combining drugs, there also are potentially serious liabilities. Examples include additive nephrotoxicity from drugs such as aminoglycosides, amphotericin, and possibly vancomycin. Inactivation of aminoglycosides by penicillins may be clinically significant when excessive doses of penicillin are given to a patient in renal failure.
- Some combinations of antimicrobials are potentially antagonistic. Such combinations should probably be avoided whenever possible, unless the clinical situation warrants the use of both drugs for different pathogens.
- Of more current relevance is the increasing use of β-lactam antimicrobials in combination. Agents that are capable of inducing β-lactamase production in bacteria such as *Enterobacter cloacae* and *P. aeruginosa* (e.g., imipenem, cephamycins) may antagonize the effects of enzyme-labile drugs such as penicillins.

FAILURE OF ANTIMICROBIAL THERAPY

- A variety of factors may be responsible for apparent lack of response to therapy. Factors include those directly related to the host, those related to the pathogen, and, although unlikely, laboratory error in identification and/or susceptibility testing. Factors directly related to the antimicrobial agents being utilized are only a small proportion of the possibilities.

Failures Caused by Drug Selection

- Factors directly related to the drug selection include an inappropriate selection of drug, dosage, or route of administration. Malabsorption of a drug product because of gastrointestinal disease (e.g., short-bowel syndrome) or a drug interaction (e.g., complexation of fluoroquinolones with multivalent cations resulting in reduced absorption) may lead to potentially subtherapeutic serum concentrations.
- Accelerated drug elimination is also a possible reason for failure which may occur in patients with cystic fibrosis or during pregnancy, when more rapid clearance or larger volumes of distribution may result in low serum concentrations, particularly for aminoglycosides.
- Inactivation of antimicrobial agents by other drugs may occur, as in the case of aminoglycoside inactivation by penicillins.
- Finally, a common cause of failure of therapy is poor penetration into the site of infection. This is especially true for the so-called "privileged" sites such as the CNS, the eye, and the prostate gland.

Failures Caused by Host Factors

- Patients who are immunosuppressed (e.g., granulocytopenia from chemotherapy, AIDS) may respond poorly to therapy because their own defenses are inadequate to eradicate the infection despite seemingly adequate drug regimens.
- Other host factors are related to the necessity for surgical drainage of abscesses or removal of foreign bodies and/or necrotic tissue. If these situations are not corrected, they result in persistent infection and, occasionally, bacteremia, despite adequate antimicrobial therapy.
- Concurrent diseases may be responsible for predisposition to or persistence of infection, including cardiac or pulmonary disease, immunosuppressive disorders, and structural abnormalities of various organ systems.

Failures Caused by Microorganisms

- Factors related to the pathogen include the development of drug resistance during therapy. Primary resistance refers to the intrinsic resistance of the pathogens producing the infection. However, acquisition of resistance during treatment has become a major problem as well.
- The increase in resistance among pathogenic organisms is believed to be due, in large part, to continued overuse of antimicrobials in the community, as well as in hospitals, and the increasing prevalence of immunosuppressed patients receiving long-term suppressive antimicrobials for the prevention of infections.

See Chapter 96, Antimicrobial Regimen Selection, authored by Betty J. Abate, PharmD, BCPS, and Steven L. Barriere, PharmD, FCCP, for a more detailed discussion of this topic.

Chapter 34

▶ CENTRAL NERVOUS SYSTEM INFECTIONS

▶ DEFINITION

- Central nervous system (CNS) infections include a wide variety of clinical conditions and etiologies: meningitis, meningoencephalitis, encephalitis, brain and meningeal abscesses, and shunt infections. The focus of this chapter is meningitis.
- CNS infections are divided into two categories: septic and aseptic. Septic or bacterial infections are the result of hematogenous spread from a primary site of infection, parameningeal seeding from a localized infection, or trauma or congenital defects in the CNS. Aseptic infection is a term broadly used to describe chemical irritants, viral, fungal, parasitic, tuberculous, sarcoid, neoplastic, and syphilitic processes of the CNS.

▶ PATHOPHYSIOLOGY

- CNS infections may be caused by a variety of bacteria, fungi, viruses, and parasites. The most common causes of bacterial meningitis include *Streptococcus pneumoniae, Haemophilus influenzae,* and *Neisseria meningitidis.*
- The critical first step in the acquisition of acute bacterial meningitis is nasopharyngeal colonization by the bacterial pathogen. The bacteria must first attach themselves to nasopharyngeal epithelial cells. The bacteria are then phagocytized across nonciliated columnar nasopharyngeal cells into the host's bloodstream.
- A common characteristic of most CNS bacterial pathogens (e.g., *H. influenzae, Escherichia coli,* and *N. meningitidis*) is the presence of an extensive polysaccharide capsule that is resistant to neutrophil phagocytosis and complement opsonization.
- Bacteria replicate freely within the CSF until either bacterial overgrowth occurs or an effective antibiotic regimen is administered that terminates the process.
- Bacterial cell death then causes the release of cell wall components such as lipopolysaccharide (LPS), lipid A (endotoxin), lipoteichoic acid, teichoic acid, and peptidoglycan depending on whether the pathogen is gram positive or gram negative. These cell wall components cause capillary endothelial cells and CNS macrophages to release cytokines (interleukin-1 [IL-1] and tumor necrosis factor [TNF]).
- Capillary endothelial cells and CNS leukocytes release products of the cyclooxygenase-arachidonic acid pathway (prostaglandins and thromboxanes) and platelet activating factor (PAF). PAF activates the coagulation cascade, and arachidonic acid metabolites stimulate vasodilatation. These lead to cerebral edema, elevated intracranial pressure, CSF

pleocytosis, disseminated intravascular coagulation (DIC), syndrome of inappropriate antidiuretic hormone secretion (SIADH), decreased cerebral blood flow, cerebral ischemia, and death.

▶ CLINICAL PRESENTATION

- Signs and symptoms of CNS infection have clinical features similar to those of a variety of infectious diseases. Fever, peripheral leukocytosis with a left shift, and malaise are common observations.
- On initial presentation, differentiation of patients with bacterial, viral, or fungal meningitis is virtually impossible.
- The clinical signs and symptoms of meningitis are variable and dependent on the age of the patient. Adult patients may present with variable complaints of fever, stiffness of the neck and/or back, nuchal rigidity, positive Brudzinski's sign, and/or positive Kernig's sign. Later in the course of the disease, the patient may experience seizures, focal neurologic deficits, and hydrocephalus.
- Young infants infected with bacterial meningitis may reveal only nonspecific symptoms such as irritability, altered sleep patterns, vomiting, high-pitched crying, decreased oral intake, or seizures. Symptoms in the elderly may resemble stroke or endocarditis.
- The diagnosis of bacterial meningitis is usually made on the basis of examination of CSF collected soon after the diagnosis is suspected. In addition to CSF examination, blood cultures should be performed because meningitis can frequently arise via hematogenous dissemination. Elevated CSF protein >50 mg/dL and a CSF glucose concentration <50% of the simultaneously obtained peripheral value suggest bacterial meningitis (Table 34–1). VIII
- Gram stain and aerobic culture of the CSF are the most important laboratory tests to diagnose bacterial meningitis. When performed before antibiotic therapy is initiated, Gram stain is both rapid and sensitive and

TABLE 34–1. Typical Components of Normal and Abnormal Cerebrospinal Fluid

Type	Normal	Bacterial	Viral	Fungal	Tuberculosis
WBC (mm^3)	<10[a]	400–100,000	5–500	40–400	100–1000
Differential	>90%[a]	>90 PMN[b]	50[c,d]	>50[c]	>80[c,d]
Protein (mg/dL)	<50	80–500	30–150	40–150	≥40–150
Glucose (mg/dL)	½–⅔ serum	<½ serum	<30–70	<30–70	<30–70

[a]Monocytes.
[b]PMN, polymorphonuclear cells.
[c]Lymphocytes.
[d]Initial CSF WBC may reveal a predominance of PMNs.
Adapted from Maxson S, Jacobs RF. Postgrad Med *1993;93(8):153–166, with permission.*

can confirm the diagnosis of bacterial meningitis in 60–90% of cases. The sensitivity of Gram stain decreases to 40–60% in patients receiving prior antibiotic therapy.

- Several rapid diagnostic methods are available for identifying potential bacterial pathogens from CSF. Latex fixation, latex coagglutination, and enzyme immunoassay (EIA) tests provide for the rapid identification of *S. pneumoniae,* group B Streptococci, *N. meningitidis,* type B *H. influenzae,* and *E. coli* (K1).

▶ DESIRED OUTCOME

- Early intervention is important to avoid mortality.
- Appropriate antimicrobial therapy should be instituted to eradicate the causative organism.
- Amelioration of the signs and symptoms associated with meningitis.
- Prevention of neurologic sequelae.

▶ TREATMENT

GENERAL PRINCIPLES

- The administration of fluids, electrolytes, antipyretics, analgesia, and other supportive measures are indicated as needed for patients presenting with acute bacterial meningitis.
- Antimicrobials are the primary treatment and are usually given for 7–14 days for *L. monocytogenes,* group B *streptococcus,* and enteric gram-negative bacilli.

PHARMACOLOGIC TREATMENT

- Appropriate antibiotic therapy (empiric or definitive) should be started as soon as possible. Isolation and identification of the causative agent can direct the selection of the most appropriate antimicrobial therapy for the patient (Tables 34–2, 34–3 and 34–4).
- With increased meningeal inflammation, there will be greater antibiotic penetration (Table 34–2). Problems of CSF penetration may be overcome by direct instillation of antibiotics by intrathecal, intracisternal, or intraventricular routes of administration (Table 34–3).
- Antibiotic factors that promote penetration into the CSF include low molecular weight, unionized molecules, lipid solubility, and low protein binding.

Dexamethasone as an Adjunctive Treatment for Meningitis

- In addition to antibiotics, **dexamethasone** is commonly used therapy for the treatment of pediatric meningitis. Dexamethasone may cause a significant improvement in CSF glucose concentrations, as well as CSF protein and lactate concentrations, as well as a significantly lower incidence of neurologic sequella commonly associated with bacterial meningitis.

TABLE 34–2. Penetration of Antimicrobial Agents into the Cerebrospinal Fluid (CSF)

Therapeutic Levels in CSF With or Without Inflammation	
Sulfonamides	Trimethoprim
Chloramphenicol	Isoniazid
Rifampin	Pyrazinamide
Ethionamide	Cycloserine
Metronidazole	
Therapeutic Levels in CSF With Inflammation of Meninges	
Penicillin G	Ampicillin ± sulbactam
Carbenicillin	Ticarcillin ± clavulanic acid
Nafcillin	Mezlocillin
Piperacillin	Cefuroxime
Cefotaxime	Ceftizoxime
Ceftriaxone	Ceftazidime
Imipenem	Aztreonam
Meropenem	Ofloxacin
Vancomycin	Ciprofloxacin
Vidarabine	Ethambutol
Flucytosine	Fluconazole
Pyrimethamine	Ganciclovir
Acyclovir	Foscarnet
Nontherapeutic Levels in CSF With or Without Inflammation	
Aminoglycosides	First-generation cephalosporins
Cefoperozone	Second-generation cephalosporins[a]
Clindamycin[b]	Ketoconazole
Amphotericin B[c]	Itraconazole[c]

[a]Cefuroxime is an exception.
[b]Achieves therapeutic brain tissue concentrations.
[c]Achieves therapeutic concentrations for *C. neoformans* therapy.

VIII

- Currently, the American Academy of Pediatrics suggests that the use of dexamethasone be considered for infants and children 2 months of age or older with proven or strongly suspected bacterial meningitis. The commonly used intravenous (IV) dexamethasone dose is 0.15 mg/kg every 6 hours for 4 days. Alternatively, dexamethasone 0.15 mg/kg every 6 hours for 2 days or dexamethasone 0.4 mg/kg every 12 hours for 2 days is equally effective and potentially less toxic regimens.
- Dexamethasone should be administered prior to the first antibiotic dose, and serum hemoglobin and stool guaiac should be monitored for evidence of gastrointestinal (GI) bleeding.

Neisseria Meningitidis (Meningococcus)

- *N. meningitidis* meningitis is most commonly found in children and young adults. Most cases usually occur in the winter or spring, at a time when viral meningitis is relatively uncommon.

TABLE 34–3. Intraventricular and Intrathecal Antibiotic Dosage Recommendations

Antibiotic	Adult Dose (mg)	Expected CSF Concentration[a] (mg/L)
Ampicillin	10–50	60–300
Methicillin	25–100	160–600
Nafcillin	75	500
Cefazolin	1–2 mg/kg, 50 mg maximum	300
Cephalothin	25–100	160–600
Chloramphenicol	25–100	160–600
Gentamicin	1–10	6–60
Tobramycin	1–10	6–60
Amikacin	5–10	60
Vancomycin	5	30
Amphotericin B	0.05–0.25 mg/d to 0.05–1 mg 1–3 times weekly	—

[a]Assumes adult CSF volume = 150 mL.

Clinical Presentation

- Approximately 10–14 days after the onset of the disease and despite successful treatment, the patient develops a characteristic immunologic reaction of fever, arthritis (usually involving large joints), and pericarditis.
- Approximately 50% of patients die within the first 24 hours as a result meningococcemia. Other patients develop chronic meningococcemia characterized by fever, arthritis, and a morbilliform rash that recurs every 48–72 hours.
- Deafness unilaterally, or more commonly bilaterally, may develop early or late in the disease course.
- Approximately 50% of patients with meningococcal meningitis have purpuric lesions, petechiae, or both. Patients may have an obvious or subclinical picture of DIC, which may progress to infarction of the adrenal glands and renal cortex and cause widespread thrombosis.

Treatment and Prevention

- Aggressive, early intervention with **high-dose intravenous crystalline penicillin G,** 50,000 units/kg every 4 hours intravenously, is usually recommended for treatment of *N. meningitidis* meningitis.
- **Chloramphenicol** may be used in place of penicillin G. Several third-generation cephalosporins (e.g., **cefotaxime**) approved for the treatment of meningitis are acceptable alternatives to penicillin G (Table 34–5).

TABLE 34–4. Bacterial Meningitis: Most Likely Bacteria and Empiric Therapy by Age Group

Age Commonly Affected	Most Likely Organisms	Empiric Therapy	Risk Factors for All Age Groups
Newborn–1 month	Gram negative enterics[a] Group B streptococcus *Listeria monocytogenes*	Ampicillin + CTX or CTR or AG	Respiratory tract infection Otitis media Mastoiditis Head trauma Alcoholism
1 month–4 years	*Haemophilus influenzae* *Neisseria meningitidis* *Streptococcus pneumoniae*	CTX or CTR ± VM	High-dose steroids Splenectomy Sickle cell disease Immunoglobulin deficiency
5–29 years	*N. meningitidis* *S. pneumoniae* *H. influenzae*	CTX or CTR ± VM	Immunosuppression
30–60 years	*S. pneumoniae* *N. meningitidiis*	CTX or CTR ± VM	
>60 years	*S. pneumoniae* Gram-negative enterics *Listeria monocytogenes*	Ampicillin + CTX or CTR or AG ± VM	

[a] *E. coli, Klebsiella* spp., *Enterobacter* spp. common.

CTX, cefotaxime; CRT, ceftriaxone, AG, aminoglycoside; VM, vancomycin (use should be based on local incidence of penicillin-resistant *S. pneumoniae* and until CTX or CTR MIC results are available).

TABLE 34–5. Antimicrobial Agents of First Choice and Alternative Choice in Treatment of Meningitis Caused by Gram-Negative Organisms

Organism	Antibiotic of First Choice[a]	Alternative Antibiotics[a]
Neisseria meningitidis (meningococcal)	Penicillin G 200,000–300,000 units/kg/day	Cefotaxime 200 mg/kg/day q 4 h max: 2 g IV q 4 h Ceftriaxone 100 mg/kg/day q 24 h[b] max: adults 2 g IV q 12 h Chloramphenicol 100 mg/kg/day q 6 h max: 1.5 g IV q 6 h
Escherichia coli	Cefotaxime	Ceftriaxone Chloramphenicol
Haemophilus influenzae		
β-Lactamase positive	Cefotaxime	Ceftriaxone
β-Lactamase negative	Ampicillin 200–400 mg/kg/day q 6 h IV max: 2 g q 4 h IV	Cefotaxime Ceftriaxone
Pseudomonas aeruginosa	Ceftazidime 85 mg/kg/d max: 2 g IV q 6 h **plus** tobramycin 5–7.5 mg/kg/day IV[c]	Imipenem 80 mg/kg/day max: 1 g IV q 6 h Piperacillin 200–300 mg/kg/day max: 3 g q 4 h IV plus tobramycin
Enterobacteriaceae	Cefotaxime	Ceftriaxone Piperacillin **plus** aminoglycoside Imipenem

[a] Recommended doses for adults and pediatric patients with normal renal and/or hepatic function.
[b] Pediatrics.
[c] Direct CNS administration may be added, see Table 34–3 for dosage.

- Close contacts of patients contracting *N. meningitidis* meningitis are at an increased risk of developing meningitis. Prophylaxis of contacts should be started without delay and, therefore, without the aid of culture and sensitivity studies.
- Adult patients should receive 600 mg of **rifampin** orally every 12 hours for four doses. Children 1 month to 12 years of age should receive 10 mg/kg of rifampin orally every 12 hours for four doses, and children younger than 1 month should receive 5 mg/kg orally every 12 hours for four doses. Alternatives to rifampin include **ciprofloxacin** (single dose) in adults and **ceftriaxone** 125–250 mg (single dose, intramuscularly).
- Patients receiving rifampin should be counseled as to the expected red-to-orange color change in urine and other body secretions.

Streptococcus Pneumoniae (Pneumococcus or Diplococcus)

- Pneumococcal meningitis occurs in the very young (1–4 months) and the very old. It is the most common cause of meningitis in adults and accounts for 12% of meningitis episodes in children 2 months to 10 years.

Treatment (Table 34–6)

- The treatment of choice until susceptibility of the organism is known is **vancomycin** (15 mg/kg every 6 hours up to 2 grams per day) plus a broad-spectrum cephalosporin (**ceftriaxone** 100 mg/kg every 24 hours intravenously in children 2 grams every 12 hours in adults). If adjunctive **dexamethasone** is given in adults, the preferred regimen is ceftriaxone plus rifampin (600 mg per day). VIII
- Vancomycin alone or in combination with ceftriaxone is probably the most effective regimen for penicillin-resistant strains.
- If the pathogen is found to be susceptible to penicillin and ceftriaxone, either agent may be used alone (**penicillin** given at 200,000–300,000 units/kg/d given every 4 hours intravenously). If the pathogen is resistant to penicillin but susceptible to ceftriaxone or cefotaxime, either alone may be continued.
- Virtually all serotypes of *S. pneumoniae* exhibiting intermediate or complete resistance to penicillin are found in the current **23 serotype pneumococcal vaccine,** and clinicians need to universally immunize appropriate patients.
- Chemoprophylaxis and vaccination for close contacts of an index case with *S. pneumoniae* meningitis are generally not recommended because the risk of acquiring secondary pneumococcal disease is similar to the infection rate in the general population. However, vaccination and chemoprophylaxis with oral penicillin reduce the incidence of pneumococcal septicemia and meningitis in young patients with sickle cell disease.

Gram-Negative Bacillary Meningitis

Currently, enteric gram-negative bacteria are the fourth leading cause of meningitis.

TABLE 34–6. Antimicrobial Agents of First Choice and Alternative Choice in Treatment of Meningitis Caused by Gram-Positive Microorganisms

Organism	Antibiotic of First Choice[a]	Alternative Antibiotics[a]
Streptococcus pneumoniae		
Penicillin susceptible	Penicillin G 200,000–300,000 units/kg/day, q 4 h IV max: 4 million units q 4 h IV	Cefotaxime 200 mg/kg/day q 4 h IV max: 2 g q 4 h Ceftriaxone 100 mg/kg/day q 24 h IV[b] max: adults 2 g q 12 Chloramphenicol 100 mg/kg/day, q 6 h max: 1.5 g q 6 h
Low-level penicillin resistance[c]	Cefotaxime or ceftriaxone	Vancomycin 30–40 mg/kg/day IV
High-level penicillin resistance[d]	Vancomycin ± ceftriaxone	Imipenem 80 mg/kg/day max: 1 g IV q 6 h
Group B *Streptococcus*	Penicillin	Cefotaxime Ceftriaxone Chloramphenicol
Staphylococcus aureus		
Penicillin resistant	Nafcillin 200 mg/kg/day q 4 h max: 2 g q 4 h IV	Vancomycin
Methicillin resistant	Vancomycin	—
Staphylococcus epidermidis		
Penicillin resistant	Nafcillin	Vancomycin
Methicillin resistant	Vancomycin	
Listeria monocytogenes	Ampicillin 200–400 mg/kg/day, q 6 h IV or Pen G max: 2 g q 4 h IV **plus** aminoglycoside	Trimethoprim 10 mg/kg/day and sulfamethoxazole 50 mg/kg/day, divided q 6 h

[a]Recommended doses for adults and pediatric patients with normal renal and/or hepatic function.
[b]Pediatrics.
[c]Incidence of low-level resistance is 10–20%
[d]Incidence of high-level resistance is 1–2%; therapeutic recommendations for this infection have not been clearly defined.

Treatment (Table 34–5)

- Meningitis caused by *P. aeruginosa* is treated with **ceftazidime** or **piperacillin** plus an aminoglycoside, usually **tobramycin.**
- If the pseudomonad is suspected to be antibiotic resistant or becomes resistant during therapy, an intraventricular aminoglycoside (preservative-free) should be considered along with IV aminoglycoside. Intraventricular aminoglycoside dosages are adjusted to the estimated CSF volume (0.03 mg of tobramycin or **gentamicin**/mL of CSF and 0.1 mg of **amikacin**/mL of CSF every 24 hours). Ventricular levels of aminoglycoside are monitored every 2 or 3 days, just prior to the next intraventricular dose, and "trough levels" should approximate 2–10 mg/L.
- Gram-negative organisms, other than *P. aeruginosa,* that cause meningitis can also be treated with a third-generation cephalosporin such as **cefotaxime, ceftizoxime, ceftriaxone,** or **ceftazidime**. In adults, daily doses of 8–12 g/d of these third-generation cephalosporins or 2 g of ceftriaxone should produce CSF concentrations of 5–20 mg/L.
- Therapy for gram-negative meningitis is continued for 21 days. CSF cultures may remain positive for 10 days or more on a regimen that will eventually be curative.

Haemophilus Influenzae

- In the past, *H. influenzae* was the most common cause of meningitis in children 6 months to 3 years. The disease is often a complication of primary infectious involvement of the middle ear, paranasal sinuses, or lungs. VIII
- Coma and seizures commonly occur early in the course of the disease. Morbiliform and petechial rashes are very uncommon, but may resemble the rash seen with meningococcal infection.

Treatment

- Approximately 30–40% of *H. influenzae* are ampicillin resistant. For this reason, many clinicians use a third-generation cephalosporin (**cefotaxime** or **ceftriaxone**) or **chloramphenicol with ampicillin** for initial antimicrobial therapy. Once bacterial susceptibilities are available, ampicillin may be used if the isolate proves ampicillin sensitive.

Prevention

- Secondary cases may occur within 30 days of the index case and so treatment of close contacts (household members, individuals sharing sleeping quarters, crowded confined populations, day care attendees, and nursing home residents) of patients is usually recommended. The goal of prophylaxis is to eliminate nasopharyngeal and oropharyngeal carriage of *H. influenzae.*
- Prophylaxis for *H. influenzae* is not recommended when at least one member of the same household as the patient is less than 4 years of age, if all contacts under 4 years old are fully immunized. Households with children less than 12 months old (regardless of vaccination status), or with children ages 1–3 years old who are not adequately vaccinated,

should all receive **rifampin** prophylaxis to eliminate nasopharyngeal carriage and the subsequent spread of disease to others. Chemoprophylaxis should be initiated as soon as possible after exposure. The patient should also receive chemoprophylaxis prior to discharge from the hospital because there have been reports of recolonization after successful antibiotic therapy.

- Adults receive 600 mg of rifampin daily for 4 days. Children 1 month to 12 years old receive 20 mg/kg (maximum 600 mg) per day for 4 days, and children less than 1 month old receive 10 mg/kg/d for 4 days.
- Vaccination with **HIB conjugate vaccines** is usually begun in children at 2 months.
- The vaccine should be considered in patients greater than 5 years of age with sickle cell disease, asplenia, or immunocompromising diseases.

Listeria Monocytogenes

- Listeria monocytogenes is a gram-positive diphtheroid-like organism and is responsible for 3% of all reported cases of meningitis. The disease affects primarily neonates, immunocompromised adults, and the elderly. In the immunocompromised patient, the CSF resembles that found in bacterial meningitis.

Treatment

- The combination of **penicillin G** or **ampicillin** with **gentamicin** results in a bactericidal effect. Patients should be treated for 2–3 weeks after defervescence to prevent the possibility of relapse.
- **Trimethoprim–sulfamethoxazole** may be an effective alternative, because adequate CSF penetration is achieved with these agents.

Mycobacterium Tuberculosis

- *Mycobacterium tuberculosis* var. *hominis* is the primary cause of tuberculous meningitis. Tuberculous meningitis may exist in the absence of disease in the lung or extrapulmonary sites. Upon initial examination, CSF usually contains from 100–1000 WBC/mm^3, which may be 75–80% polymorphonuclear cells. Over time, the pattern of WBC in the CSF will shift to lymphocytes and monocytes.
- **Isoniazid** is the mainstay in virtually any regimen to treat *M. tuberculosis.* In children, the usual dose of isoniazid is 10–20 mg/kg/d (maximum 300 mg/d). Adults usually receive 5–10 mg/kg/d or a daily dose of 300 mg.
- Supplemental doses of **pyridoxine hydrochloride (vitamin B_6)** 50 mg/d are recommended to prevent the peripheral neuropathy associated with isoniazid administration.
- As of 1993, the CDC recommends a regimen of four drugs for empiric treatment of *M. tuberculosis,* unless resistance to isoniazid in the area is <4%. This regimen should consist of **isoniazid, rifampin, pyrazinamide,** and **ethambutol** 15–25 mg/kg/d (maximum 2.5 g/d) or **streptomycin** 15–30 mg/kg/d (maximum 1 g/d) for the first 2 months, generally followed by isoniazid plus rifampin for the duration of therapy.

Therapy after the first 2 months should be individualized based on susceptibility patterns.

- Concurrent administration of rifampin is recommended at doses of 10–20 mg/kg/d (maximum 600 mg/d) for children and 600 mg/d for adults. The addition of pyrazinamide (children and adults 15–30 mg/kg/d; maximum in both 2 g/d) to the regimen of isoniazid and rifampin is now recommended. The duration of concomitant pyrazinamide therapy should be limited to 2 months to avoid hepatotoxicity.
- Patients with *M. tuberculosis* meningitis should be treated for a duration of 9 months or longer with multiple drug therapy.
- The use of steroids for tuberculous meningitis remains controversial. In some cases, administration of steroids as oral **prednisone** 40–60 mg/d or 0.2 mg/kg/d of IV **dexamethasone** has resulted in a dramatic clearing of sensorium, remission of CSF abnormalities, reduction in fever, and elimination of headaches.

Cryptococcus Neoformans

- In the United States, cryptococcal meningitis is the most common form of fungal meningitis and is a major cause of morbidity and mortality in immunosuppressed patients. Patients with HIV are at a 5–10% risk of developing cryptococcus during their lifetime.
- Fever and a history of headaches are the most common symptoms of cryptococcal meningitis, although altered mentation and evidence of focal neurologic deficits may be present. Diagnosis is based on the presence of a positive CSF, blood, sputum, or urine culture for *C. neoformans.* VIII
- CSF cultures are positive in more than 90% of cases.

Treatment

- **Amphotericin B** is the drug of choice for treatment of acute *C. neoformans* meningitis. Amphotericin B 0.5–1 mg/kg/d combined with **flucytosine** 100 mg/kg/d is more effective than amphotericin alone. In the AIDS population, flucytosine is often poorly tolerated, causing bone marrow suppression and GI distress.
- Intraventricular amphotericin B in addition to IV amphotericin B plus is generally reserved for patients who fail to respond to systemic therapy.
- Due to the high relapse rate following acute therapy for *C. neoformans,* AIDS patients require lifelong maintenance or suppressive therapy. The standard of care for AIDS-associated cryptococcal meningitis is primary therapy, generally using amphotericin B with or without flucytosine or **fluconazole** alone, followed by maintenance therapy with fluconazole for the life of the patient.

Viral Meningitis

- Meningitis typically is characterized as being either purulent or aseptic. While purulent meningitis refers to a bacterial etiology, aseptic meningitis historically was defined by diagnosis of exclusion.

- At least 70% of aseptic meningitis cases are caused by viruses; however, unusual bacterial organisms such as *M. tuberculosis, Brucella* spp., and *Borrelia burgdorferi* can cause aseptic meningitis.
- Common signs in adults include headache, mild fever (<40°C), nuchal rigidity, malaise, drowsiness, nausea, vomiting, and photophobia. Only fever and irritability may be evident in the infant, and meningitis must be ruled out as a cause of fever when no other localized findings are observed in a child.
- Laboratory examination of CSF usually reveals a pleocytosis with 10–1000 WBCs/mm^3, which are primarily lymphocytic; however, 20–75% of patients with viral meningitis may have a predominance of polymorphonuclear cells on initial examination of the CSF, especially in enteroviral meningitis.
- **Acyclovir** is the drug of choice for herpes simplex encephalitis. In patients with normal renal function, acyclovir is usually administered as 10 mg/kg every 8 hours. Herpes virus resistance to acyclovir has been reported with increasing incidence, particularly from immunocompromised patients with prior or chronic exposures to acyclovir.
- The alternative treatment for acyclovir-resistant herpes simplex virus is **vidarabine.** Vidarabine is used intravenously in a dose of 15 mg/kg/d.

VIII *See Chapter 97, Central Nervous System Infections, authored by Marnie L. Peterson, PharmD, AnhThu D. Hoang, PharmD, David H. Wright, PharmD, and John C. Rotschafer, PharmD, FCCP, for a more detailed discussion of this topic.*

Chapter 35

▶ ENDOCARDITIS

▶ DEFINITION

Endocarditis is an inflammation of the endocardium, the membrane lining the chambers of the heart and covering the cusps of the heart valves. Infective endocarditis (IE) refers to infection of the heart valves by microorganisms.

Endocarditis is often referred to as either acute or subacute depending on the clinical presentation. Acute bacterial endocarditis is a fulminating infection associated with high fevers, systemic toxicity, and death within a few days to weeks if untreated. Subacute bacterial endocarditis (SBE) is a more indolent infection, usually occurring in a setting of prior valvular heart disease.

▶ PATHOPHYSIOLOGY

- Most types of structural heart disease resulting in turbulence of blood flow will increase the risk for IE. Some of the most important include:
  - Congenital heart disease accompanied by cyanosis (such as patent ductus arteriosus and ventricular septal defects).
  - Rheumatic heart disease following rheumatic fever.
  - Mitral valve prolapse with regurgitation.
  - Degenerative valvular lesions in the elderly, such as valvular stenosis and regurgitation.
  - Presence of a prosthetic valve.
- Three groups of organisms cause most cases of IE: streptococci (50–60%), staphylococci (25%), and enterococci (10%) (Table 35–1).
- The development of IE via hematogenous spread, the most common route, requires the sequential occurrence of several factors:

    1. The endothelial surface of the heart must be damaged, which occurs with turbulent blood flow.
    2. Platelet and fibrin deposition occurs on the abnormal epithelial surface, referred to as nonbacterial thrombotic endocarditis (NBTE).
    3. Bacteremia results in colonization of the endocardial surface.
    4. Staphylococci, viridans streptococci, and enterococci are most likely to adhere to NBTE, probably because of production of specific adherence factors, such as dextran production by some oral streptococci.
    5. After colonization of the endothelial surface, fibrin, platelets, and bacteria continue to aggregate and a "vegetation" forms. The protective cover of fibrin and platelets allows unimpeded bacterial

TABLE 35–1. Etiologic Agents in Infective Endocarditis

Agent	Percentage of Cases
Streptococci	55–62
Viridans streptococci	30–40
Other streptococci	15–25
Enterococci	5–18
Staphylococci	20–35
Coagulase-positive	10–27
Coagulase-negative	1–3
Gram-negative aerobic bacilli	1.5–13
Fungi	2–4
Miscellaneous bacteria	<5
Mixed infections	1–2
"Culture negative"	<5–24

Adapted from Scheld WM, Sande M. Endocarditis and intravascular infections. In: Mandell GL, Dolin R, Bennett JE, eds. Principles and Practice of Infectious Diseases, *4th ed. New York, Churchill Livingstone, 1995;740–783.*

growth to concentrations as high as 10^9–10^{10} per gram of tissue. Bacteria within the vegetation grow slowly and are protected from antibiotics and host defenses.

▶ CLINICAL PRESENTATION

- The clinical presentation of patients with IE is highly variable (Table 35–2).
- Important clinical signs, especially prevalent in subacute illness, may include the following peripheral manifestations ("stigmata") of endocarditis:
  - Osler nodes
  - Janeway lesions
  - Splinter hemorrhages
  - Petechiae
  - Clubbing of the fingers
  - Roth spot
  - Emboli
- Without appropriate antimicrobial therapy and surgery, if required, IE is usually fatal. With proper management, recovery can be expected in most patients.
- Factors associated with increased mortality include:

  1. Congestive heart failure.
  2. Culture-negative endocarditis.

TABLE 35–2. Clinical Manifestations of Infective Endocarditis

Symptoms	Percentage of Patients	Physical Findings	Percentage of Patients
Fever	80	Fever	90
Chills	40	Heart murmur	85
Weakness	40	Changing murmur	5–10
Dyspnea	40	New murmur	3–5
Sweats	25	Embolic phenomenon	>50
Anorexia	25	Skin manifestations	18–50
Weight loss	25	Osler nodes	10–23
Malaise	25	Splinter hemorrhages	15
Cough	25	Petechiae	20–40
Skin lesions	20	Janeway lesion	<10
Stroke	20	Splenomegaly	20–57
Nausea/vomiting	20	Septic complications (pneumonia, meningitis, etc.)	20
Headache	15		
Myalgia / arthralgia	15		
Edema	15	Mycotic aneurysms	20
Chest pain	15	Clubbing	12–52
Abdominal pain	15	Retinal lesion	2–10
Delirium/coma	10–15	Signs of renal failure	10–15
Hemoptysis	10		
Back pain	10		

From Scheld WM, Sande MA. In Mandell GL, Bennett JE, Dolin R (eds): Principles and Practices of Infectious Diseases, *4th ed. New York. Churchill Livingstone, 1995:748, with permission.*

3. Endocarditis caused by resistant organisms such as fungi and gram-negative bacteria.
4. Left-sided endocarditis caused by *S. aureus*.
5. Prosthetic valve endocarditis.

LABORATORY AND DIAGNOSTIC FINDINGS

- The hallmark of IE is a continuous bacteremia caused by shedding of bacteria from the vegetation into the bloodstream. More than 95% of patients with IE have a positive blood culture when three samples are obtained during a 24-hour period.
- Two-dimensional echocardiography (TEE) is increasingly important in identifying and localizing valvular lesions in patients suspected of having IE. TEE is more sensitive for detecting vegetations (about 95%), compared to transthoracic echocardiography (TTE) (60–65%).

▶ DESIRED OUTCOME

- To relieve the signs and symptoms of disease.
- Eradicate the causative organism.
- Provide cost effective antimicrobial therapy.
- Prevent IE in high-risk patients with appropriate antimicrobials.

▶ TREATMENT

GENERAL PRINCIPLES

- The most important approach to treatment of IE includes isolation of the pathogen followed by high-dose, bactericidal antibiotics for an extended period.
- For some pathogens, such as enterococci, the use of synergistic antimicrobial combinations is essential to obtain a bactericidal effect.
- For most patients 4–6 weeks of therapy are required.
- Specific recommendations for treating IE caused by the most common organisms are discussed in this chapter.

NON-PHARMACOLOGIC THERAPY

- Surgery is an important adjunct to management of endocarditis in certain patients. The major causes of death in patients with IE are heart failure and infection of vital organs from septic embolization. In most cases, valvectomy and valve replacement are performed to remove infected tissues and restore hemodynamic function.
- The most important indications for surgery include the following:
  - Valvular dysfunction with heart failure, perivalvular necrosis, aortic dissection, or valvular orifice obstruction.
  - Local suppurative complications such as a myocardial abscess.

- Endocarditis caused by resistant organisms (e.g., most cases of endocarditis caused by *Enterobacteriaceae*, *Pseudomonas*, or fungi).
- Almost all cases of early prosthetic valve endocarditis (PVE).
- Persistent bacteremia or other evidence of failure of appropriate medical therapy.

VIRIDANS STREPTOCOCCAL ENDOCARDITIS

- Viridans streptococcus is the most common cause of IE, especially in cases involving native valves. *Streptococcus bovis* is not a viridans streptococcus, but is included here because it is penicillin sensitive and treatment regimens are the same as for viridans streptococci.
- The MIC should be determined for all viridans streptococci, and the results be used to guide therapy.
- Recommended therapy in the uncomplicated case caused by fully susceptible strains is 2 weeks of combined therapy with **penicillin G** and **gentamicin** (Table 35–3). Alternative therapy consists of penicillin G or **ceftriaxone** alone for 4 weeks.
- Therapy for the patient with penicillin allergy is relatively straightforward. **Vancomycin** is effective and is the drug of choice.
- For patients with complicated infection, or when the organism is relatively resistant (MIC of 0.1–0.5 μg/mL) combination therapy with penicillin and gentamicin is recommended for 2 weeks or penicillin alone (Table 35–4).

STAPHYLOCOCCAL ENDOCARDITIS

- *Staphylococcus aureus* is the most common organism causing IE both among IV drug abusers and in persons with venous catheters. Coagulase-negative staphylococci (CNST, usually *S. epidermidis*) are prominent causes of PVE.
- Management requires consideration of several factors:

    1. Is the organism methicillin resistant?
    2. Should combination therapy be used?
    3. Is the infection on a native valve or a prosthetic valve?
    4. Is the patient an intravenous drug abuser?
    5. Is the infection on the left or right side of the heart?

- The recommended therapy for patients with left-sided IE caused by methicillin-sensitive *S. aureus* (MSSA) is 4–6 weeks of **oxacillin** or **nafcillin,** often combined with a short course of gentamicin (Table 35–5).
- If a patient has a mild allergy to penicillin, first-generation cephalosporins are effective alternatives but they should be avoided in immediate-type hypersensitivity reactions.
- The use of cephalosporins, particularly **cefazolin,** has been somewhat controversial for MSSA endocarditis. In the majority of studies, these

TABLE 35–3. Suggested Regimens for Therapy of Native Valve Endocarditis Due to Penicillin-Susceptible Viridans Streptococci and *Streptococcus bovis* (Minimum Inhibitory Concentration ≤ 0.1 μg/mL)[a]

Antibiotic	Dosage and Route	Duration (week)	Comments
Aqueous crystalline penicillin G sodium	12–18 million U/24 h IV either continuously or in six equally divided doses	4	Preferred in most patients older than 65 years and in those with impairment of nerve VIII or renal function
or			
Ceftriaxone sodium	2 g once daily IV or IM[b]	4	
Aqueous crystalline penicillin G sodium	12–18 million U/24 h IV either continuously or in six equally divided doses	2	
With gentamicin sulfate[c]	1 mg/kg IM or IV every 8 h	2	When obtained 1 h after a 20–30 min IV infusion or IM injection, serum concentration of gentamicin of approximately 3 μg/mL is desirable; trough concentration should be <1 μg/mL
Vancomycin hydrochloride[d]	30 mg/kg per 24 h IV in two equally divided doses, not to exceed 2 g/24 h unless serum levels are monitored	4	Vancomycin therapy is recommended for patients allergic to β-lactams; peak serum concentrations of vancomycin should be obtained 1 h after completion of the infusion and should be in the range of 30–45 μg/mL for twice-daily dosing

[a]Dosages recommended are for patients with normal renal function. For nutritionally variant streptococci, see Table 35–7. IV, intravenous; IM, intramuscular.
[b]Patients should be informed that IM injection of ceftriaxone is painful.
[c]Dosing of gentamicin on a mg/kg basis will produce higher serum concentrations in obese patients than in lean patients. Therefore, in obese patients, dosing should be based on ideal body weight. (Ideal body weight for men is 50 kg + 2.3 kg per inch over 5 feet, and ideal body weight for women is 45.5 kg + 2.3 kg per inch over 5 feet.) Relative contraindications to the use of gentamicin are age >65 years, renal impairment, or impairment of the nerve VIII. Other potentially nephrotoxic agents (e.g., nonsteroidal anti-inflammatory drugs) should be used cautiously in patients receiving gentamicin.
[d]Vancomycin doseage should be reduced in patients with impaired renal function. Vancomycin given on a mg/kg basis will produce higher serum concentrations in obese patients than in lean patients. Therefore, in obese patients, dosing should be based on ideal body weight. Each dose of vancomycin should be infused over at least 1 h to reduce the risk of the histamine-release "red man" syndrome.
From Wilson WR, Karchmer AW, Dajani AS, et al. Antibiotic treatment of adults with infective endocarditis due to streptococci, enterococci, and staphylococci, and HACEK microorganisms. JAMA *1995;274:1706–1713, with permission. Copyright 1995–97, American Medical Association.*

TABLE 35–4. Therapy for Native Valve Endocarditis Due to Strains of Viridans Streptococci and *Streptococcus bovis* Relatively Resistant to Penicillin G (Minimum Inhibitory Concentration > 0.1 μg/mL and < 0.5 μg/mL)[a]

Antibiotic	Dosage and Route	Duration (week)	Comments
Aqueous crystalline penicillin G sodium	18 million U/24 h IV either continuously or in six equally divided doses	4	Cefazolin or other first generation cephalosporins may be substituted for penicillin in patients whose penicillin hypersensitivity is not of the immediate type
With gentamicin sulfate[b]	1 mg/kg IM or IV every 8 h	2	
Vancomycin hydrochloride[c]	30 mg/kg per 24 h IV in two equally divided doses, not to exceed 2 g/24 h unless serum levels are monitored	4	Vancomycin therapy is recommended for patients allergic to β-lactams

[a]Dosages recommended are for patients with normal renal function. IV, intravenous; IM, intramuscular.
[b]For specific dosing adjustment and issues concerning gentamicin (obese patients, relative contraindications), see Table 35–3 footnotes.
[c]For specific dosing adjustment and issues concerning vancomycin (obese patients, length of infusion), see Table 35–3 footnotes.
From Wilson WR, Karchmer AW, Dajani AS, et al. Antibiotic treatment of adults with infective endocarditis due to streptococci, enterococci, and staphylococci, and HACEK microorganisms. JAMA *1995;274:1706–1713, with permission. Copyright 1995–97, American Medical Association.*

TABLE 35–5. Therapy for Endocarditis due to *Staphylococcus* in the Absence of Prosthetic Material[a]

Antibiotic	Dosage and Route	Duration (week)	Comments
Methicillin-Susceptible Staphylococci			
Regimens for non-β-lactam-allergic patients			
Nafcillin sodium **or** oxacillin sodium	2 g IV every 4 h	4–6 wk	Benefit of additional aminoglycosides has not been established
With optional addition of gentamicin sulfate[b]	1 mg/kg IM or IV every 8 h	3–5 d	
Regimens for β-lactam-allergic patients			
Cefazolin (or other first generation cephalosporins in equivalent dosages)	2 g IV every 8 h	4–6 wk	Cephalosporins should be avoided in patients with immediate-type hypersensitivity to penicillin
With optional addition of gentamicin[b]	1 mg/kg IM or IV every 8 h	3–5 d	
Vancomycin hydrochloride[c]	30 mg/kg per 24 h IV in two equally divided doses, not to exceed 2 g/24 h unless serum levels are monitored	4–6 wk	Recommended for patients allergic to penicillin
Methicillin-Resistant Staphylococci			
Vancomycin hydrochloride[c]	30 mg/kg per 24 h IV in two equally divided doses, not to exceed 2 g/24 h unless serum levels are monitored	4–6 wk	

[a]For treatment of endocarditis due to penicillin-susceptible staphylococci (minimum inhibitory concentration $\leq 0.1\ \mu g/mL$, aqueous crystalline penicillin G sodium (Table 35–3, first regimen) can be used for 4–6 weeks instead of nafcillin or oxacillin. Shorter antibiotic courses have been effective in some drug addicts with right-sided endocarditis due to *Staphylococcus aureus* (see text). See text for comments on use of rifampin. IV, intravenous; IM, intramuscular.

[b]For specific dosing adjustment and issues concerning gentamicin (obese patients, relative contraindications), see Table 35–3 footnotes.

[c]For specific dosing adjustment and issues concerning vancomycin (obese patients, length of infusion), see Table 35–3 footnotes.

From Wilson WR, Karchmer AW, Dajani AS, et al. Antibiotic treatment of adults with infective endocarditis due to streptococci, enterococci, and staphylococci, and HACEK microorganisms. JAMA *1995;274:1706–1713, with permission.*

agents appear effective; however, there are reports of failures with cephalosporins despite in vitro susceptibility.

- If there is a history of immediate hypersensitivity to penicillin, vancomycin is the agent of choice. Vancomycin, however, only slowly kills *S. aureus* and is generally regarded as inferior therapy to penicillinase-resistant penicillins for MSSA.
- **Rifampin** may be added to vancomycin in refractory or complicated infections in patients with left-sided IE and, in some cases, addition of rifampin appeared to result in dramatic patient improvement. Generally, antibiotic therapy should be continued for 4–6 weeks.

Treatment of Methicillin-Resistant Staphylococcal Endocarditis

- Vancomycin is the drug of choice for methicillin-resistant staphylococci since most methicillin-resistant *S. aureus* (MRSA) and most CNST are susceptible (Table 35–5).

Treatment of Staphylococcus Endocarditis in the Intravenous Drug Abuser

- IE in the IV drug abuser is most frequently (60–80%) caused by *S. aureus,* although other organisms may be more common in certain geographic locations.
- Standard treatment for MSSA consists of 4 weeks of therapy with a penicillinase-resistant penicillin (Table 35–5).
- In contrast to treatment of left-sided IE, addition of an aminoglycoside to penicillin does not improve outcome in *S. aureus* IE in addicts with right-sided disease.

PROSTHETIC VALVE ENDOCARDITIS

- Prosthetic valve endocarditis (PVE) that occurs within 1 year of surgery is usually caused by staphylococci implanted at the time of surgery. Methicillin-resistant organisms are common. Vancomycin is the cornerstone of therapy.
- Surgery is often a more essential component of management than are antibiotics.
- Because of the high morbidity and mortality associated with PVE and refractoriness to therapy, combinations of antimicrobials are usually recommended.
- For methicillin-resistant staphylococci (both MRSA and CNST), vancomycin is used with rifampin for ≥6 weeks (Table 35–6). An aminoglycoside is added for the first 2 weeks if the organism is susceptible.
- For methicillin-susceptible staphylococci, a penicillinase-stable penicillin is used in place of vancomycin.

ENTEROCOCCAL ENDOCARDITIS

- Enterococci cause 5–18% of endocarditis cases and are noteworthy for the following reasons: (1) no single antibiotic is bactericidal; (2) MICs

TABLE 35–6. Treatment of Staphylococcal Endocarditis in the Presence of a Prosthetic Valve or Other Prosthetic Material[a]

Antibiotic	Dosage and Route	Duration (week)	Comments
Regimen for Methicillin-Resistant Staphylococci			
Vancomycin hydrochloride[b]	30 mg/kg per 24 h IV in 2 or 4 equally divided doses, not to exceed 2 g/24 h unless serum levels are monitored	≥6	
With rifampin[c]	300 mg orally every 8 h	≥6	Rifampin increases the amount of warfarin sodium required for antithrombotic therapy
And with gentamicin sulfate[d,e]	1 mg/kg IM or IV every 8 h	2	
Regimen for Methicillin-Susceptible Staphylococci			
Nafcillin sodium or oxacillin sodium	2 g IV every 4 h	≥6	First generation cephalosporins or vancomycin should be used in patients allergic to β-lactam
With rifampin[c]	300 mg orally every 8 h	≥6	
And with gentamicin sulfate[d,e]	1 mg/kg IM or IV every 8 h	2	Cephalosporins should be avoided in patients with immediate-type hypersensitivity to penicillin or with methicillin-resistant staphylococci.

[a]Dosages recommended are for patients with normal renal function. IV, intravenous; IM, intramuscular.

[b]For specific dosing adjustment and issues concerning vancomycin (obese patients, length of infusion), see Table 35–3 footnotes.

[c]Rifampin plays a unique role in the eradication of staphylococcal infection involving prosthetic material (see text); combination therapy is essential to prevent emergence of rifampin resistance.

[d]For specific dosing adjustment and issues concerning gentamicin (obese patients, relative contraindications), see Table 35–3 footnotes.

[e]Use during initial 2 weeks.

From Wilson WR, Karchmer AW, Dajani AS, et al. Antibiotic treatment of adults with infective endocarditis due to streptococci, enterococci, and staphylococci, and HACEK microorganisms. JAMA *1995;274:1706–1713, with permission. Copyright 1995–97, American Medical Association.*

to penicillin are relatively high (1–25 mg/mL); (3) they are intrinsically resistant to all cephalosporins and relatively resistant to aminoglycosides (i.e., "low-level" aminoglycoside resistance); (4) they are killed only by a combination of a cell wall active agent, such as a penicillin or vancomycin, plus an aminoglycoside; (5) resistance to all available drugs is increasing.

- Enterococcal endocarditis ordinarily requires 4–6 weeks of high-dose penicillin G or ampicillin, plus an aminoglycoside for cure (Table 35–7). A 6-week course is recommended for patients with symptoms lasting longer than 3 months, recurrent cases, and patients with mitral valve involvement.
- In addition to isolates with high-level aminoglycoside resistance, β-lactamase-producing enterococci (especially *E. faecium*) are increasingly reported. Therapy with vancomycin is usually recommended, although penicillin-beta-lactamase inhibitor combinations appear effective.
- Vancomycin resistant enterococci, particularly *E. faecium* are becoming more common.

GRAM-NEGATIVE BACILLI

- Endocarditis caused by gram-negative bacilli is relatively uncommon, although the incidence may be increasing. Patients at higher risk include IV drug abusers and those with prosthetic valves.
- The organism most commonly associated with gram-negative rod endocarditis in IV drug abusers is *Pseudomonas aeruginosa*. Other gram-negative bacilli causing IE include other pseudomonads, *Serratia marcescens*, *Escherichia coli*, *Enterobacter*, *Salmonella*, and *Haemophilus*. Generally, these infections have a poor prognosis with mortality rates as high as 60–80%.
- Overall, there is very little clinical information on which to base solid recommendations for treatment. For most cases of IE due to *P. aeruginosa* and *Enterobacteriaceae*, antibiotics and valve replacement are necessary.
- Antimicrobial therapy includes the combination of an aminoglycoside and an extended-spectrum β-lactam.
- The appropriate regimen for the treatment of gram-negative bacillary endocarditis caused by *Enterobacteriaceae* depends on the results of in vitro susceptibility testing. For *Klebsiella pneumoniae*, *E. coli*, and *Proteus mirabilis*, a third-generation cephalosporin is frequently combined with an aminoglycoside. Treatment should generally be continued for 6 weeks.

▶ EVALUATION OF THERAPEUTIC OUTCOMES

- The evaluation of patients treated for IE includes assessment of signs and symptoms, reculture of blood, in vitro microbiologic tests (e.g., MIC, minimum bactericidal concentration (MBC), or serum bactericidal

TABLE 35–7. Standard Therapy for Endocarditis Due to Enterococci[a]

Antibiotic	Dosage and Route	Duration (week)	Comments
Aqueous crystalline penicillin G sodium	18–30 million U/24 h IV either continuously or in six equally divided doses	4–6	4-week therapy recommended for patients with symptoms <3 mo in duration; 6-week therapy recommended for patients with symptoms >3 mo in duration
With gentamicin sulfate[b]	1 mg/kg IM or IV every 8 h	4–6	
Ampicillin sodium	12 g/24 h IV either continuously or in six equally divided doses	4–6	Same as above
With gentamicin sulfate[b]	1 mg/kg IM or IV every 8 h	4–6	
Vancomycin hydrochloride[b,c]	30 mg/kg per 24 h IV in two equally divided doses, not to exceed 2 g/24 h unless serum levels are monitored	4–6	Vancomycin therapy is recommended for patients allergic to ß-lactams; cephalosporins are not acceptable alternatives for patients allergic to penicillin
With gentamicin sulfate[b]	1 mg/kg IM or IV every 8 h	4–6	

[a]All enterococci causing endocarditis must be tested for antimicrobial susceptibility in order to select optimal therapy (see text). This table is for endocarditis due to gentamicin- or vancomycin-susceptible enterococci, viridans streptococci with a minimum inhibitory concentration of >0.5 μg/mL, nutritionally variant viridans streptococci, or prosthetic valve endocarditis caused by viridans streptococci or *Streptococcus bovis*. Antibiotic dosages are for patients with normal renal function. IV, intravenous; IM, intramuscular.

[b]For specific dosing adjustment and issues concerning gentamicin (obese patients, relative contraindications), see Table 35–3 footnotes.

[c]For specific dosing adjustment and issues concerning vancomycin (obese patients, length of infusion), see Table 35–3 footnotes.

From Wilson WR, Karchmer AW, Dajani AS, et al. Antibiotic treatment of adults with infective endocarditis due to streptococci, enterococci, and staphylococci, and HACEK microorganisms. JAMA *1995;274:1706–1713, with permission. Copyright 1995–97, American Medical Association.*

titers), antimicrobial serum-concentration determinations, and other tests that may be necessary in the evaluation of organ function.

SIGNS AND SYMPTOMS

- Persistence of fever may indicate ineffective antimicrobial therapy, emboli, infections of intravascular catheters that have been in place for long periods of time, or a drug reaction. In some patients, low-grade fever may persist even with appropriate antimicrobial therapy.

BLOOD CULTURES AND BACTERIAL SUSCEPTIBILITY

- With effective therapy, blood cultures should be negative within a few days, although microbiological response to vancomycin may be unusually slow.
- After the initiation of therapy, blood cultures should be rechecked, possibly daily, until they are found negative. During the remainder of therapy, frequent blood culturing is not necessary.

SERUM BACTERICIDAL TITER (SBT)

- SBTs may be useful when the causative organisms are only moderately susceptible to antimicrobials, when less well-established regimens are used, or when response to therapy is suboptimal and dosage escalation is considered. In addition, an extremely high SBT may suggest that a decrease in antimicrobial dose is acceptable when the patient is at high risk of drug toxicity.

SERUM DRUG CONCENTRATION

- Serum concentrations of the antimicrobial should generally exceed the MBC of the organism, however, in practice this principle is usually not helpful in monitoring patients with endocarditis.
- In IE caused by *P. aeruginosa*, clinical trials previously discussed suggest that higher aminoglycoside concentrations (e.g., 15–20 μg/mL) improve the outcome to therapy.

▶ PREVENTION OF ENDOCARDITIS

- Antimicrobial prophylaxis is used to prevent IE in patients believed to be at high risk.
- The use of antimicrobials for this purpose requires consideration of the types of patients who are at risk, the procedures causing bacteremia, the organisms that are likely to cause endocarditis, and the pharmacokinetics, spectrum, cost, and ease of administration of available agents. The objective of prophylaxis is to diminish the likelihood of IE in high-risk individuals who are undergoing procedures that cause transient bacteremia.

TABLE 35–8. Cardiac Conditions Associated With Endocarditis

Endocarditis Prophylaxis Recommended
High-risk category
Prosthetic cardiac valves, including bioprosthetic and homograft valves
Previous bacterial endocarditis
Complex cyanotic congenital heart disease (e.g., single ventricle states, transposition of the great arteries, tetralogy of Fallot)
Surgically constructed systemic pulmonary shunts or conduits
Moderate-risk category
Most other congenital cardiac malformations (other than above and below)
Acquired valvar dysfunction (e.g., rheumatic heart disease)
Hypertrophic cardiomyopathy
Mitral valve prolapse with valvar regurgitation and/or thickened leaflets
Endocarditis Prophylaxis Not Recommended
Negligible-risk category (no greater risk than the general population)
Isolated secundum atrial septal defect
Surgical repair of atrial septal defect, ventricular septal defect, or patent ductus arteriosus (without residua beyond 6 mo)
Previous coronary artery bypass graft surgery
Mitral valve prolapse without valvar regurgitation
Physiologic, functional, or innocent heart murmurs
Previous Kawasaki disease without valvar dysfunction
Previous rheumatic fever without valvar dysfunction
Cardiac pacemakers (intravascular and epicardial) and implanted defibrillators

From Dajani AS, Taubert KA, Wilson W, et al. Prevention of bacterial endocarditis: Recommendations by the American Heart Association. JAMA *1997;277:1794–1801, with permission. Copyright 1995–97, American Medical Association.*

PATIENTS AT RISK

- Patients with certain cardiac lesions, particularly those with a history of rheumatic heart disease and prosthetic heart valves, are at risk for developing endocarditis (Table 35–8). However, only 15–25% of patients who develop IE are in a definable high-risk category, and only a small proportion of high-risk patients (estimated to be 1 of 53–115,500 persons) will develop IE if prophylaxis is not given.

PROCEDURES CAUSING BACTEREMIA (TABLES 35–9 AND 35–10)

- For dental procedures of the gums and oral structures which cause bleeding, viridans streptococci frequently (~40%) cause bacteremia, whereas instrumentation and surgery of the gastrointestinal and genitourinary tracts more often result in enterococcal bacteremia.

ANTIBIOTIC REGIMENS

- A 3-g dose of amoxicillin is recommended for adult patients at risk, given 60 minutes prior to undergoing procedures associated with bac-

TABLE 35–9. Dental Procedures and Endocarditis Prophylaxis

Endocarditis Prophylaxis Recommended[a]
Dental extractions
Periodontal procedures including surgery, scaling and root planing, probing, and recall maintenance
Dental implant placement and reimplantation of avulsed teeth
Endodontic (root canal) instrumentation or surgery only beyond the apex
Subgingival placement of antibiotic fibers or strips
Initial placement of orthodontic bands but not brackets
Intraligamentary local anesthetic injections
Prophylactic cleaning of teeth or implants where bleeding is anticipated
Endocarditis Prophylaxis Not Recommended
Restorative dentistry[b] (operative and prosthodontic) with or without retraction cord[c]
Local anesthetic injections (nonintraligamentary)
Intracanal endodontic treatment; post placement and buildup
Placement of rubber dams
Postoperative suture removal
Placement of removable prosthodontic or orthodontic appliances
Taking of oral impressions
Fluoride treatments
Taking of oral radiographs
Orthodontic appliance adjustment
Shedding of primary teeth

[a]Prophylaxis is recommended for patients with high- and moderate-risk cardiac conditions.
[b]This includes restoration of decayed teeth (filling cavities) and replacement of missing teeth.
[c]Clinical judgment may indicate antibiotic use in selected circumstances that may create significant bleeding.
From Dajani AS, Taubert KA, Wilson W, et al. Prevention of bacterial endocarditis: Recommendations by the American Heart Association. JAMA *1997;277:1794–1801, with permission. Copyright 1995–97, American Medical Association.*

VIII

teremia. This is to be followed by 1.5 g 6 hours later (Table 35–11). For penicillin-allergic patients or those undergoing gastrointestinal surgery, alternative prophylaxis is recommended (Tables 35–11 and 35–12).

See Chapter 101, Infective Endocarditis, authored by Michael A. Crouch, PharmD, BCPS, and Ron E. Polk, PharmD, for a more detailed discussion of this topic.

TABLE 35–10. Other Procedures and Endocarditis Prophylaxis

Endocarditis Prophylaxis Recommended

Respiratory tract
- Tonsillectomy and/or adenoidectomy
- Surgical operations that involve respiratory mucosa
- Bronchosopy with a rigid bronchoscope

Gastrointestinal tract[a]
- Sclerotherapy for esophageal varices
- Esophageal stricture dilation
- Endoscopic retrograde cholangiography with biliary obstruction
- Biliary tract surgery
- Surgical operations that involve intestinal mucosa

Genitourinary tract
- Prostatic surgery
- Cystoscopy
- Urethral dilation

Endocarditis Prophylaxis Not Recommended

Respiratory tract
- Endotracheal intubation
- Bronchoscopy with a flexible bronchoscope, with or without biopsy[b]
- VIII Tympanostomy tube insertion

Gastrointestinal tract
- Transesophageal echocardiography[b]
- Endoscopy with or without gastrointestinal biopsy[b]

Genitourinary tract
- Vaginal hysterectomy[b]
- Vaginal delivery[b]
- Cesarean section
- In uninfected tissue:
  - Urethral catheterization
  - Uterine dilation and curettage
  - Therapeutic abortion
  - Sterilization procedures
  - Insertion or removal of intrauterine devices

Other
- Cardiac catheterization, including balloon angioplasty
- Implanted cardiac pacemakers, implanted defibrillators, and coronary stents
- Incision or biopsy of surgically scrubbed skin
- Circumcision

[a]Prophylaxis is recommended for high-risk patients; optional for moderate-risk patients.
[b]Prophylaxis is optional for high-risk patients.

From Dajani AS, Taubert KA, Wilson W, et al. Prevention of bacterial endocarditis: Recommendations by the American Heart Association. JAMA *1997;277:1794–1801, with permission. Copyright 1995–97, American Medical Association.*

TABLE 35–11. Prophylactic Regimens for Dental, Oral, Respiratory Tract, or Esophageal Procedures

Situation	Agent	Regimen[a]
Standard general prophylaxis	Amoxicillin	Adults: 2 g; children: 50 mg/kg orally 1 h before procedure
Unable to take oral medications	Ampicillin	Adults: 2 g intramuscularly (IM) or intravenously (IV); children: 50 mg/kg IM or IV within 30 min before procedure
Allergic to penicillin	Clindamycin	Adults: 600 mg; children: 20 mg/kg orally 1 h before procedure
	or	
	Cephalexin[b] or cefadroxil[b]	Adults: 2 g; children: 50 mg/kg orally 1 h before procedure
	or	
	Azithromycin or chlarithromycin	Adults: 500 mg; children: 15 mg/kg orally 1 h before procedure
Allergic to penicillin and unable to take oral medications	Clidamycin	Adults: 600 mg; children: 20 mg/kg IV within 30 min before procedure
	or	
	Cefazolin[b]	Adults: 1 g; children: 25 mg/kg IM or IV within 30 min before procedure

[a]Total children's dose should not exceed adult dose.
[b]Cephalosporins should not be used in individuals with immediate-type hypersensitivity reaction (urticaria, angioedema, or anaphylaxis) to penicillins.
From Dajani AS, Taubert KA, Wilson W, et al. Prevention of bacterial endocarditis: Recommendations by the American Heart Association, JAMA *1997;227:1794–1801, with permission. Copyright 1995–97, American Medical Association.*

TABLE 35–12. Prophylactic Regimens for Genitourinary Gastrointestinal (Excluding Esophageal) Procedures

Situation	Agent[a]	Regimen[b]
High-risk patients	Ampicillin **plus** gentamicin	Adults: ampicillin 2 g intramuscularly (IM) or intravenously (IV) plus gentamicin 1.5 mg/kg (not to exceed 120 mg) within 30 min of starting the procedure; 6 h later, ampicillin 1 g IM/IV or amoxicillin 1 g orally
		Children: ampicillin 50 mg/kg IM or IV (not to exceed 2 g) plus gentamicin 1.5 mg/kg within 30 min of starting the procedure; 6 h later, ampicillin 25 mg/kg IM/IV or amoxicillin 25 mg/kg orally
High-risk patients allergic to ampicillin/amoxicillin	Vancomycin **plus** gentamicin	Adults: vancomycin 1 g IV over 1–2 h plus gentamicin 1.5 to mg/kg IV/IM (not to exceed 120 mg); complete injection/infusion within 30 min of starting the procedure
		Children: vancomycin 20 mg/kg IV over 1–2 h plus gentamicin 1.5 mg/kg IV/IM; complete injection/infusion within 30 min of starting the procedure
Moderate-risk patients	Amoxicillin **or** ampicillin	Adults: amoxicillin 2 g orally 1 h before procedure, or ampicillin 2 g IM/IV within 30 min of starting the procedure
		Children: amoxicillin 50 mg/kg orally 1 h before procedure, or ampicillin 50 mg/kg IM/IV within 30 min of starting the procedure
Moderate-risk patients allergic to ampicillin/amoxicillin	Vancomycin	Adults: vancomycin 1 g IV over 1–2 h; complete infusion within 30 min of starting the procedure
		Children: vancomycin 20 mg/kg IV over 1–2 h; complete infusion within 30 min of starting the procedure

[a]Total children's dose should not exceed adult dose.
[b]No second dose of vancomycin or gentamicin is recommended.

From Dajani AS, Taubert KA, Wilson W, et al. Prevention of bacterial endocarditis: Recommendations by the American Heart Association, JAMA *1997;227:1794–1801, with permission. Copyright 1995–97, American Medical Association.*

Chapter 36

▶ FUNGAL INFECTIONS

Systemic mycoses, such as histoplasmosis, coccidioidomycosis, cryptococcosis, blastomycosis, paracoccidioidomycosis, and sporotrichosis, are caused by primary or "pathogenic" fungi that can cause disease in both healthy and immunocompromised individuals. In contrast, mycoses caused by opportunistic fungi such as *Candida albicans, Aspergillus* sp., *Trichosporon, Torulopsis (Candida) glabrata, Fusarium, Alternaria,* and *Mucor* are generally found only in the immunocompromised host.

▶ SPECIFIC FUNGAL INFECTIONS

HISTOPLASMOSIS

- Histoplasmosis is caused by inhalation of dust-borne microconidia of the dimorphic fungus *Histoplasma capsulatum.*
- In the United States, most disease is localized along the Ohio and Mississippi river valleys.

Clinical Presentation

- In the vast majority of patients, low-inoculum exposure to *H. capsulatum* results in asymptomatic infection. Patients exposed to a higher inoculum during a primary infection or reinfection may experience an acute, self-limited illness with flu-like pulmonary symptoms, including fever, chills, headache, myalgia, and nonproductive cough.
- Chronic pulmonary histoplasmosis generally presents as an opportunistic infection imposed on a preexisting structural abnormality such as lesions resulting from emphysema. Patients demonstrate chronic pulmonary symptoms and apical lung lesions that progress with inflammation, calcified granulomas, and fibrosis. Progression of disease over a period of years, seen in 25–30% of patients, is associated with cavitation, bronchopleural fistulas, extension to the other lung, pulmonary insufficiency, and often death.
- In patients exposed to a large inoculum and in immunocompromised hosts, progressive illness, disseminated histoplasmosis, occurs. The clinical severity of the four diverse forms of disseminated histoplasmosis (Table 36–1) generally parallels the degree of macrophage parasitization observed.
- Acute (infantile) disseminated histoplasmosis is seen in infants and young children and (rarely) in adults with Hodgkin's disease or other lymphoproliferative disorders. It is characterized by unrelenting fever; anemia; leukopenia or thrombocytopenia; enlargement of the liver, spleen, and visceral lymph nodes; and gastrointestinal symptoms, particularly nausea, vomiting, and diarrhea. Untreated disease is uniformly fatal in 1–2 months.

TABLE 36–1. Clinical Manifestations and Therapy of Histoplasmosis

Type of Disease and Common Clinical Manifestations	Approximate Frequency[a] (%)	Therapy and Comments
Acute Pulmonary Histoplasmosis		
Immunosuppressed Host		
Asymptomatic histoplasmosis	50–99	Asymptomatic disease: No therapy generally required
Self-limited disease	1–50	Self-limited disease: AmB[b] 0.3–0.5 mg/kg/d × 2–4 weeks (total dose 500 mg)
		or
		Ketoconazole 400 mg orally daily × 3–6 months may be beneficial in patients with severe hypoxia following inhalation of large inoculae
		Antifungal therapy generally not useful for arthritis or pericarditis. NSAIDs[c] or corticosteroids may be useful in some cases
		Mediastinal granulomas: Most lesions resolve spontaneously; surgery or antifungal therapy with AmB 40–50 mg/d × 2–3 weeks
		or
		Ketoconazole 400 mg/d orally × >30 months may be beneficial in some cases
Immunosuppressed Host		
Inflammatory/fibrotic histoplasmosis	0.02	Fibrosing mediastinitis: Antifungal therapy generally not helpful; surgery may be of benefit if disease is detected early; late disease may not respond to therapy
		Sarcoid-like: NSAIDs or corticosteroids may be of benefit for some patients

Chronic Pulmonary Histoplasmosis	0.05	Antifungal therapy generally recommended for immunosuppressed patients with either persistent cavitation, cavitary wall thickness >2mm, or progressive symptoms (including weight loss, cough, sputum production, low-grade fever) Itraconazole 200–400 mg PO qd **or** Ketoconazole 400 mg/d orally for 1 year Relapses common
Disseminated Histoplasmosis Acute (infantile)	0.02–0.05	Disseminated histoplasmosis: Untreated mortality 83–93%; relapse 5–23% in non-AIDS patients Nonimmunosuppressed patients: Ketoconazole 400 mg/d orally × 6–12 months **or** AmB 35 mg/kg IV
Subacute		Immunosuppressed patients (non-AIDS) or + endocarditis or CNS disease: AMB ≥35 mg/kg
Chronic (adult type)		Non-AIDS: Life threatening; AmB 0.5–0.75 mg/kg/d IV
Progressive disease of AIDS	25–50[d]	AIDS patients: AmB 15–30 mg/kg (1–2 g over 4–10 weeks) **or** Itraconazole 200 mg PO qd; followed by chronic suppressive therapy with itraconazole 200 mg PO qd

[a]As a percentage of all patients presenting with histoplasmosis.
[b]AmB, amphotericin B.
[c]NSAIDs, nonsteroidal anti-inflammatory drugs.
[d]As a percentage of AIDS patients presenting with histoplasmosis as the initial manifestation of their disease.

- Adult patients with AIDS demonstrate an acute form of disseminated disease that resembles the syndrome seen in infants and children.

Diagnosis

- Identification of mycelial isolates from clinical cultures can be made by conversion of the mycelium to the yeast form (requires 3–6 weeks) via commercially available exoantigen test kits, or by the more rapid (2 hours) and 100% sensitive DNA probe.
- In most patients, serologic evidence remains the primary method in the diagnosis of histoplasmosis. A four-fold rise in the CF titer is usually indicative of recent infection, although some patients with severe disease or profound immunosuppression may demonstrate a weaker antibody response.
- In the AIDS patient with progressive disseminated histoplasmosis, the diagnosis is best established by bone marrow biopsy and culture, which yield positive cultures in >90% of patients.

Treatment

- Recommended therapy for the treatment of histoplasmosis is summarized in Table 36–1.
- In AIDS patients, intensive primary (induction and consolidation therapy) antifungal therapy is followed by lifelong suppressive (maintenance) therapy.
- In patients with underlying immunosuppression, including AIDS patients with progressive disseminated histoplasmosis, **amphotericin B** remains the drug of choice for induction therapy. **Itraconazole** 400 mg daily for 6 weeks is an alternative.
- Amphotericin B dosages of 50 mg/d (up to 1 mg/kg/d) should be administered to a cumulative dose of 15–35 mg/kg (1–2 g) and until negative fungal cultures are achieved.
- Response to therapy should be measured by resolution of radiologic, serologic, and microbiologic parameters, and improvement in signs and symptoms of infection.
- Once the initial course of therapy for histoplasmosis is completed, lifelong suppressive therapy with oral azoles or amphotericin B (1–1.5 mg/kg weekly or biweekly) is recommended, because of the frequent recurrence of infection.
- Relapse rates in AIDS patients not receiving preventive maintenance is 50–90%.

BLASTOMYCOSIS

- North American blastomycosis is a systemic fungal infection caused by *Blastomyces dermatitidis.*
- Pulmonary disease probably occurs by inhalation. It may be acute or chronic and can mimic infection with tuberculosis, pyogenic bacteria, other fungi, or malignancy.

- Blastomycosis can disseminate to virtually every other body organ including skin, bones and joints, or genitourinary tract involvement without any evidence of pulmonary disease.

Clinical Presentation

- Acute pulmonary blastomycosis is generally an asymptomatic or self-limited disease characterized by fever, shaking chills, and a productive, purulent cough.
- Pulmonary blastomycosis may present as a more chronic or subacute disease, with low-grade fever, night sweats, weight loss, and a productive cough that resembles tuberculosis rather than bacterial pneumonia.
- Chronic pulmonary blastomycosis is characterized by fever, malaise, weight loss, night sweats, and cough.

Diagnosis

- The simplest and most successful method of diagnosing blastomycosis is by direct microscopic visualization of the large, multinucleated yeast with single, broad-based buds in sputum or other respiratory specimens, following digestion of cells and debris with 10% potassium hydroxide.
- Early and rapid definitive diagnosis of blastomycosis can be achieved by demonstration of *B. dermatitidis* in tissue or specimen culture or histopathology.

Treatment

- Acute pulmonary blastomycosis may not require therapy in patients with mild illness, but patients must be followed carefully for many years for evidence of reactivation or progressive disease.
- Some authors recommend **ketoconazole** therapy for the treatment of self-limited pulmonary disease, with the hope of preventing late extrapulmonary disease.
- Ketoconazole appears to be as effective as amphotericin B for non–life-threatening, nonmeningeal, mild to moderate blastomycosis in immunocompetent hosts.
- The dosage of ketoconazole should be 400 mg/d orally and increased to 600–800 mg/d in the absence of a favorable clinical response.
- Patients with CNS disease, progressive or life-threatening disease, or those experiencing toxicity while on ketoconazole should receive **amphotericin B** (40–50 mg/d) until clinical improvement is observed, followed by administration three times weekly until a total dose of 1.5–2 g is achieved.
- All patients with chronic pulmonary blastomycosis and those with extrapulmonary disease require therapy (ketoconazole 400 mg orally per day for 6 months).
- Patients with genitourinary tract disease should be treated initially with 600–800 mg/d of ketoconazole because low concentrations of drug are achieved in the urine and prostate tissue.

- CNS disease should be treated with amphotericin B for a total dose of 30–35 mg/kg.
- HIV-infected patients should receive induction therapy with amphotericin B and chronic suppressive therapy with an oral azole antifungal. Itraconazole is the drug of choice for non–life-threatening histoplasmosis.

COCCIDIOIDOMYCOSIS

- Coccidioidomycosis is caused by infection with *Coccidioides immitis.*
- The endemic regions encompass the semi-arid regions of the southwestern United States from California to Texas, known as the Lower Sonoran Zone.

Clinical Presentation

- Sixty percent of subjects are asymptomatic or have nonspecific symptoms that are often indistinguishable from ordinary upper respiratory infections, including fever, cough, headache, sore throat, myalgias, and fatigue.
- "Valley fever" is a syndrome characterized by erythema nodosum and erythema multiforme of the upper trunk and extremities in association with diffuse joint aches or fever. Valley fever occurs in approximately 25% of patients although, more commonly, a diffuse mild erythroderma or maculopapular rash is observed.
- Pulmonary coccidioidomycosis can also present as acute pneumonia or develop into a chronic, persistent pneumonia complicated by hemoptysis, pulmonary scarring, and the formation of cavities of bronchopleural fistulas.
- Disseminated infection occurs in <1% of infected patients. Dissemination may occur to the skin, lymph nodes, bone, meninges, spleen, liver, kidney, and adrenal gland.

Diagnosis

- Most patients develop a positive skin test within 3 weeks of the onset of symptoms.
- Early infection is characterized by the development of IgM, which peaks within 2–3 weeks of infection then declines rapidly.
- Recovery of *C. immitis* from infected tissues or secretions for direct examination and culture provides an accurate and rapid method of diagnosis.

Treatment

- Candidates for therapy include those with severe primary pulmonary infection or increasing CF antibody titers (particularly $\geq 1:16$ to $1:32$), immunocompromised patients, and those with persistent (>6 weeks) fever, prostration, or worsening pulmonary disease. Any patient with evidence of disseminated disease should receive therapy.
- Almost all patients with disease located outside the lungs should receive **amphotericin B** in dosages of 1–1.5 mg/kg/d, tapering to

1–1.5 mg/kg three times a week to a total dose of 0.5–1.5 g over 2–4 weeks, based on clinical response.

- A minimum of 2–3 g of amphotericin B is probably necessary for the treatment of persistent pulmonary infection or miliary coccidioidomycosis.
- **Ketoconazole** at a dosage of 400 mg orally per day is efficacious in patients with infiltrative pulmonary disease, soft tissue infection, or skeletal involvement.
- **Fluconazole** has become the drug of choice for the treatment of coccidioidal meningitis (minimum dose 400 mg/d).

CRYPTOCOCCOSIS

- Cryptococcosis is a noncontagious, systemic mycotic infection caused by the ubiquitous encapsulated soil yeast *Cryptococcus neoformans.*

Clinical Presentation

- Primary cryptococcosis in humans almost always occurs in the lungs.
- Symptomatic infections are usually manifested by cough, rales, and shortness of breath that generally resolve spontaneously.
- Disease may remain localized in the lungs or disseminate to other tissues, particularly the CNS, although the skin can also be affected.
- In the non-AIDS patient, the symptoms of cryptococcal meningitis are nonspecific. Headache, fever, nausea, vomiting, mental status changes, and neck stiffness are generally observed.
- In AIDS patients, fever and headache are common, but meningismus and photophobia are much less common than in non-AIDS patients.

Diagnosis

- Examination of CSF in patients with cryptococcal meningitis generally reveals an elevated opening pressure, CSF pleocytosis (usually lymphocytes), leukocytosis, a decreased CSF glucose, an elevated CSF protein, and a positive cryptococcal antigen.
- Antigens to *C. neoformans* can be detected by latex agglutination.
- *C. neoformans* can be detected in approximately 60% of patients by India ink smear of CSF, and cultured in more than 96% of patients.

Treatment

- Treatment of cryptococcosis is detailed in Table 36–2.
- The use of large (1–1.5 mg/kg) daily doses of **amphotericin B** results in cure rates of approximately two-thirds of patients.
- When amphotericin B is combined with **fluorocytosine** (150 mg/kg/d) for 6 weeks, a smaller dose of amphotericin B (0.3 mg/kg/d) can be used due to the in vitro and in vivo synergy between the two antifungal agents.
- The use of intrathecal amphotericin B is not recommended for the treatment of cryptococcal meningitis except in patients who fail to respond to amphotericin B alone. The dosage of amphotericin B employed is

TABLE 36–2. Therapy of Cryptococcosis[a,b]

Type of Disease and Common Clinical Manifestations	Therapy and Comments
NonImmunocompromised Host	Comparative trials for AmB vs azoles not available
Cutaneous disease	Asymptomatic disease: Drug therapy generally not required
Acute cryptococcal meningitis	AmB 0.3 mg/kg/day IV + 5-FC 150 mg/kg/day × 6 weeks
	Four weeks of therapy for patients with no underlying disease, no immunosuppression, and an uncomplicated course of disease
Recurrent or progressive disease not responsive to AmB	AmB 0.5–0.75 mg/kg/day IV ± IT AmB 0.5 mg 2–3 times weekly
HIV-Infected Patient	
Prophylactic therapy	None
	or
Acute disease treatment	FLU 200 mg PO qd
	AmB IV 0.7 mg/kg/day + 5-FC 100 mg/kg/day PO qd × 2 weeks *(induction therapy)* followed by FLU 400 mg PO qd
	or
	ITRA 400 mg PO qd × 8 weeks *(consolidation therapy)*, then *suppressive therapy*
Suppressive therapy	FLU 200 mg PO qd

[a]When more than one therapy is listed, they are listed in order of preference.
[b]See text for definitions of induction, consolidation, suppressive therapy, and prophylactic therapy.
AmB, amphotericin B; IT, intrathecal; 5-FC, flucytosine; FLU, fluconazole; ITRA, itraconazole.

usually 0.5 mg administered via the lumbar, cisternal, or intraventricular (via an Ommaya reservoir) route two or three times weekly.

- Amphotericin B with or without fluorocytosine remains the treatment of choice for acute therapy of cryptococcal meningitis in AIDS patients. Many clinicians will initiate therapy with amphotericin B 0.7 mg/kg/d IV (with or without oral fluorocytosine 100 mg/kg/d). After 2 weeks, therapy may be changed to oral fluconazole 400 mg daily or itraconazole 400 mg daily for the remaining 8 weeks of therapy.
- Relapse of *C. neoformans* meningitis occurs in approximately 50% of AIDS patients after completion of primary therapy. Fluconazole (200 mg daily) is currently recommended for chronic suppressive therapy of cryptococcal meningitis in AIDS patients.

▶ *CANDIDA* INFECTIONS

- Eight species of *Candida* are regarded as clinically important pathogens in human disease, including *C. albicans, C. tropicalis, C. parapsilosis, C. krusei, C. stellatoidea, C. guilliermondi, C. lusitaniae,* and *C. glabrata.*

MUCOCUTANEOUS CANDIDIASIS

- Mucocutaneous candidiasis can generally be divided into several categories: oropharyngeal candidiasis (thrush), esophageal candidiasis, gastrointestinal candidiasis, and vaginal candidiasis. VIII
- Oral candidiasis is often the first sign of infection in patients with AIDS.

Chronic Mucocutaneous Candidiasis

- Chronic mucocutaneous candidiasis refers to a collection of syndromes characterized by chronic or recurrent infections of the skin, nails, and mucous membranes by *C. albicans.*

Oral Candidiasis (Thrush)

- Oral candidiasis is characterized by the presence of creamy, white plaques on the tongue and buccal mucosa that generally leave a painful, raw, ulcerated surface when scraped.
- The diagnosis of oral candidiasis is based on the clinical appearance of the lesions and by scraping of lesions, using either 10% potassium hydroxide digestion of this material to reveal the presence of pseudohyphae and yeast forms or the presence of gram-positive–staining yeast forms.
- Treatment of candidiasis is presented in Table 36–3.
- Topical (local) therapy with a variety of antifungal agents, including **nystatin suspension** and **clotrimazole troches** are generally efficacious in the prophylaxis and therapy of oral candidiasis.
- In oncology patients, **ketoconazole** in dosages of 200–400 mg daily is as efficacious as nystatin in dosages of 0.5–3 MU four times daily for the treatment of oral candidiasis.

TABLE 36–3. Therapy of Candidiasis[a]

Type of Disease and Common Clinical Manifestations	Therapy and Comments[b]
Chronic mucocutaneous candidiasis	KETO 100–200 mg PO qd **or** FLU 100 mg PO qd **or** ITRA 100–200 mg PO qd
Oral candidiasis (thrush)	
Acute disease treatment	Non-AIDS: FLU 100 mg PO qd **or** KETO 400 mg PO qd **or** ITRA 200 mg PO qd AIDS: Generally not recommended due to development of resistant isolates
Resistant isolates	FLU 400–800 mg PO qd **or** ITRA-S 200–400 mg PO qd **or** AmB-S 100 mg topically qid × 2 weeks
Esophageal candidiasis	FLU 100–200 mg PO qd **or** KETO 100–200 mg PO qd **or** AmB 10–15 mg IV qd
Vaginal candidiasis	
Acute therapy	Topical agents (miconazole, clotrimazole) PV qd × 1–3 days **or** FLU 150 mg PO × 1 dose **or** KETO 100–200 mg PO
Suppression of recurrent infections	FLU 100 mg PO qd
Invasive candidiasis	
Prophylaxis	FLU 100 mg PO qd **or** KETO 400 mg PO qd **or** ITRA 200 mg PO qd
Treatment	Non-immunocompromised host: FLU 400 mg IV/PO qd **or** AmB 0.5 mg/kg/day IV Immunocompromised host: AmB 0.5–0.75 mg/kg/day (total dosages of 0.5–1 g) **or** Lipid formulation of AmB 3–5 mg/kg/day (in patients who fail therapy with traditional AmB)
Candiduria	AmB bladder wash (50 mg in 500 mL of sterile water) can be instilled twice daily into the bladder via a three-way catheter **or** FLU 100 mg PO qd

VIII

[a]Therapy is generally the same for AIDS and non-AIDS patients except where indicated.

[b]When more than one therapy is listed, they are listed in order of preference.

AmB, amphotericin B; IT, intrathecal; 5-FC, flucytosine; FLU, fluconazole; ITRA, itraconazole; ITRA-S, itraconazole oral solution; AmB-S, amphotericin B oral solution; KETO, ketoconazole.

- Fluconazole 100 mg orally appears to be as efficacious as ketoconazole 400 mg daily, clotrimazole troches 10 mg five times daily, or amphotericin B 400 mg (as 200-mg tablets plus 200-mg suspension) administered four times daily in the prophylaxis or therapy of oropharyngeal candidiasis.

Esophageal Candidiasis

- Generally, systemic antifungal agents, such as ketoconazole 200–400 mg daily or fluconazole 100–200 mg daily are required.
- A lack of response to antifungal therapy can be due to altered absorption of drugs such as ketoconazole. In patients who do not respond to oral therapy with ketoconazole or fluconazole, a low dose (10–15 mg) of IV amphotericin B is often successful.

Vaginal Candidiasis

- Vulvovaginal candidiasis is characterized by the presence of a thick, curdlike vaginal discharge, intense pruritus, and the presence of masses of epithelial cell, hyphae, and pseudohyphae on KOH smear of the vaginal discharge.
- Although treatment with 7-day topical regimens has been traditionally employed, recent studies have demonstrated success utilizing 1- and 3-day topical regimens.
- A single oral dose of fluconazole (150 mg) is generally effective.

Hematogenous Candidiasis

- "Hematogenous candidiasis" describes the clinical circumstances in which hematogenous seeding to deep organs such as the eye, brain, heart, and kidney occurs.
- Three distinct presentations of disseminated *C. albicans* have been recognized: Patients present with (1) the acute onset of fever, tachycardia, tachypnea, and occasionally chills or hypotension; (2) intermittent fevers; and (3) progressive deterioration with or without fever.
- Administration of fluconazole 400 mg daily is as efficacious as intravenous amphotericin B 0.5–0.6 mg/kg/d in non-neutropenic patients with blood cultures with *C. albicans.* Since fluconazole has poor activity against *Aspergillus* sp. and some nonalbicans strains of *Candida,* amphotericin B remains the therapy of choice in patients with suspected fungemia.
- In some patients, particularly those patients with a relatively intact immune system and in whom candidemia is clearly associated with the presence of an indwelling venous catheter, removal of the catheter will result in spontaneous resolution.
- Currently, most clinicians recommend amphotericin B in total dosages of 0.5–1 g administered over approximately 1–2 weeks in patients with *Candida* endophthalmitis and in all neutropenic patients with candidemia.
- Many clinicians advocate early institution of empiric intravenous amphotericin B in patients with neutropenia and persistent (>5–7 days) fever.

Candiduria

- Within the urinary tract, most common lesions are either *Candida* cystitis or hematogenously disseminated renal abscesses.
- In most patients, the infection is asymptomatic and clears spontaneously without specific antifungal therapy.
- Initial therapy of candidal cystitis should focus on removal of urinary catheters whenever possible. If this is not feasible, local irrigation may be used.
- Amphotericin B (50 mg in 500 mL of sterile water) can be instilled twice daily into the bladder via a three-way catheter.
- Oral therapy with fluorocytosine or fluconazole can be considered for short courses of therapy since high urinary concentrations are achieved.

► *ASPERGILLUS*

- Of over 300 species of *Aspergillus,* three are most commonly pathogenic: *A. fumigatus, A. flavus,* and *A. niger.*
- Aspergillosis is generally acquired by inhalation of airborne conidia that are small enough (2.5–3 mm) to reach alveoli or the paranasal sinuses.

SUPERFICIAL INFECTION

- Superficial or locally invasive infections of the ear, skin, or appendages can often be managed with topical antifungal therapy.

ALLERGIC BRONCHOPULMONARY ASPERGILLOSIS

- Allergic manifestations of *Aspergillus* range in severity from mild asthma to allergic bronchopulmonary aspergillosis (BPA) characterized by severe asthma with wheezing, fever, malaise, weight loss, chest pain, and a cough productive of blood-streaked sputum.
- Therapy is aimed at minimizing the quantity of antigenic material released in the tracheobronchial tree.
- Antifungal therapy is generally not indicated in the management of allergic manifestations of aspergillosis, although some patients have demonstrated a decrease in their corticosteroid dose following therapy with itraconazole.

ASPERGILLOMA

- In the nonimmunocompromised host, *Aspergillus* infections of the sinuses most commonly occur as saprophytic colonization (aspergillomas or "fungus balls") of previously abnormal sinus tissue. Treatment consists of removal of the aspergilloma. Therapy with corticosteroids and surgery is generally successful.
- Although intravenous amphotericin B is generally not useful in eradicating aspergillomas, intracavitary instillation of amphotericin B has been employed successfully in a limited number of patients. Hemoptysis generally ceases when the aspergilloma is eradicated.

INVASIVE ASPERGILLOSIS

- Patients often present with classic signs and symptoms of acute pulmonary embolus: pleuritic chest pain, fever, hemoptysis, a friction rub, and a wedge-shaped infiltrate on chest radiographs.

Diagnosis

- Demonstration of *Aspergillus* by repeated culture and microscopic examination of tissue provides the most firm diagnosis.
- In the immunocompromised host, aspergillosis is characterized by vascular invasion leading to thrombosis, infarction, and necrosis of tissue.
- Serologic tests (immunoprecipitation, immunodiffusion, and counterimmunoelectrophoresis) to detect antibody production to *Aspergillus* are generally helpful only in the diagnosis of allergic BPA and aspergilloma.

Treatment of Invasive Aspergillosis

- Antifungal therapy should be instituted in any of the following conditions: (1) persistent fever or progressive sinusitis unresponsive to antimicrobial therapy; (2) an eschar over the nose, sinuses, or palate; (3) the presence of characteristic radiographic findings, including wedge-shaped infarcts, nodular densities, or new cavitary lesions; or (4) any clinical manifestation suggestive of orbital or cavernous sinus disease or an acute vascular event associated with fever. Isolation of *Aspergillus* sp. from nasal or respiratory tract secretions should be considered confirmatory evidence in any of the previously mentioned clinical settings.
- Since *Aspergillus* is only moderately susceptible to **amphotericin B,** full doses (1–1.5 mg/kg/d) are generally recommended, with response measured by defervescence and radiographic clearing.
- **Itraconazole** should be reserved as a second-line agent for patients intolerant or not responding to high-dose amphotericin B. If itraconazole is used, a loading dose of 200 mg three times daily with food for 2–3 days should be employed, followed by itraconazole 200 mg twice daily with food for a minimum of 6 months.
- The use of prophylactic antifungal therapy to prevent primary infection or reactivation of aspergillosis during subsequent courses of chemotherapy is controversial.

See Chapter 110, Invasive Fungal Infections, authored by Peggy L. Carver, PharmD, for a more detailed discussion of this topic.

Chapter 37

▶ GASTROINTESTINAL INFECTIONS

Gastrointestinal infections are among the more common causes of morbidity and mortality around the world. In underdeveloped and developing countries, acute gastroenteritis involving diarrhea is the leading cause of mortality in infants and young children under 4 years of age. In the United States, more than 210,000 children per year are hospitalized for gastroenteritis.

▶ REHYDRATION THERAPY

- The mainstay of therapy for gastrointestinal infections is rehydration, most often, oral rehydration therapy (ORT).
- Initial assessment of fluid loss is essential for rehydration. Weight loss is the most reliable means of determining the extent of water loss. Clinical signs such as changes in skin turgor, sunken eyes, dry mucous membranes, decreased tearing, decreased urine output, altered mentation, and changes in vital signs can be helpful in determining approximate deficits (Table 37–1).
- Although ORT may be successful in reversing severe dehydration, parenteral replacement is indicated as initial treatment for the patient in shock or a comatose state, the patient unable to tolerate oral fluids, the patient with ileus, and the patient with persistent vomiting or stool output >100 mL/kg/h.
- The necessary components of ORT solutions include glucose, sodium, potassium, chloride, and water (Table 37–2).
- The rehydration phase should provide replacement of estimated fluid deficits in 4–6 hours.
- The maintenance phase should not exceed 150 mL/kg/d and is generally adjusted to equal stool output and insensible water loss.
- Guidelines for parenteral fluid replacement of severe fluid loss are shown in Table 37–3.
- Early initiation of feeding has shortened the course of diarrhea. Initially, easily digested foods, such as bananas, applesauce, and cereal, may be added as tolerated. Foods high in fiber, sodium, and sugar should be avoided.

▶ BACTERIAL INFECTIONS

- The bacterial species most commonly associated with gastrointestinal infection and infectious diarrhea in the United States are *Shigella* sp., *Salmonella* sp., *Campylobacter* sp., *Yersinia* sp., *Escherichia* sp., *Clostridium* sp., and *Staphylococcus* sp.

TABLE 37–1. Signs of Dehydration

Percent Body Weight Loss as Water	Clinical Signs
Adults and Older Children	
< 4 (mild)	Decreased tearing, thirsty, alert, restless
4–8 (moderate)	Decreased skin turgor, sunken eyes, tachycardia, reduced urine flow, postural hypotension, dry mucous membranes, thirsty
> 8 (severe)	Hypotension, muscle cramps, variable alertness, cold, sweaty, cyanotic, wrinkled skin, usually conscious
Infants and Young Children	
< 5 (mild)	Thirsty, alert, restless, moist mucous membranes, normal urine flow, tearing
5–10 (moderate)	Thirsty, restless, lethargic, irritable, tachycardia, hypotension, deep respirations, sunken fontanelle, sunken eyes, absent tearing, dry mucous membranes, reduced and dark urine
> 10 (severe)	Drowsy, limp, cold, sweaty, cyanotic, comatose, tachycardia, tachypnea, very sunken fontanelles, hypotension, sunken eyes, absent tears, dry mucous membranes, no urine production

TABLE 37–2. Comparison of Solutions Used in Oral Rehydration and Maintenance

VIII

Product	Electrolytes (mEq/L)					Carbohydrate (g/L)	Osmolarity (mOsm/L)
	Na	*K*	*Cl*	*Base*	*Other Cations*		
Infalyte (Penwalt)	50	20	40	30	—	20	251
Lytren (Mead Johnson)	50	25	45	30	—	20	583
Pedialyte (Ross)	45	20	35	30	—	25	388
Pedialyte RS (Ross)	75	20	65	30	—	25	314
Ricelyte (Mead Johnson)	50	25	45	34	—	30	200
WHO (Unicef)	90	20	80	30	—	20	333
Resol (Wyeth)	50	20	50	34	4 Ca, 4 Mg, 5 PO4	20	—
Rehydralyte (Ross)	75	20	65	30	—	25	—
EquaLYTE (Ross)	78.2	22.3	67.6	30.1	—	25	305
Less Desirable Alternatives							
Cola	0–6.5	0–4	—	13	—	100–120	390–750
Gatorade	20–24	3	17	30	—	46–58	305
Grape juice	3	31–34	—	32	—	156	1180
Jell-O (½ strength)	6–17	0.2	0–5			70–80	600
Kool-Aid	1	1	—		—	102	250–590
7-Up	5–7	2	—		—	74–102	535

TABLE 37–3. Parenteral Replacement of Fluid Deficit for Severely Dehydrated (>10% of Body Weight) Children

Type of Dehydration	Replacement Solution	% Replaced During Noted Period		
		0–12 h	*12–24 h*	*24–48 h*
Isonatremic (130–150 mEq/L)	D_5 ⅓ NS	50	50	—
Hyponatremic (<130 mEq/L)	D_5 ½ NS	75	25	—
Hypernatremic (>150 mEq/L)	D_5 ¼ NS	25	25	50

D_5, dextrose 5%; NS, normal saline (0.9% sodium chloride).

- The two most commonly recognized mechanisms of bacterial-induced infectious diarrhea involve enterotoxin-stimulated hypersecretion (secretory diarrhea) and mucosal invasion (invasive diarrhea). Antibiotic choices for bacterial infections are given in Table 37–4.

ENTEROTOXIGENIC (CHOLERA-LIKE) DIARRHEA

Cholera *(Vibrio cholerae)*

VIII
- The two species most often causing human illness are *Vibrio cholerae* and *Vibrio parahemolyticus.* Four mechanisms for transmission have been proposed, including animal reservoirs, chronic carriers, asymptomatic or mild disease victims, or water reservoirs.
- Most pathology of cholera is thought to result from an enterotoxin that increases cyclic AMP–mediated secretion of chloride ion into the intestinal lumen that results in isotonic secretion (primarily in the small intestine) exceeding the absorptive capacity of the intestinal tract (primarily the colon).
- The incubation period of *V. cholerae* is 1–3 days.
- Cholera is characterized by a spectrum from the asymptomatic state to the most severe typical cholera syndrome. In the most severe state, this disease can progress to death in a matter of 2–4 hours if not treated.
- Most signs and symptoms are a direct result of fluid and electrolyte loss. These frequently include poor skin turgor, sunken eyes, cyanosis, shallow or absent pulses, tachycardia, hypotension, and tachypnea.

Treatment

- The mainstay of treatment for cholera consists of fluid and electrolyte replacement. Rice-based rehydration formulations are the preferred **ORT** for cholera patients. Intravenous (IV) therapy is usually required only in severe cases.
- Antibiotics shorten the duration of diarrhea, decrease the volume of fluid lost, and shorten the duration of the carrier state (Table 37–4). The

TABLE 37–4. Antibiotic Selection

Organism	First Choice	Alternatives
Clostridium difficile	Metronidazole	Vancomycin
Campylobacter	Fluoroquinolone[a]	Macrolide, doxycycline
Escherichia coli	TMP–SMX, fluoroquinolone	Aminoglycoside, chloramphenicol, cephalosporin
Salmonella	Fluoroquinolone	Cephalosporin, TMP–SMX, chloramphenicol
Shigella	Fluoroquinolone	TMP–SMX, ampicillin, 3rd generation cephalosporin
Vibrio cholerae	Fluoroquinolone	Doxycycline, TMP–SMX
Yersinia enterocolitica	Fluoroquinolone	TMP–SMX, aminoglycoside, ceftriaxone

Dosing Guidelines

Drug	Children	Adults
Amikacin (IV)	15–22.5 mg/kg/day divided every 8 h	15 mg/kg/day divided every 8–12 h
Ampicillin (IV)	100–200 mg/kg/day divided every 6 h	150–200 mg/kg/day divided every 6 h
(PO)	50 mg/kg/day divided every 6 h	250–500 mg every 6 h
Bacitracin (PO)	800–1200 units/kg/day divided every 8 h	25,000 units every 6 h
Cefoperazone (IV)	100–150 mg/kg/day divided every 8–12 h	4–16 g/day divided every 6–12 h
Ceftriaxone (IV)	50–100 mg/kg/day divided every 12–24 h	1–2 g/day divided every 12–24 h
Chloramphenicol (PO)	50–75 mg/kg/day divided every 6 h	50 mg/kg/dose every 6 h
Ciprofloxacin (IV)	NR	200–400 mg every 12 h
(PO)		500–750 mg every 12 h
Clindamycin (PO)	20–30 mg/kg/day divided every 6 h	150–450 mg every 6 h
(IV)	25–40 mg/kg/day divided every 6–8 h	150–900 mg every 8 h
Doxycycline (PO)	NR	100 mg every 12–24 h
Enoxacin (PO)	NR	600–800 mg/day divided every 12–24 h
Erythromycin (PO)	30–40 mg/kg/day divided every 6–8 h	250–500 mg every 6 h
Gentamicin (IV)	3–7.5 mg/kg/day divided every 8 h	3–5 mg/kg/day divided every 8 h
Lomefloxacin (PO)	NR	400 mg every 24 h
Metronidazole (PO)	15–35 mg/kg/day divided every 8 h	500 mg every 6 h
Netilmicin (IV)	3–7.5 mg/kg/day divided every 8 h	4–6.5 mg/kg/day divided every 8 h
Norfloxacin (PO)	NR	400 mg every 12 h
Ofloxacin (PO)	NR	200–400 mg every 12 h
TMP–SMX (PO)	8–12 mg/kg/day divided every 12 h	160 mg every 12 h
Tobramycin (IV)	3–6 mg/kg/day divided every 8 h	3–5 mg/kg/day divided every 8 h
Vancomycin (PO)	10–50 mg/kg/day divided every 6 h, max 125 mg per dose	125 mg every 6 h

[a]Fluoroquinolone: ciprofloxacin, ofloxacin, lomefloxacin, enoxacin, norfloxacin (fluoroquinolones are not approved for children).
[b]TMP–SMX, trimethoprim–sulfamethoxazole.
NR, not recommended.

tetracyclines or **fluoroquinolones** are considered drugs of first choice but should be avoided during pregnancy or in young children, and **cotrimoxazole** is an appropriate alternative. Antibiotics need only be given for 3–5 days in most cases.

▶ *ESCHERICHIA COLI*

- *Escherichia coli* gastrointestinal disease may be caused by enterotoxigenic *E. coli* (ETEC), enteroinvasive *E. coli* (EIEC), enteropathogenic *E. coli* (EPEC), enteroadhesive *E. coli* (EAEC), and enterohemorrhagic *E. coli* (EHEC). ETEC is now incriminated as being the most common cause of traveler's diarrhea.
- ETEC is capable of producing two plasmid-mediated enterotoxins: heat-labile toxin (HLT) and heat-stable toxin (HST). The net effect of this toxin on the mucosa is production of a cholera-like secretory diarrhea.
- Diarrhea caused by ETEC is often characterized by abrupt onset of watery diarrhea, with or without abdominal cramping. Usually, there is no blood or pus in the stool. Most ETEC diarrhea resolves within 24–48 hours without complication.
- Most cases respond readily to **ORT**, and although antibiotic therapy is seldom necessary, prophylaxis has been shown to effectively prevent the development of ETEC diarrhea.
- Effective prophylactic agents include **tetracycline, cotrimoxazole, neomycin, furazolidone, norfloxacin,** and **ciprofloxacin.** Nonantibiotic regimens, including **bismuth subsalicylate** and **cholestyramine,** have also been recommended as effective prevention or treatment regimens.

▶ PSEUDOMEMBRANOUS COLITIS *(CLOSTRIDIUM DIFFICILE)*

- Pseudomembranous colitis (PMC) results from toxins produced by *Clostridium difficile.* It occurs most often in epidemic fashion and affects high-risk groups such as the elderly, debilitated patients, cancer patients, surgical patients, or any patient receiving antibiotics.
- PMC has been associated most often with broad-spectrum antimicrobials, including clindamycin, ampicillin, or cephalosporins.
- Symptoms can occur from several days after the start of antibiotic therapy to several weeks after antibiotics are discontinued.
- PMC is characterized by vomiting, fever, cramping, abdominal pain and tenderness, and profuse greenish diarrhea (watery or mucoid). Fevers of 103–105°F, marked leukocytosis, and hypoalbuminemia are also common. Pseudomembranous lesions, which look like whitish-yellow raised plaques, can be found anywhere in the colon.
- Diagnosis is made by colonoscopic visualization of pseudomembranes, finding cytotoxins in stools, or stool culture for *C. difficile.*
- The patient should be supported with fluid and electrolyte replacement. If the patient has not improved within 48–72 hours, has severe disease,

requires continuation of the inducing antibiotic, or is a high-risk patient (pediatric, elderly, debilitated), antibiotic therapy should be promptly initiated. *C. difficile* is usually susceptible in vitro to **vancomycin, metronidazole, bacitracin,** and **cephalosporins.**

- Metronidazole (250–500 mg four times daily orally) is the agent of choice for treatment of PMC. Vancomycin, 125–500 mg four times daily orally, is as effective but should be reserved for patients not responding to metronidazole, organisms resistant to metronidazole, patients allergic or intolerant to metronidazole, patients who are pregnant or under 10 years of age, critically ill patients, or those with diarrhea that is caused by *Staphylococcus aureus.*
- Clinical response is generally observed within the first 4 days of therapy.
- Drugs that inhibit peristalsis, such as **diphenoxylate,** are contraindicated. Some patients have become worse after use of these drugs.

▶ INVASIVE (DYSENTERY-LIKE) DIARRHEA

BACILLARY DYSENTERY (SHIGELLOSIS)

- Four species of *Shigella* are most often associated with disease, *S. dysenteriae* type I, *S. flexneri, S. bovdii,* and *S. sonnei.*
- Poor sanitation, poor personal hygiene, inadequate water supply, malnutrition, and increased population density are associated with increased risk of *Shigella* gastroenteritis epidemics, even in developed countries. The majority of cases are thought to result from fecal–oral transmission.
- *Shigella* sp. causes dysentery upon penetrating the epithelial cells lining the colon. Microabscesses may eventually coalesce, forming larger abscesses. Some *Shigella* species produce a cytotoxin, or shigatoxin, the pathogenic role of which is unclear although it is thought to damage endothelial cells of the lamina propria, resulting in microangiopathic changes that can progress to hemolytic uremic syndrome. Watery diarrhea commonly precedes the dysentery and may be a result of these toxins.
- Shigellosis is generally a self-limiting disease. Patients most often become afebrile and completely recover within 4–7 days. Approximately 10% experience a recurrence.
- Signs and symptoms are initially nonspecific: nausea, fever, malaise, abdominal tenderness of the lower quadrants, and hyperactive bowel sounds. Frequent watery stools, 10–25 per day, appear within 48 hours, and are followed by bloody diarrhea and dysentery within a few days. Stools are greenish in color and often contain mucus and/or blood, as well as many leukocytes. If untreated, bacillary dysentery usually lasts about 1 week (range 1–30 days).
- Fluid and electrolyte loss may be significant, particularly in infants and elderly patients. Stool culture will establish *Shigella* species as the causative agent.

- Treatment of bacillary dysentery generally includes correction of fluid and electrolyte disturbances and, occasionally, antimicrobials in the very young and elderly.
- Fluid and electrolyte losses can generally be replaced with oral therapy, as dysentery is generally not associated with significant fluid loss. Intravenous replacement is necessary only for those patients with severe illness.
- Because shigellosis is usually a self-limiting disease and antibiotic resistance is an increasing concern, some clinicians feel antibiotics should be reserved for the severely ill. However, because antibiotic therapy has been shown to shorten the period of fecal shedding (usually 1–4 weeks in patients not receiving antimicrobials) and attenuate the clinical illness, many clinicians prefer to treat with antibiotics (Table 37–4).
- Antispasmodics and agents that inhibit intestinal peristalsis are not used because they may prolong fever and diarrhea, worsen the dysentery, and possibly contribute to development of toxic megacolon.

SALMONELLOSIS

- Human disease caused by *Salmonella* generally falls into four categories: acute gastroenteritis (enterocolitis), bacteremia, extraintestinal localized infection, and enteric fever (typhoid and paratyphoid fever). *S. typhimurium* is the most common cause of salmonellosis.

- *Salmonella* enterocolitis appears to occur secondary to mucosal invasion of microorganisms, but it may involve enterotoxin production, or local inflammatory exudates as possible mechanisms of pathology. Organisms may invade beyond the mucosa and enter the mesenteric lymphatics which then carry bacteria to the general circulation via the thoracic duct. Bacteria not cleared by the reticuloendothelial system may cause metastatic infection in various organs.
- With enterocolitis, patients often complain of nausea and vomiting within 72 hours of ingestion followed by crampy abdominal pain, fever, and diarrhea, although the actual presentation is quite variable.
- Stool cultures inevitably yield the causative organism, if obtained early. However, recovery of organisms continues to decrease with time so that by 3–4 weeks, only 5–15% of adult patients are passing *Salmonella*.
- Some patients may continue to shed *Salmonella* for a year or longer. These "chronic carrier" states are rare for serotypes other than *S. typhi*.
- *Salmonella* can produce bacteremia without classic enterocolitis or enteric fever. The clinical syndrome is characterized by persistent bacteremia and prolonged intermittent fever with chills. Stool cultures are frequently negative.
- Extraluminal infection and/or abscess formation can occur at any site. They may follow any of the other syndromes or may be the primary presentation. Metastatic infections have been reported to involve bone, cysts, heart, kidney, liver, lungs, pericardium, spleen, and tumors.
- Enteric fever caused by *S. typhi* is called typhoid fever. If caused by any other serotype, it is referred to as paratyphoid fever. The onset of symp-

toms is gradual. Nonspecific symptoms of fever, dull headache, malaise, anorexia, and myalgias are most common. Initially, fever tends to be remittent but gradually progresses over the first week to temperatures that are often sustained over 104°F. Other frequently encountered symptoms include chills, nausea, vomiting, cough, weakness, and sore throat.

- About 80% of patients have positive blood cultures. Bacteremia persists in about one-third of patients for several weeks if not treated. Diagnostic tests other than culture are unreliable.

Treatment

- Most patients with enterocolitis require no therapeutic intervention. When required, the most important part of therapy for *Salmonella* enterocolitis is fluid and electrolyte replacement.
- Antimicrobials have not been shown to shorten the course of this self-limiting disorder. Antibiotic therapy should be considered if there is suspected transition to one of the other *Salmonella* syndromes (bacteremia, localized infection, or enteric fever) or if underlying conditions predispose to systemic spread. Both **cotrimoxazole** and **ciprofloxacin** have been used to treat *Salmonella* enterocolitis.
- **Chloramphenicol** or **ampicillin** is most frequently used for the treatment of bacteremia and localized infections. Cotrimoxazole is considered when the organism is resistant to both chloramphenicol and ampicillin. The duration of antibiotic therapy is dictated by the site.
- Chloramphenicol has been the mainstay of therapy for enteric fever in most areas of the world, but because of increasing resistance, ciprofloxacin or **ceftriaxone** are used more commonly. Ampicillin, **amoxicillin,** and cotrimoxazole are also effective, although response is not as predictable as with chloramphenicol. Therapy should be continued for10–14 days.
- Clinical response to antibiotics is often seen within 2 days; however, temperatures slowly normalize within 3–5 days.
- Live oral attenuated vaccine Ty21a and parenteral polysaccharide vaccine have been shown to confer 42–77% efficacy for a duration of 3–5 years, respectively.

CAMPYLOBACTERIOSIS

- *Campylobacter* species are now thought to be a major cause of diarrhea, comparable to *Salmonella* and *Shigella.*
- Transmission of infection appears to be by the fecal–oral route or by ingestion of contaminated food or water.
- Incubation usually averages 2–4 days.
- The most common symptoms include diarrhea of varying consistency and severity, abdominal pain, and fever. Nausea, vomiting, headache, myalgias, and malaise may also occur. Bowel movements may be numerous, bloody (dysentery-like), foul smelling, melenic, and range from loose to watery (cholera-like).

- The disease is self-limiting and signs and symptoms usually resolve in about a week, but may persist longer in 10–20% of patients.
- As with other acute diarrheal illnesses, fluid and electrolyte support is a mainstay of therapy mainly with ORT.
- Antibiotic therapy is not necessary in the majority of cases. Antibiotics should be considered in the very young and the very old and when the patient has severe bloody diarrhea, continued fever (>102°F), persistence of symptoms beyond 7 days, worsening symptoms, or a compromised immune system.
- Currently, **ciprofloxacin** is the agent of choice with **erythromycin** or **azithromycin** as alternatives.

YERSINIOSIS

- *Yersinia enterocolitica* and *Yersinia pseudotuberculosis* are associated with intestinal infection. The organisms have been isolated from a variety of food sources, including raw goat and cow milk.
- These bacteria cause a wide spectrum of clinical syndromes.
- The majority of cases present with enterocolitis that is mild and self-limiting. Symptoms, generally lasting 1–3 weeks, include vomiting, abdominal pain, diarrhea, and fever.
- A clinical syndrome seen in older children may resemble appendicitis.
- Many patients develop a reactive arthritis 1–2 weeks after recovery from enteritis.

- These diseases are generally self-limiting and are easily managed with oral rehydration solutions.
- In severe disease, bacteremia, or localizing forms of the disease, antibiotic treatment is indicated.
- *Y. enterocolitica* is generally susceptible to **third-generation cephalosporins, aminoglycosides, chloramphenicol, tetracycline, quinolones,** and **cotrimoxazole.**
- Suggested antibiotics of choice are shown in Table 37–4.

▶ ACUTE VIRAL GASTROENTERITIS

Rotavirus accounts for the majority of morbidity and even mortality among children with gastroenteritis, while Norwalk and Norwalk-like viruses account for the majority of adult cases.

ROTAVIRUSES

- The highest frequency of rotavirus-associated diarrhea appears between ages of 3 and 24 months. The exact mechanism by which the rotaviruses cause diarrhea is not known.
- Clinical manifestations of rotavirus infections vary from asymptomatic (which is common in adults) to severe nausea, vomiting, and diarrhea with dehydration. Symptoms are characterized initially by nausea and vomiting. Diarrhea occurs in most patients and lasts from 1 to 9 days, but some patients experience only loose stool with no increase in fre-

quency. Other signs and symptoms include fever, respiratory symptoms, irritability, lethargy, pharyngeal erythema, rhinitis, red tympanic membranes, and palpable cervical lymph nodes. Dehydration and electrolyte disturbances occur more frequently in children.

- Treatment of rotavirus-associated vomiting and/or diarrhea is directed at prevention or correction of dehydration.

NORWALK AND NORWALK-LIKE AGENTS

- Norwalk-like viral gastroenteritis is characterized by sudden onset of abdominal cramps with nausea and/or vomiting. Although adults frequently experience nonbloody diarrhea, children experience vomiting more often. Other frequent complaints are myalgias, headache, and malaise, which are accompanied by fever in about 50% of cases. Signs and symptoms generally last only 12–60 hours.
- The disease is generally self-limiting and does not require therapy. On occasion, oral rehydration may be required. Rarely is parenteral hydration necessary.

See Chapter 103, Gastrointestinal Infections and Enterotoxigenic Poisonings, authored by Laura J. Odell, PharmD, and Tom A. Larson, PharmD, FCCP, for a more detailed discussion of this topic.

Chapter 38

▶ HIV/AIDS

▶ DEFINITION

The Centers for Disease Control and Prevention (CDC) case definition of AIDS includes persons with serious symptomatic disease, and also all HIV-infected people who have <200 CD_4 lymphocytes/μL or a percentage of CD_4 T lymphocytes <14% of the total lymphocytes. Table 38–1 presents the classification system for adult HIV infection and a listing of the clinical conditions included in the 1993 definition.

▶ PATHOGENESIS

TRANSMISSION OF HIV

Infection with HIV occurs through three primary modes: sexual, parenteral, and perinatal. Sexual intercourse, primarily receptive anal and vaginal intercourse, is the most common vehicle for transmission of infection. The probability of HIV transmission from heterosexual or homosexual intercourse has been estimated at 0.1–0.2 per sexual contact. In general, the risk is increased when the index partner is in an advanced stage of disease. Male-to-female sexual transmission is seven to nine times more efficient than female-to-male sexual transmission.

- The use of contaminated needles or other injection-related paraphernalia by drug abusers has been the main cause of parenteral transmissions and currently accounts for one-fourth of AIDS cases reported in the United States.
- Perinatal infection, or vertical transmission, is the most common cause (>90%) of pediatric HIV infection.

HIV LIFE CYCLE

- The life cycle of HIV is depicted in Figure 38–1.
- Ultimately, most infected cells will be destroyed from a number of mechanisms including cell lysis by newly budding virions, accumulation of unintegrated viral DNA, interference of protein synthesis, syncytia formation, or apoptosis. Uninfected cells may also be destroyed through syncytia formation or the apoptosis pathway.
- Besides a decrease in the number of CD_4 lymphocytes, there are also functional abnormalities with the remaining T lymphocytes. B-cell lymphocytes also do not appear to have normal function in patients with advanced HIV infection. There is often a depressed response to pure B-cell mitogens, as well as an inability to mount a response to new antigens.

TABLE 38–1. Centers for Disease Control and Prevention 1993 Revised Classification System for HIV Infection in Adults and Conditions Included in AIDS Surveillance Case Definition

CD4+ T-cell Categories (Absolute Number and Percentage)	Clinical Categories		
	A: Asymptomatic, Acute (Primary) HIV or PGL[a]	*B: Symptomatic, Not A or C Conditions*	*C: AIDS-Indicator Conditions*
≥ 500/μL or ≥ 29%	A1	B1	C1
200–499/μL or 14–28%	A2	B2	C2
< 200/μL or < 14%	A3	B3	C3

Conditions	
Candidiasis of bronchi, trachea, or lungs	Lymphoma, Burkitt's
Candidiasis, esophageal	Lymphoma, immunoblastic
Cervical cancer, invasive	Lymphoma, primary, of brain
Coccidioidomycosis, disseminated or extrapulmonary	*Mycobacterium avium* complex or *M. kansasii*, disseminated or extrapulmonary
Cryptococcosis, extrapulmonary	*Mycobacterium tuberculosis*, any site (pulmonary or extrapulmonary)
Cryptosporidiosis, chronic intestinal (duration > 1 month)	*Mycobacterium*, other species or unidentified species, disseminated or extrapulmonary
Cytomegalovirus disease (other than liver, spleen, or nodes)	*Pneumocystis carinii* pneumonia
Cytomegalovirus retinitis (with loss of vision)	Pneumonia, recurrent
Encephalopathy, HIV-related	Progressive multifocal leukoencephalopathy
Herpes simplex: Chronic ulcer(s) (duration > 1 month); or bronchitis, pneumonitis, or esophagitis	*Salmonella* septicemia, recurrent
Histoplasmosis, disseminated or extrapulmonary	Toxoplasmosis of brain
Isosporiasis, chronic intestinal (duration > 1 month)	Wasting syndrome due to HIV
Kaposi's sarcoma	

[a]PGL = persistent generalized lymphadenopathy.

VIII

- Spontaneous secretion of immunoglobulin, increased spontaneous lymphocyte proliferation, elevated circulatory immune complexes, and numerous autoimmune phenomena are other manifestations. Monocyte and macrophage function (e.g., chemotaxis) may also be abnormal in advanced HIV infection.

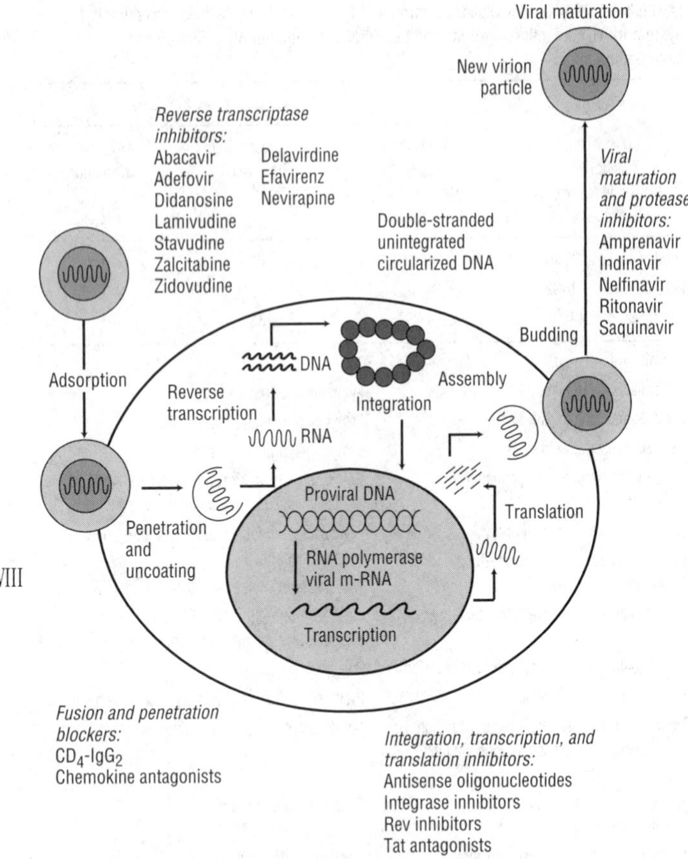

Figure 38–1. Life cycle of HIV with potential targets where replication may be interrupted and known or putative antiretroviral agents. *(From Courtney V. Fletcher, 1998, with permission.)*

VIII

▶ CLINICAL PRESENTATION

- Clinical presentations of primary HIV infection vary, but patients often have a viral syndrome or mononucleosis-like illness with fever, pharyngitis, and adenopathy. About 40–60% of patients will also exhibit an erythematous macular, or mixed maculopapular rash.
- Approximately 5% of infected individuals will develop AIDS within 3 years, and 20% within 5 years; the median time from initial infection with HIV to the development of an opportunistic or AIDS is 10 years.

- Initial clinical presentation of HIV infection varies. The classification scheme of the CDC divides HIV infection into a matrix of nine categories based on the CD_4 cell count (see section "Diagnosis") and clinical conditions (Table 38–1).
  - Category A consists of asymptomatic infection, persistent generalized lymphadenopathy, and acute retroviral syndrome.
  - Category B consists of mild to moderate symptomatic conditions that are not AIDS-defining conditions. This category includes AIDS-related complex (ARC) and conditions such as bacillary angiomatosis; oropharyngeal candidiasis; vulvovaginal candidiasis that is persistent, frequent, or poorly responsive to therapy; cervical dysplasia; unexplained constitutional symptoms (fever >38.5°C, diarrhea lasting >1 month); oral hairy leukoplakia; recurrent or multidermatomal varicella-zoster infection; idiopathic thrombocytopenia purpura; listeriosis; pelvic inflammatory disease; and peripheral neuropathy.
  - Category C includes clinical conditions from the AIDS surveillance case definition (Table 38–1), which are generally severe, life-threatening opportunistic diseases.
- Most patients with advanced HIV infection are anergic. They also have a moderate anemia (hemoglobin of 7–12 g/dL), moderate transient leukopenia (1000–3000 cells/μL), and moderate thrombocytopenia. Lymphocyte counts are frequently below 1500 cells/μL with a disproportionate decrease in T lymphocytes compared with B lymphocytes. Following lymphopenia, there is a CD_8 lymphocytosis with depletion of CD_4 lymphocytes and the appearance of atypical lymphocytes.
- HIV-related illnesses in children often present with unexplained physical signs such as hepatomegaly, failure to thrive and weight loss, unexplained fever, splenomegaly, unexplained lymphadenopathy, low birth weight (in prenatally exposed infants), eczema, and parotitis. Laboratory findings include anemia, hypergammaglobulinemia, altered mononuclear cell function, and altered T-cell subset ratios. The CDC current pediatric AIDS surveillance definition (Table 38–2) excludes children with congenital or perinatally acquired cytomegalovirus or other identified causes of congenital immunodeficiency.
- HIV itself does not produce most of the morbidity and mortality associated with AIDS. Rather, opportunistic infections, many caused by organisms that are common in the environment, are responsible for almost 90% of deaths.
- Clinical presentation of the opportunistic infections is presented in the "Infectious Complications of HIV" section.

DIAGNOSIS

- The most commonly used screening method for HIV is an enzyme-linked immunosorbent assay (ELISA, EIA) which detects antibodies against HIV-1 and is both highly sensitive and specific. False-negatives may occur if the patient is newly infected and the test is performed before antibody production is detectable.

TABLE 38–2. Centers for Disease Control and Prevention 1994 Revised Classification System for HIV Infection in Children Less Than 13 Years of Age

	Cells/μL (%)[a]			Signs/Symptoms			
Immunologic Categories	*< 12 Months*	*1–5 Years*	*6–12 Years*	*N: No*	*A: Mild*	*B: Moderate*	*C: Severe*
1. No evidence of suppression	≥ 1500 (≥ 25%)	≥ 1000 (≥ 25%)	≥ 500 (≥ 25%)	N1	A1	B1	C1
2. Evidence of moderate suppression	750–1499 (15–24%)	500–999 (15–24%)	200–499 (15–24%)	N2	A2	B2	C2
3. Severe suppression	< 750 (< 15%)	< 500 (< 15%)	< 200 (< 15%)	N3	A3	B3	C3

[a]Percentage of total lymphocytes.

- Positive ELISAs are repeated in duplicate and if one or both tests are reactive, a confirmatory test is performed for final diagnosis. Several confirmatory tests exist, including Western blot assay, indirect immunofluorescence assay (IFA), or radioimmunoprecipitation assay (RIPA). If the confirmatory test is negative, the patient is most likely not infected.
- There are three commonly used methods for determining the amount of HIV RNA: reverse transcriptase–coupled polymerase chain reaction (RT-PCR), branched DNA (bDNA) signal amplification, and nucleic acid sequence–based assay (NASBA). Each assay has its own lower limit of sensitivity and results can vary from one assay method to the other, therefore, it is recommended that the same assay method be used consistently within patients.
- Plasma HIV RNA levels indicate the magnitude of HIV replication and its associated rate of CD_4 cell destruction, while CD_4 cell counts indicate the extent of HIV-induced immune damage already suffered.
- The number of CD_4 lymphocytes in the blood is a surrogate marker of disease progression. The normal adult CD_4 lymphocyte count ranges between 500 and 1600 cells/μL or 40–70% of all lymphocytes.
- Other previously used laboratory markers of disease progression include HIV p24 antigen, β_2-microglobulin, and serum neopterin.

► TREATMENT

GOALS OF TREATMENT

- The goal of antiretroviral therapy is to achieve the maximum suppression of HIV replication (HIV RNA level that is less than the lower limit of quantitation).

GENERAL APPROACH TO TREATMENT OF HIV INFECTION

- Regular, periodic measurement of plasma HIV RNA levels and CD_4 cell counts is necessary to determine the risk of disease progression in an HIV-infected individual and to determine when to initiate or modify antiretroviral treatment regimens.
- The use of potent combination antiretroviral therapy to suppress HIV replication to below the levels of detection of sensitive plasma HIV RNA assays limits the potential for selection of antiretroviral-resistant HIV variants, the major factor limiting the ability of antiretroviral drugs to inhibit virus replication and delay disease progression.
- The most effective means to accomplish durable suppression of HIV replication is the simultaneous initiation of combinations of effective anti-HIV drugs with which the patient has not been previously treated and that are not cross-resistant with antiretroviral agents with which the patient has been treated previously.
- Each of the antiretroviral drugs used in combination therapy regimens should always be used according to optimum schedules and dosages.

- Women should receive optimal antiretroviral therapy regardless of pregnancy status.
- The same principles of antiretroviral therapy apply to both HIV-infected children and adults, although the treatment of HIV-infected children involves unique pharmacologic, virologic, and immunologic considerations.
- Persons with acute primary HIV infections should be treated with combination antiretroviral therapy to suppress virus replication to levels below the limit of detection of sensitive plasma HIV RNA assays.
- HIV-infected persons, even those with viral loads below detectable limits, should be considered infectious and should be counseled to avoid sexual and drug-use behaviors that are associated with transmission or acquisition of HIV and other infectious pathogens.
- Figure 38–2 presents the state-of-the-art for treatment of the HIV-infected individual at the time of the writing of this chapter. Treatment is recommended for all HIV-infected persons with symptomatic disease, CD_4 lymphocyte counts <500 cells/μL, or with plasma HIV RNA >20,000 copies/mL (by RT-PCR) or >10,000 copies/mL (by bDNA) regardless of the CD_4 count.
- A more aggressive treatment approach recommends treatment if viral load becomes >5000 copies/mL. The available data do not permit an absolute treatment threshold to be established based on plasma HIV RNA level. Therefore, the relative merits of a cautious approach that delays therapy for patients with values <5000 copies/mL and considers therapy for patients with values between 5000–10,000 copies/mL is as valid as an aggressive approach of offering therapy to any patient who requests it and is committed to lifelong medication compliance.

PHARMACOLOGIC THERAPY

Antiretroviral Agents

- Inhibiting viral replication with highly active antiretroviral therapy has been the most clinically successful strategy in the treatment of HIV infection. There have been two primary groups of drugs used: reverse transcriptase inhibitors and protease inhibitors (Table 38–3).

Pivotal Developments in Antiretroviral Treatment Strategies

Important findings determined from clinical trials of antiretroviral agents are as follows:

- Early studies with zidovudine alone for treatment of patients with AIDS or AIDS-related complex (ARC) resulted in a reduction in viral burden, an increase in CD_4 lymphocytes, a decrease in the incidence of opportunistic infections (from 43% of patients with placebo to 23% with zidovudine), and improved survival.
- Zidovudine used alone transiently delayed the onset of AIDS-defining events in both symptomatic and asymptomatic HIV-infected individuals

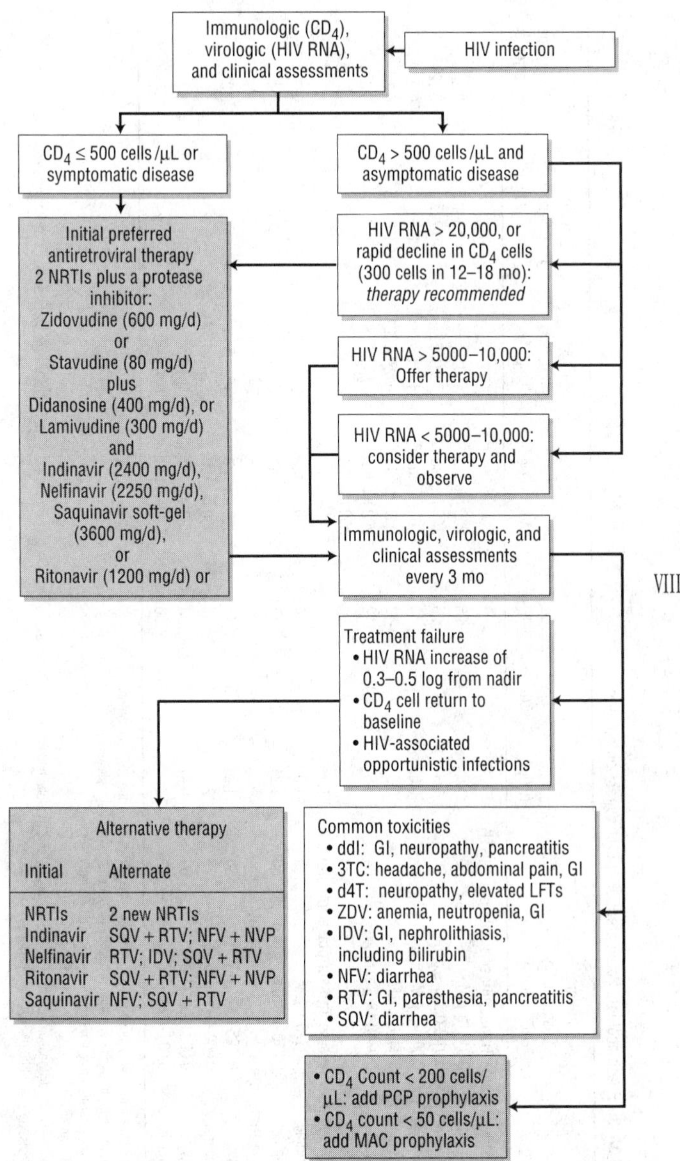

VIII

Figure 38–2. Management of HIV infection. *(From Courtney V. Fletcher, 1998, with permission.)*

TABLE 38–3. Pharmacologic Parameters of Antiretroviral Compounds

Drug	In Vitro Susceptibility (IC_{50} range)	F (%)	V_d (L/kg)	$T_{1/2}$ (h)	CL/F (L/h)	Adult Dose[a]	Plasma C_{max}/C_{min} (μM)	Ratio Fetal:Maternal Concentration	Ratio CSF:Plasma Concentration
Nucleoside Reverse Transcriptase Inhibitors (NRTI)									
Didanosine	0.01–10 μM	40	1.0	1.4	26.9	200 mg bid	4/0.02	0.3–0.5	0.22
Lamivudine	0.015–0.321 μg/mL[b]	86	1.3	5	23.1	150 mg bid	7.5/0.22	>0.7	0.12
Stavudine	0.009–4 μM	82	0.53	1.6	40	40 mg bid	4/0.004	>0.7	0.02
Zalcitabine	0.03–0.5 μM	85	0.53	2	12	0.75 mg tid	0.05/0.001	0.3–0.5	0.2
Zidovudine	0.03–0.13 μg/mL	64	1.6	1.1	112	200 mg tid 300 mg bid	2/0.2	>0.7	0.6
Non–Nucleoside Reverse Transcriptase Inhibitors (NNRTI)									
Delavirdine	0.05–0.1 μM[b]	85	1.0	4.7	4	400 mg tid	35/14	?	0.004
Nevirapine	0.010–0.1 μM	50	1.21	25	2.6	200 mg bid[c]	5.5/3.0	1	0.45
Protease Inhibitors									
Indinavir	0.025–0.1 μM[b]	60	1.2	1.5	43	800 mg q 8 h	13/0.25	?	0.03–0.94
Nelfinavir	0.009–0.06 μM	?	2	2.6	37.4	750 mg tid	5.6/0.7	?	—
Ritonavir	0.0038–0.154 μM	60	0.41	3-5	8.8	600 mg bid[c]	16/5	?	—
Saquinavir[d]	0.001–0.03 μM	12	10	3	80	1200 mg tid	0.4/0.15	?	—

[a]Dose adjustment may be required for weight, renal or hepatic disease, and drug interactions.

[b]Range given is for IC_{90} (concentration necessary to inhibit 90% of viral replication).

[c]Initial dose escalation recommended to minimize side effects.

[d]Soft-gel formulation.

F, bioavailability; V_d, distribution volume; $T_{1/2}$, elimination half-life; CL, total body clearance; C_{max}, maximum plasma concentration; C_{min}, minimum plasma concentration; CSF, cerebrospinal fluid; IC_{50}, concentration necessary to inhibit 50% of viral replication.

for up to 2 years. The duration of benefits of zidovudine therapy in terms of risk of progression to AIDS or death was demonstrated for up to 4.5 years (ACTG 019). However, the benefit decreased with increased duration of use. These benefits were evident with patients with CD_4 cells <500/μL and >500/μL.

- Zidovudine reduced the rate of maternal-to-fetal transmission of HIV from 25.5% to 8.3% (ACTG 076). The dose used was 100 mg five times daily (given at 14–34 weeks' gestation) plus a continuous infusion during labor (2 mg/kg IV over 1 hour followed by 1 mg/kg/h). The newborns received 2 mg/kg orally every 6 hours for 6 weeks. Adverse reactions associated with zidovudine were minimal. Hemoglobin concentrations were lower in the zidovudine infants, but this difference disappeared by 12 weeks of age.
- Evidence from trials of combinations of nucleoside reverse transcriptase inhibitors (NRTI) regimens in children and patients with advanced disease all support the following conclusions: (1) Progression of disease can be delayed with treatment, (2) combination therapy is more effective than monotherapy in both immunologic and virologic response, and (3) patients are more likely to respond to combination therapy when CD_4 counts are higher or baseline viral load is lower.
- The addition of a protease inhibitor to combination NRTIs has resulted in improved immunologic outcomes and mortality. A study with the combination of up to two NRTIs plus the protease inhibitor ritonavir or placebo was the first that demonstrated a reduction in both mortality and AIDS-defining clinical events with a protease inhibitor in patients with advanced HIV disease. VIII
- Non–nucleoside reverse transcriptase inhibitors (NNRTIs) also result in increased CD_4 cell count and reduced viral load when combined with two NRTIs. The combination of zidovudine plus didanosine and nevirapine (the first NNRTI to be approved) was more effective than zidovudine plus didanosine and placebo in a 48-week study.

TREATMENT DURING PREGNANCY

- Therapy is warranted particularly in light of the dramatic reduction in transmission seen with **zidovudine** monotherapy (ACTG protocol 076).
- Unfortunately, little is known about the use of antiretrovirals in pregnant women and the effect these drugs may have on the developing fetus. Currently, there are no data to indicate any adverse consequences of the administration of zidovudine to pregnant women during the second and third trimester and their newborns for 6 weeks.
- The National Institutes of Health Treatment Principles recommend that women receive optimal therapy regardless of pregnancy status. Pregnant women should be treated similar to a nonpregnant woman, and, if possible, zidovudine should be used for both the mother and the infant.

POSTEXPOSURE PROPHYLAXIS

- Postexposure prophylaxis (PEP) with a triple-drug regimen consisting of two nucleoside reverse transcriptase inhibitors and a protease inhibitor is recommended by the CDC for percutaneous blood exposure involving significant risk (i.e., large volume of blood or blood from patients with advanced AIDS).
- Two nucleoside reverse transcriptase inhibitors may be offered to the health care worker with lower risk of exposure such as those involving either the mucous membrane or skin.
- Treatment is not necessary if the source of exposure is urine or saliva.
- Treatment should ideally be initiated within 1–2 hours. The optimal duration of treatment is unknown, but at least 4 weeks of therapy is advocated.
- A similar treatment approach should be initiated for postcoital and post–injection-drug use prophylaxis.

▶ EVALUATION OF THERAPEUTIC OUTCOMES

- Following the initiation of therapy, patients are usually monitored at 3-month intervals with immunologic (i.e., CD_4 count), virologic (i.e., viral load), and clinical assessments.
- There are two general indications to change therapy: significant toxicity or treatment failure.
- Specific criteria to indicate treatment failure have not been established through controlled clinical trials. As a general guide, the following events should prompt consideration for changing therapy:
  - Less than a one log reduction in HIV RNA 1 month after the initiation of therapy, or a failure to achieve maximal suppression of HIV replications within 4–6 months.
  - A persistent decline in the CD_4 cell count or a return to the pretreatment value or an increase in HIV RNA of 0.3–0.5 $\log_{10}$ copies/mL from nadir.
  - Clinical disease progression, usually the development of a new opportunistic infection.

THERAPEUTIC FAILURE

- HIV has been shown to develop resistance to antiretroviral drugs. The guiding principles are to change to at least two new antiretroviral drugs that are not cross-resistant with agents the patient has received previously. Figure 38–2 presents some examples of alternative regimens.

▶ INFECTIOUS COMPLICATIONS OF HIV

- The development of certain opportunistic infections is directly or indirectly related to the level of CD_4 lymphocytes (Figure 38–3).

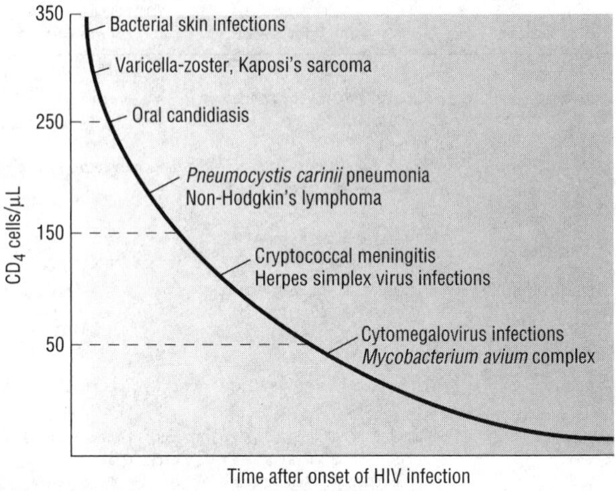

Figure 38–3. Natural history of opportunistic infections associated with HIV infection. *(From Courtney V. Fletcher, 1995, with permission.)*

VIII

- The most common opportunistic diseases and their frequencies found before death in patients with AIDS between 1990 and 1994 were *Pneumocystis carinii* pneumonia, 45%; *Mycobacterium avium* complex, 25%; wasting syndrome, 25%; bacterial pneumonia, 24%; cytomegalovirus (CMV) disease, 23%; and candidiasis, 22%.
- The spectrum of infectious diseases observed in HIV-infected individuals and recommended first-line therapies are shown in Table 38–4.

PNEUMOCYSTIS CARINII

- *Pneumocystis carinii* pneumonia (PCP) is the most common life-threatening opportunistic infection in patients with AIDS. The taxonomy of the organism is unclear, having been classified as both protozoan and fungal.

Clinical Presentation

- Characteristic symptoms include fever and dyspnea; clinical signs are tachypnea, with or without rales or rhonchi, and a nonproductive or mildly productive cough. Chest radiographs may show florid or subtle infiltrates or may occasionally be normal, although infiltrates are usually interstitial and bilateral. Arterial blood gases may show minimal hypoxia (PaO_2 80–95 mm Hg), but in more advanced disease may be markedly abnormal.
- The onset of PCP is often insidious, occurring over a period of weeks, although more fulminant presentations can occur.

TABLE 38–4. Therapies for Common Opportunistic Pathogens in HIV-Infected Individuals

Clinical Disease	Selected Initial Therapies for Acute Infection in Adults	Common Drug or Dose-Limiting Adverse Reactions
Fungi		
Candidiasis, oral	Fluconazole 200 mg PO single dose or 100 mg PO for 5 days	Elevated liver function tests, hepatotoxicity, nausea and vomiting
	or	
	Nystatin 500,000 units PO swish 4–6 times daily for 7–10 days	Taste, patient acceptance
	or	
	Clotrimazole 10 mg (1 troche) PO 5 times daily for 7–10 days	Elevated liver function tests, hepatotoxicity, nausea and vomiting
Candidiasis, esophageal	Fluconazole 200 mg PO or IV on the first day then 100 mg/days for 10–14 days	
	or	
	Ketoconazole 400 mg/days PO for 10–14 days	Elevated liver function tests, hepatotoxicity, rash, nausea and vomiting
Pneumocystis carinii pneumonia	Trimethoprim–sulfamethoxazole IV or PO 12–20 mg/kg/days as TMP component in 3–4 divided doses for 21 days[a]	Skin rash, fever, leukopenia, thrombocytopenia
	or	
	Pentamidine 3–4 mg/kg/days IV for 21 days[a]	Azotemia, hypoglycemia, hyperglycemia
	Mild episodes: Atovaquone suspension 750 mg (5 mL) PO twice daily with meals for 21 days[a]	Rash, elevated liver enzymes, diarrhea
Cryptococcal meningitis	Amphotericin B 0.5–1 mg/kg/days IV for minimum of 2 weeks *with or without* flucytosine 100–150 mg/kg/days PO in 4 divided doses	Nephrotoxicity, hypokalemia, anemia, fever, chills, bone marrow suppression, elevated liver enzymes
	followed by	
	Fluconazole 100 to 200 mg/days PO[a]	Same as above
Histoplasmosis	Amphotericin B 0.5–1 mg/kg/days IV for 6–8 weeks[a]	Same as above
	or	
	Itraconazole 200–400 mg/days PO for 3 months[a]	Elevated liver function tests, hepatotoxicity, nausea and vomiting, hypertension
Coccidioidomycosis	Amphotericin B 0.5–1 mg/kg/days IV for ≥ 6–8 weeks[a]	Same as above
Protozoa		
Toxoplasmic encephalitis	Pyrimethamine 200 mg PO once then 50–100 mg/days	Bone marrow suppression
	plus	
	Sulfadiazine 1–1.5 g PO four times daily	Allergy, rash, drug fever
	and	
	Folinic acid 10–20 mg PO daily for a minimum of 28 days[a]	
Isosporiasis	Trimethoprim–sulfamethoxazole 1–2 double-strength tablets (160 mg TMP and 800 mg SMX) PO twice daily for 2–4 weeks	Same as above

VIII

TABLE 38–4. continued

Clinical Disease	Selected Initial Therapies for Acute Infection in Adults	Common Drug or Dose-Limiting Adverse Reactions
Bacteria		
Organisms associated with T-cell defects		
Mycobacterium avium complex	Clarithromycin 500 mg PO twice daily **plus** Ethambutol 15 mg/kg/d PO to a maximum of 1000 mg/d **and**	Gastrointestinal intolerance, optic neuritis, peripheral neuritis
	Rifabutin 300 mg/d[a]	Rash, gastrointestinal intolerance, neutropenia, discolored urine, uveitis
Salmonella enterocolitis or bacteremia	Ciprofloxacin 500–750 mg PO twice daily for 14 days **or**	Gastrointestinal intolerance
	Trimethoprim (160 mg)–sulfamethoxazole (800 mg) 1 tablet PO twice daily for 14 days	Same as above
Organisms associated with B-cell defects		
Campylobacter enterocolitis	Ciprofloxacin 500 mg PO twice daily for 7 days **or**	Same as above
	Erythromycin 250–500 mg PO four times daily for 7 days	Gastrointestinal intolerance, colitis, ototoxicity
Shigella enterocolitis	Ciprofloxacin 500 mg PO twice daily for 5 days	Same as above
Viruses		
Mucocutaneous herpes simplex	Acyclovir 1–2 g/d PO in 3–5 divided doses for 7–10 days **or**	Gastrointestinal intolerance
	Valacyclovir 500 mg PO q 12 h for 7–10 days **or**	Gastrointestinal intolerance
	Famciclovir 500 mg PO q 12 h for 7–10 days	Headache, gastrointestinal intolerance
Varicella-zoster	Acyclovir 30 mg/kg/d IV in 3 divided doses **or**	Obstructive nephropathy, CNS symptomatology
	4 g/d PO for 7–10 days **or**	
	Valacyclovir 1 g PO q 8 h for 7–10 days **or**	
	Famciclovir, 500 mg PO q 8 h for 7–10 days	Obstructive nephropathy, CNS symptomatology
Cytomegalovirus	Ganciclovir 7.5–10 mg/kg/d in 2–3 divided doses for 14 days[a] **or**	Neutropenia, thrombocytopenia
	Foscarnet 180 mg/kg/d in 2 or 3 divided doses for 14 days[a]	Nephrotoxicity, hypo–hypercalcemia, hypo–hyperphosphatemia, anemia
Cytomegalovirus retinitis	Ganciclovir intraocular implant	

[a]Maintenanace therapy is recommended.

VIII

PCP Treatment

- Treatment with **trimethoprim–sulfamethoxazole** (**TMP–SMX** or **co-trimoxazole**) or parenteral **pentamidine** is associated with a 60–100% response rate. TMP–SMX is the regimen of choice for treatment and subsequent prophylaxis of PCP in patients with and without HIV.
- TMP–SMX is given in doses of 15–20 mg/kg/d (based on the TMP component) as three to four divided doses for the treatment of PCP.
- TMP–SMX is usually initiated by the intravenous route, although oral therapy (as oral absorption is high) may suffice in mildly ill and reliable patients, or to complete a course of therapy after a response has been achieved with intravenous administration.
- For treatment of HIV-associated PCP, **pentamidine isethionate** is administered intravenously usually in doses of 4 mg/kg.
- The optimum length of therapy for treatment of PCP with either agent is not known, but 21 days is commonly recommended.
- The more common adverse reactions seen with TMP–SMX are rash, fever, leukopenia, elevated serum transaminases, and thrombocytopenia. The incidence of these adverse reactions is higher in HIV-infected individuals than in those not infected with HIV.
- For pentamidine, side effects include hypotension, tachycardia, nausea, vomiting, severe hypoglycemia or hyperglycemia, pancreatitis, irreversible diabetes mellitus, elevated transaminases, nephrotoxicity, leukopenia, and cardiac arrhythmias.
- The early addition of adjunctive corticosteroid therapy to anti-PCP regimens has been shown to decrease the risk of respiratory failure and improve survival in patients with AIDS and moderate to severe PCP (PaO_2 ≤70 mm Hg or A-a gradient ≥35 mm Hg. The regimen currently recommended is 40 mg of **prednisone** orally twice daily during days 1 through 5; 40 mg once daily on days 6 through 10; and 20 mg once daily on days 11 through 21, or for the duration of therapy. In general, adjunctive corticosteroid therapy should be initiated when antipneumocystis therapy is started, as the data supporting the use of corticosteroids are based on initiation within the first 24–72 hours of the start of antipneumocystis therapy.

PCP Prophylaxis

- Currently, PCP prophylaxis is recommended for all HIV-infected individuals who have already had previous PCP. Prophylaxis is also recommended for any HIV-infected person who has a CD_4 lymphocyte count <200 cells/μL or their CD_4 cells are <20% of total lymphocytes, or unexplained fever (>100°F) for >2 weeks, or a history of oropharyngeal candidiasis. Patients on PCP prophylaxis whose CD_4 counts increase above 200 cells/μL due to antiretroviral therapy should not discontinue PCP prophylaxis at this point (Table 38–5).
- TMP–SMX is the preferred therapy for both primary and secondary prophylaxis of PCP in adults and adolescents.

TABLE 38–5. Therapies for Prophylaxis of First Episode Opportunistic Diseases in Adults and Adolescents

Pathogen	Indication	First Choice
Standard of Care		
Pneumocystis carinii	CD_4+ count <200/μL **or** Oropharyngeal candidiasis **or** Unexplained fever ≥ 2 weeks	Trimethoprim–sulfamethoxazole (TMP–SMX), 1 DS tablet PO qd
Mycobacterium tuberculosis		
Isoniazid-sensitive	TST reaction >5 mm **or** prior positive TST result without treatment **or** Contact with case of active tuberculosis	Isoniazid, 300 mg PO **plus** pyridoxine, 50 mg PO qd for 12 months **or** Isoniazid, 900 mg PO **plus** pyridoxine, 50 mg PO twice weekly for 12 months
Isoniazid-resistant	Same; high probability of exposure to isoniazid-resistant tuberculosis	Rifampin, 600 mg PO qd for 12 months
Toxoplasma gondii	IgG antibody to *Toxoplasma* and CD_4+ count <100/μL	TMP–SMX, 1 DS tablet PO qd
Mycobacterium avium complex	CD_4+ count <50/μL	Azithromycin, 1200 mg PO once weekly or clarithromycin, 500 mg PO bid
Streptococcus pneumoniae	All patients	Pneumococcal vaccine, 0.5 mL IM x 1
Varicella-zoster virus (VZV)	Significant exposure to chickenpox or shingles for patients who have no history of either condition or, if available, negative antibody to VZV	Varicella-zoster immunoglobulin (VZIG), 5 vials (1.25 mL each) IM, administered ideally within 48 h of exposure, but ≤96 h
Generally Recommended		
Hepatitis B virus	All susceptible (anti-HBc-negative) patients	Engerix B, three 20 μg IM **or** Recombivax HB, three 10 μg IM
Influenza virus	All patients (annually, before influenza season)	Whole or split virus, 0.5 mL IM each year
Indicated for Use Only in Selected Circumstances		
Candida sp.	CD_4+ count <50/μL	Fluconazole, 100–200 mg PO qd
Bacteria	Neutropenia	Granulocyte colony-stimulating factor (G-CSF), Filgrastim 5–10 μg/kg SC qd for 2–4 weeks **or** Sargramostin 250 μg/m^2 IV over 2 h qd for 2–4 weeks
Cryptococcus neoformans	CD_4+ count <50/μL	Fluconazole, 100-200 mg PO qd
Histoplasma capsulatum	CD_4+ count <100/μL, endemic geographic area	Itraconazole, 200 mg PO qd
Cytomegalovirus	CD_4+ count <50/μL and CMV antibody positivity	Oral ganciclovir, 1 g PO tid

DS, double strength.

- The recommended dose in adults and adolescents is one double-strength tablet daily.
- TMP–SMX is also the recommended drug of choice for PCP prophylaxis in children. The TMP–SMX regimen recommended (although other acceptable alternatives exist) is 150 mg/m^2/d of TMP and 750 mg/m^2/d of SMX given in divided doses twice daily, three times weekly on consecutive days (e.g., Monday, Tuesday, and Wednesday). The total daily dose of TMP–SMX in children should not exceed 320 mg of TMP with 1600 mg of SMX.

TOXOPLASMA GONDII

Toxoplasma gondii can infect any organ of the body and cause an acute infection; it has a predilection for the brain and the eye.

Clinical Presentation

- The clinical signs and symptoms of toxoplasmosis are most frequently associated with involvement of the CNS, and less commonly the lungs and eyes, although any organ can be affected. Clinical presentation often includes fever, headache, seizures (in approximately 10–25% of patients), focal neurologic abnormalities (in approximately 60–90%), and mental status changes.
- VIII Brain biopsy is required to make a definitive diagnosis of toxoplasmic encephalitis although presumptive diagnosis is commonly made in *T. gondii*–seropositive patients with typical CNS lesions.

Treatment

- The initial treatment of CNS toxoplasmosis is usually empiric.
- The combination of **pyrimethamine** and **sulfadiazine** is considered the most effective regimen for acute therapy of AIDS-related CNS toxoplasmosis.
- Pyrimethamine loading doses of 75 mg orally on the first day followed by 25 mg/d thereafter have been commonly used. Others have recommended larger loading doses of 100–200 mg followed by daily oral doses of 1–1.5 mg/kg/d (50–100 mg/d).
- The usual dose of sulfadiazine is 1–1.5 g every 6 hours (4–8 g/d).
- **Folinic acid,** in doses of 10–20 mg/d (although doses as high as 50 mg/d have been used), is usually added to the combination to reduce the pyrimethamine-induced bone marrow toxicity.
- Acute therapy with this combination should be continued for at least 3 weeks, but 6 weeks of treatment is recommended for more severely ill patients.
- The combination of pyrimethamine plus **clindamycin** appears to be less toxic than that of pyrimethamine plus sulfadiazine.
- The discontinuation of pyrimethamine and sulfadiazine after successful initial therapy is associated with a relapse rate that may approach 100%. Thus, lifelong maintenance therapy/secondary prophylaxis is

recommended for AIDS patients to prevent recrudescence of the disease. A regimen of pyrimethamine (25–75 mg/d with folinic acid) plus sulfadiazine (500–1000 mg qid) has been recommended.

CRYPTOCOCCUS NEOFORMANS

- Cryptococcal infection is the fourth most common infection in patients with AIDS and is the most common life-threatening fungal infection.

Clinical Presentation

- The usual clinical presentation of cryptococcal infection is meningitis. The clinical features of cryptococcal meningitis may be subtle, nonspecific, and not localized to the CNS. Fever, headache, and malaise are the most frequent symptoms.
- Methods for diagnosis of cryptococcal infection include serum and cerebrospinal fluid (CSF) testing for cryptococcal antigen and fungal cultures. Detection of cryptococcal antigen in serum and CSF is the most sensitive and specific test; an antigen titer >1:8 should be regarded as evidence of infection.

Treatment

- The standard therapeutic approach has been **amphotericin B** for both acute and maintenance therapy.
- **Fluconazole** is also effective for treatment of cryptococcal meningitis; however, the combination of amphotericin B and **flucytosine** was found to be superior.
- Most patients with cryptococcal meningitis should receive amphotericin B in an intravenous dose of at least 0.5 mg/kg/d for a minimum of 2 weeks as acute therapy. Flucytosine in doses of 100–150 mg/kg/d can be considered for combination with amphotericin B.
- Serum concentrations of flucytosine should be monitored and peak levels kept below 100 μg/mL to minimize hematologic adverse reactions.
- Maintenance therapy is necessary to prevent relapse. Fluconazole is superior to amphotericin or **itraconazole** for maintenance therapy and is the drug of choice to prevent relapse of cryptococcal meningitis.

MYCOBACTERIUM INFECTIONS

Clinical Presentation

- The clinical syndrome associated with mycobacterium avium complex (MAC) includes high spiking fevers, diarrhea, night sweats, malaise, weight loss, anemia, and neutropenia. Persistent diarrhea and abdominal pain, a malabsorption syndrome, and extrahepatic biliary obstruction are manifestations associated with MAC gastrointestinal infection.
- Diagnosis of MAC infection is usually based on culture of the organisms from the blood, although biopsies of the liver, bone marrow, and lymph nodes are also highly sensitive and specific.

Treatment

- Treatment regimens should contain at least two antimycobacterial agents.
- Every regimen should contain either **clarithromycin** or **azithromycin,** with clarithromycin (500 mg bid) being the preferred agent. For the second agent, numerous choices are available, although **ethambutol** (15 mg/kg/d) is preferred by many experts. Many clinicians would add a third, and some, a fourth drug to this regimen.
- Clinical responses usually occur within 2–8 weeks of the start of therapy. If a clinical and microbiologic response is observed, therapy should continue for the duration of the patient's life.
- MAC prophylaxis is now strongly recommended for all HIV-infected adults and adolescents with a CD_4 count <50 cells/μL. The first-line choices are either azithromycin or clarithromycin.

HERPESVIRUS INFECTIONS

Herpes Simplex Virus (HSV)

- The manifestations of HSV disease observed in persons with AIDS include orolabial, genital, anorectal mucocutaneous disease; esophagitis; and less commonly encephalitis. Ulcerative HSV lesions present for longer than 1 month in an individual with laboratory evidence of HIV infection, or no other apparent cause for immunodeficiency, are considered an AIDS-defining condition.

VIII

- Symptoms of anorectal lesions, the most common clinically evident HSV disease causing morbidity in homosexual men, include pain, itching, and painful defecation.
- **Acyclovir** is the drug of choice for treatment of HSV disease. For mild to moderate mucocutaneous disease, oral acyclovir in doses of 200 mg five times daily or 400 mg tid are used. Intravenous acyclovir (15 mg/kg/d) should be used in those settings where absorption of an oral drug is questionable, oral tolerance is unlikely (HSV esophagitis), or perhaps when severe mucocutaneous disease is present.
- Treatment of mucocutaneous disease should be continued until all lesions have crusted.
- Intravenous acyclovir (30 mg/kg/d) should also be used for viscerally disseminated disease and for HSV encephalitis.
- **Famciclovir** or **valacyclovir** is an alternative to oral acyclovir.
- Recurrent HSV disease can often be managed with low-dose suppressive oral acyclovir therapy, 200 mg qid, 400 mg bid, or 800 mg qd.

Varicella-Zoster Virus (VZV)

- Zoster usually begins as radicular pain followed by localized erythematous rash and characteristic vesicles. Zoster will usually remain confined to a limited number of dermatomes, but complications such as widespread cutaneous involvement and disseminated visceral zoster may occur.

- Acyclovir is the drug of choice for VZV infections. While an oral acyclovir regimen of 4 g/d has been shown effective for the treatment of zoster in immunocompetent adults, the drug has not been fully evaluated in immunocompromised patients such as those with AIDS.
- AIDS patients with disseminated cutaneous or visceral zoster should receive treatment with intravenous acyclovir in doses of 30 mg/kg/d for at least 7 days or until all lesions are crusted.

Cytomegalovirus (CMV)

- Manifestations of CMV infection include retinitis, esophagitis, hepatitis, gastrointestinal involvement, and less commonly radiculopathy, encephalitis, and pneumonitis. CMV retinitis is usually associated with a painless progressive loss of vision. Patients may initially complain of blurry vision, loss of visual acuity, or "floaters."
- **Ganciclovir** therapy for CMV disease has traditionally been divided into two phases—induction and maintenance—because high relapse rates are found after discontinuation of the drug following successful completion of a 2- to 3-week course of initial therapy. Induction regimens are typically 7.5–10 mg/kg/d intravenously in two or three equally divided doses for 14 days, or longer if there is a slow clinical response. Maintenance therapy is usually 5–6 mg/kg once daily, although doses of 10 mg/kg have been used, 5–7 days/week for an indefinite period of time.
- The recommended dose of oral ganciclovir for maintenance therapy of CMV retinitis is 1000 mg tid taken with food. VIII
- **Foscarnet** is an alternative to ganciclovir that appears less likely to cause neutropenia; however, it has a variety of potential adverse effects, including renal insufficiency and metabolic disturbances (both increases and decreases) in calcium and phosphorus.
- Prophylaxis with oral ganciclovir should be considered in HIV-infected adults and adolescents who have a CD_4 cell count <50 cells/μL; ganciclovir prophylaxis is not a recommended standard of care.

See Chapter 114, Human Immunodeficiency Virus Infection, authored by Courtney V. Fletcher, PharmD, Thomas N. KaKuda, PharmD, and Ann C. Collier, MD, for a more detailed discussion of this topic.

Chapter 39

► INTRA-ABDOMINAL INFECTIONS

► DEFINITION

Intra-abdominal infections are those contained within the peritoneum or retroperitoneal space. Two general types of intra-abdominal infection are discussed throughout this chapter: peritonitis and abscess.

- Peritonitis is defined as the acute, inflammatory response of peritoneal lining to microorganisms, chemicals, irradiation, or foreign body injury. Peritonitis may be classified as either primary or secondary. With primary peritonitis, an intra-abdominal focus of disease may not be evident. In secondary peritonitis, a focal disease process is evident within the abdomen.
- An abscess is a purulent collection of fluid separated by a more or less well-defined wall from surrounding tissue. It usually contains necrotic debris, bacteria, and inflammatory cells.

► PATHOPHYSIOLOGY

- Table 39–1 summarizes many of the potential causes of bacterial peritonitis. The causes of intra-abdominal abscess somewhat overlap those of peritonitis and, in fact, both may occur sequentially or simultaneously. Appendicitis is the most frequent cause of abscess.
- Intra-abdominal infection results from entry of bacteria into the peritoneal or retroperitoneal spaces or from bacterial collections within intra-abdominal organs. When peritonitis results from peritoneal dialysis, skin surface flora are introduced via the peritoneal catheter.
- In secondary peritonitis, bacteria most often enter the peritoneum or retroperitoneum as a result of disruption of the integrity of the gastrointestinal tract caused by diseases or traumatic injuries.
- When bacteria become dispersed throughout the peritoneum, the inflammatory process involves the majority of the peritoneal lining.
- Peritonitis often results in mortality because of the effects on multiple organ systems. Fluid shifts and endotoxins may cause hypotension and shock. Fluid loss from the vasculature with generalized peritonitis is similar to that which occurs after a 50% second-degree skin burn.
- An abscess begins by the combined action of inflammatory cells (such as neutrophils), bacteria, fibrin, and other inflammatory components. A mature abscess may have a fibrinous capsule that isolates bacteria and the liquid core from antimicrobials and immunologic defenses.

TABLE 39–1. Causes of Bacterial Peritonitis

Primary Bacterial Peritonitis
- Peritoneal dialysis
- Cirrhosis with ascites

Secondary Bacterial Peritonitis
- Miscellaneous causes
  - Diverticulitis with perforation
  - Appendicitis
  - Inflammatory bowel diseases
  - Salpingitis
  - Biliary tract infections
  - Necrotizing pancreatitis
- Neoplasms
  - Intestinal obstruction
  - Perforation
- Mechanical gastrointestinal problems
  - Any cause of small bowel obstruction
- Vascular causes
  - Mesenteric arterial or venous occlusion
  - Mesenteric ischemia without occlusion
- Trauma
  - Blunt abdominal trauma with rupture of intestine
  - Penetrating abdominal trauma
  - Iatrogenic intestinal perforation
- Intraoperative events
  - Peritoneal contamination during abdominal operation
  - Leakage from gastrointestinal anastomosis

MICROBIOLOGY

- Primary bacterial peritonitis is often caused by a single organism. In children, the pathogen is usually *Streptococcus pneumoniae* or a group A streptococcus. When peritonitis occurs in association with cirrhotic ascites, enteric organisms (such as *Escherichia coli*) are usually responsible.
- Peritonitis in patients undergoing peritoneal dialysis is most often caused by common skin organisms: *Staphylococcus epidermidis, Staphylococcus aureus,* streptococci, and diphtheroids.
- Secondary intra-abdominal infections are often polymicrobial. The mean number of isolates of microorganisms from infected intra-abdominal sites has ranged from 2.5 to 5.0, including an average of 1.4 to 2.0 aerobes and 2.4 to 3.0 anaerobes. The frequencies with which specific bacteria were isolated in intra-abdominal infections are given in Table 39–2.
- The combination of aerobic and anaerobic organisms appears to greatly increase pathogenicity. In intra-abdominal infections, facultative bacteria may provide an environment conducive to the growth of anaerobic bacteria.
- Aerobic enteric bacteria and anaerobic bacteria are both pathogens in intra-abdominal infection. Aerobic bacteria, particularly *E. coli,* appear responsible for the early mortality from peritonitis, whereas anaerobic bacteria are major pathogens in abscesses, with *Bacteroides fragilis* predominating.
- The role of *Enterococcus* as a pathogen is not clear because it fails to produce peritonitis or abscesses when given alone in experimental animal models.

TABLE 39–2. Pathogens Isolated from 255 Patients With Intra-Abdominal Infections

Aerobic Bacteria	Number of Isolates	Anaerobic Bacteria	Number of Isolates
E. coli	140	*Bacteroides* sp.	305
Klebsiella sp.	33	*Peptostreptococcus*	78
Enterobacter sp.	19	*Fusobacterium*	48
Proteus sp.	15	*Clostridium*	35
Pseudomonas sp.	33	*Prevotella*	27
Streptococcus	184	*Gemella*	26
Enterococcus	35	*Porphyromonas*	18
Staphylococcus	34		
Others	24		

▶ CLINICAL PRESENTATION

VIII

PERITONITIS

- With generalized bacterial peritonitis, the patient most often presents in acute distress. The patient lies still, usually on his or her back, possibly with hips slightly flexed. The patient exhibits voluntary guarding of the abdomen, and respirations are shallow and frequent. There is generalized abdominal tenderness on examination, and after a short period of time, the abdominal muscles become rigid ("board-like abdomen"). Because of the fluid loss into the peritoneum and vomiting, the patient may appear dehydrated, and a decreased urine output is noted. Temperature may progress from normal up to 103°F.
- If peritonitis continues untreated, the patient may go into hypovolemic shock from fluid loss into the peritoneum. This may be accompanied by generalized sepsis.
- Laboratory evaluations with peritonitis usually demonstrate leukocytosis.
- Abdominal radiographs may be useful, as free air in the abdomen (indicating intestinal perforation) or distention of the small or large bowel is often evident.
- Primary peritonitis can develop over a period of days to weeks, evident as an acute febrile illness. Usually the patient has nausea, vomiting (sometimes with diarrhea), abdominal tenderness, and hypoactive bowel sounds, although the abdominal signs are variable. The patient's temperature or WBC count may be only mildly elevated. The cirrhotic patient may have worsening encephalopathy.

- Patients with peritonitis related to chronic peritoneal dialysis (CPD) usually have abdominal pain and tenderness, possibly with nausea and vomiting, but fever is not a consistent finding. In these patients, a cloudy dialysate drainage is often noted as a first sign of peritonitis indicating the presence of bacteria and inflammatory cells.

ABSCESS

- The patient with an intra-abdominal abscess may complain of abdominal pain or discomfort, but these symptoms are not reliable.
- Plain radiographs may show air–fluid levels or may demonstrate the shift of normal intra-abdominal contents by the abscess mass. Computed tomography (CT) and magnetic resonance imaging may be used to locate some intra-abdominal abscesses.

▶ DESIRED OUTCOME

- The goals of treatment are the correction of intra-abdominal disease processes or injuries that have caused infection and the drainage of collections of purulent material (e.g., abscess).
- Secondary goals are the prevention of dissemination of infection to sites outside the abdomen and reinfection in the abdomen. Ideally, treatment would be completed without significant complications such as organ dysfunction or adverse drug reactions. VIII

▶ TREATMENT

GENERAL PRINCIPLES

- The three major modalities for the treatment of intra-abdominal infection are prompt drainage, support of vital functions, and appropriate antimicrobial therapy.
- Antimicrobials are an important adjunct to surgical procedures in the treatment of intra-abdominal infections; however, the use of antimicrobial agents without surgical intervention is usually inadequate. For some specific situations (e.g., most cases of primary peritonitis), drainage procedures may not be required, and antimicrobial agents become the mainstay of therapy.
- With generalized peritonitis, large volumes of intravenous fluids are required to restore vascular volume and improve cardiovascular function.

NONPHARMACOLOGIC TREATMENT

- Secondary peritonitis requires surgical correction of the underlying pathology. Drainage of the purulent material, either by open surgical procedure or drained percutaneously, is the critical element in the management of an intra-abdominal abscess.

- Aggressive fluid repletion and management are required for the purposes of achieving or maintaining proper intravascular volumes and adequate urine output and correcting acidosis.
- In the initial hour of treatment, a large volume of solution (4 L or more) may need to be administered to restore intravascular volume.
- In patients with significant blood loss (hematocrit of 25%), blood should be given. This is generally in the form of packed red blood cells.

PHARMACOLOGIC THERAPY

- The goals of antimicrobial therapy are to control bacteremia and to establish the metastatic foci of infection, to reduce suppurative complications after bacterial contamination, and to prevent local spread of existing infection.
- An empiric antimicrobial regimen should be started as soon as the presence of intra-abdominal infection is suspected based on the likely pathogens.
- Likely pathogens, those against which antimicrobial agents should be directed, are listed in Table 39–3.
- Table 39–4 presents recommended and alternative regimens for selected situations. These are general guidelines, not rules, because there are many factors that cannot be incorporated into such a table.

VIII Recommendations

- Most patients with severe intra-abdominal infections (where there is generalized peritonitis or septic shock or where the patient has a high fever and shaking chills) should be placed on an antianaerobic cephalosporin with or without **metronidazole,** a carbapenem, or a penicillin/β-lactamase inhibitor combination. An aminoglycoside with an antianaerobic agent such as **clindamycin** or metronidazole are alternatives.
- The selection of a specific agent or combination should be based on culture and susceptibility data for peritonitis that occurs from chronic peritoneal dialysis. If microbiologic data are unavailable, empiric therapy as listed in Table 39–4 should be initiated.
- Patients with peritonitis who are undergoing CPD may receive parenteral as well as intraperitoneal antimicrobial agents. Intraperitoneal antimicrobial agents alone are often sufficient, unless severe infection is present. Recommended concentrations of antimicrobial agents for intraperitoneal irrigation solutions are 8 mg/L for **gentamicin** and **tobramycin,** 1–3 mg/L for **clindamycin,** 50,000 U/L for **penicillin G,** 125 mg/L for **cephalosporins,** 100–150 mg/L for **ticarcillin** or **carbenicillin,** 50 mg/L for **ampicillin,** 100 mg/L for **methicillin,** 30 mg/L for **vancomycin,** and 3 mg/L for **amphotericin B.**
- The usual duration of therapy for peritonitis associated with CPD is 10–14 days but may extend to 3 weeks. Antimicrobial therapy should be continued until dialysate fluid is clear, cultures are negative for 2–3 days, and the patient is asymptomatic.

TABLE 39–3. Likely Intra-Abdominal Pathogens

Type of Infection	Aerobes	Anaerobes
Primary Bacterial Peritonitis		
Children (spontaneous)	Pneumococci, group A *Streptococcus*	—
Cirrhosis	*E. coli*, *Klebsiella*, pneumococci (many others)	—
Peritoneal dialysis	*Staphylococcus*, *Streptococcus*	—
Secondary Bacterial Peritonitis		
Gastroduodenal	*Streptococcus*, *E. coli*	—
Biliary tract	*E. coli*, *Klebsiella*, enterococci	*Clostridium* or *Bacteroides* (infrequent)
Small or large bowel	*E. coli*, *Klebsiella* sp., *Proteus* sp.	*Bacteroides fragilis* and other *Bacteroides*, *Clostridium*
Appendicitis	*E. coli*, *Pseudomonas*	*Bacteroides* sp.
Abscesses	*E. coli*, *Klebsiella*, enterococci	*B. fragilis* and other *Bacteroides*, *Clostridium*, anaerobic cocci
Liver	*E. coli*, *Klebsiella*, enterococci, staphylococci, amoeba	*Bacteroides* (infrequent)
Spleen	*Staphylococcus*, *Streptococcus*	

- Antianaerobic cephalosporins or extended-spectrum penicillins are effective in preventing most infectious complications after acute bacterial contamination, such as with abdominal trauma where gastrointestinal contents enter the peritoneum, and when the patient is seen soon after injury (within 2 hours) and surgical measures are instituted promptly.
- Acute intra-abdominal contamination, such as after a traumatic injury, may be treated with a short course (24 hours). For established infections (peritonitis or intra-abdominal abscess), an antimicrobial course of at least 7 days is justified.

▶ EVALUATION OF THERAPEUTIC OUTCOMES

- The patient should be continually reassessed to determine the success or failure of therapies.
- Unsatisfactory outcomes in patients with intra-abdominal infections may result from complications that arise in other organ systems. A complication commonly associated with mortality after intra-abdominal infection is pneumonia.
- Once antimicrobials are initiated and other important therapies described before are used, most patients should show improvement

TABLE 39–4. Recommendations for Initial Antimicrobial Agents for Intra-Abdominal Infections

Infection Type	Primary Agents	Comments/Alternatives
Primary Bacterial Peritonitis		
Cirrhosis	Cefotaxime	1. Add clindamycin or metronidazole if anaerobes are suspected 2. Other third-generation cephalosporins, extended-spectrum penicillins, aztreonam, and imipenem as alternatives 3. Aminoglycoside with antipseudomonal penicillin
Peritoneal dialysis	Regimen based on organism isolated 1. *Staphylococcus:* penicillinase-resistant penicillin or first-generation cephalosporin 2. *Streptococcus:* penicillin G 3. Aerobic gram-negative bacilli: cefotaxime, ceftazidime, or aminoglycoside plus an antipseudomonal penicillin 4. *Pseudomonas aeruginosa:* aminoglycoside plus antipseudomonal penicillin or ceftazidime	1. Alternative for resistant staphylococci is vancomycin 2. Alternative for *Streptococcus* is a first-generation cephalosporin 3. Alternatives for gram-negative bacilli are other third-generation cephalosporins, aztreonam, and extended-spectrum penicillins with β-lactamase inhibitors
Secondary Bacterial Peritonitis		
Perforated peptic ulcer	First-generation cephalosporins	1. Antianaerobic cephalosporins[a] 2. Possibly add aminoglycoside if patient condition is poor
Other	Imipenem/cilistatin, antianaerobic cephalosporins[a] Extended-spectrum penicillins with β-lactamase inhibitor	1. Aminoglycoside with clindamycin or metronidazole, add ampicillin if patient is immunocompromised or if biliary tract origin of infection 2. Aztreonam with clindamycin 3. Antianaerobic cephalosporins, an extended-spectrum penicillin with β-lactamase inhibitor

Abscess		
General	Imipenem/cilistatin, antianaerobic cephalosporins[a],or Extended-spectrum penicillins with β-lactamase inhibitor	1. Aztreonam with clindamycin, or extended-spectrum penicillins with β-lactamase inhibitor, as alternatives 2. Aminoglycoside with clindamycin or metronidazole, possibly add ampicillin
Liver	As above but add a first-generation cephalosporin	3. Use metronidazole if amoebic liver abscess is suspected
Spleen	Aminoglycoside plus penicillinase-resistant penicillin	4. Alternatives for penicillinase-resistant penicillin are first-generation cephalosporins or vancomycin
Appendicitis		
Normal or inflamed	Antianaerobic cephalosporins[a] (discontinued immediately postoperation)	1. Aminoglycoside with clindamycin or metronidazole
Gangrenous or perforated	Imipenem/cilistatin, antianaerobic cephalosporins[a] or extended-spectrum penicillins with β-lactamase inhibitor	1. Aztreonam with clindamycin, or imipenem alone 2. Aminoglycoside with clindamycin or metronidazole
Acute Cholecystitis	First-generation cephalosporin	Aminoglycoside plus ampicillin if severe infection
Cholangitis	Aminoglycoside with ampicillin with or without clindamycin or metronidazole	Use vancomycin for ampicillin if patient is allergic to penicillin
Acute Contamination from Abdominal Trauma	Antianaerobic cephalosporins[a] or extended-spectrum penicillins	Aminoglycoside with one of the following: clindamycin, metronidazole, or antianaerobic cephalosporins[a]

[a]Cefoxitin, cefotetan, ceftizoxime, and cefmetazole.

within 2–3 days. Usually, temperature will return to near normal, vital signs should stabilize, and the patient should not appear in distress, with the exception of recognized discomfort and pain from incisions, drains, and nasogastric tube.

- At 24–48 hours, aerobic bacterial culture results should return. If a suspected pathogen is not sensitive to the antimicrobial agents being given, the regimen should be changed if the patient has not shown sufficient progress.
- If the isolated pathogen is extremely sensitive to one antimicrobial, and the patient is progressing well, concurrent antimicrobial therapy may often be discontinued.
- With present anaerobic culturing techniques and the slow growth of these organisms, anaerobes are often not identified until 4–7 days after culture, and sensitivity information is difficult to obtain. For this reason, there are usually few data with which to alter the antianaerobic component of the antimicrobial regimen.
- Superinfection in patients being treated for intra-abdominal infection is often due to *Candida,* but enterococci or opportunistic gram-negative bacilli such as *Pseudomonas* or *Serratia* may be involved.
- Treatment regimens for intra-abdominal infection can be judged successful if the patient recovers from the infection without recurrent peritonitis or intra-abdominal abscess and without the need for additional antimicrobials. A regimen can be considered unsuccessful if a significant adverse drug reaction occurs, if reoperation is necessary, or if patient improvement is delayed beyond 1 or 2 weeks.

See Chapter 104, Intra-Abdominal Infections, authored by Joseph T. DiPiro, PharmD, FCCP, and David A. Rogers, MD, FACS, FAAP, for a more detailed discussion of this topic.

Chapter 40

► RESPIRATORY TRACT INFECTIONS, LOWER

Lower respiratory tract infections include infectious processes of the lungs and bronchi, pneumonia, bronchitis, and lung abscess.

► BRONCHITIS

ACUTE BRONCHITIS

- Bronchitis refers to an inflammatory condition of the tracheobronchial tree that is usually associated with a generalized respiratory infection. The inflammatory process does not extend to include the alveoli. The disease entity is frequently classified as either acute or chronic.
- Acute bronchitis most commonly occurs during the winter months. Cold, damp climates and/or the presence of high concentrations of irritating substances such as air pollution or cigarette smoke may precipitate attacks.

PATHOPHYSIOLOGY

- Respiratory viruses are by far the most common infectious agents associated with acute bronchitis. The common cold viruses, rhinovirus and coronavirus, and lower respiratory tract pathogens, including influenza virus, adenovirus, and respiratory syncytial virus, account for the majority of cases. *Mycoplasma pneumoniae* also appears to be a frequent cause of acute bronchitis. More recently, a new *Chlamydia psittaci* strain, often denoted as TWAR or *Chlamydia pneumoniae,* has been associated with acute respiratory tract infections.
- Infection of the trachea and bronchi causes an increase in bronchial secretions. Destruction of respiratory epithelium can range from mild to extensive and may affect bronchial mucociliary function. In addition, the increase in bronchial secretions, which can become thick and tenacious, further impairs mucociliary activity. Recurrent acute respiratory infections may be associated with increased airway hyperreactivity and possibly the pathogenesis of chronic obstructive lung disease.

CLINICAL PRESENTATION

- Cough is the hallmark of acute bronchitis and occurs early. The onset of cough may be insidious or abrupt and will persist despite the resolution of nasal or nasopharyngeal complaints. Frequently, the cough is initially nonproductive but progresses, yielding mucopurulent sputum.
- Initial physical examination usually reveals a variable degree of rhinitis. Chest examination may reveal rhonchi and coarse, moist rales bilaterally. Chest radiographs, when performed, are usually normal.

- Bacterial cultures of expectorated sputum are generally of limited utility due to the inability to avoid normal nasopharyngeal flora by the sampling technique. In routine cases, viral cultures are unnecessary and frequently unavailable. Cultures or serologic diagnosis of *M. pneumoniae* and culture or direct fluorescent antibody detection for *Bordetella pertussis* should be obtained in prolonged or severe cases when epidemiologic considerations would suggest their involvement.

▶ DESIRED OUTCOMES

- The goals of therapy are to provide comfort to the patient and to treat associated dehydration and respiratory compromise.

TREATMENT

- The treatment of acute bronchitis is symptomatic and supportive in nature. Bed rest and mild analgesic–antipyretic therapy are often helpful in relieving the associated lethargy, malaise, and fever. **Aspirin** or **acetaminophen** (650 mg in adults or 10–15 mg/kg per dose in children) or **ibuprofen** (200–400 mg in adults or 10 mg/kg per dose in children) is administered every 4–6 hours.
- Patients should be encouraged to drink fluids to prevent dehydration and possibly decrease the viscosity of respiratory secretions.

VIII

- In children, aspirin should be avoided and acetaminophen used as the preferred agent because of the possible association between aspirin use and the development of Reye's syndrome.
- Mist therapy and/or the use of a vaporizer may further promote the thinning and loosening of respiratory secretions.
- Persistent, mild cough, which may be bothersome, may be treated with **dextromethorphan;** more severe coughs may require intermittent **codeine** or other similar agents.
- Routine use of antibiotics in the treatment of acute bronchitis is discouraged; however, in patients who exhibit persistent fever or respiratory symptomatology for more than 4–6 days, the possibility of a concurrent bacterial infection should be suspected.
- When possible, antibiotic therapy is directed toward anticipated respiratory pathogen(s) (i.e., *Streptococcus pneumoniae, Haemophilus influenzae*) and/or those demonstrating a predominant growth upon throat culture.
- *Mycoplasma pneumoniae*, if suspected by history or positive cold agglutinins (titers ≥1 : 32), or if confirmed by culture or serology, may be treated with **erythromycin** or its analogs (e.g., **clarithromycin** or **azithromycin**).
- During known epidemics involving the influenza A virus, **amantadine** or **rimantadine** may be effective in minimizing associated symptomatology if administered early in the course of the disease.

CHRONIC BRONCHITIS

- Chronic bronchitis is a nonspecific disease that primarily affects adults.

Pathogenesis

- Current data and experience suggest that chronic bronchitis is a result of several contributing factors including cigarette smoking; exposure to occupational dusts, fumes, and environmental pollution; and bacterial (and possibly viral) infection.
- In chronic bronchitis, the bronchial wall is thickened and the number of mucus-secreting goblet cells in the surface epithelium of both larger and smaller bronchi is markedly increased. Hypertrophy of the mucus glands and dilatation of the mucus gland ducts are also observed.
- As a result of these changes, chronic bronchitics have substantially more mucus in their peripheral airways, further impairing normal lung defenses and causing mucus plugging of the smaller airways.
- Continued progression of this pathology can result in residual scarring of small bronchi, augmenting airway obstruction, and the weakening of bronchial walls.

Clinical Presentation

- The hallmark of chronic bronchitis is cough that may range from a mild "smoker's" cough to severe incessant coughing productive of purulent sputum. Expectoration of the largest quantity of sputum usually occurs upon arising in the morning, although many patients expectorate sputum throughout the day. The expectorated sputum is usually tenacious and can vary in color from white to yellow-green.
- The diagnosis of chronic bronchitis is based primarily on clinical assessment and history. By definition, any patient who reports the coughing up of sputum on most days for at least 3 consecutive months each year for 2 consecutive years suffers from chronic bronchitis.
- With the exception of pulmonary findings, the physical examination of patients with mild to moderate chronic bronchitis is usually unremarkable. Chest auscultation usually reveals inspiratory and expiratory rales, rhonchi, and mild wheezing with an expiratory phase that is frequently prolonged. Normal vesicular breathing sounds are diminished. Depending on the severity of the disease, an increase in the anteroposterior diameter of the thoracic cage (observed as a "barrel chest"), hyperresonance on percussion with obliteration of the area of cardiac dullness, and depressed diaphragms with limited mobility are often observed.
- An increased number of polymorphonuclear granulocytes in sputum often suggest continual bronchial irritation, whereas an increased number of eosinophils may suggest an allergic component. The most common bacterial isolates identified from sputum culture in patients experiencing an acute exacerbation of chronic bronchitis are outlined in Table 40–1.

TABLE 40–1. Common Bacterial Pathogens Isolated from the Sputum of Patients with an Acute Exacerbation of Chronic Bronchitis

Pathogen	Estimated Incidence[a]
Haemophilus influenzae[b]	24–26
Haemophilus parainfluenzae	20
Streptococcus pneumoniae	15
Moraxella catarrhalis[b]	15
Klebsiella pneumoniae	4
Serratia marcescens	2
Neisseria meningitidis[b]	2
Pseudomonas aeruginosa	2

[a]Expressed as percent of cultures.
[b]Often β-lactamase positive.

Desired Outcome

- The goals of therapy for chronic bronchitis are to reduce the severity of symptoms and to ameliorate acute exacerbations and to achieve prolonged infection-free intervals.

VIII Treatment

General Principles

- A complete occupational/environmental history for the determination of exposure to noxious, irritating gases, as well as cigarette smoking, must be assessed. Attempts must be made to reduce exposure to bronchial irritants.
- Humidification of inspired air may promote the hydration (liquefaction) of tenacious secretions allowing for more effective sputum production. The use of mucolytic aerosols (e.g., ***N*-acetylcysteine; DNAse**) is of questionable therapeutic value.
- Postural drainage may assist in promoting clearance of pulmonary secretions.

Pharmacologic Therapy

- Oral or aerosolized bronchodilators (e.g., **albuterol** aerosol) may be of benefit to some patients during acute pulmonary exacerbations.
- The use of antimicrobials has been controversial, although antibiotics are an important component of treatment. Agents should be selected that are effective against likely pathogens, have the lowest risk of drug interactions, and can be administered in a manner that promotes compliance (Table 40–2).
- Antibiotics commonly used in the treatment of these patients and their respective adult starting doses are outlined in Table 40–3. Duration of symptom-free periods may be enhanced by antibiotic regimens using the upper limit of the recommended daily dose for 10–14 days.

TABLE 40–2. Useful Classification System for Patients with Chronic Bronchitis and Initial Treatment Options

Baseline Status	Criteria or Risk Factors	Usual Pathogens		Initial Treatment Options
Class I				
Acute tracheobronchitis	No underlying structural disease	Usually a virus	1st	None unless symptoms persist
			2nd	Amoxicillin or a macrolide/azithromycin
Class II				
Chronic bronchitis	$FEV_1 > 50\%$ predicted value, increased sputum volume and purulence	*Haemophilus influenzae, Haemophilus* sp., *Moraxella catarrhalis, Streptococcus pneumoniae* (β-lactam resistance possible)	1st	Amoxicillin or quinolone if prevalence of *H. influenzae* resistance to amoxicillin is > 20%
			2nd	Quinolone, amoxicillin–clavulanate, azithromycin, tetracycline, or trimethoprim–sulfamethoxazole
Class III				
Chronic bronchitis with complications	$FEV_1 < 50\%$ predicted value, increased sputum volume and purulence, advanced age, at least four flares/year, or significant comorbidity	Same as class II; also *Klebsiella pneumoniae, Pseudomonas aeruginosa, K. pneumoniae,* and other gram-negative organisms (β-lactam resistance common)	1st	Quinolone
			2nd	Expanded-spectrum cephalosporin, amoxicillin–clavulanate, or azithromycin
Class IV				
Chronic bronchial infection	Same as for class III plus yearlong production of purulent sputum	Same as class III	1st	Oral or parenteral quinolone, carbapenem or expanded-spectrum cephalosporin followed by high-dose oral ciprofloxacin or routine-dose trovafloxacin

1st = first choices; 2nd = alternate treatment options.
Quinolone: ciprofloxacin, clinafloxacin, grepafloxacin, trovafloxacin.
Tetracycline: tetracycline HCl, doxycycline.
Carbapenem: imipenem/cilistatin, meropenem.
Expanded-spectrum cephalosporin: ceftazidime, cefepime.

TABLE 40–3. Oral Antibiotics Commonly Used for the Treatment of Acute Respiratory Exacerbations in Chronic Bronchitis

Antibiotic	Usual Adult Dose (g)	Dose Schedule (doses/d)
Preferred Drugs		
Ampicillin	0.5–1	4
Amoxicillin	0.5–1	2–3
Ciprofloxacin	0.5–0.75	2
Ofloxacin	0.2–0.4	2
Doxycycline	0.1	2
Minocycline	0.1	2
Tetracycline HCl	0.5	4
Amoxicillin–clavulanate	0.5	3
Trimethoprim–sulfamethoxazole	1 DS[a]	2
Lomefloxacin	0.4	1
Supplemental Drugs		
Erythromycin	0.5	4
Clarithromycin	0.25–0.5	2
Cephalexin	0.5	4
Cefaclor	0.25–0.5	3

VIII [a]DS, double-strength tablet (160 trimethoprim/800 mg sulfamethoxazole).

- **Ampicillin** is often considered the drug of choice for the treatment of acute exacerbations of chronic bronchitis. Unfortunately, the need for multiple repeat daily doses (four times daily) and the increasing incidence of penicillin-resistant β-lactamase–producing strains of bacteria have limited the usefulness of this safe and cost-effective antibiotic.
- The value of macrolides when *Mycoplasma* is involved is unquestioned. **Azithromycin** should be considered as the macrolide of choice for *Mycoplasma*.
- The **fluoroquinolones** are effective alternative agents for adults, particularly when gram-negative pathogens are involved.
- The decision to use antibiotics for the prevention and/or treatment of an acute exacerbation of chronic bronchitis should be made on an individual patient-specific basis. In those patients whose history suggests recurrent exacerbations of their disease that might be attributable to certain specific events (i.e., seasonal-winter months), a trial of prophylactic antibiotics might be beneficial. If no clinical improvement is noted over an appropriate period (e.g., 2–3 months per year for 2–3 years), one might elect to discontinue further attempts at prophylactic therapy.

BRONCHIOLITIS

- Bronchiolitis is an acute viral infection of the lower respiratory tract of infants that shows a definite seasonal pattern (peaks during the winter months and persists through early spring). The disease most commonly affects infants during the first year of life.
- Respiratory syncytial virus is the most common cause of bronchiolitis, accounting for 45–60% of all cases. Parainfluenza viruses are the second most common etiologic. Bacteria serve as secondary pathogens in only a small minority of cases.

Clinical Presentation

- The most common clinical signs of bronchiolitis are cough and coryza. As symptoms progress, infants may experience vomiting, diarrhea, noisy breathing, and an increase in respiratory rate.
- For those infants presenting to a hospital, examination reveals a rapid pulse and a respiratory rate between 40 and 80 breaths per minute. Breathing is labored with retractions of the chest wall, nasal flaring, and grunting. Chest auscultation reveals wheezing and inspiratory rales.
- As a result of limited oral intake due to coughing combined with vomiting and diarrhea, infants are frequently dehydrated.
- The diagnosis of bronchiolitis is based primarily on history and clinical findings. The ability to identify specific viral pathogens is often hindered by the limited availability of special virology laboratories. VIII
- The peripheral WBC count is usually normal or only slightly elevated.
- Hypoxemia is common and acts to increase the respiratory drive, whereas hypercarbia is seen only in the most severe cases.
- ELISA (enzyme-linked immunosorbent assays) or fluorescent antibody staining of nasopharyngeal secretions can identify viral pathogens in a few hours.

Treatment

- Bronchiolitis is a self-limiting illness and usually requires no therapy unless the infant is hypoxic or dehydrated.
- In severely affected children, the mainstays of therapy for bronchiolitis are oxygen therapy and intravenous fluids.
- Aerosolized β-adrenergic therapy appears to offer little benefit for the majority of patients, but may be useful in the child with a predisposition toward bronchospasm.
- Because bacteria do not represent primary pathogens in the etiology of bronchiolitis, antibiotics should not be routinely administered. However, many clinicians frequently administer antibiotics initially while awaiting culture results because the clinical and radiographic findings in bronchiolitis are often suggestive of a possible bacterial pneumonia.
- **Ribavirin** may offer an effective therapy for bronchiolitis although it is approved only in aerosolized form against respiratory syncytial virus. Use of the drug requires special equipment (small-particle aerosol gen-

erator) and specifically trained personnel for administration via oxygen hood or mist tent. Use of ribavirin should be reserved for more severely ill patients, including those with chronic lung disease (particularly bronchopulmonary dysplasia), congenital heart disease, prematurity, and immunodeficiency (especially severe combined immunodeficiency and HIV infection); ribavirin also should be considered in any patient requiring mechanical ventilation.

▶ PNEUMONIA

- Pneumonia occurs throughout the year, with the relative prevalence of disease resulting from different etiologic agents varying with the seasons. It occurs in persons of all ages, although the clinical manifestations are most severe in the very young, the elderly, and the chronically ill.

PATHOGENESIS

- Microorganisms gain access to the lower respiratory tract by three routes: They may be inhaled as aerosolized particles; they may enter the lung via the bloodstream from an extrapulmonary site of infection; or aspiration of oropharyngeal contents may occur.
- Lung infections with viruses suppress the bacterial clearing activity of the lung by impairing alveolar macrophage function and mucociliary clearance, thus setting the stage for secondary bacterial pneumonia.
- The vast majority of pneumonia cases acquired in the community by otherwise healthy adults are due to *S. pneumoniae* (Pneumococcus) or *M. pneumoniae* (up to 70% and 10–20% of all acute bacterial pneumonias in the United States, respectively). Community-acquired pneumonias caused by *Staphylococcus aureus* and gram-negative rods are observed primarily in the elderly, especially those residing in nursing homes, and in association with alcoholism and other debilitating conditions.
- Gram-negative aerobic bacilli and *S. aureus* are also the leading causative agents in hospital-acquired pneumonia.
- Anaerobic bacteria are the most common etiologic agents in pneumonia that follows the gross aspiration of gastric or oropharyngeal contents.
- Most pneumonias in the pediatric age group are due to viruses, especially respiratory syncytial virus, parainfluenza, and adenovirus.

CLINICAL PRESENTATION

Gram-Positive and Gram-Negative Bacterial Pneumonia

- Typically the onset of illness is abrupt or subacute, with fever, chills, dyspnea, and productive cough predominating. Pneumococcus, *Staphylococcus,* the enteric gram-negative rods, and occasionally other organisms may produce local irritation or destruction of blood vessels leading to rust-colored sputum or hemoptysis.

- On physical examination, the patient is tachypneic and tachycardiac, frequently with chest wall retractions and grunting respirations. There are diminished break sounds on auscultation over the affected area accompanied by inspiratory crackles as pus-filled alveoli open during lung expansion.
- The chest radiograph and sputum examination and culture are the most useful diagnostic tests in gram-positive and gram-negative bacterial pneumonia. Gram stain of the expectorated sputum demonstrates many polymorphonuclear cells per high-powered field in the presence of a predominant organism, which is reflected in heavy growth of a single species on culture.
- The complete blood count usually reflects a leukocytosis with a predominance of polymorphonuclear cells. However, normal or mildly elevated WBC counts do not exclude bacterial pneumonic disease. The patient may also be hypoxic as reflected by low oxygen saturation on arterial blood gas or pulse oximetry.

Legionella pneumophila

- Infection with *L. pneumophila* is characterized by multisystem involvement, including rapidly progressive pneumonia. It has a gradual onset, with prominent constitutional symptoms such as malaise, lethargy, weakness, and anorexia occurring early in the course of the illness. A dry, nonproductive cough is initially present, which, during several days, becomes productive of mucoid or purulent sputum. Fevers exceed 40°C and are typically unremitting and associated with a relative bradycardia. Pleuritic chest pain and progressive dyspnea may be seen, and fine rales are found on lung exam, progressing to signs of frank consolidation later in the course of the illness. Extrapulmonary manifestations remain evident throughout the course of the illness and include diarrhea, nausea, vomiting, myalgias, and arthralgias.
- Substantial changes in a patient's mental status, often out of proportion to the degree of fever, are seen in approximately one-fourth of patients. Obtundation, hallucinations, grand mal seizures, and focal neurologic findings have also been associated with this illness.
- Laboratory findings include leukocytosis with predominance of mature and immature granulocytes in 50–75% of patients. Urinalysis may reveal proteinuria, hematuria, and casts; liver function tests may be abnormal. Because *L. pneumophila* stains poorly with commonly used stains, routine microscopic examination of sputum is of little diagnostic value. Fluorescent antibody testing can be performed to diagnose Legionnaires' disease.

Anaerobic Pneumonia

- The course of anaerobic pneumonia is typically indolent with cough, low-grade fever, and weight loss, although an acute presentation may occur. Putrid sputum, when present, is highly suggestive of the diagnosis. Chest radiographs reveal infiltrates typically located in dependent lung segments, and lung abscesses develop in 20% of patients 1–2 weeks into the course of the illness.

Mycoplasma pneumoniae

- *Mycloplasma pneumoniae* pneumonia presents with a gradual onset of fever, headache, and malaise, with the appearance 3–5 days after the onset of illness of a persistent, hacking cough that initially is nonproductive. Sore throat, ear pain, and rhinorrhea are often present. Lung findings are generally limited to rales and rhonchi; findings of consolidation are rarely present.
- Nonpulmonary manifestations are extremely common and include nausea, vomiting, diarrhea, myalgias, arthralgias, polyarticular arthritis, skin rashes, myocarditis and pericarditis, hemolytic anemia, meningoencephalitis, cranial neuropathies, and Guillain-Barré syndrome. Systemic symptoms generally clear in 1–2 weeks, while respiratory symptoms may persist up to 4 weeks.
- Radiographic findings include patchy or interstitial infiltrates, which are most commonly seen in the lower lobes. Small unilateral, transient pleural effusions are common, but large effusions and empyema are rare. Roentgenographic abnormalities resolve slowly, and 4–6 weeks may be required for complete resolution.
- Sputum Gram stain may reveal mononuclear or polymorphonuclear leukocytes, with no predominant organism. While *M. pneumoniae* can be cultured from respiratory secretions using specialized medium, 2–3 weeks may be necessary for culture identification.
- Indirect evidence of infection by *M. pneumoniae* is the presence of elevated levels of serum cold hemagglutinins. A definitive diagnosis can also be made by demonstrating a fourfold or greater rise in serum antibodies to *M. pneumoniae;* however, this test also requires 2–4 weeks for results.

Viral Pneumonia

- The clinical pictures produced by respiratory viruses are sufficiently variable and overlap to such a degree that an etiologic diagnosis cannot confidently be made on clinical grounds alone. Serologic tests for virus-specific antibodies are often used in the diagnosis of viral infections. The diagnostic four-fold rise in titer between acute and convalescent phase sera may require 2–3 weeks to develop; however, same-day diagnosis of viral infections is now possible through the use of indirect immunofluorescence tests on exfoliated cells from the respiratory tract.
- Radiographic findings are nonspecific and include bronchial wall thickening and perihilar and diffuse interstitial infiltrates.
- Pleural effusions may be seen especially in adenovirus and parainfluenza pneumonia.

Nosocomial Pneumonia

- The strongest predisposing factor for nosocomial pneumonia is mechanical ventilation. Risk is increased by prior antibiotic use, use of H_2-receptor blocking agents, and severe illness.
- The diagnosis of nosocomial pneumonia is usually established by presence of a new infiltrate on chest radiograph, fever, and worsening respiratory status.

DESIRED OUTCOME

- Eradication of the offending organism and clinical resolution.
- Associated morbidity should be minimized (e.g., renal, pulmonary, or hepatic dysfunction).

TREATMENT

- The supportive care of the patient with pneumonia includes the use of humidified oxygen for hypoxemia, fluid resuscitation, administration of bronchodilators when bronchospasm is present, and chest physiotherapy with postural drainage if there is evidence of retained secretions.
- Important therapeutic adjuncts include adequate hydration (by intravenous route if necessary), optimal nutritional support, and fever control.
- The treatment of bacterial pneumonia initially involves the empiric use of a relatively broad-spectrum antibiotic (or antibiotics) that is effective against probable pathogens after appropriate cultures and specimens for laboratory evaluation have been obtained. VIII
- Therapy should be narrowed to cover specific pathogens once the results of cultures are known.
- Appropriate empiric choices for the treatment of bacterial pneumonias relative to a patient's underlying disease are shown in Table 40–4 for adults and Table 40–5 for children.
- Antibiotic concentrations in respiratory secretions in excess of the pathogen minimum inhibitory concentration (MIC) are necessary for successful treatment of pulmonary infections.
- The benefit of antibiotic aerosols or direct endotracheal instillation has not been consistently demonstrated.
- Prevention of pneumonia is possible through the use of vaccines against *S. pneumoniae* and *H. influenzae* type B. In addition, **amantadine** may be administered for prevention of influenza A infection, beginning as soon as possible after exposure and continuing for at least 10 days.

▶ EVALUATION OF THERAPEUTIC OUTCOMES

- With community-acquired pneumonia, time to resolution of cough, sputum production, and presence of constitutional symptoms (e.g., malaise, nausea/vomiting, lethargy) should be assessed. Progress should be noted in the first 2 days with complete resolution in 5–7 days.

TABLE 40–4. Empiric Antimicrobial Therapy for Pneumonia in Adults[a]

Clinical Setting	Usual Pathogen(s)	Presumptive Therapy
Previously healthy, ambulatory patient	*Pneumococcus, Mycoplasma pneumoniae*	Macrolide/azilide,[b] tetracycline[c]
Elderly	*Pneumococcus,* gram-negative bacilli (e.g., *Klebsiella pneumoniae*), *Staphylococcus aureus, Haemophilus influenzae*	Ticarcillin/clavulanate, piperacillin/tazobactam, cephalosporin[d]; carbapenem[e]
Chronic bronchitis	*Pneumococcus, H. influenzae, Moraxella catarrhalis*	Amoxicillin, tetracycline,[c] TMP–SMX,[f] cefuroxime, cefprozil, amoxicillin/clavulanate, macrolide/azilide,[b] quinolone
Alcoholism	*Pneumococcus, K. pneumoniae, S. aureus, H. influenzae,* possibly mouth anaerobes	Ticarcillin/clavulanate, piperacillin/tazobactam, **plus** aminoglycoside; carbapenem[e]
Aspiration		
Community	Mouth anaerobes	Penicillin or clindamycin
Hospital/residential care	Mouth anaerobes, *S. aureus,* gram-negative enterics	Clindamycin, ticarcillin/clavulanate, piperacillin/tazobactam, **plus** aminoglycoside
Nosocomial pneumonia	Gram-negative bacilli (e.g., *K. pneumonia, Enterobacter* sp., *Pseudomonas aeruginosa),* *S. aureus*	Ticarcillin/clavulanate, piperacillin/tazobactam, carbapenem[e] or expanded-spectrum cephalosporin[g] **plus** aminoglycoside

[a]See section on Treatment of Bacterial Pneumonia.
[b]Macrolide/azilide: erythromycin, clarithromycin/azithromycin.
[c]Tetracycline: tetracycline HCl, doxycycline.
[d]Cephalosporin: (e.g., cefuroxime, ceftriaxone, cefotaxime).
[e]Carbapenem: imipenem/cilistatin, meropenem.
[f]TMP–SMX, trimethoprim–sulfamethoxazole.
[g]Expanded-spectrum cephalosporin: ceftazidime, cefepime.
[h]Cephalosporin is not optimal therapy for aspiration pneumonia.
Systemically effective quinolone may prove to be a viable alternative for initial therapy in these patients.
The role of quinolones as first-line therapy for pneumonia in any of the clinical settings outlined above remains controversial. If penicillin-intolerant/resistant *S. pneumoniae* is suspected as a causative pathogen, a newer quinolone (e.g., trovafloxacin) may be an appropriate first choice.

TABLE 40–5. Empiric Antimicrobial Therapy for Pneumonia in Pediatric Patients[a]

Age	Usual Pathogen(s)	Presumptive Therapy
1 month	Group B streptococcus, *Haemophilus influenzae* (nontypable), *Escherichia coli, Staphylococcus aureus, Listeria*	Ampicillin/sulbactam, cephalosporin,[b] carbapenem[c]
	CMV, RSV, adenovirus	Ribavirin for RSV
1–3 months	*Chlamydia,* possibly *Ureaplasma,* CMV, *Pneumocystis carinii* (afebrile pneumonia syndrome)	Macrolide/azilide,[d] TMP–SMX
	RSV	Ribavirin
	Pneumococcus, S. aureus	Semisynthetic penicillin[e] or cephalosporin[f]
3 months–6 years	*Pneumococcus, H. influenzae,* RSV, adenovirus, parainfluenza	Amoxicillin or cephalosporin[f] Ampicillin/sulbactam, amoxicillin/clavulanate Ribavirin for RSV
>6 years	*Pneumococcus, Mycoplasma pneumoniae,* adenovirus	Macrolide/azilide[d] Cephalosporin,[f] amoxicillin/clavulanate

[a]See section on Treatment of Bacterial Pneumonia.
[b]Third-generation cephalosporin (e.g., ceftriaxone, cefotaxime, cefepime). Note that the cephalosporins are not active against *Listeria.*
[c]Carbapenem (imipenem/cilistatin, meropenem).
[d]Macrolide/azilide (erythromycin, clarithromycin, azithromycin).
[e]Semisynthetic penicillin (e.g., nafcillin, oxacillin).
[f]Second-generation cephalosporin (e.g., cefuroxime, cefprozil).
See text for details regarding ribavirin treatment for RSV infection.
CMV, cytomegalovirus; RSV, respiratory syncytial virus; TMP–SMX, trimethoprim–sulfamethoxazole.

- With nosocomial pneumonia, the above parameters should be assessed along with white blood cell counts, chest radiograph, and blood gas determinations.

See Chapter 98, Lower Respiratory Tract Infections, authored by Philip Toltzis, MD, Mark L. Glover, PharmD, and Michael D. Reed, PharmD, FCCP, FCP, for a more detailed discussion of this topic.

Chapter 41

▶ RESPIRATORY TRACT INFECTIONS, UPPER

▶ OTITIS MEDIA

DEFINITION

Otitis media is a nonspecific term describing an inflammation of the middle ear. Acute otitis media involves the rapid onset of signs and symptoms of inflammation in the middle ear that manifests clinically as one or more of the following: otalgia (denoted by pulling of the ear in some infants), hearing loss, fever, or irritability. Otitis media with effusion (accumulation of liquid in the middle ear cavity) differs from acute otitis media in that signs and symptoms of an acute infection are absent.

PATHOPHYSIOLOGY

- Bacterial cultures from the middle ear effusion of children over 1 month of age with acute, symptomatic otitis media have yielded strains of *Streptococcus pneumoniae* (35%), predominantly nontypable strains of *Haemophilus influenzae* (25%), and *Moxarella catarrhalis* (10%).
- β-lactam resistance occurs in about 30% of *H. influenzae* and 75% of *M. catarrhalis.*
- With otitis media, the patient has an antecedent event that results in congestion of the respiratory mucosa, causing secretions to accumulate in the middle ear.
- Bacteria present in the middle ear proliferate in the secretions, resulting in acute otitis media.
- Abnormal function of the eustachian tube can cause reflux, aspiration, or insufflation of nasopharyngeal bacteria up to the middle ear.
- In infants, the difference in angulation of the eustachian tube may cause improper drainage of the middle ear as a result of decreased gravitational effects on the eustachian tube.

CLINICAL PRESENTATION

- Acute otitis media involves the rapid onset of otalgia, hearing loss, fever, and a sudden onset of irritability.
- Clinical presentation may include nonspecific symptoms such as lethargy, anorexia, vomiting, or diarrhea.
- Redness or opacity of the tympanic membranes, the absence of light reflection, and bulging and immobility of the membrane to pneumatic otoscopy are all indicative of middle ear effusion and suggestive of otitis media.
- Otorrhea (purulent discharge) through perforation of the tympanic membrane or through tympanostomy tubes, accompanied by otalgia and fever, is also indicative of acute otitis media.

- Complications and sequella of otitis media are categorized as intracranial (meningitis and brain abscess) and intratemporal (eardrum diseases). The latter are more frequent and can result in hearing loss.

DESIRED OUTCOME

- The goals of treatment include control of pain, eradication of the infection, prevention of complications, and avoidance of unnecessary antibiotics.

TREATMENT

- Oral antibiotics are still the mainstay of therapy. However, a significant percentage of children will be cured with symptomatic treatment alone.
- The selection of the appropriate antibiotic is based on antimicrobial susceptibility, penetration into the middle ear, clinical efficacy, compliance factors, adverse effects profile, and cost.
- **Amoxicillin,** with excellent in vitro activity against *S. pneumoniae* and most *H. influenzae* isolates from the middle ear, is still the first choice in the treatment of acute otitis media in areas where the emergence of β-lactamase–producing *H. influenzae* and *M. catarrhalis* is limited.
- β-lactamase–resistant antibiotics **(trimethoprim–sulfamethoxazole [TMP–SMX], cefixime, cefuroxime, cefaclor, ceftibuten, cefprozil, cefpodoxime protexetil, loracarbef, azithromycin, clarithromycin, and erythromycin–sulfisoxazole)** should be used when there is no clinical improvement in 24–48 hours of therapy or documentation of regional resistance.
- Table 41–1 summarizes the recommended doses and dosing schedules of the primary antimicrobials used in the treatment of upper respiratory tract infections. Short dosing intervals and the recommended 10-day course of antimicrobial therapy for acute otitis media certainly represent contributory factors to noncompliance.
- Supportive therapy with analgesics, antipyretics, and local heat has been shown to be beneficial in the comfort of the child with otitis media.
- Although antihistamines and decongestants have been used for the symptomatic relief of acute otitis media, studies have not shown them to be efficacious in the resolution of effusion or relief of symptoms.

Recurrent Acute Otitis Media

- If the signs and symptoms of acute otitis media occur within 1 month of the initial episode, it is assumed that the same microorganism caused the infection. This new episode should be treated with a different antibiotic, preferably one with β-lactamase activity.
- If the new episode occurs over 1 month after the initial infection in a child who was completely free of signs and symptoms between episodes, the management of the recurrent episodes is the same as the first episode.

TABLE 41–1. Dosing Regimen and Cost of Antibiotic Use in Upper Respiratory Tract Infections

Antibiotic(s)	Daily Pediatric Oral Dose	Adult Oral Dose	Regimen	Cost ($)
Amoxicillin	40 mg/kg	250–500 mg	Every 8 h	$
Pivampicillin	40–60 mg/kg	500 mg	Every 12 h	$$
Amoxicillin–clavulanate	40 mg/kg as amoxicillin	250–500 mg	Every 8 h	$$$$
Trimethoprim–sulfamethoxazole	8–10 mg/kg trimethoprim	160/800 mg	Every 12 h	$
Cefaclor	40 mg/kg	250–500 mg	Every 8 or 12 h	$$$
Cefixime	8 mg/kg	400 mg	Every 12 or 24 h	$$$$
Cefpodoxime proxetil	10 mg/kg	100–200 mg	Every 12 or 24 h	$$$$
Cefprozil	7.5–15 mg/kg	250–500 mg	Every 12 or 24 h	$$$$
Ceftibuten	9 mg/kg	400 mg	Every 24 h	$$$$
Cefuroxime axetil	30–40 mg/kg	250–500 mg	Every 12 h	$$$$
Loracarbef	7.5–15 mg/kg	200–400 mg	Every 12 h	$$$$
Erythromycin–sulfisoxazole	40 mg/kg of erythromycin	—	Every 8 or 12 h	$$
Clarithromycin	7.5–15 mg/kg	250–500 mg	Every 12 h	$$$$
Azithromycin	10 mg/kg day 1, 5 mg/kg days 2–5 (OM) 12 mg/kg × 5 days (SP)	500 mg day 1, 250 mg days 2–5	Every 24 h	$$$

OM, otitis media; SP, streptococcal pharyngitis.
$ < $10; $$ $10–20; $$$ > $20; $$$$ > $30.

- If children exhibit more than four episodes in a 6-month period, or six episodes in a 12-month period, these patients can be managed by chemoprophylaxis with antimicrobials, and/or myringotomy and insertion of tympanostomy tubes.
- The most popular surgical approach to the treatment of recurrent episodes of otitis media is myringotomy and insertion of tympanostomy tubes.

Chronic Purulent Otitis Media

- On examination of an infant or child presenting with chronic otorrhetic discharge, the pus is suctioned and the external canal is cleansed prior to culturing the middle ear.
- After the invading pathogen(s) has been identified or speculated, therapy is initiated with an oral drug that is active against β-lactamase–producing organisms.
- **Amoxicillin with clavulanic acid, cefuroxime axetil, cefaclor, cefixime,** and **erythromycin ethylsuccinate with sulfisoxazole** are first-line agents. The use of fluoroquinolones, such as **ciprofloxacin,** can be considered in adults.

Chemoprophylaxis

- Prophylactic therapy appears to have a beneficial but limited effect on recurrent otitis media, should be initiated during the winter and early spring when recurrences are highest, and continued for 3 months or until there is a failure of therapy.
- The following regimens have been advocated: (1) **amoxicillin** (20–30 mg/kg/day) in one dose at bedtime or in two divided doses every 12 hours; (2) **sulfisoxazole** (80–100 mg/kg/day) every 24 hours; and (3) **TMP–SMX** (equivalent of 4 mg/kg/day of TMP) every 24 hours.

EVALUATION OF THERAPEUTIC OUTCOMES

- With proper treatment, symptoms of acute otitis media in most children will abate within 24–72 hours. When otalgia or fever persists or recurs during therapy, a β-lactamase–producing microorganism should be suspected and an agent with β-lactamase activity should be used.
- If treatment with the second-line agent fails, tympanocentesis to identify the pathogen may be indicated, particularly if the child is symptomatic or has an underlying disease.
- All children should be reexamined at the end of the 10-day antibiotic therapy. Even with an efficacious antibiotic treatment, effusion of the middle ear may be present in 10% of children following treatment with antibiotics. If the middle ear effusion persists beyond 3 months, several options can be considered:

    1. **Amoxicillin** 20 mg/kg/day or **TMP–SMX** 4/20 mg/kg/day continuously while the effusion persists.

2. Appropriate antimicrobial therapy of each episode of acute otitis media.
3. Myringotomy and tympanostomy tube placement.

▶ PHARYNGITIS

Pharyngitis is an inflammation of the pharynx and surrounding lymphoid tissue that may be of viral or bacterial origin.

ETIOLOGY/PATHOPHYSIOLOGY

- Viruses appear to be the cause of the majority of episodes, often as constituents of the common cold. However, a significant number are of bacterial origin, with group A β-hemolytic streptococci *(Streptococcus pyogenes)* being the most prevalent microorganism.
- In children less than 4 years of age, the etiology is usually viral.
- Bacterial pathogens constitute 10–30% of all pharyngitis and the symptomatology generally overlaps that of viral pharyngitis.
- Group A β-hemolytic streptococci is the most prevalent bacterial pathogen in symptomatic pharyngitis.

CLINICAL PRESENTATION

- Symptoms of pharyngitis include a sore throat associated with dysphagia and fever.
- In the majority of cases of acute pharyngitis, it is not possible to differentiate, on a clinical basis, between viral and bacterial etiology.
- Four findings predict a positive throat culture for group A β-hemolytic streptococci: presence of a tonsillar exudate, swollen and tender cervical lymph nodes, lack of cough, and a history of fever more than 38°C.
- If two or three of the above findings are present, a culture should be taken and treatment postponed until culture results are available. With one or no findings, no culture should be taken and no antibiotics prescribed. With all four findings, a culture should be taken and the decision to initiate antibiotic therapy made based on clinical grounds.
- A rapid diagnosis for the prevention of acute rheumatic fever is not essential, because antibiotic therapy can be initiated as late as 9 days after the onset of streptococcal pharyngitis and still be effective.

TREATMENT

- The treatment of viral pharyngitis is symptomatic.
- Appropriate antibiotic therapy for group A β-hemolytic streptococci (GAS) infection prevents acute rheumatic fever, reduces the period of contagion, limits the spread of infection, and reduces the incidence of suppurative complications.
- Many antimicrobial agents are appropriate choices in the treatment of group A β-hemolytic streptococci pharyngitis. These agents include **penicillin, amoxicillin, ampicillin,** several cephalosporins, **erythromycin,** and **erythromycin–sulfisoxazole.**

- **Penicillin** remains the mainstay of therapy for patients infected with group A β-hemolytic streptococci. Children less than 12 years old with group A β-hemolytic streptococcal pharyngitis should receive penicillin V 250 mg twice daily given orally for 10 days, or benzathine penicillin 25,000–50,000 U/kg intramuscularly as a single dose. For adults and adolescents, 500 mg should be given twice daily for 10 days.
- New macroslides, like *azithromyin,* are also effective against GAS and can be used as second-line drugs.
- For the penicillin-allergic patient, **erythromycin estolate** 20–30 mg/kg/day in two to four divided doses or **erythromycin ethylsuccinate** 40–50 mg/kg/day in two to four divided doses for 10 days are suitable alternatives. However, resistance of group A β-hemolytic streptococci to erythromycin has been observed in the United States in approximately 5% of the strains isolated.

EVALUATION OF THERAPEUTIC OUTCOMES

- Approximately 10 to 20% of children and adults with GAS pharyngitis who are treated adequately will relapse.
- For a relapse, it is appropriate to change the antimicrobial agent. **Cephalosporins** with β-lactamase activity are good alternatives. If a new strain is present, the initial antimicrobial can be reinstated.
- With persistent recurrent episodes, penicillin for 10 days with **rifampin** for the last 4 days is suggested.

▶ SINUSITIS

The predominant organisms causing sinusitis are *S. pneumoniae* (35% in adults, 29% in children), nontypable *H. influenzae* (35% in adults, 29% in children), and *M. catarrhalis* (2% in adults, 26% in children). Infrequently encountered bacteria include *S. pyogenes, S. aureus,* and anaerobic bacteria such as *Peptostreptococcus, Fusobacterium,* and *Bacteroides melan-inogenicus.*

PATHOPHYSIOLOGY

- Conditions that affect patency of the sinus ostia, normal function of the mucociliary sinus epithelium, normal immune defenses of the upper respiratory tract, or events that introduce microorganisms into the sinuses predispose to sinus infections.
- Bacterial and viral infections of the respiratory tract and allergic inflammation are conditions that cause sinus ostia obstruction and lead to retention of secretions.

CLINICAL PRESENTATION

- The most commonly encountered symptoms with sinusitis include mucopurulent nasal discharge, nasal congestion, facial pain, maxillary toothache, and fever. The persistence of nasal discharge and daytime cough for more than 10 days following a viral infection of the upper respiratory tract is indicative of sinusitis.

- The finding of the following symptoms indicates a high likelihood of sinusitis: maxillary toothache, poor response to decongestants, colored nasal discharge, as do the signs of purulent nasal secretions and abnormal sinus transillumination.
- The diagnosis of sinusitis may require transillumination of maxillary sinuses, radiography of the sinuses for adults and children over 1 year of age, and occassionally, computed tomography, or magnetic resonance imaging.
- On microscopic examination of fresh nasal secretions, a high concentration of polymorphonuclear cells with intracellular bacteria is often observed. A differentiation between chronic sinusitis and allergic rhinitis can be made when eosinophils predominate. If the smear is devoid of eosinophils, chronic sinusitis can be suspected.

TREATMENT

- Many symptoms of sinusitis will resolve without medical therapy within 48 hours. When they persist, pharmacotherapy should be directed toward symptomatic relief, restoring and improving sinus function, preventing intracranial complications, and eradicating the causative pathogen(s).

- Antibiotics are the mainstay of therapy of sinusitis. **Amoxicillin** is an appropriate agent for most uncomplicated cases of sinusitis.
- If β-lactamase–resistant strains are suspected, if the patient is allergic to penicillin, or if there is an apparent antibiotic failure, alternative regimens can be used, such as **trimethoprim–sulfamethoxazole, cefaclor, erythromycin–sulfisoxazole, amoxicillin–clavulanate, loracarbef,** and **azithromycin, clarithromycin, cefuroxime axetil,** and **cefixime.**
- Acute sinusitis is treated for 10–14 days, but duration can be extended to 30 days in protracted cases.
- Vasoconstrictor sprays or drops such as **phenylephrine** or **oxymetazoline** may facilitate drainage. The use of such agents should not exceed 72 hours owing to a tolerance effect and possible rebound congestion. Antihistamines are not effective in the treatment of acute sinusitis.

▶ EPIGLOTTITIS AND CROUP

Epiglottitis and croup are two distinct entities, both resulting from infections of the laryngeal area (Table 41–2). Noisy breathing is characteristic of these two clinical diseases. They both cause airway obstruction but at different anatomic sites.

EPIGLOTTITIS

- Epiglottitis is a true airway emergency in which acute airway obstruction can occur, and it is caused primarily by *H. influenzae* type B.

TABLE 41–2. Differentiating Clinical Features of Epiglottitis and Croup

Feature	Epiglottitis	Croup
Age	3–7 years	>3 years
Gender	Male = Female	Male > Female
Season	All seasons	Late spring and late fall
Pathogens(s)	Bacterial: *H. influenzae* B	Viral: parainfluenza (type 1, 2, and 3)
Progression	Rapid	Slow (generally at night)
Clinical presentation	Sitting, toxic, typical posture	Supine, nontoxic, barking cough
Dysphagia	Marked, occasional drooling	None
Fever	>39.4°C (103°F)	<39.4°C (103°F)
Stridor	Rare	Frequent
WBC	>18,000 mm^3	Normal
Treatment	Parenteral antibiotics, intubation	Cool mist, racemic epinephrine
Recurrence	Rare	Common

- Epiglottitis is more prevalent in children ages 2–6. The onset of the disease is rapid and the evolution is often brisk.
- Respiratory distress, drooling, dysphagia, and dysphonia (the four "Ds") are typical signs of the disease. Fever is usually high and manifests as the first symptom.
- Airway obstruction evolves rapidly and manifests by respiratory distress, on inspiratory stridor, loss of voice, and the presence of intercostal drawing.

Treatment

- The primary concern in the management of epiglottitis is establishing and maintaining the airway.
- Initial therapy may involve the use of a moist-oxygen tent to help facilitate the breathing.
- In severe cases, endotracheal intubation or a tracheostomy may be required.
- Antibiotic therapy should be instituted if epiglottitis is suspected and empirically directed against *H. influenzae* type B.
- **Cefuroxime** (50–100 mg/kg/day given every 8 hours), **cefotaxime** (150–225 mg/kg/day given every 6 hours), or **ceftriaxone** (80–100 mg/kg/day given every 12 hours) are preferred treatments if the infection is severe.

CROUP (LARYNGITIS)

- Laryngitis may be viral or bacterial in origin.
- Common causative bacteria include *S. aureus,* group A β-hemolytic streptococci, *H. influenzae* B, *M. catarrhalis,* and pneumococcus.
- Viral croup (acute laryngotracheobronchitis) is caused primarily by parainfluenza (type 1 and 2).
- Laryngitis most often occurs in children less than 3 years of age and is characterized by stridor, a barking cough, and absence of drooling.

Treatment

- Most cases of croup can be treated at home with air humidification.
- More severe cases may require **humidified oxygen, racemic epinephrine, corticosteroids,** or **antibiotics.**
- Because of its drying effect, oxygen therapy should be reserved for cyanotic children (SaO_2 <90%). In most serious cases, racemic epinephrine inhalation may provide relief. The recommended doses are 0.5 mL of a 2.25% solution of racemic epinephrine diluted in 2.5–3.5 mL of saline.
- Corticosteroids (**dexamethasone** 0.6 mg/kg orally or intramuscularly to a maximum of 10 mg) are beneficial with moderate to severe laryngitis. Inhaled **budesonide** may also be useful.
- Antibiotics should only be used for bacterial laryngotracheitis. Preferred agents are **cefuroxime, cloxacillin** with **cefotaxime,** or **vancomycin** with an **aminoglycoside** to provide activity against *S. aureus* and *H. influenzae* B.

See Chapter 99, Upper Respiratory Tract Infections, authored by Monique Richer, PharmD, MA (ed), BCPS, and Michel Deschênes, MD, for a more detailed discussion of this topic.

Chapter 42

▶ SEPSIS AND SEPTIC SHOCK

▶ DEFINITIONS

Definitions of terms related to sepsis are given in Table 42–1.

▶ PATHOPHYSIOLOGY

- Sepsis may be caused by gram-negative or gram-positive bacteria as well as fungi or other microorganisms.
- Figure 42–1 shows a schematic representation of the pathogenesis of gram-negative sepsis and septic shock.
- The major offenders in gram-negative sepsis are the *Enterobacteriaceae (Escherichia, Klebsiella, Enterobacter, Serratia,* and *Proteus)* and *Pseudomonadaceae.* Gram-positive sepsis is most often caused by staphylococci.
- The pathophysiologic focus of gram-negative sepsis has been on the lipopolysaccharide (endotoxin) component of the gram-negative cell wall. Lipid A is a part of the endotoxin molecule that is highly immunoreactive and is responsible for most of the toxic effects. Endotoxin first associates with a protein called lipopolysaccharide-binding protein in plasma. This complex then engages a specific receptor (CD14) on the surface of the macrophage, which activates it and causes release of inflammatory mediators.
- Sepsis involves a complex interaction of proinflammatory (e.g., tumor necrosis factor-α [TNF-α], interleukin [IL]-1, IL-8) and anti-inflammatory mediators (e.g., IL-4 and IL-10).
- A primary mechanism of injury with sepsis is through endothelial cells. With inflammation, endothelial cells allow circulating cells (e.g., granulocytes) and plasma constituents to enter inflamed tissues, which may result in organ damage. In addition, endothelial cells may cause vasodilatation through production of nitric oxide.
- TNF-α is believed to be an important proinflammatory mediator.
- Endotoxin activates complement, causing direct activation of Hageman factor, which activates coagulation and fibrinolysis and the release of vasoactive peptides.
- Disseminated intravascular coagulation (DIC), a frequent complication of gram-negative sepsis, is attributed to the activation of coagulation factor XII (Hageman factor) by endotoxin.
- Shock is the most ominous complication associated with gram-negative sepsis.
- Another important complication of sepsis is acute respiratory distress syndrome (ARDS). Approximately 25% of patients with gram-negative sepsis develop ARDS, and this carries a mortality rate of 60–90%.
- The hallmark of the hemodynamic effect of sepsis is the hyperdynamic state characterized by high cardiac output and an abnormally low systemic vascular resistance (SVR).

TABLE 42–1. Definitions Related to Sepsis

Condition	Definition
Infection	Microbial phenomenon characterized by inflammatory response to the presence of microorganisms or invasion of normally sterile host tissue by the microorganisms
Bacteremia	Presence of viable bacteria in the bloodstream
Fungemia	Presence of viable fungi in the bloodstream
Systemic inflammatory response syndrome (SIRS)	Systemic inflammatory response to a variety of severe clinical insults that is considered secondary to the widespread effects of proinflammatory cytokine mediators (e.g., TNFα, IL-1, IL-6). The response is manifested by two or more of the following conditions: T > 38°C or < 36°C; HR > 90 beats/min; RR > 20 breaths/min or $Paco_2$ < 32 torr; WBC > 12,000 cells/mm^3, < 4000 cells/mm^3, or > 10% immature (band) forms
Sepsis	The above systemic inflammatory response syndrome that is secondary to infection, most commonly by bacteria or fungi, but also occasionally due to infection by viruses or parasites
Severe sepsis	Sepsis associated with organ dysfunction, hypoperfusion, or hypotension. Hypoperfusion and perfusion abnormalities may include, but are not limited to, lactic acidosis, oliguria, or acute alteration in mental status
Septic shock	Sepsis with hypotension, despite aggressive fluid resuscitation, along with the presence of perfusion abnormalities (listed above). Patients who are on inotropic or vasopressor agents may not be hypotensive at the time perfusion abnormalities are measured
Multiple organ dysfunction syndrome (MODS)	Presence of altered organ function in an acutely ill patient such that homeostasis cannot be maintained without clinical intervention
Compensatory anti-inflammatory response syndrome (CARS)	Compensatory physiologic response to systemic inflammatory response syndrome that is considered secondary to the actions of anti-inflammatory cytokine mediators (e.g., IL-4, IL-10, IL-11, IL-13, TGFβ)

HR, heart rate: IL, interleukin: RR, respiratory rate; T, temperature, WBC, white blood cell count; TNFα, tumor necrosis factor; TGFβ, transforming growth factor β.

- Sepsis results in distributive shock characterized by inappropriately increased blood flow to selected tissue at the expense of other tissue independent of oxygen needs.
- The pathophysiologic spectrum of sepsis is an exaggerated inflammatory response to the presence of bacteria or endotoxin in the bloodstream.

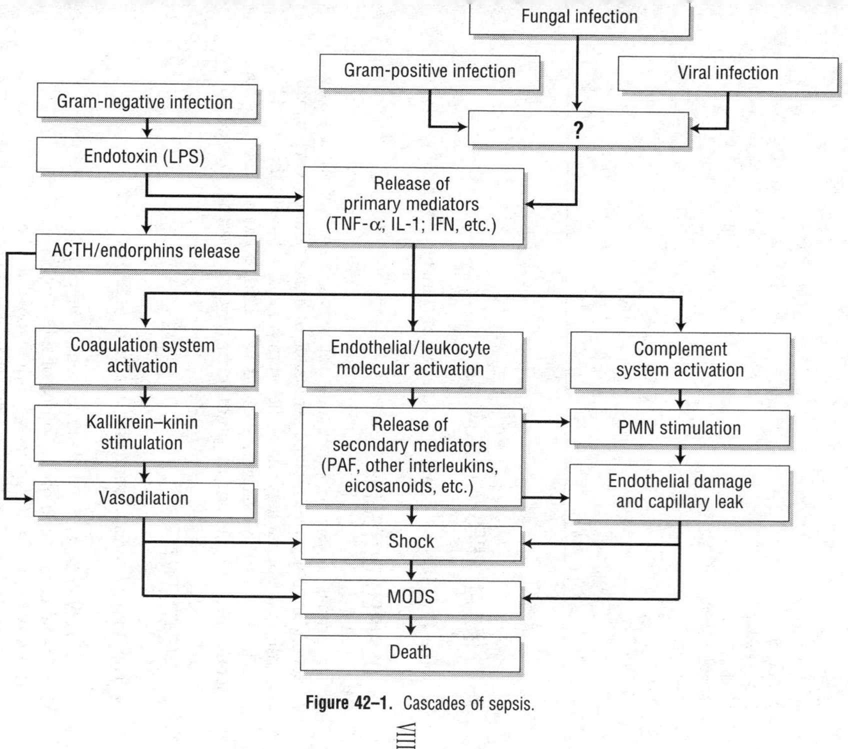

Figure 42–1. Cascades of sepsis.

VIII

TABLE 42–2. Clinical Signs and Symptoms Associated With Sepsis

Early Sepsis	Late Sepsis
Fever or hypothermia	Lactic acidosis
Rigors, chills	Oliguria
Tachycardia	Leukopenia
Tachypnea	DIC
Nausea, vomiting	Myocardial depression
Hyperglycemia	Pulmonary edema
Myalgias	Hypotension (shock)
Lethargy, malaise	Hypoglycemia
Proteinuria	Azotemia
Hypoxia	Thrombocytopenia
Leukocytosis	ARDS
Hyperbilirubinemia	GI hemorrhage
	Coma

▶ CLINICAL PRESENTATION

- Table 42–2 lists the clinical features characteristic of sepsis.

▶ DESIRED OUTCOME

- The primary objective of treatment for sepsis is survival of the patient. Secondary objectives include avoidance of organ failure (renal, hepatic, cardiac, and pulmonary) and other complications. Ideally, this would be done without the occurrence of adverse drug effects. Important outcome measures include length of intensive care unit and hospital stays.

▶ TREATMENT

- The primary considerations for treatment of sepsis are:

  1. Timely diagnosis and identification of the pathogen.
  2. Rapid elimination of the source of infection.
  3. Early initiation of aggressive antimicrobial therapy.
  4. Appropriate provision of cardiovascular and pulmonary support.
  5. Consideration of metabolic and other supportive therapies.

ANTIMICROBIAL THERAPY

- Aggressive, early antimicrobial therapy is critical in the management of septic patients. The regimen selected should be based on the likely pathogens and the local antibiotic susceptibility patterns.
- When serious sepsis is suspected, the use of a combination of antimicrobials is usually recommended to provide additive or synergistic

effects, to expand coverage, and to reduce the emergence of resistance. The antibiotics that may be used to treat sepsis are listed in Table 42–3.

- In a non-neutropenic patient with community-acquired urinary tract infection, a **third-generation cephalosporin, fluoroquinolone,** or **antipseudomonal penicillin,** each with or without an aminoglycoside, may be used. For non–urinary tract community-acquired infections, a **third- or fourth-generation cephalosporin** plus **metronidazole, piperacillin/tazobactam, ampicillin/sulbactam,** or **ticarcillin/clavulanate** should be considered.
- With nosocomial infections, aggressive therapy with activity against *Pseudomonas aeruginosa* and *Enterobacter* sp. should be instituted (e.g., piperacillin/tazobactam plus an **aminoglycoside,** ticarcillin/clavulanate with an aminoglycoside, **imipenem** or **meropenem** with or without an aminoglycoside, and **ceftazidime** or **cefepime** plus metronidazole and an aminoglycoside).
- **Vancomycin** should be added whenever the risk of methicilin-resistant staphylococci is significant.
- Aminoglycosides should be used when a synergistic regimen is desired for gram-negative bacilli and should be dosed aggressively initially to achieve high serum peak concentrations with dosage adjustment made later based on renal function. There is not sufficient information to recommend single daily dosing for aminoglycosides in pediatric patients, in burned patients, in pregnancy, in patients with preexisting renal dysfunction, and for gram-positive sepsis. VIII
- The average duration of treatment in immunocompetent individuals would be 10–14 days.

FLUID THERAPY AND PULMONARY SUPPORT

- Maintenance of adequate tissue oxygenation is important in the treatment of sepsis and is dependent on adequate perfusion and adequate oxygenation of the blood.
- Rapid restoration of intravascular fluid volume and expansion of the extravascular space is an essential therapeutic intervention in the initial management of septic shock.
- The goal of fluid replacement is to maintain a systolic blood pressure >90 mm Hg and to prevent hypoperfusion to tissues and vital organs.
- Controversy exists regarding the optimal type of fluid (crystalloid versus colloid). An increase in transitory pulmonary edema has been demonstrated during crystalloid volume expansion when compared with colloids, but it is not known whether there are any long-term sequelae. Successful fluid resuscitation in sepsis usually requires a combination of crystalloid and colloid.
- Iso-oncotic colloid solutions (plasma and plasma protein fractions), such as 5% albumin and 6% hetastarch, offer the advantage of more rapid restoration of intravascular volume with less volume infused. However, they may prolong tissue edema when capillary permeability to oncotically active solutes is increased.

TABLE 42–3. Options for Parenteral Antibiotic Therapy in the Management of Sepsis[a]

(Trade Name)	Usual Adult Dose	Pediatric Dose	Comments
Aminoglycosides			
Gentamicin (generic)	1–1.5 mg/kg q 8 h 4–7 mg/kg q 24 h	2–2.5 mg/kg q 8 h	Active against gram-negative aerobes only; single daily dose not recommended in pediatrics
Tobramycin (generic)	See Gentamicin		See Gentamicin
Amikacin (generic)	5–7.5 mg/kg q 8–12 h 10–15 mg/kg q 24 h	5–7.5 mg/kg q 8 h	See Gentamicin
Penicillins			
Penicillin G (generic)	2–4 million units q 4 h	25–50,000 units/kg q 4–6 h	Use generally limited to streptococcal infections
Ampicillin (generic)	2 g q 4–6 h	25–50 mg/kg q 6 h	Use is limited due to widespread resistance
Oxacillin (generic)	2 g q 4 h	25–50 mg/kg q 6 h	Use limited to staphylococcal infections
Nafcillin (generic)	See Oxacillin		See Oxacillin
Ticarcillin (Ticar)	3 g q 4 h	75 mg/kg q 6 h	Broad gram-negative activity
Piperacillin (Piperacil)	4 g q 6 h	75 mg/kg q 6 h	See Ticarcillin
Mezlocillin (Mezlin)	4 g q 6 h	75 mg/kg q 6 h	See Ticarcillin
β–Lactamase Inhibitor Combinations			
Ampicillin/sulbactam (Unasyn)	3 g q 6 h	See Ampicillin	Covers staphylococci and anaerobes
Ticarcillin/clavulanate (Timentin)	3.1 g q 4–6 h	See Ticarcillin	Expanded gram-negative, staphylococci, and anaerobic activity
Piperacillin/tazobactam (Zosyn)	3.375–4.5 q 6 h	See Piperacillin	See Piperacillin

Cephalosporins			
Cefotaxime (Claforan)	1–2 g q 6–8 h	50 mg/kg q 6 h	Broad gram negative and gram positive; not *Pseudomonas*
Ceftriaxone (Rocephin)	1–2 g q 24 h	50–75 mg/kg q 24 h	See Cefotaxime
Ceftizoxime (Ceftizox)	1–2 g q 6–8 h	50 mg/kg q 6 h	See Cefotaxime
Ceftazidime (various)	1–2 g q 8 h	50 mg/kg q 8 h	Very good against *Pseudomonas;* weak gram positive
Cefepime (Maxipime)	1–2 g q 8–12 h	50 mg/kg q 8 h	Antipseudomonal and antistaphylococcal
Fluoroquinolones			
Ciprofloxacin (Cipro)	400 mg q 8–12 h	Relative contraindication	Good antipseudomonal and other gram negatives
Ofloxacin (Floxin)	400 mg q 12 h	Relative contraindication	Antipseudomonal activity less than ciprofloxacin
Levofloxacin (Levoquin)	500 mg q 24 h	Relative contraindication	Active stereoisomer of ofloxacin
Carbapenems			
Imipenem/cilastatin (Primaxin)	500 mg q 6 h	10–15 mg/kg q 6 h	Very broad spectrum to include anaerobes and *Pseudomonas*
Meropenem (Merem)	500 mg q 8 h	10–15 mg/kg q 8 h	See Imipenem
Monobactam			
Aztreonam (Azactam)	1–2 g q 8 h	50 mg/kg q 6 h	Use limited to gram-negative aerobes only
Others			
Vancomycin (generic)	1 g q 12 h	10 mg/kg q 6 h	Use should be limited to methicillin-resistant staphylococci
Metronidazole (generic)	500 mg q 6–8 h	15 mg/kg q 12 h	Excellent antianaerobic activity
Clindamycin (Cleocin)	600 mg q 8 h	10 mg/kg q 6–8 h	Good antianaerobic activity; some gram-positive activity
Cotrimoxazole (various)	160/800 mg q 12 h	4/20 mg/kg q 12 h	Good gram-negative activity; not antipseudomonal

[a]Doses listed are for normal renal function.

- Fluid resuscitation in sepsis usually requires hemodynamic monitoring. Maintenance of pulmonary capillary wedge pressure in the range of 15–18 mm Hg should provide sufficient left ventricular filling pressure without excessive risk of pulmonary edema.

INOTROPE AND VASOACTIVE DRUG SUPPORT

- When fluid resuscitation is insufficient to maintain tissue perfusion, the use of inotropes and vasoactive drugs is necessary. Selection and dosage are based on the pharmacologic properties of various catecholamines and how they influence hemodynamic parameters (Table 42–4).

Suggested Protocol for the Use of Inotropes and Vasoactive Agents

- **Dopamine** is widely used in low doses (2–3 μg/kg/min) to increase renal and mesenteric perfusion. Renal blood flow is enhanced even when used with norepinephrine.
- Dopamine in moderate doses (10–20 μg/kg/min) may be used to support blood pressure.
- **Dobutamine** (2–20 μg/kg/min) is superior to dopamine for cardiac output and oxygen delivery.
- **Norepinephrine** (2–100 μg/min) is useful in septic shock for vasoconstriction of peripheral beds.
- In the patient with significant hypotension (mean arterial pressure [MAP] <60 mm Hg) and a low systemic vascular resistance index (SVRI) (<500 dynes/cm^5/m^2) that cannot be overcome by inotropic agents, an α-adrenergic agent (norepinephrine) can be useful. It often is combined with an inotrope such as dobutamine.
- **Phenylephrine** may be useful in patients with refractory hypotension.
- Prior to administering vasoactive agents, aggressive appropriate fluid resuscitation should occur. Vasoactive agents should not be considered an acceptable alternative to volume resuscitation.

TABLE 42–4. Receptor Activity of Cardiovascular Agents Commonly Used in Septic Shock

Agent	α_1	α_2	β_1	β_2	Dopaminergic
Dopamine	++/+++	?	++++	++	++++
Dobutamine	+	+	++++	++	0
Epinephrine	++++	++++	++++	+++	0
Norepinephrine	+++	+++	+++	+/++	0
Phenylephrine	++/+++	+	?	0	0

α_1, α_1-adrenergic receptor; α_2, α_2-adrenergic receptor; β_1, β_1-adrenergic receptor; β_2, β_2-adrenergic receptor; 0, no activity; ++++, maximal activity; ?, unknown activity.

INVESTIGATIONAL THERAPIES

- A wide variety of investigational strategies have been used to attempt to reverse or control the inflammatory process initiated with sepsis.
- One mechanism studied is direct inhibition of the effects of endotoxin from gram-negative bacteria by antibodies or with other binding substances such as bactericidal/permeability increasing protein or high-density lipoprotein.
- A second general approach is inhibition of inflammatory cytokines through antibodies that bind the cytokines, through competitive inhibitors for cytokine receptor binding, or through soluble receptors that bind the cytokine but do not activate the target cells.
- Another general approach is the administration of anti-inflammatory cytokines or other substances, such as IL-10, IL-4, or IL-1 receptor antagonists.

CONTROVERSIES IN THE MANAGEMENT OF SEPTIC SHOCK

- The **corticosteroids** have been the subject of controversy in the management of the septic process. Multiple clinical trials have demonstrated that they are not beneficial for sepsis but may be useful for patients with ARDS (after 5–7 days).
- Heparinization for the treatment of DIC has been recommended because the paradoxical bleeding is caused by a hypercoagulable state; however, there is little clinical evidence that **heparin** prolongs survival. VIII
- **Naloxone,** through its antagonist effect on opiates and β-endorphins, has been shown to raise and sustain systolic blood pressure in animals but has not been shown useful in humans with septic shock.

See Chapter 109, Sepsis and Septic Shock, authored by Thomas C. Hardin, PharmD, FCCP, and Joseph T. DiPiro, PharmD, FCCP, for a more detailed discussion of this topic.

Chapter 43

▶ SEXUALLY TRANSMITTED DISEASES

▶ DEFINITION

The spectrum of sexually transmitted diseases (STDs) includes the classic venereal diseases—gonorrhea, syphilis, chancroid, lymphogranuloma venereum, and granuloma inguinale—as well as a variety of other pathogens known to be spread by sexual contact (Table 43–1). Common clinical syndromes associated with STDs are listed in Table 43–2.

▶ GONORRHEA

CLINICAL PRESENTATION

- Infected individuals may be symptomatic or asymptomatic, have complicated or uncomplicated infections, and have infections involving several anatomic sites.
- Urethritis is the most common presenting manifestation in males and usually develops within 2–8 days of exposure. Dysuria and urinary frequency are seen initially, followed in 1–2 days by a profuse, purulent urethral discharge.
- The majority of symptomatic patients who are not treated become asymptomatic within 6 months, with only a few becoming asymptomatic carriers of the disease.
- The majority of gonococcal urethral or cervical infections in females are either asymptomatic or produce minimal symptoms.
- In females, symptoms typically appear within 10 days following exposure, including dysuria, urinary frequency, abnormal vaginal discharge, and abnormal uterine bleeding.
- Other sites of gonococcal infection include the rectum, oropharynx, and eye. Anorectal gonococcal infections are common in females and in homosexual males.
- Approximately 15% of women with gonorrhea develop pelvic inflammatory disease (PID). Left untreated, PID can be an indirect cause of infertility and ectopic pregnancies.
- In 0.5–3.0% of patients with gonorrhea, the gonococci invade the bloodstream and produce disseminated disease.
- The usual clinical manifestations of disseminated gonnococcal infection are tender necrotic skin lesions, tenosynovitis, and monoarticular arthritis.

DIAGNOSIS

- Diagnosis of gonococcal infections can be made by Gram-stained smears, culture (the most reliable method), or newer methods based on

TABLE 43–1. Sexually Transmitted Diseases

Disease	Pathogen
Bacterial	
Gonorrhea	*Neisseria gonorrhoeae*
Syphilis	*Treponema pallidum*
Chancroid	*Haemophilus ducreyi*
Granuloma inguinale (donovanosis)	*Calymmatobacterium granulomatis*
Salmonellosis	*Salmonella* sp.
Shigellosis	*Shigella* sp.
Campylobacter infection	*Campylobacter jejuni*
Bacterial vaginosis	*Gardnerella vaginalis, Mycoplasma hominis, Bacteroides* sp., *Mobiluncus* sp.
Group B streptococcal infections	Group B streptococcus
Chlamydial	
Nongonococcal urethritis	*Chlamydia trachomatis*
Lymphogranuloma venereum	*Chlamydia trachomatis*
Viral	
Acquired immune deficiency syndrome	Human immunodeficiency virus
Herpes genitalis	Herpes simplex virus
Viral hepatitis	Hepatitis A, B, C, D virus
Condylomata acuminata	Human papilloma virus
Molluscum contagiosum	Poxvirus
Cytomegalovirus infection	Cytomegalovirus
Mycoplasmal	
Nongonococcal urethritis	*Ureaplasma urealyticum*
Protozoal	
Trichomoniasis	*Trichomonas vaginalis*
Amebiasis	*Entamoeba histolytica*
Giardiasis	*Giardia lamblia*
Fungal	
Candidiasis	*Candida albicans*
Parasitic	
Scabies	*Sarcoptes scabiei*
Pediculosis	*Phthirus pubis*
Enterobiasis	*Enterobius vermicularis*

the detection of cellular components of the gonococcus (e.g., enzymes, antigens, DNA, or lipopolysaccharide) in clinical specimens.

- Culture of exposed body areas is the most reliable means of diagnosing gonococcal infection.
- Alternative methods of diagnosis include enzyme immunoassay (EIA), DNA probes, and nucleic acid amplification techniques.

TABLE 43–2. Selected Syndromes Associated With Common Sexually Transmitted Pathogens

Syndrome	Commonly Implicated Pathogens	Common Clinical Manifestations[a]
Urethritis	*Chlamydia trachomatis,* herpes simplex virus, *Neisseria gonorrhoeae, Trichomonas vaginalis, Ureaplasma urealyticum*	Urethral discharge, dysuria
Epididymitis	*C. trachomatis, N. gonorrhoeae*	Scrotal pain, inguinal pain, flank pain, urethral discharge
Cervicitis/vulvovaginitis	*C. trachomatis, Gardnerella vaginalis,* herpes simplex virus, human papilloma virus, *N. gonorrhoeae, T. vaginalis*	Abnormal vaginal discharge, vulvar itching/irritation, dysuria, dyspareunia
Genital ulcers, painful	*Haemophilus ducreyi,* herpes simplex virus	Usually multiple vesicular/pustular (herpes) or papular/pustular (*H. ducreyi*) lesions that may coalesce; painful, tender lymphadenopathy[b]
Genital ulcers, painless	*Treponema pallidum*	Usually single papular lesion
Genital warts	Human papilloma virus	Multiple lesions ranging in size from small papular warts to large exophytic condylomas
Pharyngitis	*C. trachomatis* (?), herpes simplex virus, *N. gonorrhoeae*	Symptoms of acute pharyngitis, cervical lymphadenopathy, fever[c]
Proctitis	*C. trachomatis,* herpes simplex virus, *N. gonorrhoeae, T. pallidum*	Constipation, anorectal discomfort, tenesmus, mucopurulent rectal discharge
Salpingitis	*C. trachomatis, N. gonorrhoeae*	Lower abdominal pain, purulent cervical or vaginal discharge, adnexal swelling, fever[d]

VIII

[a]For some syndromes, clinical manifestations may be minimal or absent.
[b]Recurrent herpes infection may manifest as a single lesion.
[c]Most cases of pharyngeal gonococcal infection are asymptomatic.
[d]Salpingitis increases the risk of subsequent ectopic pregnancy and infertility.

TREATMENT

- All currently recommended regimens are single-dose treatments with various oral or parenteral cephalosporins and fluoroquinolones (Table 43–3).
- Coexisting chlamydial infection, which is documented in up to 60% of individuals with gonorrhea, constitutes the major cause of postgonococcal urethritis, cervicitis, and salpingitis in patients treated for gonorrhea. As a result, concomitant treatment with **doxycycline** or **azithromycin** is recommended in all patients treated for gonorrhea.
- Pregnant women infected with *Neisseria gonorrhoeae* should be treated with either a **cephalosporin** or **spectinomycin,** because fluoroquinolones are contraindicated.

TABLE 43–3. Treatment of Gonorrhea

Type of Infection	Recommended Regimen[a]	Alternative Regimen
Uncomplicated urethral, endocervical, rectal, proctitis, or epididymitis infection in adults[b,c]	Ceftriaxone 125 mg IM once; or ciprofloxacin 500 mg PO once; or cefixime 400 mg PO once; or ofloxacin 400 mg PO once **plus** A treatment regimen for presumptive *C. trachomatis* coinfection (see Table 43–5)	Spectinomycin 2 g IM once; or ceftizoxime 500 mg IM once; or cefotetan 1 g IM once; or cefoxitin 2 g IM once; or cefuroxime axetil 1 g PO once; or cefpodoxime proxetil 200 mg PO once; or lomefloxacin 400 mg PO once; or enoxacin 400 mg PO once; or norfloxacin 800 mg PO once **plus** A treatment regimen for presumptive *C. trachomatis* coinfection (see Table 43–5)
Gonococcal infections in pregnancy	Ceftriaxone 125 mg IM once[d,e] **plus** Erythromycin base 500 mg PO 4 times daily for 7 days	Spectinomycin 2 g IM once **plus** A treatment regimen for presumptive *C. trachomatis* coinfection (see Table 43–5)
Disseminated gonococcal infection in adults (>45 kg)[e–h]	Ceftriaxone 1 g IM or IV every 24 h	Ceftizoxime 1 g IV every 8 h; or cefotaxime 1 g IV every 8 h until all symptoms resolve; or spectinomycin 2 g IM every 12 h
Disseminated gonococcal infection in infants[i]	Ceftriaxone 25–50 mg/kg IV or IM once daily for 7 days; or cefotaxime 25 mg/kg IV or IM twice daily for 7 days	
Uncomplicated urethritis, vulvovaginitis, cervicitis, pharyngitis, or proctitis infection in children (<45 kg)	Ceftriaxone 125 mg IM once[j]	Spectinomycin 40 mg/kg IM once (not to exceed 2 g)

(continued)

TABLE 43–3. continued

Type of Infection	Recommended Regimen[a]	Alternative Regimen
Gonococcal conjunctivitis	Ceftriaxone 1 g IM once[k]	
Ophthalmia neonatorum	Ceftriaxone 25–50 mg/kg IV or IM once (not to exceed 125 mg)	
Infants born to mothers with gonococcal infection (prophylaxis)	Ceftriaxone 25–50 mg/kg IV or IM (not to exceed 125 mg)	

[a]Recommendations are those of the CDC.
[b]Treatment failures are usually due to reinfection and necessitate patient education and sex-partner referral; additional treatment regimens for gonorrhea and chlamydia infections should be administered. Epididymitis should be treated for 10 days (see Table 43–5).
[c]Patients allergic to β-lactams should receive a quinolone. Persons unable to tolerate a β-lactam (penicillin or cephalosporin) or a quinolone should receive spectinomycin.
[d]Another recommended IM or PO cephalosporin also may be used.
[e]The fluoroquinolones, doxycycline, and erythromycin ethylsuccinate are contraindicated during pregnancy.
[f]Patients treated with one of the recommended regimens should be treated with doxycycline or azithromycin for possible coexistent chlamydial infection.
[g]Patients with gonococcal meningitis should be treated for 10–14 days and those with endocarditis for at least 4 wk with ceftriaxone 1–2 g IV every 12 h.
[h]Treatment regimen should be continued for 24–48 h after improvement begins and switched to cefixime 400 mg PO twice daily or ciprofloxacin 500 mg two times a day to complete a week of therapy.
[i]Treatment for 10–14 days is required if meningitis is present.
[j]Patients with bacteremia or arthritis should receive ceftriaxone 50 mg/kg (maximum 1 g) IM or IV once daily for 7 days. Patients with meningitis should be treated for 10–14 days, with a daily dose of ceftriaxone not to exceed 2 g.
[k]The eye should be lavaged one time with saline solution.

- Treatment of gonorrhea during pregnancy is essential to prevent ophthalmia neonatorum. The American Academy of Pediatrics recommends that either **silver nitrate** (1%), **tetracycline** (1%), or **erythromycin** (0.5%) be instilled in each conjunctival sac immediately postpartum to prevent ophthalmia neonatorum.
- Infants born to infected mothers should also receive an intramuscular or intravenous injection of ceftriaxone 50 mg/kg for 7 days.

EVALUATION OF THERAPEUTIC OUTCOMES

- Combination gonorrhea/chlamydia therapy rarely results in treatment failures, and routine follow-up of patients treated with a regimen included in the CDC guidelines is not recommended.
- Persistence of symptoms following any treatment requires culture of the site(s) of gonorrheal infection, as well as susceptibility testing if gonococci are isolated.

▶ SYPHILIS

- The causative organism of syphilis is *Treponema pallidum,* a spirochete.
- Syphilis is usually acquired by sexual contact with infected mucous membranes or cutaneous lesions, although on rare occasions, it can be acquired by nonsexual personal contact, accidental inoculation, or blood transfusion. VIII

CLINICAL PRESENTATION

Primary Syphilis

- After exposure and an incubation period of 10–90 days (average, 21 days), a painless lesion or chancre appears at the site of treponemal penetrance. Subsequently, it develops into a papule that erodes and ulcerates.
- Chancres persist only for 1–8 weeks before spontaneously disappearing.

Secondary Syphilis

- The secondary stage of syphilis develops 2–6 weeks after the onset of the primary stage in untreated or inadequately treated patients and is characterized by a variety of mucocutaneous eruptions, resulting from widespread hematogenous and lymphatic spread of *T. pallidum*.
- Often lesions appear on the palms of the hands and the soles of the feet. Mild and transitory malaise, fever, pharyngitis, headache, anorexia, and arthralgia are common.
- Signs and symptoms of secondary syphilis disappear in 4–10 weeks; however, in untreated patients, lesions may recur at any time within 4 years.

Latent Syphilis

- Persons with a positive serologic test for syphilis but with no other evidence of disease have latent syphilis.

- A large percentage of untreated patients with latent syphilis have no further sequelae; however, approximately 25–30% progress to late or tertiary syphilis.

Neurosyphilis and Late Syphilis Other Than Neurosyphilis

- Previously referred to as "tertiary syphilis," manifestations of disease 2–25 years after the onset of syphilis are referred to as neurosyphilis or late syphilis with manifestations other than neurosyphilis.
- Forty percent of patients with primary or secondary syphilis exhibit CNS infection with general paresis, eighth cranial nerve deafness, optic atrophy and blindness, progressive dementia, meningovascular complications, or tabes dorsalis.
- Patients may also develop cardiovascular syphilis, characterized by aortitis and aortic insufficiency.

DIAGNOSIS

- Because *T. pallidum* is difficult to culture in vitro, diagnosis is based primarily on dark-field or direct fluorescent antibody microscopic examination of serous material from a suspected syphilitic lesion or on results from serologic testing.
- Serologic tests used in screening for the diagnosis of syphilis are categorized as nontreponemal or treponemal. Commonly used nontreponemal tests include the Venereal Disease Research Laboratory (VDRL) slide test and the rapid plasma reagin (RPR) card test.
- Treponemal tests are used to confirm the diagnosis (i.e., the fluorescent treponemal antibody absorption [FTA-ABS]).

TREATMENT

- Treatment recommendations for syphilis from the CDC are presented in Table 43–4.
- For pregnant patients, **penicillin** is the treatment of choice at the dosage recommended for that particular stage of syphilis. To assure treatment success and prevent transmission to the fetus, some experts advocate an additional intramuscular dose of benzathine penicillin G 2.4 million units 1 week after completion of the recommended regimen.
- The majority of patients treated for primary and secondary syphilis experience the Jarisch–Herxheimer reaction beginning 2–4 hours after treatment, characterized by flu-like symptoms such as transient headache, fever, chills, malaise, arthralgia, myalgia, tachypnea, peripheral vasodilation, and aggravation of syphilitic lesions.
- The Jarisch–Herxheimer reaction should not be confused with penicillin allergy. Most reactions can be managed symptomatically with analgesics, antipyretics, and rest.

EVALUATION OF THERAPEUTIC OUTCOMES

- CDC recommendations for serologic follow-up of patients treated for syphilis are given in Table 43–4. Quantitative nontreponemal tests

TABLE 43–4. Drug Therapy and Follow-up of Syphilis

Stage/Type of Syphilis	Recommended Regimen[a]	Follow-up Serology
Primary, secondary, or latent syphilis of less than 1-y duration (early latent syphilis)	Benzathine penicillin G 2.4 million U IM in a single dose[b]	Quantitative nontreponemal tests at 3 and 6 mo for primary and secondary syphilis; at 6 and 12 mo for early latent syphilis[c]
Syphilis of more than 1-y duration (includes late latent syphilis of unknown duration and late syphilis other than neurosyphilis)	Benzathine penicillin G 2.4 million U IM once a wk for 3 successive wk	Quantitative nontreponemal tests at 6 and 12 mo for late latent syphilis[d]
Neurosyphilis	Aqueous crystalline penicillin G 12–24 million U IV (2–4 million U every 4 h) for 10–14 days[f]; or aqueous procaine penicillin G 2.4 million U IM daily plus probenecid 500 mg PO four times daily, both for 10–14 days[f]	CSF[e] examination every 6 mo until the cell count is normal; if it has not decreased at 6 mo or is not normal by 2 y, retreatment is suggested
Congenital syphilis	Aqueous crystalline penicillin G 50,000 U/kg IV every 12 h during the first 7 days of life and every 8 h thereafter for 10–14 days; or procaine penicillin G 50,000 U/kg IM daily for 10–14 days	Quantitative nontreponemal tests every 2–3 mo until nonreactive (6–12 mo)

(continued)

TABLE 43–4. continued

Stage/Type of Syphilis	Recommended Regimen[a]	Follow-up Serology
Penicillin-allergic patients[g] with primary, secondary, or latent syphilis of less than 1 y duration	Doxycycline 100 mg PO two times daily for 2 wk; or tetracycline 500 mg PO four times daily for 2 wk; or erythromycin 500 mg PO four times daily for 2 wk	Same as for non–penicillin-allergic patients
Syphilis of more than 1 y duration (except neurosyphilis)	Doxycycline 100 mg PO two times a day for 4 wk; or tetracycline 500 mg PO four times daily for 4 wk	Same as for non–penicillin-allergic patients

[a]Recommendations are those of the CDC.

[b]Some experts recommend multiple doses of benzathine penicillin G or other supplemental antibiotics in addition to benzathine penicillin G in HIV-infected patients with primary or secondary syphilis; HIV-infected patients with early latent syphilis should be treated with the recommended regimen for syphilis of more than 1 y duration.

[c]More frequent follow-up (i.e., 1, 2, 3, 6, 9, and 12 mo) recommended for HIV-infected patients.

[d]Minimal data exist on which to base specific follow-up recommendations for late syphilis.

[e]CSF, cerebrospinal fluid.

[f]Some experts administer benzathine penicillin G 2.4 million U IM after completion of the neurosyphilis regimens to provide a total duration of therapy comparable to that used for late syphilis in the absence of neurosyphilis.

[g]For nonpregnant patients; pregnant patients should be treated with penicillin after desensitization.

should be performed at 3 and 6 months in all patients treated for primary and secondary syphilis and at 6 and 12 months for early and late latent disease.

- For women treated during pregnancy, monthly quantitative nontreponemal tests are recommended until the adequacy of therapy is established. Women who do not demonstrate a four-fold decrease in titer over a 3-month period, or who show a four-fold increase in titer between tests, should be retreated.

► CHLAMYDIA

- Infections caused by *Chlamydia trachomatis* are believed to be the most common STD in the United States and the most common cause of nongonococcal urethritis (NGU).

CLINICAL PRESENTATION

- In males, the most common symptoms of chlamydial genital tract infections are dysuria, urinary frequency, and a mucoid urethral discharge occurring 7–21 days after exposure.
- In approximately 50% of men with chlamydial infections, no signs or symptoms are present.
- The majority of women with chlamydial infections are asymptomatic. In women with urethral infections, dysuria and frequency are uncommon.
- When symptomatic, the most common manifestation of infection is endocervicitis with a mucopurulent discharge.
- Similar to gonorrhea, chlamydia may be transmitted to an infant during contact with infected cervicovaginal secretions. Nearly two-thirds of infants acquire chlamydial infection after endocervical exposure, with the primary morbidity associated with seeding of the infant's eyes, nasopharynx, rectum, or vagina.

DIAGNOSIS

- Tests that allow rapid identification of chlamydial antigens in genital secretions are the direct fluorescent antibody test, the EIA, and the DNA hybridization probe.

TREATMENT

- Recommended regimens for treatment of chlamydial infections are given in Table 43–5.
- For prophylaxis of ophthalmia neonatorum, various groups have proposed the use of **erythromycin** (0.5%) or **tetracycline** (1%) ophthalmic ointment in lieu of silver nitrate. Although silver nitrate and antibiotic ointments are effective against gonococcal ophthalmia neonatorum, silver nitrate is not effective for chlamydial disease and may cause a chemical conjunctivitis.

TABLE 43–5. Treatment of Chlamydial Infections

Infection	Recommended Regimen[a]	Alternative Regimen
Uncomplicated urethral, endocervical, or rectal infection in adults	Doxycycline 100 mg PO 2 times daily for 7 days; or azithromycin 1 g once[b]	Ofloxacin 300 mg PO 2 times daily for 7 days[c]; or erythromycin base 500 mg PO 4 times daily for 7 days; or erythromycin ethylsuccinate 800 mg PO 4 times daily for 7 days; or sulfisoxazole 500 mg 4 times daily for 10 days
Urogenital infections during pregnancy	Erythromycin base 500 mg 4 times PO daily for 7 days	Erythromycin base 250 mg PO 4 times daily for 14 days; or erythromycin ethylsuccinate 800 mg PO 4 times daily for 7 days (or 400 mg PO 4 times daily for 14 days); or amoxicillin 500 mg PO 3 times daily for 7 days[d]
Conjunctivitis of the newborn	Erythromycin suspension 50 mg/kg/days PO in 4 divided doses for 10–14 days	
Pneumonia in infants	Erythromycin suspension 50 mg/kg/days PO in 4 divided doses for 10–14 days	
Acute epididymo-orchitis	Ceftriaxone 250 mg IM[e] **plus** Doxycycline 100 mg PO 2 times daily for 10 days	

[a]Recommendations are those of the CDC.
[b]Data regarding the use of azithromycin in children ≤ 15 years old are not established.
[c]Ofloxacin is contraindicated during pregnancy and should not be used in patients ≤ 17 years old.
[d]Only if GI intolerance to erythromycin; limited data exist for efficacy.
[e]The efficacy of ceftriaxone 125 mg or azithromycin has not been studied and is unknown.

VIII

- The only acceptable treatment for chlamydial ophthalmia neonatorum is systemic therapy with oral **erythromycin** 50 mg/kg/d in four divided doses for 10–14 days.

EVALUATION OF THERAPEUTIC OUTCOMES

- Treatment of chlamydial infections with the recommended regimens is highly effective; therefore, post-treatment cultures are not routinely recommended.
- Infants with pneumonitis should receive follow-up testing, because erythromycin is only 80% effective.

► GENITAL HERPES

- The term "herpes" is used to describe two distinct but antigenically related serotypes of herpes simplex virus (HSV). Herpes simplex virus type 1 (HSV-1) is most commonly associated with oropharyngeal disease, and herpes simplex virus type 2 (HSV-2) is most closely associated with genital disease.

CLINICAL PRESENTATION

- The clinical manifestations of first episodes of genital herpes usually appear within 2–14 days after exposure.
- Up to 50% of HSV-2 infections are asymptomatic, and these infections may represent the most common source of transmission of genital and neonatal herpes infections.
- More than 50% of patients with primary infections (classified as infections occurring in persons lacking antibody to either type of HSV) experience flu-like symptoms of fever, headache, malaise, and myalgias. Systemic symptoms gradually resolve over the course of a week.
- Local symptoms include development of painful pustular or ulcerative lesions on the external genitalia. Lesions usually begin as papules or vesicles that rapidly spread over the genitalia. Clusters of the lesions coalesce into large areas of ulceration, which over 2–3 weeks crust and/or reepithelialize. VIII
- Other local symptoms can include itching, dysuria, vaginal or urethral discharge, and tender inguinal adenopathy.
- First-episode nonprimary genital herpes is defined as an infection in individuals who have clinical or serologic evidence of prior HSV (usually HSV-1) infection at another body site. These infections tend to be milder than true primary infections, with a lower incidence of constitutional symptoms and a shorter duration of disease reported.
- Recurrent infection is localized to the genital area and is milder and of a shorter duration (e.g., 8–12 days). Viral shedding lasts approximately 4 days.
- Symptoms of recurrent infection tend to be more severe in women, primarily as a result of the greater genital surface area involved, and in immunocompromised patients.
- Neonatal herpes is associated with a high mortality and significant morbidity.

DIAGNOSIS

- A presumptive diagnosis of genital herpes commonly is made based on the presence of dark-field–negative, vesicular, or ulcerative genital lesions. A history of similar lesions or recent sexual contact with an individual with similar lesions also is useful in making the diagnosis.
- Tissue culture is the most specific (100%) and sensitive method (80–90%) of confirming the diagnosis of first-episode genital herpes.

- Antigen detection methods such as direct immunofluorescence, immunoperoxidase staining, and enzyme-linked immunosorbent assay provide more rapid results than culture and are less expensive.

TREATMENT

- The goals of therapy in genital herpes infection are to shorten the clinical course, prevent complications, prevent the development of latency and/or subsequent recurrences, decrease disease transmission, and eliminate established latency.
- Palliative and supportive measures are the cornerstone of therapy for patients with genital herpes. Pain and discomfort usually respond to warm saline baths or the use of analgesics, antipyretics, or antipruritics.
- To prevent bacterial superinfection, lesions must be kept clean and dry.
- Specific chemotherapeutic approaches to treating genital herpes fall into six major areas: antiviral compounds, topical surfactants, photodynamic dyes, immune modulators, vaccines, and interferons.
- Specific recommendations are given in Table 43–6.

TABLE 43–6. Treatment of Genital Herpes

Type of Infection	Recommended Regimen[a,b]	Alternative Regimen
First clinical episode of genital herpes[c]	Acyclovir 200 mg PO five times daily for 7–10 days, or until clinical resolution occurs	Acyclovir 5–10 mg/kg IV every 8 h for 5–7 days or until clinical resolution occurs[d]
First clinical episode of herpes proctitis	Acyclovir 400 mg PO five times daily for 10 days, or until clinical resolution occurs	Acyclovir 5–10 mg/kg IV every 8 h for 5–7 days or until clinical resolution occurs[d]
Recurrent infection		
Treatment	Acyclovir 200 mg PO five times daily; or 400 mg PO three times daily; or 800 mg PO twice daily for 5 days, initiated within 48 h of onset of lesions[e]	
Suppression	Acyclovir 400 mg PO twice daily[f]	Acyclovir 200 mg PO 3–5 times daily

[a] Recommendations are those of the CDC.

[b] HIV-infected patients may require more aggressive therapy.

[c] Primary or nonprimary first episode.

[d] Only for patients with severe symptoms or complications that necessitate hospitalization.

[e] Treatment should be limited to patients with severe symptoms. Treatment is most beneficial when instituted at the earliest sign of recurrence (i.e., prodrome); therapy initiated 48 h or more after the onset of symptoms has no effect.

[f] Indicated only for patients with frequent and/or severe recurrences; although safety and efficacy are documented in patients receiving daily therapy for as long as 5 y, it is recommended that therapy be discontinued after 1 y of continuous suppressive therapy to assess the patient's rate of recurrent episodes.

- Topical therapy alone or with oral therapy is considered of little or no benefit in most patients. In humans, no acyclovir regimen is known to prevent latency or alter the subsequent frequency and severity of recurrences.
- Oral acyclovir is the treatment of choice for outpatients with first-episode genital herpes. Treatment does not prevent latency or alter the subsequent frequency and severity of recurrences.
- When initiated early during the course of recurrence, oral acyclovir reduces the duration of viral shedding and diminishes the time to healing of lesions. Appreciable effects on symptomatology are not seen. Patients with prolonged episodes of recurrent infection are most likely to benefit from oral therapy instituted at the earliest sign of recurrence.
- Chronic oral therapy reduces the frequency and the severity of recurrences in 70–90% of patients experiencing frequent recurrences.
- Both intravenous and oral acyclovir have been used to prevent reactivation of infection in patients seropositive for HSV who undergo transplantation procedures or induction chemotherapy for acute leukemia.
- The safety of acyclovir therapy during pregnancy is not established, although there is no evidence of teratogenic effects in humans.

▶ TRICHOMONIASIS

- Trichomoniasis is caused by *Trichomonas vaginalis,* a flagellated, motile protozoan.
- It is estimated that 2.5–3 million cases of vaginal trichomoniasis occur annually in the United States. The peak incidence in women occurs between the ages of 16 and 35, although there is a high prevalence between ages 35 and 45.

CLINICAL PRESENTATION

- The incubation period of trichomoniasis is 3–28 days, with as many as 50% of infected women remaining asymptomatic.
- When symptomatic, females can present with mild to severe vaginal discharge, vulvar pruritis, and dysuria.
- Vaginal discharge is noted in approximately 50–75% of infected women and classically has been described as malodorous, foamy, and greenish yellow in color; however, more typically the discharge is grayish and only mildly odoriferous.
- Trichomoniasis may be responsible for causing premature rupture of the membranes and preterm delivery. It can be transmitted to neonates after passage through an infected birth canal.
- In men, the majority of trichomonal infections are asymptomatic. The most common site of infection is the urethra. In symptomatic males, urethral discharge is seen most commonly, followed by pruritis and dysuria. The discharge may range from mucoid to purulent.

- For most men, trichomonal urethritis is apparently self-limited. *T. vaginalis* has been implicated in some cases of prostatitis and epididymitis.

DIAGNOSIS

- The diagnosis of *T. vaginalis* may be complicated because approximately 97% of symptomatic women are concomitantly colonized with yeast.
- The simplest and most reliable means of diagnosis is a wet-mount examination of the vaginal discharge. Trichomoniasis is confirmed if characteristic pear-shaped, flagellating organisms are observed.

TREATMENT

- **Metronidazole** is the only antimicrobial agent available in the United States that is consistently effective in *T. vaginalis* infections.
- Treatment recommendations for *Trichomonas* infections are given in Table 43–7.
- Gastrointestinal complaints (e.g., anorexia, nausea, vomiting, diarrhea) are the most common adverse effects with the single 2-g dose of metronidazole, occurring in 5–10% of treated patients. Some patients complain of a bitter metallic taste in the mouth.
- Patients intolerant of the single 2-g dose because of gastrointestinal adverse effects can be treated with a 7-day course of 500 mg twice daily.

TABLE 43–7. Treatment of Trichomoniasis

Type	Recommended Regimen[a]	Alternative Regimen
Symptomatic and asymptomatic infections	Metronidazole 2 g PO in a single dose[b]	Metronidazole 500 mg PO 2 times daily for 7 d[c]
Treatment in pregnancy	No treatment recommended unless symptoms are severe[d]	
Neonatal infections[e]	Metronidazole 10–30 mg/kg daily for 5–8 d	

[a]Recommendations are those of the CDC.

[b]Treatment failures should be treated with metronidazole 500 mg PO two times daily for 7 d. Persistent failures should be managed in consultation with an expert. Metronidazole 2 g PO daily for 3–5 d has been effective in patients infected with *T. vaginalis* strains mildly resistant to metronidazole, but experience is limited; higher doses also have been used.

[c]Metronidazole labeling approved by the FDA does not include this regimen. Dosage regimens for treatment of trichomoniasis included in the product labeling are the single 2-g dose; 250 mg three times daily for 7 d; and 375 mg two times daily for 7 d. The 250- and 375-mg dosage regimens are currently not included in the CDC recommendations.

[d]Metronidazole is contraindicated in the first trimester of pregnancy and generally should be avoided throughout pregnancy. If used, a single 2-g dose administered after the first trimester of pregnancy is recommended by the CDC; however, a 7-d regimen is preferred by some because it produces lower peak serum concentrations.

[e]Only infants with symptomatic trichomoniasis or with urogenital trichomonal colonization that persists beyond the fourth week of life.

- To achieve maximal cure rates and prevent relapse with the single 2-g dose of metronidazole, simultaneous treatment of infected sexual partners is necessary.
- Patients who fail to respond to an initial course usually respond to a second course of metronidazole therapy.
- Patients taking metronidazole should be instructed to avoid alcohol ingestion during therapy and for 1–2 days after completion of therapy because of a possible disulfiram-like effect.
- At present, no satisfactory treatment is available for pregnant women with *Trichomonas* infections. Clotrimazole vaginal suppositories may relieve symptoms in many women.

EVALUATION OF THERAPEUTIC OUTCOMES

- Follow-up is considered unnecessary in patients who become asymptomatic after treatment with metronidazole.
- When patients remain symptomatic, it is important to determine if reinfection has occurred. In these cases, a repeat course of therapy, as well as identification and treatment or retreatment of infected sexual partners, is recommended.

▶ OTHER SEXUALLY TRANSMITTED DISEASES

- Several STDs other than those previously discussed occur with varying frequency in the United States and throughout the world. While an in-depth discussion of these diseases is beyond the scope of this chapter, recommended treatment regimens are given in Table 43–8. VIII

See Chapter 107, Sexually Transmitted Diseases, authored by Leroy C. Knodel, PharmD, for a more detailed discussion of this topic.

TABLE 43–8. Treatment Regimens for Miscellaneous Sexually Transmitted Diseases

Infection	Recommended Regimen[a]	Alternative Regimen
Chancroid *(Haemophilus ducreyi)*	Azithromycin 1 g PO in a single dose; or ceftriaxone 250 mg IM in a single dose; or erythromycin 500 mg PO four times daily for 7 days	Amoxicillin 500 mg plus clavulanic acid 125 mg three times daily for 7 days; or ciprofloxacin 500 mg PO two times daily for 3 days
Lymphogranuloma venereum	Doxycycline 100 mg PO two times daily for 21 days	Erythromycin 500 mg PO four times daily for 21 days; or sulfisoxazole 500 mg PO four times daily for 21 days or equivalent sulfonamide course
Condylomata acuminata (external genital/perianal warts)	Cryotherapy (e.g., liquid nitrogen or cryoprobe) **or** Podofilox 0.5% solution applied twice daily for 3 days, followed by 4 days of no therapy; cycle is repeated as necessary for a total of four cycles[b] **or** Podophyllin 10–25% in compound tincture of benzoin applied to lesions and washed off in 1–4 h; repeat weekly for up to six applications[c] **or** Trichloroacetic acid 80–90% applied to warts; repeat weekly for up to 6 applications **or** Electrodesiccation[d] or electrocautery	

[a]Recommendations are those of the CDC.
[b]Genital warts only.
[c]Because podophyllin is systemically absorbed and toxic, use of large amounts should be avoided. Use of podophyllin is contraindicated in pregnancy.
[d]Electrodesiccation is contraindicated in patients with cardiac pacemakers or for lesions proximal to the anal verge.
[e]Some experts caution against vaginal use; care must be taken to ensure that the treated area is dry before removing the speculum.

Chapter 44

▶ SKIN AND SOFT TISSUE INFECTIONS

▶ DEFINITION

Bacterial infections of the skin can be classified as primary (pyodermas/cellulitis) or secondary (invasion of the wound) (Table 44–1). Primary bacterial infections are usually caused by a single bacterial species and involve areas of generally normal skin (e.g., impetigo, erysipelas). Secondary infections, however, develop in areas of previously damaged skin and are frequently polymicrobic in nature.

▶ CELLULITIS

- Cellulitis is generally an acute, spreading infectious process that initially affects the epidermis and dermis and may subsequently spread within the superficial fascia. This process is characterized by inflammation, but with little or no necrosis or suppuration of soft tissue.
- A variety of bacteria are responsible for the several types of cellulitis most commonly encountered (Table 44–1).
- Cellulitis is caused by group A β-hemolytic streptococci (most commonly *Streptococcus pyogenes*) or by *Staphylococcus aureus.* Occasionally, other gram-positive cocci such as *Streptococcus pneumoniae* or, in the newborn, group B streptococci can be etiologic agents.

CLINICAL PRESENTATION

- Cellulitis is characterized by erythema and edema of the skin.
- The lesion, which may be extensive, is painful, is nonelevated, and has poorly defined margins. Tender lymphadenopathy associated with lymphatic involvement is common. Malaise, fever, and chills are also commonly present. There is usually a history of an antecedent wound from minor trauma, an ulcer, or surgery.
- Cellulitis of an incised wound may be caused by any microorganism, but the most aggressively spreading lesions are caused by group A streptococci or *Clostridium perfringens.*
- A Gram stain of a smear obtained by injection and aspiration of 0.5 mL of saline (using a small-gauge needle) into the advancing edge of the erythematous lesion may help in making the microbiologic diagnosis but often yields negative results.
- Acute cellulitis with mixed aerobic–anaerobic flora generally occurs (1) in diabetes, where the skin is near a traumatic site or surgical incision; or (2) when host defenses are compromised.

TABLE 44–1. Bacterial Classification of Important Skin and Soft Tissue Infections

Primary Infections	
Cellulitis	Group A streptococcus, *S. aureus, Haemophilus influenzae* (children); occasionally other streptococci or gram-negative bacilli
Gangrenous	Group A streptococcus, anaerobic streptococci plus a second organism, cellulitis (*Staphylococcus* sp. or gram-negative bacilli, e.g., *Proteus*)
Crepitant cellulitis	*Clostridia* sp., *Bacteroides* sp., anaerobic streptococci, gram-negative bacilli *(Klebsiella, E. coli)*
Impetigo	Group A streptococcus, *S. aureus*
Erysipelas	Group A streptococcus
Secondary Infections	
Bite wounds	*Pasteurella multocida, S. aureus, Eikenella corrodens,* anaerobic streptococci, *Fusobacterium* sp., *Bacteroides* sp.
Burn wounds	*Pseudomonas aeruginosa, Enterobacter* sp., other gram-negative bacilli, *S. aureus, Streptococcus* sp.
Diabetic foot infections	*Proteus* sp., *E. coli, S. aureus, Bacteroides fragilis,* anaerobic streptococci
Infections in IV drug abusers	*S. aureus, Streptococcus* sp., gram-negative bacilli, *Bacteroides* sp.
Decubitus ulcers	Gram-negative bacilli, *P. aeruginosa,* various gram-positive and -negative anaerobes
Lymphangitis (acute)	Group A streptococcus, *S. aureus, P. multocida*

TREATMENT

- Antimicrobial therapy of bacterial cellulitis depends on the type of bacteria either documented to be present or suspected. In some instances, the rapid identification and treatment are imperative (i.e., group A streptococci).
- Local care of cellulitis includes elevation and immobilization of the involved area to decrease local swelling.
- Surgical intervention (incision and drainage) as a mode of therapy is rarely indicated in the treatment of cellulitis.
- As streptococcal cellulitis is indistinguishable clinically from staphylococcal cellulitis, administration of a semisynthetic penicillin **(nafcillin** or **oxacillin)** is recommended until a definitive diagnosis, by skin or blood cultures, can be made (Table 44–2). If documented to be a mild cellulitis secondary to streptococci, oral **penicillin** VK 250–500 mg four times daily or intramuscular procaine penicillin for 10–14 days is adequate. More severe streptococcal infections should be treated with intravenous antibiotics. Mild to moderate staphylococcal infections may be treated orally with **dicloxacillin** 250–500 mg four times daily.

- In penicillin-allergic patients, oral or parenteral **erythromycin** is used. Alternatively, a first-generation cephalosporin such as **cefazolin** (1–2 mg every 6–8 hours) may be used cautiously for patients who have not experienced immediate or anaphylactic penicillin reactions and are penicillin skin test negative. In cases where an oral cephalosporin can be used, **cefadroxil** 500 mg twice daily or **cephalexin** 250–500 mg four times daily is recommended.
- When erythromycin or cephalosporins cannot be used due to methicillin-resistant staphylococci or severe allergic reactions to β-lactam antibiotics, intravenous **vancomycin** (for 10–14 days) should be administered. Other effective but more expensive agents include **clarithromycin, azithromycin, ceftriaxone, imipenem,** and the β-lactamase inhibitor combination antibiotics **(ampicillin/sulbactam, ticarcillin/clavulanic acid,** and **piperacillin/tazobactam).**
- For cellulitis caused by gram-negative bacilli or a mixture of microorganisms, immediate antimicrobial chemotherapy as determined by Gram stain is essential, along with appropriate surgical excision of necrotic tissue and drainage. Usually an aminoglycoside combined with an antianaerobic cephalosporin, extended-spectrum penicillin, or clindamycin will be used. Therapy should be 10–14 days in duration.

▶ ERYSIPELAS

- Erysipelas (Saint Anthony's fire) is a distinct type of superficial cellulitis with extensive lymphatic involvement. It is almost always due to *S. pyogenes* (group A streptococci). Other streptococci (in the newborn) and, rarely, *S. aureus* can cause similar skin lesions.
- Erysipelas manifests as a warm, painful, edematous, indurated lesion sharply circumscribed by an elevated border. Fever and leukocytosis are common.
- In adults, it occurs most commonly on the skin of the face and involves the bridge of the nose and cheeks.
- Mild to moderate cases of erysipelas in adults are treated with **procaine penicillin G** 600,000 units intramuscularly twice daily or **penicillin VK** 250–500 mg orally four times daily for 7–10 days. Dramatic improvement is generally expected 24–48 hours after treatment has begun.
- Penicillin-allergic patients can be treated with **erythromycin** 250–500 mg orally every 6 hours for 7–10 days. For more serious infections, aqueous penicillin G 2–8 million units daily should be administered intravenously.

▶ IMPETIGO

- Impetigo is a distinctive type of superficial cellulitis caused by group A streptococci (known as streptococcal impetigo or impetigo contagiosa). *S. aureus* may be the causative agent in approximately 10% of patients.

TABLE 44–2. Initial Treatment Regimens for Cellulitis Caused by Various Pathogens

Infection	Adult Dose and Route	Pediatric Dose and Route
Staphylococcal or unknown gram-positive infection		
Mild infection	Dicloxacillin 0.25–0.5 g PO every 6 h[a,b]	Dicloxacillin 25–50 mg/kg/days PO in 4 divided doses[a,b]
Moderate–severe infection	Nafcillin or oxacillin 1–2 g IV every 4–6 h[a,b]	Nafcillin or oxacillin 150–200 mg/kg/days (not to exceed 12 g/24 h) IV in 4 to 6 equally divided doses[a,b]
Streptococcal (documented)		
Mild infection	Penicillin VK 0.5 g PO every 6 h[a] or procaine penicillin G 600,000 units intramuscularly every 8–12 h[a]	Penicillin VK 125–250 mg PO every 6–8 h or procaine penicillin G 25,000–50,000 U/kg (not to exceed 600,000 U) IM every 8–12 h[a]
Moderate–severe infection	Aqueous penicillin G 1-2 million U IV every 4–6 h[a]	Aqueous penicillin G 100,000–200,000 U/kg/days IV in 4 divided doses[a]
Haemophilus influenzae		
Mild infection	Ampicillin 0.5 g PO every 6 h[c] or amoxicillin 0.5 g PO every 8 h[c] **or** Cefaclor 0.5 g PO every 8 h or cefuroxime axetil 0.5 g PO every 12 h[e]	Ampicillin 50–100 mg/kg/days PO in 4 divided doses[c,d] or amoxicillin 20–40 mg/kg/days PO in 3 divided doses[c,d] **or** Cefaclor 20–40 mg/kg/days (not to exceed 1 g) PO in 3 divided doses[d] or cefuroxime axetil 0.125–0.25 g (tablets) PO every 12 h[d]
Moderate–severe infection	Ampicillin 0.5–1 g IV every 6 h[c] **or** Cefuroxime 0.75–1.5 g IV every 8 h or a third-generation cephalosporin (i.e., ceftriaxone 1 g IV once daily or cefotaxime 1–2 g IV every 6–8 h)[e]	Ampicillin 50–100 mg/kg/days IV in four divided doses[c,d] **or** Cefuroxime 75 mg/kg/days IV in three divided doses[d] or a third-generation cephalosporin (i.e., ceftriaxone 75–100 mg/kg IV once or twice daily or cefotaxime 200 mg/kg/days IV in three or four divided doses)[d]
Other single gram-negative aerobes		
Mild infection	Cefaclor 0.5 g PO every 8 h[g] or cefuroxime axetil 0.5 g PO every 12 h[g]	Cefaclor 20–40 mg/kg/days (not to exceed 1 g) PO in 3 divided doses or cefuroxime axetil 0.125–0.25 g (tablets) PO every 12 h

Moderate–severe infection	Aminoglycoside[f] or IV cephalosporin (first- or second-generation depending on severity of infection or susceptibility pattern)[g]	Aminoglycoside[f] or IV cephalosporin (first- or second-generation depending on severity of infection or susceptibility pattern)
Polymicrobic infection without anaerobes	Aminoglycoside[f] + penicillin G 0.6–1 million U every 4–6 h or a semisynthetic penicillin (i.e., nafcillin 1–2 g every 4–6 h) depending on isolation of staphylococci or streptococci[b]	Aminoglycoside[f] + penicillin G 100,000–200,000 U/kg/days IV in 4 divided doses or a semisynthetic penicillin (i.e., nafcillin 150–200 mg/kg/days [not to exceed 12 g/24 h] IV in 4 to 6 equally divided doses) depending on isolation of staphylococci or streptococci[b]
Polymicrobic infection with anaerobes		
Mild infection	Amoxicillin/clavulanic acid 0.5 g PO every 8 h **or** A fluoroquinolone (i.e., ciprofloxacin or levofloxacin) plus clindamycin 0.6–0.9 g PO every 8 h or metronidazole 0.5 g PO every 8 h	Amoxicillin/clavulanic acid 20 mg/kg/days PO in 3 divided doses
Moderate–severe infection	Aminoglycoside[f] + clindamycin 0.9 g IV every 8 h or metronidazole 0.5 g IV every 8 h **or** Monotherapy with second- or third-generation cephalosporin (i.e., cefoxitin 1–2 g IV every 6 h or ceftizoxime 1–2 IV every 8 h) **or** Monotherapy with imipenem 0.5 g every 6–8 h or meropenem 1 g IV every 8 h or extended-spectrum penicillins with a β-lactamase inhibitor	Aminoglycoside[f] + clindamycin 15 mg/kg/days IV in 3 divided doses or metronidazole 30–50 mg/kg/days IV in 3 divided doses

[a]For penicillin-allergic patients, use erythromycin 0.5–1 g every 6 h (pediatric dosing 30–40 mg/kg/days in divided doses).
[b]For methicillin-resistant staphylococci, use vancomycin 0.5–1 g every 6–12 h (pediatric dosing 40 mg/kg/days in divided doses) with dosage adjustments made for renal dysfunction.
[c]In areas with a high incidence of β-lactamase–producing strains, a third-generation cephalosporin should be used until sensitivities are available.
[d]For penicillin-allergic children, use trimethoprim–sulfamethoxazole (4 mg/kg twice daily) or chloramphenicol (50–100 mg/kg/days in four divided doses).
[e]For penicillin-allergic adults, use trimethoprim–sulfamethoxazole (4–5 mg/kg twice daily) or a fluoroquinolone (ciprofloxacin 200–400 mg IV or 750 mg PO twice daily; ofloxacin 400 mg IV or PO twice daily; levofloxacin 500 mg IV or PO once daily).
[f]Gentamicin or tobramycin, 2 mg/kg loading dose, then maintenance dose determined by serum concentrations.
[g]For penicillin-allergic adults, use a fluoroquinolone.

- Impetigo manifests initially as small, fluid-filled vesicles. These lesions then rapidly develop into pus-filled blisters that readily rupture. The purulent discharges of these lesions dry to form golden-yellow crusts that are quite characteristic of impetigo. Pruritus is common, and scratching of the lesions may further spread infection through excoriation of the skin. Other systemic signs of infection are minimal.
- The drug of choice for treatment of impetigo is **penicillin.** It may be administered as either a single intramuscular dose of **benzathine penicillin G** (300,000–600,000 units in children, 1.2 million units in adults) or as oral **penicillin VK** (25,000–90,000 units/kg/day divided into four doses in children, 250–500 mg orally four times daily in adults) given for 7–10 days.
- Penicillin-allergic patients can be treated with oral **erythromycin** (30–50 mg/kg/day divided into four doses in children, 250–500 mg every 6 hours in adults) for 7–10 days.

▶ INFECTED PRESSURE ULCERS

- Many factors are thought to predispose patients to the formation of pressure ulcers: paralysis, paresis, immobilization, malnutrition, anemia, infection, and advanced age. Four factors thought to be most critical to their formation are pressure, shearing forces, friction, and moisture; however, there is still debate as to the exact pathophysiology of pressure sore formation.
- Without treatment, an initial small localized area of ulceration can rapidly progress to 5–6 cm within days.
- Pressure sores are routinely colonized by a wide variety of microorganisms; gram-negative aerobes and anaerobes are most often associated with the infections.

CLINICAL PRESENTATION

- More than 95% of all pressure sores are located on the lower part of the body (65% in the region of the pelvis and 3.4% on the lower extremities). The most common sites on the lower portion of the body are the sacral and coccygeal areas, ischial tuberosities, and greater trochanter.
- Pressure sores vary greatly in their severity, ranging from an abrasion to large lesions that can penetrate into the deep fascia involving both bone and muscle.

PREVENTION AND TREATMENT

- Prevention is the single most important aspect in the management of pressure sores. Friction and shearing forces can be minimized by proper positioning. Skin care and prevention of soilage are important, with the intent being to keep the surface relatively free from moisture. Relief of pressure (even for 5 minutes once every 2 hours) is probably the single most important factor in preventing pressure sore formation.

Medical Management

- Medical management is generally indicated for lesions that are of moderate size and of relatively shallow depth (stage 1 or 2 lesions) and are not located over a bony prominence.
- The main factors to be considered for successful topical therapy (local care) are the relief of pressure, cleaning measures (debridement), disinfection, and stimulation of granulation tissue.

Debridement

- Debridement can be accomplished by surgical or mechanical means (wet-to-dry dressing changes). None of the currently available debriding agents (e.g., **sutilains, collagenase, dextranomer**) have been documented to be superior to wet-to-dry dressings.
- **Collagenase** is thought by many to be the most effective enzymatic debriding agent. Generally, collagenase need only be applied to a clean wound once daily, unless the wound is extremely soiled.
- **Dextranomer** appears to be effective in cleansing exudative venous stasis and decubitus ulcers. It also appears to increase tissue granulation, decrease wound inflammation, and decrease pus and debris; however, its cost and application techniques limit its usefulness.

Disinfection

- A number of agents have been used to disinfect pressure sores (e.g., **acetic acid, sodium hypochlorite, hydrogen peroxide, mupirocin, bacitracin**) as well as other types of open wounds; however, objective clinical trials evaluating their efficacy are lacking. VIII
- Most pressure sores are infected with both aerobic and anaerobic microorganisms; however, disinfectants have not been shown to penetrate tissue effectively to completely eradicate these organisms.
- Although disinfectants do not sterilize a wound and may interfere with wound healing, they may be of potential benefit by cleaning the wound (by decreasing the bacterial counts), but they should be stopped when the wound is clean and granulation appears to be occurring.

Granulation/Epithelialization

- After the pressure sore has been adequately debrided and disinfected, and pressure, friction, and moisture have been kept to a minimum, granulation and reepithelialization begin. Many agents have been suggested to aid this process, but hardly any evidence of a supportive nature exists.

RECOMMENDATIONS

- Treatment of the wound begins with the removal of necrotic tissue via either debridement or surgery, along with elimination of any infection. The goal of therapy is to maintain a clean and moist environment.

Some broad major guidelines can be recommended for the treatment of pressure sores (stages 1 and 2):

- Relieve pressure.
- Avoid unnecessary friction and shearing forces.
- Prevent patient from lying in a moist environment.
- Use debridement, either pharmacologic or via minor surgical approach.
- Keep the wound clean by pharmacologic means or through use of a physical barrier.
- Use occlusive dressing (may also lead to increased healing and simplify the nursing care routine) if possible.

▶ INFECTED BITE WOUNDS

DOG BITES

- Health care providers see two distinct groups of patients seeking medical attention for dog bites. The first group of patients presents 8–12 hours after the injury and requires general wound care, repair of tear wounds, or rabies and/or tetanus therapy. The second group of patients presents more than 12 hours after the injury has occurred and usually has clinical signs of infection and seeks medical attention for infection-related complaints (i.e., pain, purulent discharge, swelling).

- The infected dog bite is usually characterized by a localized cellulitis and pain at the site of injury. The cellulitis usually spreads proximally from the initial site of injury. If *Pasteurella multocida* is present, a rapidly progressing cellulitis with a gray malodorous discharge may be encountered.
- The most frequently isolated organisms from infected and noninfected wounds are *S. aureus,* α-hemolytic streptococci, *Streptococcus* intermedius, *P. multocida, Eikenella corrodens, Capnocytophaga canimursus, Bacteroides* sp., and *Fusobacterium* sp.
- Wounds should be thoroughly irrigated with a sterile saline solution or a chlorhexidine scrub solution. Proper irrigation significantly decreases the rate of subsequent infection.
- The role of antimicrobials for noninfected dog bite wounds remains controversial. A semisynthetic penicillinase-resistant penicillin orally or **amoxicillin/clavulanic acid** should be used in high-risk patients, those with puncture wounds, patients over 50 years of age, wounds to the hands, and wounds in compromised hosts.
- **Tetracycline** or **trimethoprim–sulfamethoxazole** is recommended as an alternative form of therapy for those patients allergic to penicillins. **Erythromycin** may be considered an alternative for tetracycline in growing children or pregnant women.
- Prophylactic therapy should be given for 5 days. In addition to irrigation and antibiotics, when indicated, the injured area should be immobilized and elevated.

- Infections developing within the first 24 hours of a bite are most often caused by *P. multocida* and should be treated with **penicillin** or **amoxicillin/clavulanic** acid (**tetracycline** is an alternative for nonpregnant adult penicillin-allergic patients). Treatment should be given for 10–14 days.
- For those infections developing more than 36–48 hours after the bite, the risk of *P. multocida* being involved dramatically decreases in likelihood. Therapy in this instance includes a penicillinase-resistant penicillin (e.g., **dicloxacillin**) or a cephalosporin (e.g., **cefuroxime axetil**) and should be given for a full 10–14 days.
- If the immunization history of a patient with anything other than a clean minor wound is not known, **tetanus/diphtheria toxoids** (Td) and **tetanus immune globulin** (TIG) should be administered.
- If a patient has been exposed to rabies, the treatment objectives consist of thorough irrigation of the wound, tetanus prophylaxis, antibiotic prophylaxis, if indicated, and immunization. Postexposure prophylaxis immunization consists of both passive antibody administration and vaccine administration.

CAT BITES

- Approximately 40% of cat bites and scratches become infected. These infections are frequently caused by *P. multocida,* which has been isolated in the oropharynx of 50–70% of healthy cats. VIII
- The management of cat bites is similar to that discussed for dog bites. Antibiotic therapy with **penicillin** is the mainstay and therapy is as described for dog bites.

HUMAN BITES

- Infections can occur in up to 50% of patients with human bites.
- Infections caused by these injuries are most often caused by the normal oral flora, which includes both aerobic and anaerobic microorganisms. The most frequent aerobic organisms are streptococcal species, *S. aureus, Haemophilus parainfluenzae, Klebsiella pneumoniae,* and *E. corrodens.* The most common anaerobic organisms are *Bacteroides* sp., *Fusobacterium* sp., *Peptostreptococcus* sp., and *Peptococcus* sp. Anaerobic microorganisms have been isolated in the range of 40% of human bites and 55% of clenched-fist injuries.
- Management of bites wounds consists of aggressive irrigation, surgical debridement, and immobilization of the affected area. Primary closure for human bites is not generally recommended. If damage to a bone or joint is suspected, radiographic evaluation should be undertaken. **Tetanus toxoid** and **antitoxin** may be indicated.
- Patients with noninfected bite injuries should be given prophylactic antibiotic therapy. Initial therapy should consist of a penicillinase-resistant penicillin (e.g., **dicloxacillin**) in combination with **penicillin.** Prophylactic therapy should be given for 3–5 days as for dog bites. A first-generation cephalosporin is not recommended, as the sensitivity

to *E. corrodens* is variable. For infected bite wounds, penicillin and a **penicillinase-resistant penicillin** or **amoxicillin/clavulanic acid** should be empirically started and changed pending the culture results. Duration of therapy for infected bite injuries should be 7–14 days.

▶ BACTERIAL DIABETIC FOOT INFECTIONS

- Three key factors are involved in the causation of diabetic foot problems: neuropathy, ischemia, and immunologic defects. Any of these disorders can occur in isolation; however, they frequently occur together.
- Diabetic foot infections are typically polymicrobic (an average of 4.1–5.8 isolates per culture). Obligate anaerobes have a significant part in the bacterial flora of these infections. The most common aerobic isolates are *Proteus mirabilis,* group D streptococci, *Escherichia coli,* and *S. aureus.* The principal anaerobic isolate is *Bacteroides fragilis,* followed by *Peptococcus* and *Peptostreptococcus* sp.

TREATMENT

- The goal of therapy is preservation of as much normal limb function as possible while preventing infectious complications.
- Most infections can be successfully treated on an outpatient basis with wound care and antibiotics.
- Maximize diabetic control to ensure optimal healing.
- Restrict the patient initially to bed rest, leg elevation, and control of edema, if present.
- Rule out the possibility of osteomyelitis via x-ray and/or bone scan.
- After healing of the infected ulcer has occurred, a program for prevention should be designed.
- **Amoxicillin/clavulanate** is the agent of choice for oral outpatient treatment. **Fluoroquinolones** with **metronidazole** or **clindamycin** are reasonable alternatives.
- Serious polymicrobic infections may be treated with agents used for anaerobic cellulitis (Table 44–2).
- Monotherapy with broad-spectrum parenteral antimicrobials, along with appropriate medical and/or surgical management, is often effective in treating moderate to severe infections (including those in which osteomyelitis is present).
- Treatment of soft tissue infections in diabetic patients should generally be 10–14 days in duration. However, in cases of underlying osteomyelitis, treatment should continue for 6–12 weeks.

RECOMMENDATIONS FOR THE MANAGEMENT OF THE INFECTED DIABETIC FOOT

- Initially assess the extent of the lesion.
- Obtain deep tissue cultures for both anaerobes and aerobes.

- Debride necrotic tissue and keep wound clean with dressing changes as needed (generally two to three times daily).

See Chapter 100, Skin and Soft Tissue Infections, authored by Larry H. Danzinger, PharmD, and Douglas N. Fish, PharmD, BCPS, for a more detailed discussion of this topic.

Chapter 45

▶ SURGICAL PROPHYLAXIS

▶ DEFINITION

- *Prophylactic* antibiotics are administered prior to contamination of previously uninfected tissues or fluids. The goal is to prevent a surgical-site infection (SSI) from developing. The prevention and management of postoperative complications (non-SSI), such as catheter-related urinary tract infections and atelectasis, are important and occasionally require antibiotics, but that is not the goal of surgical prophylaxis.
- Antibiotics that are given when there is a strong possibility of, but as yet unproven, established infection are termed *presumptive. Therapeutic* antibiotics are required for established infection.
- SSIs are classified as either incisional or deep. Both types, by definition, occur by postoperative day 30. This period extends to 1 year in the case of deep infection associated with prosthesis implantation.

▶ RISK FACTORS FOR SURGICAL WOUND INFECTION

- The traditional classification system developed by the National Research Council (NRC) stratifying surgical procedures by infection risk is reproduced in Table 45–1. The NRC wound classification for a specific procedure is determined intraoperatively.

INDIVIDUALIZING RISK FOR SURGICAL WOUND INFECTION

- The Study on the Efficacy of Nosocomial Infection Control (SENIC) analyzed >100,000 surgery cases in order to identify and validate risk factors for SSI. Abdominal operations, operations lasting >2 hours, contaminated or dirty procedures by NRC classification, and more than three underlying medical diagnoses were associated with an increased incidence of SSI. When the NRC classification was stratified by the number of SENIC risk factors present, the infection rates varied by as much as a factor of 15 within the same operative category (Table 45–2).
- The SENIC risk assessment technique has been modified to include the American Society of Anesthesiologists (ASA) preoperative assessment score (Table 45–3). An ASA score of 3 or above was associated with increased SSI risk.

REDUCING SURGICAL-SITE INFECTION RISK

- Prolonged hospitalization is associated with colonization of, and occasionally infection with, nosocomial bacteria, which increases the incidence of SSI. For this reason, elective surgery is often postponed if the patient is hospitalized for an unrelated medical problem.
- Shaving the incision site with a razor the day before surgery is associated with higher infection rates. Clipping the operative site just prior to the procedure is preferred.

TABLE 45–1. National Research Council Wound Classification, Risk of Surgical Wound Infection, and Indication for Antibiotics

Classification	SSI Rate (%)	Criteria	Antibiotics
Clean	<2	No acute inflammation or transection of gastrointestinal, oropharyngeal, genitourinary, biliary, or respiratory tracts. Elective case, no technique break	Not indicated unless high-risk procedure[a] (? high-risk patient)
Clean–contaminated	<10	Controlled opening of aforementioned tracts with minimal spillage/minor technique break. Clean procedures performed emergently or with major technique breaks	Prophylactic antibiotics indicated
Contaminated	20	Acute, nonpurulent inflammation present. Major spillage/technique break during clean–contaminated procedure	Prophylactic antibiotics indicated
Dirty	40	Obvious preexisting infection present (abscess, pus, or necrotic tissue present)	Therapeutic antibiotics required

[a]High-risk procedures include implantation of prosthetic materials and other procedures where surgical wound infection is associated with high morbidity.

- Preoperative showering with an antiseptic soap may also lower infection rates.
- Unnecessary prolongation of the surgical procedure results in a higher incidence of SSI.

▶ MICROBIOLOGY

- Bacteria involved in SSI are either acquired from the patient's normal flora (endogenous) or from contamination during the surgical procedure (exogenous).

TABLE 45–2. Surgical Site Infection Incidence (%) Stratified by National Research Council Wound Classification and SENIC Risk Factors[a]

No. of SENIC Risk Factors	Clean	Clean–Contaminated	Contaminated	Dirty
0	1.1	0.6	N/A	N/A
1	3.9	2.8	4.5	6.7
2	8.4	8.4	8.3	10.9
3	15.8	17.7	11.0	18.8
4	N/A	N/A	23.9	27.4

[a]SENIC risk factors include abdominal operation, operations lasting >2 h, contaminated or dirty procedures by NRC classification, and >3 underlying medical diagnoses.

TABLE 45–3. American Society of Anesthesiologists Physical Status Classification

Class	Description
1	Normal healthy patient
2	Mild systemic disease
3	Severe systemic disease that is not incapacitating
4	Incapacitating systemic disease that is a constant threat to life
5	Not expected to survive 24 hours with or without operation

- Loss of protective flora via antibiotics can upset the balance and allow pathogenic bacteria to proliferate and increase infectious risk.
- Normal flora can become pathogenic when translocated to a normally sterile tissue site or fluid during surgical procedures.
- According to the National Nosocomial Infections Surveillance System (NNIS), the five most common pathogens encountered in surgical wounds are *Staphylococcus aureus,* enterococci, coagulase-negative staphylococci, *Escherichia coli,* and *Pseudomonas aeruginosa.*

▶ ANTIBIOTIC ISSUES

BASIC PRINCIPLES FOR THE USE OF ANTIMICROBIAL SURGICAL PROPHYLAXIS

- Antimicrobials should be delivered to the targeted tissue site prior to the initial incision.
- Bactericidal antibiotic tissue concentrations should be maintained throughout the length of the surgical procedure.
- Antimicrobials with short serum half-lives may require multiple dosing at frequent dosing intervals, especially if the surgery is prolonged or in instances of massive blood loss.
- Under ideal conditions, the antibiotic chosen for surgical prophylaxis should achieve its highest tissue concentrations at the time of initial skin incision during surgery.
- Antibiotics administered too early or after skin incision probably achieve subtherapeutic concentrations during the operation, putting the patient at high risk of infection.

ANTIMICROBIAL SELECTION

- The choice of the prophylactic antimicrobial depends on the type of surgical procedure, most likely pathogenic organisms, safety and efficacy of the antimicrobial, track record for success based on published literature, and costs.
- The antimicrobial must also take into account the susceptibility patterns of nosocomial-derived pathogens associated with the specific institution.

- Typically, gram-positive coverage is included in the choice of surgical prophylaxis, because organisms such as *S. aureus* and *S. epidermidis* are common wound pathogens.
- Intravenous antibiotic administration is favored because of its reliability in achieving suitable tissue concentrations.
- First-generation cephalosporins (particularly **cefazolin**) are the preferred choice (as good as second- or third-generation cephalosporins) for most surgical procedures. Although there are some reports of failure with cefazolin in cardiac procedures associated with methicillin-sensitive *S. aureus,* the majority of concern is due to the increasing incidence of methicillin-resistant *S. aureus* (MRSA) infections.
- **Vancomycin** is an alternative to cefazolin in institutions with a high incidence of MRSA or for patients with β-lactam allergy.
- In cases where broader gram-negative and anaerobic coverage is desired, the antianaerobic cephalosporins such as **cefoxitin, cefotetan,** and **cefmetazole** are appropriate.

▶ RECOMMENDATIONS FOR SPECIFIC TYPES OF SURGERY

Specific recommendations are summarized in Table 45–4.

GASTRODUODENAL SURGERY

- The risk of infection rises with conditions that increase gastric pH and subsequent bacterial overgrowth such as obstruction, hemorrhage, malignancy, or acid-suppression therapy (clean–contaminated). VIII
- A single dose of intravenous **cefazolin** will provide adequate prophylaxis for most cases.
- Postoperative antibiotics may be indicated if perforation is detected during surgery, depending on whether an established infection is present.

BILIARY TRACT SURGERY

- Antibiotic prophylaxis has been proven beneficial for surgery involving the biliary tract.
- Most frequently encountered organisms include *E. coli, Klebsiella,* and enterococci. Single-dose prophylaxis with **cefazolin** is currently recommended.
- Some surgeons use presumptive antibiotics for cases of acute cholecystitis or cholangitis and defer surgery until the patient is afebrile, in an attempt to decrease infection rates further, but this practice is controversial.
- Detection of an active infection during surgery (gangrenous gallbladder, suppurative cholangitis) is an indication for therapeutic postoperative antibiotics.

COLORECTAL SURGERY

- Anaerobes and gram-negative aerobes predominate in SSIs, although gram-positive aerobes are also important (Table 45–4). Therefore, the

TABLE 45–4. Most Likely Pathogens and Specific Recommendations for Surgical Prophylaxis[a]

Type of Operation	Likely Pathogens	Recommended Prophylaxis Regimen	Comments
Gastroduodenal	Enteric gram-negative bacilli, gram-positive cocci, oral anaerobes	Cefazolin 1 g × 1 IV	High-risk patients only
Biliary tract	Enteric gram-negative bacilli, enterococci, clostridia	Cefazolin 1 g × 1 IV	Bactobilia does not correlate well with pathogens
Colorectal	Anaerobes, enteric gram-negative bacilli	PO: Neomycin 1 g + erythromycin base 1 g at 1 PM, 2 PM, and 11 PM 1 day preop plus mechanical bowel prep IV: Cefoxitin or cefotetan 1 g × 1	Benefit of oral plus IV is controversial
Appendectomy	Anaerobes, enteric gram-negative bacilli	Cefoxitin or cefotetan 1 g × 1 IV	3–5 d of therapeutic antibiotics postop if established infection present
Urologic	*E. coli*	Cefazolin 1 g IV or oral antibiotic with comparable spectrum (where appropriate) × 1	Only beneficial in high-risk cases (preexisting bacteriuria, high infection rate)
Cesarean section	Enteric gram-negative bacilli, anaerobes, group B streptococci, enterococci	Cefazolin 2 g × 1 IV	Give after cord is clamped
Hysterectomy	Same as Cesarean section	Vaginal: Cefazolin 1 g × 1 IV, may repeat q 8 h × 2 doses Abdominal: Cefazolin 1 g × 1 IV	Beneficial in abdominal hysterectomy regardless of risk; lower SSI rate with cefotetan?
Head and neck	*S. aureus*, streptococci, oral anaerobes	Clindamycin 600 mg IV or cefazolin 2 g IV at induction and q 8 h × 2 more doses	Addition of gentamicin to clindamycin is controversial; ampicillin/sulbactam also studied
Cardiac	*S. aureus*, *S. epidermidis*, *Corynebacterium*, enteric gram-negative bacilli	Cefazolin 1 g q 8 h IV × 48 h beginning at induction	Second-generation cephalosporins have been advocated; controversial shorter courses also studied
Vascular	*S. aureus*, *S. epidermidis*, enteric gram-negative bacteria	Cefazolin 1 g IV at induction and q 8 h × 2 more doses	Abdominal and lower extremity procedures have highest infection rate
Orthopedic	*S. aureus*, *S. epidermidis*	Joint replacement: Cefazolin 1 g × 1 IV preop, then q 8 h × 2 more doses Hip fracture repair: Same except continue for 48 h total	Open fractures assumed contaminated with gram-negative bacilli; aminoglycosides often used (see text)
Neurosurgery	*S. aureus*, *S. epidermidis*	Cefazolin 1 g × 1 IV	Use in CSF shunting procedures is controversial

[a]One-time doses are optimally infused at induction of anesthesia except as noted. Repeat doses may be required for long procedures. CSF, cerebrospinal fluid: SSI, surgical-site infection.

risk of SSI in the absence of an adequate prophylactic regimen is substantial.

- Reducing bacteria load with a thorough bowel preparation regimen (4 L of **polyethylene glycol solution** administered orally the day before surgery) is the single most important method to prevent SSI.
- The combination of 1 g of **neomycin** plus 1 g of **erythromycin** base given orally 19, 18, and 9 hours preoperatively is the most commonly used oral regimen in the United States.
- Whether perioperative parenteral antibiotics, in addition to the standard preoperative oral antibiotic regimen, will lower SSI rates further is controversial.
- Postoperative antibiotics are unnecessary in the absence of any untoward events or findings during surgery.

APPENDECTOMY

- A cephalosporin with antianaerobic activity such as **cefoxitin** or **cefotetan** is currently recommended as a first-line agent.
- Single-dose therapy is adequate as long as the appendix is not found to be gangrenous or perforated during surgery.
- Established intra-abdominal infections require appropriate therapeutic postoperative antibiotics.

UROLOGIC PROCEDURES

- As long as the urine is sterile preoperatively, the risk of SSI after urologic procedures is very low and the benefit of prophylactic antibiotics in this setting is controversial. *E. coli* is the most frequently encountered organism.
- Specific recommendations are listed in Table 45–4.
- Urologic procedures requiring an abdominal approach such as a nephrectomy or cystectomy require prophylaxis appropriate for a clean–contaminated abdominal procedure.

CESAREAN SECTION

- Antibiotics are efficacious to prevent SSIs for women undergoing cesarean section regardless of underlying risk factors.
- Several types of bacteria have been implicated in SSIs.
- **Cefazolin** 2 g IV remains the drug of choice. Providing a broader spectrum by using **cefoxitin** against anaerobes or **piperacillin** for better coverage against *Pseudomonas* or enterococci, for example, does not lower postoperative infection rates any further in comparative studies.
- Antibiotics should be administered just after the umbilical cord is clamped, avoiding exposure of the infant to the drug.

HYSTERECTOMY

- Vaginal hysterectomies are associated with a high rate of postoperative infection when performed without the benefit of prophylactic antibiotics.

- **Cefazolin** is the drug of choice.
- Single-dose therapy should be adequate, but most reports used a 24-hour regimen.
- Abdominal hysterectomy SSI rates are correspondingly lower than vaginal hysterectomy rates. However, prophylactic antibiotics are still recommended regardless of underlying risk factors.
- Both cefazolin and antianaerobic cephalosporins (e.g., **cefoxitin, cefotetan**) have been studied extensively, and it is unclear which is superior.
- The antibiotic course should not exceed 24 hours in duration.

HEAD AND NECK SURGERY

- Many head and neck surgical procedures, such as parotidectomy or a simple tooth extraction, are clean procedures by NRC definition and are associated with very low rates of SSI. As expected, surgical prophylaxis has not been proven to be beneficial in these circumstances.
- Head and neck procedures involving an incision through a mucosal layer (and therefore breaching primary immune system barriers) carry a high risk of SSI.
- Specific recommendations for prophylaxis are listed in Table 45–4.
- Whereas typical doses of **cefazolin** are ineffective for anaerobic infections, the recommended 2-g dose produces concentrations high enough to be inhibitory to these organisms. A 24-hour duration has been used in most studies, but single-dose therapy may also be effective.

CARDIAC SURGERY

- Although most cardiac surgeries are technically clean procedures, prophylactic antibiotics have been shown to lower rates of SSI.
- The usual pathogens are skin flora (see Table 45–4) and, rarely, gram-negative enteric organisms.
- **Cefazolin** has been extensively studied and is currently considered the drug of choice.
- The accepted duration of prophylactic antibiotics after cardiac surgery is currently 48 hours. However, there is some evidence that 24 hours is sufficient.
- It may be necessary to use vancomycin in hospitals with a high incidence of SSI with MRSA. The need for **vancomycin** should be evaluated carefully, as previously discussed.

NONCARDIAC VASCULAR SURGERY

- Prophylactic antibiotics are beneficial, especially in procedures involving the abdominal aorta and the lower extremities.
- Staphylococci and gram-negative enterics are the most likely pathogens.
- Twenty-four hours of prophylaxis with IV **cefazolin** is adequate.

ORTHOPEDIC SURGERY

- Prophylactic antibiotics have been shown to be beneficial in cases involving implantation of prosthetic material (pins, plates, artificial joints).
- The most likely pathogens mirror those of other clean procedures and include staphylococci and, infrequently, gram-negative aerobes.
- **Cefazolin** is the best-studied antibiotic and is thus the drug of choice.
- Rates of SSI after total joint replacement are reduced with prophylactic antibiotics. They are also indicated for hip fracture surgery. The current accepted duration is up to 48 hours.

NEUROSURGERY

- The use of prophylactic antibiotics in neurosurgery is controversial.
- Single doses of **cefazolin** or, where required, **vancomycin** appear to lower SSI risk after craniotomy.
- Conversely, studies performed on shunting procedures do not consistently show lower infection rates with antibiotic prophylaxis.

See Chapter 112, Antimicrobial Prophylaxis in Surgery, authored by Stephen W. Janning, PharmD, and Michael J. Rybak, PharmD, FCCP, BCPS, for a more detailed discussion of this topic.

Chapter 46

▶ TUBERCULOSIS

Tuberculosis (TB) is a communicable infectious disease caused by *Mycobacterium tuberculosis.* It can produce silent, latent infection as well as an active disease state.

▶ PATHOPHYSIOLOGY

- *M. tuberculosis, Mycobacterium bovis,* and *Mycobacterium africanum* are pathogenic to normal human hosts, with *M. tuberculosis* being the most prevalent.
- Tuberculosis is invariably transmitted from person to person via micro-size droplet nuclei that are dispersed by either coughing or sneezing.
- Primary infection is initiated by the alveolar implantation of organisms in droplet nuclei that are small enough (1–5 mm) to escape the ciliary epithelial cells of the upper respiratory tract. Once implanted, the organisms multiply and are ingested by pulmonary macrophages, where they continue to multiply, albeit more slowly. Tissue necrosis and calcification of the originally infected site and regional lymph nodes may occur, resulting in the formation of a radiodense area referred to as a Ghon complex.
- After lymph node involvement, organisms may be held in check or may spread via the bloodstream to a variety of organ systems.
- Concurrent with the proliferation of organisms is the development of delayed hypersensitivity via activation and multiplication of CD4 lymphocytes.
- The arrest of mycobacterial proliferation is characterized pathologically by formation of granulomas of two types: proliferative granulomas, which are stable and can effectively limit the spread of the organism, and caseating granulomas, so named for their cheese-like appearance. They have a necrotic center, are relatively unstable, and permit the limited growth of *M. tuberculosis* within them.
- Approximately 90% of patients who experience primary disease have no further clinical manifestations other than a positive skin test either alone or in combination with radiographic evidence of stable granulomas.
- Approximately 3–5% of patients (usually children, the elderly, or the immunocompromised) experience progressive primary disease at the site of the primary infection (usually the lower lobes) and frequently by dissemination, leading to meningitis and often to involvement of the upper lobes of the lung as well. The remaining 7–10% of patients develop reactivation disease, which arises subsequent to the hematogenous spread of the organism.
- Occasionally, a massive inoculum of organisms may be introduced into the bloodstream, causing widely disseminated disease and granuloma formation known as miliary tuberculosis.

TABLE 46–1. Likelihood of Various Clinical Presentations of Tuberculous Infection in Different Patient Groups

Status at Exposure	Asymptomatic Infection	Progressive Primary Infection	Reactivation Pulmonary	Extrapulmonary Disease	Miliary Tuberculosis
<1 y old	++	+++	+/–	++	+
1–5 y	++	++	+/–	++	+
6–10 y	++	+	+	+	+
11–15 y	+++	+/–	+	+	+/–
HIV (–) adult	+++	+/–	+	+	+/–
HIV (+) adult	+	++	+	++	+

+++, predominant feature; ++, common; +, occasional; +/–, rare.

- The various forms of tuberculosis infection occur at different degrees of frequency in different populations (Table 46–1).
- HIV infection increases the risk that a patient infected with *M. tuberculosis* will develop active disease. The Centers for Disease Control and Prevention (CDC) estimate an HIV-infected individual with tuberculous infection to be over 100-fold more likely to develop active disease than an HIV-seronegative patient.

VIII

▶ CLINICAL PRESENTATION

NON–HIV-INFECTED PATIENTS

- The clinical presentation of pulmonary tuberculosis is nonspecific, indicative only of a slowly evolving infectious process (Table 46–2).

TABLE 46–2. Clinical Features of Tuberculosis in HIV-Positive versus -Negative Patients

	HIV Negative (Immunocompetent)	HIV Positive (AIDS)
Onset	Gradual	Abrupt
Presentation	Reactivation	Progressive primary
PPD result	Usually positive	Usually negative
Chest radiograph	Apical infiltrate	Diffuse, lower lobes
Extrapulmonary forms	Occasional	Common
Other pathogens present	Occasional	Common
AFB-positive sputum	Usually	Usually
Response to therapy	Excellent	Fair–good

- A patient with subclinical or early disease may be completely asymptomatic. When the population of organisms increases to a certain point, however, the patient begins to complain of generalized malaise, anorexia, weight loss, and fatigue as well as intermittent fevers with alternating chills and night sweats. Subsequently, a cough with increasing sputum production develops. Hemoptysis and shortness of breath are usually indicative of advanced disease.
- Physical examination is nonspecific, suggestive of progressive pulmonary disease. Dullness to chest percussion suggests consolidation in involved areas of the lung. Rales and increased vocal fremitus are frequently observed upon auscultation.
- Abnormal laboratory data are usually limited to moderate elevations in the white blood cell count with a lymphocyte predominance.
- Clinical features associated with extrapulmonary tuberculosis vary depending on the organ system(s) involved, but typically consist of slowly progressive compromise of organ function with low-grade fever and other constitutional symptoms.

HIV-INFECTED PATIENTS

- The clinical features of patients with HIV infection who develop tuberculosis may be markedly different from those classically observed in immunocompetent individuals (Table 46–2). In AIDS patients, tuberculosis is much more likely to present as the progressive primary form, to involve extrapulmonary sites, and to involve multiple lobes of the lung.
- Tuberculosis in AIDS patients is less likely to involve cavitary disease, be associated with a positive skin test, or be associated with fever. Nonspecific findings of tuberculosis such as malaise, weight loss, weakness, and fever are, in fact, the norm in AIDS patients.

▶ DIAGNOSIS

IDENTIFICATION OF INDIVIDUALS WITH ASYMPTOMATIC INFECTION

- The types of individuals who should be screened with purified protein derivative (PPD) are shown in Table 46–3.

TUBERCULIN SKIN TEST

- The most widely used screening method for tuberculous infection is the tuberculin skin test, which uses PPD. Three test strengths of Purified Protein Derivative Standard (PPD-S) are available:
  - First strength (1 TU), intermediate strength (5 TU), and second strength (250 TU). First-strength PPD-S is sometimes used for testing patients in whom a severe reaction may be expected (i.e., patients with known prior positive test), although few data exist to support this practice.

TABLE 46–3. Candidates for Screening with PPD Skin Test

Individuals	Initial Screening	Retest Periodically	Test If Local Outbreak
HIV infected	×	If possible	N/A
Hospital employees	×	Annually–semiannually	Yes, if exposed
Nursing home staff	×	Annually	Yes, if exposed
Nursing home residents	×	Probably not	Yes, if exposed
Workers at prisons, homeless shelters, clinics, etc.	×	Annually	Yes, if exposed
Immigrants	×	If possible	N/A
Health care students	×	Annually–biannually	Yes, if exposed
General population	No	No	Yes, if exposed

- The intermediate-strength form is almost invariably used for routine screening and diagnostic purposes.
- Second-strength PPD-S may be used in testing patients with depressed cell-mediated immunity who have had a negative result with the intermediate-strength test, but appear likely to have tuberculosis on the basis of clinical criteria.

- The Mantoux method of PPD administration, which is the most reliable technique, consists of the intradermal injection of 0.1 mL of PPD containing 5 TU. The test is read 48–72 hours after injection by measuring the diameter of the zone of induration.
- A positive reaction may remain for 5 days after the test has been administered.
- An area of induration (not erythema) of ≥10 mm for most immunocompetent patients at risk for recent infection, and ≥5 mm for HIV-infected individuals, is considered positive. For patients with AIDS or young children with recent exposure to an index case, any extent of induration might be read as positive.
- Some patients may exhibit a positive test after initial negative test, and this is referred to as a *booster effect.*

SYMPTOMATIC DISEASE

- Confirmatory diagnosis of a clinical suspicion of tuberculosis must be made via chest x-ray and microbiologic examination of sputum or other infected material to rule out active disease.
- Examination of sputum is important in providing microbiologic evidence of pulmonary tuberculosis. Multiple sputum collections during 3 consecutive days are recommended.
- Drug susceptibility tests should routinely be performed. Agar-based susceptibility testing requires at least 3 weeks to complete.

▶ DESIRED OUTCOME

- Rapid identification of new cases of TB.
- Immediate isolation of the patient with active disease to prevent spread.
- Prompt resolution of signs and symptoms of disease after initiation of treatment.
- Achievement of a noninfectious state and cure through patient adherence to the treatment regimen.

▶ TREATMENT

GENERAL PRINCIPLES

- Drug treatment is the cornerstone of TB management. A minimum of two drugs, and generally three or more, must be used simultaneously.
- Drug treatment is continued for at least 6 months and up to 2–3 years for some cases of multidrug-resistant TB (MDR-TB).
- Measures to assure adherence, such as directly observed therapy (DOT), are important.

PHARMACOLOGIC TREATMENT

Asymptomatic Infection

- Chemoprophylaxis should be initiated in patients as described in Table 46–4.
- A 6-month course of **isoniazid** (INH) administered daily is sufficient in most asymptomatic patients. Children, HIV-positive patients (or high-risk patients who refuse testing), and patients with stable abnormal chest films should still remain on therapy for 12 months. Individuals likely to be noncompliant may be treated with a regimen of 15 mg/kg (to a maximum of 900 mg) twice weekly with observation.
- If the individual has been exposed to a patient with INH-resistant *M. tuberculosis* or a patient who has failed chemotherapy, chemoprophylaxis with **rifampin** (RIF) alone or in combination with **pyrazinamide** (PZA) or **ethambutol** (EMB) should be initiated and continued for 12 months.
- If the index case has documented MDR-TB, combination therapy with PZA, EMB, PZA and a fluoroquinolone, or EMB and a fluoroquinolone, has been recommended, but neither has been proven effective.
- All patients treated with INH should also receive **pyridoxine,** 50 mg daily, to reduce the incidence of CNS effects or peripheral neuropathies.

Treating Active Disease

- Table 46–4 lists drug regimen options for initial treatment of tuberculosis in children and adults.
- If available, the drug susceptibility pattern of the source case's isolate should guide the initial drug selection for the new patient. If the source

TABLE 46–4. Antimicrobial Regimens for Chemoprophylaxis of Tuberculosis in Asymptomatic Patients

Patient Type/Situation	Drug and Regimen
Child with documented recent exposure to an index case of pulmonary tuberculosis	Skin test and INH for 3 mo; continue for 12 mo if skin test is positive
Adult with "positive" PPD skin test and no other confounding factors	INH for 6 mo
HIV-infected patient with "positive" PPD skin test, or anergic with risk factors for tuberculosis	INH for 12 mo
Positive skin test and documented exposure to INH-resistant TB	PZA/rifampin or PZA/ethambutol for 12 mo
Positive skin test and documented exposure to INH- and rifampin-resistant TB	PZA/ofloxacin for 12 mo

case cannot be identified, the drug resistance pattern in the area where the patient likely acquired TB must be taken into account.

- If the patient is being evaluated for the retreatment of TB, it is imperative to know what drugs were used previously and for how long.
- Appropriate samples should be sent for culture and susceptibility testing prior to initiating therapy.
- INH and RIF may be used for 9 months of treatment; however, the addition of 2 months of PZA shortens the duration of treatment to 6 months for patients with drug-susceptible TB.
- With rare exceptions, patients must complete 6 months or more of treatment. It has been argued that HIV-positive patients should be treated for an additional 3 months and at least 6 months from the time that they convert to smear and culture negativity. When INH and RIF cannot be used, treatment durations became 2 years or more, regardless of immune status.
- Ethambutol or **streptomycin** (SM) are typically added to INH, RIF, and PZA at the start of treatment until susceptibility information is available. If the organism is drug susceptible, a regimen of INH and RIF for 6 months, supplemented by 2 months of PZA initially, can be used in immunocompetent patients.
- If the organism is drug resistant, the aim is to introduce two *or more* active agents that the patient has not received previously.
- In the case of retreatment for TB or MDR-TB, no standard regimen can be proposed.

Drug Resistance Should Be Suspected in the Following Situations:

- Patients who have received prior therapy for TB.
- Patients from geographic areas with a high prevalence of resistance (New York, Mexico, Southeast Asia).
- Patients who are homeless, institutionalized, IV drug abusers, and/or infected with HIV.
- Patients who still have acid-fast bacilli (AFB)-positive sputum smears after 2 months of therapy.
- Patients who still have positive cultures after 4 months of therapy.
- Patients who require retreatment.

Special Populations

TUBERCULOUS MENINGITIS AND EXTRAPULMONARY DISEASE

- In general, INH, PZA, **ethionamide** (ETA), and **cycloserine** (CS) penetrate the CSF readily. Patients with CNS tuberculosis are often treated for longer periods (9–12 months). Extrapulmonary TB of the soft tissues can be treated with conventional regimens. TB of the bone is typically treated for 9–12 months, occasionally with surgical debridement.

CHILDREN

- Tuberculosis in children may be treated with regimens similar to those used in adults, although some physicians still prefer to extend treatment to 9 months (Table 46–5).

PREGNANT WOMEN

- Women with TB should be cautioned against becoming pregnant, as the disease poses a risk to the fetus as well as to the mother. It appears that INH is relatively safe when used during pregnancy, despite its ability to cross the placenta. Supplementation with **B vitamins** is particularly important during pregnancy. RIF is not frequently associated with birth defects, but those seen are occasionally severe, including limb reduction and central nervous system lesions. EMB does not appear to produce frequent physical or mental aberrations in the developing fetus, and is therefore preferable to many other agents. Ethionamide may be associated with premature delivery and congenital deformities when used during pregnancy.
- Pregnant women with active TB should probably receive INH and rifampin for a period of 9 months. If a third drug is necessary, ethambutol may be added. Therapy with INH for asymptomatic tuberculous infection may be delayed until after pregnancy.

HIV-INFECTED PATIENTS

- AIDS patients and other immunocompromised hosts may be managed with chemotherapeutic regimens similar to those used in immunocompetent individuals, although treatment is often extended (9–12 months).

TABLE 46–5. Regimen Options for the Initial Treatment of Active Tuberculosis Among Children and Adults

TB Without HIV Infection			
Option 1	*Option 2*	*Option 3*	TB With HIV Infection
Administer daily INH, RIF, and pyrazinamide for 8 wk followed by 16 wk of INH and RIF daily or 2–3 times/wk[a] in areas where the INH resistance rate is not documented to be <4%. Ethambutol or streptomycin should be added to the initial regimen until susceptibility to INH and RIF is demonstrated. Continue treatment for at least 6 mo and 3 mo beyond culture conversion. Consult a TB medical expert if the patient is symptomatic or smear or culture positive after 3 mo.	Administer daily INH, RIF, pyrazinamide, and streptomycin or ethambutol for 2 wk followed by 2 times/wk[a] administration of the same drugs for 6 wk (by DOT), and subsequently, with 2 times/wk administration of INH and RIF for 16 wk (by DOT). Consult a TB medical expert if the patient is symptomatic or smear or culture positive after 3 mo.	Treat by DOT, 3 times/wk[a] with INH, RIF, pyrazinamide, and ethambutol or streptomycin for 6 mo.[b] Consult a TB medical expert if the patient is symptomatic or smear or culture positive after 3 mo.	Options 1, 2, or 3 can be used, but treatment regimens should continue for a total of 9 mo and at least 6 mo beyond culture conversion.

DOT, directly observed therapy; INH, isoniazid; RIF, rifampin; TB, tuberculosis; HIV, human immunodeficiency virus.

[a]All regimens administered 2 times/wk or 3 times/wk should be monitored by DOT for the duration of therapy.

[b]The strongest evidence from clinical trials is the effectiveness of all four drugs administered for the full 6 mo. There is weaker evidence that streptomycin can be discontinued after 4 mo if the isolate is susceptible to all drugs. The evidence for stopping pyrazinamide before the end of 6 mo is equivocal for the 3 times/wk regimen, and there is no evidence on the effectiveness of this regimen with ethambutol for less than the full 6 mo.

From Ann Pharmacother, *1994; 28: 72–84, with permission.*

Antitubercular Agents

Isoniazid

- Isoniazid (INH) remains the mainstay for treatment of patients with both asymptomatic and symptomatic infection.
- Therapy with INH results in a transient elevation in serum transaminases in 12–15% of patients and usually occurs within the first 8–12 weeks of therapy. Risk factors for hepatotoxicity include patient age, preexisting liver disease, and pregnancy/postpartum state. INH also may result in neurotoxicity, most frequently presenting as peripheral neuropathy or, in overdose, seizures and coma. Patients with pyridoxine deficiency, such as alcoholics, children, and the malnourished, are at increased risk, as are patients who are slow acetylators of INH and those predisposed to neuropathy, such as diabetics.

Rifampin

- Adverse effects associated with RIF are infrequent and rarely necessitate withdrawal of drug. Elevations in hepatic enzymes have been attributed to RIF in 10–15% of patients, with overt hepatotoxicity occurring in <1%. More frequent adverse effects of RIF include rash, fever, and gastrointestinal distress.
- RIF's induction of hepatic enzymes may enhance the elimination of a number of, most notably, protease inhibitors. Females who use oral contraceptives should be advised to use another form of contraception during therapy.
- The red colorizing effects of RIF on urine, other secretions, and contact lenses should be discussed with the patient.

Pyrazinamide

- Hepatotoxicity is the major limiting adverse effect seen with PZA therapy. PZA also frequently causes gastrointestinal irritation with nausea and vomiting.

Ethambutol

- Retrobulbar neuritis is the major adverse effect noted in patients treated with EMB. Incidence is dose related, with occurrence rates of 5% or more. Patients usually complain of a change in visual acuity and/or inability to see the color green.
- EMB should be avoided in children who are too young to undergo testing for color blindness.

Streptomycin

- Impairment of eighth cranial nerve function is the most important adverse effect of SM. Vestibular function is most frequently affected, but hearing may also be impaired.

► EVALUATION OF THERAPEUTIC OUTCOMES

- Symptomatic patients should be isolated and have sputum samples sent for AFB stains every few days, until smears are negative. This may typically take 10–14 days. After that time, the patient may be removed from isolation and, if symptomatically improved, discharged from the hospital.

- Once on maintenance therapy, patients should have sputum cultures performed monthly until negative. It is anticipated that cultures will convert to negative within 2 months. If sputum cultures continue to be positive after 2 months, drug resistance should be suspected.
- Patients should have blood urea nitrogen, serum creatinine, aspartate transaminase/alanine transaminase, and a complete blood count determined at baseline and periodically, depending on the presence of other factors that may increase the likelihood of toxicity (advanced age, alcohol abuse, and possibly pregnancy). Hepatotoxicity should be suspected in patients whose transaminases exceed five times the upper limit of normal or whose total bilirubin exceeds 3 mg/dL. At this point, the offending agent(s) should be discontinued, and alternatives selected.
- Audiometric testing should be performed in patients who must receive SM for more than 2 months.
- Vision testing should be performed on all patients who must receive EMB for more than 2 months. All patients diagnosed with tuberculosis should be tested for HIV infection.
- The most serious problem with TB therapy is nonadherence to the prescribed regimen. The most effective way to assure adherence is with DOT. VIII

See Chapter 102, Tuberculosis, authored by Charles A. Peloquin, PharmD, and Steven C. Ebert, PharmD, for a more detailed discussion of this topic.

Chapter 47

▶ URINARY TRACT INFECTIONS AND PROSTATITIS

▶ DEFINITION

- Infections of the urinary tract represent a wide variety of clinical syndromes including urethritis, cystitis, prostatitis, and pyelonephritis.
- A urinary tract infection (UTI) may be defined as the presence of microorganisms in the urine that cannot be accounted for by contamination, and have the potential to invade the tissues of the urinary tract and adjacent structures.
- Lower tract infections, such as cystitis, involve the bladder and manifest with symptoms of dysuria, frequency, urgency, and occasionally suprapubic tenderness. Upper tract infections involve the kidney and are referred to as pyelonephritis.
- Uncomplicated UTIs are not associated with structural or neurologic abnormalities that may interfere with the normal flow of urine or the voiding mechanism. Complicated UTIs are the result of a predisposing lesion of the urinary tract such as a congenital abnormality or distortion of the urinary tract, a stone, indwelling catheter, prostatic hypertrophy, obstruction, or neurologic deficit that interferes with the normal flow of urine and urinary tract defenses.
- Recurrent UTIs are characterized by multiple symptomatic episodes with asymptomatic periods occurring between these episodes. These infections are either due to reinfection or to relapse.
- Reinfections are caused by a new organism and account for the majority of recurrent UTIs.
- Relapse represents the development of repeated infections caused by the same initial organism.

▶ PATHOPHYSIOLOGY

- UTIs can be acquired via three possible routes: the ascending, hematogenous, or lymphatic pathways.
- In females, the short length of the urethra and proximity to the perirectal area make colonization of the urethra likely. Bacteria are then believed to enter the bladder from the urethra.
- Once in the bladder, the organisms multiply quickly and can ascend the ureters to the kidney.
- Infection of the kidney by hematogenous spread of organisms usually can occur as the result of dissemination of organisms from a distant primary infection in the body.
- Three factors determine the development of infection: the size of the inoculum, virulence of the microorganism, and competency of the natural host defense mechanisms.

- Patients who are unable to void urine completely are at greater risk of developing urinary tract infections and frequently have recurrent infections.
- An important virulence factor of bacteria is their ability to adhere to urinary epithelial cells. Other virulence factors include hemolysin, a cytotoxic protein produced by bacteria that lyses a wide range of cells including erythrocytes, polymorphonuclear leukocytes, and monocytes, and aerobactin, which facilitates the binding and uptake of iron by *Escherichia coli.*

MICROBIOLOGY

- The most common cause of uncomplicated urinary tract infections is *E. coli,* accounting for more than 85% of community-acquired infections, followed by *Staphylococcus saprophyticus* (coagulase-negative staphylococcus), accounting for 5–15%.
- The urinary pathogens in complicated or nosocomial infections may include *Proteus* sp., *Klebsiella* sp., *Enterobacter* sp., *Pseudomonas* sp., staphylococci, and *Enterococcus faecalis* as well as *E. coli,* which accounts for <50% of these infections. *Candida* sp. have become common causes of urinary infection in the critically ill and chronically catheterized patient.
- The majority of urinary tract infections are caused by a single organism; however, in patients with stones, indwelling urinary catheters, or chronic renal abscesses, multiple organisms may be isolated.

▶ CLINICAL PRESENTATION

- The typical symptoms of lower tract infections include dysuria, urgency, frequency, nocturia, and suprapubic heaviness or pain. Fever is uncommonly associated with lower tract infections.
- The manifestations of upper tract infections classically include flank pain, costovertebral tenderness, or abdominal pain, and systemic symptoms such as fever, rigors, headache, nausea, vomiting, and malaise.

▶ DIAGNOSIS

- The key to the diagnosis of UTI is the ability to demonstrate significant numbers of microorganisms present in an appropriate urine specimen to distinguish contamination from infection.
- A standard urinalysis should be obtained in the initial assessment of a patient. Microscopic examination of the urine should be performed by preparation of a Gram stain of unspun or centrifuged urine. The presence of at least one organism per oil-immersion field in a properly collected uncentrifuged specimen correlates with >100,000 bacteria/mL of urine.
- Criteria for defining significant bacteriuria are listed in Table 47–1.

TABLE 47–1. Criteria for Defining Significant Bacteriuria

Criteria
$\geq 10^2$ CFU coliforms/mL or $\geq 10^5$ noncoliforms/mL in a symptomatic female
$\geq 10^3$ CFU bacteria/mL in a symptomatic male
$\geq 10^5$ CFU bacteria/mL in asymptomatic individuals on two consecutive specimens
Any growth of bacteria on suprapubic catheterization in a symptomatic patient
$\geq 10^2$ CFU bacteria/mL in a catheterized patient

From Johnson CC. *Med Clin North Am* 1991;75:242, with permission.

- The presence of >10 WBCs/mm^3 is almost always existent in symptomatic bacteriuria. Patients with pyuria may or may not have infection.
- The Griess test can be used to detect the presence of nitrate-reducing bacteria in the urine. The leukocyte esterase test is a rapid dipstick test to detect pyuria.
- The most reliable method of diagnosing urinary tract infections is by quantitative urine culture. Patients with infection usually have >105 bacteria/mL of urine, although as many as one-third of women with symptomatic infection have <105 bacteria/mL.
- A method to detect upper urinary tract infection is the antibody-coated bacteria (ACB) test, an immunofluorescent method that detects bacteria coated with immunoglobulin in freshly voided urine.

▶ DESIRED OUTCOME

- The goals of treatment for urinary tract infections are to prevent or resolve systemic consequences of infection, eradicate the invading organism, and prevent recurrence.

▶ TREATMENT

GENERAL PRINCIPLES

- The management of a patient with a UTI includes initial evaluation, selection of an antibacterial agent and duration of therapy, and follow-up evaluation.
- The initial selection of an antimicrobial agent for the treatment of UTI is primarily based on the severity of the presenting signs and symptoms, the site of infection, and whether the infection is determined to be complicated or uncomplicated.

PHARMACOLOGIC TREATMENT

- The ability to eradicate bacteria from the urinary tract is directly related to the sensitivity of the organism and the achievable concentration of the antimicrobial agent in the urine.
- Table 47–2 lists the most common agents used in the treatment of urinary tract infections along with comments concerning their general use.

TABLE 47–2. Commonly Used Antimicrobial Agents in the Treatment of Urinary Tract Infections

Oral Therapy	Comments
Sulfonamides	These agents have generally been replaced by more agents due to resistance.
Trimethoprim–sulfamethoxazole	This combination is highly effective against most aerobic enteric bacteria, except *Pseudomonas aeruginosa.* High urinary tract tissue levels and urine levels are achieved, which may be important in complicated infection treatment. Also, effective as prophylaxis for recurrent infections.
Penicillins Ampicillin Amoxicillin Amoxicillin/clavulanic acid Carbenicillin indanyl	Ampicillin is the standard penicillin that has broad-spectrum activity. Increasing *E. coli* resistance has limited its use in acute cystitis. It is the drug of choice for enterococci sensitive to penicillin. Amoxicillin–clavulanate therapy is preferred for resistance problems. Carbenicillin indanyl is only indicated for the treatment of urinary tract infections.
Cephalosporins Cephalexin Cephradine Cefaclor Cefadroxil Cefuroxime Cefixime Cefzil Cefpodoxime	There are no major advantages of these agents over other agents in the treatment of urinary tract infections and they are more expensive. They may be useful in cases of resistance to amoxicillin and trimethoprim–sulfamethoxazole. These agents are not active against enterococci.
Tetracyclines Tetracycline Doxycycline Minocycline	These agents have been effective for initial episodes of urinary tract infections. However, resistance develops rapidly and their use is limited. These agents also lead to candidal overgrowth. They are primarily useful for chlamydial infections.
Quinolones Ciprofloxacin Ofloxacin Norfloxacin Levofloxacin	The newer quinolones have a greater spectrum of activity that includes *Pseudomonas aeruginosa.* These agents are effective for pyelonephritis and prostatitis. Avoid in pregnancy and children.
Nitrofurantoin	This agent is effective as both a therapeutic and prophylactic agent in patients with recurrent UTI. Main advantage is the lack of resistance even after long courses of therapy. Adverse effects may limit use (GI intolerance, neuropathies, pulmonary reactions).
Azithromycin	Single-dose therapy for chlamydial infections.
Methanamine hippurate/ mandalate	These agents are reserved for prophylactic therapy or suppressive use between episodes of infection.
Fosfomycin	Single-dose therapy for uncomplicated infections.

(continued)

VIII

TABLE 47–2. continued

Oral Therapy	Comments
Parenteral Therapy	
Aminoglycosides Gentamicin Tobramycin Netilmicin Amikacin	Gentamicin and tobramycin are equally effective and gentamicin is less expensive. Tobramycin has better pseudomonal activity, which may be important in serious systemic infections. Amikacin is generally reserved for multiresistant bacteria.
Penicillins Ampicillin Ampicillin/sulbactam Ticarcillin/clavulanate Piperacillin Piperacillin/tazobactam	These agents are generally equally effective for susceptible bacteria. The extended-spectrum penicillins are more active against *Pseudomonas aeruginosa* and enterococci. Often they are preferred over cephalosporins. They are very useful in renally impaired patients or when an aminoglycoside is to be avoided.
Cephalosporins First, second, and third generation	Second- and third-generation cephalosporins have a broad spectrum of activity against gram-negative bacteria, but are not active against enterococci and have limited activity against *Pseudomonas aeruginosa.* Ceftazidime and cefepime are active against *P. aeruginosa.* They are useful for nosocomial infections and urosepsis due to susceptible pathogens.
Imipenem/cilastatin Meropenem	These agents have a broad spectrum of activity including gram-positive, gram-negative, and anaerobic bacteria. They are active against *Pseudomonas aeruginosa* and enterococci, but may be associated with candidal superinfections.
Aztreonam	A monobactam that is only active against gram-negative bacteria, including some strains of *Pseudomonas aeruginosa.* Generally useful for nosocomial infections when aminoglycosides are to be avoided and in penicillin-sensitive patients.
Quinolones Ciprofloxacin Ofloxacin Levofloxacin Sparfloxacin	These agents have broad-spectrum activity primarily against gram-negative pathogens including *Pseudomonas aeruginosa* and other resistant organisms. They provide urine and high tissue concentrations and are actively secreted in reduced renal function.

- Table 47–3 presents an overview of various therapeutic options for outpatient therapy for UTI.
- Table 47–4 describes empiric treatment regimens for selected clinical situations.

Uncomplicated Urinary Tract Infections in Females

- These infections are predominantly caused by *E. coli,* and antimicrobial therapy should be directed against this organism initially. Other causes include *S. saprophyticus* and occasionally *Klebsiella* and *Proteus* species.

TABLE 47–3. Overview of Outpatient Antimicrobial Therapy for Lower Tract Infections in Adults

Indications	Antibiotic	Dose[a]	Interval	Duration
Lower Tract Infection	Trimethoprim–sulfamethoxazole	2 DS tablets	Single dose	1 d
Uncomplicated		1 DS tablet	bid	3 d
	Ciprofloxacin	250 mg	bid	3 d
	Norfloxacin	400 mg	bid	3 d
	Ofloxacin	200 mg	bid	3 d
	Levofloxacin	250 mg	qd	3 d
	Lomefloxacin	400 mg	qd	3 d
	Enoxacin	200 mg	bid	3 d
	Amoxicillin	6 × 500 mg	Single dose	1 d
		500 mg	bid	3 d
	Amoxicillin–clavulanate	500 mg	tid	3 d
	Trimethoprim	100 mg	bid	3 d
	Nitrofurantoin	100 mg	qid	3 d
	Fosfomycin	3 g	Single dose	1 d
Complicated	Trimethoprim–sulfamethoxazole	1 DS tablet	bid	7–10 d
	Trimethoprim	100 mg	bid	7–10 d
	Norfloxacin	400 mg	bid	7–10 d
	Ciprofloxacin	200–500 mg	bid	7–10 d
	Ofloxacin	200–400 mg	bid	7–10 d
	Levofloxacin	400 mg	qd	7–10 d
	Lomefloxacin	250 mg	qd	7–10 d
	Amoxicillin–clavulanate	500 mg	tid	7–10 d
Recurrent infections	Nitrofurantoin	50 mg	qd	6 mo
	Trimethoprim	100 mg	qd	6 mo
	Trimethoprim–sulfamethoxazole	½ SS tablet	qd	6 mo
Acute Urethral Syndrome	Trimethoprim–sulfamethoxazole	1 DS tablet	bid	3 d
Failure of TMP–SMX	Azithromycin	1 g	Single dose	7 d
	Doxycycline	100 mg	bid	14 d
Acute Pyelonephritis	Trimethoprim–sulfamethoxazole	1 DS tablet	bid	14 d
	Ciprofloxacin	500 mg	bid	14 d
	Ofloxacin	400 mg	bid	14 d
	Norfloxacin	400 mg	bid	14 d
	Levofloxacin	250 mg	qd	14 d
	Lomefloxacin	400 mg	qd	14 d
	Enoxacin	400 mg	bid	14 d
	Amoxicillin–clavulanate	500 mg	tid	14 d

[a]Dosing interval for normal renal function. DS, double strength; SS, single strength.

TABLE 47–4. Empiric Treatment of Urinary Tract Infections/Prostatitis

Diagnosis	Pathogens	Treatment	Comments
Acute uncomplicated cystitis	*E. coli* *S. saprophyticus*	1. TMP–SMX × 3 day 2. Quinolone × 3 day	Short-course therapy more effective than single dose.
Pregnancy	As above	1. Amp–clav × 7 day 2. Cephalosporin × 7 day 3. TMP–SMX × 7 day	Avoid TMP–SMX during third trimester.
Acute pyelonephritis			
Uncomplicated	*E. coli*	1. TMP–SMX × 14 day 2. Quinolone × 14 day	Can be managed as outpatient.
Complicated	*E. coli, P. mirabilis, K. pneumoniae, Pseudomonas aeruginosa, E. faecalis*	1. Quinolone × 14 day 2. Extended-spectrum penicillin plus aminoglycoside	Severity of illness will determine duration of IV therapy. Culture results should direct therapy. Oral therapy may complete 14 day of therapy.
Prostatitis	*E. coli, K. pneumoniae, Proteus* sp., *Pseudomonas aeruginosa*	1. TMP–SMX × 4–6 wk 2. Quinolone × 4–6 wk	Acute prostatitis may require IV therapy initially. Chronic prostatitis may require longer treatment periods or surgery.

- Because the causative organisms and their susceptibilities are generally known, a cost-effective approach to management is recommended which includes a urinalysis and initiation of empiric therapy without a urine culture (Figure 47–1).
- Single-dose therapy provides high urinary concentrations for 12–24 hours and is highly effective in treating many women with acute cystitis. Cure rates have ranged from 65–100% using single doses of **sulfisoxazole** (2 g), **trimethoprim–sulfamethoxazole** (two double-strength [DS] tablets), **amoxicillin** (3 g), and **fosfomycin** (3 g).
- Single-dose therapy should not be considered when symptoms of upper tract infection are present or suspected, when stones or other urologic abnormalities are present, when there is a previous history of antibiotic resistance, or in males.
- Short-course therapy (3-day therapy with amoxicillin, trimethoprim, trimethoprim–sulfamethoxazole, or a fluoroquinolone) may be superior to single-dose therapy for uncomplicated infection and should be the treatment of choice. Follow-up urine cultures are not necessary in those patients who respond.

Symptomatic Abacteriuria

- In patients who present for the first time, cultures should be obtained for gonorrhea before treatment is started.
- Single-dose or short-course therapy with **trimethoprim–sulfamethoxazole** has been used effectively, and prolonged courses of therapy are not necessary for the majority of patients.

Asymptomatic Bacteriuria

- The management of asymptomatic bacteriuria depends on the age of the patient and, if female, whether she is pregnant.
- In children, treatment should consist of conventional courses of therapy, as described for symptomatic infections.
- In the nonpregnant female, therapy is controversial; however, it appears that treatment has little effect on the natural course of infections.
- Most clinicians feel that asymptomatic bacteriuria in the elderly is a benign disease and may not warrant treatment. The presence of bacteriuria can be confirmed by culture if treatment is considered.

Complicated Urinary Tract Infections

Acute Pyelonephritis

- The presentation of high-grade fever and severe flank pain should be treated as acute pyelonephritis, and aggressive management is warranted. Severely ill patients with pyelonephritis should be hospitalized and intravenous drugs administered initially. VIII
- At the time of presentation, a Gram stain of the urine should be performed, along with urinalysis, culture, and sensitivities.
- In the mild to moderately symptomatic patient in which oral therapy is considered, an effective agent should be administered for at least a 2-week period. Oral antibiotics that have shown efficacy in this setting include **trimethoprim–sulfamethoxazole** or **fluoroquinolones.** If a Gram stain reveals streptococci, *E. faecalis* should be considered and **ampicillin** or **amoxicillin** is probably the agent of choice.
- In the seriously ill patient, the traditional initial therapy has included an **aminoglycoside** in combination with ampicillin given intravenously. Because of the increased incidence of ampicillin resistance in the community, other agents have been proposed. These include parenteral trimethoprim–sulfamethoxazole, **aztreonam,** extended-spectrum **penicillins with β-lactamase inhibitors,** and the extended-spectrum cephalosporins (**cefotaxime, ceftriaxone,** etc.), or **imipenem.**
- If the patient has been hospitalized in the last 6 months, has a urinary catheter, or is in a nursing home, the possibility of *Pseudomonas* and *Enterococcus* infection, as well as resistant organisms, should be considered. In this setting, **ceftazidime, ticarcillin–clavulanic acid, aztreonam, imipenem,** or **piperacillin** in combination with an **aminoglycoside** is recommended. If the patient responds to initial combination therapy, the aminoglycoside may be discontinued after 3 days.
- Follow-up urine cultures should be obtained 2 weeks after the completion of therapy to ensure a satisfactory response and to detect possible relapse.

VIII

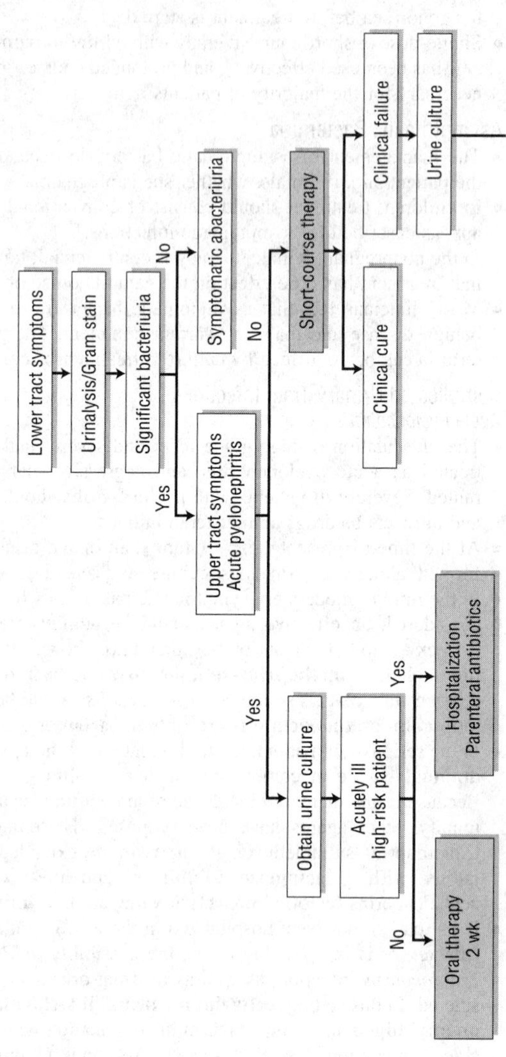

Lower tract symptoms
Urinalysis/Gram stain
Significant bacteriuria
No
Symptomatic abacteriuria
Yes
Upper tract symptoms
Acute pyelonephritis
No
Short-course therapy
Clinical cure
Clinical failure
Urine culture
Yes
Obtain urine culture
Acutely ill
high-risk patient
Yes
Hospitalization
Parenteral antibiotics
No
Oral therapy
2 wk

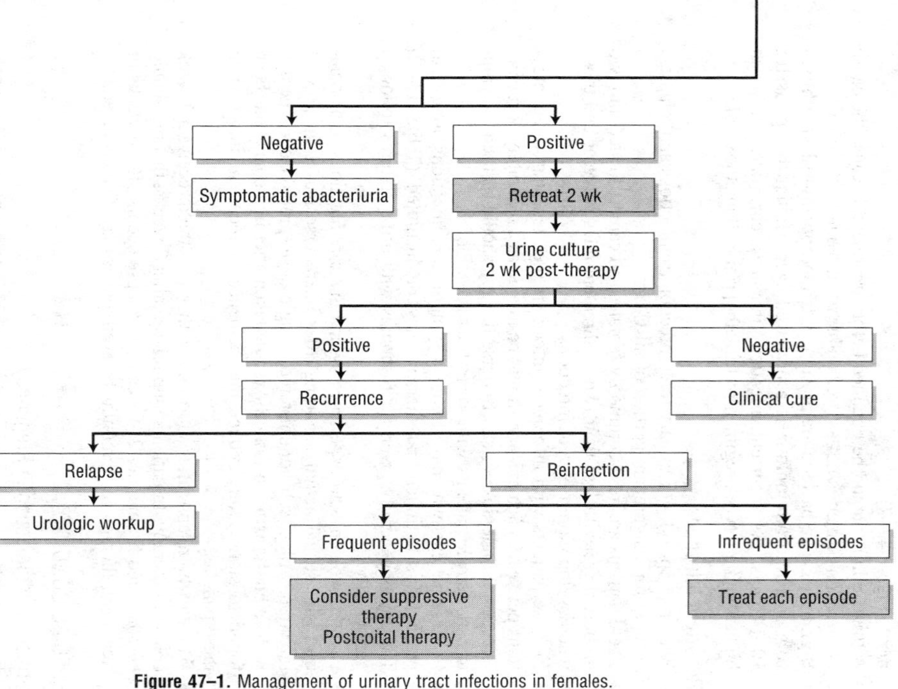

Figure 47–1. Management of urinary tract infections in females.

VIII

Urinary Tract Infections in Males

- The conventional view is that therapy in males requires prolonged treatment (Figure 47–2).
- A urine culture should be obtained before treatment, because the cause of infection in men is not as predictable as in women.
- If gram-negative bacteria are presumed, **trimethoprim–sulfamethoxazole** or a **fluoroquinolone** is a preferred agent. Initial therapy is for 10–14 days. For recurrent infections in males, cure rates are much higher with a 6-week regimen of trimethoprim–sulfamethoxazole.

Recurrent Infections

- Recurrent episodes of urinary tract infection (reinfections and relapses) account for a significant portion of all UTIs.
- These patients are most commonly females and can be divided into two groups: those with less than two or three episodes per year and those who develop more frequent infections.
- In those patients with infrequent infections (i.e., less than three infections per year), each episode should be treated as a separately occurring infection. Single-dose or short-course therapy should be used in symptomatic female patients with lower tract infection.
- In those patients who have frequent symptomatic infections, long-term prophylactic antimicrobial therapy may be instituted (Table 47–3). Therapy is generally given for 6 months with urine cultures followed periodically.

- In those women who experience symptomatic reinfections in association with sexual activity, voiding after intercourse may help prevent infection. Also, self-administered, single-dose prophylactic therapy with **trimethoprim-sulfamethoxazole** taken after intercourse has been found to significantly reduce the incidence of recurrent infection in these patients.
- Women who relapse after short-course therapy should receive a 2-week course of therapy. In patients who relapse after 2 weeks, therapy should be continued for another 2–4 weeks. If relapse occurs after 6 weeks of treatment, therapy for 6 months or even longer may be considered.

SPECIAL CONDITIONS

Urinary Tract Infection in Pregnancy

- In those patients with significant bacteriuria, symptomatic or asymptomatic, treatment is recommended in order to avoid possible complications during the pregnancy. Therapy should consist of an agent with a relatively low adverse-effect potential (a **sulfonamide, cephalexin, ampicillin, amoxicillin, amoxicillin/clavulanate, nitrofurantoin**) administered for 7 days.
- Tetracyclines should be avoided due to teratogenic effects, and sulfonamides should not be administered during the third trimester due to the possible development of kernicterus and hyperbilirubinemia. Also, the

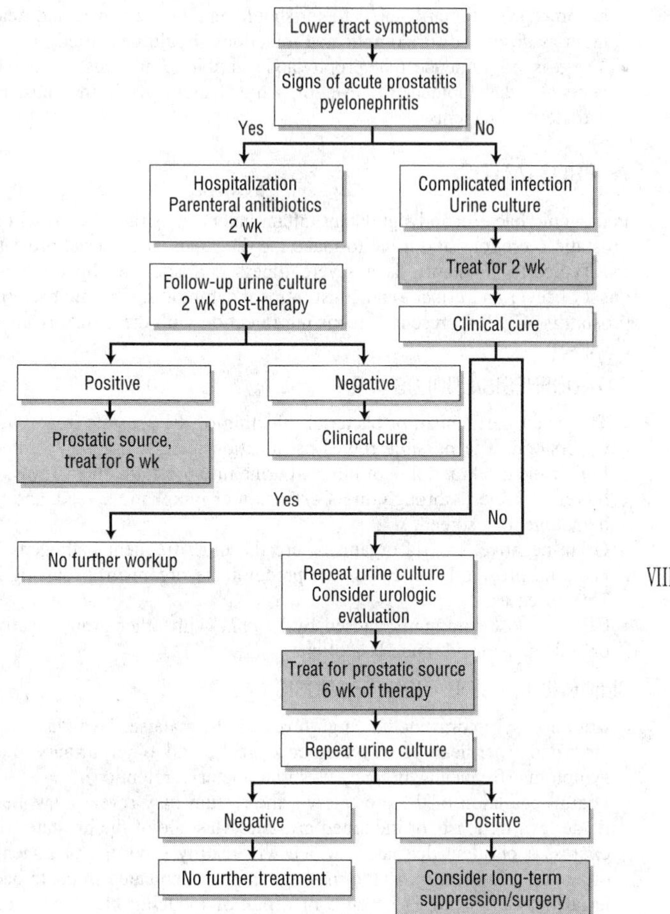

Figure 47–2. Management of urinary tract infections in males.

VIII

quinolones should not be given because of their potential to inhibit cartilage and bone development in the newborn.

Catheterized Patients

- When bacteriuria occurs in the asymptomatic, short-term catheterized patient (<30 days), the use of systemic antibiotic therapy should be withheld and the catheter removed as soon as possible. If the patient becomes symptomatic, the catheter should again be removed and treatment as described for complicated infections should be started.

- There is no evidence that prophylactic antibiotic administration prevents the development of fever or acute pyelonephritis in long-term catheterized patients.

▶ PROSTATITIS

Pathogenic bacteria and significant inflammatory cells must be present in prostatic secretions and urine to make the diagnosis of bacterial prostatitis. Typically, prostatitis is a severe illness characterized by a sudden onset of fever and urinary and constitutional symptoms. Chronic bacterial prostatitis (CBP) represents a recurring infection with the same organism (relapse).

PATHOGENESIS/ETIOLOGY

- The exact mechanism of bacterial infection of the prostate is not well understood. The possible routes of infection include ascending infection of the urethra, reflux of infected urine into prostatic ducts, invasion by rectal bacteria through direct extension or lymphatic spread, and by hematogenous spread.
- Gram-negative, enteric organisms are the most frequent pathogens in bacterial prostatitis. *E. coli* is the predominate organism, occurring in 75% of cases.
- CBP is most commonly caused by *E. coli,* with other gram-negative organisms isolated much less often.

CLINICAL PRESENTATION/DIAGNOSIS

- Common symptoms include high fever, chills, malaise, myalgia, localized pain (perineal, rectal, sacrococcygeal), and other urinary tract symptoms (frequency, urgency, dysuria, nocturia, retention).
- Digital palpation of the prostate via the rectum may reveal a swollen, tender, warm, tense, or indurated prostate. Massage of the prostate will express a purulent discharge, which will readily grow the pathogenic organism. However, prostatic massage is contraindicated in acute bacterial prostatitis (ABP) because of a risk of inducing bacteremia and associated pain.
- CBP is characterized by recurrent urinary tract infections with the same pathogen. In fact, CBP is the most common cause of recurrent UTI in males. Presenting symptoms include the vague description of voiding difficulties such as frequency, urgency, and dysuria, along with low back pain and perineal and suprapubic discomfort.
- Urinary tract localization studies are critical to the diagnosis of CBP.
- Both ABP and CBP are characterized by the presence of numerous WBC and lipid-containing macrophages (oval fat bodies) on microscopic exam of expressed prostatic secretions.

TREATMENT

- Oral or parenteral therapy with **trimethoprim–sulfamethoxazole** (TMP–SMX) has been advocated as initial therapy. Intravenous to oral sequential therapy with a TMP–SMX or a fluoroquinolone, such as **ciprofloxacin** or **ofloxacin,** would be appropriate.
- Parenteral therapy should be maintained until the patient is afebrile and less symptomatic. The conversion to an oral antibiotic can be considered if the patient has been afebrile for 48 hours or after 3–5 days of intravenous therapy. The total course of antibiotic therapy should be 4 weeks in order to reduce the risk of development of chronic prostatitis.
- The choice of antibiotics in CBP should include those agents that are capable of crossing the prostatic epithelium into the prostatic fluid in therapeutic concentrations and which also possess the spectrum of activity to be effective.
- Currently, the fluoroquinolones appear to provide the best therapeutic option in the management of CBP.

See Chapter 106, Urinary Tract Infections and Prostatitis, authored by Timothy A. Mullenix, PharmD, MS, and Randall A. Prince, PharmD, for a more detailed discussion of this topic.

Chapter 48

▶ VACCINES, TOXOIDS, AND OTHER IMMUNOBIOLOGICS

▶ DEFINITIONS

- Vaccines are substances administered to generate a protective immune response.
- Toxoids are inactivated bacterial toxins. They retain the ability to stimulate the formation of antitoxin.
- Adjuvants are inert substances, such as aluminum salts (i.e., alum), which enhance vaccine antigenicity by prolonging antigen absorption.
- Immune sera are sterile solutions containing antibody derived from human (immune globulin) or equine (antitoxin) sources.
- Antitoxins are made by immunizing animals with an antigen and then harvesting the antibodies from serum.

▶ VACCINE AND TOXOID RECOMMENDATIONS

- The recommended schedules for routine immunization of children and adults are shown in Tables 48–1 and 48–2, respectively. Table 48–3 lists the minimum age for initial vaccination and minimum interval between vaccine doses.
- Inactivated vaccines can be simultaneously administered at separate sites. Killed and live antigens may be administered simultaneously or, if they cannot be administered simultaneously, at any interval between doses with the exception of cholera (killed) and yellow fever (live) vaccines, which should be given at least 3 weeks apart. Simultaneous administration of live attenuated vaccines should be avoided, if possible, unless specified (i.e., measles, mumps, rubella [MMR]). Live vaccines should be given at least 1 month apart; however, oral polio vaccine may be given at the same time as measles, mumps, and rubella vaccine.
- Administration of live attenuated vaccines should not be done during pregnancy, and inactivated vaccines should not be given until the second trimester. However, inactivated vaccines have not been shown to be teratogenic during the first trimester.
- Those patients who are immunocompromised or with active malignant disease may receive killed vaccines or toxoids but should not be given live vaccines.
- The simultaneous administration of immune globulin (general or disease specific) and live attenuated vaccines (but not inactivated vaccines) may inhibit host antibody response owing to impairment of viral replication. Administration of killed vaccines along with immunoglobulins is not contraindicated.

TABLE 48–1. Recommended Childhood Immunization Schedule, United States, January–December 1997[a,b]

Vaccine	Age: *Birth*	*1 mo*	*2 mo*	*4 mo*	*6 mo*	*12 mo*	*15 mo*	*18 mo*	*4–6 yr*	*11–12 yr*	*14–16 yr*
Hepatitis B[c,d]	Hep B-1										
			Hep B-2		Hep B-3					Hep B[d]	
Diphtheria, tetanus, pertussis[e]			DTaP or DTP	DTaP or DTP	DTaP or DTP		DTaP or DTP[e]		DTaP or DTP	Td	
H. influenzae type b[f]			HIB	HIB	HIB[f]	HIB[f]					
Polio[g]			Polio[g]	Polio			Polio[g]		Polio		
Measles, mumps, rubella[h]						MMR			MMR[h] or	MMR[h]	
Varicella[i]						Var				Var[h]	

[a]Approved by the Advisory Committee on Immunization Practices (ACIP), the American Academy of Pediatrics (AAP), and the American Academy of Family Physicians (AAFP). This schedule indicates the recommended age for routine administration of currently licensed childhood vaccines. Some combination vaccines are available and may be used whenever administration of all components of the vaccine is indicated. Providers should consult the manufacturers' package inserts for detailed recommendations.

[b]Vaccines are listed under the routinely recommended ages. Bars indicate range of acceptable ages for vaccination. Shaded bars indicate *catch-up vaccination:* at 11–12 years of age, hepatitis B vaccine should be administered to children not previously vaccinated, and varicella vaccine should be administered to children not previously vaccinated who lack a reliable history of chickenpox.

[c]*Infants born to HBsAg-negative mothers* should receive 2.5 μg of Merck vaccine (Recombivax HB) or 10 μg of SmithKline Beecham (SB) vaccine (Engerix-B). The second dose should be administered ≥ 1 mo after the first dose.

(continued)

TABLE 48–1. continued

Infants born to HBsAg-positive mothers should receive 0.5 mL hepatitis B immune globulin (HBIG) within 12 h of birth, and either 5 μg of Merck vaccine (Recombivax HB) or 10 μg of SB vaccine (Engerix-B) at a separate site. The 2nd dose is recommended at 1–2 mo of age and the 3rd dose at 6 mo of age.

Infants born to mothers whose HBsAg status is unknown should receive either 5 μg of Merck vaccine (Recombivax HB) or 10 μg of SB vaccine (Engerix-B) within 12 h of birth. The 2nd dose of vaccine is recommended at 1 mo of age and the 3rd dose at 6 mo of age. Blood should be drawn at the time of delivery to determine the mother's HBsAg status; if it is positive, the infant should receive HBIG as soon as possible (no later than 1 wk of age). The dosage and timing of subsequent vaccine doses should be based on the mother's HBsAg status.

[d]Children and adolescents who have not been vaccinated against hepatitis B in infancy may begin the series during any childhood visit. Those who have not previously received three doses of hepatitis B vaccine should initiate or complete the series during the 11–12-year-old visit. The 2nd dose should be administered at least 1 mo after the 1st dose, and the 3rd dose should be administered at least 4 mo after the 1st dose and at least 2 mo after the 2nd dose.

[e]DTaP (diphtheria and tetanus toxoids and acellular pertussis vaccine) is the preferred vaccine for all doses in the vaccination series, including completion of the series in children who have received ≥ 1 dose of whole-cell DTP vaccine. Whole-cell DTP is an acceptable alternative to DTaP. The 4th dose (DtaP or DTP) may be administered as early as 12 mo of age, provided 6 mo have elapsed since the 3rd dose, and if the child is considered unlikely to return at 15–18 mo of age. Td (tetanus and diphtheria toxoids, adsorbed, for adult use) is recommended at 11–12 y of age if at least 5 y have elapsed since the last dose of DTP, DTaP, or DT. Subsequent routine Td boosters are recommended every 10 y.

[f]Three *H. influenzae* type b (HIB) conjugate vaccines are licensed for infant use. If PRP-OMP (PedvaxHIB [Merck]) is administered at 2 and 4 mo of age, a dose at 6 mo is not required. After completing the primary series, any HIB conjugate vaccine may be used as a booster.

[g]Two poliovirus vaccines are currently licensed in the United States: inactivated poliovirus vaccine (IPV) and oral poliovirus vaccine (OPV). The following schedules are all acceptable by the ACIP, the AAP, and the AAFP, and parents and providers may choose among them:

1. IPV at 2 and 4 mo; OPV at 12–18 mo and 4–6 y
2. IPV at 2, 4, 12–18 mo, and 4–6 y
3. OPV at 2, 4, 6–18 mo, and 4–6 y

The ACIP routinely recommends schedule 1. IPV is the only poliovirus vaccine recommended for immunocompromised persons and their household contacts.

[h]The 2nd dose of MMR is routinely recommended at 4–6 y of age or at 11–12 y of age but may be administered during any visit, provided at least 1 mo has elapsed since receipt of the 1st dose and that both doses are administered at or after 12 mo of age.

[i]Susceptible children may receive varicella vaccine (Var) at any visit after the first birthday, and those who lack a reliable history of chickenpox should be immunized during the 11–12-year-old visit. Children ≥ 13 y of age should receive two doses, at least 1 mo apart.

TABLE 48–2. Immunization Schedules in Adults

Age Group (y)	Vaccine/Toxoid[a]					
	Td[b]	*Measles*	*Mumps*	*Rubella*	*Influenza*	*Pneumococcal Polysaccharide*
18–24	X	X	X	X		
25–64	X	X[c]	X[c]	X		
≥65	X				X	X

[a]Refer also to sections in text on specific vaccines or toxoids for indications, contraindications, precautions, dosages, side effects, adverse reactions, and special considerations.
[b]Td = tetanus and diphtheria toxoids, adsorbed (for adult use), which is a combined preparation containing <2 flocculation units of diphtheria toxoid.
[c]Indicated for persons born after 1956.
From Centers for Disease Control and Prevention. MMWR 1991;40:1–95.

▶ DIPHTHERIA TOXOID ADSORBED AND DIPHTHERIA ANTITOXIN

- Two strengths of diphtheria toxoid are available (pediatric [D] and adult [d], which contains less antigen). Primary immunization with DTA is indicated for children under 6 weeks of age. Generally, diphtheria toxoid adsorbed (DTA) is given along with pertussis and tetanus vaccines (DPT) at ages 2, 4, and 6 months of age, and then at 15–18 months and 4–6 years of age. VIII
- For nonimmunized adults, a complete three-dose series of diphtheria toxoid should be administered, with the first two doses given at least 4 weeks apart and the third dose given 6–12 months after the second. The combined preparation, Td, is recommended in adults, because it contains less diphtheria toxoid than DPT with fewer reactions seen to the diphtheria preparation. Booster doses are given every 10 years.
- Diphtheria antitoxin (DA) is a sterile antitoxin derived from hyperimmunized horses and is indicated for immediate use in patients with diphtheria. Sensitivity testing by performing an intradermal or scratch test and a conjunctival test should be performed before administration.
- The usual dose of DA is 20,000–40,000 U for pharyngeal disease, 40,000–60,000 U for nasopharyngeal lesions, and 80,000–120,000 U for extensive disease of 3 or more days.

▶ TETANUS TOXOID (TT), TETANUS TOXOID ADSORBED (TTA), AND TETANUS IMMUNE GLOBULIN (TIG)

- In children, primary immunization against tetanus is usually done in conjunction with diphtheria and pertussis vaccination. The trivalent vaccine, DPT, containing TTA is given intramuscularly at 2, 4, 6, and 15–18 months of age.

TABLE 48–3. Minimum Age for Pediatric Vaccination

Vaccine	Minimum Age for First Dose[a]	Minimum Interval from Dose 1 to 2[a]	Minimum Interval from Dose 2 to 3[a]	Minimum Interval from Dose 3 to 4[a]
DTP (DT)[b]	6 wk[c]	4 wk	4 wk	6 mo
Combined DTP-HIB	6 wk	1 mo	1 mo	6 mo
DTaP[b]	15 mo			6 mo
HIB (primary series)				
HbOC	6 wk	1 mo	1 mo	[d]
PRP-T	6 wk	1 mo	1 mo	[d]
PRP-OMP	6 wk	1 mo	[d]	
OPV	6 wk[c]	6 wk	6 wk[f]	
IPV[e]	6 wk	4 wk	6 mo[f]	
MMR	12 mo[g]	1 mo		
Hepatitis B	Birth	1 mo	2 mo[h]	

DTP, diphtheria–tetanus–pertussis; DTaP, diphtheria–tetanus–acellular pertussis; HIB, *Haemophilus influenzae* type b conjugate; IPV, inactivated poliovirus vaccine; MMR, measels–mumps–rubella; OPV, live oral polio vaccine.

[a]These minimum acceptable ages and intervals may not correspond with the optimal recommended ages and intervals for vaccination.

[b]DTaP can be used in place of the fourth (and fifth) dose of DTP for children who are at least 15 mo of age. Children who have received all four primary vaccination doses before their fourth birthday should receive a fifth dose of DTP (DT) or DTaP at 4–6 y of age before entering kindergarten or elementary school and at least 6 mo after the fourth dose. The total number of doses of diphtheria and tetanus toxoids should not exceed six each before the seventh birthday.

[c]The American Academy of Pediatrics permits DTP and OPV to be administered as early as 4 wk of age in areas with high endemicity and during outbreaks.

[d]The booster dose of HIB vaccine which is recommended following the primary vaccination series should be administered no earlier than 12 mo of age and at least 2 mo after the previous dose of HIB vaccine.

[e]See text to differentiate conventional inactivated poliovirus vaccine from enhanced-potency IPV.

[f]For unvaccinated adults at increased risk of exposure to poliovirus with <3 mo but >2 mo available before protection is needed, three doses of IPV should be administered at least 1 mo apart.

[g]Although the age for measles vaccination may be as young as 6 mo in outbreak areas where cases are occurring in children <1 y of age, children initially vaccinated before the first birthday should be revaccinated at 12–15 mo of age, and an additional dose of vaccine should be administered at the time of school entry or according to local policy. Doses of MMR or other measles-containing vaccines should be separated by at least 1 mo.

[h]This final dose is recommended no earlier than 4 mo of age.

From Centers for Disease Control and Prevention. MMWR 1994;43:1–38.

- Primary vaccination provides protection for at least 10 years.
- Additional doses of TTA are recommended as part of traumatic wound management if a patient has not received a dose of TTA or TT during the preceding 5 years (Table 48–4).
- In adults or children older than 7 years of age where primary immunization against tetanus alone is needed, a series of three doses of TTA is administered intramuscularly initially, followed by repeat doses at 4–8 weeks and 6–12 months.

TABLE 48–4. Summary Guide to Tetanus Prophylaxis in Routine Wound Management[a]

	Clean, Minor Wounds		All Other Wounds[b]	
	Td[c]	*TIG*[d]	*Td*[c]	*TIG*[d]
Uncertain or <3	Yes	No	Yes	Yes
>3[e]	No[f]	No	No[g]	No

[a]Refer also to text on specific vaccines or toxoids for contraindications, precautions, dosages, side effects, adverse reactions, and special considerations. Important details are in the ACIP recommendations on diphtheria, tetanus, and pertussis (DTP) (MMWR 1991: 40 [RR-10]).

[b]Such as, but not limited to, wounds contaminated with dirt, feces, and saliva; puncture wounds; avulsions; and wounds resulting from missiles, crushing, burns, and frostbite.

[c]Td, tetanus and diphtheria toxoids, adsorbed (for adult use). For children <7 y old, DTP (DT, if pertussis vaccine is contraindicated) is preferred to tetanus toxoid alone. For persons ≥7 y old, Td is preferred to tetanus toxoid alone.

[d]TIG, tetanus immune globulin.

[e]If only three doses of fluid toxoid have been received, a fourth dose of toxoid, preferably an adsorbed toxoid, should be given.

[f]Yes, >10 y since last dose.

[g]Yes, >5 y since last dose. (More frequent boosters are not needed and can accentuate side effects.)

From Centers for Disease Control and Prevention. MMWR 1991;40:1–95.

- TT and TTA may be given to immunosuppressed patients if needed. TT or TTA may be simultaneously given with other killed and live vaccines. VIII
- TIG is used to provide passive tetanus immunization following the occurrence of traumatic wounds in nonimmunized or suboptimally immunized persons (Table 48–4). A dose of 250–500 U is administered intramuscularly. When administered with TTA, separate sites for administration should be used.
- TIG is also used for the treatment of tetanus. In this setting, a single dose of 3000–6000 U is administered intramuscularly.

► *HAEMOPHILUS INFLUENZAE* TYPE B (HIB) VACCINES

- HIB vaccines currently in use are conjugate products, consisting of either a polysaccharide or oligosaccharide of polyribosylribitol phosphate (PRP) covalently linked to a protein carrier (Table 48–5).
- HIB conjugate vaccines are indicated for routine use in all infants and children under 5 years of age.
- For infants 7–11 months who have not been vaccinated, three doses of HbOC, PRP-OMP, and PRP-T should be given: two doses, spaced 8 weeks apart, and then a booster dose at age 12–18 months (but at least 8 weeks since dose 2). For unvaccinated children ages 12–14 months, two doses should be given, with an interval of 2 months between them. In a child older than 15 months, a single dose of any of the four conjugate vaccines is indicated.

TABLE 48–5. *Haemophilus influenzae* Vaccines Currently Available in the United States

Manufacturer	Abbreviated Name	Trade Name	Protein Carrier
Connaught Labs	PRP-D	ProHIBit	Diphtheria toxoid
Lederle-Praxis	HbOC[a]	HIBTITER	CRM_{197} (diphtheria toxin)
Merck	PRP-OMP	PedvaxHIB	OMP (from *N. meningitidis*)
Pasteur Merieux	PRP-T	ActHIB/OmniHIB	Tetanus toxoid

Note: PRP-D is recommended by the American Academy of Pediatrics for infants age ≥12 mo only. HbOC, PRP-OMP, and PRP-T are recommended for infants age ≥2 mo.
[a]Available as Tetramune, a combination vaccine with DPT.

▶ HEPATITIS A VACCINE

- Hepatitis A vaccine is recommended for the following groups:
  - Travelers to areas that are not developed.
  - Men who have sex with men.
  - Persons working with primates.
  - Persons who have clotting factor disorders.
  - Illegal drug users.
  - Persons with chronic liver disease.
  - Food handlers where the vaccine is cost effective.
  - Children in highly endemic areas.
- The vaccine is available as two products with multiple formulations. The dose and regimen vary with age.
- Protective levels of anti-HAV may be present for 20 years or more.

VIII

▶ HEPATITIS B VACCINE

- Antibody conversion rates are about 90% in healthy individuals after three vaccine doses. The vaccine protects against all hepatitis B serotypes (including delta viroid) but does not cross-react with other hepatitis viruses (i.e., hepatitis A, C, E).

PRIMARY VACCINATION

- The vaccine is recommended for persons with occupational risk (health care workers, public safety workers), persons in training for health care fields, clients and staff of institutions for the developmentally disabled, hemodialysis patients, recipients of clotting factor concentrate, household contacts and sex partners of hepatitis B carriers, adoptees from countries where hepatitis B is endemic, international travelers (those spending more than 6 months in areas with high rates of hepatitis B infection or high-risk, short-term travelers), injecting drug users, sexually active homosexual/bisexual men, sexually active heterosexual men and women, and inmates of long-term correctional facilities. In addition, the American Academy of Pediatrics recommends universal immunization of all newborns.

- For neonates born to mothers who are not positive for hepatitis B surface antigen (HBsAg), the primary vaccination series is 2.5 mg of Recombivax HB or 10 mg of Engerix-B. The first dose should be given at 0–2 days of age, the second dose at 1–2 (or 2–4) months of age, and the third dose at 6–18 months of age.
- In infants born to HBsAg-positive mothers, vaccination with 5 mg of Recombivax HB or 10 mg of Engerix-B is given at 12 hours after birth (but no more than 7 days after birth), 1 month of age, and 6 months of age. A fourth dose of vaccine is administered to infants who are anti-HB nonresponders or hyporesponders and are HBsAg negative.
- For children less than 11 years of age who are not born of mothers who are HBsAg positive, 2.5 mg of Recombivax HB or 10 mg of Engerix-B is administered at 0, 1, and 6 months. Children and adolescents ages 11–19 receive 5 mg of Recombivax HB or 20 mg of Engerix-B at 0, 1, and 6 months. An alternate four-dose schedule (0, 1, 2, and 12 months) may be used for Engerix-B.
- Adults 20 years or more of age receive 10 mg of Recombivax HB or 20 mg of Engerix-B at 0, 1, and 6 months. An alternative schedule of 20 mg at 0, 1, 2, and 12 months may be used for Engerix-B only.
- Hemodialysis patients receive either 40 mg of Recombivax HB or 40 mg of Engerix-B in a 0-, 1-, and 6-month schedule. Anti-HBs should be determined, and if the value is <10 mIU/mL, one to three booster doses are administered. In addition, these persons should be tested yearly and boosted with a single dose of 40 mg if anti-HBs <10 mIU/mL.
- The preferred site of administration is the deltoid muscle in adults (immunogenicity is significantly lower in adults who receive injection in the buttock) and the anterolateral thigh in infants.
- Patients who should receive postvaccination serologic testing include immunocompromised patients (owing to any cause), persons at occupational risk of exposure, and infants born of HBsAg-positive mothers.
- In persons who do not mount a protective anti-HNs titer after the standard vaccine series, a standard dose should be administered at 0, 1, and 2 months followed by anti-HBs testing in 1–2 months.

POSTEXPOSURE PROPHYLAXIS

- Hepatitis B vaccine is also used with hepatitis B immune globulin (HBIG) in the postexposure setting. This regimen is recommended in susceptible individuals having percutaneous or permucosal exposure to blood containing HBsAg, sexual contacts of HBsAg carriers who will continue to be exposed, and infants born of mothers who are HBsAg carriers.
- The same vaccine dosage schedule used for primary immunization is used in the postexposure setting.
- The hepatitis B vaccine series should be initiated as soon as possible after HBIG administration. Table 48–6 illustrates the specifics of vaccine use.

TABLE 48–6. Recommendations for Hepatitis B Prophylaxis following Percutaneous Exposure

	Treatment When Source Is Found to Be		
Exposed Person	*HBsAg Positive*	*HBsAg Negative*	*Unknown or Not Tested*
Unvaccinated	Administer HBIG × 1[a] and initiate hepatitis B vaccine	Initiate hepatitis B vaccine	Initiate hepatitis B vaccine
Previously Vaccinated			
Known responder	Test exposed person for anti-HBs 1. If adequate, no treatment 2. If inadequate, hepatitis B vaccine booster dose	No treatment	No treatment
Known nonresponder	HBIG × 2 or HBIG × 1, plus one dose of hepatitis B vaccine	No treatment	If known high-risk source, may treat as if source were HBsAg positive
Response unknown	Test exposed person for anti-HB[b] 1. If inadequate, HBIG × 1, plus hepatitis B vaccine booster dose 2. If adequate, no treatment	No treatment	Test exposed person for anti-HBs[b] 1. If inadequate , hepatitis B vaccine booster dose 2. If adequate, no treatment

[a]Hepatitis B immune globulin (HBIG) dose 0.06 mL/kg IM.
[b]Adequate anti-HBs is ≥10 mIU.
From Centers for Disease Control and Prevention. MMWR 1991;40:1–25.

VIII

► HEPATITIS B IMMUNE GLOBULIN

- HBIG is used for postexposure, and rarely preexposure, prophylaxis for hepatitis B infection.
- Indications for the use of HBIG include passive immunization following exposure to hepatitis B virus via percutaneous, permucosal, or oral ingestion routes (e.g., needlesticks, accidental splash, sexual contact, mouth pipetting) and for infants born to mothers who are hepatitis B carriers.
- It is currently recommended by the CDC that HBIG be given as soon as possible after acute exposures (percutaneous, permucosal, oral

ingestion), preferably within 24 hours. It is not recommended that HBIG be given beyond 14 days after acute exposure.

▶ INFLUENZA VIRUS VACCINE

- Indications for current split-virus and whole-virus influenza vaccines are as follows: adults with chronic cardiovascular or pulmonary diseases, residents of nursing home facilities, health care personnel dealing with high-risk patients, healthy adults older than age 65, children with chronic metabolic diseases, women who will be in the second or third trimester during influenza season, household members of persons in high-risk groups, and HIV-infected patients. In addition, groups that can transmit influenza to high-risk people should be vaccinated (health care personnel, employees of nursing homes or chronic care facilities who have patient contact, providers of home care to high-risk patients, and household members of persons in high-risk groups).
- Individuals who should not be vaccinated are those with anaphylactic hypersensitivity to eggs or other components of the vaccine or adults with febrile illness (until the fever abates).

▶ MEASLES VACCINE

- Measles vaccine is administered for primary immunization to persons 12–15 months of age or older, usually as MMR. A second dose is recommended prior to entry into elementary school or junior high school. VIII
- The vaccine should not be given to immunosuppressed patients (except those infected with HIV), pregnant women, or patients with a history of egg allergy.
- The vaccine should not be given within 6 weeks (preferably 3 months) of IM immune globulin administration, or within 8 months of intravenous immune globulin given as replacement therapy for humoral immune deficiencies.
- The vaccine should not be given within 1 month of any other live vaccine except mumps, rubella, and oral polio.
- Measles vaccine is indicated in all persons born after 1956 or in those who lack documentation of wild virus infection either by history or antibody titers.
- For postexposure prophylaxis, the vaccine is effective if given within 72 hours of exposure. In addition, immune globulin may be administered intramuscularly at a dose of 0.25 mg/kg (maximum dose, 15 mL), if given within 6 days of exposure.

▶ MENINGOCOCCAL POLYSACCHARIDE VACCINE (MPV)

- MPV is indicated in high-risk populations such as those exposed to the disease, those in the midst of uncontrolled outbreaks, or travelers to an area with epidemic or hyperendemic meningococcal disease.

- In the United States, serotype B, a strain not contained in the current vaccine, causes the majority of disease, thus routine vaccination is not recommended.
- The vaccine should not be given to pregnant women unless there is a substantial risk of infection.

▶ MUMPS VACCINE

- The vaccine (usually given in conjunction with measles and rubella) is given beginning at age 12–15 months, with a second dose prior to entry into elementary school (or alternatively, prior to entry into junior high school). If the vaccine is given before 12 months of age, revaccination is necessary and should be given after reaching 1 year of age.
- The vaccine is also indicated in previously unvaccinated adults and in those in whom a poor history of wild virus infection or previous administration of killed mumps exists.
- Postexposure vaccination is of no benefit.
- Mumps vaccine should not be given to pregnant women or immunosuppressed patients. The vaccine should not be given within 6 weeks (preferably 3 months) of administration of immune globulin. Finally, the vaccine should not be given to neomycin-sensitive individuals.

VIII ▶ PERTUSSIS VACCINE

- Pertussis vaccine is usually administered in combination with diphtheria and tetanus toxoids (as DPT).
- The primary immunization series for pertussis vaccine consists of four doses given at ages 2, 4, 6, and 15–18 months. A booster dose is recommended at age 4–6 years.
- Adverse events reportedly having a temporal relationship to pertussis vaccine administration include prolonged crying (3%), unusual high-pitched cry (0.1%), convulsions (0.06%), and encephalopathy (0.00005%).
- The American Academy of Pediatrics and the Immunization Practices Advisory Committee continue to recommend routine pertussis vaccination.
- There are only two absolute contraindications to pertussis administration: an immediate anaphylactic reaction to a previous dose, or encephalopathy within 7 days of a previous dose, with no evidence of other cause.

▶ PNEUMOCOCCAL VACCINE

- Pneumococcal vaccine is recommended for the following immunocompetent persons:
    - Persons 65 or more years of age. If an individual received vaccine more than 5 years earlier and was under age 65 at the time of administration, revaccination should be given.

- Persons ages 2–64 years with chronic illness.
- Persons ages 2–64 years with functional or anatomic asplenia. When splenectomy is planned, pneumococcal vaccine should be given at least 2 weeks prior to surgery. Revaccination is recommended at 5 or more years in subjects older than 10 years, and at 3 or more years in subjects under 10 years old.
- Persons ages 2–64 years living in environments where the risk of invasive pneumococcal disease or its complications is increased. This does not include day-care center employees and children.

- A single revaccination should be given if 5 or more years have passed since the first dose in subjects older than 10 years. In subjects 10 years of age or younger, revaccination should be given 3 years after the previous dose.

▶ POLIOVIRUS VACCINES

- Two types of trivalent poliovirus vaccines are currently licensed for distribution in the United States, an enhanced inactivated vaccine (eIPV) and a live attenuated, oral vaccine (OPV), which has been the primary immunizing agent for poliovirus infection.
- OPV is administered beginning at 6–12 weeks of age with doses at 2 months, 4 months, and 6–18 months, and a booster at 4–6 years.
- OPV is not recommended for persons who are immunodeficient or for normal individuals who reside in a household where another person is immunodeficient. VIII
- HIV-infected patients should receive eIPV in place of the live vaccine.
- OPV should not be given during pregnancy because of the small but theoretical risk to the fetus.
- Primary immunization with eIPV consists of subcutaneous injections at 2 months, 4 months, and 12–18 months, with a booster at 4–6 years of age.
- Primary poliomyelitis immunization is recommended for all children and young adults up to age 18.
- Primary immunization of adults older than 18 years is not routinely recommended, because a high level of immunity already exists in this age group and the risk of exposure in developed countries is small. However, unimmunized adults who are at increased risk for exposure because of travel, residence, or occupation should receive primary immunization with eIPV.

▶ RUBELLA VACCINE

- The vaccine is indicated for children under 1 year of age, persons 12 years or older without evidence of wild virus infection, women of childbearing potential for whom serologic testing is unavailable, and persons at a substantial risk for exposure.

- The vaccine should not be given to immunosuppressed individuals nor used within 6 weeks (preferably 3 months) of immune globulin administration.
- Although the vaccine has been shown to be safe to the fetus, its use in pregnancy is discouraged. Women should be counseled not to become pregnant for 3 months following vaccination.

▶ VARICELLA VACCINE

- The American Academy of Pediatrics recommends routine immunization with varicella vaccine for all children at 12–18 months of age and for persons above this age if they have not had chicken pox. Persons 13 years and older should receive two doses separated by 4–8 weeks.
- The vaccine is contraindicated in immunosuppressed or pregnant patients.

▶ VARICELLA-ZOSTER IMMUNE GLOBULIN

- Varicella-zoster immune globulin (VZIG) is used for passive immunization of susceptible immunodeficient patients exposed to VZ infection.
- Use of VZIG should be considered in exposed children and certain adults who are immunocompromised and susceptible to VZ. Criteria for its use after varicella-zoster exposure are listed in Table 48–7.
- For maximum effectiveness, VZIG must be given within 48 hours and not more than 96 hours following exposure.
- Administration of VZIG is by the intramuscular route (never intravenously).

TABLE 48–7. Conditions Warranting Consideration of Varicella-Zoster Immune Globulin (VZIG) after Varicella-Zoster Virus Exposure

Conditions
Neoplastic diseases
Primary or acquired immunodeficiency
Immunosuppressive treatment
Pregnancy
Newborn of mother who had onset of chickenpox within 5 d before delivery or within 48 h after delivery
Premature infant > 28 wk gestation whose mother has no history of chickenpox
Premature infant < 28 wk gestation or < 1000 g, regardless of maternal history of chickenpox

Adapted from Centers for Disease Control and Prevention. Prevention of varicella: Recommendations of the Advisory Committee on Immunization Practices (ACIP). MMWR 1996;45:1–36.

TABLE 48–8. Indications and Dosage of Intramuscular Immune Globulin in Infectious Diseases

Primary immunodeficiency states	1.2 mL/kg IM then 0.6 mL/kg IM every 2–4 wk
Hepatitis A exposure	0.02 mL/kg IM within 2 wk
Hepatitis A prophylaxis	0.02 mL/kg IM if exposure <3 mo 0.06 mL/kg if exposure >3 mo, every 4–6 mo
Hepatitis B	0.06 mL/kg IM (HBIG is preferred in known exposures) as soon as possible
Non-A/non-B hepatitis	0.06 mL/kg IM as soon as possible (questionable effectiveness)
Measles	0.25 mL/kg IM within 6 d (maximum dose = 15 mL)
Rubella	0.55 mL/kg, single dose
Primary immunodeficiency states	1.2 mL/kg IM then 0.6 mL/kg IM every 2–4 wk

► IMMUNE GLOBULIN

- Immune globulin (IG) is available as both intramuscular (IGIM) and intravenous preparations (IGIV).
- IGIM is indicated for providing passive immunity in hepatitis A infections, as an alternative to HBIG in hepatitis B exposures (however, HBIG is significantly more effective), hepatitis C (but not hepatitis E), measles, varicella zoster, and primary immunodeficiency diseases. IGIM is not indicated for prevention of rubella, mumps, or poliomyelitis. Table 48–8 lists the suggested dosages for IGIM in various disease states.

VIII

IVIG USES

- Primary immunodeficiency states including both antibody deficiencies and combined deficiencies. Idiopathic thrombocytopenia purpura (ITP).
- Chronic lymphocytic leukemia (CLL) in patients who have had a serious bacterial infection.
- Kawasaki disease (mucocutaneous lymph node syndrome).
- Neonatal sepsis.
- Bone marrow transplant.
- Varicella-zoster.

► RHO(D) IMMUNE GLOBULIN (RDIG)

- RDIG suppresses the antibody response and formation of anti-Rho(D) in Rho(D)-negative, D^u-negative women exposed to Rho(D)-positive blood and prevents the future chance of erythroblastosis fetalis in subsequent pregnancies with a Rho(D)-positive fetus.

- RDIG, when administered within 72 hours of delivery of a full-term infant, reduces active antibody formation from 12% to 1–2%.
- RDIG is also used in the case of a premenopausal woman who is Rho(D) negative or D^u negative and has inadvertently received Rho(D)-positive or D^u positive blood or blood products.
- RDIG may be used after abortion, miscarriage, amniocentesis, or abdominal trauma.
- RDIG is administered intramuscularly only.

See Chapter 113, Vaccines, Toxoids, and Other Immunobiologics, authored by Joseph S. Bertino, Jr., PharmD, FCCP, and Daniel T. Casto, PharmD, FCCP, for a more detailed discussion of this topic.

Neurologic Disorders

Edited by Barbara G. Wells, PharmD, FASHP, FCCP, BCPP

Chapter 49

▶ EPILEPSY

▶ DEFINITIONS

Epilepsy implies a periodic recurrence of seizures with or without convulsions. A seizure results from an excessive synchronous discharge of cortical neurons and is characterized by changes in electrical activity as measured by the electroencephalogram (EEG). A convulsion implies violent, involuntary contraction(s) of the voluntary muscles.

▶ ETIOLOGY

- There is no identifiable cause for seizures in most patients, especially children.
- The most clearly established risk factors for epilepsy are severe head trauma, central nervous system (CNS) infections, and stroke. Children who are small for gestational age, neonates with seizures, and children with febrile seizures, cerebral palsy, or mental retardation are at increased risk for developing epilepsy.
- Hyperventilation, sleep, sleep deprivation, sensory stimuli, and emotional stress may initiate seizures. Hormonal changes occurring at the time of menses, puberty, or pregnancy have been associated with onset of or increase in seizure activity. Other precipitants include fever, lack of food, trauma, drugs (e.g., theophylline, alcohol, phenothiazines, antidepressants, cocaine, antiepileptic drugs [AEDs] in excessive concentrations, oral contraceptives), and drug withdrawal.
- The causes of seizures in the elderly include cerebrovascular disease, tumor, head trauma, metabolic disorders, and CNS infections.

▶ PATHOPHYSIOLOGY

- A seizure is traceable to an unstable cell membrane or its surrounding cells. Excess excitability spreads either locally (focal seizure) or more widely (generalized seizure).
- An abnormality of potassium conductance, a defect in the voltage-sensitive calcium channels, or a deficiency in the membrane adenosine triphosphatase (ATPases) linked to ion transport may result in neuronal membrane instability and a seizure.
- Normal neuronal activity depends on normal functioning of excitatory (e.g., glutamate, aspartate, acetylcholine, norepinephrine, histamine,

corticotropin-releasing factor, purines, peptides, cytokines, and steroid hormones) and inhibitory (e.g., dopamine, γ-aminobutyric acid [GABA]) neurotransmitters, and an adequate supply of glucose, oxygen, sodium, potassium, calcium, and amino acids; normal pH; and normal receptor function.

▶ CLINICAL PRESENTATION

- The International Classification of Epileptic Seizures (Table 49–1) classifies epilepsy based on clinical description and electrophysiologic findings.
- Partial seizures begin in one hemisphere of the brain, and unless they become secondarily generalized, result in an asymmetric seizure.
- Absence seizures have a characteristic 2–4 cycle/s spike and slow-wave EEG pattern.
- Partial seizures manifest as alterations in motor functions, sensory or somatosensory symptoms, or automatisms. If there is no loss of consciousness, the seizures are called simple partial. If there is loss of consciousness, they are termed complex partial, and the patients may have automatisms, memory loss, or aberrations of behavior.

TABLE 49–1. International Classification of Epileptic Seizures

I. Partial seizures (seizures begin locally)
   A. Simple (without impairment of consciousness)
      1. With motor symptoms
      2. With special sensory or somatosensory symptoms
      3. With psychic symptoms
   B. Complex (with impairment of consciousness)
      1. Simple partial onset followed by impairment of consciousness—with or without automatisms
      2. Impaired consciousness at onset—with or without automatisms
   C. Secondarily generalized (partial onset evolving to generalized tonic-clonic seizures)

II. Generalized seizures (bilaterally symmetrical and without local onset)
   A. Absence
   B. Myoclonic
   C. Clonic
   D. Tonic
   E. Tonic-clonic
   F. Atonic
   G. Infantile spasms

III. Unclassified seizures

IV. Status epilepticus

- In generalized seizures, motor symptoms are bilateral, and there is loss of consciousness.
- Absence seizures generally occur in young children or adolescents and exhibit a sudden onset, interruption of ongoing activities, a blank stare, and possibly a brief upward rotation of the eyes.
- Generalized tonic-clonic seizures may be preceded by premonitory symptoms (i.e., an aura). A tonic-clonic seizure that is preceded by an aura is likely a partial seizure that is secondarily generalized. Tonic-clonic seizures begin with a short tonic contraction of muscles followed by a period of rigidity. The patient may lose sphincter control, bite the tongue, or become cyanotic. The episode may be followed by unconsciousness, and frequently the patient goes into a deep sleep.
- Myoclonic jerks are brief shock-like muscular contractions of the face, trunk, and extremities. They may be isolated events or rapidly repetitive.
- In atonic seizures, there is a sudden loss of muscle tone that may be described as a head drop, dropping of a limb, or slumping to the ground.

▶ DIAGNOSIS

- The patient and family should be asked to characterize the seizure for frequency, duration, precipitating factors, time of occurrence, presence of an aura, ictal activity, and postictal state.
- Physical, neurologic, and laboratory examination (SMA-20, complete blood cell count [CBC], urinalysis, and special blood chemistries) may identify an etiology. A lumbar puncture may be indicated if there is fever.
- An EEG should be done as soon after the seizure as possible. Simultaneous EEG and video monitoring may be helpful.
- Imaging studies (computed tomography [CT], positron emission tomography [PET], single-photon emission CT [SPECT], and magnetic resonance imaging [MRI]) may identify structural or functional abnormalities.

▶ DESIRED OUTCOME

- The goal of treatment is to control or reduce the frequency of seizures and ensure compliance, allowing the patient to live as normal a life as possible. Complete suppression of seizures must be balanced against tolerability of side effects, and the patient should be involved in defining the balance.

▶ TREATMENT

GENERAL APPROACH

- The treatment of choice depends on the type of epilepsy (Table 49–2) and on drug-specific adverse effects and patient preferences. Figure 49–1 is a suggested algorithm for treatment of epilepsy.

TABLE 49–2. Drugs of Choice for Specific Seizure Disorders

Seizure Type	Commonly Used Initial Drugs	Alternative Drugs
Partial	Carbamazepine Phenytoin Valproic acid	Felbamate Gabapentin Lamotrigine Phenobarbital Tiagabine Topiramate Vigabatrin
Tonic-clonic	Phenytoin Valproic acid Carbamazepine	Phenobarbital Lamotrigine
Absence	Ethosuximide Valproic acid	Clonazepam Acetazolamide
Bilateral massive epileptic myoclonus, atonic, infantile spasms[a]	Clonazepam ACTH	Phenytoin Phenobarbital Benzodiazepines Acetazolamide Felbamate Topiramate Vigabatrin
Juvenile myoclonic Epilepsy (JME)	Valproic acid	Lamotrigine

IX [a]Difficult group to treat; combinations are the rule.

- Begin with monotherapy; about 70% of patients can be maintained on one drug, but all are not seizure free.
- Up to 60% of patients with epilepsy are noncompliant, and this is the most common reason for treatment failure.
- Drug therapy may not be indicated in patients who have had only one seizure or those whose seizures have minimal impact on their lives. Patients who have had two or more seizures should generally be started on AEDs. Early initiation of appropriate AED therapy enhances the likelihood of controlling seizures.
- Factors favoring successful withdrawal of AEDs include a seizure-free period of 2–4 years, complete seizure control within 1 year of onset, an onset of seizures after age 2 and before age 35 years, and a normal EEG. Poor prognostic factors include a history of a high frequency of seizures, repeated episodes of status epilepticus, a combination of seizure types, and development of abnormal mental functioning. A 2-year seizure-free period is suggested for absence and rolandic epilepsy, while a 4-year seizure-free period is suggested for simple partial, complex partial, and absence associated with tonic-clonic seizures.

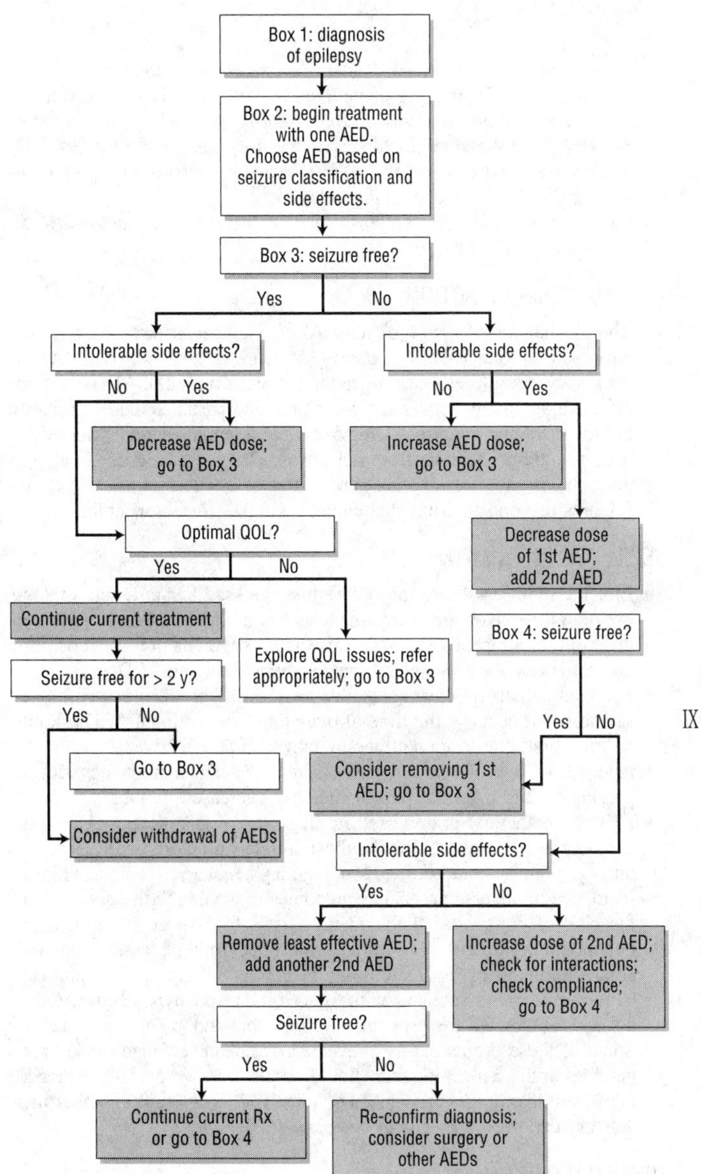

Figure 49–1. Algorithm for treatment of epilepsy.

IX

According to the American Academy of Neurology Guidelines, discontinuance of AEDs may be considered if the patient is seizure free for 2–5 years, if there is a single type of partial seizure or single type of primary generalized tonic-clonic seizure, if the neurologic exam and IQ are normal, and if the EEG normalized with treatment. AED withdrawal should always be done gradually.

- Patient knowledge of epilepsy and treatment correlates with an improved quality of life.

MECHANISMS OF ACTION

- The mechanism of action of most AEDs includes effects on ion channels (sodium and calcium), inhibitory neurotransmission (GABA), or excitatory neurotransmission (glutamate and aspartate). AEDs that are effective against generalized tonic-clonic and partial seizures probably reduce sustained repetitive firing of action potentials by delaying recovery of sodium channels from activation. Drugs that reduce T-calcium currents are effective against generalized absence seizures. Myoclonic seizures respond to drugs that enhance $GABA_A$ receptor inhibition.

EPILEPSY IN WOMEN

- Enzyme-inducing AEDs may cause treatment failures in females taking oral contraceptives; thus, treatment with a moderate or high hormonal dose oral contraceptive is necessary, and a supplemental form of birth control is advised in women taking enzyme-inducing AEDs.
- For catamenial epilepsy (seizures just before or during menses) or seizures that occur at the time of ovulation, conventional AEDs should be tried first, but hormonal therapy may also be effective.
- About 25–30% of women have increased seizure frequency during pregnancy, and a similar percentage have decreased frequency.
- AED monotherapy is preferred in pregnancy. Clearance of phenytoin, carbamazepine, phenobarbital, ethosuximide, and clorazepate increases during pregnancy, and protein binding may be altered. There is a higher incidence of adverse pregnancy outcomes in women with epilepsy, and the risk of congenital malformations is 4–6% (twice as high as in nonepileptic women). Barbiturates and phenytoin are associated with congenital heart malformations and facial clefts. Valproic acid and carbamazepine are associated with spina bifida and hypospadias. Other adverse outcomes are growth, psychomotor, and mental retardation. Some of these events can be prevented by adequate folate intake; prenatal vitamins with folic acid should be given to women of childbearing potential who are taking AEDs. Vitamin K given to the mother predelivery can prevent neonatal hemorrhagic disorder.

PHARMACOKINETICS

- AED pharmacokinetic data are summarized in Table 49–3. For populations known to have altered plasma protein binding, free rather than

TABLE 49–3. Antiepileptic Drug Pharmacokinetic Data

AED	$t_{1/2}$ (h)[a]	Time to Steady State (d)	Unchanged %	V_D (L/kg)	Clinically Important Metabolite	Removed by Dialysis (%)	Protein Binding (%)
Carbamazepine	12 M; 5–14 Co	21–28 for completion of auto-induction	<1	1–2	10,11-epoxide	<20	40–90
Ethosuximide	A 60 C 30	6–12	10–20	0.67	No	~50	0
Felbamate	16–22	5–7	50	0.73–0.82	No		~25
Gabapentin[a]	5–40[b]	1–2[b]	100	0.65–1.04	No	Y	0
Lamotrigine	25.4 M	3–15	0	1.28	No	20	40–50
Phenobarbital	A 46–136 C 37–73	14–21	20–40	0.6	No	30 (H)[c]	50
Phenytoin	A 10–34 C 5–14	7–28	<5	0.6–8.0	No	4 (H)[c]	90
Primidone	A 3.3–19 C 4.5–11	1–4	40	0.43–1.1	PB[d] PEMA[d]	30 (H)[b]	80
Tiagabine	5–13		Negligible		No		95
Topiramate	18–21	4–5	50–70	0.55–0.8 (male) 0.23–0.4 (female)	No		15
Valproic acid	A 8–20 C 7–14	1–3	<5	0.1–0.5	May contribute to toxicity	—	90–95 binding saturates
Vigabatrin	5–14[b]	1–5	50–70	0.8	No		0

A, adult; C, child; M, monotherapy; Co, combination therapy; H, hemodialysis; PB, phenobarbital; PEMA, phenylethylmalonamide.

[a]The bioavailability of gabapentin is dose dependent.

[b]Half-life depends on renal function.

total serum concentrations should be measured if the AED is highly protein bound. Conditions altering AED protein binding include chronic renal failure, liver disease, hypoalbuminemia, burns, pregnancy, malnutrition, displacing drugs, and age (neonates and the elderly). Phenytoin and valproic acid are highly protein bound; **carbamazepine** has variable binding; phenobarbital and primidone are minimally bound; and ethosuximide is not bound to plasma proteins. Unbound concentration monitoring is especially useful for phenytoin.

- Neonates may metabolize drugs more slowly, and infants and children may metabolize drugs more rapidly than adults. Lower doses of AEDs are required in the elderly. Some elderly patients have an increased receptor sensitivity to CNS drugs, making the accepted therapeutic range invalid.
- Liver disease may decrease drug metabolism and protein binding. Patients with chronic renal failure may have decreased elimination of unchanged drug as well as altered protein binding.

SERUM CONCENTRATIONS

- Seizure control may occur before the "minimum" of the accepted therapeutic range is reached, and some patients may need concentrations beyond the "maximum." The therapeutic range for AEDs may be different for different seizure types (e.g., higher for complex partial seizures than for tonic-clonic seizures).

EFFICACY

- The traditional treatment of tonic-clonic seizures is phenytoin or phenobarbital, but the use of carbamazepine and valproic acid is increasing, as efficacy is equal and side effects more favorable. Carbamazepine may cause less cognitive impairment than phenytoin.
- Most seizures in adults are partial in onset. For complex partial seizures, carbamazepine is recognized as the AED of choice. Alternatives include phenytoin, gabapentin, lamotrigine, tiagabine, topiramate, vigabatrin, phenobarbital, and valproic acid. Carbamazepine and valproic acid are equally effective for tonic-clonic seizures, but carbamazepine was superior for partial seizures, and valproic acid caused more adverse effects. The newer AEDs were first approved as adjunctive therapy for patients with refractory partial seizures, but monotherapy trials are under way.
- Absence seizures are best treated with ethosuximide or valproic acid. For a combination of absence and other generalized or partial seizures, valproic acid is preferred. If valproic acid is ineffective in treating a mixed seizure disorder that includes absence, ethosuximide should be used in combination with another AED.
- Benzodiazepines can be useful for the management of seizure types that occur primarily in children, although tolerance may develop. Recently, a rectal formulation of **diazepam** has been approved.

- Acetazolamide is effective for generalized tonic-clonic, absence, complex partial, and catamenial seizures, but tolerance is a problem, and intermittent use is preferred.

ADVERSE EFFECTS

- Chronic and acute adverse effects of AEDs are listed in Table 49–4.
- When acute organ failure occurs, it usually happens within the first 6 months of AED therapy.
- Chronic side effects can occur despite serum concentrations within the therapeutic range, and their incidence is 33% with phenytoin, 23% with phenobarbital, 15% with carbamazepine, and 12% with valproic acid.
- Carbamazepine and valproic acid may cause less cognitive impairment than phenytoin and phenobarbital. Almost all AEDs (except felbamate) are associated with depressed CNS function (e.g., drowsiness, lethargy) early in treatment, but some tolerance usually develops within 7–10 days.

DRUG–DRUG INTERACTIONS

- Drug interactions involving AEDs are shown in Tables 49–5 and 49–6.
- Phenobarbital, phenytoin, primidone, and carbamazepine are potent inducers of cytochrome P450, epoxide hydrolase, and uridine diphosphate glucuronosyltransferase enzyme systems. Valproic acid inhibits many hepatic enzyme systems and displaces some drugs from plasma albumin. Felbamate and topiramate can act as inducers with some isoforms and inhibitors or others.
- Other than vigabatrin and gabapentin, which are eliminated mostly unchanged by the renal route, other AEDs are metabolized wholly or in part by hepatic enzymes.

DOSING AND ADMINISTRATION

- Initial and maximal daily doses are shown in Table 49–7. Usually therapy is initiated at one-fourth to one-third the anticipated maintenance dose, and gradually increased over 3 or 4 weeks to an effective dose. Serum concentrations may be useful, but the therapeutic range must be correlated with clinical outcome. Some patients need and tolerate concentrations above the range.
- The initial agent should be titrated to maximum benefit or intolerable side effects. A second medication may be added if seizures continue despite good plasma concentrations. The second AED may replace or be added to the initial therapy. If the initial AED is replaced, it should be gradually tapered after the second drug has been titrated to the desired dose. If two drugs are used, they generally should have differing mechanisms of action and side-effect profiles.

SPECIFIC ANTIEPILEPTIC DRUGS

Carbamazepine

- **Carbamazepine** may act by inhibition of voltage-gated sodium channels. There is some depression of post-tetanic potentiation (PTP), but

TABLE 49–4. Antiepileptic Drug Side Effects

AED	Acute Side Effects: *Concentration Dependent*	Acute Side Effects: *Idiosyncratic*	Chronic Side Effects
Carbamazepine	Diplopia Dizziness Drowsiness Nausea Unsteadiness Lethargy	Blood dyscrasias Rash	Hyponatremia
Ethosuximide	Ataxia Drowsiness GI distress Unsteadiness Hiccoughs	Blood dyscrasias Rash	Behavior changes Headache
Felbamate	Anorexia Nausea Vomiting Insomnia Headache	Aplastic anemia Acute hepatic failure	Not established
Gabapentin	Dizziness Fatigue Somnolence Ataxia	Weight gain	Weight gain
Lamotrigine	Ataxia Diplopia Dizziness Unsteadiness Headache Somnolence Nausea Vomiting Weight gain Nervousness Abnormal thinking	Rash	Not established
Phenobarbital	Ataxia Hyperactivity Headache Unsteadiness Sedation Nausea	Blood dyscrasis Rash	Behavior changes Connective tissue disorder Intellectual blunting Metabolic bone disease Mood change Sedation
Phenytoin	Ataxia Nystagmus Behavior changes Dizziness Headache Incoordination Nausea Sedation Lethargy Cognitive impairment	Blood dyscrasias Rash Immunologic reaction	Behavior changes Cerebellar syndrome Connective tissue changes Skin thickening Folate deficiency Gingival hyperplasia Hirsutism Coarsening of facial features

TABLE 49–4. continued

	Acute Side Effects		
AED	*Concentration Dependent*	*Idiosyncratic*	Chronic Side Effects
Phenytoin (cont'd)	Fatigue Visual blurring		Acne Cognitive impairment Metabolic bone disease Sedation
Primidone	Behavior changes Headache Nausea Sedation Unsteadiness	Blood dyscrasias Rash	Behavior changes Connective tissue disorders Cognitive impairment Sedation
Tiagabine	Dizziness Fatigue Difficulties concentrating Nervousness Tremor Blurred vision Depression Speech or language problems Weakness Confusion	Not established	Not established
Topiramate	Difficulties concentrating Psychomotor slowing Speech or language problems Somnolence, fatigue Dizziness Headache Diplopia	Not established	Not established
Valproic acid	Behavior changes GI upset Sedation Unsteadiness Tremor	Acute hepatic failure Acute pancreatitis Thrombocytopenia Blood dyscrasias Rash	Behavior changes Alopecia Sedation Nausea Weight gain Hyperammonemia
Vigabatrin	Sedation Fatigue Unsteadiness	Behavioral disturbances Confusion Psychosis Rash	Behavior changes Confusion Psychosis Sedation Weight gain

GI, gastrointestinal.

TABLE 49–5. Interactions between Antiepileptic Drugs

AED	Added Drug	Effect
Carbamazepine (CBZ)	Felbamate	Incr. 10,11-epoxide
	Felbamate	Decr. CBZ
	Phenobarbital	Decr. CBZ
	Phenytoin	Decr. CBZ
Felbamate (FBM)	Carbamazepine	Decr. FBM
	Phenytoin	Decr. FBM
	Valproic acid	Incr. FBM
Lamotrigine (LTG)	Carbamazepine	Decr. LTG
	Phenobarbital	Decr. LTG
	Phenytoin	Decr. LTG
	Primidone	Decr. LTG
	Valproic acid	Incr. LTG
Phenobarbital (PB)	Felbamate	Incr. PB
	Phenytoin	Incr. or decr. PB
	Valproic acid	Incr. PB
Phenytoin (PHT)	Carbamazepine	Decr. PHT
	Felbamate	Incr. PHT
	Methsuximide	Incr. PHT
	Phenobarbital	Incr. or decr. PHT
	Valproic acid	Decr. Total PHT
	Vigabatrin	Decr. PHT
Primidone (PRM)	Carbamazepine	Decr. PRM
		Incr. PB
	Phenytoin	Decr. PRM
		Incr. PB
	Valproic acid	Incr. PRM
		Incr. PB
Tiagabine (TGB)	Carbamazepine	Decr. TGB
	Phenytoin	Decr. TGB
Topiramate (TPM)	Carbamazepine	Decr. TPM
	Phenytoin	Decr. TPM
	Valproic acid	Decr. TPM
Valproic acid (VPA)	Carbamazepine	Decr. VPA
	Lamotrigine	Decr. VPA
	Phenobarbital	Decr. VPA
	Primidone	Decr. VPA
	Phenytoin	Decr. VPA

Incr., increased; decr., decreased.

TABLE 49–6. Interactions With Nonepileptic Medications

AED	Altered by	Result	Alters	Result
Carbamazepine	Cimetidine	Incr. CBZ	Oral contraceptives (OC)	Decr. efficacy of OC
	Erythromycin	Incr. CBZ	Doxycycline	Decr. doxycycline
	Fluoxetine	Incr. CBZ	Theophylline	Decr. theophylline
	Isoniazid	Incr. CBZ	Warfarin	Decr. warfarin
	Propoxyphene	Incr. CBZ		
Phenobarbital	Acetazolamide	Incr. PB	OC	Decr. efficacy of OC
Phenytoin	Antacids	Decr. absorption of PHT	OC	Decr. efficacy of OC
	Cimetidine	Incr. PHT	Bishydroxycoumarin	Decr. anticoagulation
	Chloramphenicol	Incr. PHT	Folic acid	Decr. folic acid
	Disulfiram	Incr. PHT	Quinidine	Decr. quinidine
	Ethanol (acute)	Incr. PHT	Vitamin D	Decr. vitamin D
	Fluconazole	Incr. PHT		
	Isoniazid	Incr. PHT		
	Propoxyphene	Incr. PHT		
	Warfarin	Incr. PHT		
	Ethanol (chronic)	Decr. PHT		
Primidone	Isoniazid	Decr. metabolism of primidone	Chlorpromazine	Decr. chlorpromazine
			Corticosteroids	Decr. corticosteroids
	Nicotinamide	Decr. metabolism of primidone	Quinidine	Decr. quinidine
			Tricyclics	Decr. tricyclics
			Furosemide	Decr. renal sensitivity to furosemide
Valproic acid	Cimetidine	Incr. VPA		
	Salicylates	Incr. free VPA		

AED, antiepileptic drug; Incr., increased; decr., decreased.

IX

less than with phenytoin. It may also inhibit an increase in cyclic AMP.

- Bioavailability may be lower at higher doses. Food may enhance bioavailability.
- There is wide variability in time to peak plasma levels (2–24 hours; mean, 6 hours).
- The controlled-release and sustained-release preparations in twice daily dosing are bioequivalent to four times daily dosing of immediate-release forms.
- The liver metabolizes 98–99% of a dose of carbamazepine (mostly by CYP3A4), and the major metabolite is carbamazepine-10,11-epoxide, which is active.
- Carbamazepine can induce its own metabolism (auto-induction), and this effect begins within 3–5 days of dosing initiation and takes 21–28 days to become complete.

TABLE 49–7. Dosing and Target Serum Concentration Ranges of AEDS

	Trade Name	Manufacturer	Year Introduced	Initial Dose	Maximum Daily Dose	Target Serum Concention Range
Barbiturates						
Mephobarbital	Mebaral	Sanofi Winthrop	1935	50–100 mg/d	400–600 mg	Not defined
Phenobarbital	Various	Generic	1912	1–3 mg/kg/d (10–20 mg/kg LD)	180–300 mg	10–40 μg/mL
Primidone	Mysoline	Wyeth-Ayerst	1954	100–125 mg/d	750–2000 mg	PRM: 5–10 μg/mL PB: 20–40 μg/mL
Benzodiazepines						
Clonazepam	Klonopin	Roche	1975	1.5 mg/d	20 mg	20–80 ng/mL
Clorazepate	Tranxene	Abbott	1981	7.5–22.5 mg/d	90 mg	Not defined
Diazepam	Valium	Roche, generic	1968	PO: 4–40 mg IV: 5–10 mg	PO: 4–40 mg IV: 5–30 mg	100–1000 ng/mL
Lorazepam	Ativan	Wyeth-Ayerst, generic		PO: 2–6 mg IV: 0.05 mg/kg IM: 0.05 mg/kg	PO: 10 mg IV: 0.044 mg/kg	10–30 ng/mL
Hydantoins						
Ethotoin	Peganone	Abbott	1957	<1000 mg/d	2000–4000 mg with food	15–50 μg/mL
Mephenytoin	Mesantoin	Sandoz	1947	50–100 mg/d	200–800 mg	25–40 μg/mL
Phenytoin	Dilantin	Parke-Davis	1938	PO: 3–5 mg/kg (200–400 mg) (15–20 mg/kg LD)	PO: 500–600 mg	Total: 10–20 μg/mL Unbound? 0.5–3 μg/mL

Succinimides						
Ethosuximide	Zarontin	Parke-Davis	1960	500 mg/d	500–2000 mg	40–80 μg/mL
Methsuximide	Celontin	Parke-Davis	1957	300 mg/d	300–1200 mg	N-desmethyl metabolite 10–40 μg/mL
Other						
Carbamazepine	Tegretol	Novartis, generic	1974	400 mg/d	400–2400 mg	4–14 μg/mL
Felbamate	Felbatol	Carter Wallace	1993	1200 mg/d	3600 mg	Not defined
Gabapentin	Neurontin	Parke-Davis	1993	900 mg/d	4800 mg	Not defined
Lamotrigine	Lamictal	Glaxo-Wellcome	1994	25 mg qod if on VPA: 25–50 mg/d if not on VPA	100–150 mg if on VPA: 300–500 mg if not on VPA	Not defined
Tiagabine	Gabitril	Abbott	1997	4–8 mg/d	80 mg	Not defined
Topiramate	Topamax	Ortho McNeil	1997	25–50 mg/d	200–1000 mg	Not defined
Valproic acid	Depakene, Depakote, Depacon	Abbott	1978	15 mg/kg (500–1000 mg)	60 mg/kg (3000–5000 mg)	50–150 μg/mL
Vigabatrin	Sabril	Hoechst Marion-Roussel	1998		3000 mg	

LD, loading dose; PRM, primidone; PB, phenobarbital.

- Neurosensory side effects (e.g., diplopia, burred vision, nystagmus, ataxia, unsteadiness, dizziness, and headache) are the most common, occurring in 35–50% of patients initially.
- Carbamazepine may induce hyponatremia, a condition similar to the syndrome of inappropriate antidiuretic hormone secretion. The incidence may increase with age.
- Hematologic side effects include aplastic anemia (rare), thrombocytopenia, anemia, and leukopenia (as high as 10% incidence). Leukopenia is usually transient, but may be persistent in 2% of patients. Carbamazepine may be continued unless the WBC count drops to <2500/mm^3 and the absolute neutrophil count drops to <1000/mm^3.
- Carbamazepine may interact with other drugs by inducing their metabolism.
- Valproic acid appears to reduce the formation of the 10,11-epoxide metabolite without affecting the concentration of carbamazepine.
- The interaction of erythromycin with carbamazepine is particularly significant.
- Loading doses of carbamazepine are indicated only for critically ill patients. Oral loading has been accomplished with the suspension (7.4–10.4 mg/kg) and with the controlled-release formulation.
- The sustained-release formulation can be opened and sprinkled on food.

Ethosuximide

- **Ethosuximide** inhibits NADPH-linked aldehyde reductase necessary for the formation of gamma-hydroxybutyrate, which has been implicated in causing absence seizures. It may also inhibit the sodium-potassium ATPase system.

IX

- It is the drug of choice for treatment of absence seizures; it may be used in combination with valproic acid in refractory patients.
- It is not bound to plasma or tissue proteins.
- There is some evidence for nonlinear metabolism.
- Common side effects are nausea, drowsiness, lethargy, dizziness, hiccups, and headaches. Rash, lupus, and blood dyscrasias are reported rarely.
- Patients are started at 5–7 mg/kg/d in divided doses and increased in 1–2 weeks. Doses of 20 mg/kg/d usually result in plasma concentrations of approximately 50 μg/mL. The daily dose is usually divided into two doses.

Felbamate

- **Felbamate** appears to act as a glycine receptor antagonist.
- It is approved for use in patients 14 years and older as monotherapy and adjunctive therapy for partial seizures with and without secondary generalization and for children 2 years and older as adjunctive therapy for the Lennox–Gastaut syndrome. Because of the reports of aplastic anemia (1/3000 patients) and acute liver failure (1/10,000 patients), it is now recommended for patients refractory to other AEDs.

- It is recommended that the dose of phenytoin, carbamazepine, and valproic acid be decreased by about 30% when felbamate is added. Interactions with phenobarbital and warfarin have also been reported.
- If felbamate is used as monotherapy, the dose is initiated at 1200 mg/d (15 mg/kg in children) and then is increased by 600 mg every 2 weeks up to a maximum dose of 3600 mg/d (45 mg/kg in children).
- Frequently reported side effects are anorexia, insomnia, nausea, and headache.

Gabapentin

- **Gabapentin** is approved as adjunctive therapy for partial seizures with or without secondary generalization in adults.
- Bioavailability decreases with increasing doses.
- Common side effects are fatigue, sleepiness, dizziness, and ataxia.
- Aluminum antacids reduce the bioavailability of gabapentin by 20%. A high protein meal increased the maximum plasma concentration by 36% and the area under the curve (AUC) by 11%, but side effects were not increased.
- Dosing is initiated at 300 mg at bedtime and increased to 300 mg twice daily on the second day and 300 mg three times daily on the third day. Further titrations are then made. The manufacturer recommends doses up to 2400 or 3600 mg/d. It is eliminated by renal mechanisms, and dosage adjustments are necessary in patients with impaired renal function. If creatinine clearance is 60 mL/min, the dose is 1200 mg/d; if creatinine clearance is 30–60 mL/min, the dose is 600 mg/d; if creatinine clearance is 15–30 mL/min, the dose is 300 mg/d; if creatinine clearance is <15 mL/min, the dose is 300 mg every other day.

IX

Lamotrigine

- **Lamotrigine** blocks voltage-sensitive sodium channels, thus inhibiting the release of glutamate and aspartate.
- Lamotrigine is approved as adjunctive therapy in adults with partial epilepsy refractory to other agents. It has been used as monotherapy and appears to be effective against many generalized seizure types and in children.
- The most frequent side effects are diplopia, drowsiness, ataxia, and headache. Rashes are usually mild to moderate, but Steven–Johnson reaction has also occurred. The incidence of rash appears to be increased in patients who are also receiving valproic acid and who have rapid dosage titration.
- In patients taking enzyme-inducing drugs and not taking valproic acid, lamotrigine should be started at a dose of 50 mg/d for 2 weeks and then increased to 100 mg/d for 2 weeks. Then the dose can be titrated by 100 mg/d at weekly intervals up to 500 mg/d. Dosing is lower in patients taking valproic acid (Table 49–7).

Phenobarbital/Primidone

- **Phenobarbital** and **primidone** decrease postsynaptic excitation, possibly through GABA mechanisms.
- Phenobarbital is the drug of choice for neonatal seizures and is useful in generalized seizures (except absence) and may be useful in patients with partial seizures. Primidone shares the same indications, but is less useful in partial seizures.
- Primidone is an active AED and has two active metabolites, phenobarbital and phenylethylmalonamide (PEMA). In general, phenobarbital should be tried first and primidone reserved for refractory patients.
- Phenobarbital is a potent enzyme inducer. The half-life of primidone may become shorter after chronic therapy because the phenobarbital metabolite may induce the metabolism.
- The amount of phenobarbital excreted renally can be increased by giving diuretics and urinary alkalinizers.
- The most common side effects are fatigue, drowsiness, and depression. Phenobarbital impairs cognitive performance. In children, hyperactivity can occur.
- Ethanol increases phenobarbital metabolism, but valproic acid, phenytoin, cimetidine, and chloramphenicol inhibit its metabolism.
- Phenobarbital can usually be dosed once daily, and bedtime dosing may minimize daytime sedation. Primidone is given in divided doses.

Phenytoin

- **Phenytoin** blocks PTP and alters ion fluxes, thus altering depolarization, repolarization, and membrane stability.

- Phenytoin may be used for generalized seizures (except absence) and for partial seizures.
- Absorption may be saturable. Absorption is affected by particle size, and the brand should not be changed without careful monitoring. Food may slow absorption. Intramuscular administration of phenytoin is erratic and best avoided. Fosphenytoin can safely be administered intravenously and intramuscularly.
- Equations are available to normalize the phenytoin concentration in patients with hypoalbuminemia or renal failure.
- Phenytoin is metabolized in the liver mainly by CYP2C9, but CYP2C19 is also involved. Zero-order kinetics occurs within the usual dosage range, so any change in dose may produce disproportional changes in serum concentrations. One author suggested that if the serum concentration is <7 μg/mL, the daily dose should be increased by 100 mg; if the concentration is 7–12 μg/mL, the daily dose can be increased by 50 mg; if the concentration is >12 μg/mL, the daily dose can be increased by 30 mg or less.
- In nonacute situations, phenytoin may be initiated in doses of 3–6 mg/kg/d and titrated upward. Most adult patients can be maintained on a single daily dose, but children often require more frequent administration. Only extended-release preparations should be used for single daily dosing.

- Common but usually transient side effects are lethargy, incoordination, blurred vision, higher cortical dysfunction, and drowsiness. At serum concentrations >20 μg/mL, a significant number of patients exhibit nystagmus on lateral gaze. Ataxia frequently occurs at concentrations >30 μg/mL, and at concentrations >40 μg/mL, mental status changes may occur. At >30 μg/mL, phenytoin can exacerbate seizures. Gingival hyperplasia occurs in up to 50% of patients. Other chronic side effects include impaired cognition, vitamin deficiency, osteomalacia, folic acid deficiency, carbohydrate intolerance, hypothyroidism, and peripheral neuropathy.
- Phenytoin is prone to many drug interactions (Tables 49–5 and 49–6). If protein-binding interactions are suspected, free rather than total phenytoin concentrations are a better therapeutic guide.
- Phenytoin decreases folic acid absorption, but folic acid replacement enhances phenytoin clearance and can result in loss of efficacy. Phenytoin tablets and suspension contain phenytoin acid, while the capsules and parenteral solution are phenytoin sodium, which is 92% phenytoin. Clinicians should remember that there are two different strengths of phenytoin suspension and capsules.

Tiagabine

- **Tiagabine** is a specific inhibitor of GABA reuptake into glial cells and other neurons.
- It is approved for adjunctive use in patients with partial seizures; preliminary evidence supports its use as monotherapy.
- The most frequently reported side effect is dizziness. Other side effects are asthenia, nervousness, tremor, and diarrhea. These side effects are usually transient.
- It is oxidized by CYP3A4 enzymes, and enzyme inducers may reduce the AUC and decrease the half-life.
- Tiagabine is displaced from protein by naproxen, salicylates, and valproate.
- The dosage range in clinical trials was 32–56 mg/d. Slow titration is essential.

IX

Topiramate

- **Topiramate** affects voltage-dependent sodium channels, GABA receptors, and AMPA subtype glutamate receptors.
- It is approved as adjunctive therapy in adults with partial seizures.
- Approximately 50% of the dose is excreted renally, and tubular reabsorption may be prominently involved.
- The most common side effects are ataxia, impaired concentration, confusion, dizziness, fatigue, paresthesias, and somnolence. Nephrolithiasis occurred in 1.5% of patients.
- Enzyme inducers may decrease topiramate serum levels.
- The recommended dose is 400 mg/d in two divided doses. Starting doses are 25 to 50 mg in the evening, increasing by 25 to 50 mg/d

every week or every other week. Monotherapy doses of 1000 mg/d have been well tolerated and effective.

Valproic Acid/Divalproex Sodium

- **Valproic acid** may increase synthesis or inhibit degradation of GABA. It may also potentiate postsynaptic GABA responses, have a direct membrane-stabilizing effect, and affect potassium channels.
- The free fraction may increase as the total concentration increases, and free concentrations may be a better monitoring parameter than total concentrations, especially at higher concentrations. Protein binding is decreased in patients with head trauma.
- At least 10 metabolites have been identified (some may be active), and one may account for hepatotoxicity (4-en-valproic acid). This metabolite is increased by concurrent enzyme-inducing drugs. At least 67 cases have been reported, and most deaths were in children younger than 2 years who were mentally retarded and receiving multiple therapy.
- It is the drug of choice for most generalized seizures and is also useful for partial seizures. It may also be useful for neonatal seizures.
- Side effects are usually mild and include gastrointestinal (GI) complaints, weight gain, drowsiness, ataxia, and tremor. GI complaints may be minimized by the enteric-coated formulation or by food. Thrombocytopenia is common, but is responsive to a decrease in dose. Other hematologic toxicities include leukopenia with transient neutropenia, transient erythroblastopenia, and bone marrow changes.
- Valproic acid is an enzyme inhibitor, and it increases serum concentra-
IX tions of concurrently administered phenobarbital and may increase con-
centrations of carbamazepine 10,11-epoxide without affecting concen-
trations of the parent drug.
- Twice daily dosing is reasonable, but children and patients taking enzyme inducers may require three or four times daily dosing.
- The enteric-coated tablet, **divalproex sodium,** causes fewer GI side effects. It is metabolized in the gut to valproic acid.

Vigabatrin

- **Vigabatrin,** an irreversible inhibitor of GABA amino transaminase, increases brain GABA levels.
- It is used for partial and secondarily generalized tonic-clonic seizures in both adults and children and for infantile spasms. Data also suggest usefulness as monotherapy.
- Common side effects include sedation and fatigue. Agitation, irritability, or depression is reported in 2–4% of cases.
- Vigabatrin increases serum concentrations of phenytoin by approximately 30%.
- It can be dosed once or twice daily, and lower doses are used in impaired renal function.

▶ EVALUATION OF THERAPEUTIC OUTCOMES

- An individual therapeutic range should be established for each patient.
- Patients should be chronically monitored for seizure control, side effects, social adjustment, drug interactions, compliance, and toxicity.
- Patients should be asked to record severity and frequency of seizures in a seizure diary.

See Chapter 52, Epilepsy, authored by Nina M. Graves, PharmD, FCCP, and William R. Garnett, PharmD, FCCP, for a more detailed discussion of this topic.

Chapter 50

▶ HEADACHE: MIGRAINE AND CLUSTER

▶ MIGRAINE HEADACHE

The International Headache Society (IHS) has developed a classification system that provides precise definitions and standardized nomenclature for primary headache disorders (migraine, tension-type, and cluster headache).

PATHOPHYSIOLOGY

- The vascular hypothesis of migraine states that the aura is caused by intracerebral vasoconstriction followed by extracranial vasodilation resulting in headache pain.
- According to recent studies, the aura may be a manifestation of spreading depression, a cortical neuronal event characterized by slowly progressing waves of inhibition that may result in a 25–35% reduction in regional cerebral blood flow.
- Migraine pain is believed to result from activity within the trigeminovascular system that results in release of vasoactive neuropeptides, with subsequent vasodilation and plasma protein extravasation and pain.
- Activity within the trigeminovascular system is regulated by noradrenergic and serotonergic neurons within the brainstem.
- Factors that may induce arterial vasoconstriction include stress, excessive afferent stimulation (light, noise, smells), changes in the internal clock, and vasodilator therapy. This may cause an aura which may be followed by cerebral vasodilation and neurogenic inflammation. The initial vasospasm may occur due to increased release or production of prostaglandin, epinephrine, norepinephrine (NE), tyramine, and serotonin (5-HT).
- 5-HT receptors, especially 5-HT_1 and 5-HT_2, appear to play an important role in migraine pathophysiology. Platelet 5-HT concentrations decrease dramatically at the onset of a migraine, while free 5-HT concentrations in plasma may increase by as much as 100% during an attack.
- Numerous factors have been suggested to be etiologic in migraine (Table 50–1). Monosodium glutamate and disturbances in tyramine metabolism may also be a cause.
- Mechanisms of drug-induced headaches may include inhibition of reuptake and storage of 5-HT (reserpine), blocking neuronal reuptake of 5-HT (fluoxetine), altering platelet aggregation (ethinyl estradiol and mestranol), and vasodilation (nitroglycerin and nifedipine).

TABLE 50–1. Precipitating Factors Associated With Migraine

Psychological Factors	**Medications (continued)**
Stress	Ethinyl estradiol
Anxiety	Fluoxetine
Depression	Histamine
Environmental Factors	Hormone replacement therapy
Tobacco smoke	Indomethacin
Glare	Mestranol
Strong odors	Nicotine
Loud noise	Nifedipine
Bright or flickering lights	Nitroglycerin
Weather changes (increase in temperature or humidity)	Oral contraceptives
High altitude	Reserpine
Dietary Factors	**Hormonal Factors**
Alcohol	Menses
Tyramine-containing foods (e.g., red wine, aged cheese)	Pregnancy
Citrus fruit	Menopause
Food additives (e.g., monosodium glutamate, aspartame, sodium nitrite)	**Lifestyle**
Chocolate	Excessive or inadequate sleep
Caffeine	Fatigue
Medications	Fasting or dieting
Cimetidine	Skipping meals
Cocaine	Strenuous exercise

CLINICAL PRESENTATION

- Migraine without aura, common migraine, occurs in 85% of patients with migraines. Migraine with aura, classic migraine, occurs in approximately 10% of migraineurs. The remaining 5% are other migraine types (e.g., ophthalmologic migraine, retinal migraine, childhood periodic syndromes, complications of migraine).
- The aura begins 15–60 minutes prior to the onset of the headache and may include scintillations, teichopsia, photopsia, visual field defects, hemisensory disturbances (tingling or numbness in the extremities, hemiparesis, or aphasia), and alterations in mood or motor functions.
- Migraines usually occur in the early morning hours, reach peak intensity within 1 hour, and last 4–72 hours. Pain is usually unilateral, most often in the temple, and may be described as pounding. Physical activity may worsen the pain, and patients may seek a dark, quiet place. There may be a sensitivity to light or sound, anorexia, nausea, constipation or diarrhea, and changes in mood.

DIAGNOSIS

- Accurate diagnosis requires a history, physical examination, and laboratory tests (including an erythrocyte sedimentation rate) to rule out organic causes. Computed tomography (CT scan) or magnetic resonance imaging (MRI) should be considered in patients with an abnormal neurological examination, new onset of "worst headache ever," prolonged headaches, or papilledema. Headaches beginning late in life may suggest an organic etiology such as cerebrovascular disease, cancer, or temporal arteritis. Diagnostic criteria for migraine are shown in Table 50–2.

TABLE 50–2. Diagnostic Criteria for Migraine

Migraine Without Aura

A. At least five attacks fulfilling B through D, below
B. Headache attacks lasting 4–72 h (untreated or unsuccessfully treated)
C. Headache has at least two of the following characteristics:
   1. Unilateral location
   2. Pulsating quality
   3. Moderate or severe intensity (inhibits or prohibits daily activities)
   4. Aggravation by walking stairs or similar routine physical activity
D. During headache, at least one of the following:
   1. Nausea and/or vomiting
   2. Photophobia and phonophobia
E. At least one of the following:
   1. History, physical, and neurologic examinations do not suggest an organic disorder
   2. History and/or physical and/or neurologic examinations do suggest such disorder, but it is ruled out by appropriate investigations
   3. An organic disorder is present, but migraine attacks do not occur for the first time in close temporal relation to the disorder

Migraine With Aura

A. At least two attacks fulfilling B through C, below
B. At least three of the following four characteristics:
   1. One or more fully reversible aura symptoms indicating focal cerebral cortical and/or brainstem dysfunction
   2. At least one aura symptom develops gradually over more than 4 min, or two or more symptoms occur in succession
   3. No aura symptom lasts more than 60 min (if >60 min, then diagnosis is migraine with prolonged aura). If more than one aura symptom is present, accepted duration is proportionally increased
   4. Headache follows aura with a free interval of less than 60 min. (It may also begin before or simultaneously with the aura)
C. At least one of the following:
   1. History, physical, and neurologic examinations do not suggest an organic disorder
   2. History and/or physical and/or neurologic examinations do suggest such disorder, but it is ruled out by appropriate investigations
   3. An organic disorder is present, but migraine attacks do not occur for the first time in close temporal relation to the disorder

DESIRED OUTCOME

- Treatment is aimed at altering the attack once it is under way (abortive therapy) or preventing the attack altogether.

TREATMENT

- Factors that may provoke migraine attacks must be eliminated (Table 50–1).
- Treatment algorithms for acute and prophylactic management of migraine headache are shown in Figures 50–1 and 50–2.

Abortive Therapy

- Abortive therapies must begin at the onset of the attack. Only 50–80% of patients will receive significant relief. Table 50–3 shows medications used for abortive therapy.

Simple Analgesics

- Initial therapy for patients with infrequent migraines should be with simple analgesics. **Aspirin** is considered the drug of choice, but **acetaminophen** can also be used.

Nonsteroidal Anti-inflammatory Drugs (NSAIDs)

- **NSAIDs** may work through inhibition of prostaglandin synthesis, inhibition of platelet aggregation, and reduction of 5-HT release. They are particularly useful to treat migraines that occur before, during, or after menstruation.
- **Naproxen** was superior to placebo and more efficacious than **ergotamine** in controlling acute migraine attacks. NSAIDs with rapid onset of action (naproxen, **naproxen sodium, ibuprofen**) are preferred. **Ketorolac** may be useful in patients with drug-seeking behavior and those with nausea and vomiting. IX

Ergotamine

- **Ergotamine's** antimigraine action may result from blockade of neurogenic inflammation through stimulation of presynaptic 5-HT_1 receptors. It also has activity at α-adrenergic, β-adrenergic, and dopaminergic receptors.
- Intravenous administration is the fastest way to achieve therapeutic drug concentrations and may be preferred by some patients or for more severe attacks.
- Exceeding the maximum dosage guidelines should be avoided to prevent rebound headaches. Ergotamine addiction and dependency have been reported.
- Side effects include nausea, abdominal pain, fatigue, elevated blood pressure, severe peripheral ischemia, and ergotism (nausea, diarrhea, thirst, pruritis, vertigo, muscle cramps, paresthesias, cold skin, and decreased pulses in the extremities). Complications include myocardial infarction, hepatic necrosis, and bowel and brain ischemia.

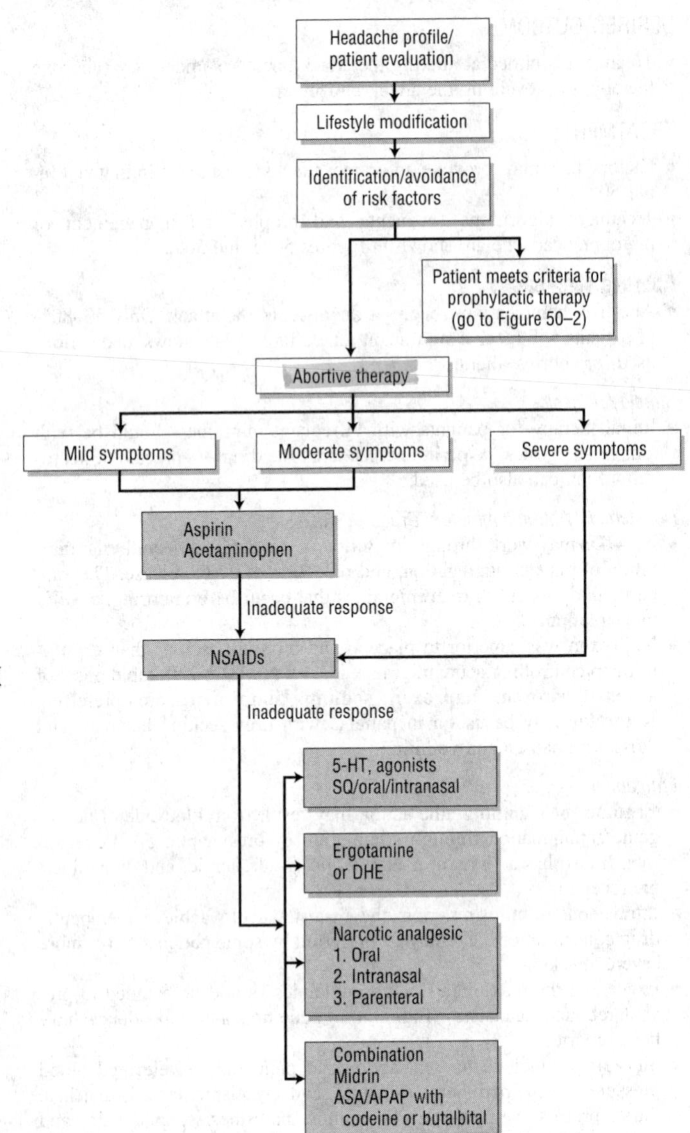

Figure 50–1. Treatment algorithm for migraine headaches.

IX

Patient meets criteria for prophylactic pharmacotherapy

Headaches recur in a predictable pattern (e.g., menstrual migraine)

NSAID at the time ofvulnerability

Ineffective

Healthy or comorbid hypertension, angina, or anxiety

β-adrenergic antagonist (verapamil if β-adrenergic antagonist contraindicated or ineffective)

Ineffective

Comorbid depression or insomnia

Tricyclic antidepressant

Ineffective

Comorbid seizure disorder or manic-depressive illness

Divalproex sodium

Ineffective

β-adrenergic antagonist (verapamil if β-adrenergic antagonist contraindicated or ineffective)

Ineffective

Other agents ineffective

Methysergide

Figure 50–2. Treatment algorithm for prophylactic management of migraine headaches.

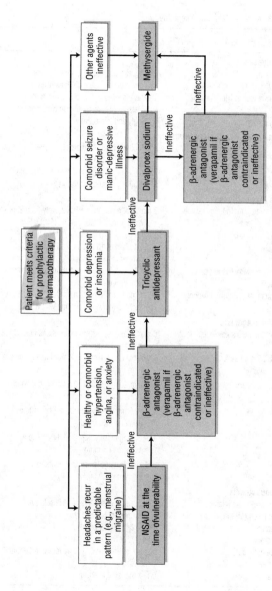

TABLE 50–3. Abortive Migraine Therapies

Medication	Dosage
Simple Analgesics	
Acetaminophen	650 mg at onset; repeat q 4 h as needed
Aspirin	650 mg at onset; repeat q 4 h as needed
Aspirin/acetaminophen with butalbital	1–2 tablets every 4–6 h, but not more than 4 tablets/d or usage more than twice per wk
Aspirin/acetaminophen with narcotics	Sparingly and infrequently
Nonsteroidal Anti-inflammatory Drugs[a]	
Ibuprofen	400–600 mg at onset; repeat in 1–2 h
Ketorolac	15–60 mg IM at onset
Naproxen	750 mg at onset; 250 mg prn up to 1375 mg/d
Naproxen sodium	550–750 mg at onset; repeat in 1–2 h
Ergotamine Preparations	
Ergotamine 1 mg with 100 mg caffeine	2 tablets at onset; then 1 tablet every 30 min prn to a maximum of 6 tablets/d or 10 tablets/wk
Ergotamine 2-mg SL tablets	1 tablet every 30 min prn to a maximum of 6 tablets/d or 10 tablets/wk. Do not swallow, crush, or chew
Ergotamine 2 mg with 100 mg caffeine suppositories	Insert 1 at onset; repeat in 1 h prn to a maximum of 2/d or 5/wk
Dihydroergotamine 1 mg/mL injection	0.5–1 mg IV or IM every h prn to a maximum of 2 mg/d, 6 mg/wk IV, or 3 mg/wk IM
5-HT$_1$ Receptor Agonists	
Sumatriptan 6 mg SC autoinjector	6 mg SC at onset; repeat in 1 hour as needed but not more than 12 mg/24 h
Sumatriptan 25-mg tablets	1 tablet at onset; repeat in 2 h prn to a maximum of 300 mg/d
Sumatriptan intranasal	5, 10, or 20 mg intranasally; repeat in 2 hours to a maximum of 40 mg/d
Zolmitriptan	1.25–2.5 mg initially; repeat in 2 hours to a maximum of 10 mg/d
Naratriptan	1 or 2.5 mg initially; repeat in 4 hours to a maximum of 5 mg/d
Rizatriptan	5–10 mg initially; repeat in 2 hours to a maximum of 30 mg/d
Miscellaneous Agents	
Isometheptene/dichloralphenazone/acetaminophen (Midrin)	2 capsules at onset; repeat 1 capsule every h to a maximum of 5/d or 12/wk
Metoclopramide	10 mg IV or PO at onset
Prochlorperazine	10 mg IV at onset
Butorphanol nasal spray	1 spray in 1 nostril only; may repeat in 60 min if necessary
Chlorpromazine	0.1–1 mg/kg IV at onset

[a]Usage should be limited to three times weekly.

- Contraindications include coronary, cerebral, or peripheral vascular disease, hypertension, liver or kidney disease, and pregnancy. Ergotamines should be used with caution in patients with prolonged auras (>60 minutes).

Sumatriptan

- **Sumatriptan** is an agonist at the 5-HT_{1D} receptor (producing vasoconstriction) and to a lesser extent at the 5-HT_{1A} receptor. It also inhibits release of tachykinnins and thus blocks neurogenic plasma protein extravasation and inflammation.
- Subcutaneous sumatriptan had equal efficacy to **dihydroergotamine (DHE)** at 3 hours postdose, but sumatriptan was more rapid in onset of action. Oral sumatriptan was more effective than oral ergotamine or aspirin plus **metoclopramide.** Headache recurs within 24–48 hours in 40% of patients; a second dose at the time of recurrence is usually effective.
- Side effects associated with oral use include bad taste, nausea, malaise, and dizziness. Subcutaneous administration has been associated with minor injection-site reactions and chest tightness/pressure.
- It is contraindicated in patients with a history of ischemic heart disease, previous myocardial infarction, uncontrolled hypertension, within 2 weeks of monoamine oxidase inhibitor therapy, and use of ergotamine derivatives within the previous 24 hours.

Midrin

- **Midrin** is a combination of a vasoconstrictor, mild sedative, and analgesic that can be used in patients who cannot take or do not respond to ergotamine or sumatriptan.
- Side effects include dizziness, insomnia, nausea, and transient numbness.

Metoclopramide

- **Metoclopramide** may be useful in preventing or treating nausea associated with migraines and increasing absorption of other abortive therapies. It may also be helpful as a single agent for pain relief.
- It should be given 15–30 minutes before the antimigraine therapy and can be repeated in 4–6 hours.

Corticosteroids

- Corticosteroids may help control prolonged migraines and reduce narcotic requirements. Patients should receive a short course with rapid dosage reduction.

Narcotics

- Parenteral narcotics can be used for pain relief and may allow patients to sleep through the attack. Use of narcotics should be minimized to prevent abuse. Transnasal **butorphanol** is an alternative to injectable narcotics.

TABLE 50–4. Prophylactic Migraine Therapies

Medication	Dose
Beta-adrenergic antagonists	
Atenolol	25–100 mg/d
Metoprolol[a]	50–300 mg/d in divided doses
Nadolol	40–240 mg/d
Propranolol[a,b]	40–320 mg/d in divided doses
Timolol[a]	10–60 mg/d in divided doses
Methysergide[a]	2–8 mg/d in divided doses
Tricyclic antidepressants	
Amitriptyline	10–200 mg at bedtime
Doxepin	10–200 mg at bedtime
Imipramine	10–200 mg at bedtime
Nortriptyline	10–150 mg at bedtime
Protriptyline	5–30 mg at bedtime
Verapamil[a]	240–360 mg/d in divided doses
Valproic acid/divalproex sodium	750–1500 mg/d in divided doses
Nonsteroidal anti-inflammatory drugs[c]	
Aspirin	1300 mg/d in divided doses
Naproxen sodium[a]	550–1100 mg/d in divided doses
Ketoprofen[a]	150 mg/d in divided doses

[a]FDA approved for prevention of migraine.
[b]Sustained-release formulation available.
[c]Daily or prolonged use limited by potential toxicity.

Prophylactic Therapy

- Prophylactic therapy should be considered if attacks occur more than two or three times monthly, attacks are severe or prolonged and produce profound impairment, symptomatic therapies have failed or produce serious side effects, or headaches occur in a predictable pattern (e.g., menstrual migraine). A trial of 2–3 months is necessary before an agent can be judged ineffective. Table 50–4 summarizes medications used for prophylactic therapy.

β-Adrenergic Blockers

- **β-blockers** are generally considered the treatment of choice for prevention of migraine. β-blockers with intrinsic sympathomimetic activity are ineffective. Nonselective β-blockers are relatively contraindicated in patients with asthma, congestive heart failure, peripheral vascular disease, atrioventricular conduction disturbances, and diabetes.

Tricyclic Antidepressants

- **Amitriptyline** appears to be the tricyclic antidepressant (TCA) of choice, but **imipramine, doxepin, nortriptyline,** and **protriptyline** have also been used.

- They are usually well tolerated, but anticholinergic effects may limit use, especially in patients with benign prostatic hyperplasia or glaucoma. Evening doses are preferred.

Methysergide

- **Methysergide,** a semisynthetic ergot alkaloid that is a potent 5-HT_2 antagonist, is effective in 60% of migraineurs.
- It is usually reserved for patients with refractory headaches because potentially serious, retroperitoneal, endocardial, and pulmonary fibrotic complications have occurred during long-term uninterrupted use.
- A 4-week medication-free period is recommended following each 6-month treatment period. Dosage should be tapered slowly to prevent rebound headaches.
- Monitoring for fibrotic changes should include periodic cardiac auscultation, chest x-ray, and urinalysis, as well as monitoring for clinical symptoms (e.g., flank pain, dysuria, chest pain, and shortness of breath).

Valproic Acid/Divalproex Sodium

- **Valproic acid** and **divalproex sodium** (a 1:1 molar combination of valproate sodium and valproic acid) can reduce the frequency, severity, and duration of headaches in up to 86% of migraineurs.
- Side effects include nausea (less common with divalproex sodium and gradual dosing titration), tremor, weight gain, hair loss, and hepatotoxicity (rare).

Nonsteroidal Anti-inflammatory Drugs (NSAIDs)

- Patients may benefit from daily administration or intermittent use of aspirin or naproxen sodium. IX
- Long-term use is discouraged because of gastrointestinal and renal toxicity. Monitoring of renal function and occult blood loss should be provided.

Verapamil

- **Verapamil** provided only modest benefit in two placebo-controlled studies. It is generally considered a second- or third-line prophylactic agent.

Pharmacoeconomic Considerations

- The estimated indirect cost of migraine-related disability is $5.6 to $17.2 billion/year. Education of headache patients regarding behavior changes and effective use of abortive and prophylactic pharmacotherapy is cost effective.

► CLUSTER HEADACHE

PATHOPHYSIOLOGY

- Pathophysiology is thought to involve activation of trigeminovascular neurons with resultant release of vasoactive neuropeptides and neurogenic inflammation. 5-HT and hypoxemia may also have a significant role.

- Hypothalamic dysfunction with resultant alterations in circadian rhythms may also be involved. Hypothalamic-induced changes in cortisol, prolactin, β-endorphin, and melatonin have been demonstrated during cluster headaches.

CLINICAL PRESENTATION

- Pain is unilateral, and attacks occur in cluster periods lasting 2 weeks to 3 months followed by pain-free intervals averaging 2 years.
- Attacks generally last 15–180 minutes, and auras are not present. Pain is excruciating and penetrating, but usually nonthrobbing. Most associated features are ipsilateral (e.g., lacrimation, nasal stuffiness, rhinorrhea, ptosis, miosis, and conjunctival injection).

TREATMENT

Abortive Therapy

Oxygen

- Inhalation of 100% **oxygen** (a cerebral vasoconstrictor) at a rate of 7 L/min for 10–15 minutes is effective in approximately 70% of patients.

Ergotamine

- Ergot preparations are effective in the same doses as for migraine headache. Repeated IV administration of **DHE** for 3–7 days can break the cycle of attacks.

IX

Sumatriptan

- Reduction in the severity of headache can occur within 15 minutes of a subcutaneous injection in 75% of patients. Oral **sumatriptan** has limited utility due to its relatively long onset of action.

Prophylactic Therapy

Verapamil

- **Verapamil** prevents cluster headaches in approximately 70% of patients. Beneficial effects often appear after 1 week of doses ranging from 240–360 mg/d for episodic attacks; higher doses may be necessary to control chronic cluster headaches.

Lithium

- Beneficial effects often appear during the first week of **lithium** therapy at a usual dose of 600–900 mg/d in divided doses. Optimal plasma levels have not been established for prevention, but therapeutic steady-state lithium levels range from 0.6–1.2 mEq/L 12 hours postdose.
- Lithium should be administered with caution to patients with renal or cardiovascular disease, dehydration, pregnancy, or concomitant diuretic use.

Ergotamine

- **Ergotamine,** given as a 2 mg at bedtime dose, often prevents nocturnal headache attacks. Daily use of 1–2 mg of ergotamine, alone or in combination with verapamil or lithium, may provide effective prophylaxis in refractory patients.

Methysergide

- In patients unresponsive to lithium, **methysergide,** 2 mg three or four times daily, is usually effective in shortening the course of headaches. Doses may be tapered after 2–3 weeks headache free.

Corticosteroids

- Corticosteroids may be useful for cluster headaches refractory to verapamil, lithium, ergotamine, and methysergide, or combinations of these agents. Therapy is initiated with 40–60 mg/d of **prednisone** and tapered over approximately 3 weeks. Relief appears within 1–2 days of initiation of therapy. Long-term use is not recommended.

▶ EVALUATION OF THERAPEUTIC OUTCOMES

- Patients should be monitored for frequency, intensity, and duration of headaches, and for any change in the headache pattern.
- Patients taking abortive therapy should be monitored for frequency of use of prescription and over-the-counter medications. Patterns of abortive medication use can be documented to establish the need for prophylactic therapy. Prophylactic therapies should also be monitored closely for adverse reactions, abortive therapy needs, and adequate dosing and compliance.

See Chapter 57, Headache Disorders: Migraine and Cluster, authored by Brian E. Beckett, PharmD, and Katherine C. Herndon, PharmD, BCPS, for a more detailed discussion of this topic.

Chapter 51

PAIN MANAGEMENT

DEFINITION

Pain is defined as an unpleasant, subjective sensory and emotional experience associated with actual or potential tissue damage or described in terms of such damage.

PATHOPHYSIOLOGY

AFFERENT PAIN TRANSMISSION

- H^+, K^+, prostaglandins, leukotrienes, histamine, and serotonin sensitize nociceptors. Receptor activation leads to action potentials that are transmitted along afferent nerve fibers to the spinal cord.
- Somatostatin, cholecystokinin, and substance P have been identified as possible neurotransmitters in afferent nociceptive neurons. Nociceptive transmission occurs in the A-delta (well-localized pain) or C fibers (dull, poorly localized, and persistent pain).
- *Gate control theory:* When large myelinated fibers are stimulated, they have an inhibitory effect on pain transmission. Therefore, perception of pain is a complex summation of non-nociceptive and nociceptive neuronal stimulation.
- Pain processes reach the brain through an array of ascending spinal cord pathways. The spinothalamic tract, a major ascending pathway, is divided into lateral and ventral pathways. The lateral pathway is associated with sharp, localized pain, and the ventral pathway with dull, nonlocalized pain and the reflexes.

PAIN MODULATION

- Three classes of opioid peptides are known: the enkephalins, dynorphins, and β-endorphins. Each has a distinct anatomical distribution. All are generically referred to as endorphins.
- There are three major classes of opiate receptors (mu, kappa, and delta) (Table 51–1).
- When a given nociceptive stimulus activates peripheral pain transmission pathways (causing pain and termed positive feedback), the brain's modulatory network (inhibiting pain and termed negative feedback) may make the sensation of pain a summation of these two processes.
- Norepinephrine and serotonin also play a role in pain regulation.

PAIN ASSESSMENT AND CLINICAL PRESENTATION

- A history and physical examination are required to evaluate underlying diseases and possible contributing factors. A baseline description of

TABLE 51–1. Opiate Receptor Effects

Opiate Receptor	Function
Mu	Analgesia Respiratory depression Miosis Reduced gastric motility Sedation Euphoria
Kappa	Analgesia Less respiratory depression than mu Less intense miosis than mu Sedation Reduced gastric motility Dysphoria Psychotomimetic effects
Delta	Analgesia

pain can be obtained by assessing PQRST characteristics (*p*alliative and *p*rovocative factors, *q*uality, *r*adiation, *s*everity, and *t*emporal factors). Mental (e.g., anxiety, depression, fatigue, anger), behavioral, cognitive, social, and cultural factors may alter pain threshold.

- Pain of a known source is often localized, well defined, and relieved by analgesics. Pain with no obvious origin is often nonlocalized, ill defined, and not easily treated. IX
- When pain is not effectively treated, there may be hypoxia, hypercapnia, hypertension, excessive cardiac activity, and emotional difficulties.
- Chronic pain includes pain that persists beyond the normal healing time, pain related to a chronic disease, pain without identifiable organic cause, and pain that involves both the chronic and acute pain associated with cancer.
- With chronic pain, there may be a psychological component, significant environmental contributions, and family involvement. Insomnia may be a factor, and dependence and tolerance to medication is a common problem.

▶ DESIRED OUTCOME

- The goal of therapy is to minimize pain and provide reasonable comfort at the lowest effective dose. When possible, patients should participate in their own therapy. With chronic pain, rehabilitation and resolution of psychosocial issues may be the goal.

► TREATMENT

ACUTE PAIN

Nonopioid Agents

- The weakest effective analgesic with the fewest side effects should be selected. Dosage, pharmacokinetic, pharmacodynamic, and side-effect profiles of FDA-approved nonopioid analgesics are shown in Tables 51–2 to 51–4.
- These drugs (except acetaminophen) reduce prostaglandins produced by the arachidonic acid cascade, thereby decreasing the number of pain impulses.
- **Aspirin** given concurrently with other **nonsteroidal anti-inflammatory drugs (NSAIDs)** is more likely to cause gastrointestinal (GI) side effects. The **salicylate salts** cause fewer GI side effects than aspirin and do not inhibit platelet aggregation. NSAIDs generally cause fewer GI problems than aspirin.

TABLE 51–2. Pharmacokinetic and Pharmacodynamic Profiles of FDA-Approved Nonopioid Analgesics

Agent	Time to Peak Concentration (h)	Elimination Half-life (h)	Analgesic Onset (h)	Analgesic Duration (h)
Aspirin	0.25–2	0.25–0.33	0.5	3–6
Choline salicylate	1.5–2	[a]	[a]	4
Magnesium salicylate	1.5–2	[a]	[a]	4
Sodium salicylate	0.67	[a]	[a]	4
Diflunisal	2–3	8–12	1	8–12
Acetaminophen	0.5–2	1–4	0.5–1	3–6
Meclofenamate	0.5–2	2.3–3.3	[a]	4–6
Mefenamic acid	2–4	2–4	[a]	6
Etodoloc	1	7	0.5–1	6–8
Diclofenac potassium	1	2	0.5	6–8
Ibuprofen	1–2	1–2.5	0.5	4–6
Fenoprofen	1–2	2–3	0.25–0.5	4–6
Ketoprofen	0.5–2	2–4	1	3–4
Naproxen	2–4	12–15	1	Up to 7
Naproxen sodium	1–2	12–13	1	Up to 7
Ketorolac (parenteral)	0.5–1	4–6	0.17	6
Ketorolac (oral)	0.5–1	4–6	0.5–1	4–6

[a]Data not available.

TABLE 51–3. FDA-Approved Nonopioid Analgesics

Class and Generic Name	Usual Dosage Range (mg)	Maximal Dose (mg/d)
Salicylates		
Acetylsalicylic acid (aspirin)[a]	325–650 every 4 h	5400
Choline[a]	870 every 3–4 h	5220
Magnesium[a]	500 every 4 h	4800
Sodium[a]	325–650 every 4 h	5400
Diflunisal	250–500 every 8–12 h	1500
***para*-Aminophenol**		
Acetaminophen[a]	325–650 every 4–6 h	4000
Fenamates		
Meclofenamate	50 every 4–6 h	400
Mefenamic acid	250 every 6 h (maximum of 7 d)	1000[b]
Acetic Acid		
Etodoloc	200–400 every 6–8 h	1200
Diclofenac potassium	50 three times a day	150[c]
Propionic Acids		
Ibuprofen[a]	200–400 every 4–6 h	3200
Fenoprofen	200 every 4–6 h	3200
Ketoprofen[a]	25–50 every 6–8 h	300
Naproxen	250 every 6–12 h	1250
Naproxen sodium[a]	220 every 8–12 h	660[d]
Naproxen delayed release[e]	375–500 every 12 h	1250
Naproxen controlled release	750–1000 every 24 h	1000
Ketorolac (parenteral)	15–30 every 6 h (maximum of 5 d)	120
Ketorolac (oral)	10 every 4–6 h (maximum of 5 d)	40

[a]Available both as an over-the-counter preparation and as a prescription drug.
[b]Up to 1250 mg on the first day.
[c]Up to 200 mg on the first day.
[d]Over-the-counter dose.
[e]Not for the initial treatment of acute pain.

IX

- If creatinine clearance is <50 mL/min, patients taking NSAIDs must be carefully monitored for further kidney damage.
- Aspirin-like compounds should not be given to children or teenagers with influenza or chicken pox, as Reye's syndrome may result.
- **Acetaminophen** has analgesic and antipyretic activity but little anti-inflammatory action. It is highly liver toxic on overdose.

Opioid Agents

- Equianalgesic doses, dosing guidelines, and major adverse effects of the opioids are shown in Tables 51–5 to 51–7. The equianalgesic doses are only a guide, and doses must be individualized. Opioid pharmacokinetics are shown in Table 51–8.

TABLE 51–4. Relative Side Effects of FDA-Approved Nonopioid Analgesics

Agent	GI Irritation	CNS Effects	Hepatic Toxicity	Renal Toxicity
Aspirin	++++++	+	++	++
Choline salicylate	+++	[a]	[a]	[a]
Magnesium salicylate	+++	[a]	[a]	[a]
Sodium salicylate	+++	[a]	[a]	[a]
Diflunisal	++	+	+	+
Acetaminophen	+	+	++	+
Meclofenamate	++	+	+	++
Mefenamic acid	++	+	+	++
Etodolac	++	+	+	++
Diclofenac potassium	++	+	+	++
Ibuprofen	++	+	+	++
Fenoprofen	++	++	+	++
Ketoprofen	++	+	+	++
Ketorolac[b]	++	+	+	+
Naproxen	++	+	+	++

[a]Data not available.
[b]Five-day use only.

IX

- Partial agonists and antagonists compete with agonists for opiate receptor sites and exhibit mixed agonist–antagonist activity. They may have selectivity for analgesic receptor sites and cause fewer side effects.
- Peak analgesic effect usually occurs 1.5–2 hours after oral administration.
- Although caution is advised, cross-sensitivity between the morphine-like agonists, meperidine-like agonists, and methadone-like agonists is less likely than among the like agents. Regarding cross-sensitivity, the mixed agonist–antagonist class acts much like the morphine-like agonists.
- In the initial stages of acute pain treatment, analgesics should be given around the clock. As the painful state subsides, as-needed schedules can be used.
- With patient-controlled analgesia (PCA), patients self-administer preset amounts of intravenous opioids via a syringe pump electronically interfaced with a timing device; thus patients can balance pain control with sedation.
- Administration of opioids directly into the central nervous system (CNS) (epidural and intrathecal) shows promise for acute pain. **Epidural morphine,** 5–10 mg, has onset of pain relief in about 24 minutes, and duration is 12–20 hours. One milligram of **hydromorphone** epidurally relieves pain in about 13 minutes and lasts for about 12 hours. **Fentanyl,** 0.1 mg

TABLE 51–5. Opioid Analgesics

Class and Generic Name	Route	Equianalgesic Dose (mg)
Morphine-like Agonists		
Morphine	IM, SC	10
	PO	30–60
Hydromorphone	IM, SC	1.3
	PO	7.5
Oxymorphone	IM, SC	1.0
	R	5
Levorphanol	IM, SC	2.0
	PO	4.0
Codeine	IM	130[a]
	PO	200[a]
Hydrocodone	PO	5–10[b]
Oxycodone	PO	5–10[b]
Meperidine-like Agonists		
Meperidine	IM, SC	75
	PO	300[a]
Fentanyl	IM	0.1–0.2
	Transdermal	25 μg/h[c]
	Transmucosal	Not available
Methadone-like Agonists		
Methadone	IM	10
	PO	10–20
Propoxyphene	PO	65[b]
Mixed Agonist–Antagonists		
Pentazocine	IM, SC	30–60
	PO	180[a]
Butorphanol	IM	2.0
	Intranasal	1.0[b] (one spray)
Nalbuphine	IM	10
Buprenorphine	IM	0.4
Dezocine	IM	10
Antagonist		
Naloxone	IV	0.4–1.2[d]
Central Analgesic		
Tramadol	PO	50–100[b]

[a]Starting doses lower (codeine, 15–30 mg; meperidine, 50 mg; pentazocine, 50 mg).
[b]Starting dose only (equianalgesia not shown).
[c]Equivalent IM morphine dose = 8–22 mg/d.
[d]Starting doses to be used in cases of opioid overdose.

TABLE 51–6. Dosing Guidelines for Opioid Analgesics

Agent(s)	Dose (titrate up or down based on patient response)	Notes
NSAIDs/acetaminophen/ aspirin	Dose to maximum before switching to another agent (see Table 51–3)	Used in mild to moderate pain May use in conjunction with opioid agents to decrease doses of each Regular alcohol use and high doses of acetaminophen may result in liver toxicity Care must be exercised to avoid overdose when combination products containing these agents are used
Morphine	PO 10–30 mg q 3–4 h[a] IM 5–10 mg q 3–4 h[a] IV 1–2.5 mg q 5 min prn[a] SR 15–30 mg q 12 h (may need to be q 8 h in some patients) Rectal 10–20 mg q 3–4 h[a]	Drug of choice in acute severe pain Use immediate-release product with SR product to control "breakthrough" pain in cancer patients
Hydromorphone	PO 2–4 mg q 3–4 h[a] IM 0.5–1 mg q 3–4 h[a] IV 0.1–0.5 mg q 5 min prn[a] Rectal 2–4 mg q 3–4 h[a]	Use in severe pain More potent than morphine, otherwise no advantages
Oxymorphone	IM 1–1.5 mg q 4–6 h[a] IV 0.5 mg initially Rectal 5 mg q 3–4 h[a]	Use in severe pain No advantages over morphine
Levorphanol	PO 2–4 mg q 6–8 h IM 2 mg q 6–8 h IV 2 mg q 6–8 h	Use in severe pain Extended half-life Useful in cancer patients
Codeine	PO 15–60 mg q 3–4 h[a] IM 15–60 mg q 3–4 h[a] IV 15–60 mg q 3–4 h[a]	Use in moderate pain Weak analgesic, use with NSAIDs, aspirin, or acetaminophen
Hydrocodone	PO 5–10 mg q 3–4 h[a]	Use in moderate to severe pain Most effective when used with NSAIDs, aspirin, or acetaminophen
Oxycodone	PO 5–10 mg q 3–4 h[a] Controlled release 10–20 mg q 12 h	Use in moderate to severe pain Most effective when used with NSAIDs, aspirin, or acetaminophen Use immediate-release product with controlled-release product to control "breakthrough" pain in cancer patients
Meperidine	PO 50–150 mg q 3–4 h[a] IM 75–100 mg q 3–4 h[a] IV 5–10 mg q 5 min prn[a]	Use in severe pain Oral not recommended Do not use in renal failure May precipitate tremors, myoclonus, and seizures Monoamine oxidase inhibitors can induce hyperpyrexia and/or seizures

TABLE 51–6. continued

Agent(s)	Dose (titrate up or down based on patient response)	Notes
Fentanyl	IM 0.05–0.1 mg q 1–2 h[a] Transdermal 25 μg/h q 72 h Transmucosal (investigational)	Used in severe pain Do not use transdermal in acute pain
Methadone	PO 10–20 mg q 6–8 h IM 5–10 mg q 6–8 h	Effective in severe chronic pain Sedation can be major problem Some chronic pain patients can be dosed 8/12 h
Propoxyphene	PO 65–100 mg q 3–4 h[a]	Use in moderate pain Weak analgesic, most effective when used with NSAIDs, aspirin, or acetaminophen Will cause carbamazepine levels to increase
Pentazocine	PO 50–100 mg q 3–4 h[b] IM 30 mg q 3–4 h[b]	Third-line agent for moderate to severe pain May precipitate withdrawal in opiate-dependent patients
Butorphanol	IM 1–4 mg q 3–4 h[b] IV 0.5–2 mg q 3–4 h[b] Intranasal 1 mg (one spray) q 3–4 h[b]	Second-line agent for moderate to severe pain May precipitate withdrawal in opiate-dependent patients
Nalbuphine	IM 10 mg q 3–6 h[b] IV 10 mg q 3–6 h[b]	Second-line agent for moderate to severe pain May precipitate withdrawal in opiate-dependent patients
Buprenorphine	IM 0.3 mg q 6 h[b] IV 0.3 mg q 6 h[b]	Second-line agent for moderate to severe pain May precipitate withdrawal in opiate-dependent patients
Dezocine	IM 5–20 mg q 3–6 h[b] IV 2.5–10 mg q 2–4 h[b]	Second-line agent for moderate to severe pain May precipitate withdrawal in opiate-dependent patients
Naloxone	IV 0.4–1.2 mg	When reversing opiate side effects in patients needing analgesia, dilute and titrate (0.1–0.2 mg q 2–3 min) so as not to reverse analgesia
Tramadol	PO 50–100 mg q 4–6 h[a]	Maximum dose is 400 mg/24 h Decrease dose in renal impairment and in the elderly

[a]May start with an around-the-clock regimen and switch to prn if or when the painful signal subsides.
[b]May reach a ceiling analgesic effect.

IX

TABLE 51–7. Major Adverse Effects of Opioid Analgesics

Effect	Manifestation
Mood changes	Dysphoria, euphoria
Somnolence	Lethargy, drowsiness, apathy, inability to concentrate
Stimulation of chemoreceptor trigger zone	Nausea, vomiting
Respiratory depression	Decreased respiratory rate
Decreased gastrointestinal motility	Constipation
Increase in sphincter tone (most evidence with morphine)	Biliary spasm, urinary retention
Histamine release (most evidence with morphine)	Urticaria, pruritus, rarely exacerbation of asthma
Tolerance	Larger doses for same effect
Dependence	Withdrawal symptoms upon abrupt discontinuation

epidurally, has an onset in 4–10 minutes and lasts 2.5–6 hours. Patients receiving epidural or intrathecal analgesics must be monitored closely, as side effects, including respiratory depression, are common. Intrathecal doses are smaller than epidural doses, and opioids administered into the CNS should be preservative free.

Morphine and Congeners

IX

- Many clinicians consider **morphine** the first-line agent for moderate to severe pain.
- Nausea and vomiting are more likely in ambulatory patients and with the initial dose.
- Respiratory depression is less likely in patients with severe pain but more likely in patients with emphysema, kyphoscoliosis, cor pulmonale, other pulmonary dysfunction, and other concurrent CNS-depressant use. Respiratory depression can be reversed by pure opioid antagonists.
- Hypovolemic patients and patients with myocardial infarction are more susceptible to morphine-induced decreases in blood pressure.
- Morphine is often considered the opioid of choice when using opioids to treat pain associated with myocardial infarction, as it decreases myocardial oxygen demand.
- In patients with increased intracranial pressure and traumatic head injury, morphine can increase intracranial pressure, cause respiratory depression, and cloud the neurologic examination results.

Meperidine and Congeners (Phenylpiperidines)

- **Meperidine** is less potent and has a shorter analgesic duration of action than morphine. In most settings, it offers no advantages over morphine.
- With high doses or in patients with renal failure, the metabolite, normeperidine, may accumulate, causing tremor, muscle twitching, and seizures.

TABLE 51–8. Opioid Analgesic Pharmacokinetics[a]

Agent	Time to Peak (h)	Half-life (h)	Analgesic Onset (min)	Analgesic Duration (h)
Morphine	0.5–1	2	15–30, 60[b]	4–5
Hydromorphone	0.5–1	2–3	15–30	4–5
Oxymorphone	0.5–1	2–3	5–15	4–6
Levorphanol	0.5–1	12–16	30–90	6–8
Hydrocodone	1.3	4	[c]	4–5
Codeine	0.5–1	2–4	15–30	4–6
Oxycodone (PO)	0.5–1	[c]	15–30	4–5
Meperidine	0.5–1	3–4	10–45	3–4
Fentanyl	[c]	1.5–6	7–8	1–2
Methadone	0.5–1	15–40	30–60	4–5 (acute) >8 (chronic)
Propoxyphene (PO)	2.0–2.5	6–12	30–60	4–6
Pentazocine	0.25–1	4–5	15–20	4–6
Butorphanol	0.5–1	2.5–3.5	<10	4–6
Nalbuphine	1	2–3	<15	4–6
Buprenorphine	1	5	15	4–5
Dezocine	0.17–1.5	0.6–5	15–30	2–4
Naloxone[d]	0.5–2	0.5–1.5	2–5	0.5–1
Tramadol	2–3	6–7	<60	6

[a]Based on intramuscular data unless otherwise indicated.
[b]Data based on intrathecal or epidural administration.
[c]Data not available.
[d]Opioid antagonist.

IX

- The effects of meperidine on the cardiovascular system, GI tract, and smooth muscle are less severe than those of morphine.
- Meperidine should not be combined with monoamine oxidase inhibitors.
- Due to its kinetic profile, fentanyl transdermal patch is not used for acute pain.

Methadone and Congeners

- With repeated doses, the analgesic duration of action of **methadone** is prolonged, but sedation may be a problem. It is usually used for chronic pain.

Mixed Opioid Agonist–Antagonists

- This class has a ceiling effect on respiratory depression and low abuse potential. They cause less constipation and less biliary spasmodic effects than morphine.

- Disadvantages include psychotomimetic effects (especially with **pentazocine** and **butorphanol**), a ceiling analgesic effect, and a propensity to initiate withdrawal in opioid-dependent patients.
- Both pentazocine and butorphanol must be used with caution in patients with myocardial ischemia. Compared to pentazocine and butorphanol, **nalbuphine** causes reduced myocardial oxygen demand in patients after myocardial infarction. It also causes little respiratory depression.
- Butorphanol, nalbuphine and **dezocine** are not controlled substances.

Opioid Antagonists

- The pure opioid antagonist **naloxone** binds competitively to opioid receptors, but does not produce an analgesic response.

Central Analgesic

- **Tramadol,** a centrally acting analgesic for moderate to moderately severe pain, binds weakly to opiate receptors and inhibits norepinephrine and serotonin reuptake.
- It causes minimal dependency and tolerance, but lowers the seizure threshold. It may have a role in therapy of chronic pain, but has few advantages over opiates for acute pain.

Combination Therapy

- The combination of an opioid and nonopioid oral analgesic often results in analgesia superior to that produced by monotherapy and may allow for lower doses of each agent. An NSAID with a scheduled opioid is often effective for pain of bone metastases.
- Agents shown to potentiate the analgesic efficacy of parenteral opioids include **hydroxyzine** and **dextroamphetamine.**

Regional Analgesia

- Regional analgesia with local anesthetics (Table 51–9) can provide complete relief of pain. They also have been applied directly to surgical wounds to decrease postoperative narcotic requirements. They have been used epidurally in acute and chronic pain.
- They cross the blood–brain barrier and cause CNS excitation and depression. Frequent administration and specialized follow-up procedures are required.

CHRONIC PAIN

- An algorithm for management of pain in cancer patients is shown in Figure 51–1.
- NSAIDs are especially effective for bone pain. **Strontium-89** and **samarium SM 153 lexidronam** are also effective.
- Around-the-clock schedules in conjunction with as-needed doses are employed when patients experience breakthrough pain.

TABLE 51–9. Local Anesthetics

Agent	Onset (min)	Duration (h)
Esters		
Procaine	2–5	0.25–1
Chloroprocaine	6–12	0.50
Tetracaine	15	2–3
Amides		
Mepivacaine	3–5	0.75–1.5
Bupivacaine	5	2–4
Lidocaine	< 2	0.5–1
Prilocaine	< 2	≥ 1
Etidocaine	3–5	5–10

- The choice of opioid is controversial, but many clinicians prefer morphine. The fentanyl patch may provide a more convenient dosing alternative in patients on stable regimens.
- For nonmalignant chronic pain, therapeutic approaches are similar to those described above, but psychological techniques may prove more successful than in acute pain.

▶ EVALUATION OF THERAPEUTIC OUTCOMES

- Hourly or daily monitoring of acute pain response and side effects may be necessary. Daily or weekly monitoring may be adequate for chronic pain. Quality of life must also be assessed on a regular basis.
- The best management of opioid-induced constipation is prevention. Patients should be counseled on proper intake of fluids and fiber, and a laxative may be added if needed.
- If acute pain does not subside within the anticipated time frame (usually 1–2 weeks), further investigation of the cause is warranted.

See Chapter 56, Pain Management, authored by Terry J. Baumann, PharmD, BCPS, for a more detailed discussion of this topic.

Mild pain	Maximum daily dose:	
Agents: Nonopioid analgesics Nonsteroidal anti-inflammatory drugs (NSAIDs)	ASA	3.6–6.0 g
	Acetaminophen	4.0 g
	Ibuprofen	3.2 g
	Naproxen	1.25 g

Principles of therapy
1. Assess the frequency/duration/occurrence/etiology of the pain.
2. If bone pain is present, use of an NSAID should be routine.
3. Always dose a medication to its maximum before reverting to the next step, unless pain is totally out of control.
4. If pain is constant or recurring, always dose around-the-clock (ATC).

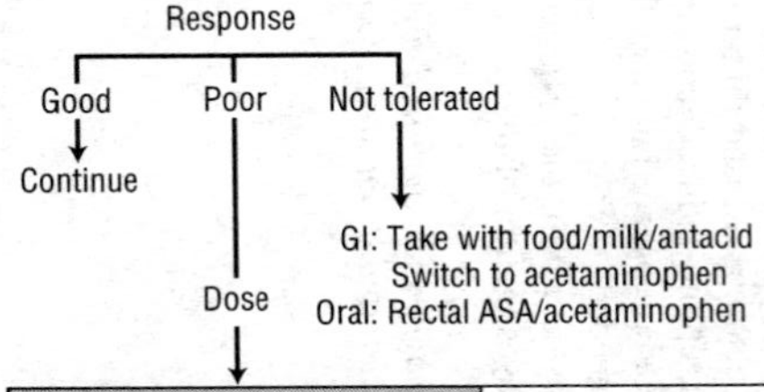

Response
- Good → Continue
- Poor → Dose → (Mild/moderate pain)
- Not tolerated →
  - GI: Take with food/milk/antacid
    - Switch to acetaminophen
  - Oral: Rectal ASA/acetaminophen

Mild/moderate pain	Maximum daily dose:	
Agents: Acetaminophen or ASA combinations with opioids	ASA	3.6–6.0 g
Adjuncts: Tricyclic antidepressants	Acetaminophen	4.0 g
Steroids	Opioids	Titrate
Anticonvulsants	Amitriptyline	10–50 mg
Radiopharmaceuticals	Imipramine	10–50 mg
	Doxepin	10–50 mg
	Prednisone	Titrate
	Dexamethasone	Titrate

Principles of therapy
1. Assess the frequency/duration/occurrence/etiology of the pain.
2. Whenever bone pain is present, use of an NSAID should be routine.
3. Pain management needs to take precedence over other therapies.
4. Fulminating sites of pain, especially in bone, need to be evaluated quickly for alternate therapy such as radiation/radiopharmaceuticals.
5. Accurate assessment and history of reported opiate allergy are extremely important. A differentiation between allergy, sensitivity and side effect needs to be made.
6. Always dose to the maximum of each agent when possible.
7. If pain is constant or recurring, always dose ATC.

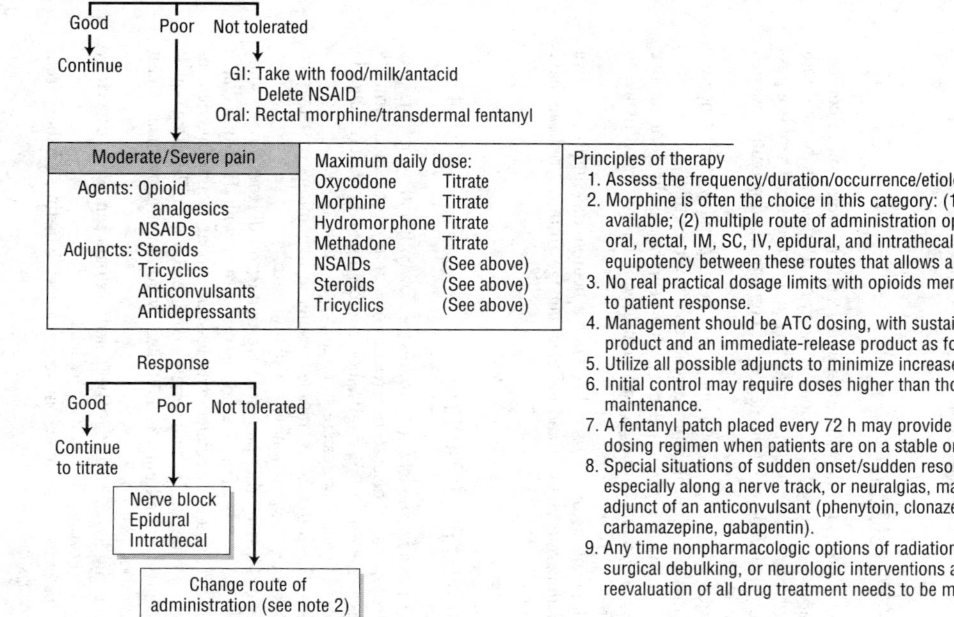

Figure 51–1. Algorithm for pain management in oncology patients. *(Adapted from the Kaiser Permanente Algorithm for Pain Management in Patients With Advanced Malignant Disease.)*

Chapter 52

► PARKINSON'S DISEASE

► DEFINITION

Idiopathic Parkinson's disease (IPD) has highly characteristic neuropathologic findings and clinical presentation including motor deficits and, in some cases, mental deterioration.

► PATHOPHYSIOLOGY

- Loss of nigrostriatal dopamine neurons results in reduction of cortical activation; virtually all the motor deficits of IPD are attributable to a loss in dopaminergic neurons projecting to the striatum. There is a positive correlation between the degree of nigrostriatal dopamine loss and disease severity.
- Activation of the D_2 receptor appears to be of primary importance for mediating both clinical improvements and adverse effects.
- Degeneration of nigrostriatal dopamine neurons results in a relative increase of striatal cholinergic interneuron activity, which contributes to the tremor of IPD.
- The pathogenesis of IPD is unknown, but neurotoxins highly selective to dopaminergic neurons and cellular damage from oxyradicals have been considered.

► CLINICAL PRESENTATION

- IPD develops insidiously and progresses slowly. Initial symptoms may be sensory, but as disease progresses, one or more classical primary features present (e.g., resting tremor, rigidity, bradykinesia, change in posture). Clinical features are summarized in Table 52–1.
- Bradykinesia in the facial muscles results in hypomimia or a masked quality to facial expression with a staring gaze.
- Only two-thirds of IPD patients have tremor on diagnosis, and some never develop this sign. Tremor is often seen with IPD onset at a younger age, and is associated with less functional decline and dementia. Tremor often begins unilaterally and often has a "pill-rolling" quality. Usually, resting tremor is abolished by volitional movement, and it is absent during sleep.
- Muscular rigidity can be cog-wheel, and dystonia can occur, especially in the feet. Postural instability may lead to falls.
- Some patients deteriorate in a manner indistinguishable from Alzheimer's disease.

TABLE 52–1. Clinical Features of Parkinson's Disease

Primary	Autonomic Symptoms
Bradykinesia	Bladder and anal sphincter disturbances
Postural instability	Constipation
Propulsion	Diaphoresis
Retropulsion	Orthostatic blood pressure changes
Resting tremor (may have postural and action components)	Paroxysmal flushing
Rigidity	Sexual disturbances
Motor Symptoms	Mental Status Changes
Decreased dexterity	Confusional state
Dysarthria	Dementia
Dysphagia	Psychosis (paranoia, hallucinosis)
Festinating gait	Sleep disturbance
Flexed posture	Other
"Freezing" at initiation of movement	Fatigue
Hypomimia	Oily skin
Hypophonia	Pedal edema
Micrographia	Seborrhea
Slow turning	Weight loss

▶ DIAGNOSIS

- To diagnose IPD, bradykinesia should be present with at least two of the following features: limb muscle rigidity, resting tremor (at 4–7 Hz and abolished by movement), or postural instability (not caused by primary visual, vestibular, cerebellar, or proprioceptive dysfunction). Other diagnostic criteria include lack of other neurological impairments and responsiveness to L-dopa. IX
- Drug-induced parkinsonism must be ruled out (e.g., induced by antipsychotics, antiemetics, or metoclopramide). The condition most commonly mistaken for IPD is progressive supranuclear palsy.

▶ DESIRED OUTCOME

- The goal of treatment is to minimize disability and side effects, while ensuring the highest possible quality of life. Families and patients should be involved in treatment decisions, and education of patients and caregivers is critical.

▶ TREATMENT

- Mechanisms for potential IPD treatments are shown in Table 52–2.
- An algorithm for treatment of IPD is shown in Figure 52–1.

TABLE 52–2. Mechanisms for Potential IPD Treatments

- Increase Endogenous Dopamine
  - Increase tyrosine hydroxylase
    - Tetrahydrobiopterin
  - L-Dopa
    - Inhibit peripheral metabolism by dopa decarboxylase
      - Carbidopa
      - Benserazide
    - Sustained-release products
    - Infusions
      - Intravenous
      - Duodenal/jejunal
    - Inhibit catechol-O-methyltransferase
      - Entacapone (peripheral only)
      - Tolcapone (peripheral and central)
    - Inhibit central and peripheral metabolism by monoamine oxidase B
      - Selegiline (deprenyl)
- Dopamine Agonists
  - D_2 specific
    - Bromocriptine
    - Lisuride
  - D_2 and D_3 specific
    - Pramipexole
    - Ropinirole
  - D_1 and D_2 nonspecific
    - Pergolide
    - Apomorphine
      - Intravenous
      - Subcutaneous infusions
      - Intranasal
      - Sublingual
  - Partial agonist
    - Terguride
- Anticholinergic Agents
  - Benztropine
  - Trihexyphenidyl
- Surgical Options
  - Autologous adrenal tissue or fetal tissue transplantation
  - Thalamotomy
  - Pallidotomy
  - Deep brain stimulation

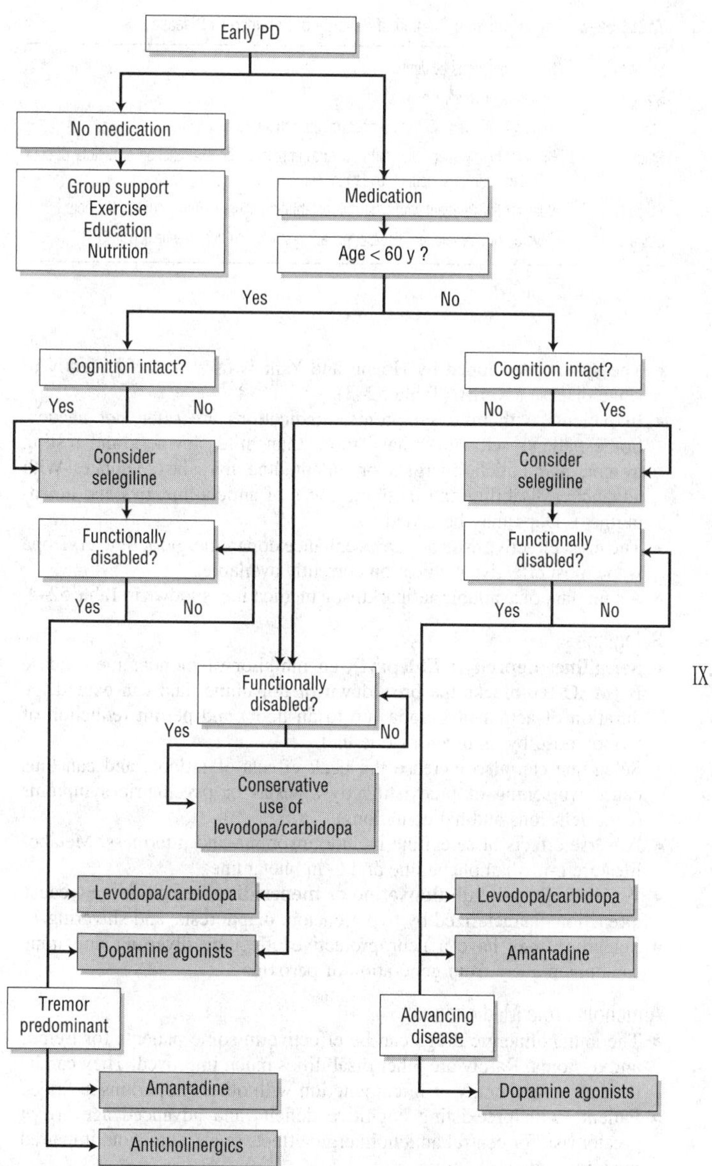

Figure 52–1. General algorithm for treating IPD.

IX

TABLE 52–3. Hoehn and Yahr Staging of Severity of Parkinson's Disease

Stage 0	No clinical signs evident
Stage I	Unilateral involvement
Stage II	Bilateral involvement but no postural abnormalities
Stage III	Bilateral involvement with mild postural imbalance on examination or history of poor balance or falls; patient leads independent life
Stage IV	Bilateral involvement with postural instability; patient requires substantial help
Stage V	Severe, fully developed disease; patient restricted to bed or wheelchair

- The system developed by Hoehn and Yahr is used most frequently to stage disease severity (Table 52–3).
- In patients with mild symptoms, medications are often not needed. Some patients will never have more than mild slowness and resting tremor, and anticholinergics or amantadine may be adequate. With advancing disability and ineffectiveness of anticholinergics and amantadine, L-Dopa may be added.
- The most effective drug therapies enhance dopaminergic activity. L-Dopa is the most effective medication currently available.
- A summary of available antiparkinson medication is shown in Table 52–4.

Selegiline

- **Selegiline (deprenyl; Eldepryl),** an inhibitor of monoamine oxidase B (MAO-B), blocks the breakdown of dopamine, and can extend the duration of action of L-dopa (up to an hour) and permit reduction of L-dopa dose by as much as one-half.
- Selegiline can also increase the peak effects of L-dopa, and can thus cause worsening of preexisting dyskinesias or psychiatric symptoms (e.g., delusions and hallucinations).
- Adverse effects of selegiline include insomnia and jitteriness. Metabolites are L-methamphetamine and L-amphetamine.
- When combined with **fluoxetine** or **meperidine,** selegiline may cause a reaction characterized by hypertension, diaphoresis, and shivering.
- Selegiline may have a neuroprotective effect by diverting dopamine catabolism away from generation of peroxide.

Anticholinergic Medications

- The anticholinergic drugs can be effective in some patients for tremor and dystonia. Rarely are other disabilities much improved. They can be used as monotherapy or in conjunction with other antiparkinson drugs.
- Patients with preexisting cognitive deficits and advanced age are at greater risk for central anticholinergic effects (e.g., confusion, impaired memory, sedation).

TABLE 52–4. Drugs Used in Parkinson's Disease

Generic Name	Trade Name	Manufacturer	Dosage Range (mg/d)	Dosage Forms (mg)	Cost Index[a]
Amantadine	Symmetrel	DuPont	200–300	100, 50/5 mL	8, 8
		Generic brands, various			3, 7
Carbidopa/L-dopa	Sinemet	DuPont	[b]	10/100, 25/100, 25/250	6, 7, 8
		Generic brands, various			
Controlled-release carbidopa/L-dopa	Sinemet CR	DuPont	[b]	25/100, 50/200	7, 14
L-Dopa	Larodopa	Roche	[b]	100, 250, 500	2, 3, 6
	Dopar	Roberts Pharm			
Selegiline	Eldepryl	Somerset	10	5	21
Tolcapone	Tasmar	Roche	300–600	100, 200	16, 17
Agonists					
Bromocriptine	Parlodel	Sandoz	[b]	2.5, 5	14, 22
Pergolide	Permax	Athena	[b]	0.05, 0.25, 1	2, 25, 82
Pramipexole	Mirapex	Pharmacia Upjohn	1.5–4.5	0.125, 0.25, 1, 1.5	6, 10, 21, 21
Ropinirole	Requip	SmithKline Beecham	[b]	0.25, 1, 2, 5	9, 9, 9, 19
Anticholinergic Drugs					
Benztropine	Cogentin	Merck	0.5–6	0.5, 1, 2	2, 2, 2
		Generic brands, various			1, 1, 1
Biperiden	Akineton	Knoll	2–16	2	2
Diphenhydramine	Benadryl	Parke-Davis	25–100	25, 50	2, 3
		Generic brands, various			1, 1
Procyclidine	Kemadrin	Glaxo-Wellcome	2.5–20	5	4
Trihexyphenidyl	Artane	Lederle	1–15	2, 5, 2/5 mL, 5 LA	1, 3, 3, 4
		Generic brands, various			1, 3

[a]Cost index calculated from June 1994 average wholesale price per 100. Approximate cost per 100 (or per pint for solutions) equivalent to index × $10.00

[b]Dosage must be individualized.

Amantadine

- **Amantadine** is often effective for relief of mild symptoms of IPD, especially tremor.
- A proposed mechanism of action is increased presynaptic dopamine synthesis, increased dopamine release, and inhibition of dopamine reuptake. Nondopaminergic mechanisms have also been proposed.
- Adverse effects include sedation, vivid dreams, dry mouth, depression, hallucinations, anxiety, dizziness, psychosis, and confusion. A frequent and reversible side effect is livedo reticularis, a diffuse mottling of the skin.
- A reduced dose should be given to patients with renal dysfunction.

L-Dopa and Carbidopa/L-Dopa

- **L-Dopa,** the most effective drug available for management of IPD, is the immediate precursor of dopamine, but unlike dopamine, it crosses the blood–brain barrier.
- There is general consensus that the proper time to initiate L-dopa therapy is when the disease interferes with occupation or activities of daily living.
- L-Dopa is converted to dopamine by L-amino acid decarboxylase (L-AAD). In the periphery, L-AAD can be blocked by concurrently administering **carbidopa,** which does not cross the blood–brain barrier. Carbidopa, therefore, increases the CNS penetration of exogenously administered L-dopa and decreases adverse effects (nausea, cardiac arrhythmias, postural hypotension) from peripheral L-dopa metabolism to dopamine.
- Starting L-dopa at 200–300 mg/d in combination with carbidopa often achieves adequate relief of disability. The usual maximal dose of L-dopa is 800 mg/d.
- Carbidopa has a usual maximal effective daily dose of 100–125 mg. Carbidopa/L-dopa is most widely used in a 25-mg/100-mg tablet, but 25-mg/250-mg and 10-mg/100-mg dosage forms are also available. Controlled-release preparations of carbidopa/L-dopa are available in 50-mg/200-mg and 25-mg/100-mg strengths.
- From 6–10% of IPD patients will develop involuntary movements or short-duration responses with each year of L-dopa treatment. Movement complications associated with long-term use of carbidopa/L-dopa and their suggested treatments are listed in Table 52–5.
- End-of-dose deterioration ("wearing off") has been related to increasing loss of neuronal storage capability for dopamine. Hence, the peripheral pharmacokinetics of L-dopa increasingly becomes the determinant of dopamine synthesis. Carbidopa/L-dopa can be given more frequently, or a sustained-release product can be tried. Dopamine agonists also can be added to a carbidopa/L-dopa regimen. Some patients taking a sustained-release form will require an increased dose of L-dopa because of decreased bioavailability, and a conventional carbidopa/L-dopa dose in the morning may be needed for its more rapid absorption.

TABLE 52–5. Motor Fluctuations and Possible Interventions in IPD

Effect	Possible Treatments
End-of-dose deterioration ("wearing off")	Increase frequency of doses; controlled-release carbidopa/L-dopa; consider agonists, selegiline, tolcapone, or amantadine; duodenal or intravenous L-dopa infusions; carbidopa/L-dopa oral solution; subcutaneous apomorphine infusions; transdermal dopamine agonists
Delayed onset of response	Give on empty stomach before meals; crush or chew and take with a full glass of water; reduce dietary protein intake; antacids; morning standard-release carbidopa/L-dopa if on sustained-release carbidopa/L-dopa; infusions of L-dopa; dopamine agonists
Drug-resistant "off" periods	Increase carbidopa/L-dopa dose and/or frequency; give on empty stomach before meals; crush or chew and take with a full glass of water; infusions of L-dopa or dopamine agonists; apomorphine intranasal spray
"Random" oscillations ("on–off")	Dopamine agonists; selegiline; tolcapone; infusions of L-dopa or dopamine agonists; consider drug holiday
Start hesitation ("freezing")	Increase carbidopa/L-dopa dose; dopamine agonists; gait modifications (tapping, rhythmic commands, stepping over objects, rocking)
Peak-dose dyskinesia ("I-D-I" response[a])	Smaller more frequent doses of carbidopa/L-dopa; controlled-release carbidopa/L-dopa
Diphasic dyskinesias ("D-I-D" response[b])	Reduce anticholinergic medication
Dystonia	Baclofen; nighttime carbidopa/L-dopa; morning standard-release carbidopa/L-dopa if on sustained-release carbidopa/L-dopa; dopamine agonists; anticholinergics
Myoclonus	Decrease nighttime L-dopa doses; clonazepam
Akathisia	Benzodiazepines; propranolol

[a]I-D-I is the "improvement-dyskinesia/dystonia-improvement" pattern of response.
[b]D-I-D is the "dyskinesia-improvement-dyskinesia" pattern of response.

IX

- MAO-B inhibitors (selegiline) and the catechol-O-methyltransferase (COMT) inhibitors **(tolcapone** and **entacapone)** extend the action of L-dopa, decreasing "off" time by about 1.5 hours and decreasing L-dopa requirements. Serious liver dysfunction and a few deaths have been reported with tolcapone. Regular liver function monitoring is required.
- Dyskinesias and dystonias are usually associated with peak antiparkinsonian benefit.
- Drug holidays are not currently used as therapeutic interventions.

- Side effects of L-dopa and the dopaminergic agonists include delirium, agitation, delusions, and hallucinations. These are especially likely in older patients and those with underlying confusion or dementia. **Clozapine** improves psychotic symptoms without worsening parkinsonian symptoms.
- There is marked intra- and intersubject variability in the time to peak plasma concentrations after oral L-dopa, and there may be more than one peak plasma concentration after a single dose. Meals delay but antacids and **cisapride** increase gastric emptying. L-Dopa is primarily absorbed in the proximal duodenum by a saturable large neutral amino acid (LNAA) transport system. Dietary LNAAs can compete for this site and can also compete with L-dopa for transport into the brain. L-Dopa is not bound to plasma proteins. The elimination half-life of L-dopa is about 1 hour, and this is extended to about 1.5 hours with the addition of carbidopa.
- L-Dopa should not be administered with MAO-A inhibitors because of a risk of hypertensive crisis or with antipsychotic agents because of possible antagonism of efficacy.

Dopamine Agonists

- The dopamine agonists **pergolide, bromocriptine,** and the nonergots **pramipexole** and **ropinirole** as adjuncts to L-dopa may prolong the effective period in patients with deteriorating response to L-dopa, in patients experiencing fluctuations in response, and in patients with limited response to L-dopa secondary to inability to tolerate higher doses. They decrease the frequency of "off" periods and provide an L-dopa–sparing effect.

- Pergolide with L-dopa may be similar or possibly more efficacious with fewer side effects than bromocriptine with L-dopa.
- Pramipexole and ropinirole seem to be more effective as monotherapy than pergolide and bromocriptine.
- The combination of L-dopa with dopamine agonists as initial therapy revealed a decreased risk for the development of response fluctuations.
- The recommended initial dose of bromocriptine, 1.25 mg once or twice daily, should be escalated slowly by 1.25–2.5 mg/d every week and maintained at the minimum effective dose. Average daily doses <30 mg may be effective for several years in many patients, but some may require doses up to 120 mg/d.
- A recommended initial dose of pergolide is 0.05 mg/d for 2 days, gradually increasing by approximately 0.1–0.15 mg/d every 3 days over a 12-day period. If higher doses are needed, the dose may be increased by 0.25 mg every 3 days until symptoms are eliminated or adverse effects occur. The mean dose in most clinical trials was approximately 3 mg/d.
- Pramipexole is initiated at a dose of 0.125 mg three times daily and increased every 5–7 days as tolerated. It is primarily renally excreted and has an 8–12-hour half-life. The initial dose must be adjusted in renal insufficiency.

- Ropinirole is initiated at 0.25 mg three times daily and increased by 0.25 mg three times daily on a weekly basis. It has a 6-hour half-life and is metabolized by CYP1A2. Fluroquinolones and smoking will likely alter ropinirole clearance.
- With dopamine agonist therapy, nausea occurs in >50% of patients. Except for postural hypotension, cardiovascular effects are infrequent. Central nervous system effects (e.g., confusion, hallucinations, and sedation) are most commonly dose limiting and occur in up to one-third of patients. Pergolide has an arrhythmogenic and bradycardic effect.

PHARMACOECONOMIC CONSIDERATIONS

- In early therapy, the sustained-release product of carbidopa/L-dopa is not indicated in the absence of response fluctuations. As symptoms progress, the addition of dopamine agonists, selegiline, or tolcapone can add considerable expense sometimes with minimal or no benefit.

▶ EVALUATION OF THERAPEUTIC OUTCOMES

- Patients and caregivers should be educated so that they can participate in treatment by recording medication administration times and duration of "on" and "off" periods.
- Symptoms, side effects, and activities of daily living must be scrupulously monitored and therapy individualized.

See Chapter 55, Parkinson's Disease, authored by Merlin V. Nelson, PharmD, MD, Richard C. Berchou, PharmD, and Peter A. LeWitt, MD, for a more detailed discussion of this topic. IX

Chapter 53

▶ STATUS EPILEPTICUS

▶ DEFINITION

Status epilepticus (SE) may be defined as recurrent seizures without an intervening period of consciousness before the next seizure or any seizure lasting longer than 30 minutes whether or not consciousness is impaired. SE may be convulsive or nonconvulsive, generalized or partial. The revised International Classification of SE is provided in Table 53–1.

▶ PATHOPHYSIOLOGY AND ETIOLOGY

- The most common causes of SE in children are epilepsy, atypical febrile seizures, encephalitis, meningitis, and metabolic disease. The most common causes of SE in adults are withdrawal of antiepileptic drugs (AEDs), alcohol withdrawal, head trauma, and underlying neurologic disorder.
- The most common causes of SE in the elderly who had their first seizure after age 60 years are cerebrovascular disease, head trauma, metabolic disorders, brain tumors, and central nervous system (CNS) infection.
- Pathophysiologic underpinnings may include:
  - A diminution of γ-aminobutyric acid (GABA)-ergic inhibition after a single, short-lived seizure.
  - Excitatory neurotransmitters, free radical formation, and toxic calcium flux may also be involved in evolution of SE.

▶ DIAGNOSIS

- A diagnosis of generalized convulsive status epilepticus (GCSE) should not be made until a trained clinician has observed at least one generalized tonic-clonic seizure in a patient with a history of repeated seizures and impaired consciousness.
- The diagnosis of nonconvulsive status epilepticus (NCSE) should not be made until 30 minutes of continuous seizure activity has been observed. For patients without a previous history of NCSE, an electroencephalogram (EEG) is required for diagnosis.
- Blood sugar and serum chemistries are essential. Hypoglycemia, hyponatremia (<120 mEq/L), hypernatremia, hypomagnesemia, hypocalcemia, and renal failure may cause seizures. A toxicology screen and complete blood cell count (CBC) should also be ordered, and women of childbearing potential should have a pregnancy test performed. AED serum concentrations should also be obtained in patients on chronic AEDs. Assessment of serum albumin and renal and hepatic function may also be useful.

TABLE 53–1. International Classification of Status Epilepticus (SE)

Convulsive		Nonconvulsive	
International	*Traditional Terminology*	*International*	*Traditional Terminology*
Primary Generalized SE		Absence[a]	Petit mal, spike-and-wave stupor, spike and slow wave, or 3/s spike and wave, epileptic fugue, epilepsia minora continua, epileptic twilight, minor SE
Tonic-clonic[b,c]	Grand mal, epilepticus convulsivus		
Tonic[a,b]			
Clonic[a]			
Myoclonic[c]			
Erratic[d]			
Secondary Generalized SE[b,c]		Partial SE[b,c]	Focal motor, focal sensory, epilepsia partialis continuans, adversive SE
Tonic			
Partial seizures with secondary generalization			
		Simple partial	Elementary
		Somatomotor	
		Dysphasic	
		Other types	
		Complex partial	Temporal lobe, psychomotor, epileptic fugue state, prolonged epileptic stupor, prolonged epileptic confusional state, continuous epileptic twilight state

[a]Most common in infants and young children.
[b]Most common in older children.
[c]Most common in adolescents and adults.
[d]most common in neonates.

- The second phase of diagnostic tests is done after seizures have stopped, and includes EEG, lumbar puncture (especially in children with fever), and brain imaging (computed tomography [CT] scan or magnetic resonance imaging [MRI]).
- Patients who do not awaken after clinical control of seizures should have an EEG performed to rule out NCSE or recurrent subclinical seizures.

▶ CLINICAL PRESENTATION

- Approximately 20% of patients present mildly obtunded, and marked clouding occurs in two-thirds of patients.
- Mutism, paucity of speech, agitation, aggressiveness, hallucinations, and emotional lability can occur.
- Motor features may include minor eyelid, face, and limb twitching.
- Systemic symptoms include hyperthermia, leukocytosis, pleocytosis, hemodynamic alterations, and respiratory defects. Rhabdomyolysis may lead to myoglobinuria and renal failure. There may be increased sweating and salivation and marked elevations in plasma prolactin, glucagon, growth hormone, and adrenocorticotropic hormone.

▶ DESIRED OUTCOME

- SE is a medical emergency, and the primary desired outcome is to stop seizure activity. However, it is similarly critical that adequate ventilation and an intact cardiovascular system be maintained and that normal blood sugar and body temperature are assured.

▶ TREATMENT

CONVULSIVE SE

- Any tonic-clonic seizure that does not automatically stop within 10 minutes should be treated during the diagnostic workup, and anyone having >3 major seizures within 24 hours should be aggressively treated. An algorithm for treatment of GCSE in hospitalized patients is shown in Figure 53–1. It is derived from limited studies, a report of an advisory committee, and clinical observations.
- Normal to high-normal blood pressure should be maintained. This may necessitate slowing the infusion rate of the AED or use of **dopamine.**
- All patients should receive **glucose** (adults, 50 mL of 50% solution; children, 2 mL/kg of 25% solution), and **thiamine** (100 mg) should be given prior to glucose in adults. Further supplementation may be suggested by serum glucose levels.
- Arterial blood gas should be determined, and if the pH is <7.2, secondary to metabolic acidosis, **sodium bicarbonate** should be given. Assisted ventilation will correct respiratory acidosis.

Benzodiazepines

- The benzodiazepines (BDZs) should be administered to patients who are actively seizing as soon as possible. If seizures have stopped, a BDZ is not indicated and a longer-acting AED should be given. Usually one or two doses of an IV BDZ will stop seizures within minutes.
- **Diazepam** is extremely lipophilic and has a large volume of distribution (1–2 L/kg). It rapidly distributes into body fat. Duration of effect is 0.25–0.5 hour; therefore, a longer-acting AED (e.g., phenytoin, phenobarbital) should be given immediately after diazepam.
- The recommended initial diazepam dose in neonates, infants and children, and adults is 0.15–0.75 mg/kg, 0.1–0.5 mg/kg, and 0.15–0.25 mg/kg, respectively. If the patient does not respond within 5 minutes, the dose should be repeated. The maximum total dose is 5 mg in children younger than 5 years, 10 mg in children 5 years of age or older, and 40 mg in adults. Therapeutic drug monitoring is impractical.
- **Lorazepam** is not approved by the Food and Drug Administration for SE, but it is currently the BDZ of choice. It requires slightly longer to reach peak drug levels in brain than diazepam, but its duration of action is 12–24 hours.
- Fewer patients treated with lorazepam require additional AEDs for seizure termination.
- The dose of lorazepam is 0.05–0.5 mg/kg in pediatric patients and 0.1 mg/kg in adults. If the seizure continues after 5 minutes, a second dose may be given. If there is no response after 5 minutes, a third (final) dose may be given. The maximum total dosage of lorazepam is 4 mg and 8 mg in pediatric patients and adults, respectively.
- Patients chronically on BDZs may require very large doses for treatment of GCSE.
- **Midazolam** is a water-soluble BDZ that moves rapidly into the CNS. It has an extremely short half-life (0.8 hour), requiring it to be given by continuous infusion. Its cost precludes its use as a first-line BDZ in the hospital.
- Diazepam and lorazepam contain propylene glycol, which may cause dysrhythmia and hypotension if administered too rapidly. Administration of diazepam and lorazepam should not exceed 5 mg/min and 2 mg/min, respectively.
- If an IV line cannot be established, lorazepam or midazolam can be given IM, and diazepam can be given rectally. Intramuscular administration of the BDZs (especially diazepam) may result in delayed or inadequate peak concentrations. Diazepam is given rectally 0.2–0.7 mg/kg, and peak concentrations occur in 6–10 minutes in children and 10–20 minutes in adults.
- With BDZ administration, a brief period of cardiorespiratory depression (30–60 seconds) may occur in 12.5% of patients and can necessitate assisted ventilation or intubation. This is especially true if BDZs are used concomitantly with barbiturates. Hypotension may occur following high doses of BDZs.

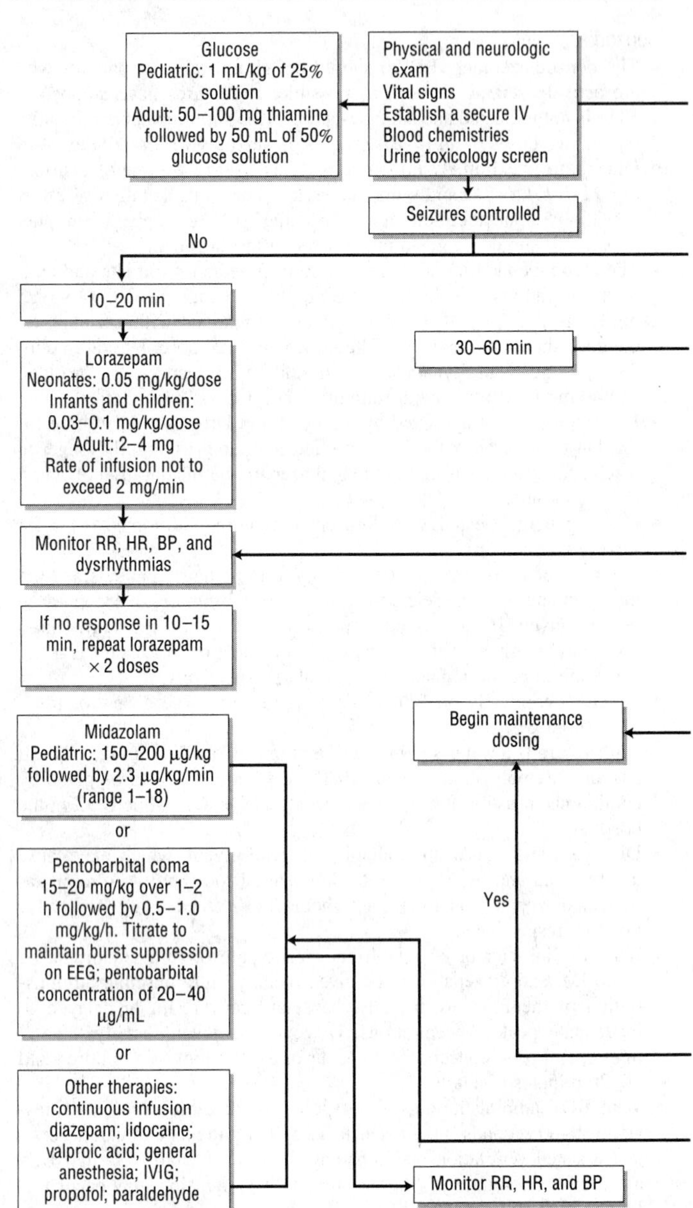

IX

Figure 53–1. Algorithm for management of generalized convulsive status epilepticus.

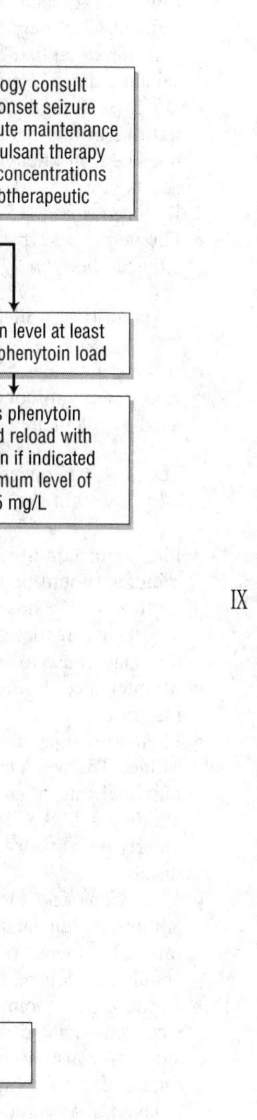

Figure 53–1. continued

IX

Phenytoin

- The hydantoins are the long-acting AEDs of choice for GCSE. Intravenous **phenytoin** is effective in terminating GCSE 40–91% of the time, and it has a relatively long half-life (20–36 hours) and lacks significant CNS depression. It cannot be delivered rapidly enough to be considered a first-line single agent. It also takes longer to control seizures than the BDZs.
- Doses <18 mg/kg do not usually achieve and maintain serum concentrations in the therapeutic range for 24 hours. Provided the patient has not been on phenytoin prior to admission, standard loading doses for adults are 15–20 mg/kg and for pediatric patients are 20 mg/kg. Reduced doses (15 mg/kg) are recommended for elderly patients.
- For very obese patients, loading doses (LD) should be calculated on adjusted body weight.

$$\text{Weight (kg)} = \text{Ideal Body Weight (IBW)} + \frac{1.33\,(\text{Weight} - \text{IBW})}{\text{IBW}}$$

- If the patient has been on phenytoin prior to admission and the admission phenytoin concentration is known, the following equation can be used to calculate a loading dose.

$$LD_{ADULT} = (\text{Concentration}_{DESIRED} - \text{Concentration}_{ADMISSION}) \times 0.75\ \text{L/kg} \times \text{weight (kg)}$$

- Phenytoin equilibrates into the brain within 20–60 minutes; thus 60 minutes should be allowed for response before administering a second partial loading dose. If seizures continue after the initial loading dose, some have recommended an additional loading dose of 5 mg/kg, but this may cause toxic serum concentrations and exacerbate seizures.
- Maintenance dosing should be started within 12–24 hours of the loading dose.
- Phenytoin injectable must be diluted to 5 mg/mL or less in normal saline. The vehicle (propylene glycol) may cause hypotension. The maximal rate of infusion is 50 mg/min in adults and 1 mg/kg/min in children <50 kg. The rate of infusion should not exceed 25 mg/min in elderly patients or those with a history of atherosclerotic cardiovascular disease.
- Vital signs and electrocardiogram (ECG) should be obtained during administration, and the rate slowed if hypotension develops, the QT interval widens, or if arrhythmias develop. In all patients, the rate should be reduced once seizures have stopped.
- Because phenytoin has a pH of approximately 13, its intravenous infusion is associated with discomfort. Catheter infiltration during an infusion can cause tissue necrosis. Intramuscular administration is not recommended, as it may cause pain and tissue necrosis, and absorption is delayed and erratic.

Fosphenytoin

- **Fosphenytoin,** the water-soluble disodium phosphate ester of phenytoin, is a phenytoin prodrug. Fosphenytoin 150 mg is equivalent to phenytoin 100 mg. It is considered safe and better tolerated than phenytoin when administered intravenously.
- The dose of fosphenytoin sodium is expressed as phenytoin sodium equivalents (PE).
- Adverse reactions include nystagmus, dizziness, pruritus, paresthesias, headache, somnolence, and ataxia.
- Pediatric and adult patients with GCSE should receive fosphenytoin loading doses of 15–20 mg PE/kg. In adults, the rate of administration should be 100–150 mg PE/min. Pediatric patients should receive fosphenytoin at a rate of 1–3 mg PE/kg/min.
- Continuous ECG, blood pressure, and respiratory status monitoring is required for all loading doses of fosphenytoin.

Phenobarbital

- Most clinicians believe that **phenobarbital** is a third-line agent for GCSE when BDZs plus phenytoin have failed. Some others (especially in pediatric institutions with large emergency departments) contend that phenobarbital should be the initial drug of choice. A third group opines that continuous infusion of midazolam should be the third-line anticonvulsant before the barbiturates.
- The Working Group on Status Epilepticus recommends that phenobarbital be given after BDZs and phenytoin have failed; phenobarbital is the long-acting AED of choice in patients with a hypersensitivity to the hydantoins or in those with cardiac conduction abnormalities.
- The barbiturates continue to be the AEDs of choice for neonatal seizures.
- There is no maximum dose beyond which further doses are likely to be ineffective.
- Patients should receive a 20–25 mg/kg load of phenobarbital, but higher doses (30 mg/kg) have been used in neonates without adverse effects. If the initial loading dose does not stop the seizures within 20–30 minutes, an additional 10–20 mg/kg dose may be given. If seizures continue, a third 10 mg/kg load may be given. Once seizures are controlled, the maintenance dose should be started within 12–24 hours. The rate of administration should not exceed 100 mg/min in adults and 2 mg/kg/min or 30 mg/min in pediatric patients.
- Medical personnel should be ready to provide respiratory support whenever phenobarbital and the BDZs are used together. If significant hypotension develops, the infusion should be slowed or stopped.

REFRACTORY GCSE

- When adequate doses of a BDZ, phenytoin, and phenobarbital have failed, the condition is termed refractory. Failure to aggressively treat early increases the likelihood of nonresponse.

Benzodiazepines

- **Midazolam** has been suggested as the third-line agent if the patient does not respond to lorazepam plus phenytoin. Pediatric patients have been given a midazolam loading dose (0.15 mg/kg) followed by 2.3 μg/kg/min (range, 1–18 μg/kg/min). The maximum total dose was 1.81 mg, and seizures were controlled by a mean time of 0.78 hour. Frequent increases in infusion rates may be necessary, and dosing should be guided by EEG.
- Refractory GCSE has also been treated with intravenous lorazepam and also with continuous infusion of diazepam.

Barbiturate Coma

- Intubation and respiratory support may be required during barbiturate coma, and continuous monitoring of vital signs is essential. While very-high-dose phenobarbital successfully stops refractory GCSE, the long half-life of phenobarbital produces coma for several days after discontinuation. Therefore, a short-acting barbiturate (e.g., **pentobarbital**) is generally preferred (Figure 53–1). Twelve hours after a burst suppression pattern is obtained, the rate of pentobarbital infusion should be titrated downward every 2–4 hours to determine if GCSE is in remission.

Valproate

- The Working Group on Status Epilepticus recommends a loading dose of 20 mg/kg rectally. An intravenous dosage form was recently approved.

Propofol

IX

- **Propofol** is very lipid soluble, has a high volume of distribution, and has a rapid onset of action. It is not approved for GCSE or NCSE. It may cause respiratory and cerebral depression, bradycardia, and metabolic acidosis.
- Normal adult doses may provide >1000 calories/d as lipid, and it is very costly.

Lidocaine

- **Lidocaine** is not recommended unless other agents have failed. The recommended initial dose is 50–100 mg (1–3 mg/kg) over 2 minutes. A lidocaine infusion is initiated at a rate of 1.5–3.5 mg/kg/h in adults or 6 mg/kg/h in infants. Seizures and obtundation may develop when concentrations exceed 8 mg/L.

NONCONVULSIVE STATUS EPILEPTICUS

Absence Status Epilepticus

- The clinical manifestations of absence SE include an altered state of consciousness and/or behavior and the classic 3 per second spike-and-wave pattern on the EEG. Correction of identifiable precipitants (e.g., structural or metabolic aberrations) may be the only therapy required. It is not considered life threatening.
- It is treated with intravenous diazepam/lorazepam or rectal **valproic acid.** Intravenous **acetazolamide** (250–500 mg) has been used, but it is

less effective than the BDZs. Intravenous phenytoin/fosphenytoin or phenobarbital may be tried in patients who are refractory.

Atypical Absence and Myoclonic Status Epilepticus

- Valproic acid remains the drug of choice for atypical absence. Refractory patients should be tried on a combination of valproic acid plus **ethosuximide** or **clonazepam.**
- Generalized myoclonic SE is rare, but may occur during absence or atypical SE.

Complex Partial Status Epilepticus

- Complex partial SE is a continuous series of repeated seizures that are focal in onset and associated with altered consciousness and periods of total unresponsiveness with stereotypical automatisms.
- Although the combination of an IV BDZ plus phenytoin is effective, phenytoin alone may be more beneficial.

▶ EVALUATION OF THERAPEUTIC OUTCOMES

- Convulsive SE is a medical emergency, and therapy must be aggressive. Drug-induced side effects are less of a concern than preventing brain damage or death. Close monitoring is required to assure that interventions are effective, that seizures do not recur, and that vital functions are supported.

See Chapter 53, Status Epilepticus, authored by Stephanie J. Phelps, PharmD, FCCP, William N. May, MD, and Douglas F. Rose, MD, for a more detailed discussion of this topic. IX

Nutritional Disorders

Edited by Cindy W. Hamilton, PharmD

Chapter 54

▶ ASSESSMENT AND NUTRITION REQUIREMENTS

▶ DEFINITION

Malnutrition is a state induced by alterations in dietary intake or nutrient utilization resulting in changes in subcellular, cellular, and/or organ function that expose the individual to increased risks of morbidity and mortality. These changes can be reversed by appropriate nutrition support.

▶ DESIRED OUTCOME

Nutrition assessment provides a basis for determining nutrition requirements, when nutrition therapy should be initiated, and the optimal type of nutritional intervention. The principles of enteral and parenteral nutrition are covered in Chapters 55 and 56.

▶ CLASSIFICATION OF NUTRITIONAL DISEASES

- Deficiency states can be categorized as those involving protein and calories (protein–energy malnutrition [PEM]) or those resulting from single nutrients (e.g., vitamins or trace minerals).
- The three types of PEM are marasmus (deficiency in total intake or food utilization), kwashiorkor (relative protein deficiency), and mixed marasmus–kwashiorkor.
- Single-nutrient deficiencies can and often do occur in combination with any PEM.

▶ NUTRITION SCREENING

- Checklists are often used to characterize a person's food and alcohol consumption habits, physical capability of buying and preparing food, and weight history. If three or more risk factors are present, a more comprehensive nutrition assessment is performed.
- The Joint Commission on Accreditation of Healthcare Organizations (JCAHO) standards call for developing and implementing a patient-specific nutrition care plan for all patients. Screening should occur within 24 hours of hospitalization to identify at-risk patients. Even stable patients should be reevaluated every 7–14 days to avoid deterioration secondary to changes in food intake.

- By identifying individuals at risk for malnutrition, nutrition screening can be a cost-effective way to help decrease complications and length of hospital stay.

▶ NUTRITION ASSESSMENT

- Nutrition assessment includes medical and dietary history, physical examination, anthropometric measurements, and laboratory data. Laboratory parameters provide objective data to confirm the diagnosis, quantify degree of malnutrition, identify end-organ changes that occur with malnutrition, and provide a baseline for evaluating response to nutrition therapy.
- Clinical evaluation (i.e., medical and dietary history, physical examination) remains the oldest, simplest, and probably most widely used method of evaluating nutrition status (Table 54–1).
- Physical examination should focus on assessment of lean body mass and physical findings of vitamin, trace mineral, and essential fatty acid (EFA) deficiency (Table 54–2).

TABLE 54–1. Pertinent Data from Medical and Dietary History for Nutrition Assessment

Nutrition Intake and Dietary Habits
Anorexia; unusual or absent taste
Actual intake; special diets
Supplemental vitamin or mineral intake
Food allergies or intolerance
Underlying Pathology with Nutritional Effects
Chronic infections or inflammatory states
Neoplastic diseases
Endocrine disorders
Chronic illnesses including pulmonary disease, cirrhosis, renal failure
Hypermetabolic states: trauma, burns, sepsis
Digestive or absorptive diseases; nausea, vomiting, diarrhea
Hyperlipidemia
End-Organ Effects
Weight changes
Skin or hair changes
Activity and energy level, exercise tolerance, fatigue
Obesity
Gastrointestinal tract symptoms: diarrhea, vomiting, constipation
Miscellaneous
Catabolic medications or therapies: steroids, immunosuppressive agents, radiation, or chemotherapy
Other medications: diuretics, laxatives
Genetic background: body habitus of parents, siblings, and family
Alcohol or drug abuse

TABLE 54–2. Physical Findings Suggestive of Malnutrition

General Appearance
Edema (especially ankle and sacral)
Cachexia or obesity
Ascites
Signs and symptoms of dehydration: skin turgor, sunken eyes, orthostasis, dry mucous membranes
Muscle wasting; loss of subcutaneous tissue
Skin and Mucous Membranes
Thin, shiny, or scaling skin
Decubitus ulcers
Ecchymoses, perifollicular petechiae
Poorly healing surgical or traumatic wounds
Pallor or redness of gums, fissures at mouth edge
Glossitis; stomatitis; cheilosis
Musculoskeletal
Retarded growth
Bone pain or tenderness, epiphyseal swelling
Muscle mass less than expected for habitus, genetic history, and level of exercise
Neurologic
Ataxia, positive Romberg test, decreased vibratory or position sense
Nystagmus
Convulsions, paralysis
Encephalopathy
Hepatic
Jaundice
Hepatomegaly

ANTHROPOMETRIC MEASUREMENTS

- Anthropometric measurements are safe, simple, and easy, but gross measures of body cell mass for both population analysis and individual long-term monitoring.
- Individual anthropometric measurements should be cautiously interpreted because (1) standards do not account for individual variations in bone size, hydration status, or skin compressibility, as well as obesity, ethnicity, and increased age; (2) technique is critical and interobserver error may be as high as 30%; and (3) parameters are slow to change, often requiring weeks before significant alterations can be observed.
- Interpretation of actual body weight (ABW) measurement should consider ideal weight for height, usual body weight, fluid status, and age. Change over time can be calculated as percentage of ideal or usual body weight (IBW or UBW). An absolute unintentional weight loss of >10 pounds in <6 months correlates with poor clinical outcome.

- Body mass index (BMI) (i.e., body weight/height [kg/m^2]) of 18.5–25 is considered normal for adults aged 18–65 years. Values >25 are associated with obesity and values <18.5 are indicative of malnutrition.
- Skinfold-thickness measurement estimates subcutaneous fat. Careful technique with pressure-regulated calipers is essential for reproducibility and reliability.
- Midarm-muscle circumference (MAMC) is a noninvasive, easy, inexpensive method of assessing skeletal muscle mass.

BIOCHEMICAL MARKERS

- Biochemical markers of lean body mass, which reflect structural and functional protein status, can be assessed by creatinine-height index (CHI) and serum visceral protein concentrations.
- CHI is the ratio of the patient's 24-hour urinary excretion of creatinine and the ideal 24-hour excretion normalized by gender, height, and body weight. Clinic utility, however, is questionable if the patient has impaired renal function, dehydration, high dietary protein intake, steroid use, old age, or stress.
- Relevant visceral protein data (Table 54–3) must be interpreted relative to individual clinical status because of the confounding effects of abnormal protein losses via renal or gastrointestinal routes, hydration status, renal and hepatic function, and metabolic stress.

TESTS OF IMMUNE FUNCTION

- The two tests of immune function most frequently used in nutrition assessment, total lymphocyte count (TLC) and delayed cutaneous hypersensitivity (DCH) reactions, are simple to perform, readily available, and inexpensive.
- DCH may be assessed as a primary response to a mitogen (e.g., phytohemagglutinin [PHA]) or, more commonly, as a secondary response using recall antigens (e.g., mumps, *Candida albicans,* streptokinase–streptodornase [SKSD], *Trichophyton,* coccidioidin, and purified protein derivative [PPD]).
- Unfortunately, tests of immune function are affected by non-nutrition factors (e.g., infection, immunosuppressive therapy, or critical illness) and are therefore nonspecific indicators of malnutrition.

OTHER TYPES OF NUTRITION ASSESSMENT

- Hand grip strength, or forearm muscle dynamometry, and stimulation of the ulnar nerve have the advantage of indicating tissue function rather than composition. Clinical utility is hampered by lack of appropriate reference standards and limited data confirming their sensitivity and specificity as nutrition assessment tools.
- Bioelectric impedance analysis (BIA) is a simple, noninvasive method of assessing body composition and fluid status. Potential limitations

TABLE 54–3. Summary of Visceral Proteins Used for Assessment of Lean Body Mass

Serum Protein	Biosynthetic Site	Normal Value (range)[a]	Half-life (d)	Function	Factors Resulting in Increased Values[b]	Factors Resulting in Decreased Values[b]
Albumin	Hepatocyte	3.5–5.0 g/dL	18–20	Maintains plasma oncotic pressure; carrier for small molecules	Dehydration, anabolic steroids, insulin, infection	Overhydration, edema, renal insufficiency, nephrotic syndrome, poor intake, impaired digestion, burns, congestive heart failure, cirrhosis, thyroid/adrenal/pituitary hormones, trauma, sepsis
Fibronectin	Hepatocyte, fibroblasts, endothelial cells	210–300 μg/mL	0.5–1.0	Glycoprotein has opsonic activity within blood; may exert chemotactic activity and facilitate wound healing	None currently described	Trauma, shock, burns, sepsis, disseminated intravascular coagulation; inappropriate specimen handling
Prealbumin (Transthyretin)	Hepatocyte	10–40 mg/dL	1–2	Binds T_3 and to a lesser extent T_4; carrier for RBP	Renal dysfunction	Cirrhosis, hepatitis, stress, inflammation, surgery, hyperthyroidism, cystic fibrosis, renal dysfunction
Retinol-binding protein (RBP)	Hepatocyte	2.0–6.0 mg/dL	0.5	Transports vitamin A in plasma; binds noncovalently to prealbumin	Renal dysfunction, vitamin A supplementation	Same as prealbumin; also vitamin A deficiency
Somatomedin C	Hepatocyte	0.4–2.0 IU/mL	0.1–0.3	Insulin-like peptide with anabolic actions on fat, muscle, cartilage, and cultured cells	None currently described	Growth hormone deficiency, psychosocial growth failure, hypothyroidism, renal failure, cirrhosis, drugs (estrogens, prednisolone)
Transferrin	Hepatocyte	200–400 mg/dL	8	Binds Fe in plasma and transports to bone	Iron deficiency, pregnancy, hypoxia, chronic blood loss, estrogens	Chronic infection, cirrhosis, enteropathies, nephrotic syndrome, burns, cortisone, testosterone

[a]Normal values represent pooled subjects; ranges vary between centers; check local values.
[b]All of the listed proteins are influenced by hydration and hepatocellular dysfunction.

include variability with electrolyte imbalance, interference by large fat masses, and lack of standards that reflect variations in individual body sizes.

- New methods to determine body composition are being used in clinical research. These clinical uses are limited by the degree of technical complexity and expensive technology.

► SPECIFIC NUTRIENT DEFICIENCIES

- Assessment of nutrition status should include evaluation of possible trace mineral, vitamin, and essential fatty acid deficiencies. Assessment includes history, physical examination, and biochemical assessment. Unfortunately, few practical methods to assess micronutrient function are available; most assays measure tissue or fluid concentration of a nutrient, not its function.
- Essential trace minerals for which deficiency states have been described are zinc, copper, manganese, selenium, chromium, iodine, molybdenum, and iron (Table 54–4).
- Iron deficiency is usually confirmed by indirect measurements because they are noninvasive, but they may be altered by chronic illness. Direct methods (e.g., marrow staining and liver biopsy) are more accurate, but invasive and thus rarely used (see Chapter 31).
- History and physical examination may be the most valuable means of screening patients for vitamin deficiency (Table 54–5). Laboratory assessment is used to confirm clinical suspicions.
- EFA, specifically linoleic acid, deficiency is rare but may appear within 1 week after initiation of fat-free parenteral nutrition or with severe PEM. Symptoms include dermatitis (e.g., dry, cracked, scaly skin), alopecia, and impaired wound healing. In severe cases, neurologic deficits, abnormal liver function, respiratory insufficiency, cardiac arrhythmias, and hemolysis may occur. Laboratory assessment of EFA deficiency is expensive and not readily available.
- Carnitine has vitamin-like properties, but there is no specific dietary requirement. Carnitine deficiency has been associated with severe protein malnutrition, inborn errors of metabolism, insufficient dietary carnitine intake in newborn infants, and kidney and liver disease. Clinical presentation includes generalized skeletal muscle weakness, fatty liver, and reactive hypoglycemia. Carnitine status may be assessed by measuring plasma, urine, or red blood cell concentrations.

► ASSESSMENT OF NUTRIENT REQUIREMENTS

- Assessment of nutrient requirements must be made in the context of patient-specific factors (e.g., age, gender, size, disease state, clinical condition, nutrition status, and physical activity).

TABLE 54–4. Assessment of Trace Mineral Status

Trace Mineral	Signs of Deficiency	Normal Serum Concentration[a]	Factors Resulting in Altered Plasma Concentrations
Chromium	Glucose intolerance, peripheral neuropathy, increased free fatty acid levels, low respiratory quotient	0.12–2.1 µg/L	Not known
Copper	Neutropenia, hypochromic anemia, osteoporosis, decreased hair and skin pigmentation, dermatitis, anorexia, diarrhea	80–155 µg/L (female) 70–140 µg/L (male)	Decreased: Serum ceruloplasmin, corticosteroid therapy, Wilson's disease Increased: Infection, rheumatoid arthritis, pregnancy, birth control pills
Iodine	Hypothyroid goiter, hypothyroidism	Assessed by T_4, TSH and free T_4 index[b]	Assays are specific to hypo- and hyperthyroid states
Manganese	Nausea, vomiting, dermatitis, color changes in hair, hypo-cholesterolemia, growth retardation	0.6–2.0 ng/mL (plasma)	Not known
Molybdenum	Tachycardia, tachypnea, altered mental status, visual changes, headache, nausea, vomiting	0.1–3.0 µg/L	Varies with assay method
Selenium	Muscle weakness and pain, cardiomyopathy	46–143 µg/dL	Decreased: Malignancy, liver failure, pregnancy Increased: Reticuloendothelial neoplasia
Zinc	Dermatitis, hypogeusia, alopecia, diarrhea, apathy, depression	70–150 µg/dL	Decreased: Infection, hypoalbuminemia, corticosteroid therapy, stress, inflammation, pregnancy Increased: Tissue injury, hemolysis, contaminated collection tubes

[a]Normal values may vary among laboratories and on assay procedures.
[b]See Chapter 18.

TABLE 54–5. Assessment of Vitamin Status

Vitamin	Signs of Deficiency	Laboratory Assay	Normal Values	Comments
Niacin (B_5)	Pellagra: dermatitis, dementia, glossitis, diarrhea, loss of memory, headaches	Urinary niacin metabolites	2.4–6.4 mg/d	Varies with age, gender, pregnancy; blood levels not done
Folate (B_9)	Megaloblastic anemia, diarrhea, glossitis	Serum folate	3–16 ng/mL	Decreased: Increased cellular or tissue turnover (pregnancy, malignancy, hemolytic anemia)
Cyanocobalamin (B_{12})	Pernicious anemia: glossitis, spinal cord degeneration, peripheral neuropathy	Serum B_{12}	100–700 pg/mL	
Thiamine (B_1)	Paresthesias, nystagmus, impaired memory, congestive heart failure, lactic acidosis, Wernicke–Korsakoff syndrome	Red blood cell transketolase activity	850–1000 μg/mL/h	
Riboflavin (B_2)	Mucositis, dermatitis, cheilosis; vascularization of cornea, photophobia, lacrimation, decreased vision; impaired wound healing; normocytic anemia	Urinary riboflavin	80–120 μg/g creatinine	Varies with age, pregnancy, exercise, nitrogen balance
Pyridoxine (B_6)	Dermatitis, neuritis, convulsions; microcytic anemia	Plasma B_6	5–30 ng/mL	Varies with age, gender

(continued)

X

TABLE 54–5. continued

Vitamin	Signs of Deficiency	Laboratory Assay	Normal Values	Comments
Pantothenic acid (B_3)	Fatigue, malaise, headache, insomnia, vomiting, abdominal cramps	Serum pantothenic acid	1.03–1.83 μg/mL	
Biotin	Dermatitis, depression, alopecia, lassitude, somnolence	Urinary biotin	6–50 μg/d	
Ascorbic acid (C)	Enlargement and keratosis of hair follicles; impaired wound healing; anemia, lethargy, depression, bleeding, ecchymosis	Plasma ascorbic acid	0.5–1.5 mg/dL	
A	Dermatitis, night blindness, keratomalacia, xerophthalmia	Serum vitamin A	30–80 μg/dL	
D	Rickets and osteomalacia, muscle weakness	Plasma 25-hydroxy-vitamin D	13–50 ng/mL	Decreased: Uremia, cirrhosis, age > 60 y, possibly in winter
E	Hemolysis	Serum vitamin E	5.0–13 μg/mL	Decreased: Low blood lipoprotein
K	Bleeding	Serum phylloquinone	0.13–1.19 ng/mL	Decreased: Hepatic disease, anticoagulants

ENERGY REQUIREMENTS

- Adult energy requirements are approximately 25 kcal/kg for healthy individuals with normal nutrition, 30 kcal/kg for malnourished or mildly metabolically stressed individuals, 30–35 kcal/kg for critically ill or hypermetabolic individuals, and ≥40 kcal/kg for patients with major burn injury. This simple approach assumes no age- or gender-related differences in energy metabolism.
- The Harris–Benedict equation (below) for calculating basal energy expenditure (BEE) has the advantage of including some patient-specific factors. BEE should be adjusted upward ranging from 20% for bed-ridden patients to 80–130% for patients with severe burn injuries.

Females: BEE (kcal/d) = 655 + 9.6 (wt in kg) + 1.8 (ht in cm) – 4.7 (age in y)

Males: BEE (kcal/d) = 66 + 13.7 (wt in kg) + 5 (ht in cm) – 6.8 (age in y)

- The most accurate clinical tool for estimating energy requirements is indirect calorimetry. This noninvasive procedure determines oxygen consumption ($V\text{O}_2$, mL/min) and carbon dioxide production ($V\text{CO}_2$, mL/min). Resting energy expenditure (REE, kcal/d) is calculated by the abbreviated Weir equation:

$$\text{REE} = [3.9(V\text{O}_2) + 1.1\,(V\text{CO}_2)] \times 1.44$$

- Data from indirect calorimetry can also be used to determine a respiratory quotient (RQ):

$$\text{RQ} = V\text{CO}_2/V\text{O}_2$$

RQ values >1.0 suggest a patient is being overfed, while values <0.7 may be indicative of a ketogenic diet, fat gluconeogenesis, or ethanol X
oxidation.

PROTEIN, FLUID, AND MICRONUTRIENT REQUIREMENTS

- The usual recommended daily protein allowance for adults is 0.8 g/kg, which varies if the following conditions are present: hypermetabolic stress (1.5–2.0 g/kg), renal failure (restriction without dialysis and 1.2–2.7 g/kg with dialysis), or hepatic failure (0.5 g/kg).
- Daily protein requirements can be individualized by measuring urinary nitrogen excretion in a 24-hour urine collection (UUN), which can be used to estimate the dietary protein required to maintain homeostasis. Nitrogen output is approximated by the following:

$$\text{Nitrogen output (g/d)} = (\text{UUN} \times 1.20) + 1$$

- Daily adult fluid requirements are approximately 30 mL/kg or 1 mL/kcal. Fluid requirements increase with increased insensible or gastrointestinal losses, fever, sweating, and increased metabolism. Fluid requirements

TABLE 54–6. Recommended Adult Daily Maintenance Doses for Electrolytes, Trace Minerals, and Vitamins

Nutrient	Enteral	Parenteral
Electrolytes		
Calcium	800–1200 mg	10–15 mEq
Chloride	1700–5100 mg	—
Fluoride	1.5–4.0 mg	—
Magnesium	280–350 mg	10–20 mEq
Phosphorus	800–1200 mg	20–45 mmol
Potassium	1875–5625 mg	60–100 mEq
Sodium	1100–3300 mg	60–100 mEq
Trace Minerals		
Chromium	50–200 µg	10–15 µg[a]
Copper	1.5–3 mg	0.5–1.5 mg
Iodine	150 µg	70–140 µg
Iron	10–15 mg	Varies with age, gender
Manganese	2–5 mg	0.15–0.8 mg
Molybdenum	75–250 µg	100–200 µg
Selenium	55–70 µg	40–80 µg
Zinc	12–15 mg	2.5–4.0 mg[b]
Vitamins		
Biotin	30–100 µg	60 µg
Cyanocobalamin (B_{12})	2.0 µg	5.0 µg
Folic acid	200 µg	400 µg
Niacin	13–19 mg NE	40 mg NE
Pantothenic acid (B_3)	4.7 mg	15 mg
Pyridoxine (B_6)	1.6–2.0 mg	4 mg
Riboflavin (B_2)	1.2–1.7 mg	3.6 mg
Thiamin (B_1)	1.0–1.5 mg	3 mg
Vitamin A	800–1000 µg RE	600 µg RE (3300 IU)
Vitamin C	60 mg	100 mg
Vitamin D	5–10 µg	5 µg (200 IU)
Vitamin E	8–10 mg TE[c]	10 mg TE (10 IU)[c]
Vitamin K	60–80 µg	0.7–2.5 mg

NE = niacin equivalent; RE = retinol equivalent; TE = tocopherol equivalent.

[a]An additional 20 µg chromium/d is recommended in patients with intestinal losses.

[b]An additional 12.2 mg zinc/L of small-bowel fluid lost and 17.1 mg zinc/kg of stool or ileostomy output is recommended; an additional 2.0 mg zinc/d for acute catabolic stress.

[c]Daily requirements may be as high as 135–150 IU, according to recent data.

Adapted from Shronts EP, Lacey JA. Metabolic support. In: Gottschlich MM, Matarese LE, Shronts EP, eds. Nutrition Support Dietetics—Core Curriculum, *2nd ed. Silver Spring, MD, Aspen, 1993: 358, with permission.*

decrease with renal failure, expanded extracellular fluid volume (e.g., congestive heart failure), or hypoproteinemia with starvation.

- Requirements for micronutrients (i.e., electrolytes, trace minerals, and vitamins) vary with route of administration (Table 54–6).

DRUG–NUTRIENT INTERACTIONS

- Concomitant drug therapy can alter serum concentrations of minerals and electrolytes (Table 54–7).
- Some drugs (e.g., chlorpromazine, corticosteroids, dopamine, furosemide, phenytoin, theophylline, and somatostatin) cause hyperglycemia, whereas others (e.g., anabolic steroids, disopyramide, clofibrate, haloperidol, insulin, oral hypoglycemics, propranolol, somatostatin) cause hypoglycemia.
- Drugs can also alter vitamin status. Sulfasalazine decreases folic acid concentrations; furosemide and antacids cause thiamine deficiency; antibiotics cause vitamin K deficiency; antineoplastics cause folic acid antagonism and malabsorption; cathartics increase requirements for vitamins D, C, and B_6; anticonvulsants impair absorption of vitamin D and folic acid; and isoniazid causes vitamin B_6 deficiency. Conversely, large doses of folic acid counter the effect of methotrexate, and vitamin K can reduce the anticoagulant effect of warfarin.

TABLE 54–7. Drug–Nutrient Interactions

	Nutrient	
Drug	*Decreased Serum Concentration*	*Increased Serum Concentration*
Antacids (aluminum)	Phosphorus	
Aminoglycosides	Magnesium	
Amphotericin B	Potassium, magnesium, zinc	
Cisplatin	Magnesium, zinc, sodium	
Cyclosporine	Magnesium	
Diuretics (thiazide)	Potassium, magnesium, zinc	
Diuretics (loop)	Potassium, calcium, magnesium, zinc	
Glucocorticoids	Potassium, calcium	
Laxatives	Potassium, calcium	
Penicillamine	Zinc, copper	
Sucralfate	Phosphorus	
Carbencillin (parenteral)		Sodium
Clindamycin (parenteral		Phosphorus
Phosphate enemas		Phosphorus
Spironolactone		Potassium
Ticarcillin (parenteral)		Sodium

▶ EVALUATION OF THERAPEUTIC OUTCOMES

- Assessment of nutrition requirements can be an acute process; however, ongoing reassessment will be required to ascertain whether nutrition goals have been achieved.
- Initially, nutrition requirements may be based on assumptions about the patient's clinical condition and nutrition needs for repletion.
- The importance of history and physical examination in both nutrition screening and nutrition assessment cannot be overemphasized.
- Those markers that show the best correlation with outcome are weight and serum albumin concentration. The cost effectiveness of more extensive biochemical evaluations remains to be determined. Assessment of other anthropometric measures is probably most useful during long-term nutrition support when they will serve as a longitudinal marker of response to therapy.

See Chapter 126, Assessment of Nutrition Status and Nutrition Requirements, authored by Kathleen M. Teasley-Strausburg, MS, RPh, BCNSP, and Jan Dalke Anderson, PharmD, BCNSP, for a more detailed discussion of this topic.

Chapter 55

ENTERAL NUTRITION

DEFINITION

Enteral nutrition and tube feeding are often used interchangeably to describe an artificial feeding method that includes use of specialized feeding formulas, tubes, and pumps.

PATHOPHYSIOLOGY

- Digestion and absorption are important and inseparably associated gastrointestinal (GI) processes that generate usable fuels for the body.
- Digestion is the stepwise conversion of complex chemical and physical nutrients via mechanical, enzymatic, and physicochemical processes into molecular forms, which can be absorbed from the GI tract.
- Nutrients ultimately reach the systemic circulation through portal venous or splanchnic lymphatic systems, provided they are not excreted by the GI or biliary tract.
- The GI tract (GIT) also actively defends the body from toxins and antigens by nonimmunologic and immunologic mechanisms. Nonimmunologic mechanisms include mechanical mechanisms and indigenous microflora that limit microbial proliferation and also antagonize exogenous microbes. Immunologic mechanisms include gut-associated lymphoid tissue, secretory immunoglobulin A, and hepatic Kupffer's cells.

CLINICAL PRESENTATION AND DIAGNOSIS

Clinical presentation of protein–energy malnutrition and nutrition assessment are discussed in Chapter 54.

DESIRED OUTCOME

The goals of enteral tube feeding are to reverse protein–calorie malnutrition, promote growth and development of infants and children, maintain adequate nutritional state, reduce disease-related morbidity and mortality, or some combination of these goals.

TREATMENT

GENERAL PRINCIPLES

- Enteral nutrition is the preferred route of nourishment if the GI tract is functioning and accessible. Advantages of enteral over parenteral nutrition include maintaining GI tract structure and function, fewer metabolic and infectious complications, and lower costs.

- Although human data are insufficient to establish whether atrophic gut changes associated with lack of enteral nutrition lead to clinically significant translocation of gut bacteria, endotoxins, and antigenic macromolecules, these considerations justify the use of at least partial enteral nutrition to maintain gut mucosal function.
- Enteral nutrition is indicated for many conditions or disease states (Table 55–1). Its use is contraindicated for patients with mechanical obstruction of GI tract, diffuse peritonitis, severe diarrhea that confounds metabolic management, severe GI hemorrhage, intractable vomiting, chronic intestinal pseudo-obstruction, or severe malabsorption.
- Assessment of length, anatomy, and motility of GI tract is required prior to initiation of enteral therapy. Minimum length of functional small bowel required for nutrient absorption is approximately 100–150 cm of jejunum, ileum, or both.

FEEDING ROUTES

- Multiple feeding routes are available for enteral nutrition support, which are distinguishable by their indications, placement options, advantages, and disadvantages (Table 55–2).
- As the site of nutrient delivery is moved further away from the mouth, tube insertion becomes more difficult and invasive but, at the same time, more permanent.
- The most frequently used short-term enteral feeding routes are those accessed by inserting a tube through the nose and threading it into the stomach or upper small bowel (e.g., nasogastric, nasoduodenal, and nasojejunal routes).

TABLE 55–1. Potential Indications for Enteral Nutrition

Neoplastic Disease	**Gastrointestinal Disease**
Chemotherapy	Inflammatory bowel disease
Radiotherapy	Short bowel syndrome
Upper gastrointestinal tumors	Esophageal motility disorder
Cancer cachexia	Pancreatitis
Organ Failure	Fistulas
Hepatic	**Neurologic Impairment**
Renal	Comatose state
Cardiac cachexia	Cerebrovascular accident
Pulmonary	Demyelinating disease
Multiple organ system failure	Severe depression
Hypermetabolic States	Failure to thrive
Closed head injury	**Other Indications**
Burns	Acquired immune deficiency syndrome
Trauma	Anorexia nervosa
Postoperative major surgery	Complications during pregnancy
Sepsis	Geriatric patients with multiple chronic disease
	Organ transplantation

TABLE 55–2. Options and Considerations in the Selection of Tube Feeding Access

Access	Indications	Tube Placement Options	Advantages	Disadvantages
Nasogastric or orogastric	Short-term use Intact gag reflex Normal gastric emptying	Manually at bedside	Ease of placement Allows for intermittent, bolus, or continuous feeding Inexpensive Multiple commercially available tubes and sizes	Potential tube displacement Increased aspiration risk Cosmetically unappealing Small-bore tube
Nasoduodenal or nasojejunal	Short-term use Delayed gastric emptying (early postoperative period or diabetic neuropathy) High risk of gastroesophageal reflux or aspiration	Manually at bedside Fluoroscopic Endoscopic	Reduced aspiration risk Allows for early postoperative feeding Multiple commercially available tubes and sizes	Manual transpyloric passage requires greater skill Potential tube displacement Continuous (and cyclic) feeding only Cosmetically unappealing Attendant risks for complication for endoscopic placement Small-bore tube
Esophagostomy or pharyngostomy	Long-term use Nasopharyngeal access contraindicated Tumors or trauma of head or neck region	Bedside with local anesthesia or during surgery	Large-bore tube Easy tube replacement	Dressing changes by patient more difficult due to location Requires stoma site care
Gastrostomy	Long-term use Normal gastric emptying Swallowing dysfunction due to neuromuscular disease or central nervous system disorders Esophageal stricture or neoplasm	Surgically Endoscopically (percutaneous endoscopic gastrostomy [PEG]) Laparoscopically Fluoroscopically	Allows for intermittent, bolus, or continuous feeding Large-bore tube Multiple commercially available tubes and sizes Low-profile buttons available	Attendant risks for complication for each method of placement Higher cost, particularly with surgical placement Aspiration risk potential Requires stoma site care
Jejunostomy	Long-term use Impaired gastric emptying (diabetic neuropathy) Facilitate postoperative enteral feeding in trauma, malnourished or upper GIT surgery Inability to access upper GIT	Surgically Endoscopically (accessing jejunum via PEG) Laparoscopically Fluoroscopically	Allows for early postoperative feeding Reduced aspiration risk Multiple commercially available tubes and sizes	Attendant risks for complication for each method of placement Continuous (and cyclic) feeding only Requires stoma site care

X

- Modern feeding tubes are generally made of pliable silicone rubber or polyurethane. They usually have a small bore, which makes them lightweight and comfortable for patients, but small-bore tubes are more likely to become clogged.
- The stomach is generally the least expensive and least labor-intensive access site for enteral feeding; however, it is not necessarily the best. Patients who have delayed gastric emptying are at risk for aspiration.
- Greater skill is required to place the feeding tube beyond the pylorus. Techniques to facilitate manual placement include use of styletted tubes or weighted tubes, placing the patient on his or her right side, and metoclopramide use.
- More permanent enteral feeding access includes esophagostomy or pharyngostomy, gastrostomy, and jejunostomy placement.

ADMINISTRATION METHODS

- Administration methods for tube feeding are continuous, continuous cyclic, intermittent, and intermittent bolus (Table 55–3). The choice depends on anatomic location of feeding tube, patient's clinical condition, environment in which patient resides, intestinal function, and patient's tolerance to tube feeding.
- Continuous tube feeding, which accounts for >80% of enteral feedings, provides maximal tolerance by minimizing abdominal distention or diarrhea. Continuous feeding is also beneficial for patients who have limited absorption capacity because of rapid GI transit time or severely impaired digestion.
- Cyclic enteral feedings allow physical and psychological breaks from the enteral infusion system, greater rehabilitation, and return to activities of daily living, especially if feeds are administered nocturnally. Cyclic feedings may require higher nutrient densities or higher infusion rates to compensate for periods when tube feedings are discontinued.

- Intermittent feeding should only be administered if the feeding tube tip is within the stomach, because the stomach is capable of handling large and more rapid volumes of feeding formula. Patients who receive intermittent feeding may be at risk for nausea, vomiting, and aspiration.
- Bolus feedings have the advantage of requiring little administration time and minimal equipment, but can result in cramping, nausea, vomiting, aspiration, and diarrhea.

EQUIPMENT AND FORMULAS

- Feeding equipment should be adaptable to multiple infusion sets and distinguishable from intravenous equipment. Feeding containers should be leak-proof, unbreakable, and easy to clean; they should be equipped with reliable closures and easy-to-read volume markings. Administration sets should be long enough to easily connect the feeding container and patient, and equipped with an infusion control regulator. Enteral feeding pumps should be lightweight, easy to operate, and low maintenance; pumps should have long-lasting batteries and alarm systems.

TABLE 55–3. Administration Methods for Tube Feeding

Method	Equipment	Indication	Infusion Example
Continuous	Infusion pump generally recommended Enteral formula container Administration set	Gastric tube feeding Postpyloric tube feeding Critically ill patient Limited absorption capacity Limited feeding tolerance via intermittent and bolus methods	Full-strength isotonic formula infused at 20 mL/h, advanced by 20-mL/h increments every 8 h to desired goal rate as tolerated
Continuous cyclic	Infusion pump generally recommended Enteral formula container Administration set	Gastric or postpyloric tube feeding Home tube feeding Rehabilitation patient Nocturnal tube feeding Potential transition to daytime oral intake Limited feeding tolerance via bolus or intermittent method	Formula infused over 10–14 h daily at desired goal rate to achieve nutrient requirements
Intermittent	Infusion pump or gravity flow Enteral formula container Administration set	Gastric tube feeding Home tube feeding Rehabilitation patient Patient unlikely to transition to oral intake Limited feeding tolerance via bolus method	240–480 mL formula infused over 20–40 min 4–6 times daily
Intermittent bolus	Large syringe (60 mL)	Gastric tube feeding Home tube feeding Rehabilitation patient Patient unlikely to transition to oral intake	240–280 mL formula infused over <10 min 4–6 times daily

- Modern enteral formulas are sophisticated and can include enhancements to optimize biological value and nutrient utilization. Macronutrient content (i.e., protein, carbohydrate, and fat) varies in nutrient complexity, which refers to the amount of hydrolysis and digestion that a substrate source requires prior to intestinal absorption. Polymeric or intact substrates have a molecular form similar to table food; other enteral formulas contain partially hydrolyzed or elemental substrates (Table 55–4).

TABLE 55–4. Enteral Formula Classification System

Category	Subcategories	Indication	Features	Product Examples
Polymeric (requires normal GIT digestive and absorptive capacity)	Lactose free	Standard oral supplement Complete tube feeding	Iso-osmolar, high-nitrogen, fiber-enhanced, and highly concentrated formulas available	Osmolite Resource IsoSource VHN Ultracal Deliver 2.0
	Lactose containing	Oral supplement Lactose tolerant	Palatable, hyperosmolar	Sustogen Meritene
	Blenderized	Complete tube feeding	May contain lactose, high viscosity, and may require infusion pump	Complete modified
Monomeric (requires less digestion and absorption)	Chemically defined	Complete tube feeding and some use as oral supplements Disease states that alter digestive or absorptive surface capacity	Nutrients hydrolyzed to varying degrees Osmolarity varies	Peptamen Reabilan HN
	Elemental	Complete tube feeding, rarely as an oral supplement Disease states that alter digestive or absorptive surface capacity Fat malabsorption	Free amino acids, >80% of kcal as oligosaccharides, <15% fat content as long-chain fat	Vivonex Plus Tolerex
Specialized (monomeric or polymeric)	Organ failure	Complete[a] tube feeding, rarely as an oral supplement Specific products for pulmonary, renal, hepatic, and endocrine failure	Composition varies; nutrient requirements modified to a specific disorder	Pulmocare Travasorb Renal Nutrihep DiabetiSource
	Immune support	Complete tube feeding, rarely as an oral supplement Enhance immune competency during critical illness or sepsis	Specific nutrients modified for immunopharmacologic function	Immun-Aid Impact
Modular (usually polymeric)	Protein Carbohydrate Fat	Can be used to compound complete[a] formulas or to supplement enteral or oral feeding	May be labor intensive Micronutrients available to make complete formulas	ProMod Polycose MCT oil
Hydration	Glucose Electrolytes	Feeding tube or oral Dehydration, severe or chronic diarrhea		Equalyte

[a]May or may not be complete nutrient composition.

- Osmolality, one of the factors that affects tolerance, is a function of size and quantity of ionic and molecular particles, and is primarily related to macronutrient and mineral content. Partially hydrolyzed or elemental substrates have higher osmolality than polymeric or intact substrate forms.
- Partially digested protein entities are the most readily absorbable forms of nitrogen. Further reductions in the molecular form of protein increases osmotic load and amino acids containing free sulfur, which in turn imparts a bitter flavor and foul odor.
- Conditionally essential amino acids (e.g., glutamine and arginine) are added to some formulas to maintain GI tract integrity and enhance nitrogen retention.
- Partially digested carbohydrates are preferred over elemental sugars as the primary source of nonprotein calories because of lower osmolality. Glucose polymers are also useful because they have minimal osmotic loads and are easily absorbed in the intestine; however, glucose polymers are not as sweet or palatable as simple glucose.
- Fat provides a concentrated calorie source and serves as a carrier for fat-soluble vitamins. Most formulas contain some long-chain triglycerides (LCTs) to provide essential fatty acids. Potential advantages of medium-chain triglycerides over LCTs are greater water solubility; more rapid hydrolysis; and minimal requirement for pancreatic lipase, bile salt, or chylomicron formation for absorption.
- Most commercially prepared formulas contain micronutrients (e.g., electrolytes, vitamins, and trace elements) to make them nutritionally complete.
- Fiber provides benefits such as trophic effects on large bowel mucosa, promotion of sodium and water absorption in the colon, energy source from resultant short-chain fatty acids, and possibly regulation of bowel motility.
- Formulas with greater solute load increase the obligatory water loss via the kidney. Patients receiving high-nitrogen enteral formulas may be at risk for significant dehydration especially if they are elderly, have altered mental status, or are otherwise unable to ingest water.

INITIATION AND TITRATION OF ENTERAL NUTRITION REGIMEN

- Although advancement of enteral feeding should be individualized, half-strength dilution can be initiated at 25–50 mL/h, regardless of the formula. The rate is increased in 25-mL/h increments every 6–8 hours to a maximal rate over 3 days.
- Many patients tolerate more rapid advancement of a full-strength feeding formula at 20–25 mL/h with increments of 20–25 mL/h every 6–8 hours.
- Hyperosmolar formulas may require slower advancement to prevent dumping syndrome.

DRUG COMPATIBILITY

- Mixing of commercially available liquid medications with selected enteral nutrition products can cause physical incompatibilities that inhibit drug absorption and clog small-bore enteral feeding tubes. Physical incompatibility is more common with formulas that contain intact (versus hydrolyzed) protein and with medications that are formulated as acidic syrups. Mixing of commercial liquid medications and enteral nutrition formulas should be avoided whenever possible (Table 55–5).
- The most significant drug–nutrient interactions result in reduced bioavailability and suboptimal pharmacologic effect (Table 55–6).

PREVENTION OF OTHER COMPLICATIONS

- Factors responsible for metabolic complications associated with enteral nutrition are analogous to those of parenteral nutrition, but GI, technical, and infectious complications are unique to the enteral route (Table 55–7).
- Patients should be monitored for complications of enteral nutrition (Table 55–8), such as dumping syndrome, which is manifested clinically as nausea, cramping, lightheadedness, and diarrhea.
- Pharmacologic intervention (e.g., opiates, **diphenoxylate,** and **loperamide**) is occasionally indicated to control severe diarrhea.

TABLE 55–5. General Considerations for Medication Administration by Enteral Feeding Tubes

1. Administer medications by mouth when feasible, and reserve enteral feeding tube as alternative route.
2. Determine location of the feeding tube tip because pre- or postpyloric drug instillation can alter effectiveness.
3. Use liquid dosage forms if available. If not, reconstitute the contents of hard or soft gelatin capsules with 10–15 mL of water and crushed compressed tablets with 15–30 mL of water.
4. Dilute hyperosmolar medications.
5. Do not crush and administer sustained-release or enteric-coated medications.
6. Adjust dosage and frequency if changing from a sustained-release drug to administer a non–sustained-release liquid form.
7. Flush the feeding tube with water prior to administering a medication. Do not mix medications. Administer each medication separately, flushing with water between and after completion of medication administration.
8. Do not add medications to the enteral formula, except for adding hypertonic electrolyte injection to enteral formulas. Be aware of specific drug–enteral product incompatibilities.

TABLE 55–6. Medications with Special Considerations for Enteral Feeding Tube Administration

Drug	Interaction	Comments
Phenytoin	↓Bioavailability during continuous tube feeding. In vitro results implicate protein (caseinate salts) and calcium chloride.	Limited clinical data provide basis for suggestions: Hold tube feeding 2 h before and after phenytoin; administer phenytoin capsules (versus suspension) during continuous feeding; and use meat-based (versus protein hydrolysate) formula. Monitor patient's clinical response and serum drug level closely.
Antibiotics (selected)	(Theoretical) ↓ bioavailability based on interaction between food and penicillin, tetracycline, isoniazid, rifampin, enoxacin, norfloxacin, and ofloxacin.	Hold tube feeding administration for specified time periods before and after drug administration. Monitor patient's clinical response closely.
Warfarin	Pharmacologic interaction between warfarin and vitamin K in enteral feeding formulas, resulting in ↓ anticoagulation effect.	Vitamin K (<200 μg/1000 kcal) is contained in most enteral products. Adjust warfarin dose based on INR and vitamin K content of the enteral formula.
Antacids	Altered pharmacologic effect of antacid if administered into small bowel. Physical incompatibility reported with aluminum-containing antacids, causing esophageal plug formation.	Administer antacids only into feeding tubes with tip in stomach. Administer aluminum-containing antacids after holding the tube feeding formula to prevent physical incompatibility.

- Nausea and vomiting may be reduced by advancing the feeding tube beyond the pylorus.
- Constipation may be reduced by using enteral formulas with enhanced fiber.
- Techniques for clearing obstructed tubes include instilling water, meat tenderizer, or pancreatic enzymes, as well as passing an endoscopic cytology brush.
- Methods for preventing bronchopulmonary aspiration of gastric contents include use of small-bore feeding tubes, avoiding accumulation of large volumes in the stomach, keeping the head of the bed at 30–45° during feeding and for 30–60 minutes after intermittent infusion, and infusing feedings into the small intestine instead of the stomach.

TABLE 55–7. Complications of Tube Feeding

Complications	Potential Causes
Metabolic	
Dehydration	Insufficient fluid intake or excessive fluid losses
Hyperglycemia	Underlying disease (diabetes mellitus)
	Drug induced (corticosteroids)
	Overfeeding
Increased serum electrolytes	Organ dysfunction (hepatic, renal, cardiac)
	Dehydration
Decreased serum electrolytes	Fluid overload due to excessive intake or organ dysfunction (hepatic, renal, cardiac)
	Extraordinary fluid losses (diarrheal, nasogastric)
	Refeeding syndrome
Decreased trace elements	Extraordinary fluid losses (diarrheal)
	Drug induced (diuretics)
Gastrointestinal	
Diarrhea	Drug related (antibiotic-induced bacterial overgrowth, antacids containing magnesium)
	Malabsorption (inadequate GIT surface area, rapid GIT transit)
	Tube feeding related (rapid formula administration, hyperosmolality, low residue or fiber, lactose intolerance, bacterial contamination)
Nausea and vomiting	Gastric dysmotility (surgery, anticholinergics, diabetic gastroparesis)
	Rapid infusion of hyperosmolar formula
Constipation	Dehydration
	Drug induced (anticholinergics)
	Inactivity
	Low-residue (fiber) content
	Obstruction/fecal impaction
Abdominal distention/cramping	Rapid formula administration
Technical	
Occluded feeding tube lumen	Insoluble complexation of enteral formula and medication(s)
	Inadequate flushing of feeding tube
	Undissolved feeding formula
Tube displacement	Self-extubation
	Vomiting or coughing
	Inadequate fixation (jejunostomy)
Aspiration	Improper patient or feeding tube position
	Gastroparesis/atony causing regurgitation
	Compromised lower esophageal sphincter
	Diminished gag reflex
Peristomal excoriation	Improper skin and tube care
	GIT secretions leaking peristomally
Infectious	
Aspiration pneumonia	Same as technical-aspiration comments
	Prolonged use of large-bore polyvinylchloride tube

TABLE 55–8. Suggested Monitoring of Enteral Nutrition (EN) to Prevent Complications

Parameter	During Initiation of EN or for a Critically Ill Patient	During Stable EN Therapy or for a Rehabilitating Patient	During Long-term Home EN Therapy
Vital signs: Temperature, respirations, pulse, blood pressure	Every 4–6 h	Every 12–24 h	Tailored to patient's clinical state, routinely done once or twice weekly
Physical exam[a]: Abdomen, lung fields, extremities, mucous membranes, skin turgor	Every 4–6 h	Every 12–24 h	Tailored to patient's clinical state, routinely done once or twice weekly
Clinical assessment: Weight, total intake/output, urine, GI and extra-ordinary fluid losses, stool frequency/consistency/volume, nausea or vomiting	Daily	Daily	Tailored to patient's clinical state, routinely done once or twice weekly
Concurrent medications and administration route	Daily	Daily	Tailored to patient's clinical state, routinely done once or twice weekly
Verification of nasal or oral tube placement with x-ray	Prior to initiating EN	N/A[b]	N/A
Ongoing assessment by tube placement	Every 6 h	Every 12 h	Tailored to patient's clinical state, routinely done once or twice weekly

(continued)

X

TABLE 55–8. continued

Parameter	During Initiation of EN or for a Critically Ill Patient	During Stable EN Therapy or for a Rehabilitating Patient	During Long-term Home EN Therapy
Gastric residual checks	Every 8–12 h	Every 8–12 h	Daily by patient and/or caregiver
Enterostomy tube site assessment for leakage and/or skin irritation/redness	Daily	Daily	Daily by patient and/or caregiver
Patient compliance with feeding procedures and feeding tube/ostomy care	N/A	Daily	Tailored to patient's clinical state, routinely done once or twice weekly
Serum electrolytes, BUN/Cr, serum glucose[c]	Daily	2–3 times/wk	Tailored to patient's clinical state, routinely done weekly
Serum calcium, magnesium, and phosphorus	4–5 times/wk	2–3 times/wk	Tailored to patient's clinical state, routinely done weekly
Liver function tests	Weekly	Monthly	Tailored to patient's clinical state, routinely done monthly
Urine glucose/acetone[c]	Every 6 h	Daily	Tailored to patient's clinical state, routinely done 2–3 times/wk
Trace elements, vitamins	Tailored to patient-specific situations	Tailored to patient-specific situations	Tailored to patient-specific situations

[a]Includes eyes, ears, nose, and throat exams for patients with nasoenteric feeding tubes.
[b]Not applicable.
[c]Frequency of glucose assessment for the nondiabetic patient.
BUN, blood urea nitrogen; Cr, creatinine.

TABLE 55–9. Suggested Monitoring of Enteral Nutrition (EN) to Promote Nutritional Efficacy

Parameter	During Initiation of EN or for a Critically Ill Patient	During Stable EN Therapy or for a Rehabilitating Patient	During Long-term Home EN Therapy
Anthropometrics			
Weight	Daily	Weekly	Weekly
Triceps skinfold	N/A[a]	N/A	Every 1–2 mo
Midarm muscle circumference	N/A	N/A	Every 1–2 mo
Muscle Function			
Level of physical endurance	N/A	Weekly	Weekly to monthly, then tailored to patient situation
Metabolic			
Albumin	Monthly	Monthly	Monthly, then tailored to patient response
Transferrin	Weekly	Weekly	Once to twice monthly, then tailored to patient response
24-h urine urea nitrogen	Weekly	Once or twice monthly	Tailored to patient-specific situations
Indirect calorimetry	Frequency tailored to patient-specific situations	Frequency tailored to patient-specific situations	Tailored to patient-specific situations
Nutritional Intake			
Calories	Daily	2–3 times weekly	Weekly, then tailored to patient situation
Protein, fluid, electrolytes, trace elements, vitamins	Daily	2–3 times weekly	Weekly, then tailored to patient situation
Skin Integrity Wound healing Pressure sore(s)	Daily	Daily	Weekly

[a]Not applicable.

▶ EVALUATION OF THERAPEUTIC OUTCOMES

- Assessing outcome includes monitoring objective measures of body composition, protein and energy balance as well as subjective outcome for physiologic muscle function and wound healing (Table 55–9). Readers can find additional details on assessment in Chapter 54.

See Chapter 129, Enteral Nutrition, authored by Douglas D. Janson, PharmD, BCNSP, for a more detailed discussion of this topic.

Chapter 56

▶ OBESITY

▶ DEFINITION

Obesity is the state of excess body fat stores, which can be defined epidemiologically or physiologically. Obesity should be distinguished from overweight, which refers to excess body weight relative to a person's height.

▶ PATHOPHYSIOLOGY

ETIOLOGY

- The etiology of obesity is usually unknown, but it is likely related to varying contributions from environmental, genetic, and physiologic factors.
- Environmental factors include reduced physical activity or work; abundant and readily available food supply; increased fat intake; increased consumption of refined simple sugars; and decreased ingestion of vegetables, fruits, and complex carbohydrates.
- Excess caloric intake is a prerequisite to weight gain and obesity, but whether the primary consideration is total calorie intake or macronutrient composition is debatable.
- Many neurotransmitters, recepters, and peptides stimulate or decrease food intake in humans and animals (Table 56–1), but the findings are not always consistent between animal models and humans.
- Activity is thought to play a role in obesity because increased physical activity is an important component in the management of obesity, but study results are controversial.
- Weight gain can be caused by medical conditions (e.g., hypothyroidism, Cushing's syndrome, hypothalamic lesion) or genetic syndromes (e.g., Prader–Willi syndrome), but these are unusual to rare causes of obesity.
- Genetic factors appear to be the primary determinants of obesity in some individuals, whereas environmental factors are more important in others. The specific gene that codes for obesity is unknown; probably there is more than one gene.

PHYSIOLOGY AND COMORBIDITIES

- The degree of obesity is determined by the net balance of energy ingested relative to energy expended over time. The single largest determinant of energy expenditure is metabolic rate, which is expressed as Resting Energy Expenditure (REE) or Basal Metabolic Rate (BMR). The two terms are frequently used interchangeably because they differ by <10%.
- There are two major types of adipose tissue: (1) white adipose tissue, which manufactures, stores, and releases lipid; and (2) brown adipose

TABLE 56–1. Effects of Various Neurotransmitters, Receptors, and Peptides on Food Intake

Neurotransmitter/ Receptor/Peptide	Action	Food Intake
Norepinephrine	$\Uparrow$ Concentration	$\Downarrow$
α_1	Stimulates receptor	$\Downarrow$
α_2	Stimulates receptor	$\Uparrow$
β_2	Stimulates receptor	$\Downarrow$
Serotonin	$\Uparrow$ Concentration	$\Downarrow$
5-HT_{1A}	Stimulates receptor	$\Uparrow$
5-HT_{1B}	Stimulates receptor	$\Downarrow$
5-HT_{2C}	Stimulates receptor	$\Downarrow$
Histamine		
H_1	Stimulates receptor	$\Downarrow$
H_3	Stimulates receptor	$\Downarrow$
Dopamine		
D_1	Stimulates receptor	$\Downarrow$
D_2	Stimulates receptor	$\Downarrow$
Leptin	$\Uparrow$ Concentration	$\Downarrow$
Neuropeptide Y	$\Uparrow$ Concentration	$\Uparrow$
Galanin	$\Uparrow$ Concentration	$\Uparrow$

tissue, which dissipates energy via uncoupled mitochondrial respiration. Obesity research includes evaluation of the activity of adrenergic receptors and their effect on adipose tissue with respect to energy storage and expenditure or thermogenesis. X

- Obesity is associated with serious health risks and increased mortality. Hypertension, hyperlipidemia, insulin resistance, and glucose intolerance are known cardiac risk factors that cluster in obese individuals. Additional comorbidities are left ventricular hypertrophy, congestive heart failure, coronary artery disease, obstructive airway disease, sleep apnea, pulmonary hypertension, polycystic ovary syndrome, increased serum urate, degenerative joint disease, acanthosis nigricans, stretch marks, hirsutism, cholelithiasis, esophageal reflux, hiatal hernia, eating disorders, depression, affective disorders, social stigma, and breast and colon cancer.

► CLINICAL PRESENTATION AND DIAGNOSIS

- There are many definitions of clinical obesity and, therefore, methods to diagnose it.
- Excess body fat can be determined by skinfold thickness, body density using underwater body weight, bioelectrical impedance and conductiv-

ity, dual-energy X-ray absorptiometry (DEXA), computerized axial tomography (CT scan), and magnetic resonance imaging (MRI). Unfortunately, methods that measure body fat directly are often expensive and time consuming.

- Normal body mass index (BMI), defined as weight (kg) divided by height (m^2), is 20 to 24.9 for males and females; overweight is >27.8 and >27.3, respectively; and severe overweight is >31.1 and >32.3, respectively.
- Central obesity is best estimated by imaging techniques (e.g., CT scan or MRI), but it is more easily estimated by a high-low waist-to-hip ratio (WHR) of ≥1.0 for men and ≥0.9 for women or waist circumference (WC) of ≥40 inches for men and ≥35 inches for women.
- Although the criteria for normal weight are unknown, life insurance data have been used to provide weight ranges or ideal body weight (IBW) for height and frame size. A person is overweight if he or she is 10% more than his or her IBW, and obese if he or she is 20% more than his or her IBW.

▶ DESIRED OUTCOME

- The goal of therapy should be reasonable and should consider factors such as comorbidities, initial body weight, patient motivation and desire, and patient age. If, for example, the primary goal is improved blood glucose, blood cholesterol, or hypertension, then the end point should be target levels of glycosylated hemoglobin, LDL cholesterol, or blood pressure; weight loss goals may be as little as 5%. If the primary goal is relief of osteoarthritis or sleep apnea, then weight loss of 10% or 20% may be more appropriate.

▶ TREATMENT

- Successful obesity treatment plans incorporate diet, exercise, behavior modification with or without pharmacologic therapy, and/or surgery (Figure 56–1).
- The primary aim of behavior modification is to help patients choose life-styles conducive to safe and sustained weight loss. Behavioral therapy is based on principles of human learning, which use stimulus control and reinforcement to substitute desirable for learned, undesirable behavior.
- Many diets exist to aid weight loss. Regardless of the program, energy consumption must be less than energy expenditure, but highly restrictive diets often yield disappointing long-term results.
- Surgery, which reduces the absorptive surface of the alimentary tract or stomach volume, remains the most effective intervention for moderate to severe obesity. Modern techniques have an operative mortality of <1% and are safer than older procedures, but there are still many poten-

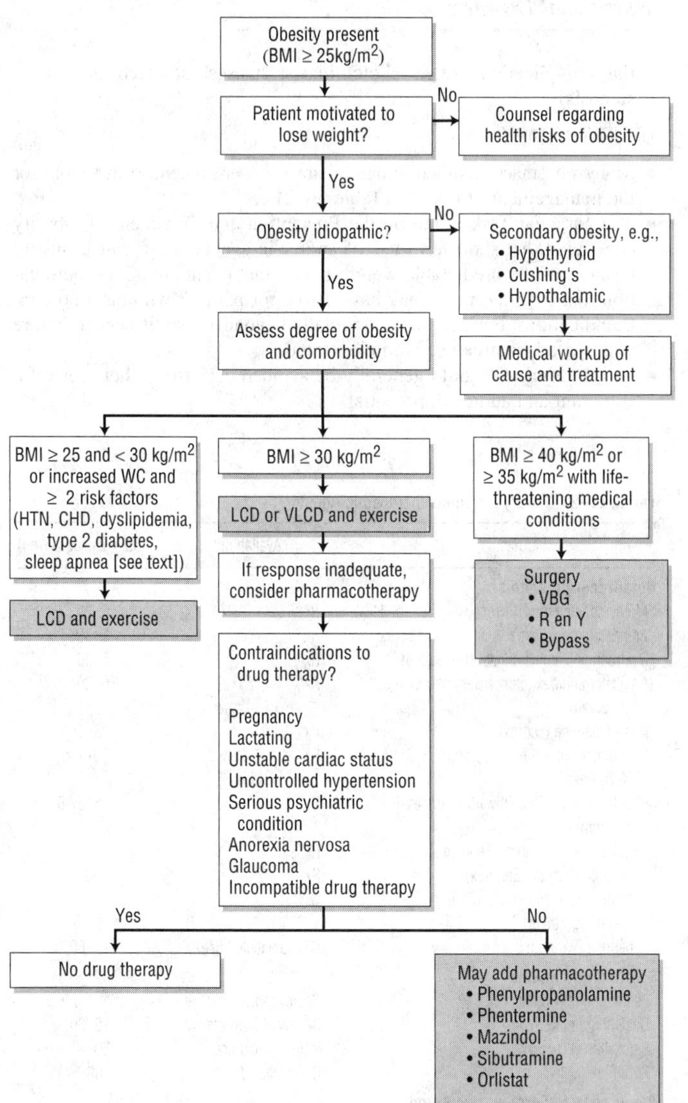

Figure 56–1. Pharmacotherapy treatment algorithm. A select population of individuals may benefit from medication therapy as an adjunct to a program of weight loss that includes diet, exercise, and behavioral modification. (BMI = body mass index; LCD = low-calorie diet; VLCD = very-low-calorie diet; VBG = vertically banded gastroplasty; R en Y = roux-en-y.)

tial complications (e.g., cholelithiasis, nausea, stomach ulceration, stenosis).

DRUG THERAPY

- Many pharmacotherapeutic agents are (or were recently) available for the management of obesity (Table 56–2).
- The National Task Force on the Prevention and Treatment of Obesity concluded that short-term use of anorectic agents is difficult to justify because of the predictable weight regain that occurs upon discontinuation, but long-term use may have a role for patients who have no contraindications. Further study, especially beyond 1 year, is needed before widespread, routine use is implemented.
- **Amphetamines** should generally be avoided because of their powerful stimulant and addictive potential.

TABLE 56–2. Obesity Pharmacotherapeutic Agents

Class	Availability	Daily Dosages (mg)
Noradrenergic Agents		
Methamphetamine HCl (desoxyephedrine HCl)	Rx[a]	5–15
Amphetamine sulfate	Rx[a]	5–30
Dextroamphetamine sulfate (Dexedrine)	Rx[a]	5–30
Amphetamine/dextroamphetamine mixtures (Adderall)	Rx[a]	5–30
Benzphetamine (Didrex)	Rx[a]	25–150
Phendimetrazine (Prelu-2, Bontril, Plegine, X-Trazine)	Rx	70–105
Phentermine (Fastin, Oby-trim, Adipex-P, Ionamin)	Rx	15–37.5
Diethylpropion (Tenuate, Tenuate Dospan)	Rx	75
Mazindol (Mazanor, Sanorex)	Rx	1–3
Phenylpropanolamine (Accutrim, Dexatrim, others)	OTC	75
Ephedrine (various)	OTC/unlabeled use	20–60
Serotonergic Agents		
Fenfluramine (Pondamin)	Removed from market	60–120
Dexfenfluramine (Redux)	Removed from market	15–30
Fluoxetine (Prozac)	Rx/unlabeled use	60
Sertraline (Zoloft)	Rx/unlabeled use	200
Noradrenergic/Serotonergic Agent		
Sibutramine (Meridia)	Rx	5–15
Gastrointestinal Lipase Inhibitor		
Orlistat (Xenical)	Rx/pending release	150–360

R_x, prescription; OTC, over the counter.
[a]High abuse potential, not recommended for routine use.

- **Phentermine** (30 mg in the morning or 8 mg before meals) has less powerful stimulant activity and lower abuse potential than amphetamines, and was an effective adjunct in placebo-controlled studies. Adverse effects (e.g., increased blood pressure, palpitations, arrhythmias, mydriasis, altered insulin or oral hypoglycemic requirements) have implications for patient selection.
- **Mazindol** (1–3 mg before breakfast or 1 mg before meals) has less powerful stimulant activity than phentermine and was an effective short-term therapy in placebo-controlled trials. As with phentermine, contraindications include monoamine oxidase inhibitor (MAOI) use, glaucoma, symptomatic cardiovascular disease, and stimulant substance abuse; however, mazindol may be safer for diabetic patients.
- **Diethylpropion** (25 mg before meals) has less powerful stimulant activity than mazindol and was more effective than placebo in achieving short-term weight loss. Diethylpropion is one of the safest noradrenergic appetite suppressants and can be used in patients with mild to moderate hypertension or angina, but it should not be used in patients with severe hypertension or significant cardiovascular disease.
- **Phenylpropanolamine** was more effective than placebo, but less effective than prescription anorectics, in a meta-analysis. Most adverse events are self-limited, but there are case reports of hypertensive crisis, intracranial hemorrhage, and seizure.
- **Ephedrine** (20 mg with or without caffeine 200 mg up to three times daily) had better appetite-suppressive and thermogenic activity than placebo in trials lasting up to 6 months. The most common side effects are tremor, agitation, nervousness, increased sweating, and insomnia; palpitations and tachycardia have also been reported.
- Serotonergic agents lack the central stimulant effects and abuse potential associated with noradrenergic compounds, but serotonergic agents can alter sleep patterns and change affect.
- **Fenfluramine** was withdrawn from the market in 1997 because of reports of cardiac valvular insufficiency and structural abnormalities. Fenfluramine was more effective than placebo, especially when combined with phentermine (Fen/Phen); the combination was also safer.
- **Dexfenfluramine** was also removed from the market because of potential cardiac valve problems.
- Patients receiving **fluoxetine** (60 mg daily) had an initial weight loss of 2–4 kg in placebo-controlled trials, but there were no differences between groups over periods of ≤1 year. Similar findings have been noted with **sertraline** (200 mg daily).
- **Sibutramine** (5–15 mg daily), marketed in 1998, was more effective than placebo, but patients tended to regain weight after 6 months of treatment. Dry mouth, anorexia, insomnia, constipation, increased appetite, dizziness, and nausea occur two to three times more often than with placebo. Sibutramine should not be used in patients with coronary artery disease, stroke, congestive heart failure, arrhythmias, or MAOI therapy.

- **Orlistat** induces weight loss by lowering dietary fat absorption and was more effective than placebo after 1 year. Soft stools, abdominal pain/colic, flatulence, and/or fecal urgency/incontinence occur in 80% of individuals, are mild to moderate in severity, and improve after 1–2 months of therapy. Orlistat interferes with the absorption of fat-soluble vitamins. Approval was delayed because of breast cancer in 0.6% of patients.
- Peptides (e.g., leptin, neuropeptide Y, galanin) are being investigated because exogenous manipulation may provide future therapeutic approaches to the management of obesity.
- Herbal, natural, and food-supplement products are used to promote weight loss (Table 56–3). The Food and Drug Administration does not strictly regulate these products, so the ingredients may be inactive and present in variable concentrations. **Chromium** failed to demonstrate effectiveness in a double-blind, placebo-controlled trial. These products are not inherently safer than prescription drugs; more than 800 reports of serious adverse events (e.g., seizures, stroke, death) were attributed to **Ma Huang.**

SEVERE ADVERSE EFFECTS

- Severe adverse effects have been reported with almost all appetite suppressants.
- Primary pulmonary hypertension (PPH) is possible with the use of some noradrenergic and serotonergic appetite suppressants, either alone or in combination (e.g., fenfluramine derivatives).

TABLE 56–3. Weight Loss Agents in Herbal, Natural, and Food Supplements[a]

Herbal/Natural/ Food Supplements	Active Moiety	Proposed Effect
Chromium picolinate	Chromium	Unclear
Ma Huang	Ephedrine derivatives	Noradrenergic
St. John's wort	Hypericin	Serotonergic/MAO inhibition
White willow bark	Salicylate	Inhibit norepinephrine breakdown
Calcium pyruvate	Pyruvate	Unclear
Guarana extract	Caffeine	Noradrenergic
Various tea extracts	Caffeine	Noradrenergic
Garcinia gambogia extract (citrin)	Hydroxycitric acid	Unclear

[a]Safety and efficacy not documented.

TABLE 57–1. Indications for TPN

1. Inability to absorb nutrients via the gastrointestinal tract because of one or more of the following:
   a. Massive small bowel resection
   b. Intractable vomiting when adequate enteral intake is not expected for 5–7 d
   c. Severe diarrhea not expected to resolve in 5–7 d
   d. Inflammatory bowel disease (Crohn's disease, ulcerative colitis): PN may benefit patients with acute exacerbations of ulcerative colitis when surgery is being considered and when preservation of lean body mass and functional capacity with enteral nutrition is impossible
   e. Bowel obstruction
2. Cancer–antineoplastic therapy, radiation therapy, bone marrow transplantation: PN (or enteral nutrition) may benefit some severely malnourished cancer patients or those in whom oral nutritional intake will be inadequate for > 1 wk. If indicated, nutrition support should be initiated in conjunction with oncologic therapy

   Specialized nutrition support is not routinely indicated for well-nourished or mildly malnourished patients undergoing surgery, chemotherapy, or radiation treatment and in whom adequate oral intake is anticipated

   PN is unlikely to benefit patients with advanced cancer unresponsive to chemotherapy or radiation therapy
3. Moderate to severe pancreatitis when adequate enteral intake is not expected for 5–7 d: PN should be used when enteral feeding exacerbates abdominal pain, ascites, or fistula output in patients with pancreatitis and limited oral intake
4. Severe malnutrition[a] with a temporary (5–7 d) nonfunctional gastrointestinal tract
5. Critical care: Moderate to severe catabolism with or without malnutrition when the gastrointestinal tract is nonfunctional for 5–7 d (e.g., major surgery, trauma, sepsis)
6. Organ failures—liver, renal, respiratory: Moderate to severe catabolism with or without malnutrition when enteral feeding is contraindicated
7. Preoperative malnutrition[a] when the gastrointestinal tract is nonfunctional and surgery is not expected for at least 7 d
8. Hyperemesis gravidarum
9. Eating disorders: PN should be considered for patients with anorexia nervosa who require nonvolitional feeding but who cannot tolerate enteral support for physical or emotional reasons

[a]Malnutrition (upon initial assessment): 0–5% weight loss over past 6 months and serum albumin <3.0 g/% 10–15% weight loss over past 6 months and serum albumin <3.5 g/%, or loss of 10 % of pre-illness weight and decreased serum albumin.

Macronutrients

- Macronutrients are generally used for energy (dextrose, fat) and as structural substrates (protein, fats) (Table 57–2).

Amino Acids

- Protein is provided as crystalline amino acids (CAAs).
- When oxidized, each gram of protein yields 4 kcal; however, including the caloric contribution from protein is controversial because amino acids are also a substrate for protein synthesis. Therefore, calories provided by a PN regimen may be calculated as total or nonprotein calories.

TABLE 57–2. Macronutrient Components of Parenteral Nutrition Solutions

Nutritional Substrate	Intravenous Source	Commercial Product (Manufacturer)	Comments
Fluid	Sterile water for injection USP	Various manufacturers	
Nitrogen	Crystalline amino acids		
	• Standard solutions	Aminosyn (Abbott) Aminosyn II (Abbott) FreAmine III (McGaw) Travasol (Travenol) Clinisol (Clintec)	Balanced profile of essential, semiessential, and nonessential L-amino acids
	• Disease-specific solutions		
	Hepatic encephalopathy	Aminosyn HF (Abbott) Hepatasol (Clintec) Hepatamine (McGaw)	Higher concentrations of BCAA, and lower concentrations of AAA and methionine
	Renal failure	Aminosyn RF (Abbott) RenAmine (Clintec) Aminess (Clintec) NephrAmine (R & D Laboratories)	Higher concentrations of EAA and histidine
	Metabolic stress/trauma	Aminosyn HBC (Abbott) BranchAmin[a] (Clintec) FreAmine HBC (McGaw)	Standard essential, semiessential, and nonessential amino acids with higher concentrations of BCAA
	Pediatrics	Aminosyn PF (Abbott) Trophamine (McGaw)	Standard essential, semiessential, and nonessential amino acids with lower concentrations of methionine, phenylalanine, glycine; plus taurine, glutamate, and aspartate

	Intravenous dipeptides		
	• L-Alanyl-L-glutamine	Investigational	
	• Glycyl-L-tyrosine	Investigational	
	• L-Alanyl-L-tyrosine	Investigational	
	• *N*-acetyl-L-tyrosine	Used in Trophamine (McGaw)	
Energy			
Carbohydrate	Dextrose	Various manufacturers	
	Glycerol	Used in Procalamine (McGaw)	Non–insulin-dependent carbohydrate
	Xylitol	Investigational	Non–insulin-dependent carbohydrate
Fat	Intravenous fat emulsion		
	• LCT emulsions	Liposyn II (Abbott)	Soybean/safflower
	{oil source}	Liposyn III (Abbott)	Soybean
		Intralipid (Clintec)	Soybean
		Neutrilipid (McGaw)	Soybean
	• LCT/MCT combination	Investigational	
	• Short-chain fatty acids	Investigational	
	• Omega-3 fatty acids	Investigational	

BCAA, branched-chain amino acids (leucine, isoleucine, valine); AAA, aromatic amino acids (includes phenylalanine and tyrosine); EAA, essential amino acids (leucine, isoleucine, valine, phenylalanine, tryptophan, methionine, threonine, and lysine); LCT, long-chain triglycerides; MCT, medium-chain triglycerides.

[a]Used as a supplement to a standard amino acid solution to increase BCAA content.

X

- Available standard products are designed for patients with "normal" organ function and nutritional requirements. Although they differ in amino acid, total nitrogen, and electrolyte content, these standard CAA products yield similar effects on protein markers.
- Higher concentrated CAA solutions (i.e., 10% and 15%) are attractive for critically ill patients who have large protein needs but are fluid restricted.
- Modified amino acid solutions are designed for patients who have altered protein requirements owing to hepatic encephalopathy, renal failure, metabolic stress/trauma, or young age. However, these solutions tend to be expensive and their clinical role in disease-specific PN regimens is controversial.
- Dipeptide amino acids are being investigated as a potential parenteral source for conditionally essential amino acids (CEAAs), but further study is required to assess their long-term safety and effectiveness.

Dextrose

- Carbohydrate, usually as dextrose monohydrate, is available in concentrations ranging from 5–70%. When oxidized, each gram of hydrated dextrose provides 3.4 kcal.
- Recommended doses for routine clinical care rarely exceed 5 mg/kg/min; higher infusion rates may contribute to metabolic complications.
- Non–insulin-dependent sources of carbohydrate are used to avoid stress-related hyperglycemia in critically ill patients. A major disadvantage of the commercially available glycerol solution is the dilute concentrations of carbohydrates and amino acids (3% of each); most patients require 3–4 L of Procalamine solution and supplemental IVLE to meet minimal energy requirements.

Lipid Emulsion

X

- Lipid emulsion may be used as a concentrated source of calories as well as a source of essential fatty acids (EFAs).
- Current IVLE products differ in source of triglycerides, fatty acid content, and concentrations (10–30%) (see Table 57–2).
- When oxidized, 1 g of fat yields 9 kcal. Because of the caloric contribution from egg phospholipid and glycerol, caloric content of IVLE is about 1 kcal/mL per 10% emulsion.
- As a caloric source, lipid emulsion is probably most useful for metabolic stress, pancreatitis or diabetes, and carbon dioxide-retaining ventilator dependency. Infusion of approximately 1–1.5 g/kg/d, not to exceed 30–40% of total calories, over 24 hours appears to be the best strategy for providing IVLE.
- Essential fatty acid deficiency (EFAD) may be prevented by giving 500 mL of 10% IVLE two to three times weekly.
- Infusions over 24 hours eliminate the need for a test dose.
- Available 10% and 20% IVLE products may be administered by central or peripheral vein, added directly to PN solution as a total nutrient

admixture (TNA) or 3-in-1 system (lipids, protein, glucose, and additives), or piggybacked with the CAA/dextrose solution.

- IVLE use is contraindicated if patients have impaired ability to clear lipid emulsion or history of severe egg allergy.

Micronutrients: Vitamins, Trace Elements, and Electrolytes

- Micronutrients are required in small amounts to support metabolic activities for cellular homeostasis such as enzymatic reactions, fluid balance, and regulation of electrophysiologic processes.
- Multiple vitamin products have been formulated to comply with guidelines established by the Nutrition-Advisory Group of the American Medical Association (NAG–AMA). These products do not contain vitamin K, which may be given intramuscularly or subcutaneously or added to the PN solution; weekly dose recommendations for adults range from 2–10 mg.
- Routine use of trace elements during short-term PN is controversial. Requirements for trace elements are age specific and depend on the clinical condition of the patient (e.g., higher doses of supplemental zinc in patients with high-output ostomies or diarrhea). Because requirements for trace elements during organ failure are not clearly defined, the recommended daily dose of a multiple trace element solution may be reduced empirically and given two to three times weekly.
- Patients who have normal organ function and serum electrolyte concentrations should receive normal maintenance doses of electrolytes on initiation of PN and daily thereafter. Requirements for specific electrolytes will vary according to the disease state, organ function, previous and current drug therapy, nutrition status, and extrarenal losses.

DESIGNING PN REGIMENS

- Peripheral PN (PPN) is a relatively safe and simple method of nutritional support. PPN candidates do not have large nutritional requirements, are not fluid restricted, and are expected to begin enteral intake within 7–10 days. Advantages of PPN include a lower risk of infectious, metabolic, and technical complications associated with central vein catheterization. Complications include limited peripheral venous access in some patients, poor tolerance of peripheral veins to hypertonic solutions, and thrombophlebitis.
- Central PN (CPN) is useful in patients who require PN for >7–10 days and who have large nutrient requirements, poor peripheral venous access, or fluctuating fluid requirements. Disadvantages of CPN include risks of catheter insertion, routine use of catheter, and care of the access site.
- Formulas (Figure 57–1) and computer programs are available for calculating volumes of solutions for PN regimens.
- If CAA/dextrose is infused separately from IVLE, two clinically useful and highly concentrated base solutions are 7% CAA/15% dextrose

(final concentrations), which can be prepared from 10% CAA and 70% dextrose stock solutions, or 8% CAA/25% dextrose (final concentrations), compounded from 15% CAA and 70% dextrose stock solutions.

COMPOUNDING AND STORING PN SOLUTIONS

- The two major PN solutions are traditional CAA/dextrose combination, with or without IVLE piggybacked into the PN line, and TNAs.
- Advantages of TNA solutions include reduced inventory (infusion pumps, tubing, and other related supplies), decreased time for compounding and administration, potential decrease in infusion-line manipulations and decreased risk of catheter contamination, and ease of delivery and storage for home PN. Disadvantages include infectious, stability, and compatibility concerns. For example, the opaque solution that results after adding IVLE confounds detection of particulate matter. TNA solutions cannot be filtered with a bacterial-retentive 0.22-μm filter.
- Bacterial growth is least likely with CAA/dextrose, greatest with IVLE, and intermediate with TNA. CAA/dextrose solutions that are not administered within 1 hour after admixing should be refrigerated and used within 24 hours. Many institutions allow expiration times up to 24 hours for IVLE infusions. TNA can be safely administered over 24 hours.

The total daily volume of a PN solution may be based upon a patient's maintenance fluid requirements or an approximation of the minimum volume may be determined by calculating the volumes of stock solutions required to provide the daily nutrients desired as illustrated below.

X

Case: A patient's estimated nutritional requirements are approximately 95–105 g protein/d and 1800–2100 nonprotein kcal/d. The patient has no history of hyperlipidemia or allergy to eggs, and is not fluid restricted. The PN solution will be compounded as an individualized regimen utilizing a single bag, 24-hour infusion of a CAA/dextrose combination with IVLE piggy-backed into the PN infusion line. The stock solutions used to compound this regimen are 10% CAA and 70% dextrose.

Step 1: Determine the volume of IVLE required (see text for IVLE dosing guidelines)

2000 kcal/d x 30 – 40% of total as fat = 600–800 kcal

The most clinically reasonable choice of IVLE product for this regimen is IVLE 20% 250 mL/d or IVLE 10% 500 mL/d.

IVLE 20% 250 mL/d x 2 kcal/mL = 500 kcal/d
IVLE 10% 500 mL/d x 1.1 kcal/mL = 550 kcal/d

2000 kcal/d	Estimated daily nonprotein calorie requirements
–500 kcal/d	IVLE calories
1500	kcal needed from dextrose

Figure 57–1. Calculations for compounding a parenteral nutrition regimen.

Step 2: Calculate the volume of 10% CAA stock solution required to provide 100 g protein

$$\frac{100 \text{ g protein}}{\mathbf{X} \text{ mL}} = \frac{10 \text{ g protein}}{100 \text{ mL}} \qquad \mathbf{X} = 1000 \text{ mL } 10\% \text{ CAA}$$

Step 3: Calculate the volume of 70% dextrose required to provide 1500 calories

$$\begin{array}{l} 1500 \text{ kcal/d} \\ \underline{\div\, 3.4 \text{ kcal/g dextrose}} \\ 441 \text{ g dextrose} \end{array} \qquad \frac{441 \text{ g dextrose}}{\mathbf{X} \text{ mL}} = \frac{70 \text{ g dextrose}}{100 \text{ mL}}$$

$$\mathbf{X} = 630 \text{ mL } 70\% \text{ dextrose}$$

Step 4: Determine the infusion rate

Total base volume:	1000 mL 10% CAA
	+ 630 mL 70% dextrose
	1630 mL base solution
	+ 50–100 mL/L for additives
Total PN volume =	1700–1800 mL/d or 70–75 mL/h

Step 5: Calculate the PN order

Choose 75 mL/h or 1800 mL/d for PN volume

$$\frac{100 \text{ g protein}}{1800 \text{ mL}} = \frac{\mathbf{X} \text{ g protein}}{100 \text{ mL}} \qquad \mathbf{X} = 5.6\% \text{ CAA (round down to } 5.5\%)$$

$$\frac{441 \text{ g dextrose}}{1800 \text{ mL}} = \frac{\mathbf{X} \text{ g dextrose}}{100 \text{ mL}} \qquad \mathbf{X} = 24.5\% \text{ CAA (round up to } 25\%)$$

Final PN order (base solution): 5.5% CAA/25% dextrose at 75 mL/h + IVLE 20% 250 mL/d

This regimen provides approximately 99 g protein/d and 2030 nonprotein calories/d

Figure 57–1. continued

- Because of their complexity, PN solutions are prone to stability and compatibility problems. CAA/dextrose solutions are generally stable for 1–2 months if refrigerated at 4°C and protected from light.
- Factors affecting TNA solution stability include pH, electrolyte charges, temperature, and time after compounding. In general, electrolytes (except phosphorus) and trace elements should be added to the dextrose solution, phosphate should be added to the CAA solution, and

the amino acid solution should be added to the IVLE before or with the dextrose solution. TNA solutions should be infused within 24–48 hours after compounding, but certain TNA solutions are stable for 10–28 days when refrigerated at 4–5°C.

- Risk factors for precipitation of calcium and phosphorus include high concentrations of calcium and phosphorus salts, use of chloride salt of calcium, decreased amino acid concentrations, increased solution temperature, increased solution pH, use of improper sequence when mixing calcium and phosphorus salts, and presence of other additives including IVLE.
- Bicarbonate should not be added to acidic PN solutions; a bicarbonate precursor salt (e.g., acetate) is usually preferred.
- Vitamins may be adversely affected by changes in solution pH, other additives, storage time, solution temperature, and exposure to light. Vitamins should be added to PN solution near the time of administration and should not be in the PN solution >24 hours.
- Advantages of using PN admixtures as drug vehicles include consolidation of dosage units, improved pharmacotherapy for certain drugs, conservation of fluid in volume-restricted patients, fewer venous catheter violations, and decreased compounding and administration time. Disadvantages are lack of compatibility and stability data in the PN solutions. Medications frequently added to PN solutions include albumin, aminophylline, hydrochloric acid, regular insulin, and histamine-2 antagonists.

ADMINISTERING PN SOLUTIONS

- PN solutions should be administered with an infusion pump.
- A 0.22-µm filter is recommended for CAA/dextrose solutions to remove particulate matter, air, and microorganisms.
- Because IVLE particles measure approximately 0.5 µm, IVLE should be administered separately and piggybacked into the PN line beyond the in-line filter.
- Routine use of in-line filters (>0.22 µm) with TNA solutions is controversial. A 1.2-µm filter may prevent catheter occlusion due to precipitates or lipid aggregates, and may also remove *Candida albicans*.
- Although protocols for initiating PN differ, many institutions gradually increase the rate over 24–48 hours to prevent hyperglycemia.
- Cyclic PN (e.g., for 12 to 18 hours/d) is useful in hospitalized patients who have limited venous access and who require other medications necessitating interruption of PN infusion, to prevent or treat hepatotoxicities associated with continuous PN therapy, and to allow home patients to resume normal lifestyles. Cyclic PN may be poorly tolerated by patients with severe glucose intolerance or unstable fluid balance.

COMPLICATIONS

- Mechanical or technical complications include malfunctions in the delivery system (e.g., infusion pump, administration sets or tubing, and

TABLE 57–3. Fluid, Electrolyte, and Acid–Base Abnormalities

Problem	Possible Causes	Intervention
Hypovolemia	Gastrointestinal fluid losses, osmotic diuresis	⇑ Fluid intake
Hypervolemia	Renal failure, excess fluid intake	⇓ Fuid intake and diuretics
Hyponatremia	Gastrointestinal losses, fluid overload, diuretics	Varies with cause
Hypernatremia	Dehydration	⇑ Fluid intake
Hypokalemia	Gastrointestinal losses, diuretics, anabolism	⇑ Potassium intake
Hyperkalemia	Renal failure	⇓ Potassium intake
Hypophosphatemia	Phosphate-binding antacids, anabolism, phosphate-free dialysate	Discontinue phosphate binders; ⇑ phosphorus intake
Hyperphosphatemia	Renal failure	⇓ Phosphorus intake
Hypomagnesemia	Diarrhea, malabsorption, anabolism	⇑ Magnesium intake
Hypermagnesemia	Renal failure	⇓ Magnesium intake
Hypocalcemia	Hypoalbuminemia, chronic renal failure	⇑ Calcium intake (with chronic renal failure only)
Hypercalcemia	Rare	⇓ Calcium intake
Metabolic acidosis	Diarrhea, high-output fistulae, renal failure, excess amino acid intake	Treat underlying causes; ⇑ acetate and ⇓ Cl in PN solution; ⇓ amino acid intake
Metabolic alkalosis	Gastric losses	Treat underlying cause; ⇑ Cl and ⇓ acetate in PN solution

Adapted from Teasley-Strausburg KM, Shronts EP. In:Teasley-Strausburg KM, ed. Nutrition Support Handbook: A Compendium of Products With Guidelines for Usage. *Cincinnati, Harvey Whitney Books, 1992:298–299, with permission.*

catheter). Catheter-related complications are potentially life threatening and include pneumothorax, catheter misdirection into the wrong vein or ill-positioned within the cardiac chambers, arterial puncture, bleeding, hematoma formation, venous thrombosis, and air embolism.

- Infectious complications can be a major hazard in patients receiving central PN. Infections commonly occur when the catheter becomes colonized by direct microbial invasion of the skin at the insertion site or at the infusion site of the catheter.
- Metabolic complications are numerous, potentially fatal if not treated, and related to fluid, electrolyte, and acid–base disorders (Table 57–3) and substrate intolerance (Table 57–4).

TABLE 57–4. Substrate Intolerance in Parenteral Nutrition

Complication	Possible Causes	Intervention
Hyperglycemia	Stress, infection, corticosteroids, pancreatitis, diabetes mellitus, peritoneal dialysis, excess dextrose administration	⇓ Dextrose load (e.g., ⇓ infusion rate or dextrose concentration [e.g., substitute fat calories]); administer insulin
Hypoglycemia (rare)	Abrupt withdrawal of dextrose, insulin overdose	⇑ Dextrose intake; ⇓ exogenous insulin
Excess carbon dioxide production	Excess dextrose intake	⇓ Dextrose intake; balance calories from fat and dextrose
Hyperlipidemia (⇑ cholesterol and triglyceride)	Stress, familial hyperlipidemia, pancreatitis	⇓ Intake of fat or discontinue if indicated
Serum amino acid imbalance	Stress, hepatic failure	Modify or ⇓ intake of amino acids
Abnormal liver function tests (⇑ AST, alkaline phosphatase, and bilirubin)	Stress, infection, cancer, excess carbohydrate intake, excess caloric intake, essential fatty acid deficiency	⇓ Dextrose load (substitute fat); ⇓ total calories; provide EFA

AST, aspartate aminotransferase (SGOT).

Adapted from Teasley-Strausburg KM, Shronts EP. Metabolic and gastrointestinal complications. In: Teasley-Strausburg KM, ed. Nutrition Support Handbook: A Compendium of Products With Guidelines for Usage. *Cincinnati, Harvey Whitney Books, 1992:298–299, with permission.*

▶ EVALUATION OF THERAPEUTIC OUTCOMES

X

- Routine evaluation should include the assessment of the clinical condition of the patient, with a focus on nutritional and metabolic effects of the PN regimen.
- A variety of biochemical and clinical measurements are necessary for effective monitoring of patients receiving PN (Table 57–5).
- Patients receiving their first dose of IVLE should be monitored for acute adverse reactions such as dyspnea, tightness of chest, palpitations, and chills. Headache, nausea, and fever have also been reported and may be associated with a rapid infusion rate. Hepatic abnormalities such as elevated transaminases, hepatomegaly, and intrahepatic cholestasis have been reported with multiple infusions, although these alterations are transient and are usually associated with excessive doses.

See Chapter 128, Parenteral Nutrition, authored by Todd W. Mattox, BCNSP, for a more detailed discussion of this topic.

TABLE 57–5. Routine Monitoring Data for Parenteral Nutrition

Every Day	Two to Three Times/wk	Every Week
Weight	Serum electrolytes (sodium, potassium, chloride, bicarbonate, calcium, magnesium, phosphorus)	Nitrogen balance
Vital signs	Serum glucose	Transferrin or prealbumin
Nutritional intake	Renal function tests (BUN, creatinine)	Triglyceride
Fluid balance		Liver function tests (alkaline phosphatase, AST, ALT, LDH, bilirubin)
Fingerstick glucose as necessary		Other tests as warranted
Serum electrolytes (sodium, potassium, chloride, bicarbonate, glucose)[a]		
Serum glucose[a]		

AST, aspartate aminotransferase (SGOT); ALT, alanine aminotransferase (SGPT); LDH, lactate dehydrogenase; BUN, blood urea nitrogen.
[a]Daily for first 3–4 days.

Oncologic Disorders

Edited by Cindy W. Hamilton, PharmD

Chapter 58

▶ BREAST CANCER

▶ DEFINITION

Breast cancer is the most common cancer and the second leading cause of cancer death in women. It is potentially curable in the early stages, but metastatic breast cancer is usually incurable.

▶ PATHOPHYSIOLOGY

- The two strongest risk factors are female gender and increasing age. Additional risk factors include endocrine factors (e.g., early menarche, nulliparity, late age at first birth, estrogen therapy), environment (e.g., diet, alcohol consumption, radiation exposure), and genetics (e.g., personal and family history, mutations of tumor suppresser genes [BRCA1 and BRCA2]).
- Spread of breast cancer via the bloodstream occurs early in the course of the disease, which results in relapse with systemic metastatic disease after local curative therapy. Tissues most commonly involved with metastases are lymph nodes, skin, bone, liver, lungs, and brain.
- The likelihood of developing metastatic disease is related to size of the primary tumor, lymph node involvement, and additional prognostic factors as described below.

▶ CLINICAL PRESENTATION

- The initial sign in >90% of women with breast cancer is a painless lump that is typically solitary, unilateral, solid, hard, irregular, and nonmobile. In approximately 10% of cases, stabbing or aching pain is the first symptom. Less commonly, nipple discharge, retraction, or dimpling may be noted. In more advanced cases, prominent skin edema, redness, warmth, and induration may be observed.
- Approximately 80% of women first detect some breast abnormalities themselves.
- It is increasingly common for breast cancer to be detected during routine screening mammography in asymptomatic women.
- Symptoms of bone pain, difficulty breathing, abdominal enlargement, jaundice, and mental status changes may occur in metastatic breast cancer.

▶ DIAGNOSIS

- Initial workup for a woman presenting with a localized lesion or other suggestive symptoms should include a careful history, physical examination of the breast, three-dimensional mammography, and possibly other breast imaging techniques such as ultrasound.
- Breast biopsy is indicated for a mammographic abnormality that suggests malignancy or mass that is palpable on physical examination.

▶ STAGING

- Stage is based on the size of the primary tumor (T_{1-4}), presence and extent of lymph node involvement (N_{1-3}), and presence or absence of distant metastases (M). Simplistically stated, these stages may be represented as:

  Early Breast Cancer
  Stage 0: Carcinoma in situ or disease that has not invaded the basement membrane.
  Stage I: Small primary tumor without lymph node involvement.
  Stage II: Metastasis to ipsilateral axillary lymph nodes.

  Advanced Breast Cancer
  Stage III: Usually a large tumor with extensive nodal involvement in which either node or tumor is fixed to the chest wall *(locally advanced disease).*
  Stage IV: Metastases to organs distant from the primary tumor.

- The approximate percent of patients presenting with each stage of breast cancer and an estimate of their 5-year disease-free survival (DFS) are shown in Table 58–1.

XI

TABLE 58–1. Estimated Stage at Presentation and 5-Year Disease-Free Survival: Breast Cancer, 1994

	Percent of Total Cases	5-Year DFS[a] (%)
Stage I	40	70–90
Stage II	40	50–70
Stage III	15	20–30
Stage IV	5	0–10[b]

[a] With current conventional local and systemic therapy.
[b] Patients in stage IV are rarely free of disease, however, 10–20% of these patients may survive with minimal disease for 5–10 y.

▶ PATHOLOGIC EVALUATION

- The pathologic evaluation of breast lesions establishes the histologic diagnosis and presence or absence of prognostic factors.
- The development of malignancy is a multistep process with invasive and preinvasive (or noninvasive) phases.

INVASIVE CARCINOMA

- Most breast carcinomas are adenocarcinomas and are classified as ductal or lobular.
- The five most common types of invasive breast cancer include infiltrating ductal carcinoma (75% of cases), infiltrating lobular carcinoma (5–10%), medullary carcinoma (5–7%), mucinous (or colloid) carcinoma (about 3%), and tubular carcinoma (2%).

NONINVASIVE CARCINOMA

- Carcinoma in situ may be a preinvasive cancer or a marker of unstable epithelium that represents an increased risk for developing aggressive cancer.
- Carcinoma in situ is diagnosed when malignant transformation is present, but the basement membrance is intact.
- In situ lesions can also be divided into ductal and lobular categories. Ductal carcimona in situ (DCIS) is much more common than lobular carcinoma in situ (LCIS).

PROGNOSTIC FACTORS

- Tumor size and the presence and number of involved axillary lymph nodes are primary factors in assessing the risk for breast cancer recurrence and subsequent metastatic disease.
- Hormone receptors are used as indicators of prognosis and to predict response to hormone therapy.

- The rate of tumor cell proliferation, nuclear grade, and tumor (histologic) differentiation are also independent prognostic research factors.
- Additional potential prognostic factors include overexpression of erb B-2 oncogen (also known as HER-2/neu) cathepsin-D, angiogenic growth factors, and mutations in the tumor suppressor p53 gene.

▶ DESIRED OUTCOME

The goal of therapy with early and locally advanced breast cancer is to cure the patient of the disease. However, once breast cancer has advanced beyond a local-regional disease, it is currently incurable. The goals of treatment of metastatic breast cancer are to improve symptoms and quality of life and prolong survival.

▶ TREATMENT

- The approaches to breast cancer treatment are evolving as a result of massive research efforts. Specific information regarding the most promising interventions can be found only in the primary literature.

EARLY BREAST CANCER

Local-Regional Therapy

- Surgery alone can cure most patients with in situ cancers and approximately half of those with stage II cancers.
- *Breast conservation* is an appropriate primary therapy for most women with stages I and II disease; it is preferable to modified radical mastectomy because it produces equivalent survival rates with cosmetically superior results. Breast conservation consists of lumpectomy (also referred to as segmental mastectomy or partial mastectomy) and is defined as excision of the primary tumor and adjacent breast tissue followed by radiation therapy to reduce the risk of local recurrence. Sampling of axillary lymph nodes is recommended for staging and prognostic information.
- *Simple* or *total mastectomy* involves removal of the entire breast without resection of the underlying muscle or axillary nodes. This procedure is used in patients with carcinoma in situ where there is a 1% incidence of axillary node involvement or in cases of local recurrence following breast conservation therapy. Simple mastectomy may be a reasonable alternative for women who wish to avoid the inconvenience of radiation therapy and preserve their option for breast reconstruction in the future.

Systemic Adjuvant Therapy

- *Systemic adjuvant therapy* is the administration of systemic therapy following definitive therapy (surgery, radiation, or both) when there is no evidence of metastatic disease but a high likelihood of recurrence owing to the presence of undetectable micrometastases. The goal of such therapy is cure of disease. XI
- The choice between chemotherapy and hormonal therapy, or both, as adjuvant therapy is evolving.
- Recent data indicate that essentially all women with stage I and stage II breast cancer derive some benefit from chemotherapy, but the absolute benefit is greater in premenopausal women.
- Tamoxifen is indicated in all postmenopausal patients with positive hormone receptors.
- The National Comprehensive Cancer Network (NCCN) practice guidelines reflect the trend toward the use of chemotherapy in all women regardless of menopausal status, and the combination of chemotherapy and hormonal therapy (Figure 58–1).

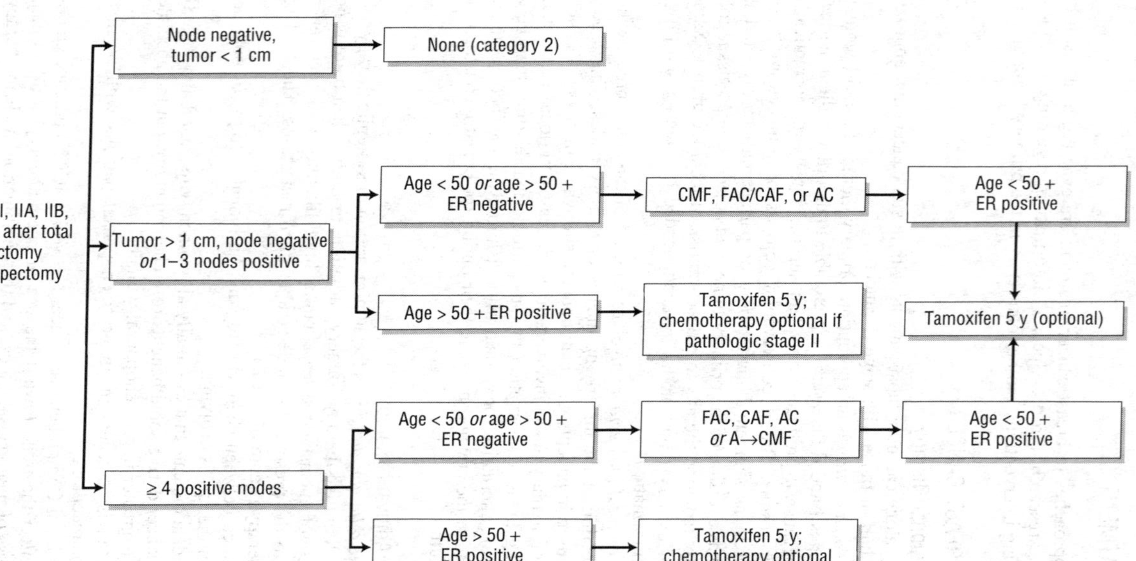

Figure 58–1. NCCN Breast Cancer (Invasive) Guidelines for Adjuvant Treatment. (See text for explanation and abbreviations.)

Adjuvant Chemotherapy

- Many combination regimens are used in the adjuvant setting (Table 58–2), which are typically derived from those that produce the highest response rate in advanced disease.
- Clinical trials are being conducted to evaluate the role of newer agents (e.g., taxanes) as adjuvant therapy, sequential therapy (e.g., **doxorubicin** followed by **cyclophosphamide, methotrexate,** and **fluorouracil** [A→CMF]), neoadjuvant or primary chemotherapy prior to surgery, dose intensity and density, and high-dose chemotherapy followed by infusion of bone marrow or peripheral blood progenitor cells.
- Chemotherapy should be initiated within 3 weeks of surgical removal of the primary tumor. The optimal duration of treatment appears to be about 12–16 weeks.
- The short-term toxic effects of chemotherapy are generally well tolerated in the adjuvant setting, especially with the availability of serotonin-antagonist antiemetics and colony-stimulating factors. Other common side effects include alopecia, weight gain, fatigue, and, in menstruating patients, cessation of menses and symptoms of menopause. Rare effects include deep vein thrombosis, secondary leukemia from cyclophosphamide-based regimens, and doxorubicin-induced cardiomyopathy.

Adjuvant Hormonal Therapy

- **Tamoxifen** is the adjuvant hormonal therapy of choice. Tamoxifen reduces the incidence of contralateral breast cancer and has beneficial estrogenic effects on the cardiovascular system and bone density.
- The optimal dose of tamoxifen appears to be 20 mg as a single daily dose. Therapy is usually initiated shortly after surgery. Most recommendations suggest 5 years of tamoxifen therapy.
- Tamoxifen is usually well tolerated. Symptoms of estrogen withdrawal (hot flashes and vaginal bleeding) may occur but decrease in frequency and intensity over time. A dose- and duration-dependent proliferation of the endometrium has been linked to a twofold increase in endometrial cancer in women receiving 20 mg/d continuously for 5 years.

LOCALLY ADVANCED BREAST CANCER (STAGE III)

- *Locally advanced disease* refers to breast carcinomas with significant primary tumor and nodal disease but no distant metastases. This stage is poorly controlled by radical surgery alone and has a poor prognosis.
- Local-regional therapy of locally advanced disease consists of surgery, radiation, or both. There is apparently no advantage to mastectomy over primary radiation therapy in patients with stage III disease. The benefit of combining mastectomy and radiation is controversial.
- Neoadjuvant or primary chemotherapy, the administration of systemic chemotherapy prior to a definitive local-regional procedure, should be

TABLE 58–2. Chemotherapy of Breast Cancer

AC
Doxorubicin 60 mg/m^2 IV, day 1
Cyclophosphamide 400–600 mg/m^2 IV, day 1
Repeat cycle every 21 days

CAF (FAC)
Cyclophosphamide 100 mg/m^2 PO, days 1–14 or 600 mg/m^2 IV, day 1
Doxorubicin 25 mg/m^2 IV, days 1, 8 or 60 mg/m^2 IV, day 1
Fluorouracil 500–600 mg/m^2 IV, days 1, 8
Repeat cycle every 28 days

or

Cyclophosphamide 500 mg/m^2 IV, day 1
Doxorubicin 50 mg/m^2 IV, day 1
Fluorouracil 500 mg/m^2 IV, day 1[a]
Repeat cycle every 21 days

CFM (CNF, FNC)
Cyclophosphamide 500–600 mg/m^2 IV, day 1
Fluorouracil 500–600 mg/m^2 IV, day 1
Mitoxantrone 10–12 mg/m^2 IV, day 1
Repeat cycle every 21 days

CMF
Cyclophosphamide 100 mg/m^2 PO, days 1–14 or 600 mg/m^2 IV, days 1, 8
Methotrexate 40 mg/m^2 IV, days 1, 8
Fluorouracil 600 mg/m^2 IV, days 1, 8
Repeat cycle every 28 days

or

Cyclophosphamide 600 mg/m^2 IV, day 1
Methotrexate 40 mg/m^2 IV, day 1
Fluorouracil 600 mg/m^2 IV, day 1
Repeat cycle every 21 days

XI

NFL
Mitoxantrone 12 mg/m^2 IV, day 1
Fluorouracil 350 mg/m^2 IV, days 1–3, given after leucovorin
Leucovorin 300 mg IV over 1 h, days 1–3

or

Mitoxantrone 10 mg/m^2 IV, day 1
Fluorouracil 1000 mg/m^2/d CI, days 1–3, given after leucovorin
Leucovorin 100 mg/m^2 IV over 15 min, days 1–3
Repeat cycle every 21 days

Sequential DOX–CMF
Doxorubicin 75 mg/m^2 IV, every 21 days for 4 cycles
Followed by CMF for 8 cycles

VATH
Vinblastine 4.5 mg/m^2 IV, day 1
Doxorubicin 45 mg/m^2 IV, day 1
Thiotepa 12 mg/m^2 IV, day 1
Fluoxymesterone 10 mg PO tid
Repeat cycle every 21 days

Vinorelbine and Doxorubicin
Vinorelbine 25 mg/m^2 IV, days 1, 8
Doxorubicin 50 mg/m^2 IV, day 1
Repeat cycle every 21 days

Single-Agent Regimens

Docetaxel
Docetaxel 60–100 mg/m^2 IV, over 1 h, every 21 days and dexamethasone 8 mg PO bid for 5 days, begin 1 day before docetaxel

Gemcitabine
Gemcitabine 725 mg/m^2 IV, over 30 min, weekly for 3 wk, followed by 1-wk rest
Repeat cycle every 28 days

Paclitaxel[b]
Paclitaxel[b] 250 mg/m^2 IV, over 3 or 24 h, every 21 days

or

Paclitaxel[b] 175 mg/m^2 IV, over 3 h, every 21 days

Vinorelbine
Vinorelbine 30 mg/m^2 IV, every 7 days

[a]Also given on day 8 with FAC.
CI, continuous infusion.

the initial choice of treatment. Neoadjuvant chemotherapy can control micrometastases, reduce tumor bulk, and allow for more limited procedures for local control.

METASTATIC BREAST CANCER (STAGE IV)

The choice of therapy for metastatic disease is based on the site of disease involvement and presence or absence of certain characteristics, as described below.

Endocrine Therapy

- Endocrine therapy is the treatment of choice for patients who are hormone receptor positive and exhibit metastatic disease in soft tissue, bone, or pleura, owing to the equal probability of response to hormonal therapy compared with chemotherapy and the lower toxicity profile of endocrine therapy.
- Patients are sequentially treated with endocrine therapy until they have rapidly growing metastatic disease, at which time cytotoxic chemotherapy can be given.
- Because most endocrine therapies are equally effective, the choice is based primarily on toxicity (Table 58–3).
- **Tamoxifen** is usually the agent of choice in both premenopausal and postmenopausal women who are also hormone receptor positive, even if they received the drug as adjuvant therapy. The maximal beneficial effects are not observed for 2 months or more. In addition to the side effects described previously, a tumor flare or hypercalcemia occurs in approximately 5% of patients after the initiation of therapy for metastatic breast cancer. This may be a positive indication that the patient will respond to endocrine therapy.
- New antiestrogens are being developed, which may maintain tamoxifen's beneficial effects on breast cells, bone, and lipids and avoid its effects on the endometrium. The new antiestrogen **toremifene** appears to be similar to tamoxifen on the basis of efficacy, safety, and cost. Unfortunately, it is not suitable for treating tamoxifen-refractory disease because of cross-resistance.
- Ovarian ablation (oophorectomy) is considered by some specialists to be the endocrine therapy of choice in premenopausal women and produces similar overall response rates to tamoxifen. Medical castration with luteinizing hormone–releasing hormone (LHRH) analogs (**leuprolide** or **goserelin**) is a reversible alternative to ovarian ablation for premenopausal women.
- Aromatase inhibitors reduce circulating estrogens by blocking peripheral conversion from an androgenic precursor, the primary source of estrogens in postmenopausal women. The prototype aromatase inhibitor, **aminoglutethimide,** is considered third-line therapy because of its toxicity profile. Newer agents, **anastrozole** and **letrozole,** are better tolerated.

TABLE 58–3. Endocrine Therapies Used for Metastatic Breast Cancer

Class	Drug	Dose	Side Effects
Antiestrogens	Tamoxifen	10–20 mg PO bid	Disease flare, hot flashes, nausea, vomiting, edema, thromboembolism, endometrial cancer
	Toremifene	60 mg PO qd	
LHRH analogs	Leuprolide	7.5 mg/m^2 SC q 28 d	Amenorrhea, hot flashes, occasional nausea
	Goserelin	3.6 mg/m^2 SC q 28 d	
Progestins	Medroxyprogesterone acetate	400–1000 mg IM qwk	Weight gain, hot flashes, vaginal bleeding, edema, thromboembolism
	Megestrol acetate	40 mg PO qid	
Aromatase inhibitors	Anastrazole	1 mg PO qd	
	Letrozole	2.5 mg PO qd	
	Aminoglutethimide	250 mg PO qid with hydrocortisone 40 mg/d	Lethargy, rash, postural dizziness, ataxia, nystagmus, nausea
Estrogens	Ethinylestradiol	1 mg PO tid	Nausea/vomiting, fluid retention, hot flashes, anorexia, thromboembolism, hepatic dysfunction
	Conjugated estrogens	2.5 mg PO tid	
Androgens	Fluoxymesterone	10 mg PO bid	Deepening voice, alopecia, hirsutism, facial/truncal acne, fluid retention, menstrual irregularities, cholestatic jaundice

- Progestins such as **megesterol acetate** (Megace) and **medroxyprogesterone acetate** (Provera) may be an alternative to first-line therapy with tamoxifen, but they cause fluid retention and edema.
- Estrogens and androgens are used rarely because they are more toxic than other alternatives.

Chemotherapy

- Women with hormone receptor–negative tumors; women with rapidly progressive lung, liver, or bone marrow involvement; or those having failed initial endocrine therapy are not likely to benefit from endocrine therapy and are usually treated with cytotoxic chemotherapy.
- *Combination chemotherapy* produces an objective response in approximately two-thirds of patients previously unexposed to chemotherapy, but complete remissions occur in <20% of patients. The median duration of response is 5–12 months; the median survival is 14–33 months.
- **Anthracyclines** are considered *first-line therapy* and are usually included in first-line combination regimens.
- The objective response rate to *single-agent therapy* is generally lower than with combination therapy and has historically ranged from 20–40%. Newer agents (e.g., **paclitaxel, vinorelbine**) yield response rates of up to 50%; **docetaxel** produces even more impressive response rates of 54–68%. Although response rates are lower in previously treated patients, these newer agents offer useful alternatives for breast cancer that is refractory to anthracyclines. Furthermore, these agents are moving to first-line regimens, often in combination with anthracyclines.
- Docetaxel appears to be associated with less neuropathy, myalgia, and hypersensitivity than paclitaxel, but docetaxel causes more febrile neutropenia, fluid retention, and skin reactions. Docetaxel is given over 1 hour every 3 weeks, whereas paclitaxel is given at different doses and infused over 3 or 24 hours (see Table 58–2).
- Very high doses of single agents or combinations with autologous bone marrow transplant produce high response rates, but the duration of response is brief. Nonetheless, 10–20% of patients who receive high-dose chemotherapy with autologous bone marrow transplantation after obtaining a complete (or near complete) response to conventional chemotherapy appear to be cured of their disease or at least achieve a prolonged disease-free interval.

PREVENTION AND EARLY DETECTION OF BREAST CANCER

- There is increasing interest in *chemoprevention* to inhibit neoplastic development. Tamoxifen 20 mg daily reduced the incidence of breast cancer by 45% in a randomized, placebo-controlled trial of 13,388 women at high risk for developing breast cancer. Questions remain regarding tamoxifen's ability to prevent breast cancer long-term mortality, which women are most likely to benefit, optimal age of initiation and duration of use, and risks of tamoxifen use for >5 years.

- The American Cancer Society recommends that all women over the age of 20 perform monthly breast self-examinations.
- Most guidelines recommend annual *mammography* for women 50 years of age and older.
- The American Cancer Society recommends a baseline mammography between 35 and 40 years of age and screening mammography every 1–2 years in the 40–50-year-old age group. However, in December 1993, the National Cancer Institute withdrew its support of screening mammography in women younger than 50. This controversy remains unresolved.

► EVALUATION OF THERAPEUTIC OUTCOMES

EARLY BREAST CANCER

- The overall goal of adjuvant therapy in early-stage disease is cure, but this goal cannot be fully evaluated for years after initial diagnosis and treatment. Since there is no clinical evidence of disease when adjuvant therapy is administered, assessment of disease response is not possible.
- Adjuvant chemotherapy is often associated with substantial toxicity. Maintaining dose intensity is important in cure of disease, and therefore optimizing supportive care with measures such as antiemetics and growth factors is highly recommended.

METASTATIC BREAST CANCER

- Optimizing quality of life is the therapeutic end point in the treatment of patients with metastatic breast cancer. Many valid and reliable tools are available for objective assessment of quality of life.
- The least toxic therapies are used initially with increasingly aggressive therapies applied in a sequential fashion and in a manner that does not significantly compromise the quality of the patient's life.
- Tumor response is measured by clinical chemistry (e.g., liver enzyme elevation in patients with hepatic metastases) or imaging techniques such as bone scans or chest x-rays.
- Assessment of the clinical status and symptom control of the patient is often adequate to evaluate response to therapy.

See Chapter 116, Breast Cancer, authored by Celeste M. Lindley, PharmD, MS, FCCP, BCPS, for a more detailed discussion of this topic.

Chapter 59

▶ COLORECTAL CANCER

▶ DEFINITION

Colorectal cancer involves the colon, rectum, and anal canal. It is one of the three most common cancers in adults and the third leading cause of cancer-related deaths in the United States.

▶ PATHOPHYSIOLOGY

- Risk increases with increasing age. Multiple factors are associated with development of colorectal cancer, including acquired and inherited genetic susceptibility, environmental elements, and lifestyle. Etiologic and clinical risk factors include high dietary fat intake, low dietary fiber intake, no postmenopausal hormone replacement therapy, chronic ulcerative colitis, Crohn's disease, familial adenomatosis polyposis, and hereditary nonpolyposis colorectal cancer.
- Development of a colorectal neoplasm is a multistep process of genetic and phenotypic alterations of normal bowel epithelium structure and function. Sequential mutations within colonic epithelium result in cellular replication or enhanced invasiveness. Genetic changes include mutational activation of oncogenes and inactivation of tumor suppressor genes.
- Adenocarcinomas account for >90% of tumors of the large intestine. Other histologic types (e.g., mucinous adenocarcinoma, signet ring adenocarcinoma, carcinoid simplex, and carcinoid tumors) occur less frequently.
- The most differentiated adenocarcinomas (i.e., grade I) generally resemble adenomas, whereas the most undifferentiated tumors (i.e., grade III) are considered "high grade" and have frequently lost characteristics of mature normal cells.

▶ CLINICAL MANIFESTATIONS

- Signs and symptoms of colorectal cancer can be extremely varied, subtle, and nonspecific. Patients with early stage colorectal cancer are often asymptomatic.
- Although rectal bleeding and abdominal pain are the most common signs, any change in bowel habits, vague abdominal discomfort, or distention may be warning signs.
- Nausea, vomiting, and abdominal discomfort are often secondary signs of a larger underlying problem such as obstruction, perforation, and/or bleeding.
- Approximately 20–25% of patients with colorectal cancer present with metastatic disease. The most common site of metastasis is the liver, followed by the lungs and then bones.

► DIAGNOSIS

- When colorectal carcinoma is suspected, a careful history and physical examination should be performed to detect risk factors and clinical manifestations.
- The entire large bowel should be evaluated by colonoscopy or sigmoidoscopy and air-contrast barium enema.
- Baseline laboratory tests should include complete blood cell count, platelet count, prothrombin time (PT), activated partial thromboplastin time (aPTT), liver function tests, and serum carcinoembryonic antigen (CEA). Red blood cell indices and workup of iron status may be useful to confirm acute or chronic blood loss and/or iron-deficiency anemia. Serum CEA can serve as a "marker" for colorectal cancer and for monitoring response to treatment, but it is too insensitive and nonspecific to be used as a screening test for early-stage colorectal cancer.
- Radiographic imaging studies may include chest x-ray, bone scan, abdominal computed tomography (CT) scan or ultrasound, intrarectal or transrectal ultrasonography, and intraluminal and hepatic magnetic resonance imaging (MRI) studies.
- Immunodetection of tumors using tumor-directed antibodies is an imaging technique for early detection of colorectal cancers. Examples of radiolabeled monoclonal antibodies include OncoScint CR/OV, CEA-Scan arcitumomab, and HumaSPECT-Tc.

STAGING

- Dukes' classification, originally published in 1932, has traditionally been used to stage colorectal cancers.
- To standardize the staging system, the American Joint Committee on Cancer and the International Union Against Cancer agreed to use the TNM classification. This system considers three aspects of cancer growth: T = *t*umor size, N = lymph *n*ode involvement, and M = presence or absence of *me*tastases.

- Stage of colorectal cancer upon diagnosis is the most important independent prognostic factor for survival and disease recurrence. For example, 5-year survival rates for colorectal cancer drop from approximately 90% for localized disease to <10% for metastatic disease. Stage of disease is also useful for determining initial treatment.

PREVENTION AND SCREENING

- Cancer prevention efforts can be primary or secondary. *Primary prevention* requires identification of etiologic factors followed by eradication or alteration of their effects on carcinogenesis. Promising strategies include dietary supplementation (e.g., fiber, calcium, and antioxidants such as vitamin A), reduction of dietary fat, and chemoprevention (e.g., α-difluoromethylornithine [DFMO] and nonsteroidal anti-inflammatory agents).

- *Secondary prevention* includes procedures that range from colonoscopic removal of precancerous polyps to total colectomy for high-risk individuals.
- American Cancer Society guidelines for average-risk individuals include annual digital rectal examination starting at age 40 years; annual occult fecal blood testing starting at age 50 years with flexible sigmoidoscopy every 5 years, colonoscopy every 10 years, or double-contrast barium enema every 5–10 years; and digital rectal examination at the same time as sigmoidoscopy, colonoscopy, or barium enema.

▶ DESIRED OUTCOME

The goal of treatment depends on the stage of disease at diagnosis. If colorectal cancer is resectable, the goal is to remove the tumor and prevent recurrence. Because metastatic colorectal cancer is incurable, the goal is to alleviate symptoms and preserve quality of life. In either case, treatment decisions require careful assessment of relative risks and benefits.

▶ TREATMENT

GENERAL PRINCIPLES

- Treatment modalities are surgery, radiation therapy, chemotherapy, and immunotherapy. These modalities can be used as primary treatment for resectable disease, adjuvant therapy to be combined with primary treatment, and options for metastatic disease. Each of these therapeutic strategies is addressed separately, later in this chapter.
- Adjuvant therapy is administered after complete tumor resection to eliminate residual local or metastatic microscopic disease.
- Adjuvant therapy is different for colon and rectal cancer because natural history and recurrence patterns are different. Rectal tumors are more difficult to resect with wide margins, so local recurrences are more frequent than with colon cancers. Adjuvant radiation therapy plus chemotherapy is considered standard for stage II/III rectal cancer, and adjuvant chemotherapy is standard for stage III colon cancer. Because most patients with stage I colorectal cancer are cured by surgical resection alone, adjuvant therapy is not indicated. By definition, adjuvant therapy is not indicated for metastatic disease.
- For the best results, chemotherapeutic agents with proven activity should be administered at maximally tolerated doses when the tumor burden is minimal and tumor growth kinetics is optimal.

TREATMENT MODALITIES

Surgery

- Surgical removal of the primary tumor is the treatment of choice for most patients.

- Surgery generally involves complete tumor resection with an appropriate margin of tumor-free bowel and a regional lymphadenectomy.
- Less than one-third of patients require permanent colostomy for rectal cancer. Other surgical complications can include infection, anastomotic leakage, obstruction, adhesions, and malabsorption syndromes. Complications unique to surgery for rectal cancer are urinary retention, incontinence, impotence, and local-regional recurrence.

Radiation Therapy

- Radiation therapy (XRT) can be administered with curative surgical resection to reduce local tumor recurrence, or in advanced or metastatic disease to reduce symptoms.
- Acute adverse effects associated with XRT include hematologic depression, dysuria, diarrhea, abdominal cramping, and proctitis. Chronic symptoms may persist for months following discontinuation of XRT and may involve diarrhea, proctitis, enteritis, small bowel obstruction, perineal tenderness, and impaired wound healing.

Chemotherapy and Biomodulators

- **Fluorouracil** (5-FU) is the most active and widely used chemotherapeutic agent for colorectal cancer. Biochemical modulating agents can be added to 5-FU to modify its activity and improve its response rates.

Fluorouracil and 5-Fluoro-2′-Deoxyuridine

- As a prodrug, 5-FU undergoes anabolism to two active metabolites, 5-fluorouridine-5′-triphosphate (FUTP) and 5-fluorodeoxyuridine-5′-monophosphate (FdUMP). FUTP is incorporated into RNA, thereby impairing protein synthesis. FdUMP bonds with thymidylate synthase (TS), the key enzyme for de novo synthesis of thymidylate, which is a major constituent for DNA synthesis, replication, and repair.
- 5-FU is typically administered by IV bolus once weekly or daily for 5 days each month, or by continuous IV infusion over 5 days. Continuous infusion appears to have more favorable clinical activity.

- 5-Fluoro-2′-deoxyuridine (FUDR; **floxuridine**) produces the same cytotoxic effect as 5-FU through conversion to FdUMP. FUDR can be administered IV, but intrahepatic use is more common.
- Toxicity patterns depend on dose, route, and schedule of administration. Leukopenia is the primary dose-limiting toxicity of IV bolus 5-FU, although diarrhea, stomatitis, nausea, and vomiting can also occur. Stomatitis can be reduced with oral cryotherapy, which involves chewing ice chips and holding them in the mouth for 35 minutes beginning 5 minutes before bolus injection of 5-FU.
- Continuous IV infusion 5-FU is generally well tolerated, but dose-limiting toxicities can be substantial. The most common toxicities are stomatitis and a distinct toxicity, palmar–plantar erythrodysesthesia (hand–foot syndrome), which is characterized by painful swelling and erythroderma of the soles of the feet, palms of the hands, and distal fin-

gers. Although reversible and not life threatening, this skin toxicity can be acutely disabling.

- Complications of hepatic infusion of 5-FU are generally mild and include nausea, vomiting, hematologic depression, hepatotoxicity, and infection.
- Common toxicities of hepatic artery infusion of FUDR include gastric ulceration and hepatobiliary toxicity, which usually require transient interruption of therapy, decreased dosage, or discontinuation of therapy. Rest periods between therapy may prevent or minimize toxicity.
- Combined 5-FU and XRT results in severe hematologic toxicity, enteritis, and diarrhea compared with either chemotherapy or XRT alone.

Levamisole

- **Levamisole** is a synthetic, oral anthelmintic drug with immunomodulatory properties (e.g., T-cell activation, augmented macrophage activity, and enhanced chemotaxis by polymorphonuclear cells and monocytes).
- Levamisole has a synergistic effect when combined in vitro with 5-FU, but the mechanism is unknown.
- Toxicities are generally mild, infrequent, and clinically tolerable. Levamisole is associated with taste abnormalities, arthralgias, myalgias, and rare (<5% of patients) central nervous system (CNS) toxicities (e.g., anxiety, irritability, somnolence, depression, insomnia, agitation, confusion, or cerebellar ataxia). Up to 40% of patients treated with levamisole plus 5-FU show laboratory abnormalities consistent with hepatic toxicity, which are mild, rarely symptomatic, and reversible on discontinuation of therapy.

Leucovorin Calcium (Folinic Acid, Citrovorum Factor)

- **Leucovorin** enhances 5-FU cytotoxicity by increasing intracellular concentrations of reduced folate.
- Leucovorin is generally nontoxic in therapeutic doses, although hypersensitivity reactions (e.g., anaphylaxis and urticaria) have been reported. Combining 5-FU with leucovorin, however, produces greater toxicity to the gastrointestinal epithelium. Dose-limiting toxicities are neutropenia and stomatitis for low-dose leucovorin and diarrhea for high-dose regimens. XI
- Diarrhea should initially be treated with bowel rest, IV fluids, and interruption of chemotherapy until symptoms are resolved. **Loperamide** and **diphenoxylate** can be used for symptomatic treatment. **Octreotide acetate** can be administered subcutaneously at a dosage of 100 μg two or three times daily or 50–150 μg/h via continuous IV infusion for refractory 5-FU–induced diarrhea.

Irinotecan (CPT-11)

- **Irinotecan** inhibits topoisomerase I, an enzyme necessary for DNA replication.

- The most common adverse effects are diarrhea, neutropenia, nausea, vomiting, asthenia, and alopecia.
- There are two patterns of diarrhea. Early-onset diarrhea occurs within 6 hours after irinotecan administration; is characterized by lacrimation, diaphoresis, abdominal cramping, flushing, and diarrhea; and responds to **atropine** 0.25–1 mg IV or subcutaneously. Late-onset diarrhea appears ≥1–12 days after drug administration; can last for 3–5 days; and can result in hospitalization or death. High-dose, oral loperamide (4 mg) should be started immediately and followed by 2 mg every 2 hours until symptom free for 12 hours.

Interferon

- **Interferon** (IFN) may enhance the cytotoxic activity of 5-FU by pharmacokinetic mechanisms (e.g., decreasing 5-FU clearance) or pharmacologic mechanisms (e.g., decreasing thymidine kinase activity).
- Toxicities of combination therapy include flu-like symptoms, lethargy, stomatitis, and leukopenia. Most toxicities resolve spontaneously or upon dose reduction or discontinuation of IFN or 5-FU.

Other Agents

- **Methotrexate** blocks purine nucleotide synthesis, which ultimately increases intracellular concentrations of a substrate that promotes 5-FU conversion to its active metabolites and provides the rationale for sequential therapy. Common toxicities include mucositis and leukopenia.
- **Trimetrexate** has the following advantages over methotrexate: (1) increased lipophilicity, (2) activity that does not require activation by folylpolyglutamate synthase, (3) intracellular uptake that does not compete with leucovorin, (4) broader spectrum of activity, and (5) activity against methotrexate-resistant cells. Dose-limiting toxicities are leukopenia; thrombocytopenia; and, in combination with 5-FU and leucovorin, diarrhea.
- *N*-(Phosphonacetyl)-L-aspartate **(PALA)** inhibits pyrimidine synthesis, but it is inactive as a single agent. The toxicity of PALA and 5-FU is generally similar to that of 5-FU alone, but a syndrome of ascites, hyperbilirubinemia, and hypoalbuminemia with elevated liver function tests has been attributed to the combination.
- Investigational agents include thymidylate synthase inhibitors (raltitrexed), oral fluorinated pyrimidines (BOF-A2 [Emitefur], capecitabine [approved for breast cancer], eniluracil, S-1, UFT [Ftorafur]), and platinum analogs (oxaliplatin). Dose-limiting toxicities generally consist of diarrhea, leukopenia, stomatitis, or some combination thereof.
- Novel investigational agents include matrix metalloproteinase inhibitors (BB-2516 [Marimastat]), farnesyl transferase, protein kinase C, growth factor and cyclin-dependent kinase inhibitors, monoclonal antibodies, tumor vaccines, and gene therapy techniques.

ADJUVANT THERAPY FOR COLON CANCER

- 5-FU and either levamisole or leucovorin reduce relapse rates by 30–40% in patients with *stage III* colon cancer. Six months of adjuvant 5-FU plus low- or high-dose leucovorin appear to be as effective as, and possibly more effective than, 12 months of levamisole. Adding levamisole to 5-FU and leucovorin does not increase efficacy but may increase toxicity.
- The impact of adjuvant therapy on patients with *stage II* colon cancer is unknown, but high-risk individuals will probably benefit and should be offered adjuvant chemotherapy in the clinical trial setting.
- Optimal doses, administration schedule, and duration of therapy have yet to be determined (Table 59–1). Although efficacy and toxicity of different regimens are similar, costs of leucovorin doses ranging from 20–500 mg/m^2 are substantially different.
- Direct hepatic infusion of 5-FU provides high local concentrations of the drug at the most common site of recurrence and minimizes systemic toxicity. The value of this approach remains unproven and controversial because of inconsistent effects on disease recurrence or survival in clinical studies.

ADJUVANT THERAPY FOR RECTAL CANCER

- The goal of adjuvant radiation therapy for rectal cancer is to decrease local tumor recurrence after surgery, preserve the sphincter, and, with preoperative radiotherapy, improve resectability.

TABLE 59–1. Recommendations for Adjuvant Therapy for Colon Cancer

Stage		
Pathologic/Duke's	*TNM*	Treatment Options
0, A, or B1	I	None
B2	II	Clinical trial; 5-FU + LV (LD or HD)[a] or 5-FU + LEV[b] for high-risk patients
B3	II	5-FU + LEV[b] or 5-FU + LV (LD or HD)[a]; 5-FU + LV + XRT[c]; clinical trial
C1–C2	III	5-FU + LEV[b] or 5-FU + LV (LD or HD)[a]; clinical trial
C3	III	5-FU + LEV[b] or 5-FU + LV (LD or HD)[a]; 5-FU + LV + XRT[c]; clinical trial

5-FU, fluorouracil; LV, leucovorin; LEV, levamisole; XRT, radiation therapy.
[a]5-FU 425 mg/m^2 IVP + LV 20 mg/m^2 IVP on d 1–5, every 4–5 wk × 6 mo **or** 5-FU 370–400 mg/m^2 IVP + LV 200 mg/m^2 IVP on d 1–5, every 5 wk × 6 mo **or** 5-FU 500 mg/m^2 IVP + LV 500 mg/m^2 IVP weekly for 6 of 8 wk × 1 y.
[b]5-FU 450 mg/m^2 IVP daily × 5 d, then weekly starting at d 28 × 1 y; LEV 50 mg PO tid × 3 d, every 2 wk × 1 y.
[c]National Comprehensive Cancer Network–specific recommendation.

TABLE 59–2. Recommendations for Adjuvant Therapy for Rectal Cancer[a]

Stage: Pathologic/Duke's	Stage: TNM	Treatment Options
A1, B1	I	None
B2, C1–C2	II	Preoperative chemotherapy[b] + XRT, postoperative 5-FU + LV × 4; or postoperative 5-FU ± LV × 2 followed by protracted 5-FU infusion or bolus 5-FU + LV + XRT, then 5-FU ± LV × 2
B3, C3	II, III	Preoperative chemotherapy[b] + XRT, surgery + intraoperative brachytherapy,[c] followed by 5-FU + LV × 4; or postoperative 5-FU ± LV × 2 followed by protracted 5-FU infusion or bolus 5-FU + LV + XRT, then 5-FU ± LV × 2

5-FU, fluorouracil; LV, leucovorin; XRT, radiation therapy.
[a]Total duration of therapy is approximately 6 mo.
[b]Preoperative chemotherapy: Bolus 5-FU, with or without leucovorin.
[c]National Comprehensive Cancer Network–specific recommendation.

- 5-FU may sensitize rectal tumor cells to cytotoxic effects of XRT. Compared with XRT alone, the combination reduces local tumor recurrence and improves survival in high-risk patients.
- Several combinations have been evaluated in clinical studies (Table 59–2), but no single regimen is clearly superior to the others. Continuous infusions of 5-FU, which may provide more effective radiosensitization, and significantly improve disease-free and overall survival compared with IV bolus injections.
- More research is needed to establish the best combination of surgery, XRT, and chemotherapy, because no single modality satisfactorily prevents recurrence and improves survival. Interest in preoperative radiation and chemotherapy has resurfaced because of advances in imaging techniques and preoperative staging.

XI TREATMENT OF METASTATIC COLORECTAL CANCER

- Site(s) of tumor involvement and symptoms help to define appropriate initial management strategy (Figure 59–1). In general, treatment options are similar for metastatic cancer of the colon and rectum.
- Surgical resection of isolated hepatic and pulmonary metastases may offer selected patients an opportunity to experience extended disease-free survival.
- Chemotherapy is the primary treatment modality for unresectable metastatic colorectal cancer (Table 59–3).
- 5-FU can be administered by IV bolus, continuous infusion, or hepatic artery infusion. *IV bolus* schedules are attractive because of low cost, ease of administration, and documented efficacy.
- *Continuous IV infusion* regimens (e.g., 8–24-hour, 4–5-day) have been developed to increase the duration of drug exposure. Even protracted

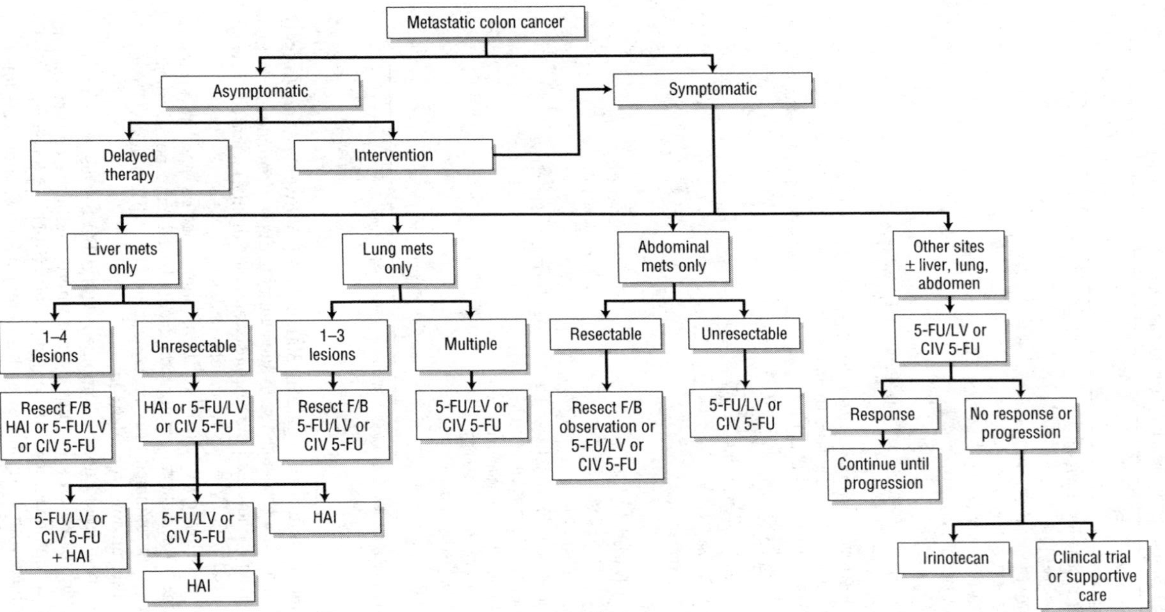

Figure 59–1. Methodic approach algorithm for patient with metastatic colorectal cancer. (5-FU, fluorouracil; LV, leucovorin; CIV, continuous intravenous infusion; HAI, hepatic arterial infusion F/B, followed by.)

TABLE 59–3. Chemotherapeutic Options for Metastatic Colorectal Cancer

Regimen	Major Dose-limiting Toxicity
Initial or Second-line Therapy	
5-FU + low-dose LV	
5-FU 370–425 mg/m^2 IVP + LV 20 mg/m^2 IVP on d 1–5 of wk 1, 4, and 8, then every 5 wk	Stomatitis, mucositis
5-FU 500–600 mg/m^2 IVP + LV 20–25 mg/m^2 IV weekly for 6 of 8 wk	Diarrhea
5-FU + high-dose LV	
5-FU 500 mg/m^2 IVP + LV 500 mg/m^2 IV weekly for 6 of 8 wk	Diarrhea
5-FU 370–400 mg/m^2 IVP + LV 200 mg/m^2 IVP on d 1–5 of wk 1, 4, and 8, then every 5 wk	Stomatitis, mucositis
5-FU 300–400 mg/m^2 IVP + LV 200 mg/m^2/d 2-h CIV, then 22-h 5-FU 300–600 mg/m^2/d, on d 1, 2 every 2 wk	Stomatitis, mucositis, hand–foot syndrome
5-FU 2600 mg/m^2/d as 24-h CIV + LV 500 mg/m^2/d over 2–24 h weekly	Stomatitis, mucositis, hand–foot syndrome
Second-line Therapy	
Irinotecan	
125 mg/m^2 IV weekly for 4 of 6 wk	Diarrhea, neutropenia
350 mg/m^2 IV every 3 wk	Diarrhea, neutropenia
Trimetrexate + 5-FU + LV	
Day 1: Trimetrexate 110 mg/m^2 IV over 1 h; 24 h later: LV 200 mg/m^2 IV over 1 h followed by 5-FU 500 mg/m^2 IVP + PO LV 15 mg every 6 h × 7, starting 6 h after 5-FU; weekly for 6 of 8 wk	Diarrhea, neutropenia
Mitomycin-C + 5-FU	Diarrhea, neutropenia

IVP, intravenous bolus injection; CIV, continuous intravenous infusion; 5-FU, fluorouracil; LV, leucovorin.

XI

continuous infusions (e.g., 250–300 mg/m^2/d IV over 24 hours for ≤10 weeks) are not associated with substantial toxicity. Continuous infusion significantly increased the response rate and slightly increased survival compared with IV bolus in a meta-analysis.

- 5-FU plus low-dose leucovorin is recommended as standard systemic treatment for metastatic colorectal cancer based on response rates, toxicity, lower estimated drug costs, and quality-of-life indices. The optimal dose remains to be defined.
- **Interferon** should not be combined with 5-FU because current doses and administration schedules do not improve efficacy or survival and produce significant toxicity compared with 5-FU and leucovorin. 5-FU combined with lower doses and different administration schedules of interferon and leucovorin are being evaluated.

- Irinotecan should be considered standard therapy for patients who have failed prior treatment with 5-FU–based regimens. Ongoing clinical trials are evaluating irinotecan as first-line therapy, in combination with other active agents, in the adjuvant setting, and in different dosing schedules.
- Randomized trials are needed to confirm the promising activity associated with adding trimetrexate or **mitomycin-C** to 5-FU and leucovorin.
- *Hepatic arterial infusion* of FUDR 0.3 mg/kg/d over 24 hours for 14 days increases local drug concentrations. **Heparin** 10,000–17,500 units/50 mL of solution is often added to prevent arterial thromboses. Prospective randomized studies consistently demonstrate significantly higher response rates compared with IV therapy and slightly higher median survival. Because of significant costs and toxicities, hepatic artery infusions should be reserved for palliative treatment of isolated liver metastases in patients who have failed systemic therapy.

▶ EVALUATION OF THERAPEUTIC OUTCOMES

- Patients who undergo curative surgical resection, with or without adjuvant therapy, require close follow-up (Table 59–4).
- The goal of monitoring is to evaluate whether the patient is benefitting from the management of their disease or to detect recurrence.
- Symptoms of recurrence such as pain syndromes, changes in bowel habits, rectal or vaginal bleeding, pelvic masses, anorexia, and weight

TABLE 59–4. General Guidelines for Follow-up After Curative Resection

Procedure or Test	Frequency
History and physical exam	Every 3–4 mo for 3 y, then every 6 mo for 2 y, then annually
Fecal occult blood testing	
CEA	
Colonoscopy or sigmoidoscopy + barium enema	Annually for several years, then every 2–3 y
Chest x-ray	Annually
Breast and pelvic examination, mammogram	Per age-specific guide lines for women
Liver function tests	As indicated by above findings
Chest, abdominal, or pelvic CT scan	
Liver ultrasound	
Liver–spleen scan	
Bone scan	
Laparotomy	

XI

loss develop in <50% of patients. More recurrences are detected in asymptomatic patients due to increased serum CEA levels that lead to further examination.

See Chapter 118, Colorectal Cancer, authored by Lisa E. Davis, PharmD, FCCP, BCPS, and Motria M. Horodysky, PharmD, BCPS, for a more detailed discussion of this topic.

Chapter 60

▶ LEUKEMIAS: ACUTE

▶ DEFINITION

Acute lymphocytic leukemia (ALL) and acute nonlymphocytic leukemia (ANLL) are hematologic malignancies characterized by unregulated proliferation of the blood-forming cells of the bone marrow. ALL and ANLL differ from each other and from chronic leukemias with respect to cell of origin, cell line maturation, life expectancy, clinical presentation, rapidity of progression of the untreated disease, and response to therapy.

▶ PATHOPHYSIOLOGY

- Both ANLL and ALL arise from a single leukemic cell. The balance between proliferation and differentiation fails, so that the cells do not differentiate past a particular stage of hematopoiesis and then proliferate uncontrollably.
- These immature proliferating cells (blasts) crowd out or inhibit normal cellular maturation in bone marrow, resulting in anemia, granulocytopenia, and thrombocytopenia. Leukemic blasts may also infiltrate other tissues such as lymph nodes, skin, liver, spleen, and kidney and the central nervous system (CNS).
- ANLL affects the immature precursors of the myeloid blood-forming cells.
- ALL is characterized by proliferation of immature lymphoblasts. Markers on the cell surface or membrane of the lymphoblast can be used to classify ALL.
- The genetic defect that leads to leukemia may be activation of a normally suppressed gene to create an oncogene that signals unregulated proliferation, differentiation, or survival. A second genetic cause is the loss or disturbance of genes such as *p*53 that suppress the development of cancer.

▶ CLINICAL PRESENTATION

- The *symptoms* of acute leukemia are nonspecific.
- Anemia often manifests as fatigue, lassitude, malaise, and pallor; palpitations or dyspnea on exertion may also be noted.
- Granulocytopenia may present as fever with or without infection.
- Thrombocytopenia may manifest as petechiae, bleeding, or bruising, often involving the gums, skin, or GI tract. Menorrhagia may be seen in premenopausal women.
- Gum hypertrophy, loss of vision, abnormal mass, or bone pain may result from leukemic infiltrates.
- Seizures, headache, diplopia, nausea, or vomiting may indicate leukemic meningitis.

- *Physical findings* are consistent with anemia (pallor, tachycardia, cardiac murmurs), granulocytopenia (infection, fever), thrombocytopenia (bruising, bleeding, petechiae, ecchymoses, purpura, menorrhagia), and leukemic infiltration (lymphadenopathy, splenomegaly, hepatomegaly, sternal tenderness, gingival hypertrophy, cranial palsies, and skin infiltration).
- On *laboratory* testing, the anemia is usually normocytic and normochromic with decreased reticulocytes. The platelet count is reduced in nearly all patients (<50,000/μL.) The WBC count is normal or elevated in about 85% of patients with ALL; it sometimes exceeds 50,000/μL. The peripheral blood smear usually demonstrates decreased normal granulocytes and increased blasts. Other laboratory findings include hyperuricemia, serum calcium imbalances, and hyperkalemia.

▶ DIAGNOSIS

- Marrow biopsy and aspirate are necessary to establish a diagnosis and follow response to therapy.
- The marrow is usually hypercellular with a predominance of blasts. Leukemia is diagnosed if >30% of the marrow cells are blasts; <5% is considered normal. If the marrow has 5–30% leukemic blasts, the term "myelodysplasia" is used, which is a preleukemic state that will eventually evolve into ANLL.
- Identification of clinical and laboratory risk factors at diagnosis may allow the clinician to better understand the disease and to tailor treatment according to the predicted response.

▶ DESIRED OUTCOME

- The short-term treatment goal is to rapidly achieve complete clinical and hematologic remission (defined as the disappearance of all clinical and bone marrow evidence of leukemia, with restoration of normal hematopoiesis).
- After complete remission is achieved, the goal is to maintain continuous complete remission, as relapse may ultimately lead to a fatal outcome.

▶ TREATMENT

GENERAL MANAGEMENT PRINCIPLES

- Neutropenia is one of the most critical complications of therapy. There are many unanswered questions regarding the role of **hematopoietic growth factors** (HGFs), such as the role in ALL, which HGF to use, and optimal dose and duration. The American Society of Oncology recommends HGF after initial induction therapy for ANLL in patients >55 years of age, but HGF does not improve the infection rate, antibiotic use, or duration of hospitalization in younger patients.

- Patients, particularly those with an initial elevated WBC count, should receive **allopurinol** to prevent urate nephropathy from rapid destruction of white cells. In adults, 300 mg once daily should be started 1–2 days prior to chemotherapy.
- Platelet transfusions are often given for peripheral counts <5000/μL or clinical signs of bleeding.
- Transfusions of packed red cells may be indicated for a hematocrit <20%, profound fatigue, or chest pain.
- Because of the GI toxicity of chemotherapy, parenteral nutrition should be used liberally.
- A triple-lumen central venous access device (e.g., Hickman catheter) is placed to facilitate simultaneous administration of chemotherapy, antibiotics, fluids, hyperalimentation, and blood products.

ACUTE LYMPHOCYTIC LEUKEMIA

Remission Induction Therapy

- **Vincristine** and **prednisone** form the foundation of induction therapy in adults (Table 60–1). Adding an **anthracycline** increases the response rate from 50% to 83% and carries a treatment-related mortality of only 3–17%.
- The value of adding more drugs to the basic three-drug regimen is unclear in adults.
- In pediatric ALL, a **glucocorticoid, vincristine,** and **asparaginase** yield a complete remission rate of near 99% in low-risk patients. In high-risk patients, the induction regimen includes additional drugs (e.g., anthracycline, **methotrexate, cytarabine,** and/or **teniposide**).

Central Nervous System Prophylaxis

- After patients achieve complete remission, they usually receive CNS prophylaxis because the CNS is a potential sanctuary from chemotherapeutic agents and undetectable leukemic cells are often present in the CNS. XI
- In adults with ALL, CNS prophylaxis usually includes cranial irradiation and intrathecal methotrexate.
- In children, low-risk ALL patients can be treated with intrathecal methotrexate alone or combined with cytarabine and hydrocortisone, with doses individualized by age. High-risk patients require both intrathecal chemotherapy and radiation or a combination of intrathecal and systemic chemotherapy.

Consolidation Therapy

- In adult ALL, consolidation therapy is started after a complete remission has been achieved and involves continued intensive chemotherapy to eradicate clinically undetectable disease. Different regimens involving non–cross-resistant drugs, high-dose therapy, or both (see Table 60–1) offer similar results.

- In pediatric ALL, a phase of dose-intensified chemotherapy usually follows induction, especially in patients with recognized poor risk factors. No specific combination is considered standard.

Maintenance Therapy

- The goal of maintenance therapy is to further eradicate residual leukemic cells and prolong remission duration.
- In adult and childhood ALL, maintenance therapy usually consists of **mercaptopurine** and methotrexate, at doses that produce minimal myelosuppression, with or without intermittent pulses of vincristine and prednisone (see Table 60–1). Most treatment programs continue maintenance therapy for at least 30 months.

ACUTE NONLYMPHOCYTIC LEUKEMIA

Remission Induction Therapy

- The most active single agents in ANLL are the anthracyclines and **cytarabine** (Table 60–2).
- **Idarubicin** has replaced **daunorubicin** in many adult protocols because of improved response and median survival. Idarubicin has not been as well tested in pediatric ANLL patients.
- In one study, addition of high-dose cytarabine to conventional "7 & 3" resulted in a higher remission rate of 89%.
- Most adults achieve a complete remission after one or two courses of chemotherapy. Patients who require additional chemotherapy have a poor prognosis, even if remission is ultimately achieved.
- The most effective pediatric regimens include an anthracycline and cytarabine with or without **thioguanine.**
- **All-*trans*-retinoic acid** (ATRA) allows induction of remission without life-threatening pancytopenia in patients with acute promyelocytic leukemia (APL), a subclass of ANLL. The complete remission rate is usually high (85–95%). Major adverse effects are headache, skin and mucous membrane reactions, bone pain, and nausea. Initiation of ATRA can lead to retinoic acid syndrome (fever, respiratory distress, interstitial pulmonary infiltrates, and weight gain), which can be avoided by adding chemotherapy to ATRA during induction.

Central Nervous System Prophylaxis

- CNS prophylaxis is not routinely given for ANLL because the risk of CNS relapse is lower than in patients with ALL.

Intensive Postremission Therapy

- Although most adults with ANLL achieve a complete remission, the duration of remission is short (4–8 months), presumably due to the presence of clinically undetectable leukemic cells. The goal of inten-

TABLE 60–1. Representative Chemotherapy Regimens for Adult Acute Lymphocytic Leukemia

Remission Induction		CNS Prophylaxis		Consolidation		Maintenance (Drug, Dose, and Schedule)
Drug and Dose	*Days*	*Drug and Dose*	*Days*	*Drug and Dose*	*Days*	
German Regimen						
PRED (PO) 60 mg/m^2	1–28	Cranial irradiation and	31,38,45,52	DEX (PO) 10 mg/m^2	1–28	MP (PO) 60 mg/m^2 qd
VCR (IV) 1.5 mg/m^2[a]	1,8,15,22	MTX (IT) 10 mg/m^2[b]		VCR (IV) 1.5 mg/m^2[a]	1,8,15,22	and MTX (PO/IV)
DNR (IV) 25 mg/m^2	1,8,15,22			DOX (IV) 25 mg/m^2	1,8,15,22	20 mg/m^2 weekly
ASP (IV) 5000 U/m^2	1–14			CTX (IV) 650 mg/m^2[c]	29	wks 10–18 and 29–130
CTX (IV) 650 mg/m^2[c]	29,43,57			ARA-C (IV) 75 mg/m^2	31–34,38–41	
ARA-C (IV) 75 mg/m^2	31–34,38–41, 45–48,52–55			TG (PO) 60 mg/m^2	29–42	
MP (PO) 60 mg/m^2	29–57					
CALGB 8811						
Course I		*Course III*		*Course II: Early Intensification*		*Course V*
CTX (IV) 1200 mg/m^2	1	Cranial irradiation		MTX (IT) 15 mg	1	VCR (IV) 2 mg d 1
DNR (IV) 45 mg/m^2	1,2,3	MTX (IT) 15 mg	1,8,15,22,29	CTX (IV) 1000 mg/m^2	1	monthly
VCR (IV) 2 mg	1,8,15,22	MP (PO) 60 mg/m^2	1–70	MP (PO) 60 mg/m^2	1–14	PRED (PO) 60 mg/m^2
PRED (PO) 60 mg/m^2	1–21	MTX (PO) 20 mg/m^2	36,43,50,57,64	ARA-C (SC) 75 mg/m^2	1–4,8–11	d 1–5 monthly
ASP (SC) 6000 U/m^2	5,8,11,15,18,22			VCR (IV) 2 mg	15,22	MTX (PO) 20 mg/m^2 d
				ASP (SC) 6000 U/m^2	15,18,22,25	1,8,15,22 monthly
For patients ≥60 yr :				*Course IV: Late Intensification*		MP (PO) 60 mg/m^2 d
CTX 800 mg/m^2	1			DOX (IV) 30 mg/m^2	1,8,15	1–28 monthly
DNR 30 mg/m^2	1,2,3			VCR (IV) 2 mg	1,8,15	
PRED 60 mg/m^2	1–7			DEX (PO) 10 mg/m^2	1–14	
				CTX (IV) 1000 mg/m^2	29	
				TG (PO) 60 mg/m^2	29–42	
				ARA-C (SC) 75 mg/m^2	29–32,36–39	

ARA-C, cytarabine; ASP, asparaginase; CTX, cyclophosphamide; DEX, dexamethasone; DNR, daunorubicin; DOX, doxorubicin; MP, mercaptopurine; MTX, methotrexate; PRED, prednisone; TEN, teniposide: TG, thioguanine; VCR, vincristine.

[a]Maximum single dose, 2 mg.

[b]Maximum single dose, 15 mg.

[c]Maximum single dose, 100 mg.

TABLE 60–2. Representative Chemotherapy Regimens for Adult Acute Nonlymphocytic Leukemia

Remission Induction	Intensive Postremission Therapy	Maintenance Therapy
Southeastern Cancer Study Group		
Cytarabine 100 $mg/m^2/d$ continuous infusion, d 1–7 Idarubicin 12 $mg/m^2/d$, d 1–3	Cytarabine 100 mg/m^2 every 12 h × 10 Thioguanine 100 mg/m^2 PO every 12 h × 10 Idarubicin 15 $mg/m^2/d$ on d 1 (3 courses)	None
CALGB		
Cytarabine 200 $mg/m^2/d$ continuous infusion, d 1–7 Daunorubicin 45 $mg/m^2/d$, d 1–3	Cytarabine 3 g/m^2 every 12 h, d 1,3,5 (4 courses)	Cytarabine 100 mg/m^2 SC every 12 h, d 1–5 Daunorubicin 45 mg/m^2, d 1 (4 courses)
Boston Group		
Daunorubicin 45 $mg/m^2/d$, d 1–3 Cytarabine 100 $mg/m^2/d$ continuous infusion, d 1–7 Cytarabine 2 $g/m^2/d$ every 12 h, d 8–10	*Cycle 1,3* Daunorubicin 60 $mg/m^2/d$, d 1 and 2 Cytarabine 200 $mg/m^2/d$ continuous infusion, d 1–5 *Cycle 2* Cytarabine 2 g/m^2 every 12 h, d 1–3 Etoposide 100 $mg/m^2/d$, d 4–5	None

sive postremission therapy (IPRT) is to eradicate residual leukemic cells and to prevent the emergence of drug-resistant disease.

- IPRT may consist of *consolidation,* which involves the administration of drugs that the patient has not previously received, or *intensification* with one or two courses of high doses of the same drugs used for remission induction, immediately after a complete remission is achieved.
- No consensus exists regarding the best drugs, doses, or duration of treatment. The three regimens in Table 60–2 offer different approaches to IPRT.
- Children with ANLL should also receive IPRT if stem cell transplant is not available.

Maintenance Therapy

- Most patients receive no further treatment after IPRT, although selected patients may go on to marrow transplantation.
- If used, the maintenance phase may employ low-dose subcutaneous cytarabine (see Table 60–2).

TREATMENT OF RELAPSED ALL AND ANLL

- Most adult patients with acute leukemia (and children with ANLL) who achieve complete remission eventually experience a leukemic relapse. After the first relapse, the median survival is 6–8 months; only 7% of patients are alive at 3 years.
- Salvage therapy for ALL has involved different schedules of drugs used during initial induction. The VAD regimen employs a 4-day continuous infusion of vincristine and **doxorubicin** with intensive **dexamethasone** therapy; IPRT follows for 24–30 months. Another regimen uses prednisone, intermediate-dose cytarabine, mitoxantrone, and **etoposide** in relapsed or refractory ALL. Combinations with high-dose cytarabine or methotrexate are also commonly employed.
- In relapsed or resistant ANLL, high-dose cytarabine, etoposide, intermediate-dose or high-dose methotrexate, **asparaginase,** carboplatin, **mitoxantrone,** and idarubicin have been useful. If the relapse occurs 6 months or more beyond the initial remission, then induction with the original chemotherapy may be successful.

MARROW TRANSPLANTATION

For both ALL and ANLL, bone marrow transplantation (BMT) is another viable treatment option once remission is induced, especially for high-risk patients and patients in relapse.

ANLL

- In the treatment of ANLL, *allogeneic* BMT given as IPRT (immediately after initial remission) improves disease-free survival and overall survival over chemotherapy alone.

- Patients who relapse after an initial remission should be offered allogeneic BMT if a donor is available. Long-term survival after autologous BMT appears to be similar to allogeneic BMT. Patients in second or later remission who do not qualify for an allogeneic BMT should be considered for autologous BMT as soon as possible after achieving remission.

ALL

- Because the initial remission is usually easily achieved in ALL and no benefit to BMT has been demonstrated in immediate postremission BMT, allogeneic BMT is not recommended after first remission.
- Once a relapse has occurred, an allogeneic BMT should be performed if a donor is available. Autologous BMT remains an option for patients when a suitable donor is not available.

▶ EVALUATION OF THERAPEUTIC OUTCOMES

- With the exception of prednisone, asparaginase, and vincristine, antineoplastic agents cause a rapid fall in peripheral platelet and WBC counts. During ANLL remission induction therapy, daily monitoring of the complete blood count and the absolute neutrophil count is necessary to determine when red cell and platelet transfusions are needed and when neutropenia is achieved. Less frequent monitoring may be sufficient during ALL induction.
- During hypoplasia, infectious and bleeding complications are major causes of death. Intense monitoring of chemistry laboratory values, microbiology reports, and the patient's physical condition are necessary to identify infections early because typical signs and symptoms of infection may be absent in the neutropenic host.
- Frequent culturing and early institution of antibiotics are required to prevent infectious deaths.
- Close monitoring of the patient's condition and laboratory values also allows appropriate institution of nutritional support.
- The primary outcome desired initially is the establishment of remission (return of hematologic values to normal and a repeat bone marrow biopsy that demonstrates no evidence of disease).
- After the appropriate postremission therapy has been completed, the patient may return on a regular basis to check hematologic values.
- Late sequelae that should be considered during long-term follow-up include complications of CNS irradiation (e.g., cortical atrophy and other endocrine dysfunctions resulting in obesity, short stature, precocious puberty, and osteoporosis; disturbed intellectual and motor func-

tion; secondary gliomas); anthracycline-induced cardiomyopathy; and secondary ANLL after etoposide or teniposide.

See Chapter 122, Acute Leukemias, authored by Steven P. Smith, PharmD, BCPS, and Susan E. Beltz, PharmD, for a more detailed discussion of this topic.

Chapter 61

▶ LEUKEMIAS: CHRONIC

▶ DEFINITION

Chronic leukemia includes at least four hematologic malignancies: chronic myelogenous leukemia (CML), chronic lymphocytic leukemia (CLL), prolymphocytic leukemia, and hairy cell leukemia. They differ from each other and from acute leukemias with respect to cell of origin, life expectancy, clinical presentation, rapidity of progression of the untreated disease, and response to therapy. This chapter focuses on the two most common types, CML and CLL.

▶ CHRONIC MYELOGENOUS LEUKEMIA

PATHOPHYSIOLOGY

- CML is a myeloproliferative disorder that results from the malignant transformation of a pluripotent stem cell leading to clonal proliferation and accumulation of both progenitor and mature myeloid and lymphoid cells. Hematologic and cytogenetic abnormalities involve the myeloid or B-lymphoid elements of bone marrow.
- The Philadelphia chromosome (Ph^1) abnormality, present in 90–95% of patients, is a shortened long arm of chromosome 22 and is found in granulocyte and erythrocyte progenitors, macrophages, megakaryocytes, and some lymphocytes. Through chromosomal translocation, the c-*abl* protooncogene is able to escape the normal genetic controls and is activated into a functional oncogene, directing the transcription of a protein known as $p210^{BCR\text{-}ABL}$, which may be essential in the development of CML.
- Carcinogenesis begins with the transformation of a single cell with an inheritable selective growth advantage, leading to the proliferation of a neoplastic, monoclonal population of pluripotent stem cells. The disease soon evolves into a Ph^1-positive chronic phase.
- Granulocytosis results from increased growth rate of the transformed clone and disruption of normal hematopoietic cell maturation.
- The silent monoclonal growth phase of CML evolves into the clinically recognized *chronic phase* when malignant cells acquire Ph^1, and immature myeloid cells begin to lose the ability to differentiate into mature functioning cells. At this stage, therapeutic intervention can control the expansion of clonal cells and normalize the WBC count.
- An *accelerated phase* emerges as the WBC count becomes increasingly difficult to manage.
- The final *acute phase* or blastic phase (blast crisis) is marked by the presence of rapidly proliferating blast cells that have lost the ability to differentiate into nonproliferating cells. CML in blastic phase is resis-

tant to treatment owing to drug resistance and the high proliferative rate of malignant cells.

CLINICAL PRESENTATION

- CML is commonly diagnosed after the patient presents with symptoms such as weight loss, fatigue, malaise, night sweats, and fever.
- On physical examination, splenomegaly and hepatomegaly are found in 30–40% of patients.

DIAGNOSIS

- The diagnosis of CML is usually made during the chronic phase following an abnormal peripheral blood smear, which may have been obtained because of presenting symptoms or during routine physical examination.
- Laboratory findings of the peripheral blood during the chronic phase include leukocytosis (WBC often >100,000/μL), thrombocytosis, basophilia, and abnormal leukocyte alkaline phosphatase levels.
- Physical symptoms of acceleration include resurgence of splenic enlargement, unexplained fever, and persistent bone pain. WBC counts and other signs and symptoms become increasingly difficult to control with conventional oral chemotherapeutic agents.
- The presence of blastic phase is confirmed by >20% blasts in the bone marrow or peripheral blood.

DESIRED OUTCOME

The goals of therapy for CML are to control the patient's signs and symptoms, delay the onset of blastic phase, and achieve cure by eradicating the Ph^1-positive cells.

TREATMENT

Conventional Chemotherapy

- Conventional cytotoxic chemotherapy can be used in chronic-phase CML to attain hematologic remission (normalization of WBC count), but it has no significant cytogenetic effects and only marginally improves median survival (Table 61–1). XI
- **Busulfan** and **hydroxyurea** are the most frequently employed chemotherapeutic agents because they can be taken orally, are inexpensive, have a reasonable side-effect profile, and rapidly normalize elevated WBC counts in the chronic phase (Table 61–2). Hydroxyurea treatment has a significant survival advantage of >1 year over busulfan therapy.
- In the daily schedule, hydroxyurea is initiated at 50 mg/kg/d in divided doses until the WBC count falls below 10,000/μL; the dose can then be decreased to a maintenance level of 20 mg/kg/d or temporarily discontinued and reinitiated at the daily maintenance dose when the WBC count climbs. Alternatively, an intermittent mainte-

TABLE 61–1. Effect of Various Treatment Modalities on Survival in CML

Therapy	Median Survival (mo)
No treatment	37 (mean)
Splenic irradiation	28 (median), 42 (mean)
Busulfan	35–47
Hydroxyurea	48–69
Combination chemotherapy	45–55
Bone marrow transplantation	40–70% alive at 5 y[a]
Interferon-α	50–60% alive at 5 y

[a]Only therapy to eliminate Ph^1 clone.

nance dose of 20 mg/kg twice daily (40 mg/kg/d) 2 d/wk effectively controls the WBC count and minimizes cutaneous toxicity.

- Busulfan may be the second-line agent because of its toxicity. Initial doses are 4–8 mg/d, which are continued until the WBC count approaches 20,000/μL and then discontinued. The WBC count continues to fall after the drug is discontinued, so WBC counts can be maintained for several weeks. Toxicities include prolonged myelosuppression, pulmonary fibrosis, and skin hyperpigmentation. Patients have more complications during allogeneic bone marrow transplant (BMT) if they have received busulfan rather than hydroxyurea.

Interferons

- Although the exact mechanism of interferon-alpha (IFN-α) in the treatment of CML is unknown, IFN-α may bind to its receptor on target cells, initiating a cascade of biochemical processes that can result in direct cytotoxicity to leukemic cells. Other mechanisms may also be operative.
- The two recombinant forms, **IFN-α-2a** (Roferon) and **IFN-α-2b** (Intron A), yield similar results. Some patients achieve cytogenetic

TABLE 61–2. Comparison of Hydroxyurea and Busulfan in Chronic-Phase CML

Effect of Therapy	Hydroxyurea	Busulfan
Rate of WBC decline	Rapid	Slower
Myelosuppression	Uncommon at usual dose	Common
Side-effect profile	Mild (skin)	Severe (lung)
Effect on platelet count	None	Decreased
Effect on splenomegaly	Significant reversal	Significant reversal
Effect on Ph^1-positive marrow	None	After prolonged myelosuppression
BMT-eligible patients	Recommended	Not recommended

BMT, bone marrow transplant.; WBC, white blood cell; PH^1, Philadelphia chromosome.

response, which leads to prolonged survival; however, the Ph[1] clone reappears when IFN is stopped.

- The optimal dose schedule appears to be 5×10^6 U/m^2/d. Higher doses are unlikely to improve response rates and increase the incidence of toxicities.
- Adverse effects consist of short-term constitutional effects and potentially dose-limiting long-term effects. The most predictable early toxicity is a flu-like syndrome involving fever, chills, myalgias, headache, and anorexia, which can be ameliorated by dosing at 50% of the final dose during the first week, giving the drug at bedtime, and coadministering acetaminophen or indomethacin. Tachycardia and hypotension are seen in about 15% of patients in the first 1–2 weeks. Long-term adverse effects include weight loss, alopecia, neurologic effects (paresthesias, cognitive impairment, depression), and immune-mediated complications (hemolysis, thrombocytopenia, nephrotic syndrome, systemic lupus erythematosus, hypothyroidism).
- The combination of hydroxyurea and IFN-α has demonstrated promise. Hydroxyurea is started at 50 mg/kg/d and titrated to maintain normal WBC counts; IFN-α is then initiated at a dose of 5×10^6 U/m^2/d. The advantage of this combination is rapid normalization of blood counts and differentials and lower incidence of IFN-α–induced symptoms; however, the cytogenetic response is not better than with IFN-α therapy alone.
- Adding low-dose **cytarabine** 20 mg/m^2/d for 10 days of each month to IFN-α and hydroxyurea results in favorable outcomes in previously untreated patients in the chronic phase, with improved major cytogenetic response rate and survival.

Treatment in Blastic Phase

- The more common myeloid form of CML is most responsive to high-dose cytarabine. The usual protocol is 3000 mg/m^2 every 12 hours for up to 12 doses, resulting in complete responses of 25–40%.
- The most effective treatment of the lymphoid form is a combination of **vincristine** (usually 2 mg IV weekly) and **prednisone** (60 mg/m^2/d PO). The addition of **doxorubicin** may enhance complete response to around 50%.

Bone Marrow Transplantation

- Allogeneic BMT is the only therapeutic option that can eradicate the Ph[1]-positive clone. It results in cure in approximately 60% of CML patients in chronic phase with an human lymphocyte antigen (HLA)-identical sibling donor.
- For patients with an HLA-matched donor, BMT is the treatment of choice and should be performed shortly after diagnosis.
- Fewer than 30% of patients have an ideal donor, but related one-antigen–mismatch transplants have survival rates that approach HLA-matched transplants. Two or more mismatches lead to high mortality rates from graft rejection and acute graft-versus-host disease (GVHD).

- T-cell depletion of the donor marrow reduces morbidity and mortality of acute GVHD but increases relapse rates owing to loss of the GVHD effect.
- Autologous BMT harvested in chronic phase and stored prior to transplantation has resulted in transient loss of the Ph^1-positive clone for several years in a few patients. Relapse rates remain very high, and methods for successfully purging CML marrow are elusive because of the similarity between CML cells and normal stem cells.

EVALUATION OF THERAPEUTIC OUTCOMES

- End points for chemotherapy are reduction in tumor bulk and relief of symptoms.
- Patients receiving chemotherapy or IFN-α should be monitored for adverse effects that can be reduced by altering the dosage regimen or by providing supportive care.
- The WBC count should be monitored to assess response to treatment. Patients with very high WBC counts (>100,000/μL) should receive **allopurinol** 300 $mg/m^2/d$ during leukopheresis.

► CHRONIC LYMPHOCYTIC LEUKEMIA

PATHOPHYSIOLOGY

- CLL is a lymphoproliferative disorder resulting in progressive accumulation of functionally incompetent lymphocytes, which usually arise from malignant transformation of a B lymphocyte with subsequent clonal proliferation.

CLINICAL PRESENTATION

- The patient complains of constitutional symptoms (e.g., fatigue, fever).

DIAGNOSIS

XI

- On physical examination, about 60% of patients have lymphadenopathy in the cervical, axillary, or inguinal areas. Intra-abdominal nodes may also be palpable. About 50% of patients have spleen and liver enlargement.
- An abnormal CBC is characterized by high numbers of mature-looking small lymphocytes (lymphocytosis).
- Bone marrow aspirate usually shows infiltration with mature-appearing lymphocytes making up 30% of nucleated cells.
- Diagnosis can be confirmed by analyzing phenotypic characteristics of the peripheral blood lymphocytes. Presence of a monoclonal B lymphocytosis may confirm the diagnosis.
- Anemia, thrombocytopenia, neutropenia, and hypogammaglobulinemia are frequently evident at diagnosis or during the course of the disease.

- The Rai staging system demonstrates the variable survival according to tumor burden and can help design appropriate management strategies (Table 61–3).

DESIRED OUTCOME

There are no curative treatments for CLL; therapy is designed to improve quality of life.

TREATMENT

General Management Principles

- Treatment is instituted if there are signs and symptoms of progressive disease, worsening of blood dyscrasias, autoimmune complications, symptomatic splenomegaly, bulky lymph nodes, severe lymphocytosis (>100,000–200,000/μL), and increased infectious complications.
  - Most stage 0 patients are managed with close observation.
  - In stage I or II disease, no consistent survival benefit has been demonstrated for drug therapy.
  - In stage III and IV disease, treatment is required with the intention of achieving a partial or complete remission. Drug therapy is usually begun with corticosteroids and an alkylating agent. Splenic radiation or splenectomy is often recommended to reduce symptoms and to improve autoimmune blood dyscrasia.
- Prednisone may be helpful in treating autoimmune thrombocytopenia and anemia. Splenomegaly, anemia, and thrombocytopenia often improve under corticosteroid therapy.

Cytotoxic Chemotherapy and Corticosteroids

- **Chlorambucil** and prednisone remain the standard treatment of CLL; response rates approach 70% with about 40% complete responses. Chlorambucil is dosed daily or intermittently every 2–4 weeks.

XI

TABLE 61–3. Rai Staging System and 10-Year Survival

	Lymphocytes >15 × 10^9/L	Lymphadenopathy	Organomegaly	Hemoglobin >11 g/dL	Platelets <100,000 × 10^9/L
Low Risk (Median Survival, 7–10 Y)					
Stage 0	+	–	–	–	–
Intermediate Risk (Median Survival, 5–6 Y)					
Stage I	+	+	–	–	–
Stage II	+	+/–	+	–	–
High Risk (Median Survival, 2–3 Y)					
Stage III	+	+/–	+/–	+	–
Stage IV	+	+/–	+/–	+/–	+

- **Cyclophosphamide** gives a similar response to chlorambucil and can be used in patients who do not tolerate chlorambucil or have a suboptimal response.
- The purine nucleoside analogs, **fludarabine** and **pentostatin,** may have an important role in the management of patients who become resistant to chlorambucil plus prednisone and may increasingly be used as initial therapy.

Other Treatments

- Experience with allogeneic BMT in CLL is limited and suggests a high complete remission rate, but few patients remain free from disease as measured by molecular studies.
- The role of IFN-α is limited; the response in advanced CLL is <20%.
- Intravenous immunoglobulin (IVIG) 400 mg/kg every 3 weeks for 1 year significantly reduces bacterial infections. However, routine use of IVIG may be difficult to justify on a quality-of-life or economic basis.

EVALUATION OF THERAPEUTIC OUTCOMES

- Patients with CLL should be monitored for signs and symptoms of disease that indicate the need for therapeutic intervention.
- When treatment is initiated, appropriate parameters should be monitored to ensure that quality of life is improved and infectious and hematologic complications are minimized.
- Patients receiving chemotherapy should be monitored for adverse effects that can be ameliorated by substituting alternate therapy or providing supportive care.

See Chapter 123, Chronic Leukemias, authored by Timothy R. McGuire, PharmD, and Peter W. Kazakoff, PharmD, for a more detailed discussion of this topic.

Chapter 62

▶ LUNG CANCER

▶ DEFINITION

Lung cancers are solid tumors that have been classified into four major cell types: (1) squamous cell carcinoma; (2) adenocarcinoma; (3) large cell carcinoma; and (4) small cell carcinoma. Histologic confirmation of cell type is essential in treatment planning because of differences in natural history, clinical features, and response to therapy.

▶ PATHOPHYSIOLOGY

- Lung carcinomas arise from pluripotent epithelial cells after exposure to carcinogens (especially tobacco smoke), which cause chronic inflammation and eventually lead to genetic and cytologic changes that progress to carcinoma.
- Activation of protooncogenes, inhibition or mutation of tumor suppressor genes, and production of autocrine growth factors also contribute to cellular proliferation and malignant transformation.
- Although cigarette smoking has been estimated to be responsible for about 83% of lung cancer cases, occupational or environmental exposure to asbestos, chloromethyl ethers, heavy metals, polycyclic aromatic hydrocarbons, and radon has also been implicated.
- The four major carcinoma cell types can be identified by light microscopy:
  - *Squamous cell* carcinoma (<30% of all lung cancers) is distinguished histologically by squamous differentiation. It (along with small cell lung cancers) has a much higher incidence among smokers and males. Most squamous cell carcinomas are slow growing and confined to the lungs but may eventually metastasize to the hilar and mediastinal lymph nodes, liver, adrenal glands, kidneys, bone, and gastrointestinal tract.
  - *Adenocarcinoma* (40%) is distinguished pathologically by a glandular or papillary pattern and mucin production. It usually metastasizes at an early stage and spreads to distant sites including the contralateral lung, liver, bone, adrenal glands, kidneys, and central nervous system (CNS).
  - *Large cell* carcinomas (15%) are anaplastic tumors that show no differentiation. They metastasize in a pattern similar to that of adenocarcinoma.
  - *Small cell* lung carcinomas (SCLCs or "oat cell" carcinomas) (25%) are distinguished by proliferation of neoplastic cells with round to oval nuclei. SCLC is a very aggressive and rapidly growing tumor with about 60–70% of patients initially presenting with metastases to the lymph nodes, opposite lung, liver, adrenal and other endocrine organs, bone, bone marrow, and CNS.

- In terms of management strategy and overall prognosis, adenocarcinoma, squamous cell carcinoma, and large cell carcinoma are frequently grouped together and referred to as non–small cell lung cancers (NSCLC).

▶ CLINICAL PRESENTATION

- The most common initial signs and symptoms include cough, dyspnea, chest pain, sputum production, and hemoptysis. Many patients also exhibit systemic symptoms such as anorexia, weight loss, and fatigue.
- Disseminated disease also may cause neurologic deficits from CNS metastases, bone pain or pathologic fractures secondary to bone metastases, or liver dysfunction from hepatic involvement.
- Paraneoplastic syndromes that commonly occur in association with lung cancers include cachexia, hypercalcemia, syndrome of inappropriate hormone secretion, and Cushing's syndrome.

▶ DIAGNOSIS

- In a patient with signs and symptoms of lung cancer, chest x-ray is the primary method of lung cancer detection. It may also be useful in measuring tumor size, establishing gross lymph node enlargement, and detecting other tumor-related findings such as pleural effusion, lobar collapse, and metastatic involvement of ribs, spine, and shoulders.
- Computed tomography (CT) scans are helpful in all of the above as well as in evaluation of parenchymal lung abnormalities, masses only suspected on the chest x-ray, and mediastinal and hilar lymph nodes.
- Pathologic confirmation of lung cancer must be established by examination of sputum cytology and/or tumor biopsy by fiber-optic bronchoscopy, percutaneous needle biopsy, or open-lung biopsy.
- All patients must also have a thorough history and physical examination with emphasis on detecting signs and symptoms of the primary tumor, regional spread of the tumor, distant metastases, paraneoplastic syndromes, and ability to withstand aggressive surgery or chemotherapy.

▶ STAGING

- The American Joint Committee has established a TNM staging classification for lung cancer based on the primary tumor size and extent (T), regional lymph node involvement (N), and the presence or absence of distant metastases (M).
- For comparison of treatments, a more simple stage grouping system is also used in which stage I refers to tumors confined to the lung without lymphatic spread, stage II refers to large tumors with ipsilateral peribronchial or hilar lymph node involvement, stage III includes other lymph node and regional involvement, and stage IV includes any tumor with distant metastases.

- The primary tumor is assessed using chest roentgenographs and fiberoptic bronchoscopy, whereas lymphatic spread is usually assessed by mediastinoscopy, gallium-67 citrate scanning, or CT.
- If there is evidence of metastatic disease, then special scans (e.g., bone, brain, liver) or biopsies (e.g., bone marrow, liver) may be necessary for staging.
- A two-stage classification is widely used for SCLC. *Limited disease* is confined to one hemithorax and the regional lymph nodes. All other disease is classified as *extensive disease.*

► TREATMENT

NON-SMALL CELL LUNG CANCER

Desired Outcome

The goal of treating NSCLC depends on the disease stage. Stage I, II, and possibly III disease can be cured with appropriate therapy. In contrast, stage IV disease is not curable, but chemotherapy can decrease symptoms and prolong survival.

General Principles

- *Surgery* is the treatment of choice for localized disease (stage I or II). If the tumor is inoperable or the patient is a poor surgical candidate, *radiation therapy* can be used; however, 5-year survival rates are usually inferior to surgery.
- For locally advanced disease (stage III), recent evidence suggests that chemotherapy (i.e., *neoadjuvant therapy*), with or without radiation therapy, followed by surgery improves survival compared with radiation followed by surgery.
- Although NSCLC has been considered to be insensitive to cytotoxic *chemotherapy,* new combinations improve response and survival rates, which are superior to best supportive care. Patients most likely to benefit from chemotherapy have a good performance status, no or minimal weight loss, and less extensive disease. XI
- No single regimen is considered standard, so selection should be based on the patient's ability to tolerate expected toxicities and likelihood of radiation therapy (and impact on chemotherapy-induced toxicities).
- The role of combination therapy is controversial because, although response rates generally exceed those of single-agent therapy, it is difficult to demonstrate consistent improvement in survival.

Cytotoxic Chemotherapy

- **Cisplatin** is included in the most widely used and recommended regimens (Table 62–1). As a single agent, cisplatin 100 mg/m^2 is superior to 70 mg/m^2, but, when combined with other agents, higher doses increase toxicity without adding survival benefit.
- New agents have single-agent activity of >20% in NSCLC and are being evaluated in various combinations, with platinum compounds,

TABLE 62–1. Combination Chemotherapy for Non–Small Cell Lung Cancer

Combination	Dosages	Schedule	Overall Response Rate (%)
CE			
DDP	60–100 mg/m² IV d 1	Every 3–4 wk	19–30
ETOP	80–120 mg/m² IV d 1–3		
DDP/VIN			
DDP	120 mg/m² IV d 1 and 29	Every 6 wk	30
VIN	3 mg/m² IV q wk × 6	Every wk × 6, then every 2 wk	
MVP			
MIT	8 mg/m² IV d 1 and 29	Every 6 wk	43
VIN	3 mg/m² IV d 1, 8, 29, and 36		
DDP	80 mg/m² IV d 1 and 29		
ICE			
IFOS	1.5 g/m² IV d 1–3	Every 3 wk	43
CARBO	300–350 mg/m² d 1		
ETOP	60–100 mg/m² d 1–3		

DDP, cisplatin; ETOP, etoposide; VIN, vindesine; MIT, mitomycin; IFOS, ifosfamide; CARBO, carboplatin.

and as multimodality therapy (with and without concurrent or sequential radiation therapy and/or postinduction surgery).

- **Vinorelbine** and cisplatin may become the standard based on the survival advantage and minimal toxicity of this combination compared with cisplatin alone. Vinorelbine is easily administered in the outpatient setting over 6–10 minutes followed by a 75–100-mL IV flush. The dose-limiting toxicity is neutropenia.
- More studies are needed to clarify the role of **paclitaxel** combined with other agents, whether the dose should be high (250 mg/m^2) or low (175 mg/m^2), and whether the dose should be infused over 1 or 3 hours or given as a continuous 24-hour infusion. The 1-hour infusion is easy to administer in the outpatient setting and causes minimal myelosuppression, but it increases the rate of peripheral sensory neuropathy. Studies are being conducted to determine whether continuous infusion or high doses are more effective; these approaches are clearly more myelosuppressive and require granulocyte colony-stimulating factor (G-CSF) support. Hypersensitivity reactions necessitate pretreatment with corticosteroids and histamine H_1 and H_2 antagonists.
- **Docetaxel,** a taxoid without the schedule-dependent efficacy and toxicity issues of paclitaxel, is given IV at 75–100 mg/m^2 over 1 hour every 3 weeks. Neutropenia is the dose-limiting toxicity, but G-CSF support is not required. An oral corticosteroid should be started 24 hours before docetaxel and continued for a total of 3–5 days to reduce the incidence and severity of fluid retention.
- The dose-limiting toxicity of **gemcitabine** is thrombocytopenia and reversible hepatotoxicity; toxicity is schedule dependent. A 30-minute

IV infusion on days 1, 8, and 15 of a 28-day cycle allows maximally tolerated dosages to be administered with acceptable toxicity in the outpatient setting.

- **Irinotecan** and **topotecan** are potent inhibitors of topoisomerase I. The dose-limiting toxicities of irinotecan are neutropenia and severe diarrhea; dose-limiting esophagitis, diarrhea, and unexpected severe pneumonitis precluded further investigation of irinotecan and chest radiation therapy.

SMALL CELL LUNG CANCER

Desired Outcome

The goal of treatment is cure or at least prolonged survival, which requires aggressive combination chemotherapy.

General Principles

- *Surgery* is almost never indicated because SCLC disseminates early in the disease. A possible exception is the rare patient who presents with a small, isolated lesion.
- In contrast with NSCLC, aggressive *combination chemotherapy* produces a fourfold to fivefold increase in median survival for patients with SCLC.
- Patients who present with limited disease, better performance status, no weight loss, female gender, age <70 years, and normal serum lactic dehydrogenase have an improved prognosis.

Cytotoxic Chemotherapy

- Combination chemotherapy is clearly superior to single-agent therapy, and the best results are generally observed when three or more active agents are combined. Some frequently used regimens are described in Table 62–2.
- Commonly used agents include cisplatin, **carboplatin, cyclophosphamide, ifosfamide, doxorubicin, etoposide, teniposide,** and **vincristine.** Newer agents undergoing investigation include docetaxel, gemcitabine, irinotecan, paclitaxel, topotecan, and vinorelbine. XI
- Alternating two active, *non–cross-resistant* regimens may prevent the growth of drug-resistant cells during treatment and prolongs survival in patients with limited, but not extensive, disease.
- Although theoretically attractive, *dose intensity* has not yet been shown to improve survival and significantly increases toxicity such as granulocytopenia, febrile neutropenia, and weight loss.
- *High-dose chemotherapy* and *peripheral blood stem cell transplantation* continue to be investigated in good-risk patients.

Radiation Therapy and Brain Metastases

- *Radiotherapy* has been combined with chemotherapy to treat tumors limited to the thoracic cavity. This combined-modality therapy may decrease the incidence and delay the onset of local tumor recurrences, but only modestly improves the survival over chemotherapy alone.

TABLE 62–2. Frequently Used Combination Regimens for Small Cell Lung Cancer

Combination	Dosages	Schedule
CAV		
CTX	1000 mg/m^2 IV d 1	Every 3 wk × 6
ADR	40 mg/m^2 IV d 1	
VCR	1 mg/m^2 IV d 1	
CAE		
CTX	1000 mg/m^2 IV d 1	Every 3 wk
ADR	45 mg/m^2 IV d 1	
ETOP	50 mg/m^2 IV d 1–5 or 80 mg/m^2 IV d 1–3	
CE		
DDP	80 mg/m^2 IV d 1	Every 3 wk
ETOP	150 mg/m^2 IV d 3–5	
(V)ICE		
IFOS	5000 mg/m^2 d 1 + Mesna	Every 3 or 4 wk
CBDCA	300 mg/m^2 d 1	
ETOP	120 mg/m^2 IV d 1 and 2, 240 mg/m^2 PO d 3	
VCR	1 mg/m^2 d 1	

CTX, cyclophosphamide; ADR, doxorubicin or Adriamycin; VCR, vincristine; ETOP, etoposide; CBDCA, carboplatin; IFOS, ifosfamide.

- Because CNS metastases often occur, *prophylactic cranial irradiation* (PCI) has been advocated in patients achieving a complete response to chemotherapy. However, neurologic and cognitive impairment lead some experts to recommend that cranial radiation be withheld until brain metastases manifest.
- As topotecan, an agent that crosses the blood–brain barrier, becomes more widely used, it will be important to evaluate the impact on the frequency of brain metastases.

► EVALUATION OF THERAPEUTIC OUTCOMES

- Response to chemotherapy should be evaluated after the second cycle and every second cycle thereafter.
  - Chemotherapy should be continued if there is a response. Although the optimal duration is unknown, it is reasonable and cost effective to continue chemotherapy for four to six cycles if patients with SCLC achieve a complete or partial response to initial chemotherapy.
  - If there is no response or progressive disease, an alternate, non–cross-resistant or investigational regimen should be considered.
- Many chemotherapy regimens are very intense and cause a wide variety of toxic effects.

  - Nausea and vomiting may be severe (especially in the cisplatin-containing regimens) and require aggressive antiemetic regimens.
  - Myelosuppression is often dose limiting, and granulocytopenia places patients at high risk of serious infections.
  - Other toxic effects include mucositis, peripheral neuropathies, nephrotoxicity, and ototoxicity.
- Patients receiving radiation therapy may experience fatigue, esophagitis, radiation pneumonitis, and cardiac toxicity.
- Patients with lung cancer frequently suffer from concomitant medical problems including chronic obstructive pulmonary diseases and cardiovascular disorders (often related to smoking), which require pharmacologic intervention and monitoring.
- Complex pharmacologic regimens (e.g., chemotherapeutic agents, antiemetics, antibiotics, analgesics, bronchodilators, corticosteroids, anticonvulsants, and cardiovascular agents) necessitate intensive therapeutic monitoring to avoid drug-related toxic effects and optimize patient management.

See Chapter 117, Lung Cancer, authored by Sally A. Felton, PharmD, and Rebecca S. Finley, PharmD, MS, for a more detailed discussion of this topic.

Chapter 63

▶ MALIGNANT LYMPHOMAS

▶ DEFINITION

Lymphomas are a heterogenous group of malignancies that arise from malignant transformation of immune cells that reside predominantly in lymphoid tissues and usually present as a solid tumor. Differences in histology have led to classification as Hodgkin's and non-Hodgkin's lymphoma, which are addressed separately in this chapter.

▶ HODGKIN'S DISEASE

PATHOPHYSIOLOGY

- Etiology has not been fully elucidated. Viruses—especially Epstein–Barr virus (EBV), which causes mononucleosis—have emerged as leading candidates for an infectious etiology.
- Hodgkin's disease is unique among lymphomas because only a small percentage of cells from involved tissue are malignant.
- The exact cellular origin of the malignant cell has yet to be determined and may not be the familiar Reed–Sternberg cell. In fact, this malignant cell appears to be of multilineage origin possibly because it represents an in vivo clonal population that occurs in response to viral stimuli (EBV) that promotes fusion of the interdigitating reticular cell, B cells, T cells, or both lymphocytes.
- The Rye classification system divides Hodgkin's disease into histologic subtypes based on the characteristics of the Reed–Sternberg cell and surrounding connective tissue. The subtypes (and incidence) are lymphocyte-predominant (9%), nodular sclerosis (56%), mixed cellularity (28%), and lymphocyte-depleted (7%).
- Hodgkin's disease appears to follow a predictable pattern of nodal spread that is not seen with non-Hodgkin's lymphomas.

CLINICAL PRESENTATION

- Most patients with lymphomas present with some form of adenopathy, which waxes and wanes for an average of 5 months before diagnosis. In Hodgkin's disease, adenopathy is usually localized to the cervical region and is painless and rubbery. Other common sites of nodal involvement include the mediastinal, hilar, and retroperitoneal regions.
- Up to 40% of patients with Hodgkin's disease present with constitutional or "B" symptoms (e.g., fever, night sweats, weight loss, and pruritus).

DIAGNOSIS AND STAGING

- The diagnosis and pathologic classification of Hodgkin's disease can only be made by biopsy of the enlarged node and histopathologic examination under a microscope.
- Staging is performed to provide prognostic information and to guide therapy.
- The staging classification (Table 63–1) has evolved from previous classifications (e.g., Rye). After careful staging, roughly half the patients have localized disease (stages I, II, and IIE), and the remainder have advanced disease, of which 10–15% are stage IV.
- Clinical staging begins with a thorough history to evaluate possible symptoms. Complete physical examination is done to determine nodal and extranodal involvement. Laboratory tests assess bone marrow, renal, and hepatic function. Chest roentgenogram and computed tomography (CT) evaluate mediastinal and abdominal involvement. Skeletal films are used to evaluate thoracic and lumbar vertebrae, pelvis, and proximal extremities.
- Pathologic staging is based on biopsy findings of strategic sites (e.g., muscle, bone, skin, spleen, abdominal nodes) using an invasive procedure (e.g., laparoscopy or laparotomy).

TABLE 63–1. Ann Arbor Staging Classification for Hodgkin's Disease

Stage I	Involvement of single lymph node region or structure (e.g., spleen, thymus)
Stage II	Involvement of ≥2 lymph node regions on the same side of the diaphragm (i.e., the mediastinum is a single site, hilar nodes are laterized). The number of anatomic sites should be indicated by a subscript (e.g., II_2)
Stage III	Involvement of lymph node regions on both sides of the diaphragm: III_1: With or without splenic hilar, celiac, or portal nodes III_2: With paraortic, iliac, or mesenteric nodes
Stage IV	Involvement of one or more extranodal sites beyond that designated E

A: No symptoms
B: Fever (>38°C for 3 consecutive d), sweats, weight loss (>10%)
X: Bulky disease
  >⅓ the width of the mediastinum
  >10 cm maximal dimension of nodal mass
E: Involvement of a single extranodal site, contiguous or proximal to a known nodal site
S: Involvement of the spleen
CS: Clinical stage
PS: Pathologic stage

Modified from Lister TA, Crowther D, Sutcliffe SB, et al. J Clin Oncol *1989;7:1630–1636.*

DESIRED OUTCOME

The current goal in the treatment of Hodgkin's disease is to maximize curability while minimizing short- and long-term treatment-related complications.

TREATMENT

Radiation Therapy

- Radiation therapy alone is the cornerstone of treatment for localized Hodgkin's disease, especially if there are no symptoms (stages IA and IIA).
- Patients with $IIIA_1$ disease (i.e., limited spleen, celiac, splenic, or portal nodes) are candidates for radiation therapy alone, but not the subset with bulky mediastinal and stage $IIIA_2$ disease.
- Most side effects are transient and seldom produce significant morbidity. Anorexia, xerostomia, odynophagia, skin burns, and changes in taste perception are common. Hypothyroidism and myelosuppression can also be seen.
- Serious toxic effects include radiation pneumonitis and fibrosis, pericarditis, cardiomyopathy, infertility, and growth retardation.
- The most common neurologic complication is Lhermitte's syndrome (i.e., numbness and tingling caused by head flexion), which occurs in up to 15% of patients.

Chemotherapy

Combination Regimens as Initial Therapy

- **MOPP** is the mainstay of treatment for advanced Hodgkin's disease (stages IIIB and IV) (Table 63–2). It produces complete remissions in 80% of patients and has a 10-year cure rate of 54%.
- Combination regimens produce more rapid and durable remissions than single-agent therapy. Patients should receive at least six cycles of MOPP and two cycles beyond that required to produce complete response. Maintenance therapy does not increase survival and may contribute to long-term complications. Delivering full doses of chemotherapy is extremely important.
- **ABVD, ChlVPP,** and other four-drug combinations (Table 63–2) are attractive alternatives to MOPP because they offer equal efficacy and differing or less severe toxicities.
- None of the alternating, hybrid, or sequential regimens provide clear advantages over fully dosed four-drug regimens.

Salvage Chemotherapy

- For patients who relapse after an initial complete response to MOPP, reinduction is possible. However, a regimen should not be used for salvage if it was not curative as first-line therapy, especially when other effective regimens with less chance of cross-resistance are available.

TABLE 63–2. Combination Chemotherapy Regimens for Hodgkin's Disease

Drug	Dose (mg/m²)	Route	Days
MOPP			
Mechlorethamine	6	IV	1, 8
Vincristine	1.4	IV	1, 8
Procarbazine	100	PO	1–14
Prednisone	40	PO	1–14
ABVD			
Doxorubicin	25	IV	1, 15
Bleomycin	10	IV	1, 15
Vinblastine	6	IV	1, 15
Dacarbazine	375	IV	1, 15
ChlVPP			
Chlorambucil	6	PO	1–14
Vinblastine	6	IV	1, 8
Procarbazine	100	PO	1–14
Prednisone	40	PO	1–14

Adapted from Longo DL. The use of chemotherapy in the treatment of Hodgkin's disease. Semin Oncol *1990;17: 7116–7135.*

- Choice of salvage treatment should be guided by estimation of the patient's tolerance for a particular set of agents.
- Patients who relapse following salvage chemotherapy are candidates for bone marrow transplantation.

Complications

- Myelosuppression is the major dose-limiting toxic effect of most combination regimens. Hematopoietic growth factors (e.g., G-CSF, GM-CSF) can decrease neutropenia and allow delivery of optimal doses on schedule. XI
- Nausea and vomiting are frequently seen with **dacarbazine, doxorubicin,** and **mechlorethamine,** although the severity has diminished with the use of the $5HT_3$ antagonists.
- Many patients experience neurotoxicity secondary to **vincristine** in MOPP therapy.
- Other acute toxic effects include alopecia, dermatitis, mucositis, phlebitis, malaise and fatigue, pulmonary reactions, cardiomyopathy, and renal dysfunction.
- Gonadal dysfunction is a major long-term complication of combination chemotherapy. **Nitrogen mustard** or **chlorambucil** consistently produces sterilization in men.
- Secondary malignancies are also major long-term complications. Solid tumors are the most common type of malignancy, and radiation therapy

is most often implicated. The risk of developing acute leukemia is highest in patients receiving both radiation therapy and chemotherapy; the risk is also higher with MOPP than with ABVD.
- Differences in toxicity patterns can be used to guide selection of combination chemotherapy. Fears of nausea, vomiting, and neurotoxicity generally lead to larger dose reductions of MOPP than ABVD. If fertility is an issue, ABVD may be a reasonable initial regimen. If not, ChlVPP may be the best choice, because it is very well tolerated, does not generally cause alopecia or neuropathy, and has leukemogenic effects that are intermediate between those of MOPP and ABVD.

Combined-Modality Treatment

- Controversy remains regarding the true role radiotherapy plays when added to chemotherapy in the treatment of Hodgkin's disease. Combined-modality therapy is beneficial only in selected patients with early disease (e.g., large mediastinal involvement).
- Radiation therapy plus ABVD increases the risk of cardiac and pulmonary complications.

▶ NON-HODGKIN'S LYMPHOMA

PATHOPHYSIOLOGY

- The etiology of non-Hodgkin's lymphoma is unknown. A relationship has been demonstrated between development of lymphoma and immunodeficient states, autoimmune disorders, infectious agents, and physical chemical exposure.
- Chromosomal translocations have become a hallmark of lymphomas. Protooncogenes alter normal cell growth function; *p*53, a tumor suppressor gene, is mutated or deleted in some non-Hodgkin's lymphomas.
- Non-Hodgkin's lymphomas are derived from monoclonal proliferation of B or, less commonly, T lymphocytes and their precursors.

CLINICAL PRESENTATION

- Patients may present with a variety of symptoms, which depend on the site of involvement, type of non-Hodgkin's lymphoma, and stage of disease at presentation, described later in this chapter.
- Indolent lymphomas usually arise in middle-aged or older individuals (median age, 55 years), and are uncommon before 40 years of age. Most patients present with advanced stages of disease, often the result of bone marrow involvement. Low-grade lymphomas usually have an indolent clinical course with waxing and waning adenopathy for months to years prior to diagnosis.
- Aggressive and highly aggressive lymphomas occur over a broader age range. Patients present at various stages of disease. Lymphoma tends to disseminate rapidly and often involves extranodal and privileged sites.
- Patients may have localized or generalized adenopathy. Involved nodes are painless, rubbery, and discrete and usually located in the cervical and

supraclavicular regions. Mesenteric or gastrointestinal involvement may cause nausea, vomiting, obstruction, abdominal pain, palpable abdominal mass, or gastrointestinal bleeding. Bone marrow involvement may cause symptoms related to anemia, neutropenia, or thrombocytopenia.

- Only 20% of patients with non-Hodgkin's lymphoma have constitutional or "B" symptoms.

DIAGNOSIS AND STAGING

- Diagnosis must be established by an appropriate biopsy of an involved lymph node.
- Diagnosis of non-Hodgkin's lymphoma is similar to that of Hodgkin's disease except as noted later in this chapter. Extent of investigative workup required prior to therapy is determined by histopathology and available treatment for the subtype of non-Hodgkin's lymphoma.
- Chest CT is usually unnecessary if chest roentgenograms are normal.
- Staging is less important in non-Hodgkin's lymphoma than in Hodgkin's disease because treatment is the same for stages II, III, and IV within a specific subtype of non-Hodgkin's lymphoma. Instead, prognosis of non-Hodgkin's lymphoma is more dependent on histologic subtype and clinical prognostic features (e.g., age ≥60 years, elevated lactic dehydrogenase, performance status ≥2, stage III or IV disease, and extranodal involvement).
- There are many systems for classifying non-Hodgkin's lymphomas, beginning with Rappaport's classification in 1956 and most recently evolving to the Revised European–American Classification of Lymphoid Neoplasms (REAL).
- Lymphomas are characterized as nodular or diffuse (depending on presence or absence of malignant cell clusters), as lymphocytic (small cells) or histiocytic (large cells), and by site of origin (B or T cell).
- Lymphomas of both B- and T-cell origin are classified as *indolent* (untreated survival measured in years), *aggressive* (untreated survival measured in months), and *highly aggressive* (untreated survival measured in weeks).

DESIRED OUTCOME

The primary treatment goals for non-Hodgkin's lymphoma are to relieve symptoms and, whenever possible, cure the patient of disease with acceptable toxicity.

TREATMENT

General Principles

- The role of radiation therapy differs for non-Hodgkin's lymphoma versus Hodgkin's disease. Only a small percentage of patients with non-Hodgkin's lymphoma are amenable to remission induction with irradiation because localized disease is rare at diagnosis. Radiation therapy is used more commonly in advanced disease, mainly as a palliative measure to control local bulky disease.

- Effective chemotherapy ranges from single-agent therapy for indolent lymphomas to aggressive, complex combination chemotherapy regimens for aggressive and highly aggressive lymphomas.
- Therapeutic approach depends on whether disease is limited (i.e., Ann Arbor stages I and II) or advanced (i.e., Ann Arbor stage III or IV, and frequently, stage II with poor prognostic features).

Limited Disease: Indolent Lymphoma

- *Radiation* therapy is the standard treatment for early-stage indolent lymphoma. There are no data to support the use of extended-field irradiation to clinically uninvolved contiguous lymph node chains, which is not surprising because spread of disease is frequently noncontiguous and less certain than with Hodgkin's disease.
- The role of adjuvant chemotherapy is unclear in localized stage I or II disease.

Limited Disease: Aggressive Lymphoma

- The current recommendation is three cycles of combination chemotherapy (i.e., CHOP) followed by involved-field radiation therapy (Table 63–3).
- If poor prognostic features are present, patients should receive treatment for advanced disease (see section on Advanced Disease).

Limited Disease: Highly Aggressive Lymphoma

- Acute leukemia-like protocols (e.g., high-dose induction, consolidation, maintenance, and CNS prophylaxis; see Chapter 60) are used in the treatment of lymphoblastic lymphoma and small noncleaved cell lymphoma.

Advanced Disease: Indolent Lymphoma

- Management of stage III and IV indolent lymphoma is controversial because standard therapeutic approaches are not curative, despite high complete remission rates.
- Therapeutic options are diverse. Complete response can be achieved in 60–90% of patients with single-agent therapy, combination chemotherapy, or combined-modality therapy; median remission durations are typically 17–24 months.

TABLE 63–3. Combination Chemotherapy for Aggressive Lymphoma (CHOP)

Drug	Dose (mg/m^2)	Route	Days
Cyclophosphamide	750	IV	1
Doxorubicin	50	IV	1
Vincristine	1.4	IV	1
Prednisone	100	PO	1–5

- Oral alkylating agents, chlorambucil 0.1–0.2 mg/kg or **cyclophosphamide** 1.5–2.5 mg/kg (adjusted to WBC and platelet counts), are the mainstay of treatment and produce minimal toxicity, but secondary acute myelogenous leukemia (AML) is a concern. **Fludarabine** and **cladribine** produce high response rates without secondary AML, but they are more myelosuppressive.
- *Combination regimens* do not improve survival, but they may eradicate the clone that is responsible for histologic transformation to aggressive or highly aggressive lymphoma.
- **Interferon** (IFN) during induction and/or maintenance can prolong the time to relapse and overall survival; however, it is unclear if the benefit applies to all or only follicular lymphomas. The most effective dose and schedule have not been determined, but lower doses appear to be as effective as higher doses.
- Because treatment regimens have not convincingly improved survival, it has been suggested that initial therapy be withheld from asymptomatic patients (i.e., "watchful waiting"). When initial therapy is delayed, the 10-year survival does not differ from that of immediate therapy. However, watchful waiting may not be appropriate for follicular mixed histologies.

Advanced Disease: Aggressive Lymphoma

General Principles

- Aggressive and highly aggressive non-Hodgkin's lymphomas are potentially curable diseases with intensive chemotherapy, even when they are widely metastatic.
- *Intensive combination chemotherapy* should be used because single-agent therapy does not consistently induce complete remission, and long-term survival is not possible without induction of complete remission.
- Dosage and administration schedules must be followed because reductions or delays compromise the ability to induce cure.
- Long-term maintenance therapy does not usually improve survival.
- Two cycles of chemotherapy following attainment of a complete response are usually recommended. Most current regimens last 6–9 months, except for MACOP-B, which requires only 12 weeks of therapy. XI
- Rapid response to chemotherapy (i.e., complete response in first three treatment cycles) is associated with a more durable remission compared with responses requiring more prolonged treatment.

Combination Regimens

- Of the *first-generation regimens*, CHOP has gained widespread popularity. Adding agents such as **bleomycin** (CHOP-Bleo, BACOP) or **methotrexate** (COMLA) does not significantly affect treatment outcome.
- *Second-generation chemotherapy* consists of six or more antineoplastic agents, with more frequent cycling of myelosuppressive agents (e.g., every 3 weeks) and administration of nonmyelosuppressive, generally

non–cross-resistant, agents during weeks of cytopenias. Response and survival rates appear to be superior to those of first-generation regimens based on results of separate trials, but there were no differences in randomized trials.

- *Third-generation treatment* regimens focus on alterations in schedules (i.e., use of more drugs and early exposure to non–cross-resistant agents) and doses (i.e., increasing dose intensity). Third-generation treatment regimens appear to be superior to the first- and second-generation regimens, but there were no significant differences in randomized trials, and third-generation regimens are more toxic.
- CHOP appears to be the therapy of choice based on response and survival rates, toxicity, and cost (see Table 63–3). Full-dose CHOP should also be considered treatment of choice in the elderly.
- Treatment of *AIDS-associated lymphoma* presents a therapeutic challenge. Standard chemotherapy regimens have been disappointing. The current approach is reduced doses of standard regimens or standard-dose regimens with hematopoietic growth factors.

Advanced Disease: Highly Aggressive Lymphoma

- Treatment of advanced-stage lymphoblastic and small noncleaved cell lymphomas is essentially the same as for limited disease.

Salvage Therapy: Indolent Lymphomas

- After relapse, patients are retreated and high remission rates are achieved; but response rates diminish with each retreatment. There is no evidence that salvage therapy improves overall survival.
- Any of the first-line options not already used can be used as salvage therapy. The most promising chemotherapy regimens not used as initial therapy include **fludarabine,** an **anthracycline,** and a steroid.
- **Rituximab** is a chimeric monoclonal antibody directed at CD20 expressed on B-cell tumors. It is indicated for relapsed or refractory indolent or follicular, CD20-positive, B-cell lymphoma and is being evaluated in combination with chemotherapy earlier in treatment. The usual dose is 375 mg/m^2 weekly for 4 weeks. Side effects are commonly seen only with the first infusion and include fever, chills, respiratory symptoms, and occasional hypotension.
- *High-dose chemotherapy* with allogeneic or autologous *transplant* is still controversial and needs further study.

Salvage Therapy: Aggressive Lymphomas

- Unfortunately, second-line salvage therapies are not capable of consistently inducing remission, possibly because nearly all effective agents are used in primary treatment regimens.
- Of the common salvage regimens, preliminary evidence favors **etoposide, methylprednisolone, high-dose cytarabine,** and **cisplatin** (ESHAP) over **cisplatin, high-dose cytarabine,** and **dexamethasone.** (DHAP). Another common regimen includes **mitoguazone, ifosfamide, methotrexate,** and **etoposide** (MIME).

- Ongoing clinical trials are evaluating investigational agents, alone and in combination, and high-dose chemotherapy, with or without stem cell rescue.

▶ EVALUATION OF THERAPEUTIC OUTCOMES

- The primary patient outcome to be identified is tumor response. Complete response is desirable because it yields the only chance for cure.
- Patients are generally monitored at 3–6 month intervals for the first year or two following treatment, with longer intervals instituted when appropriate.
- The most important predictor of a positive outcome for treatment of Hodgkin's disease is dose intensity. Patients who receive full doses of chemotherapy on time do significantly better than those who do not. Hematopoietic growth factors and other supportive care measures may facilitate this effort.
- To optimize chemotherapy administration, toxicity management is key. The clinician must identify, monitor, treat, and prevent or minimize treatment-related toxicity. A review of pertinent laboratory data and other procedures will help establish a baseline for monitoring purposes. Major organ and system toxicities to be followed include hematologic, neurologic, skin, pulmonary, gastrointestinal, renal, and cardiac.
- Myelosuppression and neutropenic fever with infection are constant concerns with aggressive chemotherapy. Appropriate patient education and monitoring are critical.
- Nutritional assessment should also be undertaken.

See Chapter 120, Malignant Lymphomas, authored by Val R. Adams, PharmD, and Ashley K. Morris, PharmD, BCPS, BCOP for a more detailed discussion of this topic.

Chapter 64

▶ PROSTATE CANCER

▶ DEFINITION

Prostate cancers are usually adenocarcinomas, which are curable when localized but not after metastatic spread occurs.

▶ NORMAL PROSTATE PHYSIOLOGY (Figure 64–1)

- Normal growth and differentiation of the prostate depend on the presence of androgens, specifically dihydrotestosterone (DHT), released primarily from the testes and the adrenal glands.
- Luteinizing hormone–releasing hormone (LHRH) from the hypothalamus stimulates the release of luteinizing hormone (LH) and follicle-stimulating hormone (FSH) from the anterior pituitary gland.
  - LH complexes with receptors on the Leydig cell testicular membrane and stimulates the production of testosterone and small amounts of estrogen.
  - FSH acts on testicular Sertoli cells to promote maturation of LH receptors and produce an androgen-binding protein.
- Circulating testosterone and estradiol influence the synthesis of LHRH, LH, and FSH by a negative feedback loop at the hypothalamic and pituitary level.
- Only 2% of total plasma testosterone is present in the active unbound state that penetrates the prostatic cell, where it is converted to DHT by 5-α-reductase. DHT subsequently binds with a cytoplasmic receptor and is transported to the cell nucleus where transcription and translation of stored genetic material occur.

▶ PATHOPHYSIOLOGY

- The only widely accepted risk factors are increased age, race-ethnicity (i.e., African-American), and family history of prostate cancer. Other factors thought to be implicated include occupational exposure, diet, benign prostatic hyperplasia, and vasectomy.
- Mutations in E-cahedrin and *p*53 are important in prostate carcinogenesis.
- The normal prostate is composed of acinar secretory cells that are altered when invaded by carcinoma; the major pathologic cell type is adenocarcinoma (>95% of cases).
- Prostate cancer can be graded. Well-differentiated tumors grow slowly, whereas poorly differentiated tumors grow rapidly and have a poor prognosis.
- Metastatic spread can occur by local extension, lymphatic drainage, or hematogenous dissemination. Skeletal metastases from hematogenous spread are the most common sites of distant spread. The lung, liver,

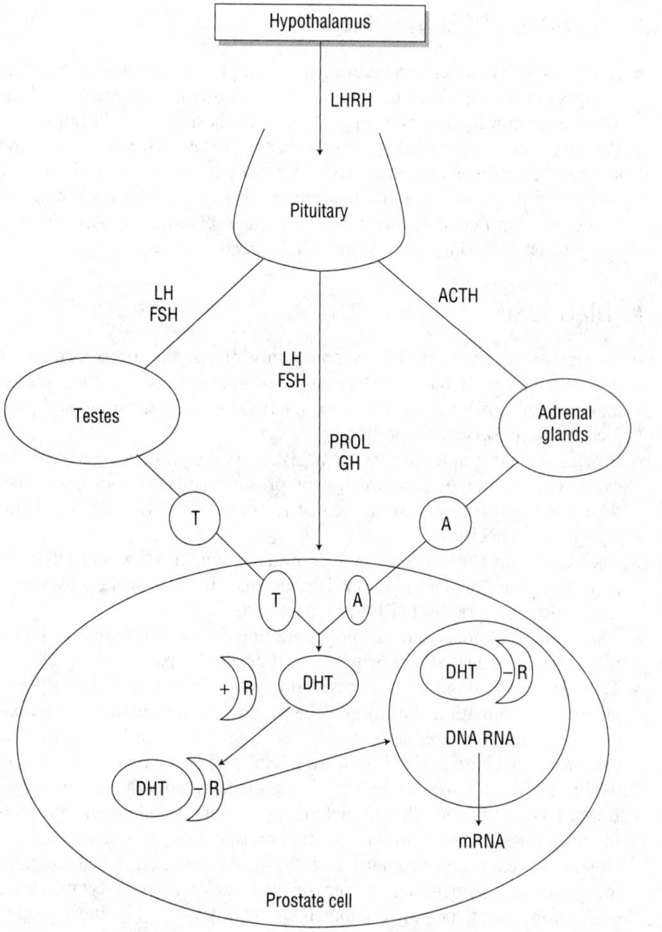

Figure 64–1. Hormonal regulation of the prostate gland. (LHRH, luteinizing hormone–releasing hormone; LH, luteinizing hormone; FSH, follicle-stimulating hormone; PROL, prolactin; ACTH, adrenocorticotropic hormone; GH, growth hormone; A, androgens; T, testosterone; R, receptor; DHT, dihydrotestosterone.)

XI

brain, and adrenal glands are the most common sites of visceral involvement, but these organs are not usually involved initially.

▶ CLINICAL PRESENTATION

- Localized prostatic carcinoma may be asymptomatic or associated with complaints arising from ureteral dysfunction or impingement, such as alterations in micturition (urinary frequency, hesitancy, dribbling).
- Patients with advanced disease commonly present with back pain and stiffness due to osseous metastases. Untreated spinal cord lesions may lead to cord compression. Pathologic fractures are rare. Lower extremity edema can occur as a result of lymphatic obstruction. Anemia and weight loss are nonspecific signs of advanced disease.

▶ DIAGNOSIS

- Digital rectal exam (DRE) is commonly employed for screening of prostate cancer. It has the advantages of specificity, low cost, safety, and ease of performance; however, DRE is not very sensitive and subject to interobserver variability.
- Prostate-specific antigen (PSA), a glycoprotein produced only in the cytoplasm of benign and malignant prostate cells, is more sensitive than DRE and likewise simple to perform, but PSA has the disadvantage of low specificity.
- The American Cancer Society recommends annual PSA and DRE for men ≥50 years of age. If either is abnormal, further workup by transrectal ultrasonography (TRUS) is indicated.
- The actual diagnosis and histologic grading can only be established by biopsy (e.g., transperianal or transrectal needle biopsy).
- The diagnostic staging workup should include a thorough history and physical examination with digital inspection of the rectum and palpation of regional lymph nodes, abdomen, and spine. On DRE, prostatic carcinoma is characterized by a rock-hard nodule or mass, whereas in benign prostatic hypertrophy (BPH) the gland is smooth and rubbery.
- Initial laboratory tests should include a complete blood chemistry, liver function tests, serum acid and alkaline phosphatase, and urinalysis.
- Bone scan, excretory urogram, and chest x-ray are performed for staging purposes. Depending on the results, skeletal films, lymph node evaluation (e.g., pelvic computed tomography [CT], indium-111-labeled capromab pendetide scan, bipedal lymphangiogram), and transrectal magnetic resonance imaging (MRI) may also be needed.

▶ DESIRED OUTCOME

The goals of treatment for localized prostate cancer are to cure the patient and prevent postprocedure complications. Advanced prostate cancer (stage D) is not currently curable, and treatment is intended to provide symptom relief and maintain quality of life.

▶ TREATMENT

GENERAL MANAGEMENT PRINCIPLES

- The initial treatment for prostate cancer depends on the stage of the disease.
- Patients with incidental carcinoma found at the time of a transurethral resection for BPH (stage A_1 or T_{1a} or T_{1b}) require only careful observation owing to high 10-year survival rate, unless the patient's life expectancy is over 10 years.
- Radical prostatectomy and radiation therapy are generally considered equivalent for localized prostate cancer (stage A_2 or B_1).
- Ongoing studies are attempting to define the best treatment for stage B_2 or C disease, because some stage C patients may have occult disease dissemination at presentation. Although external beam radiotherapy has been the primary treatment, there may also be a role for androgen deprivation before local treatment (i.e., *neoadjuvant therapy*).
- The best approach to stage D is controversial. Patients with stage D_0 and possibly D_1 prostate cancer may be carefully watched and appropriate local therapy (surgery or radiation) instituted when symptoms appear.
- The major initial treatment modality for advanced prostate cancer (stage D_2) is *androgen ablation* (e.g., orchiectomy or LHRH agonists with or without antiandrogens). Up to 80% of patients respond to initial hormonal manipulation, but most relapse within 2–4 years. After disease progression, secondary hormonal manipulations, cytotoxic chemotherapy, and supportive care are used.

ORCHIECTOMY

- Bilateral orchiectomy rapidly reduces circulating androgen levels. Many patients are not surgical candidates owing to advanced age or perceived unacceptableness. Nonetheless, orchiectomy is the preferred initial treatment for patients with impending spinal cord compression or ureteral obstruction.

LHRH AGONISTS

- LHRH agonists provide response rates similar to those of orchiectomy and estrogen and have the advantages of being reversible and causing fewer cardiovascular adverse effects than estrogens.
- There are no comparative trials of available LHRH agonists, so the choice is usually made by cost and patient and physician preference. **Leuprolide acetate** is administered daily, whereas **leuprolide depot** and **goserelin acetate implant** can be administered monthly, or every 12 or 16 weeks.

- The most common adverse effects of LHRH agonists are disease flare-up during the first week of therapy (e.g., increased bone pain, urinary symptoms), hot flashes, erectile impotence, decreased libido, and injection-site reactions.

▶ ANTIANDROGENS

- Monotherapy with **flutamide** (50–87%), **bicalutamide** (54–70%), and **nilutamide** (40%) produces objective responses (rates shown in parentheses), but antiandrogens are indicated only for advanced prostate cancer in combination with an LHRH agonist (flutamide and bicalutamide) or orchiectomy (nilutamide). In fact, antiandrogens can reduce the LHRH agonist–induced flare.
- The daily doses are flutamide 750 mg, bicalutamide 50 mg, and nilutamide 300 mg for 1 month, followed by 150 mg.
- The adverse effects of antiandrogens are gynecomastia, hot flushes, gastrointestinal (GI) disturbances, liver function test abnormalities, and breast tenderness. GI disturbances consist of diarrhea for flutamide and bicalutamide and nausea or constipation for nilutamide. Flutamide is also associated with methemoglobinemia, whereas nilutamide causes visual disturbances (impaired dark adaptation), alcohol intolerance, and interstitial pneumonitis.

COMBINED HORMONAL BLOCKADE

- The role of combined hormonal therapy, also referred to as *maximal androgen deprivation* or *total androgen blockade,* continues to be evaluated.
- Randomized trial results are mixed when candidates for *second-line therapy* are treated with combinations of antiandrogens plus either LHRH agonists or orchiectomy. Furthermore, a meta-analysis failed to show any additional survival benefit for maximal androgen blockade compared with conventional medical or surgical castration.

XI
- Some investigators consider combination androgen ablation to be the *initial hormonal therapy* of choice for newly diagnosed patients because the major benefit is seen in patients with minimal disease. In fact, some argue that treatment should not be delayed because recent combined androgen deprivation trials demonstrate survival advantage for young patients with good performance status and minimal disease, who were initially treated with hormonal therapy.
- Studies are needed to answer questions regarding the selection of modalities used as combined hormonal therapy, with careful consideration of effects on survival, time to progression, quality of life, patient preference, and economics (Table 64–1).

ESTROGENS

- Estrogens have historically been an important method of androgen ablation, but the major agent, diethylstilbestrol (DES), was removed

TABLE 64–1. Comparative Costs of Hormonal Therapy for Advanced Prostate Cancer

Drug	Dose	Average Wholesale Price/ Month of Therapy
Leuprolide depot	7.5 mg/mo	$566.85
Leuprolide depot	22.5 mg/12 wk	$1700.63
Leuprolide depot	30 mg/16 wk	$2267.50
Goserelin implant	3.6 mg q 28 d	$439.24
Goserelin implant	10.8 mg/12 wk	$1317.74
Flutamide	750 mg/d	$315.70
Bicalutamide	50 mg/d	$319.74
Nilutamide	300 mg/d for 1st mo, then 150 mg/d	$467.16, then $233.58

from the market in 1997. Alternatives (e.g., ethinyl estradiol, conjugated estrogens, chlorotrianisene, and polyestradiol phosphate) are not as extensively studied and cost more than DES.

SECONDARY TREATMENTS

- The selection of secondary or salvage therapies depends on what was used as initial therapy. Radiotherapy can be used after radical prostatectomy. Androgen ablation can be used after radiation therapy or radical prostatectomy.
- If testosterone levels are not suppressed (i.e., >20 ng/dL) after initial LHRH agonist therapy, an antiandrogen or orchiectomy may be indicated. If testosterone levels are suppressed, the disease is considered to be androgen independent and should be treated with palliative therapy.
- If initial therapy consisted of LHRH agonist and antiandrogen, then *androgen withdrawal* should be attempted. Mutations of the androgen receptor may allow antiandrogens to become agonists; withdrawal produces responses lasting 3–14 months in ≤35% of patients. XI
- Androgen synthesis inhibitors provide symptomatic, but brief, relief in approximately 50% of patients. **Aminoglutethimide** causes adverse effects in 50% of patients, such as lethargy, ataxia, dizziness, and self-limiting rash. The adverse effects of **ketoconazole** are GI intolerance, transient increases in liver and renal function tests, and hypoadrenalism.
- After hormonal manipulations are exhausted, palliation can be achieved with **strontium-89** or **samarium-153 lexidronam** for bone-related pain, analgesics, corticosteroids, local radiotherapy, or chemotherapy.

CHEMOTHERAPY

- Chemotherapy has not yet been shown to prolong survival in patients with advanced prostate cancer and consequently should be used in the clinical trial setting whenever possible.

- Single agents with modest activity include **cyclophosphamide, estramustine, fluorouracil, methotrexate, dacarbazine, mitoxantrone, doxorubicin,** and **cisplatin.**
- Active combinations include estramustine and **vinblastine** or mitoxantrone, and mitoxantrone and **prednisone.** Other possible combinations are ketoconazole and doxorubicin, and estramustine and **etoposide** or **paclitaxel.**

▶ EVALUATION OF THERAPEUTIC OUTCOMES

- The ultimate outcomes are overall and disease-free survival.
- Objective parameters include assessment of the primary tumor size, evaluation of involved lymph nodes, and response of tumor markers to treatment; however, there is no agreement about the best surrogate marker (e.g., PSA or indium-111-labeled capromab pendetide scanning).
- Clinical benefit can be documented by evaluating performance status, weight, and analgesic requirements.
- Quality-of-life assessments should be included in all clinical trials.

See Chapter 119, Prostate Cancer, authored by Jill M. Kolesar, PharmD, BCPS, and Barry R. Goldspiel, PharmD, BCPS, FASHP for a more detailed discussion of this topic.

Ophthalmic Disorders

Edited by Cindy W. Hamilton, PharmD

Chapter 65

▶ GLAUCOMA

▶ DEFINITION

The glaucomas are a group of ocular diseases characterized by changes in the optic nerve head (optic disk) and loss of visual sensitivity and field.

▶ PATHOPHYSIOLOGY

- The two major types of glaucoma are open-angle glaucoma, which accounts for most cases, and angle-closure glaucoma. Either type may be a primary, inherited disorder; secondary to disease, trauma, or drugs; or congenital (Table 65–1).
- The specific cause of glaucomatous optic neuropathy is unknown. Increased intraocular pressure (IOP) was considered to be the sole cause of visual damage, but IOP is only one of many contributing factors.
- Additional contributing factors include increased susceptibility of the optic nerve due to retinal ischemia, reduced or dysregulated blood flow, and physiologic processes of the extracellular matrix of the optic nerve head.
- Although IOP is a poor predictor of which patients will have visual field loss, the risk of visual field loss increases with increasing IOP.
- The mean normal population IOP is 15.5 ± 2.5 mm Hg, with frequency distribution skewed toward higher pressures.
- IOP is determined by the balance between the inflow and outflow of aqueous humor. *Inflow* appears to be decreased by α_2-adrenergic and adenylate cyclase–stimulating agents as well as by agents that block α-adrenergic, β-adrenergic, and dopamine receptors. *Outflow* is increased by cholinergic agents. Aqueous humor *formation* is ultimately influenced by blood pressure and IOP changes; carbonic anhydrase is also involved in aqueous humor formation.
- The increased IOP in open-angle glaucoma is caused by a decreased facility for aqueous outflow through the trabecular meshwork.
- Angle-closure glaucoma results from mechanical blockage of the trabecular meshwork by the iris.
- Many drugs (Table 65–2) have been associated with increased IOP. The potential to produce or worsen glaucoma depends on the type of glaucoma and whether or not the patient is adequately controlled.

TABLE 65–1. Classification of Glaucoma

I. Primary glaucoma
   A. Open angle
   B. Angle closure
      1. With pupillary block
      2. Without pupillary block

II. Secondary glaucoma
   A. Open angle
      1. Pretrabecular
      2. Trabecular
      3. Post-trabecular
   B. Angle closure
      1. With pupillary block
      2. Without pupillary block

III. Congenital glaucoma

TABLE 65–2. Drugs that May Induce or Potentiate Glaucoma

Open-angle Glaucoma

Ophthalmic corticosteroids (high risk)

Systematic, nasal, or inhaled corticosteroids

Fenoldapam

Ophthalmic anticholinergics

Vasodilators (low risk)

Cimetidine (low risk)

Angle-closure Glaucoma

Topical anticholinergics (high risk)

Topical sympathomimetics (high risk)

Antihistamines

Systemic anticholinergics

Heterocyclic antidepressants

Phenothiazines

Ipratropium

Benzodiazepines

Theophylline (low risk)

Vasodilators (low risk)

Systemic sympathomimetics (low risk)

CNS stimulants (low risk)

Tetracyclines (low risk)

Carbonic anhydrase inhibitors (low risk)

Monoamine oxidase inhibitors (low risk)

Topical cholinergics (low risk)

▶ CLINICAL PRESENTATION

- Characteristic visual field loss occurs in glaucoma, but loss of central visual acuity does not occur until late in the disease. Visual field defects may include general peripheral visual field constriction, isolated scotomas or blind spots, nasal visual field depression or nasal step, enlargement of the blind spot, large arc-like scotomas, and reduced contrast sensitivity.
- Patients with untreated angle-closure glaucoma typically experience intermittent prodromal symptoms (e.g., blurred or hazy vision with halos around lights and, occasionally, headache). Acute angle closure produces symptoms associated with a cloudy, edematous cornea; ocular pain; nausea, vomiting, and abdominal pain; and diaphoresis.

▶ DIAGNOSIS

- IOP, optic disk changes, and perimetry are the primary diagnostic (and monitoring) parameters; however, increased IOP is not necessary for the diagnosis of glaucoma.
- Optic disk findings associated with glaucoma include cup:disk ratio >0.5, progressive increase in cup size, cup:disk ratio asymmetry >0.2, vertical elongation of the cup, excavation or deepening of the cup, increased exposure of lamina cribrosa, pallor of the cup, splinter hemorrhages, cupping to the edge of the disk, and notching of the cup.

▶ DESIRED OUTCOME

The ultimate goal of drug therapy in patients with glaucoma is to preserve visual function by reducing the IOP to a level at which no further optic nerve damage occurs.

▶ TREATMENT OF OPEN-ANGLE GLAUCOMA

- Treatment is indicated for all patients with characteristic optic disk changes or visual field defects, but treatment of ocular hypertension remains controversial.
- Controversy exists as to whether the initial therapy of glaucoma should be surgical trabeculectomy, argon laser trabeculectomy, or medical therapy. XII
- Drug therapy of patients with documented glaucomatous change is initiated in a stepwise manner, starting with a single well-tolerated topical agent (e.g., β blocker, **dipivefrin,** or carbonic anhydrase inhibitor) (Table 65–3).
- Topical **cholinesterase inhibitors** and oral carbonic anhydrase inhibitors (CAIs) (Table 65–4) are considered last-line agents for patients who fail less toxic combination topical therapy.

TABLE 65–3. Topical Agents Used in the Treatment of Glaucoma

Drug	Form	Strength%[a]	Brand Name	Dose Frequency[a]	Mechanism of IOP Reduction
β-Adrenergic Blockers					Decreased aqueous flow
Betaxolol	Solution	0.5	Betoptic	q 12 h	
	Suspension	0.25	Betoptic S	q 12 h	
Carteolol	Solution	1	Ocupress	q 12 h	
Levobunolol	Solution	0.25, 0.5	Betagan	q 12–24 h	
Metipranolol	Solution	0.3	OptiPranolol	q 12 h	
Timolol	Solution	0.25, 0.5	Timoptic, others	q 12–24 h	
	Gelling solution	0.25	Timoptic XE	q 24 h	
Adrenergic Agonists					
α/β agonists					Increased aqueous outflow
Epinephrine HCl	Solution	0.25, 0.5, 1, 2	Epifrin, Glaucon	q 12 h	
Epinephrine bitartrate	Solution	2		q 12 h	
Epinephrine borate	Solution	0.5, 1, 2	Epinal	q 12 h	
Dipivefrin	Solution	0.1	Propine	q 12 h	
α_2 agonists					Decreased aqueous inflow
Apraclonidine	Solution	1	Iopidine	pre- and post-op	
	Solution	0.5	Iopidine	q 8–12 h	
Brimonidine	Solution	0.2	Alphagen	q 8–12 h	

Parasympathomimetics					
Direct acting					Increased aqueous outflow
Pilocarpine	Solution	0.25–10	Numerous	q 4–12 h	
Pilocarpine	Gel	4	Pilopine HS	q 24 h	
Carbachol	Solution	0.75, 1.5, 2.25	IsoptoCarbachol	q 8–12 h	
Cholinesterase inhibitors					Increased aqueous outflow
Physostigmine	Solution	0.25, 0.5	Isopto Eserine	q 8–12 h	
Demecarium	Solution	0.125	Humorsol	q 8–72 h	
Echothiophate	Solution	0.23–0.25	Phospholine Iodide	q 12–24 h	
Isoflurophate	Ointment	0.25	Floropryl	q 8–72 h	
Carbonic Anhydrase Inhibitor					Decreased aqueous inflow
Dorzolamide	Solution	2	Trusopt	q 8–12 h	
Brinzolamide	Suspension	1	Azopt	q 8–12 h	
Prostaglandin Analog					Increased uveoscular outflow
Latanoprost	Solution	0.005	Xalatan	q 24 h	

[a]Use of nasolacrimal occlusion (NLO) may allow use of lower concentrations at longer intervals.

TABLE 65–4. Systemic Carbonic Anhydrase Inhibitors Used in the Treatment of Glaucoma

Drug	Form	Strength (mg)	Brand Name	Dose	IOP Reduction (h)		
					Onset	*Peak*	*Duration*
Acetazolamide	Injection	500	Diamox	500 mg IV or IM	2 min	0.25–0.5	2–5
	Tablets	125, 250	Diamox	125–250 mg bid–qid	1–1.5	2–4	8–12
	Capsules	500	Diamox Sequels	500 mg bid	2	8–12	12–24
Dichlorphenamide	Tablets	50	Daranide	25–50 mg bid–qid	0.5–1	2–4	6–12
Methazolamide	Tablets	50	Neptazane	25–100 mg bid–tid	2–4	6–8	10–12

IOP, intraocular pressure.

▶ TREATMENT OF ANGLE-CLOSURE GLAUCOMA

- Iridectomy, the definitive treatment of angle-closure glaucoma, produces a hole in the iris that permits aqueous flow to move directly from the posterior chamber to the anterior chamber.
- Drug therapy of an acute attack typically consists of hyperosmotic agents and a secretory inhibitor (e.g., β blocker, α_2 agonist, or CAI), with or without **pilocarpine.** An osmotic agent is often used because it rapidly decreases IOP (Table 65–5).
- Although traditionally the drug of choice, pilocarpine use is controversial as initial therapy. Once the IOP is controlled, pilocarpine should be given every 6 hours until iridectomy is performed.

▶ EVALUATION OF THERAPEUTIC OUTCOMES

- Monitoring of therapy should be individualized: IOP should be measured initially every 1–2 weeks until the patient is stabilized, and then every 1–3 months. The disk should be visualized and the visual field measured every 6–12 months (more frequently after any change in drug therapy).
- Because of the poor relationship between IOP and optic nerve damage, no specific target IOP exists. Typically, a 25–30% reduction is desired.
- The target IOP also depends on disease severity and is generally <21 mm Hg for early visual field loss or optic disk changes, with progressively lower targets for greater damage. Targets as low as <10 mm Hg are desired for very advanced disease, progressive damage at higher IOPs, low-tension glaucoma, and pretreatment pressures in the low to mid-teens.
- Compliance with glaucoma therapy is commonly inadequate, and should always be considered a possible cause of drug therapy failure.

See Chapter 86, Glaucoma, authored by Timothy S. Lesar, PharmD, for a more detailed discussion of this topic.

TABLE 65–5. Osmotic Agents Used in the Treatment of Glaucoma

Drug	Molecular Weight	Strength (%)	Dose (g/kg)	Route	Distribution[a]	Ocular Penetration[b]	Intraocular Pressure Reduction (h)		
							Onset	*Peak*	*Duration*
Mannitol	182	5, 10, 15, 20, 25	1–2	IV	Extracellular	Poor	0.25	0.5–1	6–9
Urea	60	30	1–1.5	IV	Total	Good	0.25	1–2	5–6
Glycerin	92	50, 75	1–1.5	PO	Extracellular	Moderate	0.25	0.5–1.5	4–6
Isosorbide	146	45	1–2	PO	Total	Good	0.25	0.5–1.5	4–6

[a]Distribution in body water.
[b]Poor intraocular penetration is preferred for intraocular pressure reduction.

Chapter 66

▶ ALZHEIMER'S DISEASE

▶ DEFINITION

Alzheimer's disease (AD) is a progressive dementia for which no cause is known and no cure exists. Disability progresses until AD sufferers become totally dependent. It accounts for 60% of all cases of late-life cognitive dysfunction.

▶ PATHOPHYSIOLOGY

NEUROFIBRILLARY TANGLES AND NEURITIC PLAQUES

- AD affects the brain structures associated with memory, higher learning, reasoning, behavior, and emotion (cortex and limbic areas).
- The brains of AD patients have a drastically increased number of neurofibrillary tangles (NFTs) and neuritic plaques (NPs) in comparison to normal brains. These lesions occur particularly in the hippocampus, amygdala, and cerebral cortex in areas where cholinergic and other brain neuronal pathways have been destroyed.
- NFTs are intracellular and are comprised of paired neurofilaments with a helical shape that aggregate in dense bundles. The paired helical filaments are comprised of an abnormally phosphorylated form of tau protein. Affected cells function improperly and eventually die.
- NPs (also called amyloid or senile plaques) are extracellular and are comprised of a core of beta amyloid protein (βAP) surrounded by a snarled mass of broken neurites. NP formation seems to precede accumulation of NFTs. The number of NPs does not necessarily determine disease severity.

BETA AMYLOID PROTEIN

- βAP deposition may initiate the process of NP formation. Proteases cleave the amyloid precursor protein to form the βAP.
- The apolipoprotein E4 allele on chromosome 19 influences susceptibility to late-onset cases. Almost all early-onset cases of AD can be attributed to alterations on chromosomes 1, 14, and 21.

APOLIPOPROTEIN E

- A gene on chromosome 19 is responsible for the production of apolipoprotein E (apo E), which exists in three main isoforms (Apo E2, Apo E3, and Apo E4).
- In Caucasians, inheriting a single copy of E4 increases AD risk, whereas inheriting the Apo E2 allele protects against AD. In African-Americans the converse may be true.

INFLAMMATORY MEDIATORS

- Inflammatory mediators—α-antichymotrypsin (ACT), α_2-macroglobulin, cytokines, and components of the complement cascade—are present near areas of plaque formation, suggesting that the immune system may foster disease progression.

NEUROTRANSMITTER ABNORMALITIES

- Most profoundly damaged are the cholinergic pathways, especially a large system of neurons located at the base of the forebrain in the nucleus basalis of Mynert. Cholinergic cell loss does not appear to be the disease-producing event, but a consequence of disease pathology.
- Serotonergic neurons of the raphe nuclei and noradrenergic cells of the locus ceruleus are lost, whereas monoamine oxidase type-B (MAO-B) activity is increased.
- Glutamate and other excitatory amino acid neurotransmitters have been implicated as potential neurotoxins in AD.

OTHER FACTORS

- The ability of estrogen to interact with nerve growth factor may explain its ability to promote synaptic growth. Estrogen also acts as an antioxidant and may prevent formation of neuritic plaques. In one study, the relative risk of developing AD was 0.4 (95% CI = 0.22–0.85) for estrogen users versus nonusers.
- Repeated or severe head trauma may also predispose to AD.
- Preliminary in vitro evidence suggests that zinc may accelerate NP formation from soluble βAP. Although the use of zinc supplements should be discouraged in AD, at present, zinc is not considered a cause of AD.

▶ CLINICAL PRESENTATION

- Most cases of AD occur after age 65. Cognitive symptoms include memory loss (e.g., poor recall, agnosia, losing things); dysphasia (anomia, circumlocution, aphasia); dyspraxia; disorientation; and impaired calculation, judgment, and problem-solving. Impaired memory, especially for recent events, is usually the presenting complaint.
- Noncognitive symptoms include depression, psychotic symptoms, and disruptive behaviors (e.g., aggression, hyperactivity, wandering, uncooperativeness).
- As AD progresses, there is decreased socialization.
- At moderate severity, patients may be unable to use objects properly, draw complex figures or conceptualize their orientation in space (constructional apraxia), plan, do household chores, or initiate activities.
- In severe stages, patients may become lost in their homes, unable to recognize family, or speak. Judgment is very impaired. They may wander and become combative, become incontinent, and require placement in a long-term care facility.

- Depression, frustration, and irritability may occur early. Anxiety, hostility, and delusions are common in moderate stages. Disruptive behaviors and psychosis occur in moderate to severe stages.
- Choking, aspiration, or infection results in death within 3 to 20 years of AD onset.

▶ DIAGNOSIS

- If memory loss affects social or occupational functioning or is noticed by others, patients should visit a neurologist, as early diagnosis is critical.
- AD remains a diagnosis of exclusion.
- The Neurological and Communicative Disorders and Stroke and the Alzheimer's Disease and Related Disorders Association (NINCDS–ADRDA) developed criteria for AD (Table 66–1) that reduce erroneous diagnosis to less than 10%.
- All patients should have a thorough history (from patient and caregiver) and physical exam. History should include review of drug, alcohol, or other substance use; family medical history; and history of trauma, depression, or head injury.
- Medication use (anticholinergics, sedatives) must be ruled out as contributing to symptoms.
- The Folstein Mini-Mental Status Exam (MMSE) can establish a history of deficits in two or more areas of cognition.
- Other causes of dementia must be excluded (e.g., cerebral vascular disease, subcortical stroke, alcoholism, vitamin B_{12} deficiency, head trauma, Parkinson's disease, Huntington's disease, Pick's disease, Creutzfeldt–Jakob disease, hypothyroidism).
- Routine laboratory tests, physical and neurologic exams, and brain imaging tools help establish the diagnosis.
- AD is staged using a scale such as the Global Deterioration Scale (GDS; Table 66–2) which is useful in monitoring cognitive decline.

▶ DESIRED OUTCOME

- The primary goal of treatment in AD is to maintain patient functioning as long as possible. Secondary goals are to treat the psychiatric and behavioral sequelae.

▶ TREATMENT

- The primary approach in treating AD is nonpharmacologic (e.g., education, guidance for activities of daily living, installation of latches on doors to prevent wandering).
- Figure 66–1 is an algorithm for treatment of cognitive and noncognitive symptoms.

TABLE 66–1. NINCDS–ADRDA Criteria and Diagnostic Workup for Probable Alzheimer's Disease

I. History of progressive cognitive decline of insidious onset
   In-depth interview of patient and caregivers
II. Deficits in at least two or more areas of functioning
   Confirmation with use of dementia rating scale (Mini-Mental Status Exam [MMSE[a]] or Blessed Dementia Scale)
III. No disturbance of consciousness
IV. Age between 40 and 90 (usually >65)
V. No other explainable cause of symptoms
   Normal laboratory tests including hematology, full chemistries, B_{12} and folate, thyroid function tests, VDRL (to rule out venereal disease or syphilis)
   Normal electrocardiogram and electroencephalogram
   Normal physical exam, including thorough neurologic exam
   CT or MRI scanning: No focal lesions signifying other possible causes of dementia are present. Abnormalities that are common, but not diagnostic for AD, include general cerebral wasting, widening of sulci, widening of the ventricles, and lesions of white matter surrounding the ventricle deep in the brain.

[a]The Folstein Mini-Mental Status Exam is a commonly used scale measuring orientation, recall, short-term memory, concentration, constructional praxis, and language. The MMSE is scored from 0 to 30, with a score of 10 to ~28 typical of very early to moderate Alzheimer's disease. *Adapted from McKhann G, Drachman D, Folstein M, et al.* Neurology *1984; 34:939–944.*

PHARMACOTHERAPY OF COGNITIVE SYMPTOMS

Cholinesterase Inhibitors

- **Tacrine (Cognex)** has been largely replaced by a safer, better-tolerated cholinesterase inhibitor.
- **Donepezil (Acricept)** is first-line treatment for cognitive impairment in mild to moderately severe (MMSE 10–26) AD. A Folstein MMSE or similar assessment should be performed before initiating treatment.
- Donepezil is a piperidine with specificity for inhibition of acetylcholinesterase as compared with butyrylcholinesterase. This may account for the lower incidence of peripheral side effects (e.g., nausea, vomiting, diarrhea) compared with tacrine. Donepezil has similar efficacy to tacrine, but patients are more likely to continue taking donepezil than tacrine, and therefore, donepezil is more "effective."
- Unlike tacrine, donepezil pharmacokinetics are linear at therapeutic doses. Its half-life (70 hours) enables once-daily dosing.
- Donepezil 5 mg/d and 10 mg/d are effective doses, with a trend for superiority with the 10-mg/d dose. A trial at the higher dose is reasonable in patients with no side effects. Donepezil 5 mg/d should be the initial dose. If improvement has not been observed within 4–6 weeks, and the drug is well tolerated, then 10 mg/d may be tried. It should be taken in the evening, just prior to retiring, and may be taken with or without food. As long as there is no rapid decline, it is reasonable to continue treat-

TABLE 66–2. Stages of Cognitive Decline: The Global Deterioration Scale (GDS)

Stage 1	Normal	No subjective or objective change in intellectual functioning.
Stage 2	Forgetfulness	Complaints of losing things or forgetting names of acquaintances. Does not interfere with job or social functioning. Generally a component of normal aging.
Stage 3	Early confusion	Cognitive decline causes interference with work and social functioning. Anomia, difficulty remembering right word in conversation, and recall difficulties are present and noticed by family members. Memory loss may cause anxiety for patient.
Stage 4	Late confusion (early AD)	Patient can no longer manage finances or homemaking activities. Difficulty remembering recent events. Begins to withdraw from difficult tasks and give up hobbies. May deny memory problems.
Stage 5	Early dementia (moderate AD)	Patient can no longer survive without assistance. Frequently disoriented with regard to time (date, year, season). Difficulty selecting clothing. Recall for recent events is severely imapired; may forget some details of past life (school attended or occupation). Functioning may fluctuate from day to day. Patient generally denies problems. May become suspicious or tearful. Loses ability to drive safely.
Stage 6	Middle dementia (moderately severe AD)	Patient needs assistance with activities of daily living (bathing, dressing, toileting). Patient experiences difficulty interpreting surroundings; may forget names of family and caregivers; forgets most details of past life; has difficulty counting backwards from 10. Agitation, paranoia, and delusions are common.
Stage 7	Late dementia	Patient loses ability to speak (may only grunt or scream), walk, and feed self. Incontinent of urine and feces. Consciousness reduced to stupor or coma.

Adapted from Reisberg B, Ferris SH, DeLeon MJ, Crook T. The global deterioration scale for assessment of primary degenerative dementia. Am J Psychiatry *1982; 139: 1136–1139.*

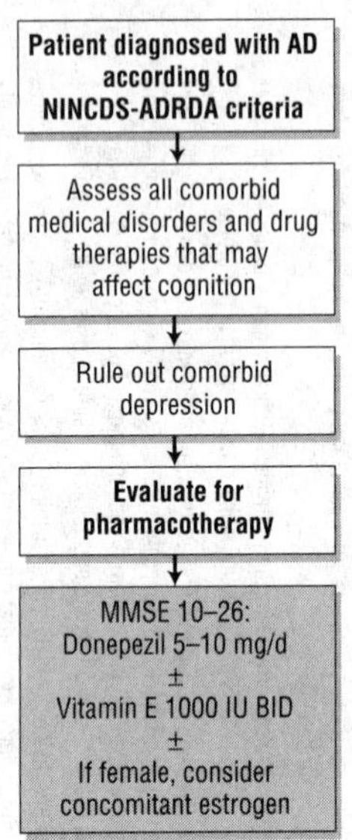

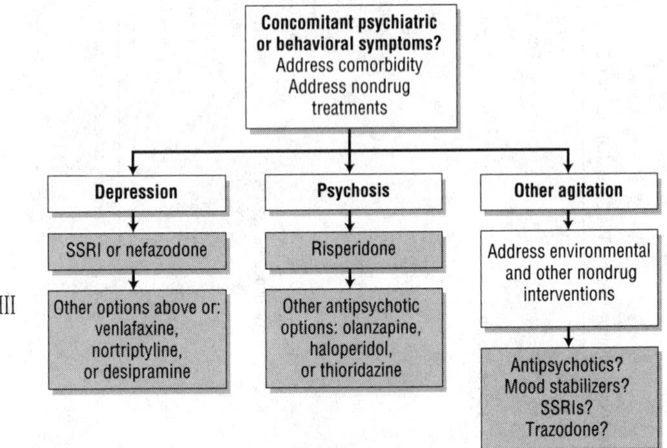

XIII

Figure 66–1. Proposed treatment algorithm for Alzheimer's disease (AD).

ment. If rapid decline occurs, tapering and discontinuation may be tried, but close monitoring for rapid decline upon discontinuation is indicated.

- Common donepezil side effects are nausea, vomiting, diarrhea, and insomnia.
- Tacrine is not recommended for patients who have not benefitted from or tolerated donepezil.
- In vitro studies suggest that **ketoconazole** (a CYP 3A3/4 inhibitor) and **quinidine** (a CYP 2D6 inhibitor) inhibit donepezil metabolism. However, in vitro studies have also shown donepezil to have low affinity for CYP 2D6 and 3A4, thus making clinically significant drug interactions through these isoenzymes unlikely.

Other Drugs

- Both **vitamin E** and **selegiline** were superior to placebo, but the combination was slightly inferior to either treatment alone. In another study, the only demonstrated effect with selegiline 10 mg/d was a mild decrease in Brief Psychiatric Rating Scale scores.
- Most epidemiologic studies have shown a lower incidence of AD in women who took **estrogen replacement therapy (ERT)** postmenopausally; one study showed higher MMSE scores in estrogen-treated AD patients. If female AD patients are not at risk for either endometrial or breast cancer, a trial of estrogen is reasonable. Doses are the same as for ERT, and estrogen may be used in combination with either donepezil or vitamin E.
- Epidemiologic studies have shown a lower incidence of AD or higher MMSE scores in AD if nonsteroidal anti-inflammatory drugs (NSAIDs) were taken regularly. Patients who used NSAIDs for >2 years had a relative risk of AD of 0.4 compared to a relative risk of 0.65 in those taking NSAIDs for less than 2 years. However, because of limited evidence and potential for side effects, NSAIDs are not recommended for general use in prevention or treatment of AD at present.
- In one study, **Egb 761,** an extract of ginkgo biloba, was significantly superior to placebo in treatment of mixed dementias, but there was a significant placebo response. Egb 761 was not different from placebo in the Clinical Global Impression of Change scale. Adverse effects and long-term toxicities are not well understood. The content of herbals is poorly standardized, and it is recommended that it be used with caution.

PHARMACOTHERAPY OF NONCOGNITIVE SYMPTOMS

- Most AD patients manifest noncognitive symptoms (e.g., psychotic symptoms, disruptive behaviors, depression, wandering) at some point in their illness. Medications and recommended doses for noncognitive symptoms are shown in Table 66–3.
- General guidelines are as follows: (1) use reduced doses, (2) monitor closely, (3) document carefully, and (4) periodically attempt to reduce medication.
- Anticholinergic and sedative drugs may worsen cognition.

TABLE 66–3. Medications Used in Treating Noncognitive Symptoms of Dementia

Drug	Suggested Dosage in Dementia (mg/d)	Indications
Antipsychotics		
Haloperidol	0.5–5	Psychosis (hallucinations, delusions, suspiciousness), disruptive behaviors (agitation, aggression)
Risperidone	0.5–2	
Thioridazine	10–100	
Antidepressants		
Citalopram	10–30	Depression: Poor appetite, insomnia, hopelessness, anhedonia, withdrawal, suicidal thoughts, agitation
Desipramine	50–150[a,b]	
Nortriptyline	25–150[a,b]	
Fluoxetine	5–20	
Sertraline	50–200	
Paroxetine	10–40	
Trazodone	75–400[a]	
Anticonvulsants		
Carbamazepine	100–1000[a,b]	Disruptive behaviors, mood instability
Valproic Acid	1000–2500[a,b]	
Others		
Selegiline	10	Disruptive behaviors, agitation, anxiety, depression
Buspirone	10–45[a]	Disruptive behaviors
Oxazepam	10–60[a]	Disruptive behaviors

[a]Administer in divided doses.
[b]Dosage adjustment should be guided by drug serum concentrations.

Depression

- Depression and dementia have many symptoms in common, and the diagnosis of depression can be difficult, especially later in the course of AD.
- There appears to be significant placebo response in treatment of depression in AD patients. Antidepressant response may not be as dramatic as in nondemented patients. Up to 12 weeks of treatment may be required to achieve antidepressant response.
- Selective serotonin reuptake inhibitors (SSRIs) are often considered to be preferred antidepressants in this population, but other acceptable agents include secondary amine tricyclic antidepressants (TCAs), **venlafaxine, nefazodone,** and **trazodone.** Orthostasis and sedation can be a disadvantage with trazodone.

Antipsychotics

- If delusions and problem behaviors are not particularly disturbing, they may not require treatment.
- Antipsychotics are used to treat disruptive behaviors and psychosis in AD patients, but they are moderately effective at best. Symptoms responding include assaultiveness, extreme agitation and hyperex-

citability, hallucinations, delusions, suspiciousness, hostility, and uncooperativeness. Symptoms not responding include withdrawal, apathy, cognitive deficits, and incontinence.

- AD patients are more sensitive to side effects than are other patient groups. Especially problematic are extrapyramidal side effects, orthostatic hypotension, anticholinergic effects, and worsening cognition.
- An attempt to taper and discontinue antipsychotics should be made at least every 3 months.
- **Haloperidol** is the most widely used antipsychotic, but **thioridazine** in low doses is also commonly used.
- **Risperidone** has also been found useful. The beginning dose, 0.25 mg/d, can be increased to 1 mg/d if needed, titrating to 2 mg/d if there is inadequate response.

Miscellaneous Therapies

- Benzodiazepines, particularly **oxazepam,** have been used to treat anxiety, agitation, and aggression but generally show inferior efficacy compared to antipsychotics.
- **Buspirone** has shown benefit in treating agitation and aggression in small studies.
- Selegiline may decrease anxiety, depression, and agitation.
- Should antipsychotics fail to manage noncognitive behaviors, a trial of buspirone or selegiline might be a reasonable alternative.

Pharmacoeconomic Considerations

- Patients receiving tacrine ≥80 mg/d were found less likely to enter a nursing home. The estimated average annual cost savings with tacrine treatment was $2243 and $4052 for 80–160-mg/d and 160-mg/d doses, respectively.

▶ EVALUATION OF THERAPEUTIC OUTCOMES

- A thorough assessment at baseline should define goals and document cognitive status, physical status, functional performance, mood, thought processes, and behavior. Both the patient and caregiver should be interviewed. A list of symptoms to be treated and potential side effects should be documented. The MMSE (or a variation) should be used to assess multiple spheres of cognition.
- Periodic assessment for efficacy, compliance, side effects, need for dosage adjustment, or change in treatment should occur at least monthly. XIII
- Six months to 1 year may be required to determine whether therapy is beneficial.

See Chapter 61, Alzheimer's Disease, authored by M. Lynn Crismon, PharmD, FCCP, BCPP, and Andrea E. Eggert, PharmD, BCPP, for a more detailed discussion of this topic.

Chapter 67

▶ ANXIETY DISORDERS

▶ DEFINITION

Anxiety disorders include a constellation of disorders in which anxiety and associated symptoms are irrational or experienced at a level of severity that impairs functioning. The characteristic features are anxiety and avoidance behavior.

▶ PATHOPHYSIOLOGY

- *Noradrenergic model.* This model suggests that the autonomic nervous system of anxious patients is hypersensitive and overreacts to various stimuli. The locus coeruleus may have a role in regulating anxiety, as it activates norepinephrine (NE) release and stimulates the sympathetic nervous system. Chronic noradrenergic overactivity downregulates α_2 adrenoreceptors in patients with generalized anxiety disorder (GAD).
- *Benzodiazepine (BZD) receptor model.* Benzodiazepine receptors are linked to γ-aminobutyric acid, type A ($GABA_A$) receptors and chloride ion channels. GABA is the major inhibitory neurotransmitter in the central nervous system (CNS). Anxiety symptoms may be related to underactivity of GABA systems.
- *Serotonin model.* GAD symptoms may reflect excessive serotonin (5-HT) transmission or overactivity of the stimulatory 5-HT pathways.
- *Peptide theory.* The role of cholecystokinin (CCK) and other peptides is under investigation. CCK increases the activity of catecholamines in the LC and coexists with GABA-producing neurons.

▶ CLINICAL PRESENTATION

- The *Diagnostic and Statistical Manual of Mental Disorders,* 4th edition (DSM-IV) classifies anxiety disorders into several categories (Table 67–1).

GENERALIZED ANXIETY DISORDER

- The DSM-IV diagnostic criteria for GAD are shown in Table 67–2. The illness has a gradual onset, usually in the early 20s. The course of illness is chronic, with multiple spontaneous exacerbations and remissions.

PANIC DISORDER

- Between late adolescence and the late 30s, symptoms usually begin as a series of unexpected panic attacks. These are followed by at least 1 month of persistent concern about having another panic attack.
- During an attack, there must be four or more of the following symptoms: palpitations or an accelerated heart rate; sweating, trembling, or shaking; shortness of breath; feeling of choking; chest pain or discom-

TABLE 67–1. DSM-IV Classification of Anxiety Disorders

A. Generalized anxiety disorder
B. Panic disorder
  With agoraphobia
  Without agoraphobia
C. Agoraphobia without a history of panic disorder
D. Phobic disorders
  Social phobia
  Specific phobia
E. Obsessive–compulsive disorder
F. Post-traumatic stress disorder
G. Acute stress disorder

Adapted from the Diagnostic and Statistical Manual of Mental Disorders, *4th ed. Washington, DC, American Psychiatric Association, 1994:435–436.*

fort; nausea; dizziness; derealization or depersonalization; fear of losing control; fear of dying; numbness or tingling; and chills or hot flushes. Symptoms reach a peak within 10 minutes and usually last no more than 20 minutes.

- Many patients eventually develop agoraphobia, which is avoidance of specific situations (e.g., crowded places, bridges) where they fear a panic attack might occur. Patients may become homebound.

SOCIAL PHOBIA

- The essential feature is a marked and persistent fear of social or performance situations in which embarrassment may occur. The fear and

TABLE 67–2. DSM-IV Diagnostic Criteria for Generalized Anxiety Disorder

A. Excessive anxiety and worry (apprehensive expectation), occurring more days than not for at least 6 months, about a number of events or activities (such as work or school performance).
B. The person finds it difficult to control worry.
C. Anxiety and worry, associated with three (or more) of the following six symptoms (with at least some symptoms present more days than not for the past 6 months):
  1. Restlessness or feeling keyed up or on edge
  2. Being easily fatigued
  3. Difficulty concentrating or mind going blank
  4. Irritability
  5. Muscle tension
  6. Sleep disturbance
D. Anxiety and worry, not confined to features of another psychiatric illness (e.g., having a panic attack, being embarrassed in public).
E. Constant worry causing significant distress, and significant impairment in social, occupational, or other important areas of functioning.
F. Excessive anxiety and worry, not caused by a drug substance (e.g., drugs of abuse or medications), or a general medical disorder, and not occurring exclusively as part of another psychiatric disorder (e.g., mood disorder).

Adapted from the Diagnostic and Statistical Manual of Mental Disorders, *4th ed. Washington, DC, American Psychiatric Association, 1994:435–436.*

avoidance of the situation must interfere with daily routine or social/occupational functioning.

SPECIFIC PHOBIA

- The primary characteristic is a marked and persistent fear of a specific object or situation such as thunderstorms, animals, or heights. These patients are not seriously impaired, as they simply avoid the feared object.

▶ DIAGNOSIS

- Evaluation of the anxious patient requires a complete physical and mental status exam, appropriate laboratory tests, and a medical, psychiatric, and drug history.
- Anxiety symptoms may be associated with medical illnesses (Table 67–3) or drug therapy (Table 67–4).
- Anxiety symptoms may be present in several major psychiatric illnesses (e.g., mood disorders, schizophrenia, organic mental syndromes, substance withdrawal).

▶ DESIRED OUTCOME

- The desired outcomes of treatment for patients with anxiety disorders are to minimize anxiety symptoms, impairment of social/occupational functioning, and drug-related problems; ensure compliance with the drug regimen; and usually ultimately to discontinue medication.
- The goals of therapy of panic disorder include a complete resolution of panic attacks (not always achievable), marked reduction in anticipatory anxiety and phobic fears, and resumption of normal activities.

TABLE 67–3. Common Medical Disorders Associated With Anxiety Symptoms

Cardiovascular
Angina, arrhythmias, hypertension, mitral valve prolapse, myocardial infarction
Endocrine and Metabolic
Anemia, Cushing's disease, hyperthyroidism, hypothyroidism, hypoglycemia, hypokalemia, insulinoma, pheochromocytoma
Gastrointestinal
Colitis, irritable bowel syndrome, peptic ulcer
Neurologic
Akathisia, essential tremor, seizures, migraine, pain, Parkinson's disease
Respiratory
Asthma, chronic obstructive lung disease, hyperventilation, pneumonia, pulmonary embolus

TABLE 67–4. Drugs Associated With Anxiety Symptoms

CNS Depressant Withdrawal
Anxiolytics/sedatives, barbiturates, ethanol, narcotic agonists
CNS Stimulants
Prescription drugs
Albuterol, amphetamines, cocaine, diethylpropion, isoproterenol, methylphenidate
Nonprescription drugs
Caffeine, ephedrine, phenylephrine, phenylpropanolamine, pseudoephedrine
Miscellaneous
Anticholinergic (toxicity), cycloserine, digitalis (toxicity), dapsone, dopamine, isoniazid, levodopa, lidocaine, antipsychotics, nicotinic acid, selective serotonin reuptake inhibitor antidepressants, steroids, theophylline

► TREATMENT

NONPHARMACOLOGIC THERAPY

- For patients with GAD, nonpharmacologic modalities include short-term counseling, stress management, cognitive therapy, meditation, supportive therapy, and exercise.
- Patients with panic disorder must be educated to avoid substances (e.g., caffeine, drugs of abuse, nonprescription stimulants) that may precipitate a panic attack. Typically, patients require exposure, cognitive, and/or cognitive–behavioral therapies to alleviate their avoidance behavior.

PHARMACOLOGIC THERAPY

Generalized Anxiety Disorder

General Therapeutic Principles

- For patients experiencing functional disability, antianxiety medication is indicated.
- **Buspirone,** autonomic blocking agents, and antidepressants are additional anxiolytic options (Table 67–5). Antipsychotics and antihistamines are usually not indicated.

Benzodiazepine Therapy XIII

- The BZDs are the drugs of choice for treating GAD (Table 67–6). It is theorized that BZDs ameliorate anxiety through potentiation of GABA activity.
- The dose must be individualized, and duration of therapy usually should not exceed 4 months. Some patients require longer treatment.
- The elderly have an enhanced sensitivity to BZDs.

TABLE 67–5. Nonbenzodiazepine Antianxiety Agents

Class/Generic Name	Brand Name	Manufacturer	Usual Dosage Range (mg/d)[a]
Diphenylmethanes			
Diphenhydramine[b]	Benadryl	Parke-Davis	25–200
Hydroxyzine[b,c]	Vistaril	Pfizer	50–400
	Atarax	Roerig	
β-Blocker			
Propranolol[b]	Inderal	Wyeth-Ayerst	80–160
Azapirones			
Buspirone[c]	BuSpar	Bristol-Myers Squibb	15–60[d]

[a]Elderly patients are usually treated with approximately one-half of the dose listed.
[b]Available generically.
[c]FDA-approved for anxiety.
[d]The dosage range in elderly patients appears to be the same, but is not established.

PHARMACOKINETICS

- BZD pharmacokinetic properties are shown in Table 67–7.
- **Diazepam** and **clorazepate** have high lipophilicity and are rapidly absorbed and distributed into the CNS. They have a shorter duration of effect after a single dose than would be predicted based on half-life, as they are rapidly distributed to the periphery.

TABLE 67–6. Benzodiazepine Antianxiety Agents

Generic Name	Brand Name	Manufacturer	Approved Dosage Range (mg/d)[a]	Approximate Equivalent Dose (mg)
Alprazolam[b]	Xanax	Pharmacia & Upjohn	0.75–4	0.5
Chlordiazepoxide[b]	Librium	Roche	25–100	10
Clorazepate[b]	Tranxene	Abbott	7.5–60	7.5
Diazepam[b]	Valium	Roche	2–40	5
Halazepam	Paxipam	Schering	20–160	20
Lorazepam[b]	Ativan	Wyeth-Ayerst	0.5–10	1
Oxazepam[b]	Serax	Wyeth-Ayerst	30–120	15

[a]Elderly patients are usually treated with approximately one-half of the dose listed. See Table 67–9 for antipanic dosage range.
[b]Available generically.

TABLE 67–7. Pharmacokinetics of Benzodiazepine Antianxiety Agents

Generic Name	Peak Plasma Level (h)	Elimination Half-life Parent (h)	Metabolic Pathway	Clinically Significant Metabolites	Protein Binding (%)
Alprazolam	1–2	12–15	Oxidation	—	80
Chlordiazepoxide	1–4	5–30	*N*-dealkylation	Desmethylchlordiazepoxide	96
			Oxidation	Demoxepam	—
				N-DMDZ[a]	—
Clorazepate	1–2	Prodrug	Oxidation	*N*-DMDZ	97
Diazepam	0.5–2	20–80	Oxidation	*N*-DMDZ	98
Halazepam	1–3	14	Oxidation	*N*-DMDZ	97
Lorazepam	2–4	10–20	Conjugation	—	85
Oxazepam	2–4	5–20	Conjugation	—	97

[a]*N*-desmethyldiazepam half-life = 36–200 h.

- **Lorazepam, oxazepam,** and **prazepam** are less lipophilic and have a slower onset, but a longer duration of action. They are not recommended for immediate relief of anxiety.
- Intramuscular diazepam and **chlordiazepoxide** should be avoided due to variability in rate and extent of drug absorption. IM lorazepam provides rapid and complete absorption.
- Clorazepate and prazepam are prodrugs. Prazepam is converted to desmethyldiazepam (DMDZ) in the liver, and clorazepate is converted to DMDZ in the stomach through a pH-dependent process that may be impaired by concurrent antacid use.
- BZDs with a long-elimination half-life ($t_{1/2}$) may be dosed once daily at bedtime and may provide hypnotic and anxiolytic effects.
- Intermediate- or short-acting BZDs are preferred for chronic use in the elderly and those with liver disorders because of minimal accumulation and achievement of steady state within 1–3 days.

ADVERSE EVENTS

- The most common side effect to BZDs is CNS depression. Tolerance usually develops to this effect. Other side effects are disorientation, psychomotor impairment, confusion, aggression, excitement, and impaired memory (anterograde amnesia).

ABUSE, DEPENDENCE, WITHDRAWAL, AND TOLERANCE

- Those with a history of drug abuse are at the greatest risk for becoming BZD abusers.
- BZD dependence is defined by the appearance of a predictable abstinence syndrome (i.e., anxiety, insomnia, agitation, muscle tension, nausea, diaphoresis, nightmares, hallucinations, and seizures) upon abrupt discontinuation.

BENZODIAZEPINE DISCONTINUATION

- After BZDs are abruptly discontinued, three events can occur:
  - Rebound symptoms are an immediate, but transient, return of original symptoms with an increased intensity compared with baseline.
  - Recurrence or relapse is the return of original symptoms at the same intensity as before treatment.
  - Withdrawal is the emergence of new symptoms and a worsening of preexisting symptoms.
- The onset of withdrawal symptoms is 24–48 hours after discontinuation of short-$t_{1/2}$ and 3–8 days after discontinuation of long-$t_{1/2}$ drugs.
- Discontinuation strategies include:
  - Twenty-five percent per week reduction in dosage until 50% of the dose is reached, then dosage reduction by one-eighth every 4–7 days.
  - A BZD with a long $t_{1/2}$ (e.g., diazepam) may be substituted for a drug with a short $t_{1/2}$ (e.g., lorazepam, oxazepam, alprazolam). The substituted drug should be given for several weeks before gradual tapering begins.

DRUG INTERACTIONS

- Drug interactions with the BZDs are summarized in Table 67–8. The combination of BZDs with **alcohol** or other CNS depressants may be fatal.

TABLE 67–8. Pharmacokinetic Drug Interactions With the Benzodiazepines

Drug	Effect
Alcohol	Decreased Cl of chlordiazepoxide and diazepam
Antacids	Decreased rate of diazepam and chlordiazepoxide absorption
Cimetidine	Decreased Cl of alprazolam, diazepam, chlordiazepoxide, and clorazepate, and increased $t_{1/2}$
Disulfiram	Decreased Cl of chlordiazepoxide and diazepam
Fluoxetine	Decreased Cl of diazepam
Fluvoxamine	Decreased Cl of alprazolam and prolonged $t_{1/2}$
Isoniazid	Decreased metabolism of diazepam
Itraconazole	Potentially decreased Cl of alprazolam
Ketaconazole	Potentially decreased Cl of alprazolam
Nefazodone	Decreased Cl of alprazolam, AUC doubled, and $t_{1/2}$ prolonged
Omeprazole	Decreased Cl of diazepam
Oral contraceptives	Increased free concentration of chlordiazepoxide and slightly decreased Cl; decreased Cl and increased $t_{1/2}$ of diazepam and alprazolam
Rifampin	Increased metabolism of diazepam
Theophylline	Decreased alprazolam concentrations

AUC, area under the plasma concentration curve; Cl, clearance; $t_{1/2}$, elimination half-life.

- Alprazolam dose should be reduced by 50% if **nefazodone** or **fluvoxamine** is added.
- As **cimetidine** inhibits the metabolism of oxidatively metabolized BZDs, **ranitidine** and **famotidine** are preferred H_2 receptor blockers for patients taking BZDs.

Buspirone Therapy

- Buspirone is a 5-HT_{1A} partial agonist. It lacks anticonvulsant, muscle relaxant, sedative, hypnotic, motor impairment, and dependence properties. It is as efficacious as BZDs.
- It is 95% protein bound and has a mean $t_{1/2}$ of 2.5 hours. It is metabolized oxidatively to active and inactive metabolites. Clearance is unaffected by age, but decreased in patients with cirrhosis and renal impairment.
- Side effects include dizziness, nausea, headaches, and nervousness. Gynecomastia, galactorrhea, and extrapyramidal symptoms are rare.

DRUG INTERACTIONS

- Buspirone may increase **cyclosporine** and **haloperidol** levels and elevate blood pressure in patients taking a **monoamine oxidase inhibitor (MAOI).**
- **Disulfiram** may cause mania, and **clomipramine** may cause hypertension and anxiety when coprescribed with buspirone.

DOSAGE AND ADMINISTRATION

- The initial dose is 7.5 mg two times daily. The usual therapeutic dose of buspirone is 20–30 mg/d, with a maximum of 60 mg/d.
- The onset of anxiolytic effects requires a week or more; maximum benefit may require 4–6 weeks.
- It is not useful in situations requiring rapid antianxiety effects or as-needed therapy.
- When switching from a BZD to buspirone, the BZD should be tapered slowly.

Adrenergic Blocking Agents

- The usefulness of **propranolol** and other beta-blockers may be limited to patients whose physical symptoms, especially cardiovascular ones, have not responded to BZDs.
- Propranolol is initially dosed at 10 mg twice daily and gradually titrated to response.
- To avoid rebound anxiety and cardiovascular effects, propranolol should be tapered prior to discontinuation. XIII

Antidepressants

- Although not first-line agents, **imipramine** (mean dose, 143 mg) and **trazodone** (mean dose, 235 mg) are effective after 3–8 weeks in GAD patients. Low doses of selective serotonin reuptake inhibitors (SSRIs) are also effective.

Evaluation of Therapeutic Outcome

- Initially, anxious patients should be monitored once to twice weekly for reduction in anxiety symptoms, improvement in functioning, and side effects.
- A Visual Analog Scale, the State-Trait Anxiety Inventory, or the Zung Self-Rating Scale may assist in the evaluation of drug response.

Panic Disorder

General Therapeutic Principles

- Antipanic drugs are shown in Table 67–9. An algorithm for pharmacologic therapy of panic disorder is shown in Figure 67–1.
- Most patients without agoraphobia improve with pharmacotherapy alone, but if agoraphobia is present, cognitive–behavioral therapy typically is initiated concurrently.
- In a meta-analysis, SSRIs and **clomipramine** were more effective than imipramine and alprazolam.

Antidepressants

- **Imipramine** is effective in 75% of patients within 3–4 weeks. Maximal improvement may require 6–10 weeks.
- Stimulatory side effects (e.g., insomnia, jitteriness, excess energy) occur in 20–30% of imipramine-treated patients. This occurs with other antidepressants also and may affect compliance and hinder dose increases. Dose reduction may eliminate these effects.
- With antidepressants, antipanic effect requires 3–5 weeks, and antiphobic effects 6–10 weeks.
- High-dose **alprazolam** is effective and well tolerated except for sedation. **Diazepam** and **lorazepam** may also be effective in adequate doses.
- The onset of antipanic response to BZDs occurs in 1–2 weeks, but improvement continues for 4–6 weeks.
- Some clinicians view SSRIs as first-line agents because of their tolerability.

DOSING AND ADMINISTRATION

- Initial doses should be low and increased to the therapeutic range. Imipramine should be initiated with 10 mg/d at bedtime and slowly increased by 10 mg every 2–4 days as tolerated to 100–200 mg/d. Most patients require 150 mg/d of imipramine or a combined imipramine–desipramine plasma level of 100–150 ng/mL.
- SSRIs should also be initiated at low doses (e.g., 2.5–5 mg/d of **fluoxetine**).
- For side effects, precautions, and dietary and drug restrictions in patients taking MAOIs, see Chapter 69.
- If breakthrough panic attacks occur at the end of a dosing interval with alprazolam, **clonazepam** may be an alternative.
- Usually patients are treated for 8–12 months before discontinuation is attempted. Twenty to 40% require chronic therapy. Many patients can be tapered off medication during the second year of therapy.

TABLE 67–9. Drugs Used in the Treatment of Panic Disorder

Class/Generic Name	Brand Name	Manufacturer	Starting Dose (mg)	Antipanic Dosage Range (mg)[a]
Benzodiazepines				
Alprazolam[b]	Xanax	Pharmacia & Upjohn	0.25–0.5 tid	4–10[c]
Clonazepam[b]	Klonopin	Roche	0.25 bid	3–4[c]
Diazepam[b]	Valium	Roche	2–5 tid	30–40
Lorazepam[b]	Ativan	Wyeth-Ayerst	0.5–1 tid	3–4
Tricyclic Antidepressants				
Desipramine[b]	Norpramin	Hoechst Marion Roussel	10–25 qd	150–300
Imipramine[b]	Tofranil	Ciba-Geigy	10–25 qd	150–300
Monoamine Oxidase Inhibitor				
Phenelzine	Nardil	Parke-Davis	15 bid	45–90
Serotonin Reuptake Inhibitors				
Fluoxetine	Prozac	Dista	2.5–5 qd	2.5–20
Fluvoxamine	Luvox	Solvay	25 qd	150–300
Paroxetine	Paxil	SmithKline Beecham	10 qd	10–60[c]
Sertraline	Zoloft	Roerig	12.5–25 qd	25–200[c]

[a]Dosage used in clinical trials but not FDA approved.
[b]Available generically.
[c]Dosage is FDA approved.

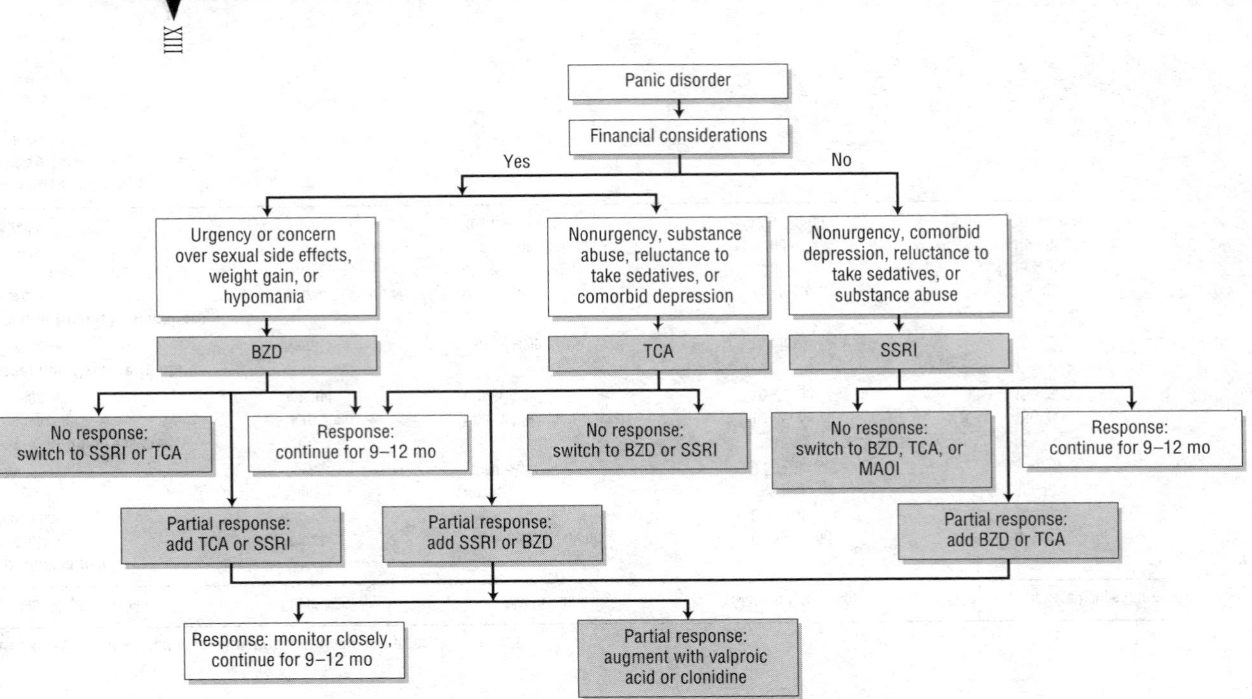

Figure 67–1. Algorithm for the treatment of panic disorders.

- In patients taking alprazolam doses greater than 3 mg/d, dose reduction should proceed by 0.5 mg every 2 weeks until 3 mg/d is reached, then 0.25 mg every 2 weeks until 1 mg is reached, then 0.125 mg every 2 weeks.
- Tricyclic antidepressants (TCAs) should be reduced by 25 mg every 2–4 weeks.
- **Phenelzine** should be reduced by 15 mg every 2–4 weeks.

Evaluation of Therapeutic Outcomes

- Patients with panic disorder should be seen twice weekly for 2 weeks to adjust medication doses based on symptom improvement and side effects. Once stabilized, they can be seen weekly until antipanic response is achieved, then monthly. The Sheehan Disability Scale can be used to measure disability.
- Patients should be encouraged to maintain a diary to document symptoms.
- During discontinuation, patients should be monitored closely for withdrawal symptoms and relapse.

Social Phobia

- Generalized social phobia may respond to MAOIs, BZDs, or SSRIs.
- Patients respond to **phenelzine** (antipanic doses) in 8–12 weeks.
- **Clonazepam,** 1.5–2 mg/d or **alprazolam** 3 mg/d have shown efficacy after 2 weeks.
- **Propranolol** may be used to manage performance anxiety in doses of 40 mg, 1 hour before the performance.
- **Fluoxetine** (10–80 mg/d), **sertraline** (50–200 mg/d), **paroxetine** (20–60 mg/d), and **fluvoxamine** (150 mg/d) reduced avoidance and social anxiety.

See Chapter 67, Anxiety Disorders, authored by Cynthia K. Kirkwood, PharmD for a more detailed discussion of this topic.

Chapter 68

▶ BIPOLAR DISORDER

▶ DEFINITION

Bipolar disorder, previously known as manic–depressive illness, is a cyclical disorder with recurrent fluctuations in mood, energy, and behavior. Diagnosis requires the occurrence of a manic, hypomanic, or mixed episode during the course of the illness.

▶ PATHOPHYSIOLOGY

- Medical conditions, medications, and somatic treatments that may induce mania are shown in Table 68–1.
- Several theories of neurotransmitter alterations in the central nervous system (CNS) are proposed.
  - The monoamine hypothesis suggests a functional deficit of norepinephrine (NE), dopamine (DA), and/or serotonin (5-HT) in depression and an excess of catecholamines (NE and DA) in mania.
  - The permissive hypothesis posits that there is low CNS 5-HT in both mania and depression. Superimposed low NE would cause depression and high NE would cause mania.
  - The dysregulation hypothesis states that mood disorders may be caused by a dysregulation between neurotransmitter systems.
  - A γ-aminobutyric acid (GABA) deficiency hypothesis is related to the sensitization-kindling theory for mood disorders. GABA is the main inhibitory neurotransmitter in the CNS.
  - Glutamate, an excitatory neurotransmitter, may also be involved in mood disorders.
  - An acetylcholine (ACh) deficiency hypothesis or cholinergic–adrenergic imbalance has also been proposed to cause bipolar disorder.
- Initially psychosocial or physical stressors may trigger episodes, but later the episodes may occur spontaneously due to behavioral sensitivity and electrophysiologic kindling.
- Excessive thyroid activity may precipitate a manic episode by potentiating β-adrenergic activity.
- High serum and cerebrospinal fluid (CSF) calcium concentrations were found in patients with depression, but low CSF levels were reported in mania.
- Secondary messenger theories suggest a role for altered cAMP, phospholipase C, G proteins, and sodium–potassium-activated adenosine triphosphatase activity.
- Circadian rhythm desynchronization may cause diurnal variations in mood and seasonal recurrences of episodes. Incidence of depression peaks in the spring and of mania during the summer months.

TABLE 68–1. Medical Conditions, Medications, and Somatic Treatments That Induce Mania

Endocrine or Metabolic Disorders
Addison's disease
Carcinoid tumors
Cushing's disease
Hyperthyroidism
Vitamin B_{12} deficiency

Infections
Acquired immune deficiency syndrome
Encephalitis
Neurosyphilis
Postinfection (viral, encephalitis, influenza)

Neurologic Disorders
Epilepsy (temporal lobe)
Huntington's disease
Multiple sclerosis
Postcerebrovascular accident
Postconcussion
Right frontotemporal lesions
Subarachnoid hemorrhage
Subcortical lesions
Surgical trauma

Medications
Alcohol
α_2-Adrenergic agonist withdrawal
Anticonvulsants
Antidepressants: TCAs, MAOIs, SSRIs
Baclofen ingestion or withdrawal
Benzodiazepine ingestion or withdrawal
Bronchodilators: Albuterol, isoetharine, isoproterenol, metaproterenol, metaraminol, salmeterol, terbutaline
Calcium replacement
Cimetidine
Decongestants/sympathomimetics: Ephedrine, epinephrine, methoxamine, midodrine, norepinephrine, phenylephrine, phenylpropanolamine, pseudoephedrine, ritodrine
Disulfiram
Dopamine-augmenting agents: Amantadine, bromocriptine, levodopa
Hallucinogens: LSD, phencyclidine
Isoniazid
NSAIDs: Indomethacin, tolmetin
Procainamide
Quinacrine
Steroids: Anabolic, corticosteroids, ACTH
Stimulants: Amphetamines, cocaine, methylphenidate, pemoline
Xanthines: Caffeine, theophylline
Yohimbine

Somatic Therapies
Bright visible spectrum light therapy
Electroconvulsive therapy
Hemodialysis
Sleep deprivation

► CLASSIFICATION, DIAGNOSIS, AND CLINICAL PRESENTATION

The *Diagnostic and Statistical Manual of Mental Disorders,* 4th edition (DSM-IV) divides bipolar disorders into four subtypes: (1) bipolar I, (2) bipolar II, (3) cyclothymic disorder, and (4) bipolar disorder not otherwise specified (NOS). XIII

- Bipolar I is characterized by one or more manic or mixed episodes and is usually accompanied by major depressive episodes.
- Bipolar II disorder is characterized by one or more major depressive episodes and at least one hypomanic episode (Table 68–2).

TABLE 68–2. Mood Disorders Defined by Episodes

Disorder	Episode(s)
Major depressive disorder, single episode	Major depressive episode
Major depressive disorder, recurrent	Major depressive episode + major depressive episode
Bipolar disorder, type I	Major depressive episode + manic or mixed episode
Bipolar disorder, type II	Major depressive episode + hypomanic episode
Dysthymic disorder	Chronic subsyndromal depressive episodes
Cyclothymic disorder	Chronic fluctuations between subsyndromal depressive and hypomanic episodes (2 y for adults and 1 y for children and adolescents)
Mood disorder due to a general medical condition	Disturbance in mood that is secondary to a general medical condition: With depressive features Major depressive-like episode With manic features With mixed features
Substance-induced mood disorder	Disturbance in mood that is due to the effects of a substance (e.g., medication, toxin, drug of abuse, somatic treatments such as ECT or light therapy): With depressive features With manic features With mixed features
Bipolar disorder not otherwise specified	Mood states do not meet criteria for any specific bipolar disorder

Adapted from Mood disorders. In: Diagnostic and Statistical Manual of Mental Disorders, *4th ed (DSM-IV). Washington, DC, American Psychiatric Press, 1994:317–390.*

- Cyclothymic disorder is characterized by at least 2 years of numerous episodes of both hypomanic and depressive symptoms, but they do not meet the criteria for a manic or major depressive episode.

XIII
- The diagnostic workup includes longitudinal psychiatric data; family history; a thorough medical, drug, and alcohol history; a complete physical examination; and appropriate laboratory tests.
- The majority of bipolar patients with depression or mixed episodes are nonsuppressors to the dexamethasone suppression test (DST). A blunted thyroid-stimulating hormone (TSH) response to the thyrotropin-releasing hormone (TRH) administration has been reported in mania.

MAJOR DEPRESSIVE EPISODE

- The clinical presentation and diagnostic criteria for bipolar depression are the same as those for major depressive episode, as discussed in Chapter 69.
- Bipolar depression is often characterized by hypersomnia, fatigue, psychomotor retardation, decreased sexual activity, carbohydrate craving, and weight gain.

MANIC EPISODE

- DSM-IV diagnostic criteria include at least 1 week of abnormal and persistently elevated mood (expansive or irritable) and at least three of the following (four if the mood was only irritable): inflated self-esteem, decreased need for sleep, pressured speech, racing thoughts (flight of ideas), distractibility, increased activity, and excessive involvement in activities that are pleasurable but have a high risk for serious consequences. There is marked impairment in functioning or the need for hospitalization.
- Seasonal changes, stressors, antidepressants, bright light, or electroconvulsive therapy (ECT) can precipitate a manic episode.
- Approximately two-thirds of bipolar patients have psychotic symptoms at some point, primarily paranoid or grandiose delusions.

HYPOMANIC EPISODE

- Hypomanic episodes are characterized by elevated, expansive, or irritable mood and associated symptoms, such as increased psychomotor activity, decreased need for sleep, pressure of speech, flight of ideas, and distractibility but no marked impairment in social or occupational functioning, no delusions, and no hallucinations.
- During a hypomanic episode, some patients may be more productive and creative.

MIXED EPISODE

- Mixed episodes are characterized by symptoms of a manic episode and a major depressive episode occurring nearly every day for at least a 1-week period. Symptoms cause impairment in social or occupational functioning or require hospitalization.

COURSE OF ILLNESS

- Recurrences may become more frequent over time. Rapid cyclers have XIII
  four or more episodes per year (major depressive, manic, mixed, or hypomanic).
  - Rapid-cycling and mixed states are associated with a poorer prognosis and nonresponse to antimanic agents.
  - Risk factors for rapid cycling include antidepressant or stimulant use, hypothyroidism, and premenstrual mood changes.

▶ DESIRED OUTCOME

- The goal of treatment is to minimize target symptoms, toxicity, and adverse effects of medications while optimizing medication compliance and social/occupational functioning.

▶ TREATMENT

GENERAL APPROACH

- An algorithm for treatment of bipolar disorder is shown in Figure 68–1.
- Hypomanic episodes may not require treatment unless there is a history of manic episodes.
- Acute manic episodes can be treated with **lithium, carbamazepine** (CBZ), or **valproic acid** (VPA) along with adjunctive **benzodiazepines (BZDs)** for anxiety/insomnia. Severe episodes with psychosis and agitation require antipsychotics ± BZDs along with lithium, CBZ, or VPA.
- If there is no response within 2–4 weeks, a second mood stabilizer can be added to the regimen. If patients are nonresponsive, the mood stabilizer should be switched to another agent or ECT may be used.
- After remission, adjunctive agents are tapered and discontinued over 2–6 months.
- After response, patients with only one manic episode should continue on a mood stabilizer for 12 months.
- Lifelong mood stabilizer therapy is recommended for bipolar type I patients with two manic episodes, one severe manic episode, a strong family bipolar history, >one manic episode per year, or rapid onset of manic episodes.
- Long-term prophylaxis for bipolar type II patients is recommended after three hypomanic episodes or if the patient required an antidepressant but became hypomanic.
- Breakthrough episodes may require short-term BZDs or antipsychotics for mania or antidepressants for depression.
- Depressed patients on lithium should be evaluated for lithium-induced hypothyroidism.
- Monotherapy is preferred for maintenance, but combinations of drugs may be necessary, especially for patients with mixed episodes, rapid cycling, or partial or no response to monotherapy (e.g., lithium plus CBZ, lithium plus VPA, CBZ plus VPA).
- Table 68–3 includes recommendations for baseline and routine laboratory testing for patients taking lithium, CBZ, and VPA.

Lithium

- **Lithium** is 50–70% effective in aborting an acute manic or hypomanic episode within 7–14 days. Prophylactic lithium therapy is approximately 70–80% effective in preventing or attenuating recurrences of mania, hypomania, and depression.

- Maintenance lithium therapy may be more effective in patients with fewer prior episodes, a history of euthymia between episodes, a family history of good response to lithium, and plasma concentrations between 0.8–1.0 mEq/L (versus 0.4–0.6 mEq/L).
- Lithium is rapidly absorbed, exhibits no protein binding, is not metabolized, and is excreted unchanged. The $T_{1/2}$ is approximately 18–20 hours in young adults (36 hours in the elderly).

Adverse Effects

- Adverse effects of the mood stabilizers are shown in Table 68–4. Common early side effects to lithium are muscle weakness, lethargy, polydipsia, nocturia, headache, memory impairment, decreased ability to concentrate, and fine tremor. Tremor may be treated by lowering or dividing the dose, switching to an extended-release product, or adding a β-adrenergic antagonist (e.g., **propranolol** 20–120 mg/d, **atenolol** 50 mg/d, or **metoprolol** 20–80 mg/d).
- A long-term side effect in some patients is vasopressin-resistant nephrogenic diabetes insipidus (urine volumes of 5–6 L/d), which is treated with loop or thiazide diuretics, **triamterene,** or **amiloride.**
- Lithium causes minimal nephrotoxicity if patients are maintained on the lowest effective dose, toxicity is avoided, and adequate hydration is maintained.
- Five to 15% of lithium-treated patients, especially women, develop goiter and/or reversible hypothyroidism which is not dose related. If TSH is >5.0 mIU/mL, **L-thyroxine** 0.05 mg/d can be added (followed by a TSH level in 1 month) and increased up to 0.2 mg/d or higher (to achieve TSH >0.1 and <5.0).

TOXICITY

- Mild toxicity (GI upset, fatigue, impaired memory) may occur at plasma concentrations of 1.2–1.5 mEq/L. Moderate toxicity (agitation, confusion, ataxia, dysarthria, nystagmus, course tremors) may occur at plasma concentrations >1.5 mEq/L. If concentrations are >3.0 mEq/L, the syndrome may progress to clonic-tonic twitching, seizures, irreversible brain damage, coma, and death.

SPECIAL CONSIDERATIONS FOR PREGNANCY AND LACTATION

- Lithium may have a lower incidence of causing fetal cardiovascular defects (Epstein's anomaly) if taken during the first trimester than previously thought. Neonatal lithium effects include hypotonia, bradycardia, cyanosis, low Apgar scores, hypothyroidism, and goiters.

Drug–Drug Interactions

- Several drug–drug interactions of the mood stabilizers are summarized in Table 68–5.

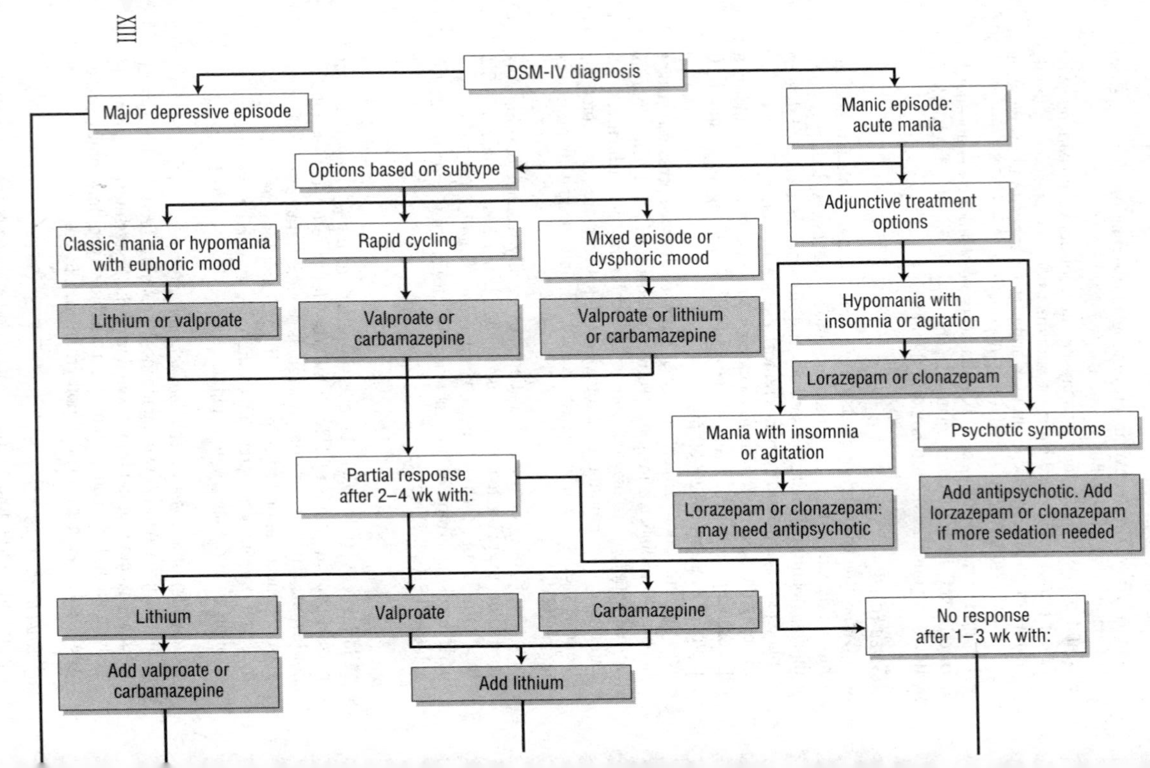
DSM-IV diagnosis
Major depressive episode
Manic episode: acute mania
Options based on subtype
Adjunctive treatment options
Classic mania or hypomania with euphoric mood
Rapid cycling
Mixed episode or dysphoric mood
Lithium or valproate
Valproate or carbamazepine
Valproate or lithium or carbamazepine
Hypomania with insomnia or agitation
Lorazepam or clonazepam
Mania with insomnia or agitation
Psychotic symptoms
Lorazepam or clonazepam: may need antipsychotic
Add antipsychotic. Add lorzazepam or clonazepam if more sedation needed
Partial response after 2–4 wk with:
Lithium
Valproate
Carbamazepine
Add valproate or carbamazepine
Add lithium
No response after 1–3 wk with:

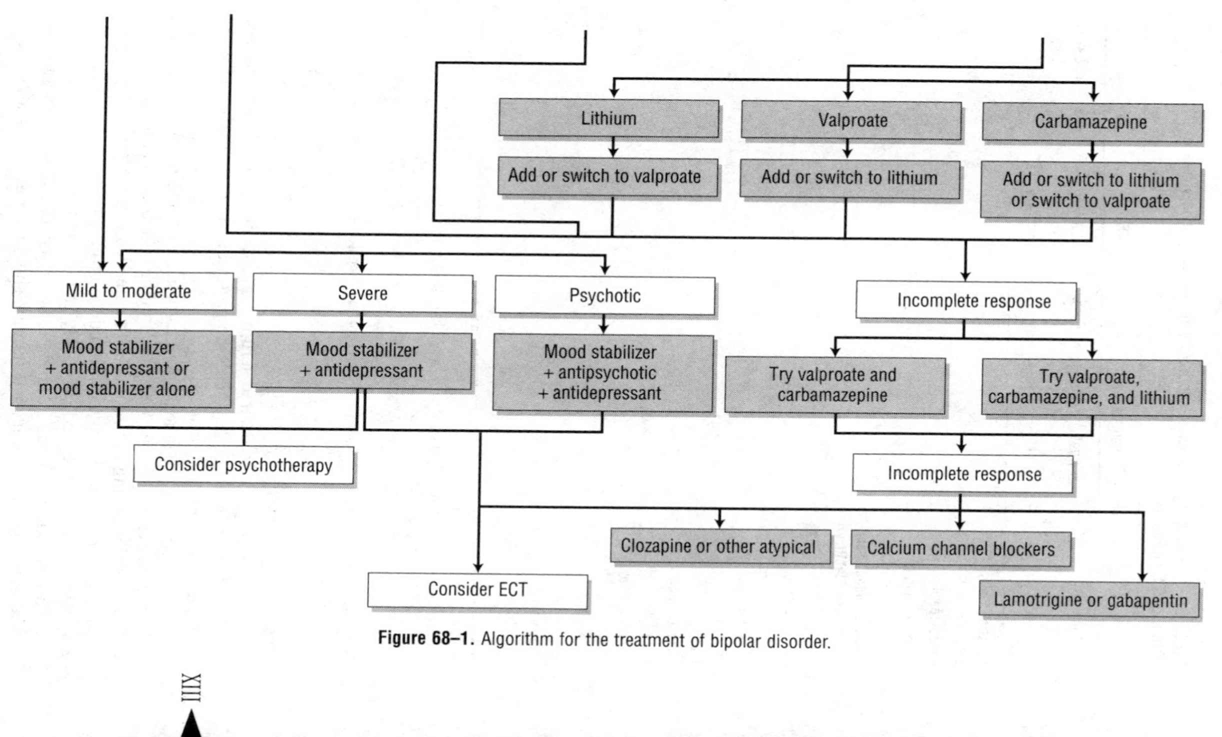

Figure 68–1. Algorithm for the treatment of bipolar disorder.

XIII

TABLE 68–3. Baseline and Routine Laboratory Testing for Patients Treated With Mood Stabilizers

	Carbamazepine		Lithium		Valproate	
Test	*Baseline*	*Follow-up Every 6–12 mo*	*Baseline*	*Follow-up Every 6–12 mo*	*Baseline*	*Follow-up Every 6–12 mo*
Baseline Tests						
Complete physical exam	+		+		+	
General chemistry screen	+		+		+	
Urine toxicology for substance abuse	+		+		+	
Recommended Tests for Mood Stabilizers						
Pregnancy test if needed	+		+		+	
Cardiac: ECG	+[a]		+[a]			
Hematologic						
CBC with differential	+	+[b]	+	+	+	+[b]
Platelet	+	+			+	+
Hepatic						
Liver enzymes	+	+[c]			+	+[c]
Metabolic						
Serum electrolytes	+	+	+	+		
Total T_4, T_4 uptake, and TSH	+	+	+	+		
Renal						
Serum creatinine			+[d]	+[d]		
Urinalysis/osmolality/ specific gravity			+	+[e]		

[a]If >40 y or preexisting cardiac disease.
[b]CBZ and VPA: CBC monthly during first 2 mo, then every 3–6 mo; discontinue CBZ if platelets <100,000/mm³ or WBC <3000/mm³.
[c]CBZ and VPA: Liver function tests (LFTs) monthly during first 2 mo, then every 3–6 mo; VPA: <10 y should have LFTs every 1–3 mo.
[d]24-h urine volume and creatinine clearance for impaired renal functioning q 3 mo.
[e]If urine volume >3 L/d.

Dosing and Administration

- Dosing strategies and desired serum concentrations are shown in Table 68–6. Lower initial doses should be prescribed in the elderly and when lithium excretion is impaired.
- Divided dosing regimens and gradual titration (300–600-mg/d increases every 2–3 days) helps to minimize nausea and tremor.
- Single-daily dosing at bedtime with extended-release products may be tried in patients with polyuria to reduce urine volume.
- Dosage is adjusted based on steady-state serum concentrations drawn 12 hours plus or minus 30 minutes after the last dose. A therapeutic trial at the desired serum concentration should last at least 4 to 6 weeks.

TABLE 68–4. Adverse Effects of Mood Stabilizers

System	Carbamazepine	Lithium	Valproate
Cardiac			
Arrhythmias	+		
Atrioventricular block	+		
Sinoatrial block		+	
T-wave flattening/inversion		+	
Widening of QRS		+	
Dermatologic			
Acne		+	
Exfoliative dermatitis (rare)	+	+	
Hair loss/thinning		+	+
Rash (maculopapular)	+	+	+
Erythema multiforme (rare)	+		+
Stevens–Johnson syndrome (rare)	+		+
Psoriasis		+	
Endocrine/Metabolic			
Female abnormalities			
Gynecomastia			+
Dysmenorrhea			+
Galactorrhea			+
Irregular menses			+
Polycystic ovaries			+
Hyperammonemia			+
Hyperandrogenism			+
Hyperparathyroidism		+	
Hyponatremia	+		+
Hypothyroidism		+	
Parotid gland swelling			+
Weight gain		+	
Gastrointestinal			
Abdominal pain	+	+	+
Abdominal bloating		+	
Constipation	+		
Diarrhea	+	+	+
Dyspepsia	+	+	+
Metallic taste		+	
Nausea	+	+	+
Vomiting (high doses)	+	+	+
Hematologic			
Agranulocytosis (rare)	+		
Aplastic anemia (rare)	+		

(continued)

TABLE 68–4. continued

System	Carbamazepine	Lithium	Valproate
Hematologic (continued)			
Anticoagulation			+
Eosinophilia	+		
Hemolytic anemia (rare)	+		
Leukocytosis		+	
Leukopenia	+		
Thrombocytopenia (rare)	+		+
Thrombocytosis		+	
Hepatic			
↑ Liver function tests (mild)	+		+
Hepatotoxicity (rare)			+
Neurologic/Neuromuscular			
Ataxia	+	+	+
Cognitive slowing	+	+	
Diplopia	+		
Dizziness	+		+
Headache	+		
Muscle weakness		+	
Nystagmus (high doses)	+	+	
Sedation	+	+	+
Tremor		+	+
Renal			
Nephrogenic diabetes insipidus (NDI)		+	
Nephrotoxicity (rare)		+	
Polyuria/polydipsia		+	
Syndrome of inappropriate antidiuretic hormone secretion (SIADH)	+		+
Toxicity in Overdoses	+	+	Relatively safe
Teratogenicity	Class C	Class D	Class D
Craniofacial defects	+		
Developmental delays	+		+
Finger hypoplasia	+		
Neural tube defects	+		+
Cardiac defects		+	+
Cardiac malformations		+	
Hypothyroidism/goiter		+	
Hypotonia/cyanosis		+	

TABLE 68–5. Drug Interactions With Mood Stabilizers

Drugs That Affect Serum Levels of Mood Stabilizers	Carbamazepine	Lithium	Valproate
ACE inhibitors		↑	
Calcium channel blockers	↑	?↓	
Carbamazepine			↓
Cimetidine	↑		↑
Ethosuximide			↓
Danazol	↑		
Diuretics[a]		↑	
Fluoxetine	↑	↑	↑
Fluvoxamine	↑		↑
Isoniazid	↑		
Ketoconazole	↑		
Lamotrigine	↑		↑
Macrolide antibiotics[b]	↑		
Metronidazole	↑		
NSAIDs[c]		↑	
Omeprazole	↑		
Phenobarbital/primidone	↑		↓
Phenytoin	↓		↓
Propoxyphene	↑		
Rifampin			↑
Salicylates			↑
Sodium bicarbonate		↓	
Sodium chloride		↓	
Sodium depletion[d]		↑	
Theophylline		↓	
Valproic acid/valproate	↑		

Carbamazepine (CBZ) Drug Interactions

CBZ causes ↓ serum levels of the following medications due to induction of cytochrome P450 liver enzyme:

Anticonvulsants (e.g., carbamazepine, lamotrigine, phenytoin, phenobarbital, primidone, valproic acid)

Benzodiazepines (e.g., alprazolam, diazepam, midazolam, triazolam)

Bupropion

Cyclosporine

Doxycycline

(continued)

XIII

TABLE 68–5. continued

CBZ causes ↓ serum concentrations of the following, cont'd:

Fentanyl

Glucocorticoids (prednisolone)

Mebendazole

Methadone

Neuroleptics (e.g., clozapine, haloperidol, phenothiazines)

Neuromuscular blocking agents

Oral anticoagulants (warfarin)

Oral contraceptives (estrogens and progestins)

Theophylline

Thyroid supplements (induces metabolism of T_3 and T_4)

Tricyclic antidepressants (e.g., amitriptyline, desipramine, imipramine, nortriptyline)

Adverse Reactions Reported With Combination Therapy

	Neurotoxicity	*Impaired Thyroid Function*	*Cardiotoxicity*	*Bone Marrow Suppression*
Lithium + SSRIs	+			
Lithium + calcium channel blockers	+		+	
Lithium + CBZ[e]	+	+		
Lithium + clonazepam	+			
Lithium + ECT	+			
Lithium + methyldopa	+			
Lithium + neuroleptics[f]	+			
CBZ + calcium channel blockers	+			
CBZ + clozapine[g]				+
CBZ + danazol	+			
CBZ + haloperidol	+			
CBZ + lamotrigine	+			
CBZ + isoniazid	+			
CBZ + macrolide antibiotics	+			

TABLE 68–5. continued

	Neurotoxicity	*Impaired Thyroid Function*	*Cardiotoxicity*	*Bone Marrow Suppression*
CBZ + monoamine oxidase inhibitors[h]	+			
VPA + clozapine[i]	+			
VPA + lamotrigine[j]	+			
VPA + traditional neuroleptics	+			

[a]Diuretics: Distal tubule (chlorthalidone, metolazone, thiazides); potassium-sparing (spironolactone, triamterene); carbonic anhydrase inhibitors (acetazolamide); loop diuretics (ethacrynic acid, furosemide) are less likely to $\uparrow$ lithium levels; amiloride has minimal effect.

[b]Macrolide antibiotics: Clarithromycin, erythromycin, troleandomycin; azithromycin, and dirithromycin are less likely to $\uparrow$ CBZ levels.

[c]NSAIDs: Diclofenac, ibuprofen, indomethacin, ketorolac, mefenamic acid, naproxen, phenylbutazone, and piroxicam $\uparrow$ lithium levels by 30%–60%; sulindac and aspirin have minimal effects on lithium clearance.

[d]Sodium depletion: Diuretics; low-sodium diets; excessive exercise/sweating; protracted diarrhea/vomiting; salt deficiency.

[e]CBZ causes hyponatremia, which may cause lithium toxicity.

[f]Increased risk with higher doses and in elderly patients.

[g]CBZ + clozapine is not recommended due to increased risk of bone marrow suppression.

[h]CBZ may cause a hypertensive crisis with MAOIs (wait 14 days between MAOI and starting CBZ therapy).

[i]Additive side effects (drowsiness, weight gain); VPA may increase levels of clozapine's metabolites.

[j]VPA increases lamotrigine plasma levels; need to lower lamotrigine starting dose and increase more slowly; reports of rash and tremor; possibly synergistic effects.

- When mania begins to resolve, the dose should be adjusted downward to decrease the risk of toxicity.

Blood Level Monitoring

- When the desired serum concentration has been achieved, serum levels should be checked every 1–2 weeks for 2 months or until lithium concentrations are stabilized. Maintenance concentrations are usually obtained every 3–6 months.
- Lithium levels should be obtained monthly during pregnancy and weekly the month before delivery.

Divalproex Sodium (DVPX), Sodium Valproate, and Valproic Acid (VPA)

- **Divalproex sodium** is approved by the U.S. Food and Drug Administration (FDA) for the treatment of manic episodes, and it may be more effective than lithium for rapid cycling, mixed mania, secondary bipolar disorder, and comorbid substance abuse. XIII
- Predictors of positive response include rapid cycling, a high level of dysphoria or depression during the manic episode (mixed episode), concomitant panic attacks, mania associated with organic features, a history of head trauma, and mental retardation.

TABLE 68–6. Dosing Strategies and Serum Concentrations of Mood Stabilizers

	Carbamazepine	Lithium	Valproate
Acute Mania			
Initial dosing	100–200 mg bid with meals	900 mg/d or 15 mg/kg/d in divided doses with meals	500–750 mg/d or 5–10 mg/kg/d in divided doses with meals; oral loading of 20 mg/kg/d with DVPX
Target dose	400–2400 mg/d or 10–15 mg/kg/d; give bid or if ≤1200 mg in single hs dose	900–2400 mg/d; give bid or ≤1200 mg in single hs dose	1000–3000 mg/d or 20–60 mg/kg/d for mania; lower doses used for hypomania; give bid or single hs dose
Drug serum concentrations			
Adults	4–15 μg/mL[a] (not well established)	0.8–1.5 mEq/L	50–150 mg/mL (not well established)
Elderly or medically ill patients	4–8 μg/mL	0.6–0.8 mEq/L	45–75 μg/mL
Maintenance Therapy[b]			
Dose	400–1800 mg/d	600–1800 mg/d	15–45 mg/kg/d
Drug serum concentrations			
Adults	4–12 μg/mL	0.6–1.2 mEq/L	50–125 μg/mL
Elderly or medically ill patients	4–6 μg/mL	0.4–0.6 mEq/L	40–60 μg/mL

[a]CBZ serum levels decrease during the first 2–4 wk due to autoinduction of metabolism by the cytochrome P450 liver enzymes; higher doses of CBZ may be required to maintain adequate CBZ concentrations.
[b]There is no evidence that dosage reduction should be done for maintenance therapy of bipolar disorder, but lower doses are often tried when the patient is stablized.

- **Sodium valproate** is rapidly converted to VPA (a branched-chain fatty acid) in the stomach, whereas DVPX delayed-release tablets are converted in the small intestine. VPA is 90–95% protein bound, and the $t_{1/2}$ is 5–20 hours.

Adverse Effects

- Frequent adverse effects (Table 68–4) include transient GI complaints and sedation, which are minimized by giving with food, lowering initial doses, gradually increasing doses, or switching to DVPX.
- Other adverse effects include ataxia, lethargy, fine tremor, alopecia, changes in texture of hair, prolonged bleeding due to inhibition of platelet aggregation, transient increases in liver enzymes, and weight gain. Thrombocytopenia may occur at higher doses.
- Rare cases of hepatitis have been reported, and liver function tests should be obtained at baseline and at 6- to 12-month intervals.
- VPA is not recommended during the first trimester of pregnancy because of the risk of neural tube defects.

Drug–Drug Interactions

- Several drug–drug interactions of VPA are summarized in Table 68–5.

Dosing and Administration

- Dosing strategies are summarized in Table 68–6. Higher initial "loading" doses of DVPX (20 mg/kg/d or 1200–1500 mg/d in divided doses) in manic patients results in therapeutic serum levels within 5 days and a rapid onset of antimanic response.
- Serum VPA levels are usually obtained every 1–2 weeks during the first 2 months, then every 3–6 months.

Carbamazepine

- **CBZ** (a tricyclic structure) has acute antimanic (60% response), antidepressant (50–60% response), and prophylactic (60–75% response), effects comparable with lithium.
- Predictors of response include severe manic episodes, anxiety, dysphoria, schizoaffective/psychotic features, abnormal EEG, early-onset manic episodes, and a negative family history for mood disorders.
- CBZ is 70–80% protein bound and is metabolized to an active metabolite (10,11-epoxide). Its $t_{1/2}$ is 20–60 hours, but after autoinduction of metabolism is 12–20 hours.

Adverse Effects

- Adverse effects of CBZ are summarized in Table 68–4. Transient CNS toxicity (e.g., drowsiness, dizziness, fatigue, ataxia, vertigo, blurred vision, diplopia, nystagmus, dysarthria, confusion, and headache) occurs in up to 60% of patients. These may be minimized by low initial doses, gradual dose increases, or giving a larger bedtime dose. XIII
- GI side effects occur in up to 15% of patients initially and can be minimized by administering the drug with food or reducing the daily dose.

- Serious hematologic dyscrasias, except leukopenia, are rare. Decreased white blood cell (WBC) counts occur in 25% of patients but return to normal with CBZ discontinuation. Patients with low- or below-normal pretreatment WBC and neutrophil counts should be monitored closely (e.g., every 2 weeks for the first 1–3 months). If the WBC falls below $3000/mm^3$, then the dose of CBZ should be decreased or discontinued.

Drug–Drug Interactions

- CBZ drug–drug interactions are summarized in Table 68–5. CBZ induces the hepatic microsomal P450 enzymes (i.e., 1A2, 3A4, 2C9/10, and 2D6) and increases the elimination of many concurrently prescribed agents (e.g., anticonvulsants, antidepressants, and antipsychotics).
- Drugs that inhibit the 3A4 isoenzyme system may cause CBZ toxicity (e.g., **cimetidine, erythromycin, isoniazid, verapamil, diltiazem, propoxyphene, nefazodone, ketoconazole, itraconazole, fluvoxamine,** and **fluoxetine**).

Dosing and Administration

- Dosing strategies are summarized in Table 68–6. If there is no response after 2 weeks, the dose can be gradually increased to obtain serum concentrations of 6–12 μg/mL. Treatment-resistant patients may require serum concentrations up to 12–14 μg/mL.
- When patients are symptom free, lower initial doses are used (e.g., 100–200 mg/d, with increases every 3–5 days up to 600–1200 mg/d).
- During the first month of therapy, serum concentrations may decrease due to autoinduction of hepatic oxidative enzymes, requiring a dose increase. Autoinduction may begin by day 3 and continue up to 30 days after the last dose change.
- CBZ serum levels are usually obtained every 1–2 weeks during the first 2 months, then every 3–6 months for maintenance therapy.

Alternate Treatments

Antipsychotics

- Manic episodes may be treated with a mood stabilizer, an antipsychotic, or a combination of an antipsychotic and a mood stabilizer for additive or synergistic effects.
- Antipsychotics should be used only in patients with psychotic symptoms, and they may have a more rapid onset of action than lithium.
- Higher doses (e.g., **haloperidol** 5–10 mg IM or 10–25 mg orally every 4–6 hours as needed) may be required. Once mania is controlled, the antipsychotic should be tapered and discontinued.

Benzodiazepines

- BZDs may be used instead of antipsychotics to calm agitated manic patients.
- The oral dose of **lorazepam** in acute mania is approximately (0.05 mg/kg) 1–4 mg three times daily with the largest dose given at bedtime. Gradual increases up to 40–80 mg/d can be made. IM or IV doses are

lower. The dose of **clonazepam** is 0.5–2 mg three times daily and can be titrated up to 20 mg/d.

Antidepressants

- Bipolar patients in a depressive episode may require antidepressants along with mood stabilizers, but they may precipitate a manic episode in some patients.
- **Bupropion** and selective serotonin reuptake inhibitors (SSRIs) are considered first-line and monoamine oxidase inhibitors (MAOIs) and **venlafaxine** second-line agents for bipolar depression.

Others

- **Verapamil** (80–480 mg/d) and **nimodipine** (30–120 mg/d) are alternative mood stabilizers in patients who cannot be treated with lithium, CBZ, or VPA.
- **Lamotrigine** has been shown to have mood-stabilizing effects in treatment-resistant bipolar type I and type II patients and may have augmenting effects when combined with VPA. Usual doses are 50–250 mg/d, but some patients may require 500–700 mg/d.

Pharmacoeconomic Considerations

- A recent study found that DVPX, both conventional titration and the rapid loading dose (20 mg/kg/d), was associated with shorter lengths of hospital stay, particularly in patients with rapid-cycling or mixed states. Other studies have reported cost savings for DVPX and for the combination of CBZ and lithium compared to lithium alone.

► EVALUATION OF THERAPEUTIC OUTCOMES

- Patients with bipolar disorder should be seen regularly (every 1–2 weeks for acute or frequent episodes or 1–3 months for stable patients with infrequent episodes) and monitored for response of target symptoms and presence of side effects.
- Patients should receive regular laboratory monitoring and compliance monitoring.

See Chapter 66, Bipolar Disorder, authored by Martha P. Fankhauser, MS Pharm, FASHP, and William H. Benefield, Jr., PharmD, FASCP, BCPP, for a more detailed discussion of this topic.

Chapter 69

▶ DEPRESSIVE DISORDERS

▶ DEFINITION

Depressive disorders include major depressive disorder and dysthymic disorder. The essential feature of major depressive disorder is a clinical course that is characterized by one or more major depressive episodes without a history of manic, mixed, or hypomanic episodes. Dysthymic disorder is a chronic disturbance of mood involving depressed mood and at least two other symptoms, and it is generally less severe than major depressive disorder.

▶ PATHOPHYSIOLOGY

- *Biogenic amine hypothesis.* Depression may be caused by inadequate monoamine neurotransmission, most notably norepinephrine (NE).
- *Permissive hypothesis.* Low serotonin (5-HT) activity may permit the expression of the affective state, but the type is governed by the level of NE. Low NE levels cause depression, and high NE levels cause mania.
- *Postsynaptic changes in receptor sensitivity.* Changes in sensitivity of NE or 5-HT_2 receptors may relate to onset of depression.
- *Dysregulation hypothesis.* This theory emphasizes a failure of homeostatic regulation of neurotransmitter systems, rather than absolute increases or decreases in their activities.
- *The role of dopamine (DA).* Recent reviews suggest that increased DA neurotransmission in the nucleus accumbens may be related to the mechanism of action of antidepressants.

▶ CLINICAL PRESENTATION

- Emotional symptoms may include diminished ability to experience pleasure, loss of interest in usual activities, sadness, pessimistic outlook, crying spells, hopelessness, anxiety (present in almost 90% of depressed outpatients), feelings of guilt, and psychotic features (e.g., auditory hallucinations, delusions).
- Physical symptoms may include fatigue, pain (especially headache), sleep disturbance, appetite disturbance (decreased or increased), loss of sexual interest, or gastrointestinal or cardiovascular complaints (especially palpitations).
- Intellectual or cognitive symptoms may include decreased ability to concentrate or slowed thinking, poor memory for recent events, confusion, and indecisiveness.
- Psychomotor disturbances may include psychomotor retardation (slowed physical movements, thought processes, and speech) or psychomotor agitation.

▶ DIAGNOSIS

- Major depression is characterized by one or more episodes of major depression, as defined by the *Diagnostic and Statistical Manual of Mental Disorders,* 4th edition (DSM-IV; Table 69–1).
- When a patient presents with depressive symptoms, it is necessary to investigate the possibility of a medical, psychiatric, and/or drug-induced cause (Table 69–2).
- Depressed patients should have a medication review, physical examination, mental status examination, a complete blood count with differential, thyroid function tests, and electrolyte determinations.

▶ DESIRED OUTCOME

- The goals of treatment of the acute depressive episode are to eliminate or reduce the symptoms of depression, minimize adverse effects, ensure compliance with the therapeutic regimen, and facilitate a return to a premorbid level of functioning.
- Seventy percent of patients with a single depressive episode experience a relapse. For about 20–35% of patients, depression is chronic with considerable residual symptoms. Older persons are less likely to fully recover.

TABLE 69–1. DSM-IV Criteria for Major Depressive Episode

A. Five (or more) of the following symptoms have been present during the same 2-week period and represent a change from previous functioning; at least one of the symptoms is either (1) depressed mood or (2) loss of interest or pleasure.
   1. Depressed mood most of the day, nearly every day
   2. Markedly diminished interest or pleasure in all, or almost all, activities
   3. Significant weight loss (not dieting) or weight gain or decrease or increase in appetite nearly every day
   4. Insomnia or hypersomnia nearly every day
   5. Psychomotor agitation or retardation nearly every day (observable)
   6. Fatigue or loss of energy nearly every day
   7. Feelings of worthlessness or excessive or inappropriate guilt (may be delusional) nearly every day
   8. Diminished ability to think or concentrate or indecisiveness
   9. Recurrent thoughts of death, recurrent suicidal ideation without a specific plan, or a suicide attempt or a specific suicide plan

B. The symptoms cause clinically significant distress or impairment in social, occupational, or other important areas of functioning.

C. The symptoms are not due to the direct physiologic effects of a substance or a general medical condition (e.g., hypothyroidism).

Modified from American Psychiatric Association, Diagnostic and Statistical Manual of Mental Disorders, *4th ed. (DSM-IV). Washington, DC, American Psychiatric Association, 1994:327, with permission.*

TABLE 69–2. Common Medical Disorders, Psychiatric Disorders, and Drug Therapy Associated With Depression

Medical Disorders		Psychiatric Disorders
Endocrine diseases Hyperthyroidism Hypothyroidism Addison's disease Cushing's disease Deficiency states Pernicious anemia Wernicke's encephalopathy Severe anemia Infections Encephalitis Influenza Mononucleosis Tuberculosis AIDS Collagen disorder Systemic lupus erythematosus	Metabolic disorders Electrolyte imbalance Hypokalemia Hyponatremia Hepatic encephalopathy Cardiovascular disease Cerebral arteriosclerosis Congestive heart failure Myocardial infarction Neurologic disorders Alzheimer's disease Huntington's disease Multiple sclerosis Parkinson's disease Poststroke Malignant disease	Alcoholism Anxiety disorders Eating disorders Schizophrenia **Drug Therapy** Alcohol Antihypertensives Reserpine Methyldopa Propranolol hydrochloride Guanethidine sulfate Hydralazine hydrochloride Clonidine hydrochloride Diuretics **Hormonal Therapy** Oral contraceptives Steroids/ACTH

▶ TREATMENT

NONDRUG TREATMENT

- Electroconvulsive therapy (ECT) is a safe and effective treatment for all subtypes of major depressive disorder. It is considered when a rapid response is needed, risks of other treatments outweigh potential benefits, there has been a poor response to drugs, and the patient expresses a preference for ECT. A rapid therapeutic response (10–14 days) has been reported. Relative contraindications include increased intracranial pressure, cerebral lesions, recent myocardial infarction, recent intracerebral hemorrhage, bleeding, or otherwise unstable vascular condition. Adverse effects of ECT include cognitive dysfunction (e.g., confusion, memory impairment), prolonged apnea, treatment emergent mania, headache, nausea, and muscle aches. Relapse rates during the year following ECT are high unless maintenance antidepressant medications are prescribed.
- The efficacy of psychotherapy and antidepressant medication is considered to be additive. Psychotherapy alone is not recommended for the acute treatment of patients with severe and/or psychotic major depressive disorders. For uncomplicated nonchronic major depressive disorder, combined treatment may provide no unique advantage. Cognitive therapy, behavioral therapy, and interpersonal psychotherapy appear to be equal in efficacy.

GENERAL THERAPEUTIC PRINCIPLES

- In general, antidepressants are equal in efficacy when administered in comparable doses.
- Factors that influence the choice of antidepressant include the patient's past history of response, history of familial response, subtype of depression, concurrent medical history, potential for drug–drug interactions, side-effect profile of various drugs, and drug cost.
- Sixty percent to 70% of patients with varying types of depression improve with drug therapy.
- Melancholic depression appears to respond well to tricyclic antidepressants (TCAs), selective 5-HT reuptake inhibitors (SSRIs), and ECT.
- A preferential response to monoamine oxidase inhibitors (MAOIs) has been reported in patients with atypical depression.
- Patients who fail to respond to a TCA may well respond to an SSRI and vice versa.
- Psychotically depressed individuals generally require either ECT or combination therapy with an antidepressant plus an antipsychotic agent.

DRUG CLASSIFICATION

- Table 69–3 shows the commonly accepted classification of available antidepressant drugs and their suggested therapeutic plasma concentration ranges, initial doses, and usual dosage ranges.
- TCAs are effective in treating all depressive subtypes, especially the severe melancholic subtype.
- Table 69–4 shows the relative potency and selectivity of the antidepressants for inhibition of NE and 5-HT reuptake and relative side-effect profiles.
- The MAOIs increase the concentrations of NE, 5-HT, and DA within the neuronal synapse through inhibition of the monoamine oxidase enzyme system.
- The triazolepyridines, **trazodone** and **nefazodone,** are antagonists at the 5-HT_2 receptor and inhibit the reuptake of 5-HT. They have negligible affinity for cholinergic and histaminergic receptors.
- **Bupropion's** most potent neurochemical action is blockade of DA reuptake.
- **Mirtazapine,** a tetracyclic agent, is an antagonist of α_2-adrenergic autoreceptors and heteroreceptors on both NE and 5-HT presynaptic axons and an antagonist of postsynaptic 5-HT_2 and 5-HT_3 receptors. The net effect is increased noradrenergic activity and increased serotonergic activity, especially at 5-HT_{1A} receptors.

ADVERSE EFFECTS

- Adverse-effect profiles of the various antidepressants are summarized in Table 69–4.

TABLE 69–3. Adult Dosages for Currently Available Antidepressant Medications[a]

Generic Name	Trade Name	Manufacturer	Suggested Therapeutic Plasma Concentration Range (ng/mL)	Initial Dose (mg/d)	Usual Dosage range (mg/d)
Tricyclic Antidepressants					
Tertiary amines					
Amitriptyline	Elavil	Stuart	120–250[b]	50–75	100–300
	Endep	Roche			
	Generic	Various			
Clomipramine	Anafranil	Novartis		25	100–250
Doxepin	Adapin	Lotus Biochemical	110–250[b]	50–75	100–300
	Sinequan	Roerig			
	Generic	Various			
Imipramine	Tofranil	Novartis	200–300[b]	50–75	100–300
	Generic	Various			
Trimipramine	Surmontil	Wyeth-Ayerst		50–75	100–300
Secondary amines					
Desipramine	Norpramin	Marion Merrell Dow	125–300	50–75	100–300
	Generic	Various			
Nortriptyline	Pamelor	Novartis	50–150	25–50	50–150
	Generic	Various			
Protriptyline	Vivactil	Merck	70–240	10–20	15–60
Dibenzoxazepine					
Amoxapine	Asendin	Lederle	200–400[c]	50–150	100–400
	Generic	Various			

Tetracyclic					
Maprotiline	Ludiomil	Novartis	200–300[b]	50–75	100–225
	Generic	Various			
Mirtazapine	Remeron	Organon		15	25–40
Triazolopyridines					
Nefazodone	Serzone	Bristol-Myers Squibb		200	300–600
Trazodone	Desyrel	Apothecon		50–150	150–400
	Generic	Various			
Aminoketone					
Bupropion	Wellbutrin	Glaxo Wellcome	50–100	200	300–450
Monoamine Oxidase Inhibitors					
Phenelzine	Nardil	Parke-Davis		15	15–90
Tranlycypromine	Parnate	SmithKline Beecham		20	20–60
Selective Serotonin Reuptake Inhibitors					
Citalopram	Celexa	Forest		20	20–60
Fluoxetine	Prozac	Dista		10–20	10–80
Fluvoxamine	Luvox	Solvay		50	50–300
Paroxetine	Paxil	SmithKline Beecham		20	20–50
Sertraline	Zoloft	Roerig		50	100–200
Serotonin/Norepinephrine Reuptake Inhibitor					
Venlafaxine	Effexor	Wyeth-Ayerst		75	75–375

[a] Doses listed are total daily doses; elderly patients are usually treated with approximately one-half of the dose listed.
[b] Parent drug plus demethylated metabolite.
[c] Parent drug plus hydroxymetabolite.

TABLE 69–4. Relative Potencies of Norepinephrine and Serotonin Reuptake Blockade and Side-effect Profile of Antidepressant Drugs

	Reuptake Antagonism		Anticholinergic Effects	Sedation	Orthostatic Hypotension	Seizures	Conduction Abnormalities
	Norepinephrine	*Serotonin*					
Tricyclic Antidepressants							
Tertiary amines							
Amitriptyline	++	++++	++++	++++	+++	+++	+++
Clomipramine	++	+++	++++	++++	++	++++	+++
Doxepin	++	++	+++	++++	++	+++	++
Imipramine	+++	+++	+++	+++	++++	+++	+++
Trimipramine	++	++	++++	++++	+++	+++	+++
Secondary amines							
Desipramine	++++	+	++	++	++	++	++
Nortriptyline	+++	++	++	++	+	++	++
Protriptyline	+++	++	++	+	++	++	+++
Dibenzoxazepine							
Amoxapine[a]	+++	++	+++	++	++	+++	++
Tetracyclic							
Maprotiline	+++	+	+++	+++	++	++++	++
Mirtazapine	++++	++	+	++	++		+

Triazolopyridines							
Nefazodone	0	++	0	+++	+++	++	+
Trazodone	0	++	0	++++	+++	++	+
Aminoketone							
Bupropion	+	+	+	0	0	++++	+
Monoamine Oxidase Inhibitors							
Phenelzine	++	++	+	++	++	+	
Tranylcypromine	++	+	+	+	++	+	+
Selective Serotonin Reuptake Inhibitors							
Citalopram	0	++++	+	+	0	++	0
Fluoxetine	0	+++	0	0	0	++	0
Fluvoxamine	0	++++	0	0	0	++	0
Paroxetine	0	++++	+	+	0	++	0
Sertraline	0	++++	0	0	0	++	0
Serotonin/Norepinephrine Reuptake Inhibitor							
Venlafaxine	++++	++++	+	+	0	++	+

++++, high; +++, moderate; ++, low; +, very low; 0, none.

[a] Also blocks dopamine receptors.

Tricyclic Antidepressants and Other Heterocyclics

- Anticholinergic side effects (e.g., dry mouth, blurred vision, constipation, urinary retention, tachycardia, and memory impairment) and sedation are more likely to occur with the tertiary amine TCAs than with the secondary amine TCAs.
- A common and potentially serious adverse effect of the TCAs is orthostatic hypotension with resultant syncope. This occurs as a result of α_1-adrenergic antagonism.
- Additional side effects include cardiac conduction delays and heart block, especially in patients with preexisting conduction disease.
- Other side effects that may lead to noncompliance include weight gain, excessive perspiration, and sexual dysfunction.
- Abrupt withdrawal of TCAs (especially high doses) may result in symptoms of cholinergic rebound (e.g., dizziness, nausea, diarrhea, insomnia, restlessness).
- **Amoxapine** is a demethylated metabolite of **loxapine** and, as a result of its postsynaptic receptor DA-blocking effects, may be associated with extrapyramidal side effects (EPS).
- **Maprotiline,** a tetracyclic drug, causes seizures at a higher incidence than do standard TCAs, and is contraindicated in patients with a history of seizure disorder. The ceiling dose is considered to be 225 mg/d.

Venlafaxine

- **Venlafaxine** may cause a dose-related increase in diastolic blood pressure, and baseline blood pressure is not a useful predictor of this phenomenon. Dosage reduction or discontinuation may be necessary if sustained hypertension occurs.

Selective Serotonin Reuptake Inhibitors

- The SSRIs produce fewer sedative, anticholinergic, and cardiovascular adverse effects than the TCAs and are not associated with weight gain. The primary adverse effects include nausea, vomiting, diarrhea, and sexual dysfunction. Headache, insomnia, and fatigue are also reported commonly.

Triazolopyridines

- **Trazodone** and **nefazodone** cause minimal anticholinergic and gastrointestinal effects. Sedation and orthostatic hypotension are the most frequent dose-limiting side effects.
- Priapism occurs rarely with trazodone use (1 in 6000 male patients).

XIII

Aminoketone

- The occurrence of seizures with **bupropion** is dose-related and may be increased by predisposing factors (e.g., history of head trauma or CNS tumor). At the ceiling dose (450 mg/d), the incidence of seizures is 0.4%.

Piperazino-azepine

- **Mirtazapine's** most common adverse effects are somnolence, weight gain, dry mouth, and constipation. In preclinical trials, liver function tests were elevated 1.6 times more frequently in the mirtazapine group than in the placebo group.

Monoamine Oxidase Inhibitors

- The most common adverse effect of MAOIs is postural hypotension (more likely with **phenelzine** than **tranylcypromine**), which can be minimized by divided-daily dosing. Anticholinergic side effects are common but less severe than with the TCAs. Phenelzine causes mild to moderate sedating effects, but tranylcypromine is often stimulating, and the last dose of the day is administered in early afternoon. Sexual dysfunction in both genders is common. Phenelzine has been associated with hepatocellular damage and weight gain.
- Hypertensive crisis is a potentially fatal adverse reaction that can occur when MAOIs are taken concurrently with certain foods, especially those high in tyramine (Table 69–5), and with certain drugs (Table 69–6). Symptoms of hypertensive crisis include occipital headache, stiff neck, nausea, vomiting, sweating, and sharply elevated blood pressure. The hypertensive crisis can be treated with 10–20 mg of **nifedipine** sublingually or swallowed or 5 mg of **phentolamine** intravenously. Education of patients taking MAOIs regarding dietary and medication restrictions is critical.

TABLE 69–5. Dietary Restrictions for Patients Taking Monoamine Oxidase Inhibitors

Aged cheese[a]	Liver (chicken or beef, more than 2 d old)
Sour cream[b]	Fermented foods
Yogurt[b]	Canned figs
Cottage cheese[b]	Raisins
American cheese[b]	Pods of broad beans (fava beans)[a]
Mild Swiss cheese[b]	Yeast extract and other yeast products[a]
Wine (especially Chianti and sherry)[c]	Meat extract (Marmite)
Beer	Soy sauce
Herring (pickled, salted, dry)[a]	Chocolate[b]
Sardines	Coffee[d]
Snails	Ripe avocado
Anchovies	Sauerkraut
Canned, aged, or processed meats	Licorice
Monosodium glutamate	

[a] Clearly warrants absolute prohibition (e.g., English Stilton, blue, Camembert, cheddar).
[b] Up to 2 oz daily is acceptable.
[c] 3 oz white wine or a single cocktail is acceptable.
[d] Up to 2 oz daily is acceptable; larger amounts of decaffeinated coffee are acceptable.

XIII

TABLE 69–6. Medication Restrictions for Patients Taking Monoamine Oxidase Inhibitors

Amphetamines	Levodopa
Appetite suppressants	Local anesthetics containing sympathomimetic vasoconstrictors
Asthma inhalants	Meperidine
Buspirone	Methyldopa
Carbamazepine	Methylphenidate
Cocaine	Other antidepressants[a]
Cyclobenzaprine	Other MAOIs
Decongestants (topical and systemic)	Reserpine
Dextromethorphan	Stimulants
Dopamine	Sympathomimetics
Ephedrine	Tryptophan
Epinephrine	
Guanethidine	

[a]Tricyclic antidepressants may be used with caution by experienced clinicians in treatment-resistant populations.

PHARMACOKINETICS

- The pharmacokinetics of the antidepressants are summarized in Table 69–7.
- Substantial amounts of TCAs pass into breast milk; breast feeding is not advised.
- The major metabolic pathways of the TCAs are demethylation, hydroxylation, and glucuronide conjugation. Metabolism of the TCAs appears to be linear within the usual dosage range, but dose-related kinetics cannot be ruled out in the elderly.
- The SSRIs, with the possible exception of citalopram, may have a nonlinear pattern of drug accumulation with chronic dosing.
- Factors reported to influence TCA plasma concentrations include disease states (e.g., renal or hepatic dysfunction), genetics, age, cigarette smoking, and concurrent drug administration. Similarly, hepatic impairment, renal impairment, and age have been reported to influence the pharmacokinetics of SSRIs.
- In acutely depressed patients, there is a correlation between antidepressant effect and plasma concentrations for some TCAs. Table 69–3 shows suggested therapeutic plasma concentration ranges. The best established therapeutic range is for **nortriptyline,** and these data suggest a therapeutic window.
- Some indications for plasma level monitoring include inadequate response, relapse, serious or persistent adverse effects, use of higher than standard doses, suspected toxicity, elderly patients, children and adolescents, pregnant patients, patients of African or Asian descent (because of slower metabolism), cardiac disease, suspected noncompli-

TABLE 69–7. Pharmacokinetic Properties of Antidepressants

Generic Name	Elimination Half-life (h)[a]	Time of Peak Plasma Concentration (h)	Plasma Protein Binding (%)	% Bioavailable	Clinically Important Metabolites
Tricyclic antidepressants					
Tertiary amines					
Amitriptyline	9–46	1–5	90–97	30–60	Nortriptyline; 10-Hydroxynortriptyline
Clomipramine	20–24	2–6	97	36–62	
Doxepin	8–36	1–4	68–82	13–45	Desmethyldoxepin
Imipramine	6–34	1.5–3	63–96	22–77	2-Hydroxyimipramine; desipramine; 2-hydroxydesipramine
Trimipramine	7–40	3	94–96	18–63	None
Secondary amines					
Desipramine	11–46	3–6	73–92	33–51	2-Hydroxydesipramine
Nortriptyline	16–88	3–12	87–95	46–70	10-Hydroxynortriptyline
Protriptyline	54–198	6–12	90–94	75–90	None
Dibenzoxazepine					
Amoxapine	8–30[b]	1–2	90	[c]	8-Hydroxyamoxapine
Tetracyclic					
Maprotiline	28–105	4–24	88	79–87	Desmethylmaprotiline
Mirtazapine	20–40	2	85	50	None known
Triazolopyridines					
Nefazodone	2–4	1	99	20	Meta-chlorophenylpiperazine; hydroxynefazodone; triazole-dione
Trazodone	6–11	1–2	92	[c]	Meta-chlorophenylpiperazine

(continued)

TABLE 69–7. continued

Generic Name	Elimination Half-Life (h)[a]	Time of Peak Plasma Concentration (h)	Plasma Protein Binding (%)	% Bioavailable	Clinically Important Metabolites
Aminoketone					
Bupropion	10–21	3	82–88	[c]	Bupropion threo-amino alcohol; bupropion morpholinol
Monoamine Oxidase Inhibitors					
Phenelzine	1.5–4	[c]	[c]	[c]	
Tranylcypromine	1.5–3	[c]	[c]	[c]	
Selective Serotonin Reuptake Inhibitors					
Citalopram	33	2–4	80	≥80	Demethyl- and didemethylcitalopram
Fluoxetine	4–6 days[d]	4–8	94	95	Norfluoxetine
Fluvoxamine	15–26	2–8	77	53	None
Paroxetine	24–31	5–7	95		None
Sertraline	27	6–8	99	36[e]	*N*-desmethylsertraline
Serotonin/Norepinephrine Reuptake Inhibitor					
Venlafaxine	5	2	27–30		O-desmethylvenlafaxine

[a] Biologic half-life in slowest phase of elimination.
[b] Amoxapine, 8 h; 8-hydroxyamoxapine, 30 h.
[c] No data available.
[d] 4–6 days with chronic dosing; norfluoxetine, 4–16 days.
[e] Increases 30–40% when taken with food.

ance, suspected pharmacokinetic drug interactions, and changing brands.

- Plasma concentrations should be obtained at steady state, usually after a minimum of 1 week at constant dosage. Sampling should be done during the elimination phase, usually in the morning, 12 hours after the last dose. Samples collected in this manner are comparable for patients on once-daily, twice-daily, or thrice-daily regimens.

DRUG–DRUG INTERACTIONS

- Drug interactions of the TCAs are summarized in Tables 69–8 and 69–9. Table 69–10 summarizes the drug interactions on non-TCAs.
- The very slow elimination of **fluoxetine** and norfluoxetine makes it critical to ensure a 5-week washout after fluoxetine discontinuation before starting an MAOI. Potentially fatal reactions may occur when any SSRI or TCA is coadministered with an MAOI.
- Increased plasma concentrations of TCAs and symptoms of toxicity may occur when fluoxetine, **sertraline, fluvoxamine, paroxetine,** and possibly **citalopram** are added to a TCA regimen. Dosage reduction of **alprazolam** and **triazolam** is required if either drug is coadministered with **nefazodone.**
- As nefazodone is an in vitro inhibitor of cytochrome P450 IIIA4, it should not be coadministered with **astemizole** or **terfenadine.**

SPECIAL POPULATIONS

Elderly Patients

- The SSRIs are often selected as first-choice antidepressants in elderly patients, and they may enable one to avoid adverse effects commonly associated with the TCAs.
- In healthy elderly patients, cautious use of a secondary amine TCA (**desipramine** or nortriptyline) may be appropriate because of their defined therapeutic plasma concentration ranges, well-established efficacy, and well-known adverse-effect profiles.
- Trazodone, nefazodone, and bupropion may also be chosen because of their milder anticholinergic and less frequent cardiovascular side effects.

Children and Adolescents

- Data supporting efficacy of antidepressants in children and adolescents are sparse. The SSRIs are better tolerated than the TCAs and are relatively safer on overdose (suicide is the second leading cause of death in adolescents).
- Several cases of sudden death have been reported in children and adolescents taking desipramine. A baseline electrocardiogram (ECG) is recommended before initiating a TCA in children and adolescents, and an additional ECG is advised when steady-state plasma concentrations are achieved. Plasma concentration monitoring is critical.

TABLE 69–8. Pharmacokinetic Drug Interactions Involving Tricyclic Antidepressants

Elevates Plasma Concentrations of TCAs	Lowers Plasma Concentrations of TCAs
Cimetidine	Barbiturates
Diltiazem	Carbamazepine
Ethanol, acute ingestion	Ethanol, chronic ingestion
SSRIs	Phenytoin
Haloperidol	**Elevates Plasma Concentrations of Interacting Drug**
Labetalol	Hydantoins
Methylphenidate	Oral anticoagulants
Oral contraceptives	**Lowers Plasma Concentrations of Interacting Drug**
Phenothiazines	Levodopa
Propoxyphene	
Quinidine	
Verapamil	

Pregnancy

- As a general rule, nondrug approaches to the treatment of depression in the pregnant patient are preferred.
- The TCAs are usually given preference, and nortriptyline or desipramine may be the treatment of choice because of the experience that has been gained with these agents, and because therapeutic plasma concentration ranges have been established. When TCAs are withdrawn during pregnancy, they should be tapered gradually to avoid withdrawal symptoms. If possible, drug tapering is usually begun 5–10 days before the estimated day of confinement.

DOSING

- Dosing recommendations are shown in Table 69–3. The usual initial adult dose of most TCAs is 50 mg at bedtime, and the dose may be increased by 25 to 50 mg every third day.
- Bupropion is usually initiated at 100 mg twice daily, and this dose may be increased to 100 mg three times daily after 3 days. An increase to 450 mg/d (the ceiling dose), given as 150 mg three times daily, may be considered in patients with no clinical response after several weeks at 300 mg/d.
- XIII A 6-week antidepressant trial at a maximum dosage is considered an adequate trial. Patients must be told about the expected lag time of 2–4 weeks before the onset of antidepressant effect.
- Elderly patients should receive half the initial dose given to younger adults, and the dose is increased at a slower rate. They may require 6–12 weeks of treatment to achieve the desired antidepressant response.
- To prevent relapse, antidepressants should be continued at full therapeutic doses for 4–9 months after remission. Some investigators rec-

TABLE 69–9. Pharmacodynamic Drug Interactions Involving Tricyclic Antidepressants

Interacting Drug	Effect
Alcohol	Increased CNS depressant effects
Amphetamines	Increased effect of amphetamines
Androgens	Delusions, hostility
Anticholinergic agents	Excessive anticholinergic effects
Bethanidine	Decreased antihypertensive efficacy
Clonidine	Decreased antihypertensive efficacy
Disulfiram	Acute organic brain syndrome
Estrogens	Increased or decreased antidepressant response; increased toxicity
Guanadrel	Decreased antihypertensive efficacy
Guanethidine	Decreased antihypertensive efficacy
Insulin	Increased hypoglycemic effects
Lithium	Possible additive lowering of seizure threshold
Methyldopa	Decreased antihypertensive efficacy; tachycardia; CNS stimulation
Monoamine oxidase inhibitors	Increased therapeutic and possibly toxic effects of both drugs; hypertensive crisis; delirium; seizures; hyperpyrexia; serotonin syndrome
Oral hypoglycemics	Increased hypoglycemic effects
Phenytoin	Possible lowering of seizure threshold and reduced antidepressant response
Sedatives	Increased CNS depressant effects
Sympathomimetics	Increased pharmacologic effects of direct-acting sympathomimetics; decreased effects of indirect-acting sympathomimetics
Thyroid hormones	Increased therapeutic and possibly toxic effects of both drugs; CNS stimulation; tachycardia

ommend lifelong maintenance therapy for persons at greatest risk for recurrence (e.g., persons >50 years of age at onset of the first episode, persons >40 years of age and with two or more prior episodes, and persons of any age with three or more prior episodes).

REFRACTORY PATIENTS

- Most "treatment-resistant" depressed patients have received inadequate therapy. Issues to be considered in patients who have not responded to treatment include: (1) Is the diagnosis correct? (2) Does the patient have a psychotic depression? (3) Has the patient received an adequate dose and duration of treatment? (4) Do adverse effects preclude adequate dosing? (5) Has the patient been compliant with the prescribed regimen? (6) Was treatment outcome measured adequately? (7) Is there a coexisting or preexisting medical or psychiatric disorder? XIII

TABLE 69–10. Drug Interactions of Nontricyclic Antidepressants

Non-TCA	Interacting Drug/Drug Class	Effect
Dibenzoxazepine		
Amoxapine	Many drugs that interact with TCAs	Similar response to that seen with TCA interaction
Tetracyclic		
Maprotiline	Many drugs that interact with TCAs	Similar response to that seen with TCA interaction
Mirtazapine	MAOIs	Theoretically central serotonin syndrome could occur
Triazolopyridines		
Nefazodone	Alprazolam	Increased plasma concentrations of alprazolam
	Astemizole	Theoretically increased plasma concentrations of astemizole with potentially serious cardiovascular adverse effects
	Digoxin	Increased C_{max}, C_{min}, and AUC of digoxin by 29%, 27%, and 15%, respectively
	Haloperidol	Decreased clearance of haloperidol by 35%
	MAOIs	Hypertensive crisis; serotonin syndrome; delirium; coma; seizures; hyperpyrexia
	Propranolol	Decreased C_{max} and AUC of propranolol; increased C_{max}, C_{min}, and AUC of m-CPP metabolite of nefazodone
	Terfenadine	Theoretically increased plasma concentrations of terfenadine with potentially serious cardiovascular adverse effects
	Triazolam	Increased plasma concentrations of triazolam; increased psychomotor impairment
Trazodone	CNS depressants	Increased CNS depression
	Digoxin	Increased serum concentrations of digoxin
	Ethanol	Additive impairment in motor skills
	Fluoxetine	Increased plasma concentrations of trazodone
	MAOIs	Theoretically central serotonin syndrome could occur
	Neuroleptics	Increased hypotension
	Phenytoin	Increased serum concentrations of phenytoin
	Tryptophan	Agitation, restlessness, poor concentration, nausea
	Warfarin	Decreased hypoprothrombinemic response
Aminoketone		
Bupropion	MAOIs	Increased toxicity of bupropion
	Medications that lower seizure threshold	Increased incidence of seizures
	Levodopa	Increased incidence of adverse experiences
Selective Serotonin Reuptake Inhibitors		
Citalopram	Cimetidine	Reduced oral clearance of citalopram
	Fluvoxamine	Increased plasma concentrations of citalopram
	TCAs	Possible increased AUC of TCA
Fluoxetine	Alprazolam	Increased plasma concentrations and half-life of alprazolam; increased psychomotor impairment
	Anticoagulants	Possible increased risk of bleeding
	β-Adrenergic blockers	Increased metoprolol serum concentrations and bradycardia; possible heart block

TABLE 69–10. continued

Non-TCA	Interacting Drug/Drug Class	Effect
Fluoxetine, cont'd	Buspirone	Decreased therapeutic response to buspirone
	Carbamazepine	Increased plasma concentrations of carbamazepine with symptoms of carbamazepine toxicity
	Dextromethorphan	Visual hallucinations (one patient only)
	Haloperidol	Increased haloperidol concentrations and increased extrapyramidal side effects
	Lithium	Neurotoxicity: Confusion, ataxia, dizziness, tremor, absence seizures
	MAOIs	Severe or fatal reactions: Confusion, nausea, double vision, hypomania, hypertension, tremor, serotonin syndrome
	Phenytoin	Increased plasma concentrations of phenytoin and symptoms of phenytoin toxicity
	TCAs	Markedly increased TCA plasma concentration with symptoms of TCA toxicity
	Terfenadine	Arrhythmias, shortness of breath, and orthostasis
	Trazodone	Headaches, dizziness, sedation
	Tryptophan	Agitation, restlessness, poor concentration, nausea
	Valproate	Increased valproate serum concentrations
Fluvoxamine	Alprazolam	Increased AUC of alprazolam by 96%, increased alprazolam half-life by 71%, and increased psychomotor impairment
	Astemizole	Theoretically increased plasma concentrations of astemizole with potentially serious cardiovascular effects
	β-Adrenergic blockers	Fivefold increase in propranolol serum concentrations; bradycardia and hypotension with combined fluvoxamine and metoprolol
	Carbamazepine	Possible carbamazepine toxicity, although a controlled study did not support this
	Clozapine	Increased clozapine serum concentrations and increased risk for seizures and orthostatic hypotension
	Diazepam	Decreased clearance of diazepam and its active metabolite
	Diltiazem	Bradycardia
	Haloperidol	Increased haloperidol plasma concentrations
	Lithium	Increased serotonergic effects; seizures, nausea, tremor
	MAOIs	Potential for hypertensive crisis, serotonin syndrome, seizures, delirium
	Methodone	Increased methodone plasma concentrations with symptoms of methodone toxicity
	TCAs	Increased TCA plasma concentration
	Terfenadine	Theoretically increased plasma concentrations of terfenadine with potentially serious cardiovascular effects
	Theophylline	Increased serum concentrations of theophylline with symptoms of theophylline toxicity
	Tryptophan	Increased serotonergic effects and severe vomiting

(continued)

TABLE 69–10. continued

Non-TCA	Interacting Drug/Drug Class	Effect
Fluvoxamine, cont'd	Warfarin	Increased hypoprothrombinemic response to warfarin
Paroxetine	Cimetidine	Increased paroxetine serum concentrations
	Desipramine	Increased plasma concentrations and half-life of desipramine
	MAOIs	Potential for hypertensive crisis, serotonin syndrome, seizures, delirium
	Warfarin	Possible increased risk for bleeding
Sertraline	Carbamazepine	Increased plasma concentrations of carbamazepine
	Diazepam	Small decrease in clearance of diazepam
	MAOIs	Serotonin syndrome, myoclonus, violent shaking
	TCAs	Increased plasma concentrations of secondary amine TCAs (desipramine, nortriptyline)
	Tolbutamide	Decreased clearance of tolbutamide (16%)
	Warfarin	Increased protime
Serotonin/Norepinephrine Reuptake Inhibitor		
Venlafaxine	Cimetidine	Reduced clearance of venlafaxine by 43%; AUC and peak serum concentration of venlafaxine increased by 60%
	MAOIs	Potential for hypertensive crisis, serotonin syndrome, seizures, delirium

- The current antidepressant may be stopped and a trial with an unrelated agent initiated. Alternatively, the current antidepressant may be augmented (potentiated) by the addition of **lithium, liothyronine,** or an anticonvulsant such as **carbamazepine** or **valproic acid.**
- Switching medications is often preferred over augmentation as an initial strategy.
- A third approach is to use two different classes of antidepressants concurrently (e.g., TCA plus an MAOI). Concurrent use of a TCA and an MAOI should be undertaken only by a clinician experienced in the use of such combinations. When this is undertaken, the MAOI is slowly added to the TCA. Desipramine is not recommended to be used in combination with an MAOI. When the combination is discontinued, the MAOI should be stopped first. The combination of an SSRI and MAOI should never be used. An algorithm for treatment of depression including refractory patients is shown in Figure 69–1.

XIII

PHARMACOECONOMIC CONSIDERATIONS

- Drug costs account for about 10–12% of the direct costs of treating depression. When evaluating the costs of treatment, more must be considered than the cost of medications.
- Several studies have shown that the SSRIs are a more economical approach to treatment of depression (compared to TCAs) when all treatment costs are considered.

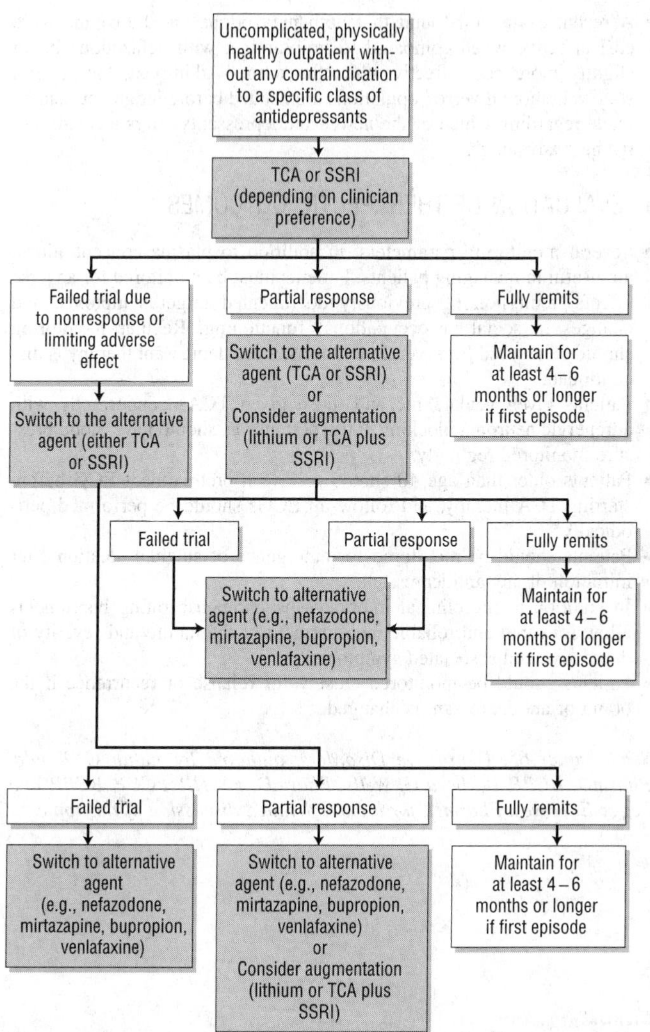

XIII

Figure 69–1. Algorithm for the treatment of uncomplicated major depression.

- A recent evaluation found that both nefazodone and fluoxetine were cost effective when compared to imipramine, with nefazodone being slightly more cost effective than fluoxetine. Additional, longer-term studies in more diverse populations are needed before judgments can be made regarding which of the newer antidepressants offers a cost-effectiveness advantage.

▶ EVALUATION OF THERAPEUTIC OUTCOMES

- Several monitoring parameters, in addition to plasma concentrations, are useful in managing patients. Patients must be monitored for adverse effects, remission of previously documented target symptoms, and changes in social or occupational functioning. Regular monitoring should be assured for several months after antidepressant therapy is discontinued.
- Patients given venlafaxine and those given TCAs concurrently with adrenergic neuronal blocking antihypertensives should have blood pressure monitored regularly.
- Patients older than age 40 should receive a pretreatment ECG before starting TCA therapy, and follow-up ECGs should be performed periodically.
- Patients should be monitored for emergence of suicidal ideation after initiation of any antidepressant.
- In addition to the clinical interview, psychometric rating instruments allow for rapid and reliable measurement of the nature and severity of depressive and associated symptoms.
- Patients should be monitored closely for relapse or recurrence if the brand of antidepressant is changed.

See Chapter 65, Depressive Disorders, authored by Judith C. Kando, PharmD, BCPP, Barbara G. Wells, PharmD, FASHP, FCCP, BCPP, and Peggy E. Hayes, PharmD, for a more detailed discussion of this topic.

Chapter 70

▶ SCHIZOPHRENIA

▶ DEFINITION

Schizophrenia is a chronic heterogeneous syndrome of disorganized and bizarre thoughts, delusions, hallucinations, inappropriate affect, and impaired psychosocial functioning.

▶ PATHOPHYSIOLOGY

- *Dopaminergic hypothesis.* Psychosis may result from hyper- or hypoactivity of dopaminergic processes in specific brain regions. This may include the presence of a dopamine (DA) receptor defect.
- *Glutamatergic dysfunction.* Glutamatergic tracts interact with dopaminergic tracts. A deficiency of glutamatergic activity relative to dopaminergic activity is proposed to be at least partially responsible for psychotic symptomatology.
- *Serotonin (5-HT) abnormalities.* Increased peripheral serotonin concentrations have been found in schizophrenics in some studies.
- *Norepinephrine (NE) abnormalities.* Increased concentrations of NE have been observed in the limbic structures of patients with chronic paranoid schizophrenia.
- *Dysregulation hypothesis.* Aberrant homeostatic control mechanisms cause erratic neurotransmission.
- Increased ventricular size, small decrease in brain size, and brain asymmetry has been reported.

▶ CLINICAL PRESENTATION

- Symptoms of the acute episode may include: out of touch with reality; hallucinations (especially hearing voices); delusions (fixed false beliefs); ideas of influence (actions controlled by external influences); disconnected thought processes (loose associations); ambivalence (contradictory thoughts); flat (no emotional expression), inappropriate, or labile affect; autism (withdrawn and inwardly directed thinking); uncooperativeness, hostility, and verbal or physical aggression; impaired self-care skills; and disturbed sleep and appetite.
- When the acute psychotic episode remits, the patient typically has residual features (e.g., anxiety, suspiciousness, lack of volition, lack of motivation, poor insight, impaired judgment, social withdrawal, difficulty in learning from experience, and poor self-care skills).

▶ DIAGNOSIS

- The *Diagnostic and Statistical Manual of Mental Disorders,* 4th edition (DSM-IV) specifies the following criteria for the diagnosis of schizophrenia.

  - Persistent dysfunction lasting longer than 6 months.
  - Two or more symptoms including hallucinations, delusions, disorganized speech, grossly disorganized or catatonic behavior, and negative symptoms. The symptoms must have been present for at least 1 month.
  - Significantly impaired functioning (work, interpersonal, or self-care).
- DSM-IV classifies symptoms as positive or negative.
  - Positive symptoms include delusions, disorganized speech (association disturbance), hallucinations, behavior disturbance (disorganized or catatonic), and illusions.
  - Negative symptoms include alogia (poverty of speech), avolition, affective flattening, anhedonia, and social isolation.
- Positive and negative symptoms may provide a framework for subtypes of schizophrenia that may correlate with prognosis, cognitive functioning, structural abnormalities in the brain, and response to typical antipsychotic (AP) drugs.
- The disorganized subtype is now considered to be a third subtype characterized by disorganized speech, disorganized behavior, and poor attention.

▶ DESIRED OUTCOME

- The goals of treatment include: alleviation of target symptoms, avoidance of side effects, improvement in psychosocial functioning and productivity, compliance with the prescribed regimen, and involvement of the patient in treatment planning.

▶ TREATMENT

- A thorough mental status examination (MSE), physical and neurologic examination, a complete family and social history, and laboratory workup (complete blood count, electrolytes, hepatic function, renal function, cardiac function, thyroid function, and urine drug screen) must be performed prior to treatment.

GENERAL THERAPEUTIC PRINCIPLES

- All typical APs are equal in efficacy in groups of patients when used in equipotent doses. High-potency drugs (e.g., **haloperidol [HPD]**) are as effective in treating acute agitation as low-potency, highly sedating APs (e.g., **chlorpromazine [CPZ]**).

- Selection of medication should be based on the need to avoid certain side effects and in view of concurrent medical or psychiatric disorders. Patient or family history of response is also helpful in the selection of an AP.
- Traditional dosage equivalents (expressed as CPZ-equivalent dosages—the equipotent dosage of any AP compared with 100 mg of CPZ) may assist in determining the range of effective dosage when switching from a typical AP to another typical AP drug (Table 70–1).

TABLE 70–1. Available Antipsychotics: Doses and Dosage Forms

Generic Name	Trade Name	Traditional Equivalent Dose (mg)[a]	Usual Dosage Range (mg/d)	Manufacturer's Maximum Dose (mg/d)	Dosage Forms[b]
Typical (Traditional) Antipsychotics					
Chlorpromazine	Thorazine	100	100–800	2000	T,L,LC,I,C-ER,S
Fluphenazine	Prolixin, Permitil	2	2–20	40	T,L,LC,I
Haloperidol	Haldol	2	2–20	100	T,LC,I
Loxapine	Loxitane	10	10–80	250	C,LC,I
Molindone	Moban	10	10–100	225	T,LC
Mesoridazine	Serentil	50	50–400	500	T,LC,I
Perphenazine	Trilafon	10	10–64	64	T,LC,I
Thioridazine	Mellaril	100	100–800	800	T,LC
Thiothixene	Navane	4	4–40	60	C,LC,I
Trifluoperazine	Stelazine	5	5–40	80	T,LC,I
Atypical Antipsychotics					
Clozapine	Clozaril	NA	50–500	900	T
Olanzapine	Zyprexa	NA	10–20	20	T
Quetiapine	Seroquel	NA	250–500	800	T
Risperidone	Risperdal	NA	2–8	16	T
Sertindole	Serlect	NA	4–20	N	N
Ziprasidone	Zeldox	NA	40–160	N	N

[a]NA, this parameter does not apply to atypical antipsychotics.

[b]T, tablet; C, capsule; ER, extended release; I, injection; L, liquid solution, elixir, or suspension; LC, liquid concentrate; R, rectal suppositories; N, not appproved by FDA..

- **Olanzapine (OLZ), quetiapine,** and **risperidone (RSP)** have become the agents of first choice in the treatment of schizophrenia.
- Atypical APs have little or no acutely occurring extrapyramidal side effects (EPS). Other attributes variously ascribed include enhanced efficacy for negative symptoms, absence of tardive dyskinesia (TD), and lack of effect on serum prolactin (PRL).
- Predictors of good response include a prior good response to the drug selected, absence of alcohol or drug abuse, acute onset and short duration of illness, presence of acute stressors or precipitating factors, later age of onset, affective symptoms, family history of affective illness, compliance with the prescribed regimen, and good premorbid adjustment.
- A suggested pharmacotherapeutic algorithm is outlined in Figure 70–1.

MECHANISMS OF ACTION

- Typical APs are putative DAergic antagonists, with an affinity for D_2 receptors that is greater than for D_1 receptors. The D_2 receptor is associated with typical AP efficacy and is the main receptor involved in the pathogenesis of EPS. D_1 receptors may have a modulating effect for EPS. Some D_1 as well as D_2 blockade may be necessary to produce EPS.
- The primary therapeutic effects of typical APs are thought to occur in the limbic system, including the ventral striatum, whereas EPS are thought to be related to DA blockade in the dorsal striatum.
- Typical APs, especially the low-potency APs (e.g., CPZ and **thioridazine [TRD]**), also block muscarinic, α_1-adrenergic, and histaminic receptors resulting in a variety of side effects including dry mouth, constipation, sinus tachycardia, and orthostatic hypotension.
- The mechanism of action of the atypical APs may be relative D_1, D_4, or D_5 specificity; relative selectivity for limbic DAergic receptors; 5-HT_2, 5-HT_6, and 5-HT_7 antagonism; or α_1-adrenergic antagonism. Some believe that the ratio between 5-HT_2 and D_2 blockade is important in producing an atypical profile.

PHARMACOKINETICS

- Pharmacokinetic parameters are summarized in Table 70–2.
- APs are highly lipophilic and highly bound to membranes and plasma proteins.
- They have large volumes of distribution and are largely metabolized through the cytochrome P450 pathways (**clozapine [CLZ],** 1A2 and to a lesser extent 2D6 and 3A4; RSP, 2D6; OLZ, 1A2 and 2D6; **quetiapine,** 3A4; **ziprasidone,** 3A4).
- They have fairly long elimination half-lives, most in the range of 20–40 hours. After dosage stabilization, most APs can be dosed once daily. Exceptions are quetiapine and ziprasidone, which have short half-lives.
- For HPD, the approximate therapeutic Cp range is 3–15 ng/mL, and at a daily dose of 10 mg, about 50% of patients will be within this range.

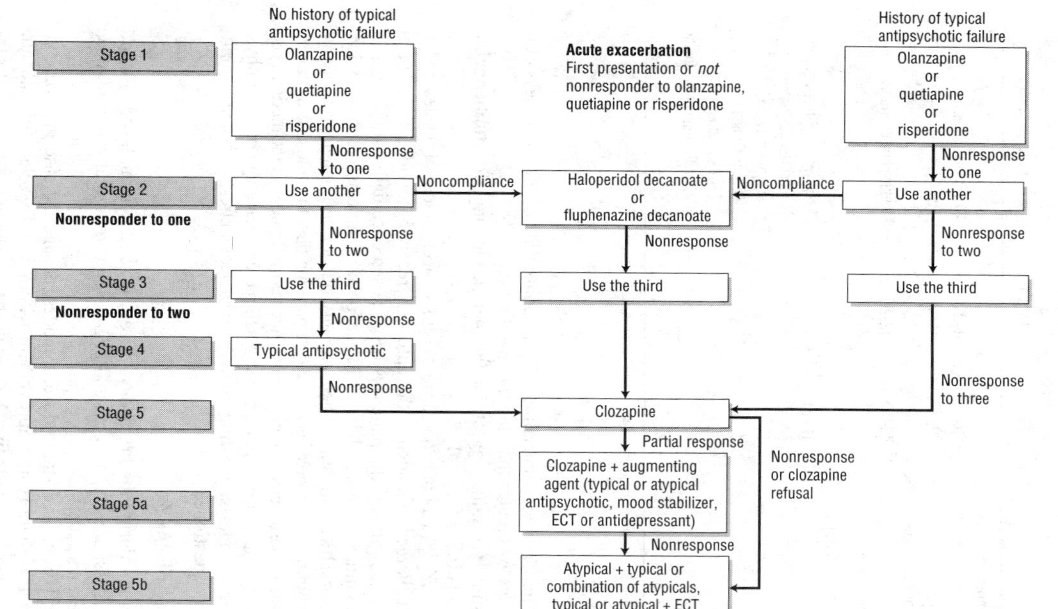

Figure 70–1. Suggested pharmacotherapeutic algorithm for schizophrenia. For updates of algorithm, see the Texas Medication Algorithm Project website at www.mhmr.state.tx.us/meds/tmap.htm.

XIII

TABLE 70–2. Pharmacokinetic Parameters of Selected Antipsychotics

Drug	Bioavailability (%)	Half-life (h)	Active Metabolites
Typical Antipsychotics			
Chlorpromazine	10–30	8–35	7-hydroxy, others
Fluphenazine	20–50	14–24	
Fluphenazine decanoate	—	14.2 ± 2.2[a] d	—
Haloperidol	40–70	12–36	Reduced haloperidol
Haloperidol decanoate	—	21 d	—
Atypical Antipsychotics			
Clozapine	12–81	11–105	None with significant activity
Olanzapine	80	20–70	N-glucuronide; 2-OH-methyl; 4-N-oxide
Quetiapine	9 ± 4	6.88	7-OH-quetiapine
Risperidone	68	3–24	9-OH-risperidone
Sertindole	74	24–200	None with significant activity
Ziprasidone	59	4–10	None

[a]Based on multiple-dose data. Single-dose data indicate half-life of 6–10 days.

HPD may possess a curvilinear Cp response relationship, with less efficacy at Cps greater than the therapeutic range.

- Preliminary results suggest that the therapeutic range for **fluphenazine (FPZ)** is 0.5–3.0 ng/mL
- For CLZ, a 12-hour postdose serum concentration of at least 250 ng/mL is recommended if the patient is receiving divided doses or at least 350 ng/mL if the patient is being dosed once daily.
- Cp monitoring should be considered only in patients receiving CLZ, FPZ, or HPD and only when patients do not respond to reasonable doses within a 6-week period, when patients develop unusual or severe adverse experiences, when patients are taking concomitant medications that may cause drug interactions, when patients have age or pathophysiologic changes suggesting altered pharmacokinetics, or when compliance is questioned.

INITIAL THERAPY

XIII

- The goals during the first 7 days are decreased agitation, hostility, combativeness, anxiety, tension, and aggression and normalization of sleep and eating patterns.
- After 1 week at a stable dose, a modest dosage increase may be considered. If there is no improvement within 3 to 4 weeks at therapeutic doses, then an alternative AP should be considered (i.e., move to the next treatment stage in the algorithm; Figure 70–1).
- Fixed-dose studies of low versus high daily doses do not reveal any differences in time to AP response or length of hospitalization.

- Rapid neuroleptization is the administration of repeated doses of a high-potency AP (e.g., HPD 5 mg IM) every 30–60 minutes over a period of less than 24 hours. The goal is to obtain a rapid calming effect (not sedation) in severely agitated patients.
- Intramuscular administration of **lorazepam** is equivalent to intramuscular APs in the management of acute agitation or aggression.

STABILIZATION THERAPY

- During weeks 2 and 3, the goals should be to increase socialization and improve self-care habits and mood. Improvement in formal thought disorder may take an additional 6–8 weeks.
- Most patients require a dose of 500–800 mg of CPZ equivalents daily or atypical antipsychotics in usual labeled doses. Dose titration may continue every 1–2 weeks, and most patients can be switched to once-daily dosing.
- If symptom improvement is not satisfactory after 6–12 weeks, a different strategy (per algorithm) should be tried.

MAINTENANCE THERAPY

- Medication should be continued for at least 12 months after remission of the first psychotic episode. Patients who have had multiple acute psychotic episodes and who respond well to medication should be treated for at least 5 years. Then low-dose strategies or complete drug withdrawal may be attempted.
- APs (especially CLZ) should be tapered slowly before discontinuation to avoid rebound cholinergic withdrawal symptoms.
- In general, when switching from one AP to another, the first should be tapered and discontinued over 1–2 weeks after the second AP is initiated.

Depot Antipsychotic Medications

- The principles for conversion from oral APs to depot formulations are as follows:
  - Stabilization on an oral dosage form of the same agent (or at least a short trial of 3–7 days to be sure the medication is tolerated adequately) is recommended.
  - For **FPZ decanoate,** the simplest conversion is the Stimmel method, which uses 1.2 times the oral daily dose for stabilized patients, rounding up to the nearest 12.5-mg interval, administered in weekly doses for the first 4–6 weeks (1.6 times the oral daily dose for patients who are more acutely ill). Subsequently, FPZ decanoate may be administered once every 2–3 weeks. Oral FPZ may be overlapped for 1 week. XIII
  - For **HPD decanoate,** a factor of 10–15 times the oral daily dose is commonly recommended, rounding up to the nearest 50-mg interval, administered in a once-monthly dose with oral HPD overlap for the first month.

- Depot APs should be administered by a deep, "Z-tract" intramuscular method.

MANAGEMENT OF THE REFRACTORY PATIENT

- Only CLZ has shown superiority in randomized clinical trials for the management of treatment-resistant schizophrenia.
- Symptomatic improvement with CLZ often occurs slowly, and as many as 60% of patients may improve if CLZ is used for up to 6 months.
- Because of the risk of orthostatic hypotension, CLZ is usually titrated more slowly than other APs. If a 12.5-mg test dose does not produce hypotension, then CLZ 25 mg at bedtime is recommended, increased to 25 mg twice daily after 3 days, and then increased in 25–50-mg/d increments every 3 days until a dose of at least 300 mg/d is reached. A CLZ serum concentration is recommended before exceeding 600 mg/d.
- Augmentation therapy involves the addition of a non-AP drug to an AP in a poorly responsive patient, while combination treatment involves using two APs simultaneously.
- Augmentation should be used only in inadequately responding patients. Responders usually improve rapidly. If there is no improvement, the augmenting agent should be discontinued.
- Mood stabilizers (e.g., **lithium, valproic acid,** and **carbamazepine**) used as augmentation agents may improve labile affect and agitated behavior. Lithium is the best studied.
- Selective 5-HT reuptake inhibitors (SSRIs) have been used for augmentation with mixed results, and **propranolol** has been used for anti-aggressive effects. If propranolol is used, a 20-mg test dose should be given to assess tolerability. If well tolerated, it can be initiated at 20 mg three times daily. Increments can then be 60 mg/d every 3 days. Six to 8 weeks may be needed to evaluate response.
- Combining a typical AP with an atypical AP and combining different atypicals have been suggested, but no empirical data exist to support or refute these strategies. If there is no improvement within 6–12 weeks, one of the drugs should be tapered and discontinued.

ANTIPSYCHOTIC ADVERSE EFFECTS

- Table 70–3 presents the relative incidence of common categories of AP side effects.

Autonomic Nervous System

- Anticholinergic (ACh) side effects include impaired memory, dry mouth, constipation, tachycardia, blurred vision, inhibition of ejaculation, and urinary retention. Elderly patients are especially sensitive to these side effects.
  - Dry mouth can be managed with increased intake of fluids, oral lubricants **(Xerolube),** ice chips, or use of sugarless chewing gum or hard candy.

TABLE 70–3. Relative Side Effects Incidence of Commonly Used Antipsychotics

	Sedation	EPS	Anticholinergic	Orthostasis
Chlorpromazine	++++	+++	+++	++++
Clozapine	+++++	+	+++++	++++
Fluphenazine	++	+++++	++	++
Haloperidol	+	+++++	+	+
Loxapine	+++	++++	++	+++
Molindone	+	+++	++	++
Olanzapine	++	++	+++	++
Perphenazine	++	++++	++	++
Quetiapine	+++	++	—	++
Risperidone	+	++	+	++
Sertindole	++	+	—	++
Thioridazine	++++	++	++++	++++
Trifluoperazine	++	++++	++	++
Thiothixene	++	++++	++	++
Ziprasidone	++	++	+	++

+, Very low; ++, low; +++, moderate; ++++, high; +++++, very high.

- Constipation can be treated with increases in fluid and dietary fiber intake, and also with exercise.

Central Nervous System

Extrapyramidal System

DYSTONIA

- Dystonias are prolonged tonic contractions, with rapid onset (usually within 24–96 hours of dosage administration or dosage increase); they may be life threatening, as in the case of pharyngeal–laryngeal dystonias.
- Dystonias are rare with atypical APs, with the exception of reports of dystonia associated with overlapping during a switch from CLZ to RSP.
- Treatment includes intramuscular or intravenous AChs (Table 70–4) or benzodiazepines. **Benztropine mesylate** 2 mg or **diphenhydramine** 50 mg may be given intramuscularly or intravenously, or **diazepam** 5–10 mg slow intravenous push or **lorazepam** 1–2 mg intramuscularly may be given. Relief usually occurs within 15–20 minutes of intramuscular injection or within 5 minutes of intravenous administration. The XIII dose should be repeated if no response in seen within 15 minutes of intravenous injection or 30 minutes of intramuscular injection.
- Prophylactic ACh medications are reasonable when using high-potency typical APs (e.g., HPD, FPZ), in young men, and in patients with a history of dystonia. The AChs, not **amantadine,** should be used for prophylaxis.

TABLE 70–4. Agents Used To Treat EPS

Generic Name	Equivalent Dose (mg)	Dosage Range (mg/d)
Antimuscarinics		
Benztropine[a]	1	1–8[b]
Biperiden[a]	2	2–8
Orphenadrine	50	50–250
Procyclidine	2	7.5–20
Trihexyphenidyl	2	2–15
Anithistaminic		
Diphenhydramine[a]	50	50–400
Dopamine agonist		
Amantadine	N/A	100–400
Benzodiazepines		
Lorazepam[a]	N/A	1–8
Diazepam	N/A	2–20
Clonazepam	N/A	2–8
β Blockers		
Propranolol	N/A	20–160

[a]Injectable dosage form can be given intramuscularly for relief of acute dystonia.
[b]Dosage may be titrated to 12 mg with care; nonlinear pharmacokinetics have been demonstrated.

AKATHISIA

- Diagnosis is made by combining subjective complaints (feelings of inner restlessness) with objective symptoms (pacing, shuffling, or tapping feet).
- Treatment with AChs is disappointing, and reduction in AP dose may be the best intervention. Another alternative is to switch to a low-potency agent or atypical AP. However, akathisia has been reported with RSP and OLZ.
- Diazepam (5 mg three times daily) is commonly used, but some researchers have failed to show efficacy.
- Propranolol (up to 160 mg/d), **nadolol** (up to 80 mg/d), and **metoprolol** (100 mg/d or less) were reported to be effective.

PSEUDOPARKINSONISM

- Symptoms are (1) akinesia, bradykinesia, or decreased motor activity, including mask-like facial expression, micrographia, slower speech, and decreased arm swing; (2) tremor (predominantly at rest and decreasing with movement); (3) rigidity, which may present as stiffness. Cogwheel rigidity is seen as the patient's limbs yield in jerky, rachet-like fashion when moved passively by the examiner; and (4) stooped, unstable posture and slow, shuffling, or festinating gait.
- Accessory symptoms include seborrhea, sialorrhea, hyperhidrosis, fatigue, dysphagia, and dysarthria. A variant is rabbit syndrome, a perioral tremor.

- The onset of symptoms is usually 1–2 weeks after initiation of AP therapy or dose increase.
- **Benztropine** has a longer half-life, which allows once- to twice-daily dosing. Dose increases above 6 mg/d must be slow, because of nonlinear pharmacokinetics. **Trihexyphenidyl,** diphenhydramine, and **biperiden** usually require three-times-daily dosing.
- **Amantadine** is as efficacious as AChs but has less effect on memory.
- An attempt should be made to taper and discontinue these agents 6 weeks to 3 months after symptoms resolve.

TARDIVE DYSKINESIA

- TD is sometimes irreversible and is characterized by abnormal involuntary movements (AIMs) occurring with chronic AP therapy.
- The classic presentation is buccolingual-masticatory (BLM) movements. Symptoms may become severe enough to interfere with chewing, speech, respiration, or swallowing. Facial movements include frequent blinking, brow arching, grimacing, upward deviation of the eyes, and lip smacking. Involvement of the extremities occurs in later stages (restless choreiform and athetotic movements of limbs). The final area of involvement is truncal movements. Movements may worsen with stress and decrease with sedation.
- The Abnormal Involuntary Movement Scale (AIMS) and the Dyskinesia Identification System: Condensed User Scale (DISCUS) can be used to screen, but neither are diagnostic.
- Dosage reduction may have significant effect on outcome, with a complete disappearance of symptoms in some patients.
- Prevention of TD is best accomplished by: (1) using APs only when there is a clear indication and at the lowest effective dose for the shortest duration possible; (2) using atypical APs as first-line agents; (3) using the DISCUS or other scales to assess for early signs of TD, at least quarterly; (4) discontinuing APs or switching to an atypical AP at the earliest symptoms of TD, if possible; and (5) using APs only short term to abort aggressive behavior in nonpsychotic patients.
- **α-Tocopherol (vitamin E),** 1200–1600 IU, may reduce movements in patients with early TD.
- To date, there are no reports of TD with CLZ monotherapy, and it decreased AIMs by ≥50% in trials lasting 22–52 weeks.

Sedation

- Administration of most or all of the daily dose at bedtime can decrease daytime sedation and may eliminate the need for hypnotics.

Seizures

- There is an increased risk of drug-induced seizures in all patients treated with APs. The highest risk for AP-induced seizures is with the use of CPZ or CLZ, followed by **trifluoperazine** and **perphenazine.** Seizures are more likely with initiation of treatment and with the use of higher doses and rapid dose increases.

- When an isolated seizure occurs, a dosage decrease is first recommended, and anticonvulsant therapy is usually not recommended.
- If a change in AP therapy is required, atypical APs (other than CLZ), **molindone,** TRD, HPD, and FPZ are recommended.

Thermoregulation

- Hyperpyrexia can lead to heat stroke. Hypothermia is also a risk, particularly in elderly patients. These problems are more common with the use of low-potency APs and may also occur with CLZ and OLZ.

Neuroleptic Malignant Syndrome (NMS)

- Neuroleptic malignant syndrome (NMS) occurs in 0.5–1% of patients receiving APs. It may be more frequent in patients receiving high-potency, injectable, or depot APs and in patients who are dehydrated or have organic mental disorders. It may also occur with atypical APs including CLZ.
- Symptoms develop rapidly over 24–72 hours and include body temperature exceeding 38°C, altered level of consciousness, autonomic dysfunction (tachycardia, labile blood pressure, diaphoresis, tachypnea, urinary or fecal incontinence), and rigidity.
- Laboratory evaluation frequently shows leukocytosis, increases in creatine kinase (CK), aspartate aminotransferase (AST), alanine aminotransferase (ALT), lactate dehydrogenase (LDH), and myoglobinuria.
- Treatment should begin with AP discontinuation and supportive care.
- **Bromocriptine,** used in theory to reverse DA blockade, reduces rigidity, fever, or CK in up to 94% of patients. **Amantadine** has been used successfully in up to 63% of patients. **Dantrolene** has been used as a skeletal muscle relaxant, with effects on temperature, respiratory rate, and CK in up to 81% of patients.
- Rechallenge with the lowest effective AP dose may be considered only for those patients in greatest need of reinstitution of APs following observation for at least 2 weeks without APs.

Psychiatric Side Effects

- Akathisia has resulted in impulsivity, violence, and suicide. Akinesia results in symptoms of apathy and withdrawal. Delirium and psychosis are reported with large doses of APs or combinations of AChs with APs. APs can cause confusion and disorientation in the elderly.
- Exacerbation of and new-onset obsessive–compulsive symptoms have been reported with CLZ.

Endocrine System

- Galactorrhea and menstrual irregularities are common. These effects may be dose related and are more common with the use of high-potency APs.
- Possible management strategies for galactorrhea include switching to an atypical AP, adding bromocriptine in doses up to 15 mg daily, or adding amantadine in doses up to 300 mg daily.

- Weight gain is frequent with AP therapy including OLZ and CLZ.
- APs may affect glucose levels.

Cardiovascular System

- Incidence of orthostatic hypotension (defined as a >20-mm Hg drop in systolic pressure) is greatest with low-potency APs and CLZ, especially with intramuscular or intravenous administration.
  - Tolerance to this effect usually occurs within 2–3 months. Reducing the dose or changing to a high-potency AP may also help.
  - For severe hypotensive episodes, volume expansion through the use of intravenous fluids should be attempted before the use of pressor agents.
  - Pure α-adrenergic pressor agents (e.g., **phenylephrine, metaraminol**) or **norepinephrine,** which has β_1-adrenergic properties, can be used. **Epinephrine,** with α- and β-adrenergic effects, should not be used, and **isoproterenol** should also be avoided.
- Electrocardiogram (ECG) changes
  - APs have direct myocardial depression and quinidine-like effects on cardiac conduction, and they also antagonize sympathetic nervous system activity in the hypothalamus and stabilize cardiac tissue through local anesthetic properties. Low-potency agents, such as TRD and CLZ, are more likely to have cardiac effects.
  - ECG changes include increased heart rate, flattened T waves, ST-segment depression, prolongation of QT and PR intervals, and torsades de pointes.
  - In patients older than 40 years, a pretreatment ECG is recommended.

Ophthalmic

- Impairment in visual accommodation results from paresis of ciliary muscles. Photophobia may also result. If severe, **pilocarpine** ophthalmic solution may be necessary.
- Exacerbation of narrow-angle glaucoma can occur.
- Opaque deposits in the cornea and lens may occur with chronic **phenothiazine** treatment, especially with CPZ. Although visual acuity is not usually affected, periodic slit-lamp examinations are recommended in patients receiving phenothiazines long term. Baseline and periodic slit-lamp examinations are also recommended for quetiapine-treated patients due to lenticular changes in animal studies.
- Retinitis pigmentosis can result from use of TRD doses greater than 800 mg daily (the recommended maximum dose) and can result in permanent visual impairment or blindness.

Hepatic System

- Liver function test (LFT) abnormalities are common. If aminotransferases are greater than three times the upper limit of normal, the AP should be changed to a chemically unrelated AP.
- Cholestatic hepatocanalicular jaundice can occur in up to 2% of patients receiving phenothiazines, and the onset is usually within the first 2 weeks of therapy. Symptoms resolve within 2–8 weeks of discontinuation of the AP.

Genitourinary System

- Urinary hesitancy and retention is commonly reported, especially with low-potency APs, and men with benign prostatic hypertrophy are especially prone. Urinary incontinence is reported more frequently in older patients, especially women.
- Erectile dysfunction, considered an ACh effect, occurs in 25–60% of patients, most frequently with TRD.
- Anorgasmia and decreased libido in women have also been proposed to be ACh effects.
- α-Adrenergic blockade is proposed to be the mechanism behind priapism and retarded and retrograde ejaculation.
- Potential interventions include lowering AP dose, changing to a high-potency or atypical AP, or discontinuing ACh medications.

Hematologic System

- Transient leukopenia may occur with AP therapy, but it typically does not progress to clinically significant parameters.
- If the white blood cell (WBC) count is <3000/mm^3 or the absolute neutrophil count (ANC) is <1000/mm^3, the AP should be discontinued, and the WBC count monitored closely until it returns to normal.
- Agranulocytosis reportedly occurs in 0.01% of patients receiving typical APs, and of the typical APs, it may occur most frequently with CPZ and piperazine phenothiazines. The onset is usually within the first 8 weeks of therapy. It may initially manifest as a local infection (e.g., sore throat, leukoplakia, and erythema and ulcerations of the pharynx). These symptoms should trigger an immediate WBC count.
- The 18-month treatment risk of developing agranulocytosis with CLZ appears to be approximately 0.91%. Increasing age and female gender are associated with greater risk. The greatest risk appears to be between months 1 and 6 of treatment. WBC count monitoring is mandated in the product labeling. If the total WBC count drops to <2000/mm^3 or the ANC is <1000/mm^3, CLZ should be discontinued. **Filgrastim** has been used to decrease time to resolution and decrease intensive care bed costs. In cases of mild to moderate neutropenia (granulocytes between 2000–3000/mm^3 or ANC between 1000–1500/mm^3), which occurs in up to 2% of patients, CLZ should be discontinued with daily monitoring of complete blood counts until values return to normal.

Dermatologic System

- Allergic reactions are rare and usually occur within 8 weeks of initiating therapy, manifesting as maculopapular, erythematous, or pruritic rashes. Drug discontinuation and topical steroids are recommended.
- Contact dermatitis, including the oral mucosa, may occur. Swallowing of the oral concentrate quickly may decrease problems.
- Erythema and severe sunburns can occur. Patients should be educated to use maximal blocking sunscreens, hats, protective clothing, and sunglasses when in the sun.

- Blue-gray or purplish discoloration of skin exposed to sunlight may occur in patients receiving higher doses of low-potency phenothiazines (especially CPZ) long term.

Sudden Death Syndromes

- The cause of death may be ventricular arrhythmias, laryngeal–pharyngeal dystonia leading to aspiration and hypoxia, hyperpyrexia, NMS, seizures, and toxic megacolon.

USE IN PREGNANCY AND LACTATION

- Case reports implicating limb malformations are rare but should be considered in deciding whether to use APs during the first trimester of pregnancy. HPD and other high-potency agents appear to be the preferred APs, but there is a lack of published reports.
- Other potential, but largely unknown, risks of APs throughout pregnancy are behavioral teratogenicity, receptor changes, perinatal effects (e.g., tonicity, strength, sucking), EPS, jaundice, respiratory depression, and intestinal obstruction.
- APs appear in breast milk with milk-to-plasma ratios of 0.5 to 1.

DRUG INTERACTIONS

- Most AP drug interactions are relatively minor and often involve additive CNS or sedative effects.
- AP pharmacokinetics can be significantly affected by concomitantly administered enzyme inducers or inhibitors. Smoking is a potent inducer of hepatic enzymes and may increase AP clearance by as much as 50%. The published literature may be consulted for a listing of drug interactions.

PHARMACOECONOMIC CONSIDERATIONS

- In 1990 prices, the economic cost of schizophrenia in the United States was $38 billion with direct health care treatment costs accounting for 53% of the total.
- Studies have shown that CLZ use in treatment-resistant patients is associated with a decrease in total patient care costs of nearly $10,000 per patient annually.
- Retrospective studies have shown decreased hospitalization days in the year after RSP use with resulting decreased direct costs ranging from $4,000 to $6,000 annually.

▶ EVALUATION OF THERAPEUTIC OUTCOMES

- Clinicians should use standardized psychiatric rating scales to rate response objectively.

- The Brief Psychiatric Rating Scale (BPRS) is recognized as the primary instrument to determine AP efficacy in phase II and III trials. Other scales [e.g., Comprehensive Psychiatric Rating Scale (CPRS), Positive and Negative Syndrome Scale (PANSS)] are also used.

See Chapter 64, Schizophrenia, authored by M. Lynn Crismon, PharmD, FCCP, BCPP, and Peter G. Dorson, PharmD, BCPP, for a more detailed discussion of this topic.

Chapter 71

▶ SLEEP DISORDERS

▶ DEFINITION

Abnormalities in the normal physiology of sleep often cause patients to complain of three types of sleep problems: (1) insomnia; (2) excessive daytime sleepiness; and (3) sleep behaviors.

▶ NEUROCHEMISTRY AND SLEEP PHYSIOLOGY

- The reticular activating system (RAS) is responsible for maintaining wakefulness. Norepinephrine (NE) and acetylcholine in the cortex and histamine and neuropeptides (e.g., substance P, corticotropin-releasing factor) in the hypothalamus modulate neuronal activity during wakefulness.
- As the RAS decelerates, information transfer to the cortex ceases and serotonin (5-HT) neurotransmission in the raphe nuclei reduces sensory input to inhibit motor activity. NE is involved in dreaming, whereas 5-HT is active during nondreaming sleep.
- Polysomnography (PSG) is a procedure that measures multiple electrophysiologic parameters simultaneously during sleep, such as an electroencephalogram (EEG), electrooculogram (EOG), and electromyogram (EMG). Two EOGs, one EEG, and one EMG are the minimal recording used in scoring sleep stages.
- The two types of sleep are nonrapid eye movement (NREM) (stages 1 through 4) and rapid eye movement (REM). During NREM sleep, skeletal muscle tone and eye movements are low compared to wakefulness, and respiratory activity is slow and regular.
  - Stage 1 sleep represents a transition between wakefulness and sleep that lasts 0.5–7 minutes. The EEG reveals low-voltage (3–7 Hz), desynchronized activity.
  - Stage 2 sleep is characterized by a low-voltage EEG, frequent "sleep spindles" (10–16 Hz spindle-shaped waves), and "K-complexes" (high-voltage spikes).
  - Stage 3 and 4 are called delta sleep and consist of high-amplitude, slow waves. Most delta sleep occurs during the first half of the night.
- REM sleep is marked by the onset of a low-voltage, mixed frequency EEG and bursts of bilaterally conjugate REMs. During REM sleep, muscle tone is low, but autonomic functions (e.g., heart rate, perspiration, penile erection) are active.
- Within 90 minutes of falling asleep, the first REM period begins and lasts only 5–7 minutes. The cycle through all stages typically lasts 70–120 minutes and occurs 4–6 times during the night. REM periods lengthen progressively throughout the night.
- In elderly individuals, the sleep pattern is altered, with a considerable decrease in delta sleep, REM sleep, and total sleep time. Correspondingly,

there is an increase in the number of awakenings and total time spent awake at night. In elderly persons, the incidence of sleep pathology may be as high as 40%.

▶ CLASSIFICATION OF SLEEP DISORDERS

- The *Diagnostic and Statistical Manual of Mental Disorders,* 4th edition (DSM-IV) classifies sleep disorders into three categories:
  - Primary sleep disorders result from endogenous abnormalities in the sleep–wake timing or generating processes and are further classified as dyssomnias (abnormalities in the amount, timing, or quality of sleep) or parasomnias (abnormal behaviors associated with sleep, such as somnambulism, sleep terrors, and nightmares). Primary sleep disorders include primary insomnia, primary hypersomnia, narcolepsy, breathing-related sleep disorder, and circadian rhythm sleep disorder.
  - Sleep disorders that are related to another mental disorder.
  - Other sleep disorders include sleep disorders due to a medical condition and substance-induced sleep disorders.

▶ INSOMNIA

CLINICAL PRESENTATION

- Patients complain of difficulty falling asleep, maintaining sleep, or not feeling rested in spite of a sufficient opportunity to sleep.
- Transient (2–3 nights) and short-term (less than 3 weeks) insomnia are typical of individuals without a history of sleep problems. Long-term or chronic insomnia (exceeding 3 weeks) may be related to medical or psychiatric disorders, or may be psychophysiologic.

DIAGNOSIS

- Common identifiable causes of insomnia are situational (e.g., stress, jet lag, shift work), medical (e.g., cardiovascular, respiratory, pain, endocrine, gastrointestinal, neurologic), psychiatric (e.g., mood disorders, anxiety disorders, substance abuse), and medications (e.g., central adrenergic blockers, diuretics, selective 5-HT reuptake inhibitors, steroids, stimulants). Evaluation of the patient with transient insomnia should focus on possible acute stresses, environmental disruptions, and drug-related causes. In patients with chronic disturbances, a complete diagnostic evaluation should include physical and mental status examinations and routine laboratory tests, as well as medication and substance abuse histories to rule out medical and psychiatric etiologies.

TREATMENT

Nonpharmacologic Therapy

- Behavioral and educational interventions include cognitive therapy, relaxation therapy, stimulus control therapy, light therapy, sleep deprivation, and sleep hygiene education. Stimulus control procedures include establishing a regular time to wake up and go to sleep, sleeping only as much as necessary to feel rested, avoiding long periods of wakefulness in bed, avoiding trying to force sleep, and avoiding daytime naps. Sleep hygiene recommendations include regular exercise (not close to bedtime); creating a comfortable sleep environment; discontinuing or reducing the use of alcohol, caffeine, and nicotine; avoiding excessive fullness or hunger at bedtime; and avoiding drinking large quantities of liquids in the evening.

- Individuals with insomnia should avoid all products containing caffeine and chocolate for at least 8 hours before bedtime. Alcoholics frequently have insomnia for months to years after cessation of drinking.

Hypnotic Agents

Nonbenzodiazepine Hypnotic Agents

- For safety reasons, the barbiturates have few indications for use as hypnotics.
- **Chloral hydrate** (500–2000 mg) offers no clinical advantage and may be complicated by gastrointestinal irritation, drug interactions, and fatalities in overdose. It also interacts with other sedatives.
- The antidepressants (e.g., **amitriptyline, doxepin, trazodone**) are alternatives for patients who should not receive benzodiazepines (BZs). Trazodone 50–100 mg is an effective hypnotic in patients with antidepressant-induced insomnia.
- Antihistamines (e.g., **diphenhydramine,** 25–100 mg; **doxylamine** 25–100 mg) are less effective than the BZs, and their use may be complicated by anticholinergic side effects.
- **Zolpidem,** an imidazolpyridine chemically unrelated to BZs or barbiturates, acts selectively at the BZ_1 receptor and has minimal anxiolytic and no muscle relaxant or anticonvulsant effects. It is comparable in effectiveness to BZ hypnotics, reducing latency to sleep, and increasing total sleep time and efficiency. It has little effect on sleep stages. Its half-life is approximately 2.5 hours, it is metabolized to inactive metabolites, and its duration of effect is 6–8 hours. Common side effects are drowsiness, amnesia, dizziness, headache, and gastrointestinal complaints. Zolpidem is not associated with tolerance or rebound insomnia after 35 days of use, and it may have no significant effects on next-day psychomotor performance. The usual dose is 10 mg, which can be increased up to 20 mg nightly. In elderly patients and those with hepatic impairment, the dose is 5 mg nightly.
- **Melatonin,** available without a prescription, may be useful in neurologically devastated children and the elderly and in individuals experiencing jet lag. Manufacturing and purity concerns are an issue, as it is not regulated by the FDA. XIII

Benzodiazepine Hypnotics

- In the United States, five BZs are marketed with a therapeutic indication for insomnia (Table 71–1). BZs decrease the duration of stages 1 and 4 sleep and increase stage 2 sleep.

TABLE 71–1. Pharmacokinetics of Benzodiazepine Hypnotic Agents

Generic Name	t_{max} (h)[a]	Parent $t_{1/2}$ (h)	Daily Dose Range (mg)	Metabolic Pathway	Clinically Significant Metabolites
Estazolam	2	12–15	1–2	Oxidation	—
Flurazepam	1	8	15–30	Oxidation	Hydroxyethylflurazepam Flurazepam aldehyde
				N-dealkylation	*N*-DAF[b]
Quazepam	2	39	7.5–15	Oxidation *N*-dealkylation	2-Oxo-quazepam *N*-DAF[b]
Temazepam	1.5	10–15	15–30	Conjugation	—
Triazolam	1	2	0.125–0.25	Oxidation	—

[a]Time to peak plasma concentration.
[b]*N*-desalkylflurazepam, mean half-life ($t_{1/2}$) 47–100 hours.

BENZODIAZEPINE PHARMACOKINETICS

- The pharmacokinetic properties of BZ hypnotics are summarized in Table 71–1.
- **Flurazepam** and **triazolam** are rapidly absorbed. **Temazepam** is less lipophilic and has a slower onset of effect. **Estazolam** and **quazepam** are similar to flurazepam in onset of effect.
- The duration of effect of triazolam is short, whereas that of temazepam and estazolam is intermediate, and flurazepam and quazepam have a long duration of effect.
- Temazepam is eliminated via conjugation; the other four are metabolized by hepatic microsomal oxidation followed by glucuronidation.
- Drugs that inhibit cytochrome P450 IIIA4 (e.g., **erythromycin, nefazodone, fluvoxamine, ketaconazole**) reduce the clearance of triazolam and increase its plasma concentration.
- **Desalkylflurazepam (DAF)** accounts for most of the pharmacologic effects of flurazepam.
- DAF helps alleviate daytime anxiety or early morning awakening, but daytime drowsiness and impaired psychomotor performance may be a problem.

BENZODIAZEPINE ADVERSE EFFECTS

XIII
- **Tolerance** to the carryover central nervous system (CNS) effects (e.g., drowsiness, psychomotor incoordination, decreased concentration, cognitive deficits) may develop in some individuals.
- Anterograde amnesia occurs more frequently with triazolam than temazepam; however, flurazepam demonstrated more anterograde amnestic effects than triazolam in one study. Using the lowest dose possible minimizes amnestic effects.

- Triazolam is associated with a higher reported rate of confusion, bizarre behavior, agitation, and hallucinations than the other BZ hypnotics.
- Daytime anxiety and rebound insomnia are associated with the use of triazolam.
- Rebound insomnia can be minimized by utilizing the lowest effective dose and tapering the dose upon discontinuation.
- The rapidly eliminated BZs are associated with less daytime sedation and fewer performance deficits; however, they may increase the chance of daytime anxiety.
- There is an association between falls and hip fractures and the use of long-elimination half-life BZs; thus, use of flurazepam and quazepam should be avoided in elderly patients.

GENERAL THERAPEUTIC PRINCIPLES FOR USE OF BENZODIAZEPINE HYPNOTICS

- Hypnotic therapy is indicated in individuals with transient or short-term insomnia. If the stressor is expected to last more than 1 week, intermittent hypnotic use (three or four nights per week) should be prescribed for no more than 3 weeks.
- For chronic insomnia, if treatment of an underlying disorder fails to result in improvement, intermittent pharmacotherapy may be indicated.
- Tolerance and dependence can be avoided by using hypnotics at the lowest possible dose, intermittently, and for the shortest duration possible. Withdrawal symptoms can be diminished by gradually tapering the dosage.
- Patients with difficulty initiating sleep and those who require daytime alertness should receive the short-acting BZ hypnotics. Those with difficulty maintaining sleep or early morning awakening may benefit from intermediate-elimination half-life agents if daytime performance is required. Long half-life agents should be considered if management of daytime anxiety is required.
- BZs should not be given to persons with sleep apnea or a history of substance abuse or to pregnant individuals.
- Patients taking BZs should be instructed to avoid **alcohol,** as even alcohol on the day after ingestion of a long-elimination half-life BZ can result in additive CNS impairment.

► SLEEP APNEA

- Apnea is the cessation of airflow at the nose and mouth lasting at least 10 seconds. The goals of therapy are to reduce apneic episodes and improve O_2 saturation. XIII

OBSTRUCTIVE SLEEP APNEA

Clinical Presentation

- Obstructive sleep apnea (OSA) is potentially life-threatening and is characterized by repeated episodes of nocturnal breathing cessation with loud snoring and gasping. It is caused by an occlusion of the upper airway. Most individuals with OSA are overweight.

- The apneic episode is terminated by a reflex action to the fall in O_2 saturation that causes a brief arousal during which breathing resumes.
- OSA patients usually complain of excessive daytime sleepiness. Other symptoms are morning headache, poor memory, and irritability.

Treatment

- Patients with severe apnea (greater than 20 apneas/hour on PSG) and moderate apnea (5–20 apneas/hour on PSG) have shown significant improvement and reduction in mortality with treatment.
- Nonpharmacologic approaches are the treatment of choice (e.g., weight loss, tonsillectomy, nasal septal repair, nasal continuous positive airway pressure [CPAP], uvulopalatopharyngoplasty, upper airway resection).
- The most important pharmacologic interventions are avoidance of all CNS depressants. Other pharmacologic interventions should be reserved for patients with mild forms of OSA and in patients who have failed other treatments.
- **Protriptyline** 10–30 mg/d reduces the frequency of apneas and increases O_2 saturation.
- **Fluoxetine** 20 mg/d was effective in reducing apneas in some patients.

CENTRAL SLEEP APNEA

Clinical Presentation

- Central sleep apnea (CSA), less than 10% of all apneas, is characterized by repeated episodes of apnea caused by temporary loss of respiratory effort during sleep.
- Hypercapnic patients complain of morning headache and daytime sleepiness, while nonhypercapnic patients complain of insomnia and nocturnal awakenings with shortness of breath or gasping.

Treatment

- For hypercapnic patients, primary treatment is ventilatory support with O_2 and CPAP; **acetazolamide, theophylline,** and **medroxyprogesterone** have shown mixed results. In refractory cases, diaphragmatic pacing, tracheostomy, or positive pressure ventilation are helpful.
- In nonhypercapnic patients, treatment may consist of BZs (**triazolam** or **temazepam**) to reduce arousals and **acetazolamide,** CPAP, and O_2 to stabilize breathing patterns.

▶ NARCOLEPSY

CLINICAL PRESENTATION

- The essential feature is excessive daytime sleepiness with sleep attacks that may last up to 30 minutes. Other features are hypersomnia, fatigue, impaired performance, disturbed nighttime sleep, cataplexy, hypnagogic hallucinations, hypnopompic hallucinations, and sleep paralysis.

TREATMENT

- The goal of therapy is to maximize alertness during waking hours or at selected times. Cataplexy can be treated on an as-needed basis in some patients.
- Patients should be encouraged to have good sleep habits and take at least two naps during the day if possible.
- The psychostimulants (Table 71–2) can be used for excessive daytime sleepiness and antidepressants for cataplexy. **Amphetamines** and **methylphenidate** have a fast onset of effect and durations of 3–4 hours and 6–10 hours, respectively. Divided daily doses are recommended. Amphetamines are associated with more likelihood of abuse and tolerance.
- **Pemoline** has a delayed onset of effect, but its duration is 8–10 hours. Liver function must be monitored at 1 month, then yearly.
- The tricyclic antidepressants (TCAs) are effective in reducing cataplexy and sleep paralysis. **Imipramine, protriptyline,** and **nortriptyline** are effective in 80% of patients.

TABLE 71–2. Drugs Used to Treat Narcolepsy

Generic Name	Trade Name (Manufacturer)	Daily Dosage Range (mg)
Excessive Daytime Somnolence		
Dextroamphetamine	Dexedrine (SmithKline Beecham) Generics (various)	5–60
Dextroamphetamine/ amphetamine salts[a]	Adderall (Richwood)	5–60
Methamphetamine[b]	Desoxyn (Abbott)	5–15
Methylphenidate	Ritalin (Ciba) Generics (various)	30–80
Pemoline	Cylert (Abbott)	37.5–112.5
Adjunct Agents for Cataplexy		
Imipramine	Tofranil (Geigy) Generics (various)	50–250
Protriptyline	Vivactil (Merck) Generics (various)	5–30
Nortriptyline	Aventyl (Lilly) Pamelor (Sandoz) Generics (various)	50–200
Selegiline	Eldepryl (Somerset)	20–40
γ-Hydroxybutyrate	(Orphan Medical)	60 mg/kg/ night

[a]Dextroamphetamine sulfate, dextroamphetamine saccharate, amphetamine aspartate, and amphetamine sulfate.
[b]Not available in some states.

- **Selegiline** improves hypersomnolence and cataplexy.
- **Hydroxybutyrate** is a therapeutic option without anticholinergic side effects.

▶ EVALUATION OF THERAPEUTIC OUTCOMES

- An algorithm for management of dyssomnias is shown in Figure 71–1. Patients with short-term or chronic insomnia should be evaluated after 1 week of therapy to assess for drug effectiveness, adverse events, and compliance with nonpharmacologic recommendations. Patients should be instructed to maintain a sleep diary, including a daily recording of awakenings, medication ingestions, naps, and an index of sleep quality.
- Patients with sleep apnea should be evaluated after 2–4 weeks of treatment for improvement in alertness, daytime symptoms, and weight reduction. The bed partner can report on snoring and gasping.
- Monitoring parameters for pharmacotherapy of narcolepsy include reduction in daytime sleepiness, cataplexy, hypnagogic and hypnopompic hallucinations, and sleep paralysis. Patients should be evaluated monthly until an optimal dose is achieved, then every 6–12 months to assess for adverse drug events (e.g., mood changes, sleep disturbances, cardiovascular abnormalities). If symptoms increase during therapy, PSG should be performed.

See Chapter 69, Sleep Disorders, authored by Donna M. Jermain, PharmD, BCPP, for a more detailed discussion of this topic.

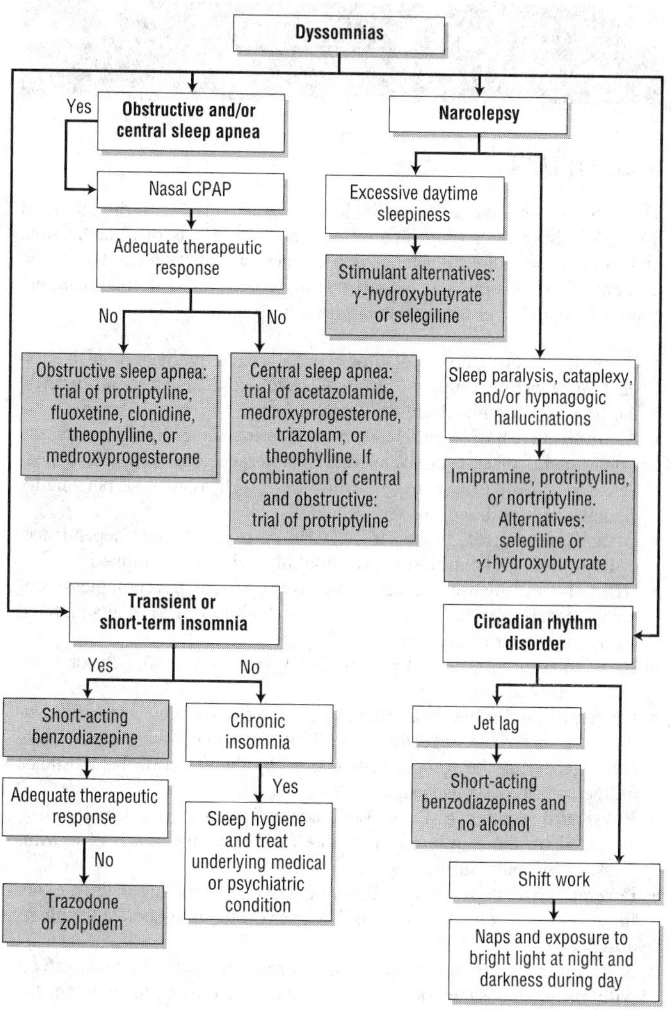

Figure 71–1. Algorithm for treatment of dyssomnias. *(Adapted and reprinted with permission from Jermain DM.* Sleep disorders. *In: Pharmacotherapy self-assessment program, 2nd ed. Kansas City, MO. American College of Clinical Pharmacy, 1995; 139–154.)* XIII

Chapter 72

▶ SUBSTANCE-RELATED DISORDERS

▶ DEFINITION

The substance-related disorders include disorders related to the taking of a drug of abuse (including **alcohol**), to the side effects of a medication, and to toxin exposure. Substance dependence or addiction can be viewed as a chronic illness that can be successfully controlled with treatment, but cannot be cured, and is associated with a high relapse rate.

- **Drug addiction:** Chronic disorder characterized by the compulsive use of a substance resulting in physical, psychological, or social harm to the user and continued use despite that harm.
- **Alcoholism:** Chronic, progressive, and potentially fatal biogenetic and psychosocial disease characterized by tolerance and physical dependence manifested by a loss of control, as well as diverse personality changes and social consequences.
- **Drug dependence:** Relates to physical or psychological dependence, or both. Impaired control over drug-taking behavior is implied.
- **Drug abuse:** Any use of drugs that causes physical, psychological, economic, legal, or social harm to the individual user or to others affected by the drug user's behavior.
- **Drug misuse:** Any use of a drug that varies from a socially or medically accepted use.
- **Intoxication:** Refers to the development of a substance-specific syndrome after recent ingestion, and it is associated with maladaptive behavior during the waking state caused by the effect of the substance on the central nervous system (CNS).
- **Physical dependence:** Physiologic adaptation to a drug, usually characterized by the development of tolerance and emergence of a withdrawal syndrome during abstinence.
- **Psychological dependence:** Emotional state of craving a drug either for its positive effect or to avoid negative effects associated with its absence.
- **Tolerance:** Physiologic adaptation to drugs, so as to diminish effects with constant dosages or to require increased dosage to maintain the intensity and duration of effects.

▶ PATHOPHYSIOLOGY

MECHANISMS OF TOLERANCE, DEPENDENCE, AND WITHDRAWAL

- Drugs disturb physiologic systems, and systems then adapt to reduce those effects. Such compensatory adaptation leads to development of tolerance. When the drug is withdrawn, the compensatory changes dominate, and withdrawal symptoms result.

- Withdrawal may be acute and last only a few days. With opiate and alcohol withdrawal, this may be followed by a protracted withdrawal syndrome lasting several months or longer and precipitated by environmental stimuli associated with drug use.
- There are two types of physiologic tolerance: (1) dispositional tolerance (metabolic or pharmacokinetic tolerance), which results from changes in pharmacokinetic handling; and (2) pharmacodynamic tolerance (cellular or functional tolerance), which results from adaption at the site of action.

Central Nervous System Depressants

- **Barbiturates:** The primary mechanism of barbiturate tolerance appears to be dispositional, as they induce their own metabolism.
- **Benzodiazepines (BZs):** Tolerance to BZs appear to be primarily pharmacodynamic, perhaps through a decrease in the number or sensitivity of BZ receptors.
- **Opiates:** Tolerance to opiates appears to be pharmacodynamic. Chronic use of exogenous opiates causes a decrease in production of enkephalin and a down-regulation of opiate receptors. Thus, larger doses are required to achieve the same degree of inhibition of noradrenergic activity. Opiate withdrawal can be conceptualized as a syndrome of noradrenergic hyperactivity.
- **Alcohol:** Alcohol disrupts neuronal membrane function and membrane-mounted proteins. It potentiates γ-aminobutyric acid type A ($GABA_A$) receptor function and inhibits the function of *N*-methyl-D-aspartate (NMDA) receptors. The principle mechanism of tolerance appears to be pharmacodynamic. Withdrawal appears to be mediated by sympathetic nervous system overactivity.

Central Nervous System Stimulants

- **Cocaine:** Tolerance to stimulants, including cocaine, is pharmacodynamic.
- **Phencyclidine (PCP):** Tolerance to PCP may be dispositional.

Marijuana

- Tolerance to **marijuana** appears to be more pharmacodynamic than dispositional.

▶ CLINICAL PRESENTATION, PATTERNS OF USE, AND DIAGNOSIS

- The *Diagnostic and Statistical Manual of Mental Disorders,* 4th Ed. (DSM-IV) categorizes substance-related disorders as substance use disorders and substance-induced disorders. Substance use disorders include dependence and abuse; substance-induced disorders include intoxication, withdrawal, dementia, psychosis, mood disorders, and anxiety.

- To meet the criteria for substance dependence, at least 3 of the following must be present at any time in a 12-month period: (1) tolerance; (2) withdrawal syndrome or use of a drug to relieve or avoid withdrawal; (3) the substance is taken in larger amounts or over a longer period of time than intended; (4) persistent desire or unsuccessful efforts to reduce or control substance use; (5) time is spent to obtain or use the substance or recover from its effects; (6) social, occupational, or recreational activities are given up because of substance use; and (7) substance use is continued despite knowledge of resultant problems.
- The essential feature of substance abuse is a maladaptive pattern of substance use with repeated adverse consequences related to repeated use.

▶ CENTRAL NERVOUS SYSTEM DEPRESSANTS

ALCOHOL

- Table 72–1 relates the effects of **alcohol** to the blood alcohol concentration (BAC). Table 72–2 lists signs and symptoms of alcohol intoxication and withdrawal.

TABLE 72–1. Specific Effects of Alcohol Related to the Blood Alcohol Concentration (BAC)

BAC (%)[a]	Effect
0.02–0.03	No loss of coordination, slight euphoria, and loss of shyness; depressant effects are not apparent.
0.04–0.06	Feeling of well-being, relaxation, lower inhibitions, sensation of warmth; euphoria; some minor impairment of reasoning and memory, lowering of caution.
0.07–0.09	Slight impairment of balance, speech, vision, reaction time, and hearing; euphoria; judgment and self-control are reduced, and caution, reason, and memory are impaired.
0.10–0.125	Significant impairment of motor coordination and loss of good judgment; speech may be slurred; balance, vision, reaction time, and hearing will be impaired; euphoria; it is illegal to operate a motor vehicle at this level of intoxication.
0.13–0.15	Gross motor impairment and lack of physical control; blurred vision and major loss of balance; euphoria is reduced and dysphoria is beginning to appear.
0.16–0.20	Dysphoria (anxiety, restlessness) predominates, nausea may appear; the drinker has the appearance of a sloppy drunk.
0.25	Needs assistance in walking; total mental confusion; dysphoria with nausea and some vomiting.
0.30	Loss of consciousness.
≥0.40	Onset of coma; possible death due to respiratory arrest.

[a]Grams of ethyl alcohol per 100 mL of whole blood.

TABLE 72–2. Signs and Symptoms of Alcohol Intoxication and Withdrawal

Intoxication	Withdrawal
Slurred speech	Tremor
Ataxia	Tachycardia
Nystagmus	Diaphoresis
Sedation	Labile blood pressure
Flushed face	Anxiety
Mood change	Nausea and vomiting
Irritability	Hallucinations
Euphoria	Seizures
Loquacity	Hyperthermia
Impaired attention	Delirium

- There are 14 grams of alcohol in 12 oz of beer, 4 oz of wine, or 1.5 oz of 80-proof whiskey. This amount will increase the BAC by about 25 mg/dL in a healthy 70-kg male. Deaths generally occur when BACs are >500 mg/dL.
- Absorption of alcohol begins in the stomach within 5–10 minutes of ingestion, but it is absorbed primarily from the duodenum. Peak concentrations are achieved 30–90 minutes after finishing the last drink.
- Alcohol is metabolized (by a zero-order process except at very high and very low concentrations) to acetaldehyde by alcohol dehydrogenase, which is metabolized to carbon dioxide and water by aldehyde dehydrogenase.
- In the post-absorptive phase in the nontolerant individual, the BAC is lowered from between 15 and 22 mg/dL/h.
- Forty percent to 50% of traffic fatalities are associated with alcohol intoxication (BAC >100 mg/dL). Only 2–3% of noninjured drivers have levels this high.
- Most clinical labs report BAC in mg/dL. In legal cases, results are reported in percent (grams of alcohol per 100 mL of whole blood). Thus, a BAC of 150 mg/dL = 0.15%.
- Alcohol withdrawal.
  - **Phase I:** Begins within hours of the last drink, lasts for 3–5 days, and XIII
    consists of tremor, tachycardia, diaphoresis, labile blood pressure, anxiety, nausea, and vomiting. Most patients do not progress beyond phase I even if untreated.
  - **Phase II:** Includes perceptual disturbances, most commonly auditory or visual.
  - **Phase III:** Includes seizures (usually tonic–clonic) lasting 30 seconds to 4 minutes and progressing to status epilepticus in about

3% of cases. Seizures occur in 10–15% of untreated withdrawal patients.
- **Phase IV (delirium tremens):** Occurs in <1% of patients. It manifests as acute autonomic hyperactivity and delirium including severe hyperthermia. The mortality rate for patients who progress to phase IV is 20%.

BENZODIAZEPINES AND OTHER SEDATIVE–HYPNOTICS

- BZs with faster onset (e.g., **diazepam**) tend to be preferred by the recreational drug user because they are reinforcing. BZs generally cause little respiratory depression.
- Withdrawal from short-acting BZs (e.g., **oxazepam, lorazepam alprazolam**) has an onset within 12–24 hours of the last dose; other sedatives (e.g., diazepam, **chlordiazepoxide, clorazepate, phenobarbital, amobarbital**) have elimination half-lives (or active metabolites with elimination half-lives) of 24 to greater than 100 hours. So, withdrawal may be delayed for several days after discontinuation.
- Dependence on sedative–hypnotics is summarized in Table 72–3.
- Likelihood and severity of withdrawal is a function of dose and duration of exposure. Gradual tapering of dosage is associated with less withdrawal and rebound anxiety than abrupt discontinuation.

FLUNITRAZEPAM

- **Flunitrazepam (Rohypnol)** is a BZ that is not approved for use in the United States. It is ingested orally, frequently with alcohol, **marijuana,** cocaine, or **heroin.** Onset of effects is within 30 minutes, and duration is for up to 8 hours or more. It is sometimes called the "date-rape drug," as it has been given to female party participants in hope of lowering inhibitions.
- Adverse effects include decreased blood pressure, memory impairment, drowsiness, visual disturbances, confusion, gastrointestinal (GI) disturbances, and urinary retention.
- Intoxication is manifested as slurred speech, poor coordination, and swaying.
- It causes dependence, and the withdrawal syndrome includes muscle pain, anxiety, restlessness, confusion, irritability, hallucinations, delirium, convulsions, and cardiovascular collapse. Withdrawal seizures can occur 1 week or more after cessation of use.

GAMMA HYDROXY BUTYRATE (GHB)

- **GHB** is a CNS depressant not approved for use in the United States. It is sold as a liquid or powder and is called "Georgia Home Boy," "Liquid Ecstasy," "Liquid X," "Liquid E," "GHB," "Soap," "Scoop," "Easy Lay," "Salty Water," "G-Riffick," "Cherry Menth," and "Organic Quaalude." It is another drug called a "date-rape drug."
- It increases dopamine levels in the brain and has effects through the endogenous opioid system. Effects include amnesia, hypotonia, abnormal

TABLE 72–3. Dependence on Sedative–Hypnotics[a]

Generic Name	Common Trade Names (Manufacturer)	Oral Sedating Dose (mg)	Physical Dependence Dose and Time Needed to Produce Dependence	Time Before Onset of Withdrawal (h)	Peak Withdrawal Symptoms (d)
Benzodiazepines					
Diazepam	Valium (Roche)	5–10	40–120 mg × 42–120 d	12–24	5–8
Chlordiazepoxide	Librium, Libritabs (Roche)	10–25	75–600 mg × 42–120 d	12–24	5–8
Clorazepate	Tranxene (Abbott)	7.5–15	45–180 mg × 42–120 d (est.)	12–24	5–8
Alprazolam	Xanax (Upjohn)	0.25–8	8–16 mg × 42 d (est.)	8–24	2–3
Flunitrazepam	Rohypnol (Roche)	1–2	8–10 mg × 42 d (est.)	24–36	2–3
Barbiturates					
Secobarbital	Seconal, Seco-8 (Lilly)	100	800–2200 mg × 35–37 d	6–12	2–3
Pentobarbital	Nembutal (Abbott)	100	800–2200 mg × 35–37 d	6–12	2–3
Equal parts of secobarbital and amobarbital	Tuinal (Lilly)	100	800–2200 mg × 35–37 d	6–12	2–3
Amobarbital	Amytal (Lilly)	65–100	800–2200 mg × 35–37 d	8–12	2–5
Nonbarbiturate Sedative–Hypnotics					
Ethchlorvynol	Placidyl (Abbott)	200	1–1.5 g × 30 d	6–12	2–3
Chloral hydrate	Noctec (various)	250	Exact dose unknown: 12 g/d chronically has led to delirium upon sudden withdrawal	6–12	2–3
Meprobamate	Equanil, Miltown, Meprotabs (various)	400	1.6–3.2 g × 270 d	8–12	3–8

[a]Withdrawal symptoms are tremor, tachycardia, diaphoresis, nausea, vomiting, blood pressure lability, delirium, seizures, and hallucinations.

TABLE 72–4. Signs and Symptoms of Opioid Intoxication and Withdrawal

Intoxication	Withdrawal
Euphoria	Lacrimination
Dysphoria	Rhinorrhea
Apathy	Mydriasis
Motor retardation	Piloerection
Sedation	Diaphoresis
Slurred speech	Diarrhea
Attention impairment	Yawning
Miosis	Fever
	Insomnia
	Muscle aching

sequence of rapid eye movements (REM) and non-REM sleep, and anesthesia.

- Manifestations of acute GHB toxicity include decreased cardiac output, respiratory depression, coma, seizures, and vomiting.

OPIATES

- **Hydromorphone** has become widely used among the opiate-using population. It has a profile similar to **heroin,** but with the advantage of purity.
- Opiates are commonly combined with stimulants (e.g., cocaine [speed-ball]) or alcohol.
- **Heroin** can be snorted, smoked, and given intravenously.
- Complications of heroin use include overdoses, anaphylactic reactions to impurities, nephrotic syndrome, septicemia, endocarditis, and acquired immunodeficiency syndrome (AIDS).
- Signs and symptoms of opioid intoxication and withdrawal are shown in Table 72–4. Onset of the acute phase of withdrawal ranges from a few hours after stopping heroin to 3–5 days after stopping **methadone.** Duration of withdrawal ranges from 3–24 days. Opioid withdrawal is not fatal unless there is a significant concurrent medical problem. Occurrence of delirium suggests withdrawal from another drug (e.g., alcohol).

▶ CENTRAL NERVOUS SYSTEM STIMULANTS

CAFFEINE

- **Caffeine** is rapidly and completely absorbed from the gastrointestinal tract, and reaches peak blood levels within 30–45 minutes of ingestion. The half-life of caffeine is 3.5–5 hours. It increases the heart rate and force of contraction and has a strong diuretic effect. Regular use is associated with tolerance.

- Signs and symptoms of excessive caffeine intake include restlessness, anxiety, insomnia, flushed face, diuresis, gastrointestinal disturbances, muscle twitching, rambling thought or speech, tachycardia, arrhythmia, increased energy, and psychomotor agitation.
- The caffeine withdrawal syndrome begins within 18–24 hours of discontinuation and includes headache; drowsiness; fatigue; and sometimes, impaired psychomotor performance; difficulty concentrating; nausea; excessive yawning; and craving. When caffeine is reintroduced, relief of withdrawal symptoms occurs within 30–60 minutes.

COCAINE

- **Cocaine** is perhaps the most behaviorally reinforcing of all drugs of abuse. Ten percent of people who begin to use the drug "recreationally" will go on to heavy use.
- It blocks reuptake of catecholamine neurotransmitters and causes a depletion of brain dopamine.
- Systemic effects include CNS stimulation, euphoria, decreased fatigue, and increased alertness.
- The hydrochloride salt is inhaled or injected. It can be converted to **cocaine base** (crack or rock) and smoked to achieve almost instant absorption and intense euphoria. Tolerance to the high develops quickly.
- In the presence of alcohol, cocaine is metabolized to cocaethylene, a longer acting compound than cocaine. The risk of death from cocaethylene is greater than from cocaine.
- The elimination half-life of cocaine is 1 hour, and the duration of effect is very short.
- Adverse events include ulceration of nasal mucosa and nasal septal collapse, tachycardia, heart failure, hyperthermia, shock, convulsions, psychosis (e.g., hallucinations, paranoid thinking, and looseness of associations), and sudden death due to arrhythmias (rare).
- Signs and symptoms of cocaine intoxication and withdrawal are shown in Table 72–5.
- Withdrawal is not life-threatening, and symptoms include fatigue, sleep disturbance, nightmares, and depression. Symptoms begin within hours of discontinuing the drug and last up to several days.

AMPHETAMINES AND OTHER STIMULANTS

- **Methamphetamine** (speed, meth, crank) can be taken orally, XIII intranasally, by intravenous injection, and by smoking. The **hydrochloride salt** (ice, crystal, glass) is a clear crystal that can be smoked.
- Systemic effects, including toxic effects and adverse events, are similar to those of cocaine. Inhalation or intravenous injection results in an intense rush that lasts a few minutes.
- Amphetamines increase release and block reuptake of catecholamines and blocks their degradation by monoamine oxidase.

TABLE 72–5. Signs and Symptoms of Cocaine Intoxication and Withdrawal

Intoxication	Withdrawal
Motor agitation	Fatigue
Elation/euphoria	Sleep disturbance
Grandiosity	Nightmares
Loquacity	Depression
Hypervigilance	Increased appetite
Tachycardia	
Mydriasis	
Elevated or lowered blood pressure	
Sweating or chills	
Nausea and vomiting	

▶ OTHER DRUGS OF ABUSE

NICOTINE

- More than 430,000 deaths annually, or 20% of the total deaths in the United States, are caused by smoking.
- **Nicotine** is a ganglionic cholinergic-receptor agonist with pharmacologic effects that are dose dependent. Effects include central and peripheral nervous system stimulation and depression, respiratory stimulation, skeletal muscle relaxation, catecholamine release by the adrenal medulla, peripheral vasoconstriction, and increased blood pressure, heart rate, cardiac output, and oxygen consumption. Low doses of nicotine produce increased alertness and improved cognitive functioning. At higher doses, nicotine stimulates the "reward" center in the limbic system.
- Chronic nicotine ingestion may lead to physical and psychological dependence, tolerance, and withdrawal symptoms including anxiety, craving for tobacco, decreased blood pressure and heart rate, depression, difficulty concentrating, drowsiness, irritability, restlessness, gastrointestinal disturbances, headache, hostility, increased appetite and weight gain, increased skin temperature, and insomnia. Withdrawal symptoms may begin within 24 hours and may last for days, weeks, or longer. Craving may last for years.

MARIJUANA

- **Marijuana** (reefer, pot, grass, weed) is the most commonly used illicit drug. The principal psychoactive component is **Δ^9-tetrahydrocannabinol (THC). Hashish,** the dried resin of the top of the plant, is more potent than the plant itself.

- Chronic exposure is not usually associated with a significant withdrawal syndrome on discontinuation, but many users exhibit compulsive drug-seeking behavior. However, sudden discontinuation by heavy users can cause a withdrawal syndrome.
- Physiologic effects include sedation, difficulty in performing complex tasks, and disinhibition. Endocrine effects include amenorrhea, decreased testosterone production, and inhibition of spermatogenesis. Signs and symptoms of marijuana intoxication are tachycardia, conjunctival congestion, increased appetite, dry mouth, euphoria, sensory intensification, apathy, and hallucinations.
- Chronic use is associated with all the risks of tobacco smoking.
- THC is detectable on toxicologic screening for up to 4–5 weeks in chronic users.
- Heredity plays a significant role in determining susceptibility to marijuana abuse.
- Smoking marijuana while shooting up cocaine may cause severe increases in heart rate and blood pressure.
- Long-term use of marijuana, like other major drugs of abuse, causes changes in the brain that may increase users' vulnerability to addiction to other abusable drugs.

DESIGNER DRUGS

- A designer drug is a chemical compound that is similar in structure and effect to another drug of abuse but differs slightly chemically.

Fentanyl Analogs

- Fentanyl analogs include **alpha-methylfentanyl** (China White) and **3-methylfentanyl** (TMF) (synthetic heroin, tango, cash, goodfella).
- They have a rapid onset and short duration of action (30–90 minutes) and are used for their euphoric effects. They cause respiratory depression and can cause sudden death.
- They can be smoked, snorted, and injected.

Meperidine Analogs

- Examples are **MPPP** (1-methyl-4-phenyl-4-propionoxypiperidine) and **PEPAP** (1-[2- phenylethyl]-4-acetyloxypiperidine. An impurity, **MPTP** (l-methyl-4-phenyl-1,2,3,6,-tetrahydro-pyridine), is a potent neurotoxin and has caused irreversible brain damage.

Methamphetamine Analogs

- The analogs of current concern include **MDA** (3,4-methylenedioxy-amphetamine) and **MDMA** (3,4-methylenedioxy-methamphetamine). XIII
- Physiologic effects of MDA are similar to those of amphetamine, and it produces a heightened need for interpersonal relationships.
- MDMA (ecstasy, Adam) stimulates the CNS and produces a mild hallucinogenic effect. It can cause muscle tension, nausea, faintness, chills, sweating, panic, anxiety, depression, hallucinations, and paranoid thinking. It increases heart rate and blood pressure and has been shown to destroy serotonin (5-HT)-producing neurons in animals.

PHENCYCLIDINE (PCP) AND KETAMINE

- **PCP** (angel dust, crystal) is often misrepresented as **lysergic acid diethylamide (LSD)** or THC.
- PCP is commonly smoked with marijuana but may also be taken orally or IV.
- PCP blocks the reuptake of 5-HT, norepinephrine (NE), and dopamine (DA); blocks activity of the NMDA receptor; and binds at an opiate receptor associated with psychotomimetic properties.
- Signs and symptoms of PCP intoxication include very unpredictable behavior, increased blood pressure, tachycardia, ataxia, slurred speech, euphoria, agitation, anxiety, hostility, and psychosis. Psychosis may last for weeks. At toxic doses, coma and seizures may occur.
- **Ketamine** (special K, jet, green), chemically related to PCP, is a veterinary anesthetic that can cause hallucinations, delirium, and vivid dreams.
- It is usually injected, but can be evaporated to crystals, powdered and smoked, snorted, or swallowed. Marijuana cigarettes can be soaked in ketamine solution.
- Side effects are increased blood pressure and heart rate, respiratory depression, apnea, muscular hypertonus, and dystonic reactions. In overdose, seizures, polyneuropathy, increased intracranial pressure, and respiratory and cardiac arrest may occur.

HALLUCINOGENS

- Signs and symptoms of hallucinogen intoxication are summarized in Table 72–6. There is not a withdrawal syndrome after discontinuation of hallucinogenic drugs.

TABLE 72–6. Signs and Symptoms of Hallucinogen Intoxication

Psychologic	Physical
Perceptual intensification	Mydriasis
Depersonalization	Tachycardia
Derealization	Diaphoresis
Illusions	Palpitations
Hallucinations	Blurred vision
Synesthesias	Tremor
	Incoordination
	Dizziness
	Weakness
	Drowsiness
	Paresthesias

- **LSD** and similar drugs stimulate presynaptic 5-HT_{1A} and 5-HT_{1B}, as well as postsynaptic 5-HT_2 receptors in brain.
- Signs and symptoms of LSD intoxication include intensified perceptions, depersonalization, derealization, hallucinations, mydriasis, tachycardia, diaphoresis, palpitations, blurred vision, tremor, incoordination, dizziness, drowsiness, and paresthesias. Flashbacks may occur within a few days or more than a year after LSD use.
- LSD is sold as tablets, capsules, and a liquid. It is also added to absorbent paper and divided into small decorated squares, each square being one dose.
- Physiologic effects of LSD include dilated pupils, higher body temperature, increased heart rate and blood pressure, sweating, loss of appetite, sleeplessness, dry mouth, and tremors. It is not considered addictive, but may produce tolerance.
- There is cross-tolerance among LSD, **psilocybin,** and **mescaline.**

INHALANTS

- Organic solvents inhaled by abusers include **gasoline, glue, aerosols, amyl nitrite, typewriter correction fluid,** and **nitrous oxide. Toluene** is a component of several solvents.
- Physiologic effects include CNS depression, headache, nausea, hallucinations, and delusions. With chronic use, the drugs are toxic to virtually all organ systems. Death may occur from arrhythmias or suffocation by plastic bags.

▶ DESIRED OUTCOME

- The goals of treatment are cessation of use of the drug and termination of associated drug-seeking behaviors. The goals of treatment of the withdrawal syndrome are prevention of progression of withdrawal to life-threatening severity, thus enabling the patient to be sufficiently comfortable and functional in order to participate in a treatment program. The ultimate goal of treatment is to allow the patient to return to normal social and occupational functioning.

▶ TREATMENT

INTOXICATION

- When possible, drug therapy should be avoided. However, drug therapy XIII
may be indicated if patients are agitated, combative, hallucinatory, or delusional (Table 72–7).
- Toxicology screens are useful and when they are desired, blood or urine should be collected immediately upon the patient's arrival.
- **Flumazenil** is not indicated in all cases of suspected BZ overdose, and it is specifically contraindicated in cases in which cyclic antidepressant involvement is known or suspected because of the risk of seizures. It

TABLE 72–7. Treatment of Substance Intoxication

Drug Class	Pharmacologic Therapy	Nonpharmacologic Therapy
Benzodiazepines	Flumazenil 0.1–0.2 mg/min IV up to 1 mg	Support vital functions
Alcohol, barbiturates, and sedative–hypnotics (nonbenzodiazepines)	None	Support vital functions
Opiates	Naloxone 0.4–2.0 mg IV every 3 min	Support vital functions
Cocaine and other CNS stimulants	Lorazepam 2–4 mg IM q 30 min to 6 h prn agitation Haloperidol 2–5 mg IM (or other antipsychotic agent) every 30 min to 6 h prn psychotic behavior	Monitor cardiac function
Hallucinogens, marijuana, and inhalants	Lorazepam and/or haloperidol as above	Reassurance; "talk-down therapy"; support vital functions
Phencyclidine	Lorazepam and/or haloperidol as above	Minimize sensory input

should be used with caution when BZ physical dependence is suspected, as it may precipitate BZ withdrawal.

- In opiate intoxication, **naloxone** may be used to revive unconscious patients with respiratory depression. However, it may also precipitate physical withdrawal in dependent patients.
- Cocaine intoxication is treated pharmacologically only if the patient is agitated and psychotic.
- Many patients with hallucinogen, marijuana, or inhalant intoxication respond to simple reassurance. When necessary, short-term antianxiety and/or antipsychotic therapy can be used.
- PCP intoxication is more unpredictable, and sensory input should be minimized; thus, "talk-down therapy" is not recommended. Antianxiety and/or antipsychotic drug therapy may be necessary.

WITHDRAWAL

- Treatment of withdrawal from some common drugs of abuse is summarized in Table 72–8.

Alcohol

- Most clinicians agree that the BZs are the drugs of choice in treatment of alcohol withdrawal.
- The long-acting drugs (e.g., **chlordiazepoxide, diazepam**) control withdrawal effectively with few rebound effects after discontinuation.

TABLE 72–8. Treatment of Withdrawal from Some Common Drugs of Abuse

Drug or Drug Class	Pharmacologic Therapy
Benzodiazepines	
Short- to-intermediate-acting	Chlordiazepoxide 50 mg tid–qid or lorazepam 2 mg tid–qid; taper over 5–7 d
Long-acting	Chlordiazepoxide 50 mg tid–qid or lorazepam 2 mg tid–qid; taper over additional 5–7 d
Barbiturates	Pentobarbital tolerance test (see text); initial detoxification at upper limit of tolerance test; decrease dosage by 100 mg every 2–3 d
Opiates	Methadone 20–80 mg PO daily; taper by 5–10 mg daily or clonidine 2 μg/kg tid × 7 d; taper over additional 3 d
Mixed-substance withdrawal	
Drugs are cross-tolerant	Detoxify according to treatment for longer acting drug used
Drugs are not cross-tolerant	Detoxify from one drug while maintaining second drug (cross-tolerant drugs), then detoxify from second drug
CNS stimulants	Supportive treatment only; pharmacotherapy often not used; bromocriptine 2.5 mg tid or higher may be used for severe craving associated with cocaine withdrawal

A dosage regimen for detoxification with chlordiazepoxide is 50 mg tid × 1 d, then 50 mg bid × 1 d, then 25 mg tid × 1 d, then 25 mg bid × 1 d, then 25 mg daily × 1 d, then discontinue.

- The short- to intermediate-acting BZs (e.g., **oxazepam, lorazepem**) are also used for alcohol detoxification. An example regimen is lorazepam, 2 mg tid × 2 d, then 2 mg bid × 2 d, then 2 mg daily × 1 d, then discontinue.
- Lorazepam 2–4 mg IM or IV, or diazepam 10 mg IV, may be required to bring alcohol withdrawal under better control.
- Patients with severe withdrawal symptoms may require higher doses and longer tapering periods. Monitoring parameters should include vital signs, tremor, sweating, and other withdrawal symptoms.
- Front-loading refers to giving frequent, high doses of medication to treat early signs and symptoms. Diazepam is given in 20-mg doses every 2 hours until resolution of withdrawal symptoms. A total of 60 mg is typically given, and further doses are not required. This approach XIII
may decrease the rate of seizures.
- In symptom-triggered therapy, medication is given only when symptoms occur. This approach avoids oversedation and may shorten the treatment period.
- Alcohol withdrawal seizures do not require anticonvulsant treatment unless they progress to status epilepticus. **Phenytoin** does not prevent or treat withdrawal seizures.

- Patients with seizures should be treated supportively, and an increase in the dosage and lengthening of the tapering schedule of the BZ used in detoxification or a single injection of a BZ may be necessary to prevent further seizures. Patients with a history of withdrawal seizures can be given a higher initial dose of a BZ and a slower tapering period of 7–10 days.

Benzodiazepines

- Detoxification is approached by initiating treatment at usual doses (Table 72–8) and maintaining this dose for 5 days. The dose is then tapered over an additional 5 days. **Alprazolam** withdrawal may require a more gradual taper.
- In patients with a history of long exposure to BZs, protracted minor abstinence symptoms (e.g., anxiety, insomnia, irritability, muscle spasms) may remain for several weeks.

Barbiturates and Other Sedative-Hypnotic Drugs

- Level of tolerance is determined by giving 200 mg of **pentobarbital** orally and observing for 2–3 hours for signs of a mild intoxication, including sedation, slurred speech, and ataxia. This can be repeated one or more times if necessary until one or more signs of intoxication are seen. The total dose required can be used as an approximate initial daily starting dose for detoxification. This dose is then reduced in decrements of 100 mg every third day at first, then every other day if the patient tolerates initial dosage reductions.

Opiates

- Unnecessary detoxification with drugs should be avoided if possible (e.g., if symptoms are tolerable).
- Conventional drug therapy for opiate withdrawal has been **methadone,** a synthetic opiate. Treatment of withdrawal from heroin usually requires no more than 20 mg of methadone/day. If **LAAM** is used instead of methadone, dosing is three times weekly.
- **Clonidine** can attenuate the noradrenergic hyperactivity of opiate withdrawal without interfering significantly with activity at the opiate receptors. Monitoring should include blood pressure checks, supine and standing, at least daily.

Caffeine

- Caffeinism is treated by reducing or discontinuing the drug. It may be necessary to wean the patient off the drug. Decaffeinated beverages may be slowly substituted for the caffeinated type. Relapses are less likely to occur when the drug is discontinued all at once.

Withdrawal from Other Substances

- Treatment of cocaine withdrawal is mostly supportive, but **bromocriptine** has been used usually short term to reduce craving.

Mixed Substance Withdrawal

- If the drugs used are cross-tolerant (e.g., alcohol and diazepam), treatment for withdrawal from diazepam, the longer acting of the two, also concurrently treats alcohol withdrawal. If the drugs are not cross-tolerant (e.g., alcohol and opiates), withdrawal from each drug must be treated separately. In a young healthy individual, withdrawal from both drugs can be treated concurrently. Otherwise, when detoxification from one drug is completed, the second drug can be tapered and discontinued.

SUBSTANCE DEPENDENCE

- The treatment of drug dependence or addiction is primarily behavioral. The goal of treatment is complete abstinence, and treatment is a lifelong process. Most drug-dependence treatment programs embrace a treatment approach based on Alcoholics Anonymous (AA).

Alcohol

- Compliance with other aspects of treatment may correlate better with abstinence than use of **disulfiram.**
- Disulfiram deters a patient from drinking by producing an aversive-reaction if the patient drinks. It inhibits the liver enzyme aldehyde-dehydrogenase in the biochemical pathway for alcohol metabolism, allowing acetaldehyde to accumulate. This results in flushing, nausea, vomiting, headache, palpitations, fever, and hypotension. Severe reactions include respiratory depression, arrhythmias, myocardial infarction, and cardiovascular collapse. Inhibition of the enzyme continues for as long as 2 weeks after discontinuation of disulfiram. Disulfiram reactions have occurred with the use of alcohol-containing mouthwashes and aftershaves. The usual dosage is 250–500 mg/d.
- Prior to starting disulfiram, baseline liver function tests (LFTs) should be obtained, and patients should be monitored for hepatotoxicity. LFTs should be repeated at 2 weeks, 3 months, and 6 months, then twice yearly. The prescriber should wait at least 24 hours after the last drink before starting disulfiram, usually at a dose of 250 mg/d.
- **Naltrexone** in doses of 50 mg daily has been associated with reduced craving and fewer drinking days. It should not be given to patients currently dependent on opiates as it can precipitate a severe withdrawal syndrome.
- Naltrexone is hepatotoxic, and it is contraindicated in patients with hepatitis or liver failure. LFTs should be monitored monthly for the first 3 months, then every 3 months.
- Side effects include nausea, headache, dizziness, nervousness, fatigue, insomnia, vomiting, anxiety, and somnolence.

Nicotine

- The components of a successful program include (1) skill building (teaching patients how to resist cues to smoke); (2) social support; and

TABLE 72–9. Important Information from the Smoking Cessation *Clinical Practice Guideline*

1. Clinicians should ask and record the tobacco use status of every patient.
2. Smoking cessation treatment should be offered to ALL smokers at EVERY office visit.
3. Smoking cessation treatment as brief as 3 minutes is effective.
4. The more intense the treatment, the more effective it is in producing long-term abstinence from tobacco.
5. Nicotine replacement therapy (NRT) combined with social support and skills training delivered by clinicians is the most effective combination of treatments.
6. Health care systems should be modified to identify and intervene routinely with all tobacco users at every visit.

(3) nicotine replacement. Key points from the smoking cessation clinical practice guideline is shown in Table 72–9.

- **Nicotine replacement therapy (NRT)** doubles the probability of a successful quit attempt. NRT is available as gum, patches, nasal spray, or inhalers. An algorithm for assessing the appropriateness of NRT in patients wishing to quit is shown in Figure 72–1.
- Interventions are more successful when they include social support and training in general problem-solving skills, stress management, and relapse prevention. Providing at least 4–7 sessions significantly increased cassation rates.
- The Agency for Health Care Policy and Research recommends use of NRT in the forms of transdermal nicotine patches because of better compliance and ease of use, but efficacy is similar for the patch and gum.
- NRT may be contraindicated for individuals with severe arrhythmia, severe or worsening angina pectoris, a myocardial infarction within the past 4 weeks, or active peptic ulcers.
- Side effects of the patch and gum include nausea and light headedness, which may warrant a dose reduction. Fifty percent of patients using the patch report skin irritation which may be treated with **hydrocortisone cream 1%** or **triamcinolone cream 0.5%** or switching to a different brand of patch. Twenty-three percent of patients using the patch report insomnia. If insomnia is severe and lasts more than a few weeks, the patient may opt to take off the patch at bedtime.

- Using the patch for longer than 8 weeks is not associated with better success rates. The duration of therapy with the gum should be at least 1–3 months on a fixed schedule.
- Generally, the maximum dose (i.e., 21 mg/d for **Habitrol** and **Nicoderm,** 22 mg/d for **Prostep,** and 15 mg/d for **Nicotrol** 16-hour patch) is recommended for smokers who smoke 10–15 cigarettes or more per day. Traditionally, a gradual fading procedure in which the patch dose

is stepped down at 2–3 week intervals is used, but no empirical support exists for gradual fading.

- Two milligrams of the gum is the optimal dose for most patients. Providers may consider using 4-mg gum for those who smoke at least 20 cigarettes a day or those who have failed on the 2-mg gum. Clinical studies found greater efficacy in patients who chewed more than nine pieces per day.
- **Bupropion** inhibits neuronal reuptake and potentiates the effects of NE and DA. Withdrawal symptoms may be decreased by bupropion's inhibition of NE reuptake. The manufacturer recommends a dosage of 150 mg once daily for 3 days, and then twice daily for 7–12 weeks or longer, with or without NRT. Patients are instructed to stop smoking during the second week of treatment and are encouraged to use counseling and support services along with the medication.

See Chapter 62, Substance-Related Disorders: Overview and Stimulants, Depressants, and Hallucinogens, and Chapter 63, Substance-Related Disorders: Alcohol, Nicotine, and Caffeine, authored by Paul L. Doering, MS, for a more detailed discussion of this topic.

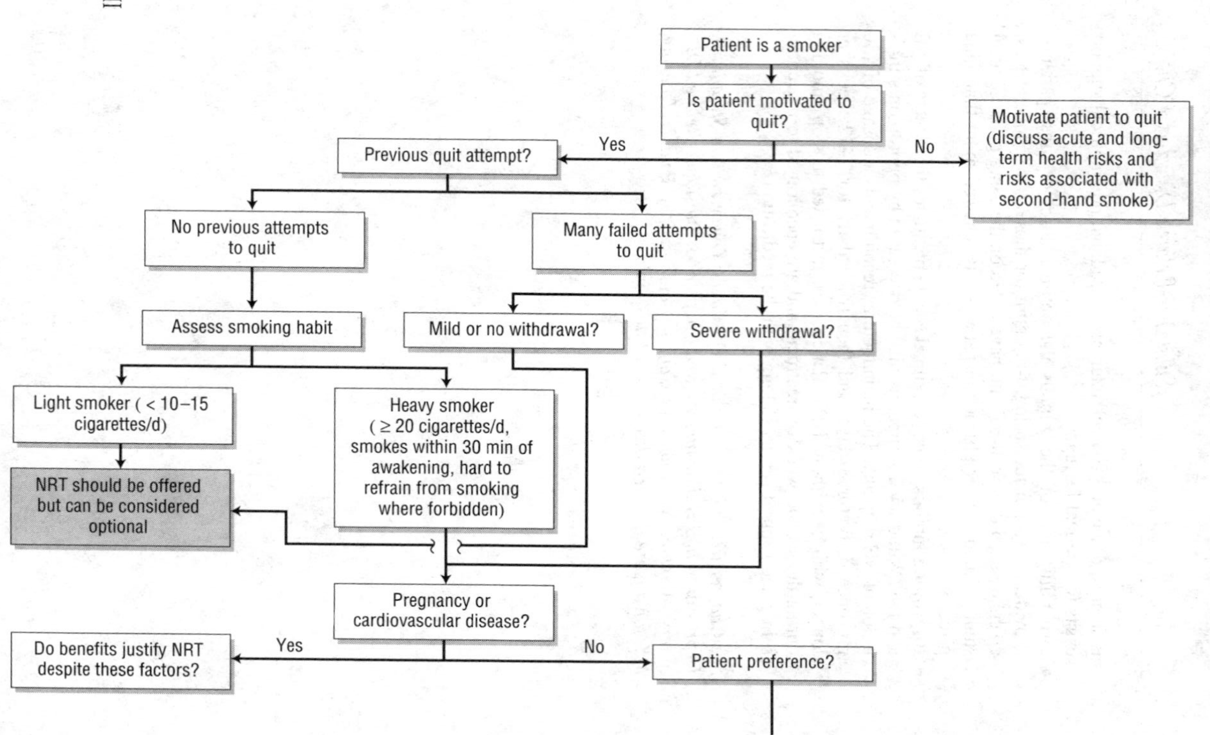

Patient is a smoker
Is patient motivated to quit?
Yes
No
Motivate patient to quit (discuss acute and long-term health risks and risks associated with second-hand smoke)
Previous quit attempt?
No previous attempts to quit
Many failed attempts to quit
Assess smoking habit
Mild or no withdrawal?
Severe withdrawal?
Light smoker (< 10–15 cigarettes/d)
Heavy smoker (≥ 20 cigarettes/d, smokes within 30 min of awakening, hard to refrain from smoking where forbidden)
NRT should be offered but can be considered optional
Pregnancy or cardiovascular disease?
Yes
No
Do benefits justify NRT despite these factors?
Patient preference?

XIII

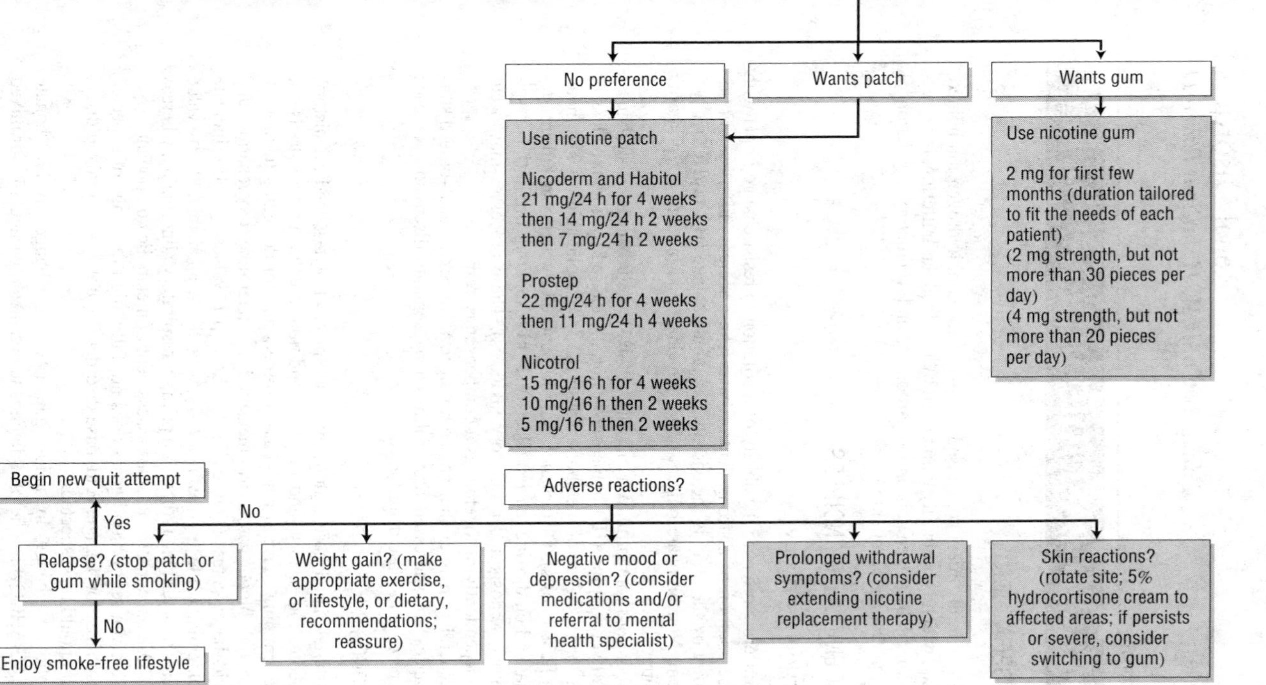

Figure 72–1. Algorithm for assessing appropriateness of nicotine replacement therapy (NRT) in patients wishing to quit smoking.

Renal Disorders

Edited by Cindy W. Hamilton, PharmD

Chapter 73

▶ ACID–BASE DISORDERS

▶ DEFINITION

Acid–base disorders are caused by disturbances in hydrogen ion homeostasis, which is ordinarily maintained by extracellular buffering, renal regulation of hydrogen ion and bicarbonate, and ventilatory regulation of carbon dioxide elimination.

▶ GENERAL PRINCIPLES

PATHOPHYSIOLOGY

- Buffering refers to the ability of a solution to resist change in pH with the addition of a strong acid or base. The principal buffer system utilized by the body is the carbonic acid/bicarbonate (H_2CO_3/HCO_3^-) system. Noncarbonate buffers (e.g., phosphate and protein) act primarily intracellularly.
- There are four primary types of acid–base disturbances. Disturbances in hydrogen ion (H^+) homeostasis initially caused by a gain or loss of H^+ or HCO_3^- are of metabolic origin (i.e., metabolic acidosis and metabolic alkalosis). Disturbances initially caused by a rise or fall in arterial carbon dioxide tension ($Paco_2$) are of respiratory origin (i.e., respiratory acidosis and respiratory alkalosis). These processes may occur independently or together as a compensatory response.
- General principles that are common to all types of acid–base disturbances are addressed first, followed by separate discussions of each type of acid–base disturbance.

DIAGNOSIS

- Arterial blood gases, along with serum electrolytes, medical history, medication history, and clinical condition, are the primary tools for determining cause of acid–base disorders and for designing therapy.
- Arterial blood gases are measured to determine oxygenation and acid–base status (Figure 73–1). Low pH values (<7.35) indicate acidemia, while high values (>7.45) indicate alkalemia. $Paco_2$ value helps to determine if there is a primary respiratory abnormality, whereas HCO_3^- concentration enables assessment of metabolic component.
- If a given set of blood gases does not fall within the range of expected responses for a single acid–base disorder (Figure 73–2), a mixed disorder should be suspected.
- Ratio of change in anion gap (AG) to change in bicarbonate ($\Delta AG/\Delta HCO_3$) is a helpful diagnostic parameter, particularly for mixed

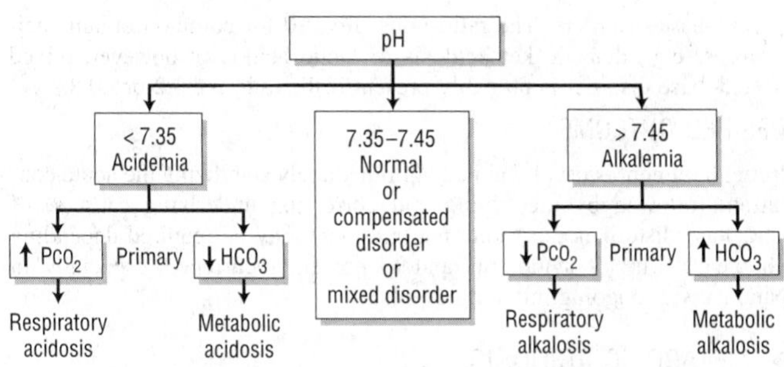

Figure 73–1. Analysis of arterial blood gases.

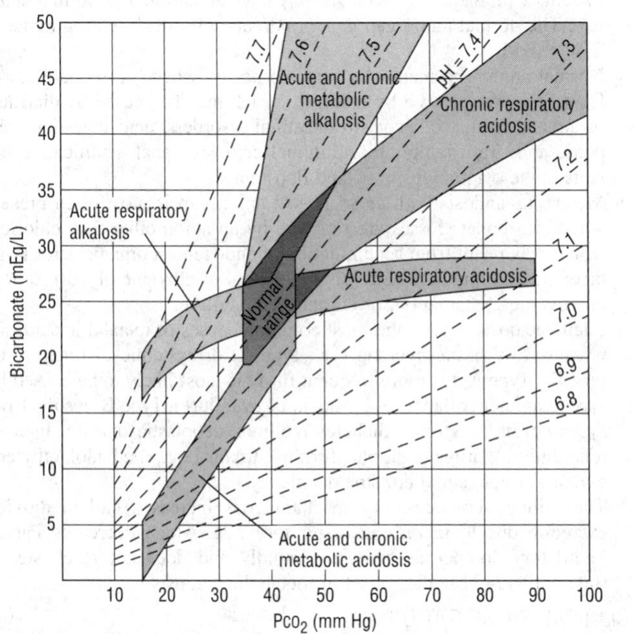

Figure 73–2. Acid–base nomogram. (met, metabolic; alk, alkalosis; resp, respiratory; acid, acidosis.) *(From CMAJ 1973;109:291–293, with permission.)*

XIV

acid–base disorders. The ratio is usually 1.0 for common organic acidoses (e.g., diabetic ketoacidosis or lactic acidosis); however, mixed acid–base disorder is probably present if the ratio is >1.2 or <0.8.

DESIRED OUTCOME

Initial treatment is usually aimed at immediately stabilizing the acute condition, followed by identifying and correcting underlying cause(s) of acid–base disturbances. Additional treatment may be required depending on the severity of symptoms and to prevent recurrence, especially in patients with ongoing initiating events.

▶ METABOLIC ACIDOSIS

PATHOPHYSIOLOGY

- Metabolic acidosis is characterized by decreased pH and low serum bicarbonate concentrations, which can result from adding organic acid to extracellular fluid (ECF) (e.g., lactic acid, ketoacids), loss of bicarbonate stores (e.g., in diarrhea), or accumulation of endogenous acids due to impaired renal function (e.g., phosphates, sulfates).
- Patients with metabolic acidosis may have an elevated or normal anion gap. The normal anion gap is approximately 9 mEq/L with a range of 3–11 mEq/L.
- Normal anion gap metabolic acidosis occurs when bicarbonate losses from ECF are replaced by chloride, which may be caused by diarrhea, pancreatic fistula, other gastrointestinal disorders, acid ingestion, carbonic anhydrase inhibitors, dilutional acidosis, renal acidification defects, ureterosigmoidostomy, and ileostomy.
- Metabolic acidosis with an increased anion gap is most often present when bicarbonate losses are replaced by an anion other than chloride, which may result from accumulation of endogenous organic acids (e.g., lactic acid), toxin ingestion (e.g., methanol or ethylene glycol), salicylate overdose, starvation, or chronic renal failure.
- Lactic acidosis, one of the most common causes of metabolic acidosis, is caused by tissue hypoxia (i.e., type A) or systemic disorders (i.e., type B). Type A, the more frequent form, is most likely to be caused by cardiovascular collapse (e.g., shock, heart failure). Type B results from systemic diseases (e.g., diabetes mellitus, neoplastic disease, liver or renal failure), drugs (e.g., phenformin), toxins (e.g., methanol, ethylene glycol), or congenital enzyme deficiency.
- The primary compensatory mechanism is increased carbon dioxide excretion due to increasing respiratory rate, which decreases $Paco_2$. Ventilatory compensation begins rapidly and does not reach steady state until 12–24 h after onset of metabolic acidosis.

CLINICAL PRESENTATION

- Hyperventilation is often the first sign of metabolic acidosis. In severe acidosis (pH <6.8), central nervous system (CNS) function may be disrupted and the respiratory center is depressed. Respiratory compensation may occur as Kussmaul's respirations (i.e., deep, rapid respirations characteristic of diabetic ketoacidosis).

- Peripheral vasodilation is characterized by flushing, rapid heart rate, and wide pulse pressure. Cardiac output may be initially increased, but it falls as hypotension worsens.
- Gastrointestinal symptoms include loss of appetite, nausea, and vomiting. Severe acidosis (pH <7.1) interferes with carbohydrate metabolism and insulin use, resulting in hyperglycemia.
- Effect on serum potassium concentrations depends on type of acidosis, ranging from consistent increases with mineral acids to smaller increments with organic acids (e.g., lactic acidosis).

DIAGNOSIS

- Diagnosis of lactic acidosis should be considered in all forms of metabolic acidosis with an increased anion gap. Lactate concentrations of ≥4.0–5.0 mEq/L with simultaneous decreases in bicarbonate and arterial pH are highly suggestive of lactic acidosis.

TREATMENT

- Treatment should be aimed at correcting the underlying disorder, but alkalinization may be required in acute, life-threatening situations or in chronic metabolic acidosis.
- **Sodium bicarbonate** has been recommended to raise arterial pH to 7.15–7.20, but no controlled clinical trials demonstrate reduced morbidity and mortality compared with general supportive care. Although excessive sodium bicarbonate is potentially detrimental, sodium bicarbonate administration may be necessary for acute situations (e.g., cardiac arrest; see Chapter 6).
- Less severe or chronic metabolic acidosis can be corrected gradually with oral bicarbonate or a substrate (see Chapter 78).
- Treatment of renal tubular acidosis depends on whether it is type I (i.e., classic, distal, or gradient limited), type II (i.e., proximal or quantity limited), or another type. Alkali administration ranges from 1–3 mEq/kg/d for type I to 10–25 mEq/kg/d for type II. **Potassium** supplementation (e.g., potassium citrate, which would provide both potassium and alkali) may also be necessary for type II renal tubular acidosis.
- Treatment of diabetic ketoacidosis is covered in Chapter 17.

► METABOLIC ALKALOSIS

PATHOPHYSIOLOGY

- Metabolic alkalosis, a common condition in hospitalized patients, is characterized by a primary increase in plasma bicarbonate concentration.
- Bicarbonate concentration elevation can be generated by net loss of hydrogen ion from ECF space, net addition of bicarbonate or its

precursors (i.e., carbonate, citrate, acetate) to ECF space, or loss of chloride-rich bicarbonate-poor fluid (i.e., gastric HCl).

- Initiating events can be categorized as sodium chloride responsive or resistant, depending on response to saline volume expansion. Sodium chloride-responsive disorders are associated with urinary chloride concentrations of <10 mEq/mL, whereas sodium chloride-resistant disorders are associated with concentrations of >20 mEq/mL.
  - The most common initiating event is loss of chloride-rich, bicarbonate-poor fluid (e.g., diuretic use, nasogastric suctioning, or vomiting); these are sodium chloride-responsive disorders.
  - Many sodium chloride-resistant disorders are associated with excess mineralocorticoid activity, which may result from primary adrenal overproduction (e.g., hyperaldosteronism) or oversupply of endogenous mineralocorticoids (e.g., licorice ingestion), and oversecretion of mineralocorticoid secondary to increased renin activity. These disorders are also caused by persistent hypokalemia.
  - Miscellaneous causes include large doses of penicillins (e.g., ticarcillin).
- The immediate compensatory response is chemical buffering, which involves movement of intracellular hydrogen ions to the ECF in exchange for potassium and sodium. The second phase is respiratory compensation (i.e., hypoventilation to raise the $Paco_2$).

CLINICAL PRESENTATION

- No unique signs or symptoms are associated with metabolic alkalosis.
- Patients may complain of symptoms related to the underlying disorder (e.g., muscle weakness with hypokalemia or postural dizziness with volume depletion).

DIAGNOSIS

- Patient history (e.g., vomiting, gastric drainage, or diuretic use) is especially useful in the diagnosis of metabolic alkalosis because of the lack of unique signs and symptoms.

TREATMENT

- Treatment of underlying cause(s) may not correct metabolic alkalosis.
- Therapy depends on whether the disorder is sodium chloride responsive or resistant (Figure 73–3).
- Initial therapy of sodium chloride–responsive disorders is directed at expanding intravascular volume and replenishing chloride stores by administering sodium chloride and potassium solutions. If patients are volume expanded or intolerant to sodium volume loads (e.g., heart failure), a carbonic anhydrase inhibitor may be beneficial (e.g., **acetazolamide** 250 mg or 375 mg once or twice daily).
- Other agents sometimes used to treat sodium chloride–responsive metabolic alkalosis include **hydrochloric acid, ammonium chloride,** and **arginine monohydrochloride.**

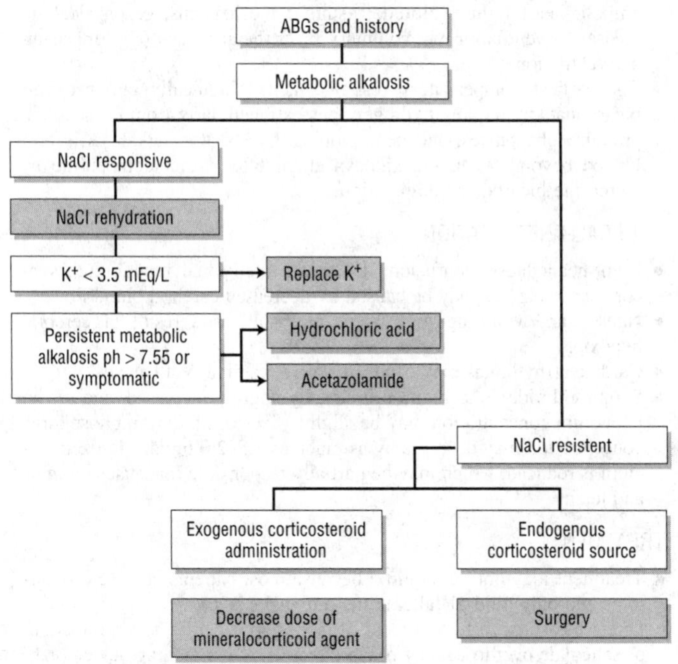

Figure 73–3. Treatment algorithm for patients with primary metabolic alkalosis.

- Standard doses of histamine H_2-receptor antagonists and omeprazole have been used to decrease the volume and hydrogen ion content in gastric fluids if metabolic alkalosis is caused by nasogastric suction.
- Treatment of sodium chloride-resistant disorders involves removal of excess mineralocorticoid activity.

▶ RESPIRATORY ALKALOSIS

PATHOPHYSIOLOGY

- Respiratory alkalosis, one of the most common acid–base disturbances, is characterized by an initial decrease in $Paco_2$, which raises pH.
- $Paco_2$ decreases when ventilatory excretion exceeds metabolic production usually because of hyperventilation. XIV
- Potential causes of respiratory alkalosis include increases in neurochemical stimulation via central (e.g., anxiety, pain, fever, brain tumor, vascular accident, salicylates), or peripheral (e.g., pulmonary

emboli, heart failure, altitude, asthma) mechanisms, or physical increases in ventilation via voluntary or artificial means (e.g., mechanical ventilation).

- The earliest compensatory response is to chemically buffer excess bicarbonate by moving hydrogen ions extracellularly from intracellular proteins, phosphates, and hemoglobin. If respiratory alkalosis is prolonged beyond >6 h, the kidneys attempt to further compensate by increasing bicarbonate elimination.

CLINICAL PRESENTATION

- Light-headedness, confusion, decreased intellectual functioning, syncope, and seizures may be caused by decreased cerebral blood flow.
- Nausea and vomiting may occur, probably as a result of cerebral hypoxia.
- Cardiac arrhythmias may occur in severe respiratory alkalosis.
- Serum chloride concentration is usually slightly increased, and serum potassium concentration may be slightly decreased. Serum phosphorus concentration may decrease by as much as 1.5–2.0 mg/dL. Ionized calcium is reduced, which may be partially responsible for muscle cramps and tetany.

TREATMENT

- Treatment may not be required because most patients have few symptoms and only mild pH alterations (i.e., pH <7.50).
- Direct measures (e.g., treatment of pain, hypovolemia, fever, infection, or salicylate overdose) may prove effective. A rebreathing device (e.g., paper bag) may help control hyperventilation.
- If the patient is receiving mechanical ventilation, respiratory alkalosis may often be corrected by decreasing the number of mechanical breaths per minute, using a capnograph and spirometer to more precisely adjust ventilator settings, or increasing dead space in the ventilator circuit.

► RESPIRATORY ACIDOSIS

PATHOPHYSIOLOGY

- Respiratory acidosis is initially caused by primary retention of carbon dioxide that lowers blood pH and results in a compensatory increase in plasma bicarbonate concentration.
- Respiratory acidosis results from a disorder that restricts ventilation or increases CO_2 production, such as perfusion abnormalities (e.g., massive pulmonary embolism, cardiac arrest), airway and pulmonary abnormalities (e.g., airway obstruction, severe pulmonary edema, severe pneumonia), neuromuscular abnormalities (e.g., trauma, stroke, brainstem or cervical cord injury, myasthenia gravis, narcotic or sedative overdose), or mechanical ventilator problems (e.g, malfunction).

- The early compensatory response to acute respiratory acidosis is buffering by noncarbonate systems. If respiratory acidosis is prolonged >12–24 h, renal excretion of hydrogen ion also increases, which generates new bicarbonate.

CLINICAL PRESENTATION

- Neuromuscular symptoms include altered mental status, abnormal behavior, seizures, stupor, and coma. Hypercapnia may mimic stroke or CNS tumor by producing headache, papilledema, focal paresis, and abnormal reflexes. CNS symptoms are caused by increased cerebral blood flow and are variable depending in part on acuity of onset.
- The degree of altered cardiac contractility and heart rate depends on severity of acidosis, whether it is metabolic or respiratory, and rapidity of onset.
- Serum sodium and chloride concentrations remain normal or increase slightly. Serum potassium concentration increases secondary to intracellular movement.

TREATMENT

- If carbon dioxide excretion is acutely and severely impaired, and life-threatening hypoxia is present (Po_2 <40 mm Hg), adequate ventilation should be provided, which may involve maintaining a patent airway (e.g., emergency tracheotomy, bronchoscopy, or intubation), clearing excessive secretions, administering oxygen, and mechanical ventilation.
- The underlying cause of acute acidosis should be treated aggressively (e.g., bronchodilators, stopping respiratory depressants such as narcotics and benzodiazepines).
- Bicarbonate administration is rarely necessary and potentially harmful.
- In a patient with chronic respiratory acidosis (e.g., chronic obstructive pulmonary disease), treatment is essentially similar for acute respiratory acidosis with a few important exceptions. Because the drive to breathe depends on hypoxemia rather than hypercarbia, oxygen therapy should be initiated carefully and only if Pao_2 is <50 mm Hg. Underlying causes of acute exacerbation should be treated (e.g., with antibiotics).
- Chronic respiratory acidosis is discussed in Chapter 81.

▶ MIXED ACID–BASE DISORDERS

PATHOPHYSIOLOGY

- Failure of compensation is responsible for mixed acid–base disorders such as respiratory acidosis and metabolic acidosis, or respiratory alkalosis and metabolic alkalosis. In contrast, excess compensation is responsible for metabolic acidosis and respiratory alkalosis, or metabolic alkalosis and respiratory acidosis. XIV

- Respiratory and metabolic acidosis may develop in patients with cardiorespiratory arrest, in chronic lung disease patients who are in shock, and in metabolic acidosis patients who develop respiratory failure.
- The most common mixed acid–base disorder is respiratory and metabolic alkalosis, which occurs in critically ill surgical patients with respiratory alkalosis caused by mechanical ventilation, hypoxia, sepsis, hypotension, neurologic damage, pain, or drugs; and with metabolic alkalosis caused by vomiting or nasogastric suctioning and massive blood transfusions. It may also occur in patients with hepatic cirrhosis, hyperventilation, diuretic use, or vomiting; and in patients with chronic respiratory acidosis and an elevated plasma bicarbonate concentration who are placed on mechanical ventilation and undergo a rapid fall in $PaCO_2$ to hypocapnic levels.
- Metabolic acidosis and respiratory alkalosis may be seen in patients with advanced liver disease, salicylate intoxication, and pulmonary–renal syndromes.
- Metabolic alkalosis and respiratory acidosis may occur in patients with chronic obstructive pulmonary disease and respiratory acidosis who are treated with salt restriction or diuretics.

DIAGNOSIS

- Because it is often difficult to correctly identify mixed metabolic alkalosis and respiratory acidosis (see Figure 73–2), it is helpful to observe the patient's response to discontinuation of diuretics and administration of sodium and potassium chloride. This treatment will correct the metabolic alkalosis component if it is a simple metabolic alkalosis, but will only minimally affect $PaCO_2$ if it is a mixed disorder.

TREATMENT

- Mixed respiratory and metabolic acidosis should be treated by responding to both the respiratory and metabolic acidosis. Improved oxygen delivery must be initiated to improve hypercarbia and hypoxia. Mechanical ventilation may be needed to reduce $PaCO_2$. During the initial stage of therapy, appropriate amounts of sodium bicarbonate should be given to reverse the metabolic acidosis.
- The metabolic component of mixed respiratory and metabolic alkalosis should be corrected by administering sodium chloride and potassium chloride solutions. The respiratory component should be treated by readjusting the ventilator or by treating the underlying disorder causing hyperventilation.
- Treatment of mixed metabolic acidosis and respiratory alkalosis should be directed at the underlying cause.
- In metabolic alkalosis and respiratory acidosis, pH may not deviate significantly from normal, but treatment may be required to maintain PaO_2 and $PaCO_2$ at acceptable levels. Treatment should be aimed at decreasing plasma bicarbonate with sodium and potassium chloride therapy,

allowing the renal excretion of retained bicarbonate from the diuretic-induced metabolic alkalosis.

► EVALUATION OF THERAPEUTIC OUTCOMES

- Patients should be monitored closely because acid–base disorders can be serious and even life threatening.
- Arterial blood gases are the primary tools for evaluation of therapeutic outcome. They should be monitored closely to ensure resolution of simple acid–base disorders without deterioration to mixed disorders due to compensatory mechanisms. For example, arterial blood gases should be obtained every 2–4 h during the acute phase of respiratory acidosis and less frequently (every 12–24 h) as the acidosis improves.

See Chapter 49, Acid–Base Disorders, authored by Robert A. Kilroy, PharmD, BCPS, and Gary R. Matzke, PharmD, FCP, FCCP, for a more detailed discussion of this topic.

Chapter 74

▶ DIALYSIS

▶ DEFINITION

Dialysis is one of the primary treatment modalities for patients with renal failure. Two of the principle functions of the kidney (i.e., removal of endogenous waste products and maintenance of water [fluid] balance) can be accomplished by a well-designed dialysis prescription based on the diffusion of solutes (movement from an area of high to low concentration, or from blood to dialysate) and ultrafiltration of water (movement from an area of high to low pressure, or from blood to dialysate) across a semi-permeable membrane (dialysis filter).

▶ PATHOPHYSIOLOGY, CLINICAL PRESENTATION, AND DIAGNOSIS

- Hemodialysis (Table 74–1) and peritoneal dialysis (Table 74–2) are the predominant treatment options for acute and chronic renal failure (see Chapters 77 and 78). Each type of dialysis has unique advantages and disadvantages that facilitate individualization of therapy. Therefore, the two types are discussed separately in this chapter.
- In patients with chronic renal failure, dialysis should be initiated electively rather than urgently to allow time to educate the patient, create a suitable access, and prevent complications. Because of the progressive nature of chronic renal failure, the need should be anticipated when creatinine clearance (CrCl) drops below 25 mL/min.
- The primary criterion for initiation of dialysis is the patient's clinical status (i.e., presence of persistent anorexia; nausea and vomiting, especially with weight loss; declining serum albumin; uncontrolled hypertension or heart failure; and neurologic deficits or pruritis). Although serum creatinine and blood urea nitrogen (BUN) are not criteria per se, dialysis should be initiated when at least one sign or symptom occurs together with a CrCl <9 mL/min/1.73 m^2 in a nondiabetic or <14 mL/min/1.73 m^2 in a diabetic.

▶ DESIRED OUTCOME

The ultimate goal of dialysis is to provide the optimal dose of dialysis for each individual patient; that is, the amount of therapy above which there is no cost-effective increment in quality-adjusted life expectancy.

TABLE 74–1. Advantages and Disadvantages of Hemodialysis (HD)

Advantages

1. Higher solute clearance, which allows intermittent treatment.
2. Better defined parameters of adequacy of dialysis, which allows early detection of underdialysis.
3. Low technique failure rate.
4. Although intermittent heparinization is required, better correction of hemostasis parameters.
5. Closer monitoring of the patient because of in-center hemodialysis.

Disadvantages

1. Multiple visits each week to the HD center, which translates to loss of control by the patient.
2. Disequilibrium, dialysis hypotension, and muscle cramps; may require months for patient to adjust to HD.
3. Bioincompatibility-induced activation of complement and cytokines, which may predispose to dialysis-related amyloidosis.
4. Infections, which may be related to the choice of HD membranes, with complement-activating membranes being more deleterious.
5. Vascular access-associated infection and thrombosis.
6. More rapid decline of residual renal function compared with PD.

TABLE 74–2. Advantages and Disadvantages of Peritoneal Dialysis (PD)

Advantages

1. More hemodynamic stability (blood pressure) due to slow ultrafiltration rate.
2. Increased clearance of larger solutes, which may explain good clinical status despite lower urea clearance.
3. Better preservation of residual renal function.
4. Convenient IP administration of drugs.
5. Suitable for elderly and very young patients who may not tolerate HD well.
6. Freedom from the "machine," which gives the patient a sense of independence (for CAPD).
7. Less blood loss and iron deficiency, which results in easier management of anemia or reduced requirements for epoietin and parenteral iron.
8. No systemic heparinization requirement.
9. Use of SC (versus IV) epoietin, which may reduce overall dose and be more physiologic.

Disadvantages

1. Predispositon to malnutrition due to protein and amino acid losses through peritoneum, and reduced appetite due to continuous glucose load and sense of abdominal fullness.
2. Risk of peritonitis.
3. Catheter malfunction, and exit site and tunnel infection.
4. Inadequate ultrafiltration and solute dialysis in patients with large body size, unless large volumes and frequent exchanges are employed.
5. Patient burnout and high rate of technique failure.
6. Risk of obesity with excessive glucose absorption.
7. Mechanical problems such as hernias, dialysate leaks, hemorrhoids, or back pain.
8. Not suitable for patients with extensive abdominal surgery.
9. No convenient access for IV iron administration.

▶ TREATMENT: HEMODIALYSIS

GENERAL PRINCIPLES

- Hemodialysis consists of perfusion of heparinized blood and physiologic salt solution on opposite sides of a semipermeable membrane. Waste products (e.g., urea and creatinine) move from blood into the dialysate by passive diffusion along concentration gradients.
- Diffusion rate depends on the difference between solute concentrations in blood and dialysate, solute characteristics, dialysis filter composition, and blood and dialysate flow rates.
- Ultrafiltration or convection, the primary mode for removal of excess body fluids, also occurs during hemodialysis. If the filter pore size is large enough, drugs and endogenous waste products in plasma water are also removed.
- Hemodialysis consists of an external vascular circuit through which blood is transferred in sterile polyethylene tubing to the dialysis filter via a mechanical pump. The patient's blood then passes through the dialyzer on one side of the semipermeable membrane material and is returned to the patient. The dialysate solution is pumped through the dialyzer countercurrent to the flow of blood on the other side of the semipermeable membrane. The dialysate circuit is not sterile and is a potential source of infection.
- Permanent access to the bloodstream for hemodialysis may be accomplished by several techniques. Native arteriovenous fistula (AV fistula) has the longest survival of all blood access devices and lowest complication rate. Synthetic vascular grafts are the access of choice for most patients. Temporary vascular access for acute dialysis is usually achieved by inserting a dual-lumen catheter into a large vein.
- In conventional or standard hemodialysis, low-permeability (low-flux) membranes are made of natural products (i.e., cellulose). Each session usually lasts 4–5 h.
- Rapid high-efficiency dialysis (RHED) has the advantages of increased clearance of low molecular weight solutes (e.g., urea), shorter procedure times, and increased blood and dialysate flow rates. However, clearance of middle and high molecular weight solutes, including many drugs, is not increased because the membrane pore size is still small.
- High-flux dialysis (HFD) shares the advantages of RHED, but the HFD membrane pores are more open and therefore have higher clearance rates for middle molecules. HFD filters have the disadvantages of being more expensive than low- or medium-flux filters, and requiring more precise ultrafiltration controllers to avoid large rapid fluid shifts.

HEMODIALYSIS PRESCRIPTION

- There is no clear agreement on the optimal dose of dialysis that should be prescribed, but mortality rates and duration of hospitalization have decreased in centers where the dose of dialysis has been proactively increased.

- The two key goals are to achieve the desired dry weight and to remove exogenous wastes.
- Many nephrologists recommend a target urea reduction ratio (URR) of ≥65 or a *Kt/V* of >1.2 for nondiabetic patients receiving standard dialysis, and a URR of >70 or a *Kt/V* of ≥1.4–1.5 for diabetics and/or patients receiving RHED or HFD therapy.
- URR can be calculated as follows:

$$URR = BUN_{pre} - BUN_{post}/BUN_{pre} \times 100$$

where BUN_{pre} is predialysis BUN and BUN_{post} is postdialysis BUN.

- *Kt/V* is a unitless parameter that represents the fraction of urea distribution volume that is cleared of urea during a dialysis session, which can be estimated as follows:

$$Kt/V = -\ln[(BUN_{post}/BUN_{pre}) - 0.008t] + [(4 - 3.5BUN_{post}/BUN_{pre})UF/Wt]$$

where *K* is dialyzer clearance of urea (in L/h), *V* is patient's distribution volume (in L), *t* is duration of dialysis (in h), and UF is ultrafiltration volume removed (in L).

- Post-treatment BUN samples should be obtained 15–30 minutes after the end of the treatment to assure re-equilibration of urea.

COMPLICATIONS OF HEMODIALYSIS

- Hemodialysis is associated with many complications (Table 74–3). The incidence is 30–40% lower in patients receiving RHED or HFD compared with standard hemodialysis.
- Anemia, hyperparathyroidism, and other complications of chronic renal failure are addressed in Chapter 78.
- Type A dialyzer reactions are similar to drug-induced anaphylactic reactions and may be due to hypersensitivity to ethylene oxide (a common dialyzer sterilant), heparin, formaldehyde, or glutaraldehyde (common reuse sterilants). This type of reaction has also been associated with bradykinin system activation by some dialyzer membranes (predominantly AN69), particularly in patients receiving angiotensin-converting enzyme (ACE) inhibitors. These reactions can be managed by immediately stopping the dialysis procedure and resuscitative therapy (e.g., **epinephrine, antihistamines,** and **steroids**). XIV
- Type B dialyzer reactions are more common than Type A but less severe. Chest and back pain are the most frequently reported symptoms. Although patients can continue dialysis, they should be switched

TABLE 74–3. Common Complications During Hemodialysis

	Incidence (%)	Etiology/Predisposing Factors	Management
Hypotension	15–50	Excessive ultrafiltration Target weight too low Acetate dialysate→vasodilation Autonomic neuropathy Inability to compensatorily increase cardiac output	Place in Trendelenburg position Decrease ultrafiltration rate 10–20 mL hypertonic saline (23.4%) 100–200 mL bolus of normal saline Midodrine or caffeine
Cramps	≤50	Hypotension Idiopathic dehydration Sodium level in dialysate too low	100–200 mL bolus of normal saline 10–20 mL hypertonic saline (23.4%) Prophylactic vitamin E 400 IU q hs
Itching	50–90	Uremic toxins ⇑ calcium–phosphorus product Dry skin Allergy to heparin, plasticizers in dialysis tubing, sterilizer used, or any other medication	Activated charcoal 6 g daily Hyperphosphatemia therapy Topical emollients Oral antihistamine Delivery of adequate dialysis Biocompatible dialyzers UVB light therapy
Chest or back pain	2.5	Type B dialyzer reaction	Biocompatible dialyzer or reuse program
Nausea and vomiting	5–15	Hypotension May be an early sign of disequilibrium syndrome	Treat hypotension Prochlorperazine 10 mg po or 2.5 mg IV
Headache	5	Usually unknown mechanism Acute caffeine withdrawal due to dialytic removal Acetate dialysate→vasodilatation	Acetaminophen 650 mg po (PRN)

to a more biocompatible dialyzer and/or placed on a reprocessing program to minimize future reactions.

- Patients with end-stage renal disease (ESRD) demonstrate immune abnormalities, some of which may be aggravated by bioincompatible filters (e.g., cellulose and cuprophane).
- Disequilibrium syndrome is characterized by systemic and neurologic symptoms and EEG changes. In mild cases, symptoms are nonspecific (e.g., nausea, vomiting, headache, or restlessness). Severe disequilibrium is characterized by seizures, obtundation, or coma. The risk can be minimized by adjusting dialysate sodium (at least 140 mEq/L) and glucose (at least 200 mg/dL) levels, and by reducing ultrafiltration rate and target urea reduction ratio.
- XIV Dialysis-related amyloidosis is common in patients who receive dialysis for >8–10 years secondary to accumulation of β_2 microglobulin. Clinical manifestations are carpal tunnel syndrome, pain and stiffness of other major joints, and soft-tissue swelling. There is no adequate, definitive treatment for this syndrome.

▶ TREATMENT: PERITONEAL DIALYSIS

GENERAL PRINCIPLES

- In peritoneal dialysis (PD), the dialysate-filled compartment is the peritoneal cavity, into which dialysate is instilled via a permanent peritoneal catheter that traverses the abdominal wall. The peritoneal membrane functions as the semipermeable membrane.
- Access to the peritoneal cavity is via placement of an indwelling catheter, which is manufactured from a silastic material that is soft, flexible, and biocompatible.
- PD dialysate solutions contain dextrose 1.5–4.25%. The osmolarity of the solutions, which ranges from 350–480 mOsm/L and exceeds that of serum (280 mOsm/L), provides the drawing force for water and solute movement across the peritoneal membrane. Dextrose is not an ideal osmotic agent, in part because it alters peritoneal mesothelial cells and leukocyte function.
- Commercial PD solutions also contain electrolytes to minimize their removal by reducing the diffusion gradient, such as sodium 132 mEq/L, chloride 102 mEq/L, lactate 35 mEq/L, magnesium 1.5 mEq/L, and calcium 3.5 or 2.5 mEq/L.
- PD is much less efficient per unit time than hemodialysis (see Tables 74–1 and 74–2), and must therefore be a more frequent or virtually continuous procedure. Quantity of dialysis delivered may be regulated by altering the number of daily exchanges, volume of each exchange, or dextrose concentration.
- Continuous ambulatory PD (CAPD) is the most common PD procedure. Others include continuous cycling (CCPD) and nightly intermittent (NIPD).
- In a basic CAPD prescription, dialysate flows into the peritoneal cavity under gravity, dwells within the peritoneal cavity, and then is drained out of the peritoneal cavity into the original container. Typically a patient instills a 2–3 liters exchange of dialysate three times a day during the day and then a single exchange, often using a higher dextrose concentration, for an overnight, 8–12-hours dwell.

DESIGN AND ASSESSMENT

- The peritoneal equilibration test (PET) is a diagnostic test that determines the peritoneal membrane clearance and ultrafiltration characteristics, and quantitates the ability to transfer solutes and water across the membrane.
  - PET test results determine which variant of PD is appropriate for an individual. Table 74–4 illustrates the prognostic interpretation where APD is nightly automated PD; DAPD is daily ambulatory PD; standard dose PD is CAPD or standard CCPD; and high dose is CAPD with >9 liters dialysate/d, or CCPD with >8 liters dialysate overnight and >2 liters dialysate during the day.

TABLE 74–4. Prognostic Value of PET Results

Creatinine or Dextrose Transport	Ultrafiltration Rate	Predicted Solute Clearance	Preferred Type[a]
High	Poor	Adequate	APD, DAPD
High average	Adequate	Adequate	Standard dose PD
Low average	Good	Adequate/inadequate	Standard to high dose PD
Low	Excellent	Inadequate	High dose PD, hemodialysis

[a] See text for discussion of terms.

From Twardowski ZJ. Blood Purif 1989;7:95–108, p 102, with permission.

- PET also predicts the daily dialysis requirement.

- Assessment of adequacy of dialysis requires more than a simple examination of BUN profile. The recommended criteria are *Kt/V* and weekly creatinine clearance, which should be measured at mo 1, 4, and 6 and then every 4 months.
- To calculate *Kt/V* for PD, a dialysate-to-plasma (D/P) urea concentration is determined, and *Kt* is estimated as:

$$Kt = \text{D/P} \times \text{volume drained (L/d)}$$

The urea volume of distribution can be approximated as 0.6 L/kg. *Kt/V* values should exceed 2.0/wk for CAPD, 2.1/wk for CCPD, and 2.2/wk for NIPD.

- The total weekly CrCl should be ≥60 L/wk/1.73 m^2 for CAPD, ≥63 L/wk/1.73 m^2 for CCPD, and ≥66 L/wk/1.73 m^2 for NIPD.

COMPLICATIONS OF PERITONEAL DIALYSIS

- Mechanical complications include kinking of catheter, inflow and outflow obstruction, excessive catheter motion at the exit site, pain from catheter-tip impingement on viscera, and inflow pain.
- PD patients have numerous metabolic and nutritional abnormalities (e.g., exacerbation of diabetes mellitus due to absorption of dextrose from the peritoneal cavity, electrolyte abnormalities especially hypercalcemia or hypocalcemia, malnutrition, fluid overload, chemical peritonitis, and fibrin formation in dialysate).

Peritonitis

- Infectious complications (e.g., peritonitis and catheter related) are a major cause of morbidity and mortality, and the leading cause of technique failure and transfer from PD to hemodialysis.
- Peritonitis is defined as an elevated dialysate white blood cell count >100/mm^3, with ≥50% polymorphonuclear neutrophils. A patient with cloudy fluid and symptoms (i.e., abdominal pain) is given a provisional diagnosis.

TABLE 74–5. Organisms Causing Peritonitis

Organisms	% Episodes
Gram positive	40–50
S. epidermidis	30–45
S. aureus	10–20
Streptococci	10–15
Enterococci	3–5
Diphtheroids	<5
Gram negative	20–35
E. coli	5–12
P. aeruginosa	5–8
Enterobacter	2–3
Acinetobacter	2–3
Klebsiella	2–3
Proteus	2–3
Mixed gram positive and negative	10–15
Fungi	5–10
Sterile culture, presumed bacterial	5–20
Other	5

- Most infections (40–50%) are caused by gram-positive bacteria (Table 74–5), of which *Staphylococcus epidermidis* predominates.
- Patients with cloudy fluid and symptoms require prompt initiation of empiric therapy (Figure 74–1). In asymptomatic patients with only cloudy fluid, it is reasonable to delay initiation of therapy until cell count, differential, and gram stain results are available.
- Initial empiric therapy should include agents effective against both gram-positive and -negative organisms, usually a combination of a first-generation **cephalosporin** and an **aminoglycoside.** The IP route is preferred.
- Within 24–48 h after culture of dialysate fluid, 70–90% of samples yield a specific microorganism, which is usually gram positive. Antimicrobial therapy is modified accordingly (Figures 74–2 and 74–3).
- If gram stain reveals yeast, oral **flucytosine** (2 g loading dose, then 1 g q d) and oral or IP **fluconazole** (100–200 mg q d) should be initiated.

Prophylaxis and Treatment of Exit-Site Infections

- Exit-site infection is defined by the presence of purulent drainage with or without erythema of the skin at the catheter–epidermal interface.
- The most common causative organisms are *S. aureus* (40–50% of episodes) followed by *S. epidermidis, P. aeruginosa,* and other enteric gram-negative bacilli (15–20% each). XIV
- The use of topical antibiotics and disinfectants is controversial for the treatment of established infections.

Empiric therapy	Continuous dose	Intermittent dose (in 1 exchange/d)	
		Residual urine output (mL/d)	
		Anuria (< 500)	Nonanuria (> 500)
Cefazolin or Cephalothin	500 mg/L load, then 125 mg/L in each exchange	500 mg/L (or 15 mg/kg)	Increase dose by 25%
Gentamicin Netilmicin Tobramycin	8 mg/L load, then 4 mg/L in each exchange	0.6 mg/kg body weight	1.5 mg/kg initial loading dose.[a]
Amikacin	25 mg/L load, then 12 mg/L in each exchange	2 mg/kg body weight	5 mg/kg initial loading dose.[a]

[a]Patients with residual urine output may require 0.6 mg/kg body weight as maintenance doses with increased dosing frequency based on serum and/or dialysate levels.

Figure 74–1. Assessment and therapy of peritonitis. *(From Keane WF, Alexander SR, Bailie GR, et al.* Perit Dial Int *1996; 16:557–573, with permission.)*

- Gram-positive infections should be treated with an oral penicillinase-resistant **penicillin** or first-generation **cephalosporin.**
- Gram-negative infections should be treated with oral **quinolones.**
- Nasal carriage of *S. aureus* is associated with exit-site/tunnel infections and peritonitis. Prophylaxis is recommended for adults with positive nasal cultures, which may consist of **mupirocin** intranasally twice daily for 5 days every 4 weeks, mupirocin at exit site daily, or **rifampin** 300 mg PO twice daily for 5 days every 12 weeks.

INTRAPERITONEAL DRUG THERAPY

- Drug dosing in renal insufficiency is covered in Chapter 75.
- For management of systemic infections, potential benefits of the IP route include use of an established access, ability to treat infections in outpatient settings and associated cost savings, possible avoidance of IV drug-related toxicities, and improved patient acceptance.

XIV

- For insulin, possible advantages of the IP route include avoidance of erratic absorption, convenience, avoidance of subcutaneous injection-site complications, and prevention of peripheral hyperinsulinemia.
- Instillation of heparin 500 U/L to each exchange may prevent fibrin formation.

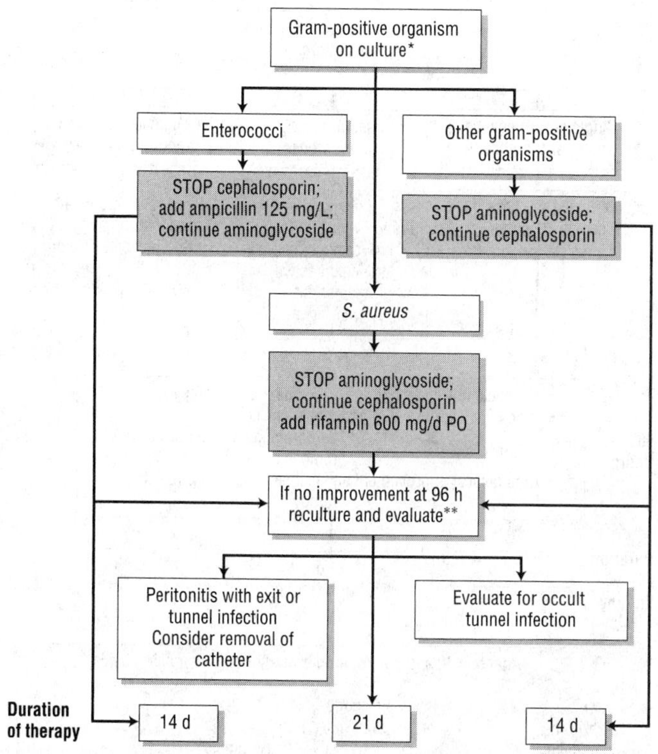

Figure 74–2. Management of gram-positive peritonitis.*Choice of therapy should always be guided by sensitivity patterns. **If MRSA is cultured and the patient is not clinically responding, clindamycin or vancomycin should be used. *(From Keane WF, Alexander SR, Bailie GR, et al.* Perit Dial Int *1996; 16:557–573, with permission.)*

- Other drugs that have been administered by the IP route include calcitriol for secondary hyperparathyroidism; deferoxamine for aluminum bone disease and hyperaluminumism; metoclopramide, cisapride, and erythromycin for diabetic gastroparesis; lithium for bipolar affective disorder; streptokinase and urokinase for recurrent peritonitis; amino acids for nutritional disorders; growth hormone for growth retardation; and epoietin and iron dextran for anemia.

XIV

See Chapter 44, Hemodialysis and Peritoneal Dialysis, authored by Gary R. Matzke, PharmD, FCP, FCCP, and George R. Bailie, MS, PharmD, PhD, FCCP, for a more detailed discussion of this topic.

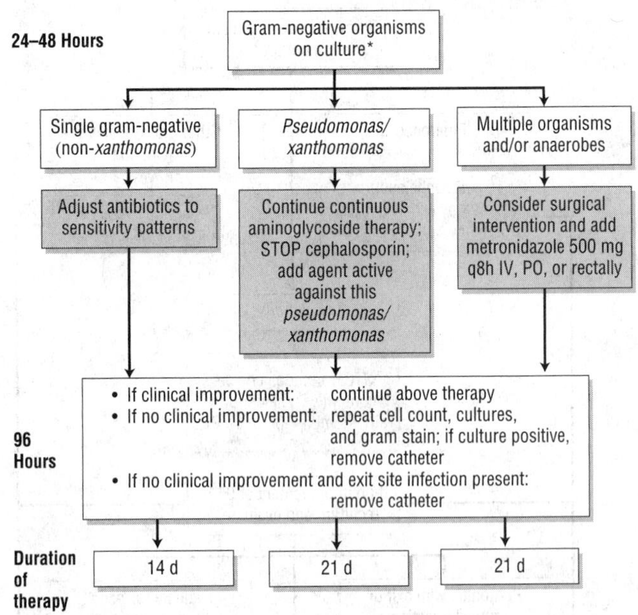

Agents with anti-*pseudomonas* or anti-*xanthomonas* activity

Agent	**Dosage**
Ceftazidime	125 mg/L IP
Piperacillin	4 g every 12 h IV (adults) 150 mg/kg every 12 h (children)
Ciprofloxacin	500 mg BID PO (avoid in children)
Aztreonam	LOAD: 1000 mg/L MAINT: 250 mg/L IP
Imipenem	LOAD: 500 mg/L MAINT: 200 mg/L IP
Sulfamethoxazole/ trimethoprim	LOAD: 1600/320 PO Q 1–2d
Aminoglycosides	Increase dose to 6–8 mg/L IP in each exchange**

* Choice of treatment should always be guided by sensitivity patterns.
** See Figure 74–1 for intermittent dosing discussion.

Figure 74–3. Management of gram-negative peritonitis. *(From Keane WF, Alexander SR, Bailie GR, et al.* Perit Dial Int *1996; 16:557–573, with permission.)*

XIV

Chapter 75

▶ DRUG DOSING IN RENAL INSUFFICIENCY

▶ DEFINITION

The primary reason to individualize drug therapy for patients with renal insufficiency is to minimize the toxicities associated with drug accumulation, which may occur owing to reduced renal clearance. Additional reasons are changes in bioavailability, protein binding, distribution volume, and metabolic activity.

▶ PATHOPHYSIOLOGY, CLINICAL PRESENTATION, DIAGNOSIS, AND TREATMENT

- The pathophysiology, clinical manifestations, diagnosis, and treatment of acute and chronic renal failure are discussed in Chapters 77 and 78, respectively.

▶ GENERAL PRINCIPLES

- Drug therapy individualization for patients with renal insufficiency may require only a simple proportional dose adjustment based on creatinine clearance. Alternatively, complex adjustments may be required for medications that are extensively metabolized or undergo dramatic changes in protein binding and/or distribution.
- Patients may also demonstrate an altered pharmacodynamic response to a given medication because of the physiologic and biochemical changes associated with progressive renal insufficiency.

BIOAVAILABILITY

- There is little quantitative information regarding influence of impaired renal function on drug absorption and bioavailability.
- Factors that may theoretically affect bioavailability include alterations in gastrointestinal (GI) transit time, gastric pH, edema of the GI tract, vomiting and diarrhea, and concomitant drug therapy, especially antacid or H_2 antagonist administration.
- Increased bioavailability has been reported for propranolol, tolamolol, bufuralol, oxprenolol, dextropropoxyphene, and dihydrocodeine in patients with renal insufficiency. However, clinical consequences have been demonstrated only with dextropropoxyphene and dihydrocodeine.

DISTRIBUTION

- Volume of distribution of many drugs is significantly increased in patients with end-stage renal disease (ESRD) (Table 75–1). Changes

TABLE 75–1. Effect of ESRD on the Volume of Distribution of Selected Drugs

	Volume of Distribution (L/kg)	
	Normal	*ESRD*
Amikacin	0.20	0.29
Azlocillin	0.21	0.28
Bretylium	3.58	4.48
Cefazolin	0.13	0.17
Cefonicid	0.11	0.14
Cefoxitin	0.16	0.26
Cefuroxime	0.20	0.26
Clofibrate	0.14	0.24
Cloxacillin	0.14	0.26
Dicloxacillin	0.08	0.18
Erythromycin	0.57	1.09
Furosemide	0.11	0.18
Gentamicin	0.20	0.32
Isoniazid	0.6	0.8
Minoxidil	2.6	4.9
Nalmefene	7.9	14.7
Naproxen	0.12	0.17
Phenytoin	0.64	1.4
Trimethoprim	1.36	1.83
Vancomycin	0.64	0.85

may result from altered protein or tissue binding, or pathophysiologic alterations in body composition (e.g., fractional contribution of total body water to total body weight).

- Generally, plasma protein binding of acidic drugs (warfarin, phenytoin) is decreased in uremia (Table 75–2), whereas binding of basic drugs (quinidine, lidocaine) is usually normal or slightly decreased.
- Ideally, unbound (versus total) drug concentrations should be monitored, especially for drugs that have a narrow therapeutic range, are highly protein bound (free fraction <20%), and have marked variability in the free fraction (e.g., phenytoin and disopyramide).
- Methods for calculating volume of distribution may be influenced by renal disease. Of the commonly used terms (i.e., volumes of central compartment [V_c], terminal phase [V_β, V_{area}], and distribution at steady state [V_{SS}]), V_{SS} may be the most appropriate for comparing patients with renal insufficiency versus those with normal renal function because V_{SS} is independent of drug elimination.

TABLE 75–2. Efffects of ESRD on Protein Binding of Acidic Drugs

	Unbound Drug (%)		
	Normal	*ESRD*	Change from Normal (%)
Abecarnil	4	15	275
Azlocillin	62.5	75	20
Cefazolin	16	29	81
Cefoxitin	27	59	119
Ceftriaxone	10	20	100
Clofibrate	3	9	200
Cloxacillin	5	20	300
Diazoxide	6	16	167
Dicloxacillin	3	9	200
Diflunisal	12	44	267
Doxycycline	12	28	133
Furosemide	4	6	50
Methotrexate	57.2	63.8	12
Metolazone	5	10	100
Moxalactam	48	64	33
Naproxen	0.2	0.8	300
Pentobarbital	34	41	21
Phenylbutazone	5.5	16	191
Phenytoin	10	21.5	115
Piretanide	6	12	100
Salicylate	8	20	150
Sulfamethoxazole	34	58	71
Valproic acid	8	23	188
Warfarin	1	2	100
Zomepirac	1.3	3.8	192

METABOLISM

- The kidney contributes to the biotransformation of many drugs. Several cytochrome P450 enzymes present in the kidney metabolize endogenous substances (e.g., vitamin D) and drugs. Chronic renal impairment may also have a detrimental effect on drug metabolism within the liver.
- Drug metabolism may be increased, decreased, or unaffected by renal failure (Table 75–3).
- Patients with severe renal insufficiency may experience accumulation of metabolite(s), which may contribute to pharmacologic activity or toxicity (Table 75–4).

TABLE 75–3. Effect of ESRD on Nonrenal (Hepatic) Clearance

	Decreased		
Acyclovir	Aztreonam	Bufuralol	Captopril
Cefmenoxime	Cefmetazole	Cefonicid	Cefotaxime
Cefotiam	Cefsulodin	Ceftizoxime	Cilastatin
Cimetidine	Ciprofloxacin	Cortisol	Encainide
Erythromycin	Imipenem	Isoniazid	Metoclopramide
Methylprednisolone	Moxalactam	Nicardipine	Nimodipine
Nitrendipine	Procainamide	Quinapril	Verapamil
Zidovudine			
	Unchanged		
Acetaminophen	Chloramphenicol	Clonidine	Codeine
Diflunisal	Indomethacin	Insulin[a]	Isradipine
Lidocaine	Morphine	Metoprolol	Nisoldipine
Nortriptyline	Pentobarbital	Propafenone	Quinidine
Theophylline	Tocainide	Tolbutamide	
	Increased		
Bumetanide	Cefpiramide	Fosinopril	Nifedipine
Phenytoin	Sulfadimidine		

[a]May be unchanged or decreased.

RENAL EXCRETION

- Differences in pharmacokinetic parameters among patients with similar reductions in glomerular filtration rate may be due to differences in their types of renal disease. Therefore, dosage-adjustment methodologies need to be developed that consider the impact of altered tubular and glomerular function.
- In the absence of clinically useful techniques to quantitate tubular function, clinical measurement or estimation of creatinine clearance remains the guiding factor for calculating drug dosage.

► CALCULATION OF DRUG DOSAGE

- Most dosage adjustment guidelines propose the use of a fixed dose or interval for patients with broad ranges of renal function. However, these categories encompass up to a tenfold range in renal function, the drug regimen may not be optimal for all patients.
- The optimal dosage regimen for patients with renal insufficiency requires an individualized assessment and depends on an accurate characterization of the relationship between the pharmacokinetic parameters of the drug and renal function, and an accurate assessment of the patient's renal function.
- Consideration must be given to stability of renal function and type of dialysis.

TABLE 75–4. Pharmacologic Activity of Selected Drug Metabolites

Parent Drug	Metabolite	Pharmacologic Activity of Metabolites
Acetaminophen	*N*-acetyl-*p*-benzo-quinoneimine	Hepatotoxicity
Allopurinol	Oxipurinol	Suppression of xanthine oxidase
Azathioprine	Mercaptopurine	(All) immunosuppressive activity
Cefotaxime	Desacetyl cefotaxime	Similar antimicrobial spectrum, but one-fourth to one-tenth as potent
Chlorpropamide	2-Hydroxychlorpropamide	Similar in vitro insulin-releasing activity
Clofibrate	Chlorophenoxyisobutyric acid	Hypolipidemic effect and muscle toxicity
Codeine	Morphine-6-glucuronide	Possibly more active than parent, which may prolong narcotic effect
Imipramine	Desmethylimipramine	Similar antidepressant activity
Meperidine	Normeperidine	Less analgesic activity than parent, but more CNS-stimulatory effects
Morphine	Morphine-6-glucuronide	Possibly more active than parent compound, which may prolong narcotic effect
Procainamide	*N*-acetyl procainamide	Distinct antiarrhythmic activity, but different mechanism
Sulfonamides	Acetylated metabolites	No antibacterial activity, but increased toxicity if elevated concentrations
Theophylline	1,3-Dimethyl uric acid	Cardiotoxicity
Zidovudine	Zidovudine triphosphate	Antiretroviral activity

STABLE RENAL INSUFFICIENCY

- If the relationship between creatinine clearance (CrCl) and the kinetic parameters of a drug (i.e., total body clearance [CL], elimination rate constant [k], and V_{SS}) have been characterized, these data should be used to individualize drug therapy (Table 75–5). The kinetic parameter/dosage adjustment factor (Q) is the ratio of the patient's predicted CL or k to the value derived from the relationship for individuals with normal creatinine clearance of 120 mL/min/1.73 m^2.

Estimation of Kinetic Parameters

XIV

- If relevant data are not available for patients with renal insufficiency, kinetic parameters must be estimated based on fraction of the drug that is eliminated renally unchanged (f_e) in subjects with normal renal function.

TABLE 75–5. Relationship Between Renal Function and Pharmacokinetic Parameters of Selected Drugs

Drug	Total Body Clearance
Acyclovir	CL = 3.37 (CrCl) + 0.41
Amikacin	CL = 0.6 (CrCl) + 9.6
Cefmetazole	CL = 1.18 (CrCl) – 0.29
Ceftazidime	CL = 1.15 (CrCl) + 10.6
Ciprofloxacin	CL = 2.83 (CrCl) + 363
Digoxin	CL = 0.88 (CrCl) + 23
Gentamicin	CL = 0.983 (CrCl)
Netilmicin	CL = 0.65 (CrCl) + 3.72
Ofloxacin	CL = 1.04 (CrCl) + 38.7
Piperacillin	CL = 1.36 (CrCl) + 1.50
Procainamide	CL = 3 (CrCl) + 0.23 (ABW)
Teicoplanin	CL = 7.09 (CrCl) – 16.2
Tobramycin	CL = 0.801 (CrCl)
Vancomycin	CL = 0.69 (CrCl) + 3.7

- If the decrease in CL and k are proportional to CrCl, renal disease does not alter drug metabolism, any metabolites are inactive and nontoxic, and the drug obeys first-order (linear) kinetic principles and is adequately described by a one-compartment model, then the Q factor for dosage adjustment can be calculated as:

  $$Q = 1 - [f_e(1 - KF)]$$

  where KF is the ratio of the patient's CrCl to the assumed normal value of 120 mL/min/1.73 m^2. Estimated total body clearance can be calculated as:

  $$CL_T = CL_{\text{norm}} \times Q$$

  where CL_{norm} is the mean value in patients with normal renal function from the literature.
- The best method for adjusting the dosage regimen depends on whether the desired goal is maintenance of a similar peak, trough, or average steady-state drug concentration.

- The principal choices are to decrease the dose, prolong the dosing interval, or both. Prolonging the interval is generally preferred because it saves costs by reducing nursing and pharmacy time as well as associated supplies.

- The prolonged dosing interval (τ_f) or reduced maintenance dose *(DF)* may be calculated from the following relationships, where τ_n is the normal dosing interval and D_n is the normal dose:

$$\tau_f = \tau_n / Q$$

$$D_f = D_n \times Q$$

- If V_d is significantly altered or a specific concentration is desired, estimation of a dosage regimen becomes more complex. The dosing interval (τ_f) is calculated as:

$$\tau_f = (-1/k_f)(\ln\,[C_{\min}/C_{\max}])$$

and the dose as:

$$\text{Dose} = V_d \times (C_{\max} - C_{\min})$$

CONTINUOUS RENAL REPLACEMENT THERAPY

- Drug therapy individualization for patients receiving continuous renal replacement therapy (CRRT) is complicated by higher residual nonrenal clearance of some drugs in patients with acute versus chronic renal insufficiency. Furthermore, there are marked differences in drug removal between intermittent hemodialysis and the three primary types of CRRT (i.e., continuous arteriovenous or venovenous hemofiltration [CAVH or CVVH], hemodialysis [CAVHD or CVVHD], and hemodiafiltration [CAVHDF or CVVHDF]).
- During CAVH/CVVH, drug clearance is a function of membrane permeability for the drug, which is called the sieving coefficient (SC) and the rate of ultrafiltrate formation (UFR). SC (Table 75–6) is often approximated by the fraction unbound (f_u) because this information may be more readily available. Thus, clearance by CAVH/CVVH can be calculated as:

$$\text{CL} = \text{UFR} \times f_u$$

- Clearance by CAVHDF/CVVHDF can be calculated as the product of the combined ultrafiltrate and dialysate volume (V_{df}) and drug concentration in this fluid (C_{df}), divided by the plasma concentration going into the filter (C_p^{mid}) at the midpoint of the V_{df} collection period:

$$\text{CL} = (V_{df} \times C_{df}) / C_p^{mid}$$

XIV

- After the total clearance has been calculated (Table 75–7), the optimal dosage regimen can be calculated using the approach described for patients with stable renal function.

TABLE 75–6. Predicted and Measured Sieving Coefficients of Selected Drugs

Drug	Predicted	Measured
Amikacin	0.95	0.88
Amphotericin	0.01	0.32–0.4
Ampicillin	0.8	0.6–0.69
Cefoperazone	0.10	0.27–0.69
Cefotaxime	0.62	0.55–1.1
Cefoxitin	0.30	0.32
Ceftazidime	0.90	0.38–0.78
Ceftriaxone	0.10	0.71–0.82
Clindamycin	0.25	0.49–0.98
Digoxin	0.75	0.96
Erythromycin	0.25	0.37
5-Flurocytosine	0.96	0.98
Gentamicin	0.95	0.81–0.75
Imipenem	0.80	0.78
Metronidazole	0.80	0.80
Mezlocillin	0.68	0.68
Nafcillin	0.20	0.47
N-acetyl procainamide	0.80	0.92
Netilmicin	—	0.85
Oxacillin	0.05	0.02
Phenobarbital	0.60	0.86
Phenytoin	0.10	0.45
Procainamide	0.80	0.86
Theophylline	0.47	0.85
Tobramycin	0.95	0.78–0.86
Vancomycin	0.90	0.5–0.8

PERITONEAL DIALYSIS

- Peritoneal dialysis has the potential to affect drug disposition; however, drug therapy individualization is often less complicated because of the continuous nature of chronic ambulatory peritoneal dialysis (CAPD).
- Factors that influence drug dialyzability include drug-specific characteristics (e.g., molecular weight, solubility, degree of ionization, protein binding, and volume of distribution) and intrinsic properties of the peritoneal membrane (e.g., blood flow, pore size, and peritoneal membrane surface area).

TABLE 75–7. Clearance of Selected Drugs by CAVH/CVVH and/or CAVHD/CVVHD

	CAVH/CVVH		CAVHD/CVVHD		
Drug	*SC*	*Clearance*	*SC*	*DFR 1 L/h Clearance*	*DFR 2 L/h Clearance*
Amikacin	0.93 ± 0.16	10.1			
Amrinone	0.80–1.4	2.4–14.4			
Cefuroxime		11.0 ± 5.2	0.90 ± 0.30	14.0 ± 2.2	16.2 ± 3.4
Ceftazidime			0.86 ± 0.07	13.1 ± 1.3	15.2 ± 1.3
Cilastatin	0.77	4.0 ± 2.3	0.68 ± 0.08	10.0 ± 3.0	18.0 ± 4.0
Ciprofloxacin				16.3	19.9
Digoxin				6.4–10.0	11
Gentamicin		3.5 ± 1.9		5.2 ± 1.8	
Imipenem	0.80	13.3	1.05 ± 0.19	16.0 ± 7.0	
Phenytoin	0.37 ± 0.08	1.0		6.5	
Theophylline				14.8	
Tobramycin		3.5 ± 1.9		11.1–29	14.9
Vancomycin	0.80	6.7–13.3	0.66 ± 0.08	12.1 ± 5.7	16.6 ± 5.7

Clearance is in mL/min. SC, sieving coefficient; DFR, dialysate flow rate; NR, not reported.

- In general, peritoneal dialysis is less effective in removing drugs than hemodialysis and, in fact, does not contribute substantially to total body clearance (Table 75–8).

CHRONIC HEMODIALYSIS

- The impact of hemodialysis on drug therapy depends on drug characteristics, dialysis prescription (e.g., dialysis membrane composition, filter surface area, blood and dialysate flow rates, and reuse of the dialysis filter), and clinical indication for dialysis.
- High-flux dialysis (HFD) (Chapter 74) allows free passage of most solutes with molecular weights ≤20,000, and therefore is more likely to remove high molecular weight drugs (e.g., vancomycin) as well as drugs with low molecular to midmolecular weights (i.e., 100–1000) than conventional dialysis (Table 75–9).
- The dialysate recovery clearance approach has become the benchmark for determination of dialyzer clearance. It can be calculated as:

$$CL_D^r = R/AUC_{0\text{-}t}$$

XIV

where R is total amount of drug recovered unchanged in dialysate and $AUC_{0\text{-}t}$ is area under the prefilter plasma concentration–time curve during

TABLE 75–8. Comparison for Selected Drugs of Residual Drug Clearance in ESRD (Cl_{ESRD}) to Clearance by Continuous Ambulatory Peritoneal Dialysis (Cl_{CAPD}), Intermittent Peritoneal Dialysis (Cl_{IPD}), and Hemodialysis (Cl_{HD})[a]

Drug	Cl_{ESRD}	Cl_{CAPD}	Cl_{IPD}	Cl_{HD}
Aztreonam	1.44	0.13	0.13	2.6
Cefazolin	0.30	0.06		2.1
Cefotaxime	7.13 ± 0.74	0.40 ± 0.08		1.6
Ceftazidime	0.74 ± 0.20	0.10 ± 0.02	0.50	2.3
Gentamicin	0.24	0.17	0.75	2.1
Mezlocillin	6.0		0.44	1.7
Pipericillin	3.90 ± 0.77	0.22		4.4
Ticarcillin	0.96		0.43	2.0
Vancomycin	5.0	0.85 ± 0.22		0.8

[a]All data (mean or mean ± SD) are in L/h.

hemodialysis. To determine AUC_{0-t}, at least two and preferably three to four plasma concentrations should be obtained during dialysis.

- Total clearance during dialysis can be calculated as the sum of the patient's residual clearance during the interdialytic period (CL_{RES}) and dialyzer clearance (CL_D):

$$CL_T = CL_{RES} + CL_D$$

TABLE 75–9. Drug Disposition During Dialysis Depends on Dialyzer Characteristics

	Hemodialysis Clearance (mL/min)		Half-Life During Dialysis (h)	
Drug	*Conventional*	*High-Flux*	*Conventional*	*High-Flux*
Ceftazidime	55–60	155[a]	3.30	1.2[a]
Cefuroxime	NR	103[b]	3.75	1.6[b]
Gentamicin	58.2	116[b]	3.0	4.3[b]
Netilmicin	46	87–109	5.0–5.2	2.9–3.4
Vancomycin	9–21	31–60[c] 40–150[b] 72–116[d]	35–38	12.0[c] 4.5–11.8[b] NR

NR = not reported.
[a]Polyamide dialyzer.
[b]Polysulfone dialyzer.
[c]Polyacrylonitrile dialyzer.
[d]Polymethylmethacrylate.

- Half-life between dialysis treatments and during dialysis can then be calculated from the following relationships using an estimate of the drug's distribution volume (V), which can be obtained from the literature:

$$t_{1/2,\ \mathrm{offHD}} = 0.693\ [V/\mathrm{CL}_{RES}] \text{ and}$$

$$t_{1/2,\ \mathrm{onHD}} = 0.693\ [V/(\mathrm{CL}_{RES} + \mathrm{CL}_D)]$$

- Key pharmacokinetic parameters can be estimated (based on population data) or calculated, used to simulate the plasma concentration–time profile of the drug for the patient, to ascertain how much drug to administer and when.
- Plasma concentrations of the drug over the interdialytic interval of 24–48 hours can be predicted. The concentration at the end of the 30-minute infusion ($C_{\max}$) would be:

$$C_{\max} = [(\mathrm{dose}/t')1 - e^{-kt'}]/\mathrm{CL}_{RES}$$

The plasma concentration prior to the next dialysis session (C_{bD}) can be calculated as:

$$C_{bD} = C_{\max} \times e^{-(\mathrm{CL}_{RES}/V) \times t}$$

- The hemodialysis clearance of most drugs is dialysis filter dependent, and a value can be extrapolated from the literature. The concentration after dialysis can be calculated as:

$$C_{aD} = C_{bD} \times e^{-(\mathrm{CL}_{RES} + \mathrm{Cl}_D)/Vt}$$

- The postdialysis dose can be calculated as follows if the elimination half-life is prolonged relative to the infusion time and thus minimal drug is eliminated during the infusion period:

$$\mathrm{Dose} = V_d \times (C_{\max} - C_{\min})$$

See Chapter 47, Renal Insufficiency, authored by Reginald F. Frye, PharmD, PhD, and Gary R. Matzke, PharmD, FCP, FCCP.

Chapter 76

▶ ELECTROLYTE HOMEOSTASIS

▶ DEFINITION

An electrolyte is any salt that dissociates in water. Electrolytes are involved in movement of body water, acid–base balance, and many other life-sustaining functions. Homeostatic mechanisms preserve serum concentrations within relatively narrow ranges. Electrolyte imbalances can result from many causes and can produce substantial morbidity and mortality. This chapter reviews disorders of sodium, potassium, calcium, magnesium, and phosphorus homeostasis.

▶ DESIRED OUTCOME

The goals of therapy for disorders of electrolyte homeostasis are to promptly identify and correct reversible underlying causes; institute treatment, if indicated, to relieve symptoms and prevent serious complications; and to normalize the serum electrolyte concentration.

▶ DISORDERS OF SODIUM AND WATER HOMEOSTASIS

HYPONATREMIA (SERUM SODIUM <135 mEq/L)

Pathophysiology

- Depending on serum osmolality, hyponatremia is classified as isotonic, hypertonic, or hypotonic (Figure 76–1).
- *Hypotonic hyponatremia* may be further classified as hypovolemic, hypervolemic, or isovolemic hyponatremia.
  - *Hypovolemic hyponatremia* is associated with a deficit of extracellular fluid (ECF) volume and sodium, with a proportionally greater deficit of sodium than water.
  - *Isovolemic hyponatremia* is associated with a normal total body sodium content and small increases in ECF volume.
  - *Hypervolemic hyponatremia* (also referred to as dilutional hyponatremia) is associated with an elevated total body sodium content and an expanded ECF volume.

Clinical Presentation

- In *hypovolemic hyponatremia,* most of the clinical manifestations are due to hypovolemia (e.g., poor skin turgor, tachycardia, and hypotension) and not hypotonicity.
- In contrast, the hypotonicity of *isovolemic* and *hypervolemic hyponatremia* may result in symptoms related to cellular swelling; cerebral edema with increased intracranial pressure is the most severe.
- There is considerable overlap between serum sodium values and symptoms. If sodium falls rapidly (>0.5 mEq/L/h) to very low levels (<120

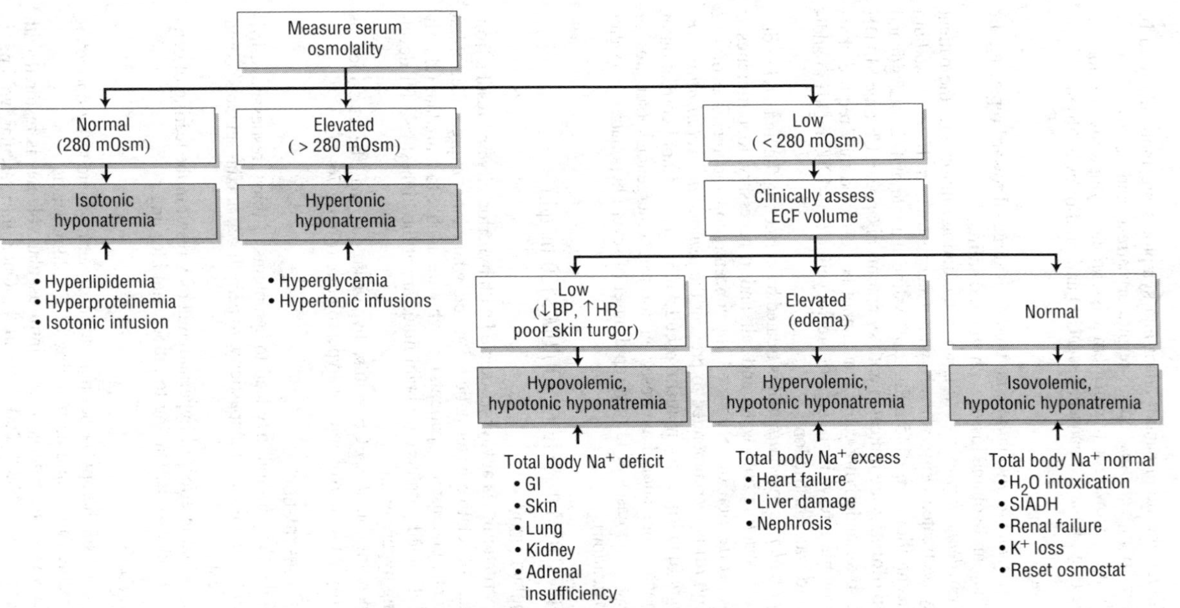
Measure serum osmolality
Normal (280 mOsm)
Elevated (> 280 mOsm)
Low (< 280 mOsm)
Isotonic hyponatremia
Hypertonic hyponatremia
Clinically assess ECF volume
• Hyperlipidemia
• Hyperproteinemia
• Isotonic infusion
• Hyperglycemia
• Hypertonic infusions
Low (↓BP, ↑HR poor skin turgor)
Elevated (edema)
Normal
Hypovolemic, hypotonic hyponatremia
Hypervolemic, hypotonic hyponatremia
Isovolemic, hypotonic hyponatremia
Total body Na^+ deficit
• GI
• Skin
• Lung
• Kidney
• Adrenal insufficiency
Total body Na^+ excess
• Heart failure
• Liver damage
• Nephrosis
Total body Na^+ normal
• H_2O intoxication
• SIADH
• Renal failure
• K^+ loss
• Reset osmostat

Figure 76–1. Diagnostic approach to hyponatremia.

XIV

mEq/L), the brain cannot adapt and symptoms are more likely to be severe (e.g., seizures, coma, respiratory arrest, and death). If sodium falls more slowly or hyponatremia is chronic, symptoms are nonspecific (e.g., lethargy, nausea, headache) and mild or even absent.

Treatment

- In *hypovolemic hyponatremia,* therapy is directed toward replacing the sodium and volume losses with **normal saline**.
- If *isovolemic hyponatremia* is not acute and asymptomatic, the patient may be treated conservatively with water restriction. If serum sodium concentrations are <115 mEq/L, 3% saline at a rate of 1–2 mL/kg/h and **loop diuretics** are indicated until symptoms disappear. Chronic SIADH due to an underlying cause that cannot be corrected may require pharmacologic intervention (e.g., **demeclocycline** 600–1200 mg/d) in addition to water restriction.
- *Hypervolemic hyponatremia* is treated by correcting the underlying disease, restricting both water and salt, and, if necessary, loop diuretics.
- Slow correction of serum sodium concentration (an increase of <12 mEq/L/d) is recommended to prevent the *osmotic demyelinization syndrome* (quadriparesis, mutism, pseudobulbar palsy. Rapid correction of hyponatremia should be reserved for true emergencies (seizures or coma) or in cases of known rapid onset of severe hyponatremia (water intoxication).

HYPERNATREMIA (SERUM SODIUM >150 mEq/L)

Pathophysiology

- Hypernatremia is always associated with hypertonicity and results from a state of relative water deficit. Patients who cannot express their thirst (infants, unconscious patients) or who are unable to ambulate (elderly and disabled patients) to obtain fluids are at the highest risk for developing hypernatremia.
- Depending on the ECF status, hypernatremia may be classified as hypovolemic, isovolemic, or hypervolemic (Figure 76–2).

Clinical Presentation

- Cellular dehydration may lead to symptoms of thirst, restlessness, irritability, tremulousness, spasticity, hyperreflexia, ataxia, seizures, coma, and death.
- The shrinking effect of hypernatremia may result in the tearing of cerebral blood vessels, leading to intracranial bleeding.

Treatment

- The goal of therapy is normalization of serum tonicity by correcting reversible causes and normalizing ECF volume status.
- In *hypovolemic hypernatremia,* intravascular volumes is restored with isotonic 0.9% NaCl 200–300 mL/h. Once intravascular volume is replaced, the free-water deficit can be replaced with 5% dextrose or

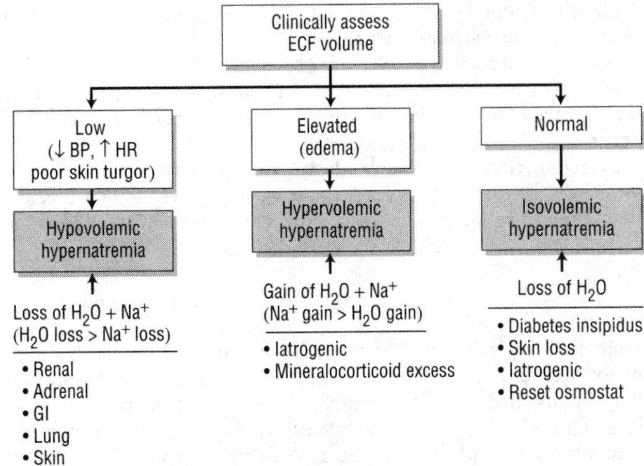

Figure 76–2. Diagnostic approach to hypernatremia.

0.45% NaCl solution. Serum sodium concentration should be decreased slowly to avoid neurologic damage. An acceptable rate is 2 mOsm/h (1 mEq/L sodium per h) over 48–72 hours.

- *Isovolemic hypernatremia* is corrected by replacing the water deficit as described above with 5% dextrose or 0.45% NaCl solution. Patients with central diabetes insipidus (DI) will respond to administration of **vasopressin** preparations. Antidiuretics (e.g., chlorpropamide, carbamazepine) have also been used.
- *Hypervolemic hypernatremia* should be treated by replacement of water deficit in conjunction with diuretics to eliminate sodium excess.

▶ DISORDERS OF POTASSIUM HOMEOSTASIS

HYPOKALEMIA (SERUM POTASSIUM <3.5 mEq/L)

Pathophysiology

- Hypokalemia with normal body potassium stores can result from laboratory error or redistribution from plasma back into cells (e.g., metabolic alkalosis, insulin).
- Hypokalemia with decreased total body stores can occur from gastrointestinal (GI) loss (e.g., vomiting, diarrhea) or renal loss (e.g., diuretics, mineralocorticoid excess).

XIV

Clinical Presentation

- Muscular symptoms can include myalgia, weakness, cramps, akathisia, and paralysis.

- Metabolic symptoms may be related to abnormal carbohydrate metabolism (e.g., glucose intolerance).
- ECG effects are characterized by ST segment lowering or flattening, inversion of the T wave, and elevated U wave. A widening of the PR interval and QRS complex and overall slowing of conduction may also occur.
- Cardiac arrhythmias include bradyarrhythmias, heart block, atrial flutter, paroxysmal atrial tachycardia with block, atrioventricular dissociation, premature ventricular contractions, and ventricular fibrillation. Hypokalemia lowers the threshold for digitalis cardiotoxicity.

Treatment

- Potassium replacement therapy is indicated for: (1) symptomatic hypokalemia; (2) malnutrition; (3) potassium loss associated with vomiting or diarrhea; (4) renal potassium acidosis with hypokalemia; (5) heart failure and digitalis therapy; (6) myocardial infarction with low serum potassium; (7) diabetic ketoacidosis treated with insulin; and (8) adrenocortical hyperactivity.
- **Sustained-release potassium** products are good choices for oral administration because they disperse potassium in the gut gradually, thereby minimizing gastric irritation and ulceration associated with enteric-coated products. **Liquid potassium preparations** are inexpensive but are poorly tolerated because of unpleasant taste, aftertaste, nausea, heartburn, and diarrhea. Salt substitutes are an effective, inexpensive alternative; potassium-rich food sources (i.e., bananas, orange juice) are generally not recommended for chronic supplementation because they often contain less chloride than other potassium sources and may add unwanted calories.
- When *metabolic alkalosis* accompanies hypokalemia, the administration of the **chloride salt** is essential for correction of both the alkalosis and the potassium deficit. **Nonchloride salts** (e.g., phosphate, gluconate) are indicated only for hypokalemia associated with *metabolic acidosis.*
- **IV potassium** (usually 10–20 mEq/h) is indicated when the oral route is not feasible or in the presence of life-threatening hypokalemia (paralysis, arrhythmias). Rates of administration >10–20 mEq/h should be accompanied by ECG monitoring. The maximally tolerated concentration for peripheral-vein administration is 40–60 mEq/L.
- For patients on *diuretic therapy* with serum potassium <3.0 mEq/L (or symptoms), 50–60 mEq/d KCl oral solution or wax matrix can be used. Potassium-sparing diuretics can also be used but should be avoided if the patient has diabetes, chronic renal failure, advanced age, or angiotensin-converting enzyme inhibitor use.
- For edematous patients (i.e., heart failure, cirrhosis with ascites, severe aldosteronism), oral therapy with 40–80 mEq/d should be used for mild

deficits and up to 100–120 mEq/d with careful monitoring for more severe deficits.

HYPERKALEMIA (SERUM POTASSIUM >5.5 mEq/L)

Pathophysiology

- Hyperkalemia associated with normal total body stores may result from redistribution of potassium from the intracellular to the extracellular space (e.g., acidosis, insulin deficiency, cellular injury), and pseudohyperkalemia, an in vitro phenomenon in which the measured serum potassium level is falsely elevated because of potassium release from red blood cells.
- Hyperkalemia associated with elevated total body potassium stores is due to excessive potassium ingestion, reduced potassium excretion (e.g., renal impairment, use of ACE inhibitors), or both.

Clinical Presentation

- Hyperkalemia is manifested clinically as muscle weakness and abnormalities of cardiac conduction. At concentrations ≥6.5 mEq/L muscle twitching, weakness, nausea, and cramping can occur.
- The earliest ECG changes (serum potassium 5.5–6 mEq/L) are peaked T waves and shortening of the QT interval. At 6–7 mEq/L, the PR interval and QRS duration are prolonged. At >7–8 mEq/L, there is widening of the QRS complex and decreased amplitude, and eventual loss of the P wave. At >9–10 mEq/L, the QRS complex merges with the T wave, resulting in a sine-wave pattern. At 10–12 mEq/L, ventricular fibrillation or asystole may occur.

Treatment (Table 76–1)

- Moderate to severe hyperkalemia (>6.5 mEq/L) with symptoms or ECG changes requires immediate treatment.
- **Calcium** administration rapidly reverses ECG manifestations and arrhythmias. Calcium does not lower serum potassium concentrations and, because it is short acting, must be repeated if signs or symptoms recur.
- Promoting intracellular movement of potassium effectively lowers extracellular serum levels (e.g., **IV glucose** and **insulin** infusion, inhaled or IV **β-adrenergic agonist** therapy, or **sodium bicarbonate**).
- **Sodium polystyrene sulfonate** is a cation-exchange resin that removes potassium from the body. It has a slow onset of action and should not be used as monotherapy for patients with ECG changes. Each gram of resin may bind as much as 1 mEq of potassium and release 1–2 mEq of sodium; 40 grams given orally in four divided doses may decrease serum potassium concentrations by 1.0 mEq/L in 24 hours in patients with renal failure. It should be administered with sorbitol to prevent constipation.

TABLE 76–1. Treatment of Hyperkalemia

Medication	Dose	Route of Administration	Mechanism of Action	Expected Result	Onset/Duration
Albuterol	10–20 mg	Nebulized over 10 min	Stimulates Na^+/K^+-ATPase pump	Redistribution of K^+ into the cell	30 min/1–2 h
Calcium chloride	1 g (13.5 mEq)	IV over 5–10 min	Raises threshold potential and reestablishes cardiac excitability	Reverses ECG effects	1–2 min/10–30 min
Dextrose 50%	50 mL (25 g)	IV over 5 min	Increases insulin release	Redistribution of K^+ into cell	30 min/2–6 h
Dextrose 10%	1000 mL (100 g)	IV over 1–2 h	Increases insulin release	Redistribution of K^+ into cell	30 min/2–6 h
Sodium bicarbonate	50–100 mEq	IV over 2–5 min	Increases serum pH	Redistribution of K^+ into cell	30 min/2–6 h
Insulin (regular)	1 unit per 3–5 g dextrose	IV with 10% dextrose SC	Enhances potassium intracellular uptake	Redistribution of K^+ into cell	30 min/2–6 h
Sodium polystyrene sulfonate	15–60 g	Orally or rectally	Exchanges resin Na^+ for K^+	Increase in K^+ elimination	1 h/variable
Hemodialysis	2–4 h	—	Removes from plasma	Increase in K^+ elimination	Immediate/variable

- If hyperkalemia persists, especially if the patient has renal failure, hemodialysis is indicated.

▶ DISORDERS OF CALCIUM HOMEOSTASIS

HYPERCALCEMIA (TOTAL SERUM CALCIUM >10.5 mg/dL)

Pathophysiology

- The most common causes of hypercalcemia are cancer and hyperparathyroidism.

Clinical Presentation

- Mild to moderate hypercalcemia (<13 mg/dL) may be asymptomatic.
- Symptoms of hypercalcemia associated with *malignancy* may have an acute presentation because the onset of hypercalcemia is rapid. A symptom complex characterized by anorexia, nausea and vomiting, constipation, polyuria, polydipsia, and nocturia is common. Patients infrequently present in hypercalcemic crisis, manifested by the acute onset of severe hypercalcemia, acute renal failure, and obtundation. If untreated, hypercalcemic crisis may progress to oliguric renal failure, coma, malignant ventricular arrhythmias, and death.
- Disorders associated with long-standing hypercalcemia (i.e., *hyperparathyroidism*) are more likely to present with metastatic calcification, nephrolithiasis, and chronic renal insufficiency.
- ECG changes associated with hypercalcemia include shortening of the QT interval, and coving of the ST-T wave; very high serum calcium concentrations may cause T wave widening.

Treatment (Figure 76–3)

- Patients with hypercalcemic crisis or symptomatic hypercalcemia should be treated immediately. Asymptomatic patients with mild hypercalcemia may be carefully observed, especially if the underlying condition is treated.
- In patients with functioning kidneys, treatment involves rehydration with IV **normal saline** 200–300 mL/h. Fluid status should be assessed by intake/output or by central venous pressure monitoring.
- After rehydration has been accomplished, loop diuretics such as **furosemide** (40–80 mg IV every 1–4 hours) may be instituted to inhibit calcium resorption and prevent volume overload.
- Saline rehydration and furosemide often decrease serum calcium by 2–3 mg/dL within 24–48 hours.
- Serum potassium and magnesium levels should be monitored during furosemide diuresis.
- **Calcitonin** (4 MRC units/kg SC or IM every 12 hours, or constant IV infusion of 10–12 MRC units/h) rapidly (within 1–2 hours) reduces serum calcium levels and can be used as short-term therapy when saline rehydration is contraindicated.

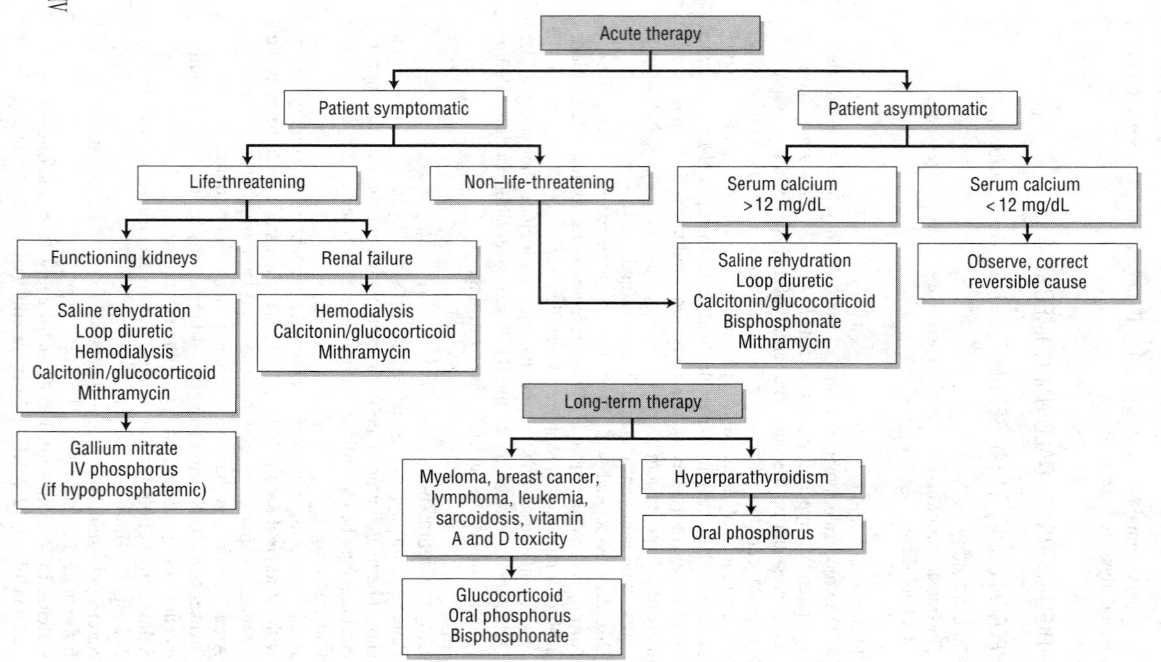

Figure 76–3. Approach to the hypercalcemic patient.

- The bisphosphonates are effective in the treatment of hypercalcemia associated with malignancy. **Pamidronate** (60–90 mg by IV infusion during 24 hours) is preferred because it may be more effective and requires only a single dose. The dose of **etidronate** is 7.5 mg/kg/d by slow IV infusion over 3 hours for 3 days, but calcitonin therapy may be necessary if rapid reduction is required. **Alendronate** and **risedronate** are newer bisphosphonates.
- **Gallium nitrate** (200 mg/m^2/d by continuous IV infusion for 5 consecutive days) is indicated for the treatment of symptomatic hypercalcemia of malignancy not responsive to hydration therapy.
- **Mithramycin** (25 μ/kg IV over 1–3 hours) has an onset within 12 hours and a peak effect within 48–96 hours. Doses may be repeated every 3–4 days as needed, along with frequent determinations of complete blood count, liver function, and renal function. It should be limited to short-term therapy (2–3 weeks) in patients who have not responded to saline rehydration and avoided in patients with thrombocytopenia, liver disease, or renal disease.
- **Glucocorticoids** (40–60 mg/d of **prednisone** or equivalent) are usually effective for hypercalcemia due to multiple myeloma, leukemia, lymphoma, sarcoidosis, and hypervitaminoses A and D, but the onset is slow.

HYPOCALCEMIA (TOTAL SERUM CALCIUM <8.5 mg/dL)

Pathophysiology

- Vitamin D deficiency states resulting in hypocalcemia include nutritional deficiency, GI disease, gastric surgery, chronic pancreatitis, small-bowel disease, and intestinal resection and bypass surgery.
- Symptomatic hypocalcemia most commonly occurs because of parathyroid gland dysfunction secondary to surgical procedures involving the thyroid, parathyroid, and neck.
- Hypoalbuminemia is a common cause of laboratory hypocalcemia.
- Hypomagnesemia may be associated with severe symptomatic hypocalcemia that is unresponsive to calcium replacement therapy.

Clinical Presentation

- The hallmark sign of acute hypocalcemia is tetany, which manifests as paresthesias around the mouth and in the extremities, muscle spasms and cramps, carpopedal spasms, and, rarely, laryngospasm and bronchospasm.
- Cardiovascular manifestations result in ECG changes characterized by a prolonged QT interval and symptoms of decreased myocardial contractility often associated with heart failure.

Treatment

- Hypocalcemia associated with hypoalbuminemia requires no treatment because ionized plasma calcium concentrations are normal.
- Acute, symptomatic hypocalcemia requires parenteral administration of soluble calcium salts.

- The initial goal is to administer 100–300 mg of elemental calcium IV over 5–10 min (not >60 mg/min).
- The initial bolus is only effective for 1–2 hours and should be followed by elemental calcium 0.5–2.0 mg/kg/h by continuous IV infusion usually for 2–4 hours and then by a maintenance dose of 0.3–0.5 mg/kg/h.
- **Calcium gluconate** (2–3 grams) is preferred over **calcium chloride** (1 grams) for peripheral administration because the latter is more irritating to veins.

- If hypomagnesemia is present, **magnesium** supplementation is indicated.
- Chronic hypocalcemia from hypoparathyroidism and vitamin D deficient states may be managed by oral calcium supplementation (e.g., 1–3 g/d of elemental calcium). If serum calcium does not normalize, a **vitamin D** preparation should be added.
- Treatment of vitamin D-deficient hypocalcemia should be individualized depending upon the underlying cause (see Chapter 78).

▶ DISORDERS OF MAGNESIUM HOMEOSTASIS

HYPERMAGNESEMIA (SERUM MAGNESIUM >2 mEq/L)

Pathophysiology

- Hypermagnesemia most commonly occurs in renal insufficiency, when glomerular filtration is <30 mL/min.
- Hypermagnesemia may also be associated with use of magnesium-containing laxatives or antacids in patients with renal failure, antacids or parenteral fluids in patients with multiple-system organ failure, or IV solutions in obstetric patients.

Clinical Presentation

- Hypermagnesemia may cause diminished or absent deep tendon reflexes, muscle weakness, and respiratory depression, depending on the serum magnesium concentration.
- CNS depression may result in lethargy and sedation, which may progress to stupor and coma, especially at high serum concentrations (≥6 mEq/L).
- Hypotension and cutaneous vasodilation may occur at serum levels >3 mEq/L. Sinus bradycardia, first-degree heart block, nodal rhythms, or bundle branch block may occur at ≥5–10 mEq/L. Complete heart block progressing to asystole and cardiac arrest may occur at ≥14–15 mEq/L.

Treatment

- Administration of IV calcium (100–200 mg of elemental calcium) is indicated to antagonize the neuromuscular and cardiovascular effects of magnesium. Repeated doses may be necessary in life-threatening situations.

- Hemodialysis is the treatment of choice for patients with renal dysfunction.
- For patients with adequate renal function and moderate hypermagnesemia, IV saline and furosemide should be administered as described for hypercalcemia.

HYPOMAGNESEMIA (SERUM MAGNESIUM <1 mEq/L)

Pathophysiology

- Dietary magnesium deprivation rarely leads to significant magnesium depletion unless it is prolonged.
- Malabsorption syndromes associated with hypomagnesemia include intestinal mucosal diseases (e.g., celiac sprue, Whipple's disease, radiation enteritis), massive intestinal resection, and pancreatic insufficiency.
- Magnesium losses exceeding intake may occur in GI disorders secondary to loss of intestinal fluids.
- Renal magnesium wasting may be due to intrinsic tubular disorders or drug-, hormone-, ion-, or nutrient-induced renal tubular magnesium losses.
- The most common cause of drug-induced hypomagnesemia is chronic diuretic therapy, especially in elderly patients, alcohol abusers, and patients consuming diets low in magnesium. Aminoglycosides, amphotericin B, foscarnet, pentamidine, cisplatin, and cyclosporine are also associated with magnesium wasting.

Clinical Presentation

- Manifestations of hypomagnesemia include neuromuscular hyperactivity (muscle twitching and tremor, muscle weakness, hyperreflexia, paresthesias), psychiatric effects (depression, delirium, agitation, confusion, hallucinations), and cardiac effects (premature ventricular beats, ventricular fibrillation or tachycardia, torsades de pointes).
- ECG changes are nonspecific and include wide QRS complexes and tall, peaked T waves in moderate deficiency. Prolonged PR, QRS, and QT intervals; ST-segment depression; and flat, broad T waves with prominent U waves occur in severe deficiency.
- Hypocalcemia is a prominent manifestation of magnesium deficiency, so serum calcium concentration should be assessed.

Treatment (Table 76–2)

- Patients who are symptomatic or have serum magnesium levels <1 mEq/L (1.2 mg/dL) should receive parenteral magnesium therapy.
- Patients with asymptomatic hypomagnesemia and levels >1 mEq/L (1.2 mg/dL) are treated with oral magnesium supplements.
- Patients with renal insufficiency are treated with lower doses and must have serum levels monitored frequently.
- Magnesium replacement must be continued for ≥3–5 days because 50% of the dose is excreted in the urine.

TABLE 76–2. Guidelines for Treatment of Magnesium Deficiency in Adults

1. Serum magnesium <1 mEq/L (1.2 mg/dL) with life-threatening symptoms (seizure, arrhythmia)

   Day 1

   2 g $MgSO_4$[a] mixed with 6 mL 0.9% NaCl in 10-mL syringe IV push over 1 min.
   Follow with 0.5 mEq Mg^{2+}/kg LBW[b] IV infusion over 5–6 h, then 0.5 mEq Mg^{2+}/kg LBW IV infusion over 17–18 h.

   Days 2–5

   0.5 mEq Mg^{2+}/kg LBW/d divided in maintenance IV fluids.
2. Serum magnesium <1 mEq/L (1.2 mg/dL) without life-threatening symptoms

   Day 1

   1 mEq Mg^{2+}/kg LBW/d as continuous IV infusion, or divided into five doses and given IM every 4 h.

   Days 2–5

   0.5 mEq Mg^{2+}/kg LBW/d as continuous IV infusion or divided and given IM every 6–8 h.
3. Serum magnesium >1 mEq/L (1.2 mg/dL) and <1.5 mEq/L (1.8 mg/dL) without symptoms

   As in no. 2 above,
   Milk of Magnesia 5 mL four times daily as tolerated,
   Magnesium-containing antacid 15 mL three times daily as tolerated, or
   Magnesium oxide tablets 300 mg four times daily, increase to two tablets four times daily as tolerated.

[a] 1 g $MgSO_4$ = 8.1 mEq Mg^{2+}.
[b] LBW = lean body weight.

- Rapid IV bolus injection is avoided because of flushing, sweating, and a sensation of warmth. Direct IV administration of 50% magnesium sulfate may produce pain and venosclerosis; therefore, it should be diluted to 20% before administration. Intramuscular injections are painful and therefore reserved for situations in which peripheral venous access is not readily available.

▶ DISORDERS OF PHOSPHORUS HOMEOSTASIS

HYPERPHOSPHATEMIA (SERUM PHOSPHORUS >4.5 mg/dL)

Pathophysiology

- The most common cause of hyperphosphatemia is decreased phosphorus excretion secondary to decreased glomerular filtration rate (GFR).
- Hypoparathyroidism results in increased renal tubular reabsorption of phosphorus and may result in hyperphosphatemia.
- Iatrogenic causes include sodium phosphate enemas, laxatives containing phosphate salts, and IV phosphorus for treatment of hypercalcemia.
- Rhabdomyolysis and chemotherapy of acute leukemia and lymphoma may release large amounts of phosphorus from intracellular stores.

Clinical Presentation

- The major effect of hyperphosphatemia is related to the development of hypocalcemia and damage resulting from calcium phosphate deposits.
- Metastatic calcification leading to band keratopathy, "red eye," pruritus, vascular calcification, and periarticular calcification is most common in renal failure.
- Soft-tissue calcifications in the conjunctiva, skin, heart, cornea, lung, gastric mucosa, and kidney may also occur in chronic renal failure.
- Hyperphosphatemia associated with chronic renal disease may result in azotemic osteodystrophy (see Chapter 78).

Treatment

- The most effective way to treat hyperphosphatemia is to decrease phosphate absorption from the GI tract with phosphate binders (e.g., antacids containing divalent cations). Because of concerns over aluminum toxicity, calcium salts are the preferred phosphate binders for chronic renal failure.
- Severe symptomatic hyperphosphatemia manifesting as hypocalcemia and tetany is treated by the IV administration of calcium salts.

HYPOPHOSPHATEMIA (SERUM PHOSPHORUS <2.5 mg/dL)

Pathophysiology

- Phosphate depletion may be caused by dietary deficiency or chronic ingestion of phosphate-binding substances (e.g., sucralfate, calcium carbonate, and aluminum/magnesium-containing antacids).
- Excess renal excretion can occur with the marked diuretic phase that accompanies recovery from extensive third-degree burns.
- Rapid refeeding of malnourished patients with high-carbohydrate, high-calorie nutritional diets with inadequate amounts of supplemental phosphorus may result in severe symptomatic hypophosphatemia.
- Severe and prolonged respiratory alkalosis may cause profound hypophosphatemia because of intracellular shifts of phosphorus.
- Patients with diabetic ketoacidosis (DKA) may present with hyperphosphatemia, but DKA treatment may ultimately result in hypophosphatemia.
- Malnutrition, poor dietary intake, diarrhea, vomiting, and phosphate-binding antacids may contribute to the hypophosphatemia of alcoholism.

Clinical Presentation

- CNS manifestations of severe hypophosphatemia include a progressive syndrome of irritability, apprehension, weakness, numbness, paresthesias, dysarthria, confusion, obtundation, seizures, and coma.
- Skeletal muscle dysfunction in severe hypophosphatemia may result in myalgia, weakness, and potentially fatal rhabdomyolysis. Respiratory muscle weakness and diaphragmatic contractile dysfunction may cause acute respiratory failure.

TABLE 76–3. Phosphorus Replacement Therapy

Moderate Hypophosphatemia (serum phosphorus 1.0–2.5 mg/dL)
Oral therapy
1.5–2 g (50–60 mmol) phosphorus per d, divided into three or four doses
Parenteral therapy
0.15 mmol/kg LBW infused in 250–1000 mL D_5W over 12 h; repeat until serum phosphorus >2 mg/dL
Severe Hypophosphatemia (serum phosphorus <1 mg/dL)
Parenteral therapy
0.25 mmol/kg LBW in 250–500 mL D_5W by infusion over 4–6 h; repeat until serum phosphorus >2 mg/dL

- Congestive cardiomyopathy, hemolysis, increased risk of infection, and platelet defects may also occur.

Treatment

- The route and dose of **phosphorus** replacement therapy is determined by the severity of hypophosphotemia (Table 76–3).
- Patients should be closely monitored with frequent serum phosphorus determinations and assessment of serum calcium concentration, especially if phosphorus is given IV or if renal dysfunction is present.
- Patients with moderate hypophosphatemia and concomitant renal dysfunction should receive reduced daily oral doses (i.e., 1 gram or approximately 30 mmol of phosphorus).
- Phosphorus 12–15 mmol/L should be routinely added to IV hyperalimentation solution to prevent hypophosphatemia.

See Chapter 48, Electrolyte Homeostasis, authored by Nathan J. Schultz, PharmD, BCPS, and Ralph A. Slaker, PharmD, for a more detailed discussion of this topic.

Chapter 77

▶ RENAL FAILURE: ACUTE

▶ DEFINITIONS

- *Acute renal failure* is an abrupt decline in renal function characterized by the inability of the kidneys to excrete metabolic waste products (nitrogenous wastes and water) and maintain acid–base balance. The most commonly used definition is an increase in the serum creatinine concentration of 0.5 mg/dL when the baseline creatinine is <3.0 mg/dL, or an increase of 1.0 mg/dL when the baseline is ≥ 3.0 mg/dL.
- *Azotemia* is an elevation in nitrogenous waste products (e.g., creatinine and urea nitrogen).
- *Uremia* is the clinical syndrome resulting from azotemia characterized by anorexia, nausea, vomiting, and mental status changes.

▶ PATHOPHYSIOLOGY

CLASSIFICATION

The classification of acute renal failure into broad categories based on precipitating factors facilitates diagnosis and patient management.

Prerenal Azotemia

- Prerenal acute renal failure results from hypoperfusion of the renal parenchyma, with or without systemic arterial hypotension.
  - Renal hypoperfusion with hypotension may be caused by a decline in intravascular volume (e.g., hemorrhage, dehydration) or a decline in effective blood volume (e.g., heart failure, liver failure).
  - Renal hypoperfusion without hypotension most commonly results from bilateral renal artery occlusion or unilateral occlusion in a patient with a single functioning kidney.

Functional Acute Renal Failure

- Functional acute renal failure is a reversible decline in glomerular ultrafiltrate production secondary to a reduced glomerular hydrostatic pressure without damage to the kidney itself.
- The decline in glomerular hydrostatic pressure is a consequence of changes in glomerular afferent (vasoconstriction) and efferent (vasodilation) arteriolar circumference.
- This condition occurs in individuals who have reduced effective blood volume (e.g., heart failure, cirrhosis, severe pulmonary disease, hypoalbuminemia) or renovascular disease (e.g., renal artery stenosis) and cannot compensate for changes in afferent or efferent arteriolar tone.
- Disorders that result in afferent arteriolar vasoconstriction include hypercalcemia and the administration of cyclosporine and NSAIDs.

Decreases in efferent arteriolar resistance usually result from administration of ACE inhibitors.

Acute Intrinsic Renal Failure

- Acute intrinsic renal failure results from damage to the kidney itself such as:
  - Small vessel vasculitis (e.g., polyarteritis nodosa, hemolytic uremic syndrome, malignant hypertension) or cholesterol emboli.
  - Acute glomerular inflammation (acute glomerulonephritis) from systemic lupus erythematosus, antiglomerular basement membrane disease, or other precipitating causes.
  - Renal tubular injury (acute tubular necrosis [ATN]) secondary to ischemia from severe hypotension or vasoconstricting drugs, exogenous toxins (e.g., contrast agents, heavy metals, aminoglycosides, amphotericin B, foscarnet), and endogenous toxins (e.g., myoglobin, hemoglobin, uric acid).
  - Acute interstitial nephritis from medications or infections.

Postrenal Obstruction

- The most common cause of obstructive uropathy is bladder outlet obstruction, which may be caused by benign prostatic hyperplasia or cervical cancer.

PHYSIOLOGY

- Pathophysiologic processes can affect the four basic components of the kidney: the vasculature, glomeruli, tubules, and interstitium surrounding the other three parts. The clinical manifestations of acute renal failure differ depending on which components are involved.
- Many texts divide the clinical course of ATN into an initial, oliguric, and recovery phase, but this approach is questionable because recovery from ATN does not begin at a defined time from onset of renal failure. Rather, recovery from ATN occurs 10–14 days after the last insult to the kidney.

▶ CLINICAL PRESENTATION

- A change in voiding habits (increased urinary frequency or nocturia) suggests a urinary concentrating defect.
- A decrease in the force of the urinary stream suggests an obstructive process.
- Cola-colored urine, indicating blood in the urine, is common in acute glomerulonephritis. If the accompanying proteinuria is heavy, the patient may note excessive foaming of the urine in the toilet.
- Bilateral flank pain suggests swelling of the kidneys secondary to either acute glomerulonephritis or acute interstitial nephritis.
- Recent onset of severe headaches suggests the development of hypertension as a result of acute renal failure.
- A recent increase in weight secondary to salt and water retention suggests the onset of renal failure.

▶ DIAGNOSIS

- Rapid determination of the etiology of acute renal failure is essential because a delay may result in a more severe nephrologic injury.

MEDICAL HISTORY AND PHYSICAL EXAMINATION

- The medical history, previous laboratory data, and recent drug history may suggest whether the renal failure is acute or chronic.
- Many physical findings suggest the diagnosis of acute renal failure (Table 77–1).
- Significant renal injury can occur before serum creatinine increases, so clinicians must pay attention to subtle changes in weight, blood pressure, and urine output to diagnose the onset of acute renal failure.
- Acute anuria (<50 mL urine/24 h) is secondary either to complete urinary obstruction or a catastrophic event (e.g., shock). Oliguria (≤400 mL urine/24 h) suggests prerenal azotemia, functional acute renal failure, or acute intrinsic renal failure. Nonoliguric renal failure (>400 mL urine/24 h) usually results from acute intrinsic renal failure or incomplete urinary obstruction.

LABORATORY EVALUATION

- Urinalysis revealing a high urinary specific gravity, in the absence of glucosuria or mannitol administration, suggests an intact urinary concentrating mechanism and prerenal azotemia or functional acute renal failure. Proteinuria and hematuria suggest glomerular injury. Glucosuria, aminoaciduria, and phosphaturia suggest acute proximal tubular dysfunction. A benign urine sediment suggests prerenal azotemia, functional acute renal failure, or urinary obstruction. The presence of red blood cells and red blood cell casts indicates a glomerular injury. The finding of white blood cells and white blood cell casts results from interstitial inflammation (i.e., interstitial nephritis), which can be secondary to an allergic, granulomatous, or infectious process.
- Simultaneous measurement of serum and urinary chemistries helps determine the etiology (Table 77–2). The equation for the calculation of the fractional excretion of sodium (FE_{Na}) is:

$$FE_{Na} = (U_{Na} \times S_{Cr} \times 100)/(U_{Cr} \times S_{Na})$$

  where U_{Na} = urine sodium, S_{Cr} = serum creatinine, U_{Cr} = urine creatinine, and S_{Na} = serum sodium.
- A low urinary sodium concentration and low FE_{Na} (<1%) in a patient with oliguria suggest prerenal azotemia or functional acute renal failure; a FE_{Na} >1–2% suggests acute intrinsic renal failure. XIV
- A highly concentrated urine (>500 mOsm/L) suggests stimulation of antidiuretic hormone, indicating prerenal azotemia secondary to hypovolemia or a decrease in effective blood volume; the urine creatinine to serum creatinine ratio usually exceeds 40.

TABLE 77–1. Physical Examination Findings in Acute Renal Failure

Physical Examination Finding	Clinical Implication If Present	Possible Diagnoses	Category of Acute Renal Failure	Possible Confounding Factors
Vital Signs				
Orthostatic hypotension	Intravascular volume status	Volume depletion	Prerenal azotemia	Antihypertensive therapy Neuropathies (diabetes mellitus)
Skin				
Tenting	Volume status	Volume depletion	Prerenal azotemia	Advanced age
Rash	Allergic reaction	Hypersensitivity reaction	Acute interstitial nephritis	Contact dermatitis
Petechiae	Platelet dysfunction	Thrombotic thrombocytopenic purpura Hemolytic uremic syndrome Sepsis	Acute intrinsic renal failure—vasculitis	Bone marrow suppression Antiplatelet drugs
Splinter hemorrhages Janeway lesions Osler's nodes	Embolic phenomenon	Endocarditis	Acute intrinsic renal failure—acute Glomerulonephritis	Small vessel vasculitis
Edema	Volume status	Total body volume overload	Prerenal azotemia *not* likely	Right heart failure, deep venous thrombosis
HEENT				
Hollenhorst plaque	Embolic phenomenon	Cholesterol emboli	Acute intrinsic renal failure—vascular	Plaque must be in aorta to affect kidney
Roth spots	Embolic phenomenon	Endocarditis	Acute intrinsic renal failure—acute glomerulonephritis	Other systemic infection

Heart				
S_3 heart sound	Left ventricular dysfunction	Heart failure	Prerenal azotemia	Preexisting compensated heart failure (HF)
New murmur (particularly diastolic murmurs)	Valvular dysfunction	Endocarditis	Acute intrinsic renal failure—acute glomerulonephritis	Preexisting valvular disease Hyperdynamic state
Lung				
Rales	Pulmonary congestion	Pulmonary edema with volume overload or left ventricular dysfunction	Prerenal azotemia	Compensated HF
Abdomen				
Renal artery bruit	Arterial integrity	Renal artery stenosis	Prerenal azotemia	Generalized atherosclerosis
Ascites	Elevated venous pressure	Liver failure or right heart failure	Prerenal azotemia Hepatorenal syndrome	Peritoneal membrane disorder (tumor)
Bladder distention	Bladder capacity	Bladder outlet obstruction	Postobstruction renal failure	
GU				
Prostatic enlargement	Prostate enlargement	Prostatic hypertrophy or cancer	Postobstruction renal failure	Nonenlarged prostate does not exclude obstruction
GYN				
Abnormal bimanual exam	Uterine size Cervical status	Bilateral ureteral obstruction or cervical cancer	Postobstruction renal failure	

TABLE 77–2. Diagnostic Parameters for Differentiating Causes of Acute Renal Failure[a]

Lab Test	Prerenal Azotemia	Acute Intrinsic Renal Failure	Postrenal Obstruction
Urine sediment	Normal	Casts, cellular debris	Cellular debris
Urinary RBC	None	2–4+	Variable
Urinary WBC	None	2–4+	1+
Urine sodium	<20	>40	>40
FE_{Na} (%)	<1	>1–2	Variable
Urine osmolality/ serum osmolality	>1.5	<1.3	<1.5
Urine creatinine/ plasma creatinine	>40:1	<20:1	<20:1
BUN/S_{Cr}	>20	15	15

[a]Common laboratory tests are listed that are used to classify the cause of acute renal failure. Functional acute renal failure, which is not included in this table, would have laboratory values similar to those seen in prerenal azotemia. However, the urine osmolality to plasma osmolality ratios may not exceed 1.5 depending on the circulating levels of antidiuretic hormone. The laboratory results listed under acute intrinsic renal failure are those seen in acute tubular necrosis, the most common cause of acute intrinsic renal failure.

- Estimation of glomerular filtration rate is difficult because this patient population is usually not in a steady-state situation. Methods of estimating the glomerular filtration rate and creatinine clearance from serum creatinine determinations (e.g., Cockcroft–Gault, Jelliffe equations) assume the patient has stable renal function. Creatinine clearance can be estimated in patients with acute renal failure using equations specially designed for nonsteady-state conditions.

DIAGNOSTIC PROCEDURES

- In hospitalized patients with previously normal renal function, insertion of a urinary catheter into the bladder is usually adequate to exclude postrenal obstruction as the cause.
- For outpatients presenting with acute renal failure, renal ultrasound is instrumental in determining whether the renal failure is acute or chronic and whether obstruction is present.
- A plain film radiograph of the abdomen will document the presence of two kidneys and also provide a check for renal stones.
- If the possibility of renal artery obstruction exists, a radioisotope scan or renal angiography may be required.
- Cystoscopy with retrograde pyelography may be helpful if the possibility of obstruction exists.
- Intravenous pyelography is rarely used in the work-up of acute renal failure.

- A percutaneous renal biopsy may be indicated if the etiology of the acute renal failure is unclear despite a careful history, physical examination, and the above diagnostic tests.

▶ DESIRED OUTCOME

The goals of therapy are to identify and remove the underlying cause; prevent progression to irreversible renal injury; and provide adequate metabolic, electrolyte, and fluid control until recovery. Unfortunately, little can be done to hasten recovery.

▶ TREATMENT

PREVENTION OF ACUTE RENAL FAILURE

- Preventive therapy should be instituted in patients at risk for developing acute renal failure due to nephrotoxic drug therapy or procedures.
- The *least nephrotoxic alternative* should be used whenever possible. Examples of this approach include substituting β-lactam antibiotics for aminoglycosides, fluconazole or lipid-based amphotericin B for amphotericin B, and low- for high-osmolality contrast media.
- *Adequate hydration* (e.g., with 0.45% or 0.9% NaCl) prior to nephrotoxic events improves renal perfusion, lowers tubular workload by reducing the need for urinary concentration, and dilutes the nephrotoxin concentration within the tubule.
- *Sodium loading* prior to nephrotoxic events (e.g., amphotericin therapy) enhances the tubular glomerular reflex and decreases the amount of the nephrotoxin delivered to the distal nephron.

TREATMENT OF ESTABLISHED ACUTE RENAL FAILURE

- Knowledge of volume status is critical because rapid fluid resuscitation can improve renal perfusion, rescue hypoxic tubules, and prevent ATN if oliguric prerenal azotemia is present. However, fluids would be harmful if oliguric ATN is established.
- **Diuretics** are the most common therapy used to change from oliguria to nonoliguria. Although diuretics do not improve patient outcome in established acute renal failure, secondary considerations, such as increased urine output and reduced need for renal replacement therapy, have been documented with diuretic use. Both classes of first-line therapy, loop diuretics and **mannitol**, have unique advantages and disadvantages.
  - A typical starting dose of mannitol (20%) is 12.5–25 g IV over 3–5 minutes. Disadvantages include IV route, risk of hyperosmolality, and need for monitoring because mannitol can contribute to acute renal failure.
  - In equipotent doses, the parenteral loop diuretics have similar efficacy in acute renal failure. The equipotency ratio of parenteral

bumetanide:torsemide:furosemide in patients with normal renal function is 1:20:40, but in renal failure this ratio changes to 1:11:11.
  - Nearly all studies in acute renal failure were conducted with furosemide, and it is commonly used for reasons of familiarity and cost. The initial dose is 40–80 mg IV. If there is no response, a higher dose can be given an hour later. Furosemide or equivalent should be followed with intermittent dosing or continuous infusion.
  - Combination therapy with a loop diuretic and a diuretic from a different pharmacologic class and with a different mechanism of action can be effective in overcoming diuretic resistance. **Metolazone** is commonly used because, unlike other thiazides, it produces effective diuresis at glomerular filtration rates <20 mL/min.
- Low-dose **dopamine** (0.5–2 μg/kg/min IV infusion) may increase urine output, but it should be used cautiously because it has not been shown to improve patient outcome.
- Exposure to nephrotoxins (e.g., contrast dye, aminoglycosides, NSAIDs, high-dose dopamine and other vasoconstrictors) should be *minimized* to avoid prolonging the recovery from acute ischemic renal disease, which usually takes 14–21 days.

RENAL REPLACEMENT THERAPIES

- The indications for renal replacement therapy in acute renal failure are *a*cid–base abnormalities, *e*lectrolyte imbalance, *i*ntoxications, fluid *o*verload, and *u*remia (AEIOU).
- The advantages and disadvantages of intermittent and continuous renal replacement therapies are listed in Table 77–3 (see also Chapter 74.)
- In contrast with chronic renal failure, acute renal failure causes more instability in terms of volume, electrolyte, and azotemic status. Therefore, renal replacement therapies are more common for acute renal failure.

▶ EVALUATION OF THERAPEUTIC OUTCOMES

- Close monitoring of the patient's status is essential during the recovery period, which may occur quickly, within a few months, or never.
- Azotemic control can be assessed in the physical examination by looking for signs of uremia. A friction rub on chest examination can be a sign of a pericardial effusion caused by uremia. Fluid status should be assessed by checking lung sounds (e.g., rales) and inspecting for edema.
- Measurements of daily weight and fluid intake/output help gauge day-to-day recovery, especially in patients receiving continuous hemofiltration or hemodiafiltration. Urine output may be the best single test to assess recovery from acute renal failure.
- Critically ill patients with acute renal failure frequently receive continuous hemodynamic monitoring via a Swan–Ganz catheter to assess fluid status and determine fluid replacement needs.

TABLE 77–3. Advantages and Disadvantages of Common Renal Replacement Therapies for Acute Renal Failure

	Intermittent Hemodialysis	Intermittent Hemofiltration	Peritoneal Dialysis	Slow Continuous Ultrafiltration (SCUF)	Continuous Arteriovenous Hemofiltration (CAVH)	Continuous Venovenous Hemofiltration (CVVH)	Continuous Arteriovenous Hemodiafiltration (CAVHD)	Continuous Venovenous Hemodiafiltration (CVVHD)
Solute control	Usually adequate	Inadequate	Inadequate	Inadequate	Inadequate	Adequate	Adequate	Adequate
Volume control	Variable	Adequate	Adequate	Adequate	Adequate	Adequate	Adequate	Adequate
Hemodynamic stability	Variable	Well tolerated	Well tolerated	Well tolerated	Well tolerated	Well tolerated	Well tolerated	Well tolerated
Access	Venous	Venous	Peritoneal	Arterial and venous	Arterial and venous	Venous	Arterial and venous	Venous
Anticoagulation	Short duration	Short duration	None	Continuous	Continuous high dose	Continuous low dose	Continuous high dose	Continuous low dose
Technical complexity	High	High	Low	Low	Low	Moderate	Moderate	High
Workload	Intermittent	Intermittent	Low	Low	Low	Moderate	Moderate	High
Drug dosing ease	Many published recommendations	Difficult	Difficult	Negligible drug removal	Difficult	Many published recommendations	Difficult	Difficult
Convective clearance (small and middle molecules)	Mixed	Minimal	Moderate	Moderate	Large	Large	Large	Large
Dialytic clearance (small molecules)	Large	None	Large	None	None	None	Large	Large
Common complications	Hypotension	Hypotension	Hyperglycemia, atelectasis, peritonitis	Arterial bleeding, hypotension	Arterial bleeding, filter clotting	Hypotension	Arterial bleeding, ↑ serum lactate	↑ Serum lactate, hypotension

- Urine collection and measurement of urinary creatinine may be beneficial to assess changes in renal function. Urinalysis also can help discern the cause of acute renal failure, so attention should be given to the presence of urinary sediment, specific gravity, and sodium concentration in order to decide on a therapy to treat the cause of the acute renal failure. Blood urea nitrogen and creatinine measurements are useful, but creatinine clearance calculations may be unreliable in patients with changing serum creatinine values.
- Therapeutic drug monitoring should be performed frequently, not only because these patients are not at steady state, but also because of the paucity of data regarding drug disposition in acute renal failure (see Chapter 75).
- Serum electrolytes should be monitored daily with particular attention given to potassium, phosphorus, and calcium in early acute renal failure.
- Arterial blood gas determinations can help determine the respiratory status of critically ill patients and assess whether the kidney is able to compensate for any acid–base disturbances.
- Peritoneal and vascular access sites should be monitored routinely for signs of infection (erythema or purulent drainage).
- Patients should also be monitored for other complications of acute renal failure such as hyperkalemia (Chapter 76), cardiovascular complications (Chapters 5 and 7), stress ulcers (Chapter 27), nausea and vomiting (Chapter 25), and neurologic sequelae.

See Chapter 41, Acute Renal Failure, authored by Bruce A. Mueller, PharmD, FCCP, BCPS, and William L. Macias, MD, PhD, for a more detailed discussion of this topic.

Chapter 78

▶ RENAL FAILURE: CHRONIC

▶ DEFINITION

Chronic renal failure is a progressive process that may occur even when the primary renal insult has been corrected or treated, or become inactive. Adaptive mechanisms may play a major role as evidenced by the common histologic appearance of kidneys from patients with end-stage renal disease (ESRD).

▶ OVERVIEW

PATHOPHYSIOLOGY

- Many diseases of the kidney, either idiopathic or secondary to systemic illness, ultimately result in ESRD.
- Diabetes and hypertension are the most common causes of ESRD in the United States. Hyperlipidemia is a major risk factor for progression of renal disease.
- As renal disease progresses, adaptations take place in functioning (remnant) nephrons that blunt the drop in total glomerular filtration rate (GFR). Changes in other renal functions (e.g., hydroxylation of vitamin D), however, are not preserved.
- Although there are multiple primary causes of renal injury, adaptive hyperfiltration ultimately contributes to glomerular hypertension, which plays a significant role in progressive loss of renal function. When creatinine clearance (CrCl) falls to 25–40 mL/min, injury usually progresses to ESRD regardless of the primary etiology of kidney disease.
- Although exact pathogenic mechanisms have not been identified, hemodynamic changes at the glomerulus influence and/or regulate progression of renal disease. Increased glomerular capillary plasma flow and glomerular capillary hydraulic pressure lead to glomerular hyperfiltration. Glomerular hyperfiltration and hypertension lead to progressive glomerular sclerosis and development of overt proteinuria. Systemic hypertension is not required for development of glomerular hyperfiltration and hypertension but, when present, may amplify the pathologic effects of intrarenal changes.

CLINICAL MANIFESTATIONS

- Clinical course of progressive renal disease can be divided into four stages. Accompanying signs and symptoms and laboratory parameters are described in Figure 78–1.

DESIRED OUTCOME

The ultimate goal of therapy is to prevent progression of renal disease. Additional goals include the prevention and management of complica-

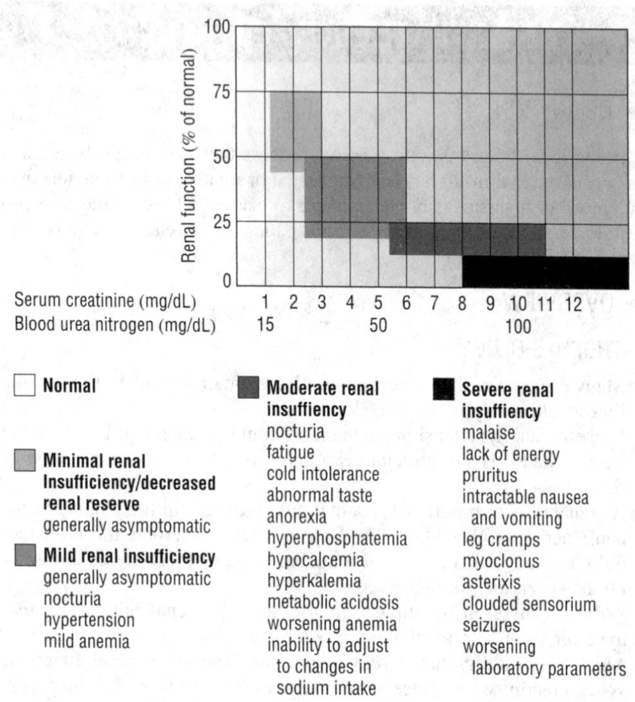

Figure 78–1. Stages of chronic renal disease.

tions such as anemia, secondary hyperparathyroidism, hyperlipidemia, hypertension, and renal osteodystrophy.

TREATMENT

Diabetics

- Early detection of microalbuminuria in the diabetic patient facilitates therapeutic intervention that can slow progression of renal disease and other vascular complications (Figure 78–2).
- Adequate blood pressure control can reduce the rate of decline in GFR and albuminuria in hypertensive patients with either type I or II diabetes mellitus.
- **Angiotensin-converting enzyme inhibitors** (ACEI) have been shown to decrease proteinuria and preserve GFR independent of blood pressure control. ACEI, nondihydropyridine calcium channel blockers

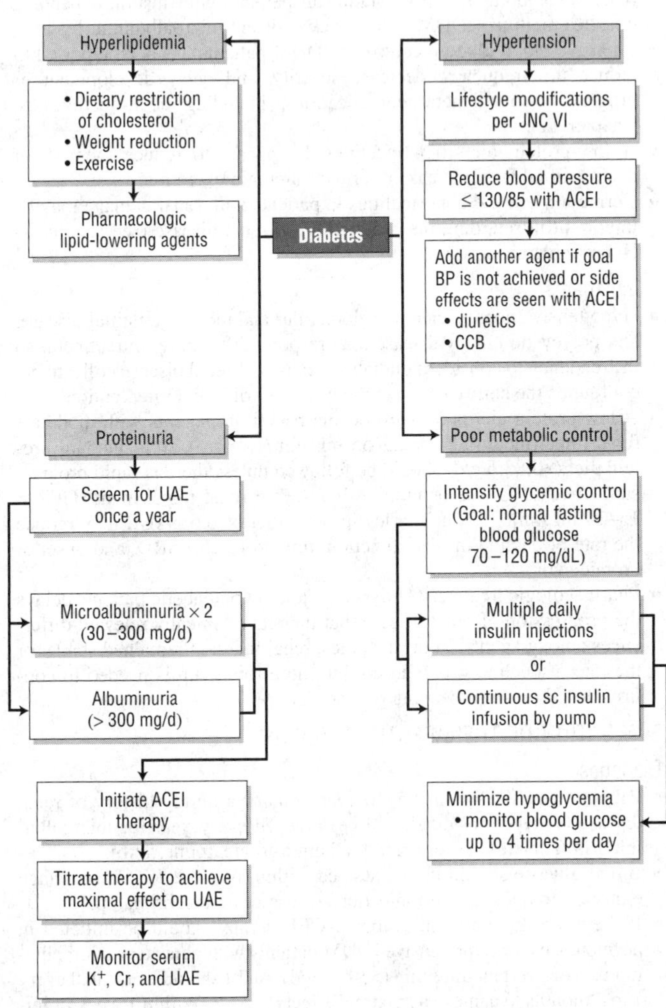

Figure 78–2. Therapeutic strategies to prevent progression of renal disease in diabetic individuals. UAE, urinary albumin excretion; CCB, calcium channel blocker; sc, subcutaneous; ACEI, angiotensin-converting enzyme inhibitor; JNC VI, sixth report of the Joint National Committee on Prevention, Detection, Evaluation, and Treatment of High Blood Pressure.

XIV

(CCBs), or both should be started in patients with insulin-dependent diabetes mellitus (IDDM) who have persistent microalbuminuria.

- Intensive blood glucose control in IDDM patients has been reported to reduce the frequency, decrease severity, and delay development or progression of diabetic complications, including nephropathy (see Chapter 17).
- A low-protein diet (0.5–0.85 g/kg/d) appears to reduce the risk of decline in GFR or increase in urinary albumin excretion.
- Correction of lipid abnormalities in patients with renal damage may be important in retarding the progression of renal disease (see section on Hyperlipidemia).

Nondiabetics

- Hypertensive nephrosclerosis, glomerular and tubulointerstitial disease, and polycystic kidney disease may respond differently to treatment, so the tendency to consider nondiabetic causes of renal disease collectively confounds the ability to detect the benefit of different interventions.
- A low-protein diet is of questionable benefit in patients with moderate renal impairment (GFR = 25–55 mL/min/1.73 m^2), so a standard protein diet (>0.8 g/kg/d) should be followed unless there is rapid progression of renal failure or uremia. For severe renal impairment (GFR = 13–24 mL/min/1.73 m^2), a low-protein diet of 0.6 g/kg/d may reduce the rate of decline in renal function, time to reach ESRD, and onset of uremic symptoms.
- Pharmacologic treatment of hypertension in nondiabetic patients delays the progression of renal disease, but there are clinically relevant differences among agents. In most studies, renal function remained stable, or the rate of decline was reduced, but more follow-up is needed to confirm that short-term benefits persist.

EVALUATION OF THERAPEUTIC OUTCOME

Diabetics

- Patients with IDDM for >5–10 years, and/or a family history of renal disease or hypertension should be screened every year for microalbuminuria (annual UAE or urinary albumin-to-creatinine ratio).
- Blood glucose should be maintained within, or close to, normal range either by frequent insulin injections or use of an insulin pump.
- If there are no contraindications, ACEI therapy should be initiated in normotensive or hypertensive IDDM patients with persistent microalbuminuria or overt albuminuria (>300 mg/d). ACEI should be titrated every 1 to 3 months to achieve a maximal effect on UAE. Within 1 week of initiating or increasing a dose of an ACEI, serum creatinine and potassium should be evaluated to detect abrupt reductions in GFR or hyperkalemia.

Nondiabetics

- Nutritional management should be monitored frequently, regardless of the prescribed protein intake, to avoid malnutrition. Nutrition goals are serum albumin >4 g/dL and transferrin >200 mg/dL.

- Blood pressure control should target normotensive levels (130/80–85 mm Hg). If proteinuria >1 g/d is present and there are no contraindications, blood pressure should be reduced to 125/75 mm Hg. If a patient has proteinuria >3 g/d and chronic renal failure, ACEI and perhaps calcium channel blockers should be considered as first-line therapy.

▶ HYPERTENSION

TREATMENT

- All hypertensive agents do not preserve renal function to the same degree despite equal blood pressure control (Table 78–1). Antihypertensive agents that maintain renal blood flow, reduce glomerular pressure, and proteinuria are preferred.
- Regardless of the regimen, hypertension should be controlled (see Chapter 9). If proteinuria is present, ACEI and nondihydropyridine CCBs may be superior to other antihypertensive agents in decreasing proteinuria and glomerular hypertension.
- Experimental data indicate that angiotensin 1 (AT-1) receptor antagonists slow the progression of renal data in animal models, but more clinical experience is needed to determine the role of AT-1 antagonists in humans.
- Hyperkalemia can complicate ACEI use, especially in diabetics or those using nonsteroidal anti-inflammatory agents. Except for **fosinopril,** the half-lives of ACEI (or active metabolites) are prolonged in renal failure and lower doses may suffice. In patients with renal insufficiency, dosage alterations are unnecessary with most CCBs.
- Other antihypertensive drugs may also be required to lower blood pressure in patients with ESRD, but they have not been shown to retard progression of renal failure. Diuretics are indicated for fluid overloads. Drugs that interfere with renin release may be useful (e.g., β blockers or the combined α- and β-blocker, labetolol). Sympathetic nervous system active agents (e.g., clonidine in particular, but also prazosin, terazosin, doxazosin, guanabenz, or guanfacine) may be required in patients unresponsive to dialytic therapy plus ACEI, CCB, or β-blocker therapy. Adding vasodilators (e.g., minoxidil or hydralazine) may be useful in patients resistant to previously mentioned agents; most patients require a β blocker or a central α adenoreceptor agonist to suppress minoxidil-induced reflex tachycardia.

EVALUATION OF THERAPEUTIC OUTCOME

- Dialysis normalizes blood pressure in 50–60% of patients with ESRD by achieving "dry weight" and controlling total body sodium. If dialysis does not control blood pressure, drug therapy should be initiated beginning with an ACEI or CCB.
- Precipitous falls in blood pressure to normotensive levels may be acutely deleterious to renal function in patients with impaired renal function. Target blood pressure should be achieved slowly to allow adaptation to reduced perfusion pressures.

TABLE 78–1. Effects of Antihypertensive Agents on Renal Blood Flow (RBF) and Glomerular Filtration Rate (GRF)

Antihypertensive Agent	Mechanism of Action	Effects on Renal Hemodynamics
Diuretics	Sodium and volume depletion	⇓ GFR and RBF
	⇑ Vasodilatory prostaglandins (IV loop diuretics)	⇑ RBF
	Renal vasoconstriction (IV thiazide)	⇓ GFR and RBF
β-Adrenergic blockers	⇓ Cardiac output	⇓ GFR and RBF
	⇑ Renal vascular resistance (nonselective agents)	⇓ GFR and RBF
	⇓ Renal vascular resistance (β_1-selective agents)	No change in GFR and RBF ⇓ Or no change in microalbuminuria
Centrally acting antiadrenergic drugs	⇓ Renal vascular resistance (α-methyldopa)	No change in GFR and RBF
	⇓ Renal perfusion pressure (clonidine, α_2-adrenergic agonist)	⇓ GFR and RBF
Peripherally acting antiadrenergic drugs	Direct vasodilation (postsynaptic α_1-adrenoreceptor blocking agents)	No change in GFR and RBF
Direct vasodilator agents	⇓ Renal vascular resistance (hydralazine, minoxidil)	⇑ RBF and no effect on GFR
	Arterial vasodilation plus dilatation of venous capacitance vessels (nitroprusside) (diazoxide—less venous dilatation)	⇓ GFR and RBF (acute effect)
ACEI	Dilation of efferent arteriole	⇑ RBF and GFR (only in patients with hypertension, renal insufficiency, and ⇑ renin states)
	Dilatation of efferent arteriole plus inhibition of angiotensin II	⇓ GFR (acute)
Calcium channel blockers	⇓ Renal vascular resistance by vasodilation of afferent arterioles (hypertensive patients)	⇑ RBF ⇑/no change in GFR
	⇓ Renal vasoconstriction (isolated perfused kidney)	⇑ RBF and GFR

- Drug dosages should be adjusted because of the effects of ESRD and dialysis (see Chapter 75).

▶ END-STAGE RENAL DISEASE

PATHOPHYSIOLOGY

- No single toxin is responsible for all of the abnormalities associated with ESRD. The clinical picture likely results from an interplay of multiple factors.
- Organic compounds known to accumulate in uremia include metabolic by-products of protein metabolism, and biologically and endogenous active substances (e.g., parathyroid hormone and atrial natriuretic peptide, gastrin, growth hormone, glucagon, somatostatin, prolactin, calcitonin, and insulin).
- Uremia can affect virtually every major organ system.

CLINICAL PRESENTATION

- Renal osteodystrophy (bone disease) is a common manifestation of chronic renal disease (discussed later in this chapter).
- Hematologic complications of chronic renal failure include normochromic, normocytic anemia secondary to decreased erythropoietin production (discussed later in this chapter), and prolonged bleeding time and a bleeding diathesis due to platelet dysfunction.
- Sodium retention leads to volume expansion, which can result in volume overload and cardiovascular (e.g., pulmonary edema) and pulmonary complications (e.g., noncardiogenic pulmonary edema).
- Common gastrointestinal (GI) complications of chronic renal failure include anorexia, hiccups, and a metallic taste in the mouth. Nausea, vomiting, diarrhea, abdominal distention, and GI bleeding may also occur.
- Neuromuscular irritability may result in leg cramps, restless leg syndrome, and reversal of the sleep–wake cycle.
- Endocrine and metabolic abnormalities include clinical symptoms of hypothyroidism (i.e., low energy, cold intolerance, constipation), hyperglycemia secondary to peripheral resistance to insulin, and primary hypogonadism and hypothalamic abnormalities resulting in sexual dysfunction and sterility.
- Common dermatologic manifestations include dry, flaking skin and generalized pruritus.
- Infectious diseases are common and result in significant morbidity and mortality.

TREATMENT

- Dialysis, discussed in Chapter 74.

► RENAL OSTEODYSTROPHY AND SECONDARY HYPERPARATHYROIDISM

PATHOPHYSIOLOGY

- Calcium and phosphorus balance is mediated through a complex interplay of hormones and their effects on bone, GI tract, kidney, and parathyroid gland. Phosphate retention inhibits renal activation of vitamin D, which in turn reduces gut absorption of calcium. Low blood calcium concentration stimulates parathyroid hormone (PTH) secretion. As functional renal mass declines, serum calcium balance can only be maintained at the expense of increased bone resorption.
- Secondary hyperparathyroidism can result in osteitis fibrosa cystica, which is characterized by high bone-formation rate.
- Aluminum toxicity, which can contribute to renal osteodystrophy and other complications, is less frequent than it used to be because of the use of deionizers and reverse-osmosis filters for purification of dialysate water, and because of decreased use of aluminum phosphate binders.

CLINICAL MANIFESTATIONS

- Excess PTH promotes progression of osteitis fibrosa cystica and may adversely affect lipid metabolism, myocardial and skeletal muscle, and neurologic and immune function. Common signs and symptoms include fatigue, and musculoskeletal and GI complaints.
- Hyperphosphatemia can lead to metastatic calcification of joints, vessels, and soft tissue.
- Although bone symptoms are rare in mild to moderate renal impairment, bone pain and skeletal fractures are characteristic of advanced renal osteodystrophy.

DIAGNOSIS

- Transiliac bone biopsy is the gold standard for evaluation of renal osteodystrophy, but is infrequently performed because it is invasive.
- Bone mineral densitometry studies are used to monitor therapeutic intervention.
- Serum calcium, phosphorous, PTH, alkaline phosphatase, and osteocalcin are useful biochemical markers.

TREATMENT

XIV
- Dietary phosphorus restriction (6.5–12.0 mg/kg/d) should be initiated in patients with CrCl <50 mL/min.
- By the time ESRD develops, most patients require a combination of phosphate-binding medication, calcium supplements, and vitamin D

therapy to prevent development of secondary hyperparathyroidism, renal osteodystrophy, and metastatic calcification.

Phosphate-binding Agents

- Phosphate-binding agents decrease phosphorus absorption from the gut and should be administered with meals to maximize this effect.
- Many phosphate-binding medications are available (Table 78–2), but none is ideal.
- Oral calcium compounds are first-line agents for controlling both serum phosphorus and calcium concentrations. Calcium salts have the potential advantage of partially correcting metabolic acidosis and increasing ionized calcium concentrations, thereby decreasing PTH secretion. Calcium carbonate can normalize phosphate concentrations, but large doses (average 6–14 g/d) may be required. Calcium acetate binds approximately twice as much phosphorus as calcium carbonate, but it is more expensive and causes more nausea and diarrhea. The chloride salt is astringent and unpalatable, and absorbed chloride may contribute to systemic acidosis. The citrate salt binds phosphate poorly in vitro and markedly increases intestinal aluminum absorption owing to the formation of soluble aluminum citrate complexes.
- If necessary, magnesium- or aluminum-containing phosphate binders can be added to calcium-containing phosphate binders to optimize phosphorus control. Magnesium-containing antacids are effective phosphate binders, but they cause diarrhea and hyperkalemia. Aluminum binders are quite effective; however, they cause constipation and toxicity due to aluminum accumulation.

Vitamin D Therapy

- Vitamin D therapy should be added if patients do not achieve normocalcemia or have biochemical features of progressive bone disease despite the use of calcium-containing binders.
- Only **dihydrotachysterol** and 1,25-dihydroxyvitamin D_3 **(calcitriol)** do not require hydroxylation in the kidney to become optimally physiologically active. Calcitriol has largely replaced dihydrotachysterol because it inhibits PTH secretion directly and stimulates intestinal absorption of calcium.
- Controversy exists regarding the most effective method of administration, optimal dose, and dosage interval of calcitriol.

EVALUATION OF THERAPEUTIC OUTCOME

- The goals are intact or *N*-terminal PTH concentrations of 2.0–3.0 times normal, total calcium concentrations (corrected for albumin) of 9–11 mg/dL ([4 − albumin) × 0.8] + serum calcium), and serum phosphorus concentrations of 4.5–6.0 mg/dL. XIV
- A calcium (mg/dL)-phosphorus product (mg/dL) >70 should be avoided to lessen the risk of metastatic calcification.

TABLE 78–2. Phosphate-binding Agents Used in the Treatment of Hyperphosphatemia of Renal Failure

Agents	Examples	Starting Doses	Comments
Calcium carbonate (40% calcium)	Os-Cal 500, Caltrate 600, Nephro-Calci, CalCarb HD, Calci-Mix, Calci-Chew, Tums, and calcium carbonate	0.5–1 g (elemental calcium) tid with meals	Dissolution characteristics and phosphate-binding effect vary among products.Usual daily maintenance dosage: 2.4–5.6 g (elemental calcium) or 6–14 g (calcium carbonate)
Calcium acetate (25% calcium)	Phos-Lo	2 tablets tid with meals	Comparable efficacy to calcium carbonate with half the dose of elemental calcium
Calcum citrate (21% calclum)	Citracal	0.5–1 g (elemental calcium) tid with meals	Citrate enhances absorption of aluminum. Should not be co-administered with aluminum binders, antacids, or sulcralfate Contains aspartame
Aluminum carbonate	Basaljel	400–500 mg tid with meals	Second-line agent after calcium binders Do not use concurrently with citrate-containing products
Aluminum hydroxide	Amphogel, AlternaGel	300–600 mg tid with meals	Second-line agent after calcium binders Do not use concurrently with citrate–containing products
Magnesium carbonate	Mag-Cad	70 mg tid with meals	Reduce magnesium concentration in dialysate to avoid hypermagnesemia Monitor serum magnesium concentration and keep within normal range Diarrhea is a common side effect
Magnesium hydroxide	Milk of Magnesia	300–400 mg tid with meals	Reduce magnesium concentration in dialysate to avoid hypermagnesemia Monitor serum magnesium concentration and keep within normal range Diarrhea is a common side effect

▶ ANEMIA OF CHRONIC RENAL FAILURE

PATHOPHYSIOLOGY

- The primary cause of anemia in patients with chronic renal failure and ESRD is erythropoietin (EPO) deficiency (Chapter 31). Other contributing factors include blood loss; iron, folic acid, or vitamin B_{12} deficiency; severe osteitis fibrosa; systemic infection or inflammatory illness; aluminum toxicity; or hypersplenism.

CLINICAL MANIFESTATIONS

- Signs and symptoms of fatigue, exertional dyspnea, dizziness, headache, pallor, angina, heart failure, and decreased cognition are commonly seen even though some adaptation to a decreased hematocrit (HCT) occurs during the progression of ESRD anemia.

TREATMENT

- **Epoetin** is the therapy of choice for long-term correction and maintenance of HCT levels in predialysis and dialysis patients. It is reasonable to begin epoetin therapy in patients with hematocrits <33%.
- Epoetin can be administered IV, subcutaneously, or intraperitoneally. The subcutaneous method is preferable, especially if patients do not have permanent IV access.
- ESRD anemia can be treated with total weekly epoietin doses of 80–180 U/kg.
- The major side effect of epoetin is elevated blood pressure, which occurs in approximately 23% of patients.
- Although **iron** management may be initiated with oral agents that have relatively high bioavailability and low cost, many centers use parenteral iron exclusively.

EVALUATION OF THERAPEUTIC OUTCOMES

- Iron balance (ferritin, >100 ng/mL; transferrin saturation, >20%) should be monitored to maximize erythropoietic response.
- Once epoetin is initiated, hematocrit/hemoglobin response may be delayed for approximately 2 weeks. Following initiation of epoetin or dose change, steady-state hematocrit levels will not be attained until one red blood cell (RBC) life span has occurred (approximately 1–4 months), so epoetin doses should not be adjusted more often than every 3–4 weeks.
- Goal hematocrit is 33–36%.
- Patients should be monitored for potential complications, such as hypertension, which, if present, should be treated before starting epoietin.

▶ HYPERLIPIDEMIA

- Chronic renal failure with or without nephrotic syndrome is frequently accompanied by abnormalities in lipoprotein metabolism.
- It has not been proven that patients with renal disease, including nephrotic syndrome, are more or less prone to the atherogenic effects of abnormal lipoprotein patterns. In the absence of solid data in this population, it seems prudent to follow guidelines set forth by the National Cholesterol Education Program Expert Panel (see Chapter 8).

See Chapter 42, Chronic Renal Insufficiency and End-Stage Renal Disease, authored by Wendy L. St. Peter, PharmD, BCPS, and Matthew J. Lewis, PharmD, BCPS, for a more detailed discussion of this topic.

Respiratory Disorders

Edited by Terry L. Schwinghammer, PharmD, FCCP, BCPS

Chapter 79

▶ ALLERGIC RHINITIS

▶ DEFINITION

Allergic rhinitis is inflammation of the nasal mucous membrane caused by exposure to inhaled allergenic materials that elicit a specific immunologic response. There are two types:

- Seasonal (hay fever): occurs in response to specific allergens present seasonally (e.g., pollens).
- Perennial: occurs year-round in response to nonseasonal allergens (e.g., dust mites, animal dander, molds), usually resulting in more subtle chronic symptoms.

▶ PATHOPHYSIOLOGY

- The initial reaction occurs when airborne allergens enter the nose and are processed by lymphocytes, which produce antigen-specific IgE, thereby sensitizing genetically predisposed hosts. On reexposure, IgE bound to mast cells interacts with the airborne allergen and triggers the release of preformed inflammatory mediators and newly formed inflammatory mediators from the arachidonic acid cascade. Preformed and rapidly released mediators include histamine, neutrophil and eosinophil chemotactic factor, kinins, and *N*-α-tosyl L-arginine methylesterase. Newly generated mediators include leukotrienes, prostaglandins, thromboxanes, and platelet-activating factor. These mediators cause vasodilatation, increased vascular permeability, and production of nasal secretions. Histamine is probably the most important mediator.
- Several hours after the initial reaction a late-phase reaction may occur, which involves an influx of inflammatory cells (e.g., eosinophils, monocytes, macrophages, basophils) and activation of the lymphocyte population. Late-phase symptoms (nasal congestion) begin 3–5 h after antigen exposure and peak at 12–24 h.

▶ CLINICAL PRESENTATION

- Symptoms include rhinorrhea, sneezing, nasal congestion, postnasal drip, allergic conjunctivitis, and pruritic eyes, ears, or nose.
- Patients may complain of loss of smell or taste, with sinusitis or polyps the underlying cause in many cases. Postnasal drip with cough can also be bothersome.

- Rhinitis symptoms may lead to insomnia, malaise, fatigue, and poor work efficiency.
- Structural facial and dental problems can result from chronic allergic rhinitis.
- Allergic rhinitis is a risk factor for asthma; approximately 90% of asthmatics younger than 16 y have allergies.
- Acute and chronic sinusitis and epistaxis are complications of allergic rhinitis.

▶ DIAGNOSIS

- Physical exam may reveal dark circles under the eyes (allergic shiners), a transverse nasal crease, adenoidal breathing, edematous nasal turbinates, clear nasal secretions, tearing, conjunctival injection, and periorbital swelling.
- Microscopic exam of nasal scrapings typically reveals numerous eosinophils. The peripheral eosinophil count may be elevated, but it is nonspecific and has limited usefulness.
- Further support for the diagnosis is provided by presence of specific IgE by allergen skin testing or in vitro assays such as the radioallergosorbent test (RAST). RAST is rarely justified in clinical practice because it is more expensive and less sensitive than skin tests. Total IgE levels are elevated in only 30–40% of allergic rhinitis patients, and it is also elevated in some nonallergic conditions, thus limiting its usefulness.

▶ DESIRED OUTCOME

- The goal of treatment is to prevent or minimize target symptoms while side effects are minimized and cost-effectiveness of therapy is assured.
- Patients should be knowledgeable about proper timing and monitoring of their illness.
- Allergic rhinitis should have minimal effect on social and occupational functioning.

▶ TREATMENT

AVOIDANCE

- Avoidance of offending allergens is difficult. Mold growth can be reduced by keeping household humidity below 50% and removing obvious growth with bleach or disinfectant.
- Patients sensitive to animals benefit most by removal of pets from the home, if feasible. Exposure to dust mites can be reduced by encasing mattresses and pillows with impermeable covers and washing bed linens in hot water. Washable area rugs are preferable to wall-to-wall carpeting.

- High-efficiency particulate air (HEPA) filters can remove lightweight particles such as pollens, mold spores, and cat allergen, thereby reducing allergic respiratory symptoms.
- In patients with seasonal allergic rhinitis, windows should be kept closed and time spent outdoors during pollen season should be minimized. Filter masks can be helpful when gardening or mowing the lawn.

ANTIHISTAMINES

- Antihistamines prevent the histamine response in sensory nerve endings and blood vessels. They are more effective in preventing the histamine response than in reversing it.
- Symptom relief is caused in part by anticholinergic properties, which are responsible for the drying effect that reduces nasal, salivary, and lacrimal gland hypersecretion. Antihistamines antagonize capillary permeability, wheal-and-flare formation, and itching.
- Antihistamines are well absorbed orally and are metabolized hepatically. Therapeutic effect is more prolonged than predicted by half-life.
- Drowsiness is the most frequent side effect (Table 79–1), and some tolerance to sedation occurs within 24 h of the first dose. Sedative effects can be beneficial in patients who have difficulty sleeping because of rhinitis symptoms.
- Development of "second-generation" peripheral-acting antihistamines (astemizole, loratadine, fexofenadine) is a major advance, as minimal sedation is associated with these agents. Cetirizine is also peripherally acting, but its sedation rate is higher than with the other newer agents.
- Astemizole is contraindicated in patients taking ketoconazole, itraconazole, and erythromycin. Co-administration of any of these drugs results in increased plasma concentrations of astemizole, which may cause arrhythimias (QT prolongation and torsades de pointes), which may be fatal.
- Many patients respond to and tolerate the older agents well, and because some are available generically, they may be less expensive than the newer agents.
- Anticholinergic symptoms can be troublesome, especially for elderly men and those on concurrent anticholinergic therapy (Table 79–1). Caution should also be used in patients with increased intraocular pressure, hyperthyroidism, and cardiovascular disease.
- Other side effects include loss of appetite, nausea, vomiting, and epigastric distress. Taking medication with meals or a full glass of water may prevent gastrointestinal side effects.
- Antihistamines are more effective when taken approximately 1–2 h before the anticipated exposure to the offending allergen.
- Table 79–2 lists recommended doses of commonly prescribed oral agents.
- Intranasal **azelastine** has been shown to be comparable to oral chlorpheniramine and cetirizine for seasonal allergic rhinitis. It produces

TABLE 79–1. Relative Side-Effect Profile of Oral Antihistamines

Agent	Relative Sedative Effect	Relative Anticholinergic Effect
Alkylamine Class		
Brompheniramine maleate	Low	Moderate
Chlorpheniramine maleate	Low	Moderate
Dexchlorpheniramine maleate	Low	Moderate
Ethanolamine Class		
Carbinoxamine maleate	High	High
Clemastine fumarate	Moderate	High
Diphenhydramine hydrochloride	High	High
Ethylenediamine Class		
Pyrilamine maleate	Low	Low to none
Tripelennamine hydrochloride	Moderate	Low to none
Phenothiazine Class		
Methdilazine hydrochloride	Low	High
Promethazine hydrochloride	High	High
Trimeprazine	Moderate	High
Piperidine Class		
Azatadine maleate	Moderate	Moderate
Cyproheptadine hydrochloride	Low	Moderate
Diphenylpyraline hydrochloride	Low	Moderate
Phenindamine tartrate	Low to none	Moderate
"Second-generation" Peripherally Selective Class		
Astemizole	Low to none	Low to none
Cetirizine	Low to moderate	Low to none
Fexofenadine	Low to none	Low to none
Loratadine	Low to none	Low to none

rapid relief of symptoms but can cause drowsiness, because approximately 40% of the dose is absorbed systemically.

- The ophthalmic antihistamines **levocabastine** or **olopatadine** can be used with allergic conjunctivitis, which is often associated with allergic rhinitis. However, systemic antihistamines are usually effective for allergic conjunctivitis, and addition of these products is not usually necessary. They may be a logical addition to nasal steroids when ocular symptoms occur.

DECONGESTANTS

- Topical and systemic decongestants are sympathomimetic agents that act on adrenergic receptors in the nasal mucosa to produce vasoconstriction, shrink swollen mucosa, and improve ventilation.
- Use of topical decongestants results in little or no systemic absorption (Table 79–3).

TABLE 79–2. Oral Dosages of Commonly Prescribed Antihistamines and Decongestants

Drug	Dosage and Interval	
	Adults	*Children*
Antihistamines		
Chlorpheniramine maleate, plain	4 mg q 6 h	6–12 y: 2 mg q 6 h 2–6 y: 1 mg q 6 h
Chlorpheniramine maleate, sustained release	8–12 mg at HS or 8–12 mg q 8 h	6–12 y: 8 mg at HS < 6 y: not recommended
Diphenhydramine HCl	25–50 mg q 8 h	5 mg/kg/d divided q 8 h (up to 25 mg per dose)
Clemastine fumarate	1.34 mg twice daily to 2.68 mg three times daily	Not recommended
Astemizole	10 mg once daily	< 6 y: 0.2 mg/kg daily
Loratadine	10 mg once daily	10 mg once daily
Fexofenadine	60 mg twice daily	Not recommended
Cetirizine	5 to 10 mg once daily	> 6 y: 5 mg once daily
Decongestants		
Pseudoephedrine	60 mg q 4–6 h 120 mg q 12 h for sustained release	6–12 y: 30 mg q 4–6 h 2–5 y: 15 mg q 4–6 h
Ephedrine sulfate	25–50 mg q 4 h	2–3 mg/kg/d divided q 4 h (up to 25 mg q 4 h)
Phenylpropanolamine	25 mg q 4 h or 50 mg q 8 h for sustained release	6–12 y: 12.5 mg q 4 h 2–5 y: 6.25 mg q 4 h

- Prolonged use of topical agents (more than 3–5 days) results in rhinitis medicamentosa, which is rebound vasodilation with associated congestion. Patients tend to use the spray more often with less response. Abrupt cessation is an effective treatment, but the rebound congestion may last for several days or weeks. Nasal steroids have been used successfully, but they take several days to work. Weaning the patient off the topical decongestant can be accomplished by decreasing the dosing interval or concentration over several weeks. Combining the weaning process with nasal steroids may be helpful.
- Other side effects of topical decongestants include burning, stinging, sneezing, and dryness of the nasal mucosa.
- Duration of therapy with topical decongestants should always be limited to 3–5 days.
- Oral decongestants have a slower onset of action than topical agents, but they may last longer and cause less local irritation. Also, rhinitis medicamentosa is not a problem. Pharmacokinetic parameters are summarized in Table 79–4.

TABLE 79–3. Duration of Action of Topical Decongestants

Drug	Duration (h)
Short acting	
Phenylephrine hydrochloride	Up to 4
Intermediate acting	
Naphazoline hydrochloride	4–6
Tetrahydrozoline hydrochloride	
Long acting	
Oxymetazoline hydrochloride	Up to 12
Xylometazoline hydrochloride	

- The therapeutic index for phenylpropanolamine and ephedrine is low. Both can cause hypertension at near-therapeutic doses. Pseudoephedrine appears to be the safest of the three—doses up to 180 mg produce no measurable change in blood pressure or heart rate, although higher doses can. Hypertensive patients should generally avoid these drugs, especially phenylpropanolamine and ephedrine.
- Monoamine oxidase inhibitors should be avoided in any patient taking decongestants.

NASAL CORTICOSTEROIDS

- Topical steroids are effective, have minimal side effects, and may inhibit early as well as late-phase response (Table 79–5). In a consensus report by the International Rhinitis Management Working Group, nasal steroids are recommended as initial therapy along with avoidance of allergens in patients with seasonal allergic rhinitis and perennial rhinitis.
- Beneficial effects on the nasal mucosa include reducing inflammation by blocking mediator release, suppressing neutrophil chemotaxis, reducing intracellular edema, causing mild vasoconstriction, and inhibiting mast cell-mediated late-phase reactions.

TABLE 79–4. Pharmacokinetic Variables of Systemic Decongestants

Drug	Half-life (h)	Mechanism of Metabolism or Elimination
Pseudoephedrine	3–8	Partially metabolized; majority excreted unchanged in urine
Ephedrine	3–6	Majority excreted unchanged in urine
Phenylpropanolamine	3–4	Majority excreted unchanged in urine

TABLE 79–5. Dosages of Topical Steroids

Drug	Dosage and Interval
Beclomethasone diproprionate	>12 y: 1 inhalation (42 μg) per nostril 2–4 times a day (maximum, 336 μg/d)
	6–12 y: 1 inhalation per nostril 3 times per day
Budesonide	>6 y: 2 sprays (64 μg) per nostril in AM and PM, or 4 sprays per nostril in AM (maximum, 256 μg)
Flunisolide	Adults: 2 sprays (50 μg) per nostril twice daily (maximum, 400 μg)
	Children: 1 spray per nostril 3 times a day
Fluticasone	Adults: 2 sprays (100 μg) per nostril once daily; after a few days decrease to 1 spray per nostril
	Adolescents: (>12 y): 1 spray per nostril once daily (maximum, 200 μg/d)
Triamcinolone acetonide	>12 y: 2 sprays (110 μg) per nostril once daily (maximum, 440 μg/d)

- Side effects include sneezing, stinging, headache, epistaxis, and infections with *Candida albicans* (rare).
- Some patients improve within a few days, but peak response may require 2–3 weeks. The dosage may be reduced once a response is achieved.
- Blocked nasal passages should be cleared with a decongestant before administration of corticosteroids to ensure adequate penetration of the spray.

CROMOLYN SODIUM

- **Cromolyn sodium,** a mast cell stabilizer, is available as a nonprescription nasal solution for symptomatic prevention and treatment of allergic rhinitis.
- It prevents mast cell degranulation and release of mediators, including histamine.
- The most common side effect is local irritation (sneezing and nasal stinging).
- The dose in individuals older than 6 year is one spray in each nostril 3–4 times daily at regular intervals.
- For seasonal rhinitis, initiate treatment just before the start of the allergen's season, and continue throughout the season.
- In perennial rhinitis, the effects may not be seen for 2–4 weeks; antihistamines or decongestants may be needed during this initial phase of therapy.
- Nasal passages should be cleared before administration, and inhaling through the nose during administration enhances distribution to the entire nasal lining.

IPRATROPIUM BROMIDE

- **Ipratropium bromide** nasal spray is an anticholinergic agent useful in perennial allergic rhinitis.
- It exhibits antisecretory properties when applied locally and provides symptomatic relief of rhinorrhea associated with allergic rhinitis.
- The 0.03% solution is given as two sprays (42 μg) 2–3 times daily. Side effects are mild and include headache, epistaxis, and nasal dryness.

IMMUNOTHERAPY

- Immunotherapy is the slow, gradual process of injecting increasing doses of antigens responsible for eliciting allergic symptoms in a patient with the intent of increasing tolerance to the allergen when natural exposure occurs.
- The effectiveness of immunotherapy probably results from diminished IgE production, increased IgG production, changes in T lymphocytes, reduced inflammatory mediator release from sensitized cells, and diminished tissue responsiveness.
- Because immunotherapy is expensive, has potential risks, and requires a major time commitment from patients, it should only be considered in selected patients. Good candidates include patients who have a strong history of severe symptoms unsuccessfully controlled by avoidance and drug therapy and patients who have been unable to tolerate the side effects of drug therapy. Poor candidates include patients with medical conditions that would compromise the ability to tolerate an anaphylactic-type reaction, patients with impaired immune systems, and patients with a history of noncompliance.
- In general, very dilute solutions (1:100,000 to 1:1,000,000,000 wt/vol) are given 1–2 times per week. The concentration is increased until the maximum tolerated dose is achieved. This maintenance dose is continued every 2–6 weeks, depending on clinical response. Better results are obtained with year-round rather than seasonal injections.
- Common mild local adverse reactions include induration and swelling at the injection site. More severe reactions (generalized urticaria, bronchospasm, laryngospasm, vascular collapse) occur rarely. Severe reactions are treated with epinephrine, antihistamines, and systemic corticosteroids.

► EVALUATION OF THERAPEUTIC OUTCOMES

- Patients should be monitored regularly for reduction in severity of identified target symptoms and the presence of side effects.
- Patients should be questioned about their satisfaction with the management of their allergic rhinitis. Management should result in minimal disruption to their life.

- The Medical Outcomes Study 36-item Short Form Health Survey (SF-36) and the Rhinoconjunctivitis Quality of Life Questionnaire measure not only improvement in symptoms but also parameters such as sleep quality, nonallergic symptoms (e.g., fatigue, poor concentration), emotions, and participation in a variety of activities.

See Chapter 87, Allergic Rhinitis, authored by J. Russell May, PharmD, for a more detailed discussion of this topic.

Chapter 80

▶ ASTHMA

▶ DEFINITION

An Expert Panel of the National Institutes of Health National Asthma Education and Prevention Program (NAEPP) has defined asthma as a chronic inflammatory disorder of the airways in which many cells and cellular elements play a role. In susceptible individuals, inflammation causes recurrent episodes of wheezing, breathlessness, chest tightness, and coughing. These episodes are usually associated with airflow obstruction that is often reversible either spontaneously or with treatment. The inflammation also causes an increase in bronchial hyperresponsiveness to a variety of stimuli.

▶ PATHOPHYSIOLOGY

- Hyperreactivity of the airways to physical, chemical, and pharmacologic stimuli is the hallmark of asthma.
- The increased bronchial responsiveness is at least in part due to an inflammatory response within the airway. The histologic examination at autopsy is characterized by marked hypertrophy and hyperplasia of the airway smooth muscle, increased airway wall thickness with an exudative inflammatory reaction and edema, and mucous gland hypertrophy and mucus hypersecretion.
- Inflammation of the airways and the release of mediators of inflammation contribute significantly to the development and maintenance of bronchial hyperreactivity. Airway inflammation is associated with epithelial cell damage and increased mucosal permeability. This facilitates access of noxious stimuli from the lumen to the airway smooth muscle, submucosal mast cells, and the cholinergic irritant receptors located in the junction between cells. Inflammation can also account for mucus hypersecretion.
- Involvement of leukocytes within the airways and surrounding tissues is important in the pathogenesis of asthma.
  - Mast cell degranulation in response to allergens results in release of mediators such as histamine; eosinophil and neutrophil chemotactic factors; leukotrienes C_4, D_4, and E_4; prostaglandins; and platelet-activating factor. Histamine is capable of inducing smooth muscle constriction and bronchospasm and is thought to play a role in mucosal edema and mucus secretion.
  - The granules within eosinophils contain major basic protein (MBP), which is responsible for damage to airway epithelium and has been found in very high quantities in the sputum of patients with asthma.
  - Neutrophils can also be a source for a variety of mediators (platelet-activating factors, prostaglandins, thromboxanes, and leukotrienes)

that contribute to bronchial hyperresponsiveness and airway inflammation.
- Alveolar macrophages produce and release a number of inflammatory mediators, including platelet-activating factor, leukotriene B_4, leukotriene C_4, and leukotriene D_4. Production of neutrophil chemotactic factor and eosinophil chemotactic factor attract neutrophils and eosinophils, which in turn further facilitate the inflammatory process.
- The presence of T lymphocytes has been correlated to bronchial hyperresponsiveness. The T_{H2} subset of T lymphocytes produces and releases interleukin (IL)-4, IL-5, IL-6, and IL-10. Conversely, T_{H1} cells secrete IL-2, IFN-γ, and tumor necrosis factor beta (TNF-β), with both T_{H1} and T_{H2} cells producing IL-3, granulocyte-macrophage colony-stimulating factor (GM-CSF), and IFN-α.

- The 5-lipoxygenase pathway of arachidonic acid breakdown is responsible for production of leukotrienes. Leukotrienes C_4, D_4, and E_4 (cysteinyl leukotrienes) constitute the slow-reacting substance of anaphylaxis (SRS-A). These leukotrienes are liberated during inflammatory processes in the lung and produce bronchoconstriction, mucus secretion, microvascular permeability, and airway edema.
- The exudative inflammatory process and sloughing of epithelial cells into the airway lumen impairs mucociliary transport. The bronchial glands are increased in size and the goblet cells are increased in size and number, suggesting an increased production of mucus. Expectorated mucus from patients with asthma tends to have a high viscosity.
- The airway is innervated by parasympathetic, sympathetic, and nonadrenergic inhibitory nerves. The normal resting tone of human airway smooth muscle is maintained by vagal efferent activity, and bronchoconstriction can be mediated by vagal stimulation in the small bronchi. All airway smooth muscle contains noninnervated β_2-adrenergic receptors that produce bronchodilation. The importance of α-adrenergic receptors in asthma is unknown.

▶ CLINICAL PRESENTATION

CHRONIC ASTHMA

- Classic asthma is characterized by episodic dyspnea associated with wheezing, but the clinical presentation of asthma is diverse. Patients may complain of a feeling of tightness in the chest or occasionally a burning sensation. A chronic persistent cough may be the only symptom.
- Asthma has a widely variable presentation from chronic daily symptoms to only intermittent symptoms. The interval between symptoms may be weeks, months, or years. It is a disease characterized by recurrent exacerbations and remissions.
- The severity is primarily determined by the number of medications required to adequately control symptoms. Patients can present with

mild intermittent symptoms that require no medications or only occasional use of inhaled bronchodilators to severe chronic asthma symptoms despite receiving multiple medications.

ACUTE SEVERE ASTHMA

- Uncontrolled asthma can progress to an acute state where inflammation, airway edema, excessive accumulation of mucus, and severe bronchospasm result in a profound airway narrowing that is poorly responsive to usual bronchodilator therapy.
- Patients present with severe dyspnea, inspiratory as well as expiratory wheezing, anxiety, tachypnea, tachycardia, and in severe cases, cyanosis.
- They exhibit supraclavicular and intercostal retractions, a hyperinflated chest, and coughing. In severe obstruction, air movement in and out of the lungs is substantially decreased, so that wheezing may actually decrease.

► DIAGNOSIS

- The diagnosis of asthma is based primarily on a good history of recurrent episodes of dyspnea and/or wheezing.
- The patient may have a family history of allergy or asthma or have symptoms of allergic rhinitis. A history of exercise or cold air precipitating the dyspnea or an association of increased symptoms during specific allergen seasons would also point to asthma.
- In the older child and adult patient in whom spirometric evaluations can be performed, abnormal pulmonary functions that improve 15% or more following bronchodilator administration help confirm the diagnosis. Failure of pulmonary functions to improve acutely does not necessarily rule out asthma. If baseline spirometry is normal, challenge testing with exercise, histamine, or methacholine can be used to elicit bronchial hyperreactivity.
- Studies for atopy such as serum IgE and sputum and blood eosinophils are not necessary to make the diagnosis of asthma, but they may help differentiate asthma from chronic bronchitis in adults.

► DESIRED OUTCOME

- The NAEPP has provided the following goals for asthma management: Prevent chronic and troublesome symptoms (e.g., coughing or breathlessness in the night, in the early morning, or after exertion); maintain near "normal" pulmonary function; maintain normal activity levels (including exercise); prevent recurrent exacerbations of asthma; minimize adverse effects from asthma medication; and meet patients' and families' expectations of care.
- In patients with an acute severe asthma exacerbation, the goals of therapy are to relieve airway obstruction as quickly as possible (within min-

utes), relieve hypoxemia immediately, restore lung function to normal as soon as possible (within hours), plan avoidance of future relapses, and develop a written action plan for treating future exacerbations.

► TREATMENT

The stepwise approaches for managing asthma recommended by the NAEPP are contained in Figures 80–1 and 80–2.

NONPHARMACOLOGIC MANAGEMENT

- Patient education and the teaching of patient self-management skills should be the cornerstone of the treatment program. Self-management programs have been shown to improve patient adherence to medication regimens, improve self-management skills, and improve use of health care services.
- Use of objective measurements of airflow obstruction with a home peak flow meter is integral to many of the programs. Because routine peak-flow monitoring may not improve patient outcomes, the NAEPP now advocates the routine use of peak flow meters for only those patients with moderate and severe persistent asthma.
- Avoidance of known allergenic triggers can result in an improvement in symptoms, a reduction in medications, and a decrease in bronchial hyperreactivity. Obvious environmental triggers (e.g., animals) should be avoided, and patients who smoke should be encouraged to stop.
- Oxygen therapy is indicated in patients requiring emergency therapy for acute severe asthma. Patients hospitalized with acute severe asthma should be given adequate maintenance hydration to mobilize secretions, but excessive hydration should be avoided to prevent excessive lung fluid in patients with inflammation and bronchial edema.

PHARMACOLOGIC MANAGEMENT

β_2 Agonists (Table 80–1)

- The β_2 agonists are the most effective bronchodilators available. β_2-adrenergic receptor stimulation activates adenyl cyclase, which produces an increase in intracellular cyclic AMP. This increase results in a decrease in unbound intracellular calcium, producing smooth muscle relaxation, mast cell membrane stabilization, and skeletal muscle stimulation.
- Aerosol administration enhances bronchoselectivity and provides a more rapid response and a greater degree of protection against provocations that induce bronchospasm (e.g., exercise and allergen challenges) than does systemic administration.
- Inhaled short-acting selective β_2 agonists are indicated for the treatment of intermittent episodes of bronchospasm and are the first treatment of choice for acute severe asthma.
- In acute severe asthma, β_2 agonists should be given in high doses by jet nebulization in frequent intervals or, alternatively, via metered dose

Treatment (preferred treatments are in bold print).			
	Long-term control	Quick relief	Education
STEP 4 Severe Persistent	Daily medications: • **Anti-inflammatory: inhaled corticosteroid (high dose) AND** • Long-acting bronchodilator: either **long-acting inhaled β_2 agonist,** sustained-release theophylline, or long-acting β_2-agonist tablets **AND** • Corticosteroid tablets or syrup long term (2 mg/kg/d, generally do not exceed 60 mg/d).	• Short-acting bronchodilator: **inhaled β_2 agonists** as needed for symptoms. • Intensity of treatment will depend on severity of exacerbation. • Use of short-acting inhaled β_2 agonists on a daily basis, or increasing use, indicates the need for additional long-term control therapy.	Steps 2 and 3 actions plus: • Refer to individual education/ counseling
STEP 3 Moderate Persistent	Daily medication: • Either **Anti-inflammatory: inhaled corticosteroid (medium dose) OR Inhaled corticosteroid (low-medium dose)** and add a long-acting bronchodilator, especially for nighttime symptoms: either **long-acting inhaled β_2 agonist,** sustained-release theophylline, or long-acting β_2-agonist tablets. • If needed Anti-inflammatory: **inhaled corticosteroids (medium-high dose) AND Long-acting bronchodilator**, especially for nighttime symptoms; either **long-acting inhaled β_2 agonist,** sustained-release theophylline, or long-acting β_2-agonist tablets.	• Short-acting bronchodilator: **inhaled β_2 agonists** as needed for symptoms. • Intensity of treatment will depend on severity of exacerbation. • Use of short-acting inhaled β_2 agonists on a daily basis, or increasing use, indicates the need for additional long-term control therapy.	Step 1 actions plus: • Teach self-monitoring • Refer to group education if available • Review and update self-management plan
STEP 2 Mild Persistent	One daily medication: • **Anti-inflammatory:** either **inhaled corticosteroid** (low doses) or **cromolyn or nedocromil** (children usually begin with a trial of cromolyn or nedocromil). • Sustained-release theophylline to serum concentration of 5–15 μg/mL is an alternative, but not preferred, therapy. Zafirlukast or zileuton may also be considered for patients ≥ 12 y of age, although their position in therapy is not fully established.	• Short-acting bronchodilator: **inhaled β_2 agonists** as needed for symptoms. • Intensity of treatment will depend on severity of exacerbation. • Use of short-acting inhaled β_2 agonists on a daily basis, or increasing use, indicates the need for additional long-term control therapy.	

STEP 1 Mild Intermittent	• No daily medication needed.	• Short-acting bronchodilator: **inhaled β_2 agonists** as needed for symptoms. • Intensity of treatment will depend on severity of exacerbation. • Use of short-acting inhaled β_2 agonists more than 2 times a week may indicate the need to initiate long-term control therapy.	• Teach basic facts about asthma • Teach inhaler/spacer/holding chamber technique • Discuss roles of medications • Develop self-management plan • Develop action plan for when and how to take rescue actions, especially for patients with a history of severe exacerbations • Discuss appropriate environmental control measures to avoid exposure to known allergens and irritants

↓ **Step down**

Review treatment every 1–6 mo; a gradual stepwise reduction in treatment may be possible.

↑ **Step up**

If control is not maintained, consider step up. First, review patient medication technique, adherence, and environmental control (avoidance of allergens or other factors that contribute to asthma severity).

Note:

- **The stepwise approach presents general guidelines to assist clinical decision making; it is not intended to be a specific prescription. Asthma is highly variable; clinicians should tailor specific medication plans to the needs and circumstances of individual patients.**
- Gain control as quickly as possible; then decrease treatment to the least medication necessary to maintain control. Gaining control may be accomplished by either starting treatment at the step most appropriate to the initial severity of the condition or starting at higher level of therapy (e.g., a course of systemic corticosteroids or higher dose of inhaled corticosteroids).
- A rescue course of systemic corticosteroids may be needed at any time and at any step.
- Some patients with intermittent asthma experience severe and life-threatening exacerbations separated by long periods of normal lung function and no symptoms. This may be especially common with exacerbations provoked by respiratory infections. A short course of systemic corticosteroids is recommended.
- At each step, patients should control their environment to avoid or control factors that make their asthma worse (e.g., allergens, irritants); this requires specific diagnosis and education.
- Referral to an asthma specialist for consultation or comanagement is *recommended* if there are difficulties achieving or maintaining control of asthma or if the patient requires step 4 care. Referral may be *considered* if the patient requires step 3 care.

Figure 80–1. Stepwise approach for managing asthma.

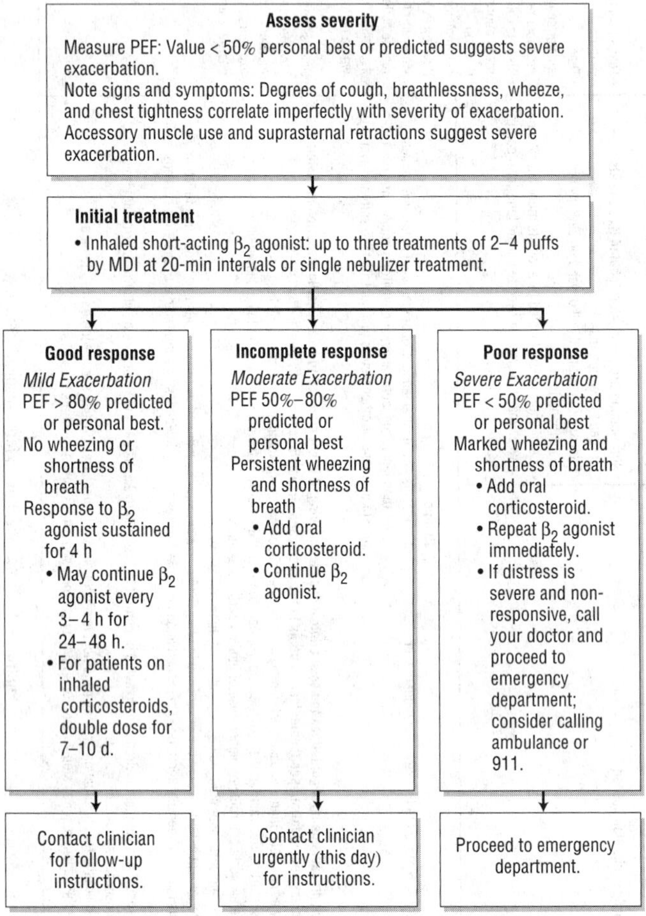

Assess severity

Measure PEF: Value < 50% personal best or predicted suggests severe exacerbation.
Note signs and symptoms: Degrees of cough, breathlessness, wheeze, and chest tightness correlate imperfectly with severity of exacerbation.
Accessory muscle use and suprasternal retractions suggest severe exacerbation.

↓

Initial treatment

- Inhaled short-acting β_2 agonist: up to three treatments of 2–4 puffs by MDI at 20-min intervals or single nebulizer treatment.

↓

Good response

Mild Exacerbation
PEF > 80% predicted or personal best.
No wheezing or shortness of breath
Response to β_2 agonist sustained for 4 h
- May continue β_2 agonist every 3–4 h for 24–48 h.
- For patients on inhaled corticosteroids, double dose for 7–10 d.

↓

Contact clinician for follow-up instructions.

Incomplete response

Moderate Exacerbation
PEF 50%–80% predicted or personal best
Persistent wheezing and shortness of breath
- Add oral corticosteroid.
- Continue β_2 agonist.

↓

Contact clinician urgently (this day) for instructions.

Poor response

Severe Exacerbation
PEF < 50% predicted or personal best
Marked wheezing and shortness of breath
- Add oral corticosteroid.
- Repeat β_2 agonist immediately.
- If distress is severe and non-responsive, call your doctor and proceed to emergency department; consider calling ambulance or 911.

↓

Proceed to emergency department.

Figure 80–2. Home management of acute asthma exacerbations.

TABLE 80–1. Relative Selectivity, Potency, and Duration of Action of the β-Adrenergic Agonists

	Selectivity			Duration of Action		
Agent	β_1	β_2	*β_2 Potency*[a]	*Bronchodilation (h)*	*Protection*[b] *(h)*	*Oral Activity*
Isoproterenol	++++	++++	1	0.5–2	0.5–1.0	No
Metaproterenol	+++	+++	15	3–4	1–2	Yes
Isoetharine	++	+++	6	0.5–2	0.5–1.0	No
Albuterol	+	++++	2	4–8	2–4	Yes
Bitolterol	+	++++	5	4–8	2–4	No
Pirbuterol	+	++++	5	4–8	2–4	Yes
Terbutaline	+	++++	4	4–8	2–4	Yes
Formoterol	+	++++	0.24	>12	>12	Yes
Salmeterol	+	++++	0.50	>12	>12	Unknown

[a]Relative molar potency: 1 = most potent.
[b]Protection refers to the duration of time that bronchoconstriction may be prevented.

inhaler (MDI) plus a spacer device by trained personnel; dosing guidelines are presented in Table 80–2. Initially, the patient should receive dosages every 20 minutes for the first 1 or 2 hours, and then the dosage should be adjusted based on response (see Figures 80–1 and 80–2). During the recovery phase, the dose is generally lowered first and then the dosing interval is extended.

- These agents are the treatment of choice for exercise-induced asthma (EIA). They provide complete protection for at least 2 hours after inhalation; the long-acting agents (e.g., salmeterol) provide significant protection for 8–12 hours initially, but the duration decreases with chronic regular use.
- Their short duration limits usefulness in patients who require chronic maintenance bronchodilators to prevent and control symptoms, particularly those with nocturnal asthma. These patients can be treated with long-acting inhaled β_2 agonists (preferred), oral sustained-release β_2 agonists, or sustained-release theophylline.
- In chronic asthma, long-acting inhaled β_2 agonists are indicated as additional long-term control for patients with symptoms who are already on standard doses of anti-inflammatories prior to advancing to medium- or high-dose inhaled corticosteroids. Twice-daily inhaled salmeterol is indicated for the chronic maintenance therapy of asthma, but it is ineffective for acute severe asthma because it can take up to 20 minutes for onset and 1–4 hours for maximum bronchodilation. Patients should be counseled to continue to use their short-acting inhaled β_2 agonists for acute exacerbations.

Methylxanthines

- The mechanism by which **theophylline** produces bronchodilation is unknown but may involve inhibition of the release of intracellular

TABLE 80–2. Dosages of Drugs for Acute Severe Exacerbations of Asthma in the Emergency Department or Hospital

Medications	Dosages: *Adults*	Dosages: *Children*	Comments
Inhaled β_2 agonists			
Albuterol nebulizer solution (5 mg/mL)	2.5–5 mg every 20 min for 3 doses, then 2.5–10 mg every 1–4 has needed, or 10–15 mg/h continuously	0.15 mg/kg (minimum dose 2.5 mg) every 20 min for 3 doses, then 0.15–0.3 mg/kg up to 10 mg every 1–4 h as needed, or 0.5 mg/kg/h by continuous nebulization	Only selective β_2-agonists are recommended For optimal delivery, dilute aerosols to minimum of 4 mL at gas flow of 6–8 L/min
MDI (90 µg/puff)	4–8 puffs every 30 min up to 4 h, then every 1–4 h as needed	4–8 puffs every 20 min for 3 doses, then every 1–4 h as needed	In patients in severe distress, nebulization is preferred; use holding-chamber type spacer
Bitolterol nebulizer solution (2 mg/mL)	See albuterol dose	See albuterol dose; thought to be as potent to one-half as potent as albuterol on a mg basis	Has not been studied in acute severe asthma. Do not mix with other drugs
MDI (370 µg/puff)	See albuterol dose	See albuterol dose	Has not been studied in acute severe asthma
Pirbuterol MDI (200 µg/puff)	See albuterol dose	See albuterol dose; one-half as potent as albuterol on a mg basis	Has not been studied in acute severe asthma

Systemic β agonists			
Epinephrine 1:1000 (1 mg/mL)	0.3–0.5 mg every 20 min for 3 doses SC	0.01 mg/kg up to 0.5 mg every 20 min for 3 doses SC	No proven advantage of systemic therapy over aerosol
Terbutaline (1 mg/mL)	0.25 mg every 20 min for 3 doses SC	0.01 mg/kg every 20 min for 3 doses, then every 2–6 h as needed SC	Not recommended
Anticholinergics			
Ipratropium bromide nebulizer solution (0.25 mg/mL)	500 μg every 30 min for 3 doses, then every 2–4 h as needed	250 μg every 20 min for 3 doses, then 250 μg every 2–4 h	May mix in same nebulizer with albuterol. Do not use as first-line therapy, only add to β_2-agonist therapy
MDI (18 μg/puff)	4–8 puffs as needed	4–8 puffs as needed	Not recommended as dose in inhaler is low and has not been studied in acute asthma
Corticosteroids[a]			
Prednisone, methylprednisolone, prednisolone	120–180 mg in 3 or 4 divided doses for 48 h, then 60–80 mg/d until PEF reaches 70% of personal best	1 mg/kg every 6 h for 48 h, then 1–2 mg/kg/d in 2 divided doses until PEF reaches 70% of normal predicted	For outpatient "burst" use 1–2 mg/kg/d; max 60 mg for 3–7 d. It is unnecessary to taper after the course

[a]No advantage has been found for very-high-dose corticosteroids in acute severe asthma, nor is there any advantage for intravenous administration over oral therapy. The usual regimen is to continue the frequent multiple daily dosing until the patient achieves an FEV_1 or PEF of 50% of personal best or normal predicted value and then lower the dose to twice daily dosing. This usually occurs within 48 h. The final duration of therapy following a hospitalization or emergency department visit may be from 7–14 d. If patients are then started on inhaled corticosteroids, studies indicate that there is no need to taper the systemic steroid dose. If the follow-up therapy is to be given once daily, studies indicate that there may be an advantage to giving the single daily dose in the afternoon at around 3:00 PM.

calcium and/or inhibition of phosphodiesterases (PDEs). PDE inhibition may result in decreased mast cell mediator release, decreased eosinophil basic-protein release, decreased T-lymphocyte proliferation, decreased T-cell cytokine release, and decreased plasma exudation. Theophylline also inhibits pulmonary edema by decreasing vascular permeability, enhances mucociliary clearance, and strengthens contraction of a fatigued diaphragm.

- Methylxanthines are ineffective by aerosol and therefore must be taken systemically (orally or IV).
- Theophylline is primarily eliminated by metabolism via the hepatic cytochrome P450 mixed-function oxidase microsomal enzymes (primarily the CYP1A2 and CYP3A3 isozymes) with 10% or less excreted unchanged in the kidney. The hepatic P450 enzymes are susceptible to induction and inhibition by various environmental factors and drugs, as listed in Table 80–3.
- Because of a relatively large intrapatient variability in theophylline clearance, no patient should be treated with theophylline without routine monitoring of serum theophylline concentrations. A range of 5–15 μg/mL has been recommended by the NAEPP and others as an effective and safe range of steady-state concentrations for most patients.
- Figure 80–3 gives recommended dosages, monitoring schedules, and dosage adjustments for theophylline.

TABLE 80–3. Factors Affecting Theophylline Clearance

Decreased Clearance	% Decrease	Increased Clearance	% Increase
Cimetidine	25–60	Rifampin	53
Macrolides: Erythromycin, TAO, clarithromycin	25–50	Carbamazepine	50
Allopurinol	20	Phenobarbital	34
Propranolol	30	Phenytoin	70
Quinolones: Ciprofloxacin, enoxacin, pefloxacin	20–50	Charcoal broiled meat	30
Thiabendazole	65	High-protein diet	25
Ticlopidine	25	Smoking	40
Zileuton	35	Sulfinpyrazone	22
Systemic viral illness	10–50		

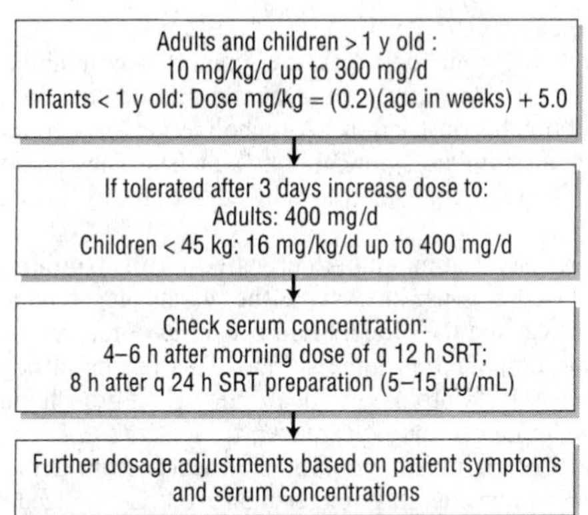

Figure 80–3. Algorithm for slow tiration of theophylline dosage and guide for final dosage adjustment based on serum theophylline concentration measurement. For infants <1 y of age, the initial daily dosage can be calculated by the following regression equation: Dose (mg/kg) = (0.2)(age in wk) + 5.0. Whenever side effects occur, dosage should be reduced to a previously tolerated lower dose. SRT, sustained-release theophylline.

- Sustained-release oral preparations are favored for outpatient therapy, but each product has different release characteristics and the products are variably susceptible to altered absorption from food or gastric pH changes. In general, preparations unaffected by food that can be administered a minimum of every 12 hours in most patients are preferable.
- In acute severe asthma exacerbations, addition of aminophylline to optimal inhaled β_2 agonists has been shown to provide no further benefit and is no longer recommended.
- In the outpatient setting, chronic theophylline administration can reduce asthma symptoms, reduce the amount of as-needed inhaled β_2 agonists used, and reduce the oral steroid requirement in steroid-dependent asthmatics.
- Sustained-release theophylline once nightly is effective for nocturnal asthma.
- Significant disadvantages to chronic theophylline therapy include the lack of effect of theophylline on underlying bronchial hyperreactivity and the dangers inherent in giving a drug that can produce severe neurologic toxicity, including seizures, permanent neurologic deficit, and death at serum concentrations only two-fold greater than optimal therapeutic concentrations.
- Due to its high risk/benefit ratio, theophylline is considered as a second- or third-line drug in the therapy of asthma.

Anticholinergics

- Anticholinergic bronchodilators are competitive inhibitors of muscarinic receptors; they only produce bronchodilation in cholinergic-mediated bronchoconstriction. Anticholinergics are effective bronchodilators but are not as potent as β_2 agonists. They attenuate, but do not block, allergen- or exercise-induced asthma in a dose-dependent fashion.
- Only quaternary ammonium derivatives (**ipratropium bromide**) should be used because they have the advantage of poor absorption across mucosae and the blood–brain barrier as compared to the tertiary ammonium compound atropine sulfate. This results in negligible systemic effects with a prolonged local effect (i.e., bronchodilation) with no decrease in mucociliary clearance.
- The time to reach maximum bronchodilation from aerosolized anticholinergics is considerably longer than from aerosolized short-acting β_2 agonists (2 hours versus 30 minutes). This is of little clinical consequence because some bronchodilation is seen within 30 seconds, 50% of maximum response occurs within 3 minutes, and 80% of maximum is reached within 30 minutes. Ipratropium bromide has a duration of action of 4–8 hours.
- Ipratropium bromide consistently produces a 10–20% improvement in FEV_1 over β_2 agonists alone in acute severe asthma, but there is significant interpatient variability in response. Regular administration of ipratropium bromide has not improved outcomes in chronic asthma over β_2 agonists alone.
- Anticholinergics have a limited role in the treatment of asthma. Ipratropium bromide is not indicated for long-term control of asthma and is only indicated as adjunctive therapy in acute severe asthma not completely responsive to β_2 agonists alone.

Cromolyn Sodium and Nedocromil Sodium

- The exact mechanism of action for these agents is unknown but is believed to result, at least in part, from mast cell membrane stabilization. As such, they inhibit the response to allergen challenge as well as EIA. Neither drug has a bronchodilatory effect.
- **Cromolyn** and **nedocromil** are effective only by inhalation and are available as MDIs, and cromolyn also comes as a nebulizer solution.
- Both drugs are remarkably nontoxic. Cough and wheezing have been reported after inhalation of each agent and bad taste and headache after nedocromil.
- Cromolyn and nedocromil are indicated for the prophylaxis of chronic mild persistent asthma in both children and adults regardless of etiology; approximately 60–75% of patients (adults and children) are adequately controlled.
- They are particularly effective for allergic asthmatics on a seasonal basis or just prior to an acute exposure (i.e., animals or mowing the lawn).

- Cromolyn is the second drug of choice for the prevention of EIA and may be used in conjunction with a β_2 agonist in more severe cases not completely responding to either agent alone.
- The NAEPP has suggested that cromolyn and nedocromil be the anti-inflammatories of first choice for childhood asthma due to their efficacy and safety. Nedocromil therapy may allow some patients to decrease inhaled steroid dosage.
- Most patients will experience an improvement in 1–2 weeks, but it may take longer to achieve maximum benefit. Patients should initially receive cromolyn or nedocromil four times daily and then only after stabilization of symptoms may the frequency be reduced to two or three times daily.

Glucocorticoid Therapy (Table 80–4)

- The mechanisms of action of glucocorticoids in asthma include increasing the number of β_2-adrenergic receptors and improving the receptor responsiveness to β_2-adrenergic stimulation, reducing mucus production and hypersecretion, and inhibiting the inflammatory response at all levels.
- Inhaled glucocorticoids are considered first-line therapy for persistent asthma in adults and children; comparative doses are included in Table 80–5. The response to inhaled corticosteroids is delayed; symptoms improve in most patients within the first 1–2 weeks and reach maximum improvement in 4–8 weeks. Improvement in FEV_1 and peak expiratory flow rates requires 3–6 weeks for maximum improvement. Systemic toxicity is low with low to moderate doses, but the risk of systemic effects increases with high doses. Local adverse effects include dose-dependent oropharyngeal candidiasis and dysphonia, which can be reduced by the use of a spacer device. In general, spacer devices also substantially increase deposition of drug to the site of action within the airways, further decreasing asthma symptoms and improving spirometry in patients with moderate to severe asthma.
- Acute severe asthma (status asthmaticus) is treated with high-dose systemic (parenteral or oral) glucocorticoids combined with frequent administration of inhaled β_2 agonists. From 4–12 hours may be required before any clinical response is noted. Recommended doses are listed in Table 80–2. After resolution of severe obstruction (achievement of 50% of predicted normal FEV_1, which generally occurs in the first 48 hours), the steroid dose is reduced to 1 mg/kg/d in children or 60 mg/d in adults as one or two doses administered orally. The duration of treatment is dependent on the patient's response and past history. Tapering the steroid dosage after hospitalization is unnecessary.
- Glucocorticoids are also recommended for the treatment of impending episodes of severe asthma unresponsive to bronchodilator therapy. **Prednisone,** approximately 1–2 mg/kg/d (up to 40–60 mg/d), is administered orally in two divided doses for 3–10 days.

TABLE 80–4. Glucocorticoid Comparison Chart

Systemic	Relative Anti-inflammatory Potency	Relative Sodium-retaining Potency	Duration of Biologic Activity (h)	Plasma Elimination Half-life (h)
Hydrocortisone	1	1.0	8–12	1.5–2.0
Prednisone	4	0.8	12–36	2.5–3.5
Methylprednisolone	5	0.5	12–36	3.3
Dexamethasone	25	0	36–54	3.4–4.0
Aerosol	**Topical Potency (Skin Blanching)**	**Receptor Binding Affinity**	**Receptor Complex Half-life (h)**	**Oral Bioavailability (%)**
Flunisolide	330	1.8	3.5	21
Triamcinolone acetonide	330	3.6	3.9	10.6
Beclomethasone dipropionate	600	13.5	7.5	20
Budesonide	980	9.4	5.1	11
Fluticasone propionate	1200	18	10.5	<1

TABLE 80–5. Comparative Dosages of Inhaled Corticosteroids for Adults (≥12 y) and Children[a]

Drug	Low Dose	Medium Dose	High Dose
Beclomethasone dipropionate MDI (42 μg/puff; 84 μg/puff)	≥12 y: 168–504 μg <12 y: 84–336 μg	≥12 y: 504–840 μg <12 y: 336–672 μg	≥12 y: >840 μg <12 y: >672 μg
Budesonide Turbuhaler DPI (200 μg/dose)	≥12 y: 200–400 μg <12 y: 100–200 μg	≥12 y: 400–600 μg <12 y: 200–400 μg	≥12 y: >600 μg <12 y: >400 μg
Flunisolide MDI (250 μg/puff)	≥12 y: 500–1000 μg <12 y: 500–750 μg	≥12 y: 1000–2000 μg <12 y: 750–1500 μg	≥12 y: >2000 μg <12 y: >1500 μg
Triamcinolone acetonide MDI (100 μg/puff)	≥12 y: 400–1000 μg <12 y: 400–600 μg	≥12 y: 1000–2000 μg <12 y: 600–1200 μg	≥12 y: >2000 μg <12 y: >1200 μg
Fluticasone propionate MDI (44, 110, 220 μg/puff); DPI (50, 100, 250 μg/dose)	≥12 y: 88–264 μg <12 y: 88–176 μg	≥12 y: 264–660 μg <12 y: 176–440 μg	≥12 y: >660 μg <12 y: >440 μg

[a]Based on dosages recommended for mild, moderate, and severe persistent asthma from the guidelines.
MDI, metered-dose inhaler; DPI, dry powder inhaler.

- Because short-term (1–2 weeks) high-dose steroids (1–2 mg/kg/d prednisone) do not produce serious toxicities, the ideal use is to administer the glucocorticoids for a short course and then maintain the patient on appropriate long-term control therapy with long periods between systemic glucocorticoid treatment.
- In patients who require chronic systemic glucocorticoids for control of asthma, the lowest possible dose required to control symptoms should be used. Toxicities of systemic glucocorticoid therapy may be decreased by alternate-day therapy or use of topical inhaled glucocorticoids.

Leukotriene Modifiers

- Leukotriene modifiers act by inhibiting the action of cysteinyl leukotrienes LTC_4, LTD_4, and LTE_4. Although they are FDA approved for prophylaxis and chronic treatment of asthma in adults and children ≥12 years of age (zafirlukast, zileuton) or ≥6 years of age (montelukast), their precise role in the treatment of asthma is not clearly defined. They may be used as alternatives to low-dose inhaled corticosteroids in mild persistent asthma. They may also be appropriate as adjuncts to inhaled corticosteroids in patients with more severe asthma. These agents are not used to treat acute episodes of asthma and must be taken on a regular basis, even during symptom-free periods.
- **Zafirlukast (Accolate)** is a leukotriene-receptor antagonist that reduces the proinflammatory effects of leukotrienes LTD_4 and LTE_4 (increased microvascular permeability and airway edema) and their bronchoconstriction. The recommended dose is 20 mg twice daily, taken at least 1 hour before or 2 hours after meals. Adverse effects include headache (13%), infection (3.5%), nausea (3%), and diarrhea (3%). Rare elevations in alanine aminotransferase (ALT) have been reported (1.5%). Co-administration with warfarin results in a clinically significant increase in prothrombin time (PT) and international normalized ratio (INR).
- **Montelukast (Singulair)** is also a leukotriene-receptor antagonist. The recommended adult dose is 10 mg once daily, taken in the evening without regard to food. For children 6–14 years the dose is one 5-mg chewable tablet daily in the evening. Adverse effects include headache (18%), influenza (4%), and abdominal pain (3%). Rare elevations in ALT (2.1%) and aspartate aminotransferase (AST, 1.6%) have been reported.
- **Zileuton (Zyflo)** directly inhibits 5-lipoxygenase, thereby inhibiting formation of leukotrienes. The recommended dose is 600 mg four times daily, taken with meals and at bedtime. It may cause elevated hepatic enzymes; the frequency of ALT elevations ≥3 times the upper limit of normal was 1.9%. Hepatic transaminases should be monitored before treatment, once a month for the first 3 months, every 2–3 months for the remainder of the first year, and then periodically thereafter. Zileuton also inhibits hepatic CYP3A4 isozymes, significantly increasing concentrations of theophylline and warfarin. When

zileuton therapy is initiated. In patients receiving theophylline, the theophylline dose should be reduced by 50% and monitored closely with serum concentrations.

Methotrexate

- Low-dose **methotrexate** (5–25 mg/wk) may act as an anti-inflammatory agent when used for the treatment of asthma. It may also have immunomodulatory effects by inhibiting chemotaxis of neutrophils, inhibiting leukotriene B_4-induced adherence to endothelium, and inhibiting the proinflammatory activity of IL-1.
- At best, methotrexate therapy results in moderate reduction in systemic steroid dosage (14–35%) in patients with severe steroid-dependent asthma and does not induce a remission in the disease.
- Methotrexate should be considered experimental and reserved for only severe steroid-dependent asthmatics under the care of specialists

► EVALUATION OF THERAPEUTIC OUTCOMES

CHRONIC ASTHMA

- Control of asthma is defined as achieving a minimal need for as-needed short-acting β_2 agonists (ideally none), no acute episodes, no limitation of activity, no emergency care visits, no nocturnal symptoms, normal pulmonary functions, minimal or no adverse effects from medicine, and satisfaction of the patient and family with the care.
- Monitoring consists of quantitating the use of as-needed short-acting inhaled β_2 agonists, days of limited activity, and number of symptoms.
- In moderate to severe asthmatics, daily peak flow monitoring once daily upon awakening is recommended.
- The NAEPP recommends yearly spirometric studies.
- Patients should also be asked about exercise tolerance and nocturnal symptoms.
- All patients on inhaled drugs should have their inhalation technique evaluated periodically, monthly initially and then every 3–6 months once optimal technique is established.
- After initiation of anti-inflammatory therapy or a change in dosage, most patients should begin experiencing a decrease in symptoms within 1–2 weeks and achieve maximum symptomatic improvement within 4–8 weeks. Improvement in baseline FEV_1 or PEF should follow a similar time frame, but a decrease in bronchial hyperreactivity as measured by diurnal variation in PEF and exercise tolerance may take longer and slowly improve over 1–3 months.

ACUTE SEVERE ASTHMA

- Patients at risk for acute severe exacerbations should monitor morning peak flows at home.

- In children una/ to perfın .Fs, supraclavicular retractions, increased respira/y rate and heart rate, and inability to speak more than one or two words between breaths are signs of severe obstruction.
- Upon admissi/ peak flow or clinical symptoms should be monitored every 2–4 ho
- Oxygen sat/ tion by pulse oximetry and peak flow should be measured in patients not completely responding to initial intensive inhaled β agonist therapy.

See Cha/ 24, Asthma, auth/d by H. William Kelly, PharmD, FCCP, BCPS, Alan K. Kamada, PharmD, for a more detailed discussion of this to/

TABLE 81–1. Clinical Features of COLD

	Predominant Emphysema	Predominant Chronic Bronchitis
Age (y)	60±	50±
Dyspnea	Severe	Mild
Cough	After dyspnea starts	Before dyspnea starts
Sputum	Scanty, mucoid	Copious, purulent
Bronchial infection	Less frequent	More frequent
Respiratory insufficiency episode	Often terminal	Repeated
Chest film markings	Increased diameter Flattened diaphragms	Increased bronchovascular markings Large heart
$Paco_2$ (mm Hg)	35–40	50–60
Pao_2 (mm Hg)	65–75	45–60
Hematocrit (%)	35–45	50–60
Pulmonary hypertension		
Rest	None to mild	Moderate to severe
Exercise	Moderate	Worsens
Cor pulmonale	Rare	Common
Diffusion capacity	Decreased	None to slightly decreased

Adapted from Ingram RH. Chronic bronchitis, emphysema, and airways obstruction. In: Wilson JD, Braunwald E, Isselbacher KJ, et al, eds. Harrison's Textbook of Internal Medicine. *New York, McGraw-Hill, 1994:1197–1206, with permission.*

- A rapid assessment of obstruction can be done by placing the stethoscope over the trachea and instructing the patient to forcefully expire. Forced expiration lasting >4 seconds correlates with obstruction in pulmonary function tests.
- The use of the scalene or sternocleidomastoid muscles of the neck to assist respiration may not be apparent unless severe obstruction is present.
- As the degree of obstruction worsens and the arterial oxygen tension (Pao_2) continues to drop, pulmonary hypertension from vasoconstriction ensues. This leads to right ventricular strain and ultimately cor pulmonale. On physical examination this is manifested by jugular venous distention, hepatomegaly, hepatojugular reflux, and peripheral edema.
- On cardiac examination, a heave may be felt (or even seen in thin patients) upon palpation of the epigastric area. Auscultation of the area may reveal a gallop rhythm suggestive of right ventricular hypertrophy.
- In the face of chronic hypoxemia, cyanosis of the lips, mucous membranes, or extremities may be seen. Clubbing of the fingers is rarely seen in chronic bronchitis.

EMPHYSEMA

- Patients with predominant emphysema are characteristically older than those with chronic bronchitis. The chief complaint is often increasing dyspnea, even at rest, with minimal cough.
- These patients have been classically termed "pink puffers" (type A) because of their obvious tachypnea and flushed appearance, which is due to their respiratory centers being quite responsive to hypoxemia as a stimulus to breathe.
- These patients are frequently thin and will present with "pursed lip" breathing. They also are tachypneic at rest and often sit with their chests forward and hands resting on their knees; this position requires the least energy for breathing. Accessory muscles of the chest and neck are frequently used to assist in the work of breathing.
- Percussion of the chest is hyperresonant, and auscultation reveals diminished breath sounds with rhonchi and minimal wheezes. Excursion of the diaphragms is limited because of persistent hyperinflation of the lungs.
- Hypoxemia is not a significant problem in the predominant emphysema patient until late in the disease state. As a result, cor pulmonale is not common until the terminal stages.

▶ DIAGNOSIS

PULMONARY FUNCTION TESTS

- In patients with chronic bronchitis and/or emphysema, there are reductions in forced expiratory volume after 1 second (FEV_1), forced vital capacity (FVC), FEV_1/FVC%, and forced expiratory flow ($FEF_{25-75\%}$).
- Measurement of diffusion capacity using carbon monoxide (DCO) can help distinguish predominant bronchitis from emphysema. In emphysema, the diffusion capacity is diminished because of loss of surface area available for gas diffusion. In bronchitis the diffusion capacity is normal or only slightly decreased.

ARTERIAL BLOOD GASES

- The predominant chronic bronchitis patient has a low arterial oxygen tension (Pao_2 = 45–60 mm Hg) and an elevated arterial carbon dioxide tension ($Paco_2$ = 50–60 mm Hg).
- The predominantly emphysematous patient has by comparison a higher Pao_2 and usually normal $Paco_2$ with similar degrees of pulmonary dysfunction.
- Because these changes in Pao_2 and $Paco_2$ are subtle and progress over many years, the pH is usually near normal because the kidneys compensate by retaining bicarbonate.

CHEST ROENTGENOGRAM

- Characteristic findings of severe emphysema include flattened diaphragms that move <3 cm between inspiration and expiration, loss of peripheral vascular markings, bullous lesions, and increased retrosternal air space, indicating extensive air trapping.

- In the patient with predominant chronic bronchitis, the only changes are increased bronchovascular markings in the lower lung field and an increased cardiac silhouette in the presence of right ventricular failure with prominent pulmonary arteries.

ELECTROCARDIOGRAM

- Common findings when cor pulmonale develops are right-axis deviation, prominent R waves in V1 and V2, S wave in V5 or V6 $\geq$ 7 mm, and tall peaked P waves in lead II.

OTHER LABORATORY TESTS

- In the predominant chronic bronchitic patient, the hemoglobin and hematocrit are elevated secondary to erythropoiesis caused by hypoxemia.
- In exacerbations of chronic bronchitis, the white cell count may or may not rise and a left shift may or may not be present.
- Examination of sputum (e.g., Gram stain) is helpful in exacerbations of chronic bronchitis to identify potential bacterial pathogens that may have precipitated the exacerbation and aid in the selection of antimicrobial therapy. Sputum should also be examined for eosinophils to rule out an allergic component that would be consistent with asthmatic bronchitis.

DIAGNOSIS OF ACUTE RESPIRATORY FAILURE IN COLD

- The diagnosis of acute respiratory failure in COLD is made on the basis of an acute drop in Pa_{O_2} of 10–15 mm Hg or any acute increase in Pa_{CO_2} that decreases the serum pH to 7.30 or less.
- Additional acute clinical manifestations include restlessness, confusion, tachycardia, diaphoresis, cyanosis, hypotension, irregular breathing, miosis, and unconsciousness.
- The most common cause of acute respiratory failure in COLD is acute exacerbation of bronchitis with an increase in the volume and viscosity of sputum. This serves to worsen obstruction and further impair alveolar ventilation, resulting in worsening hypoxemia and hypercapnia. Additional causes are pneumonia, pulmonary embolism, left ventricular failure, pneumothorax, and central nervous system depressants.

▶ DESIRED OUTCOME

The goals of therapy are to improve the chronic obstructive state, treat and prevent acute exacerbations, reduce the rate of progression of the disease, improve the physical and psychological well-being of the patient so that daily activities can be resumed or maintained, reduce the number of days lost from work, reduce hospitalizations, and reduce mortality.

▶ TREATMENT

GENERAL PRINCIPLES

- Smoking cessation is a critical first step that will slow the rate of decline in pulmonary function tests, decrease symptoms, and improve the patient's quality of life.
- Comprehensive pulmonary rehabilitation programs include exercise training along with smoking cessation, breathing exercises, optimal medical treatment, psychosocial support, and health education. Supplemental oxygen and adequate nutrition are important adjuncts in a training program.
- Many individuals with COLD obtain some degree of improvement in their obstruction from bronchodilators, even though tests of reversibility using an inhaled sympathomimetic followed by pulmonary function tests do not indicate a positive response.
- An algorithm to provide guidance in the choice of therapy for COLD is shown in Figure 81–1. The decision regarding which bronchodilator class to use first (i.e., anticholinergics, sympathomimetics, or methylxanthines) is based on likely patient adherence, individual response, and potential adverse effects. For purposes of this chapter, agents are presented in the sequence in which they are currently commonly used.

ANTICHOLINERGICS

- Anticholinergics have emerged as first-line therapy for stable COLD patients. When given by inhalation, **atropine** and **ipratropium bromide** produce bronchodilation by competitively inhibiting cholinergic receptors in bronchial smooth muscle. This activity blocks acetylcholine, with the net effect being a reduction in cyclic guanosine monophosphate (GMP), which normally acts to constrict bronchial smooth muscle.
- Anticholinergic agents produce greater improvement in pulmonary function tests than the sympathomimetics in patients with COLD, pointing out the relative importance of the cholinergic system as a mediator of bronchial tone. These agents maintain their effectiveness during years of regular continuous use.
- Ipratropium bromide is preferred over atropine sulfate because it has fewer systemic side effects. It is available as a metered dose inhaler (MDI) and a solution for inhalation and provides a peak effect in 1.5–2 hours with a duration of 4–6 hours. Systemic absorption is minimal because of its quaternary ammonium structure. Side effects include dry mouth and a metallic taste.
- Although the recommended dose is two puffs 4 times a day, many clinicians prescribe two to three times that dose to produce maximal bronchodilation.
- Spacer devices improve aerosol delivery from MDIs in patients who are unable to adequately coordinate MDI actuation with inhalation (e.g., elderly COLD patients).

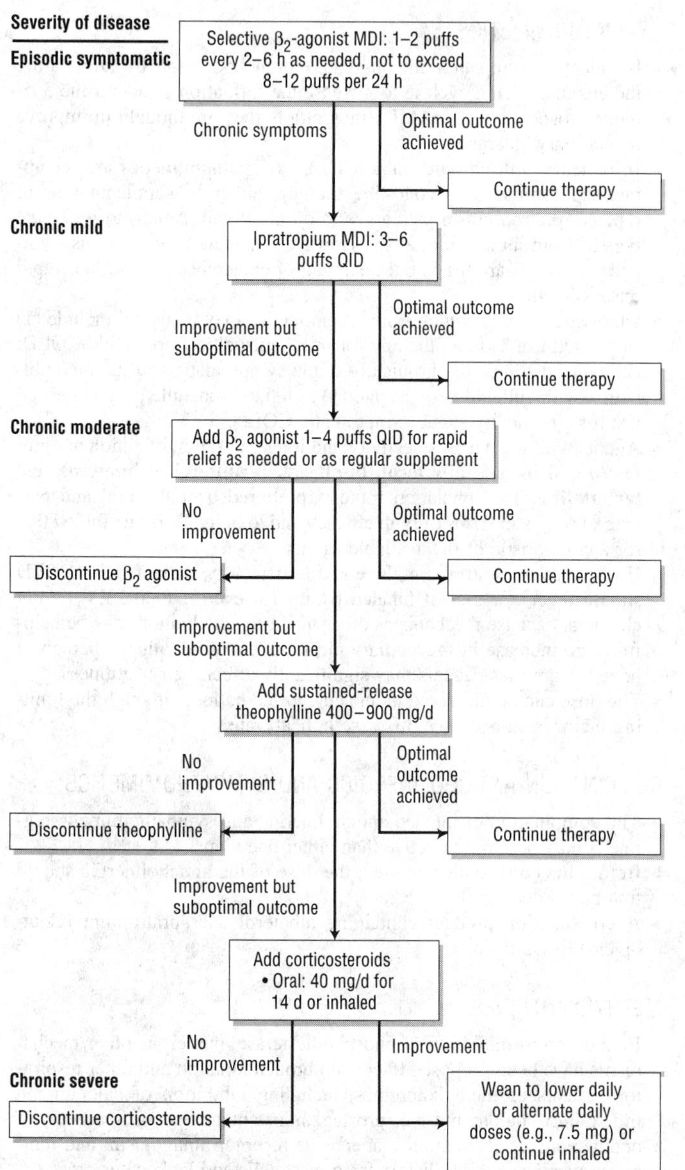

Figure 81–1. COLD treatment algorithm.

SYMPATHOMIMETICS

- β_2-selective sympathomimetics cause bronchodilation by stimulating the enzyme adenyl cyclase to increase the formation of adenosine 3′,5′ monophosphate (3′,5′-cAMP). In addition, they are thought to improve mucociliary clearance.
- In patients with chronic stable COLD, sympathomimetics are recommended for use as second-line therapy, either to supplement or to replace ipratropium in patients who do not obtain satisfactory clinical benefit from ipratropium alone. However, in acute exacerbations, sympathomimetics are the initial treatment of choice because of their rapid onset of action.
- Other situations in which sympathomimetics may be useful include (1) as-needed use as monotherapy for mild, episodic symptomatic COLD; (2) as-needed use for chronically stable symptomatic COLD in combination with anticholinergics; and (3) as a fixed schedule plus as-needed use for chronically stable symptomatic COLD.
- Agents with greater β_2 selectivity and longer duration of action are preferred and include **albuterol, bitolterol, pirbuterol, salmeterol,** and **terbutaline.** The inhalation route is preferred over the oral and parenteral routes in terms of both efficacy and toxicity. Refer to Table 80–1 for a comparison of the available agents.
- If response to ipratropium alone is unsatisfactory, patients with COLD should receive a trial of inhaled β_2 agonist even if their FEV_1 is not changed, because mechanisms other than bronchodilation may be helpful (e.g., increase in mucociliary clearance). An individual's perceived benefit from these agents may significantly affect their usefulness.
- The dose can be increased in an acute exacerbation, although the limiting factor is an excessive increase in heart rate.

COMBINATION ANTICHOLINERGICS AND SYMPATHOMIMETICS

- The combination of inhaled anticholinergic and sympathomimetic regimens may be more effective than either one alone.
- Before the combination is used, the dose of the anticholinergic should first be titrated.
- A combination product containing albuterol and ipratropium (Combivent) is available.

METHYLXANTHINES

- In addition to inhibition of phosphodiesterase, numerous other mechanisms have been proposed to explain bronchodilation and other respiratory effects of methylxanthines, including inhibition of calcium ion influx into smooth muscle, prostaglandin antagonism, stimulation of endogenous catecholamines, adenosine receptor antagonism, and inhibition of release of mediators from mast cells and leukocytes.

- **Theophylline** (1,3-dimethylxanthine), the most commonly used methylxanthine, can be an effective bronchodilator in many patients with chronic, stable disease, but it is now considered third-line therapy after anticholinergics and sympathomimetics. When methylxanthines are used, parameters other than objective measurements, such as FEV_1, should be monitored to assess efficacy. Subjective parameters, such as reduced dyspnea and enhanced exercise tolerance, are important in assessing the acceptability of methylxanthines for COLD patients.
- Sustained-release theophylline improves patient compliance and achieves more consistent serum concentrations than rapid-release theophylline and **aminophylline** preparations, but there are considerable variations in sustained-release characteristics.
- Theophylline has been shown to be of value in acute exacerbations of COLD. Oral or intravenous loading doses of theophylline or aminophylline should be given to achieve therapeutic serum theophylline concentrations rapidly. Intravenous therapy should be reserved for severe acute decompensation in patients unable to take oral medication; the administration rate should not exceed 25 mg/min to avoid cardiac arrhythmias or cardiovascular collapse. Recommended loading doses (based on actual body weight) are 5 mg/kg theophylline and 6 mg/kg aminophylline for patients who have not taken any theophylline in the previous 24 hours. If a theophylline concentration cannot be obtained rapidly in patients already taking theophylline, a partial loading dose of 2.5 mg/kg theophylline or 3 mg/kg aminophylline may be given.
- The desired therapeutic range in older COLD patients is 10–15 μg/mL in order to minimize the likelihood of toxicity.
- Initial maintenance dose recommendations for various conditions are included in Table 81–2. Serum concentrations should be obtained 12–24 hours after the initiation of the loading dose and every 24 hours thereafter until the patient is stable.
- When switching to oral therapy, the oral sustained-release preparation can be initiated at the time the IV infusion is stopped. The total

TABLE 81–2. Maintenance Doses of Intravenous Aminophylline in Exacerbations of COLD

Usual loading dose, mg/kg	6
Maintenance dose, mg/kg/h	
Smokers	0.8
Nonsmokers	0.5
Elderly	0.3
Cor pulmonale	0.3
Heart failure	0.1–0.2
Liver disease	0.1–0.2

24-hour IV dose may be divided in thirds or in halves depending on the desired interval and strength of preparation available. Follow-up trough serum concentrations should be obtained several days later to ensure the appropriateness of the dose and dosing interval. Once a dose is established, it is not necessary to routinely monitor serum concentrations unless the patient's disease worsens or toxicity is suspected.

- Administration of oral sustained-release theophylline preparations at bedtime has been demonstrated to reduce overnight declines in FEV_1 and morning respiratory symptoms.

CORTICOSTEROIDS

- The anti-inflammatory mechanisms whereby corticosteroids exert their beneficial effect in COLD include reduction in capillary permeability to decrease mucus, inhibition of release of proteolytic enzymes from leukocytes, and inhibition of prostaglandins.
- Corticosteroids may be initiated during an acute exacerbation when the patient is deteriorating or not improving as expected, despite adequate anticholinergic and/or sympathomimetic therapy and possibly methylxanthines.
- Patients taking chronic oral steroids who present in acute distress are commonly started on parenteral steroids. Therapy is initiated with **methylprednisolone** or its equivalent 0.5–1.0 mg/kg IV every 6 hours. It generally requires 3–6 hours for a beneficial effect to be observed.
- As soon as symptoms have stabilized, the patient may be switched to 40–60 mg of **prednisone** daily. Steroids should be stopped in 7–14 days, if possible, to minimize HPA suppression.
- If prolonged therapy is needed, a low morning daily dose (e.g., prednisone, 7.5 mg/d) or alternate-day therapy should be employed.
- In patients requiring continuous steroid therapy, giving short bursts of higher doses of oral prednisone during periods of worsening clinical status may be effective in decreasing hospitalizations.
- Although inhaled corticosteroids may be of some benefit in COLD, asthmatic patients tend to gain greater benefit than COLD patients.

LONG-TERM OXYGEN

- Stable outpatients receiving optimal pharmacotherapy should have long-term oxygen therapy instituted if either of two conditions exists: (1) a resting PaO_2 of <55 mm Hg; or (2) evidence of right heart failure, polycythemia, or impaired neuropsychiatric function with a PaO_2 of <60 mm Hg. Oxygen therapy may also be used during exercise or at night.
- The most practical means of administering long-term oxygen is with the nasal cannula, which provides 24–28% oxygen. The goal is to raise the PaO_2 above 60 mm Hg. Patients known to retain carbon dioxide should be cautioned to not raise the PaO_2 so high that they depress their respiratory drive.
- The use of an oxygen concentrator may cost between $200 and $400 per month. Portable oxygen tanks may cost about $300 per month.

ANTIBIOTICS

- Antibiotics are reasonable in patients who exhibit signs suggestive of bronchial infection, such as fever, leukocytosis, increased sputum quantity, increased viscosity of sputum, change in sputum color, and/or change in chest radiograph. Sputum Gram stain may be helpful in determining the need for oral antibiotic therapy, but an appropriate sputum sample is often difficult to obtain. Patients may not have fever, chills, or a leukocytosis in the early stage of infectious exacerbations. Sputum cultures obtained initially are of little practical value.
- Therapy should be initiated within 24 hours of symptoms to prevent unnecessary hospitalization.
- The bacterial organisms usually responsible for exacerbations are *Streptococcus pneumoniae, Haemophilus influenzae,* and *Moraxella catarrhalis.*
- **Amoxicillin** and **amoxicillin/clavulanate** are used most frequently in patients not allergic to penicillins. Other acceptable oral alternatives include **tetracyclines, cephalosporins, cotrimoxazole, macrolides,** and newer **fluoroquinolones** with greater gram-positive activity (e.g., **levofloxacin**).
- Therapy should generally be continued for at least 7–10 days. **Azithromycin** for 3–5 days is also effective.
- If the patient deteriorates or does not improve as anticipated, hospitalization may be necessary and more aggressive attempts should be made to identify potential pathogens responsible for the exacerbation. Parenteral antibiotics may be required.
- COLD patients should receive one dose of pneumococcal vaccine and a yearly influenza vaccination. If a patient has been exposed to influenza before vaccination, a course of amantadine or rimantadine may be considered.

▶ EVALUATION OF THERAPEUTIC OUTCOMES

- The pharmacologic plan for a given patient requires weighing the risk/benefit ratio carefully and having a comprehensive plan to assess subjectively and objectively the efficacy and toxicity of the chosen therapy.
- Objective outcome measures include improvement in the FEV_1:FVC and peak flow; improvement in the distance covered in a 6- or 12-minute walk; and objectively observed reduction in dyspnea, medication use, and nocturnal symptoms.
- Disease-specific quality of life measures developed to assess the overall efficacy of therapies for COLD include the Chronic Respiratory Questionnaire (CRQ) and the St. George's Respiratory Questionnaire (SGRQ). These instruments measure the impact of therapies on disease variables such as dyspnea and level of activity, but they do not measure the impact on survival.

- Subjective parameters, such as perceived improvement in exercise tolerance should also be considered; although objective improvement may be minimal with some therapies, clinical benefit to the individual may be meaningful.

See Chapter 25, Chronic Obstructive Lung Disease, authored by Sherri L. Konzem, PharmD, and Mark A. Stratton, PharmD, BCPS, FASHP, for a more detailed discussion of this topic.

Appendices

Edited by Barbara G. Wells, PharmD, FASHP, FCCP, BCPP

Appendix 1

▶ ALLERGIC AND PSEUDOALLERGIC DRUG REACTIONS

TABLE A1–1. Classification of Allergic Drug Reactions

Type	Descriptor	Characteristics	Typical Onset	Drug Causes
I	Anaphylactic (IgE mediated)	Allergen binds to IgE on basophils or mast cells resulting in release of inflammatory mediators	Within 30 min	Penicillin immediate reaction Blood products Polypeptide hormones Vaccines Dextran
II	Cytotoxic	Cell destruction occurs because of cell-associated antigen that initiates cytolysis by antigen-specific antibody (IgG or IgM). Most often involves blood elements	Typically 5–12 h	Penicillin, quinidine, phenylbutazone, thiouracils, sulfonamides, methyldopa
III	Immune complex	Antigen–antibody complexes form and deposit on blood vessel walls and activate complement. Result is a serum-sickness-like syndrome	3–8 h	May be caused by penicillins, sulfonamides, radiocontrast agents, hydantoins
IV	Cell mediated (delayed)	Antigens cause activation of lymphocytes, which release inflammatory mediators	24–48 h	Tuberculin reaction

TABLE A1–2. Top 10 Drugs or Agents Reported to Cause Skin Reactions

	Reactions per 1000 Recipients
Amoxicillin	51.4
Trimethoprim–sulfamethoxazole	33.8
Ampicillin	33.2
Iopodate	27.8
Blood	21.6
Cephalosporins	21.1
Erythromycin	20.4
Dihydralazine hydrochloride	19.1
Penicillin G	18.5
Cyanocobalamin	17.9

TABLE A1–3. Procedure for Performing Penicillin Skin Testing

A. Percutaneous (prick) skin testing

Materials	**Volume**
Pre-Pen 6×10^{-6} M	1 drop
Penicillin G 10,000 U/mL	1 drop
β-Lactam drug 3 mg/mL	1 drop
0.03% albumin-saline control	1 drop
Histamine control (1 mg/mL)	1 drop

1. Place a drop of each test material on the volar surface of the forearm.
2. Prick the skin with a sharp needle inserted through the drop at a 45° angle gently tenting the skin in an upward motion.
3. Interpret skin responses after 15 min.
4. A wheal at least 2×2 mm with erythema is considered positive.
5. If the prick test is nonreactive, proceed to the intradermal test.
6. If the histamine control is nonreactive, the test is considered uninterpretable.

B. Intradermal skin testing

Materials	**Volume**
Pre-Pen 6×10^{-6} M	0.02 mL
Penicillin G 10,000 U/mL	0.02 mL
β-Lactam drug 3 mg/mL	0.02 mL
0.03% albumin-saline control	0.02 mL
Histamine control (0.1 mg/mL)	0.02 mL

1. Inject 0.02–0.03 mL of each test material intradermally (amount sufficient to produce a small bleb).
2. Interpret skin responses after 15 min.
3. A wheal at least 6×6 mm with erythema and at least 3 mm greater than the negative control is considered positive.
4. If the histamine control is nonreactive, the test is considered uninterpretable.

Antihistamines may blunt the response and cause false-negative reactions.

TABLE A1–4. Treatment of Anaphylaxis

1. Place patient in recumbent position and elevate extremities.
2. Monitor vital signs often (or continuously if possible).
3. Apply tourniquet proximal to site of antigen injection; remove every 10–15 min.
4. Administer epinephrine 1:1000 into nonoccluded site: 0.3–0.5 mL subcutaneously or intramuscularly in adults and 0.01 mL/kg subcutaneously or intramuscularly in children.
5. Administer aqueous epinephrine 1:1000 into site of antigen injection; 0.15–0.25 mL subcutaneously in adults and 0.005 mL/kg subcutaneously in children.
6. Establish and maintain airway with oropharyngeal airway device, endotracheal intubation, transtracheal catheterization, or cricothyrotomy.
7. Administer oxygen at 6–10 L/min.
8. Institute rapid fluid replacement with 0.9% sodium chloride, lactated Ringer's, or colloid solution (e.g., 5% albumin or 4% hetastarch).
9. For hypotension in adults, administer norepinephrine, 32 μg/min (use 8 mg in 500 mL dextrose 5%) with the rate adjusted to maintain low-normal blood pressure. Alternatively, administer dopamine at 2–10 μg/kg/min intravenously.
10. If refractory hypotension is present, administer cimetidine 300 mg or ranitidine 50 mg, intravenously over 3–5 min.
11. If bronchospasm is present, administer aminophylline 6 mg/kg intravenously over 20 min.
12. Administer hydrocortisone sodium succinate 100 mg intravenously (push) and 100 mg intravenously in saline every 2–4 h to block the late-phase reaction.
13. Administer diphenhydramine 1–2 mg/kg intravenously (up to 50 mg) over 3 min to block histamine-1 receptors.
14. For adults taking a β-adrenergic blocker, administer atropine (0.5 mg intravenously) every 5 min until heart rate is greater than 60 beats/min, or isoproterenol 2–20 μg/min intravenously titrated to heart rate of 60 beats/min, or glucagon 0.5 mg/kg intravenously (push) followed by 0.07 mg/kg/h continuously intravenously.

TABLE A1–5. Protocol for Oral Penicillin Desensitization

	Phenoxymethyl Penicillin			
Step[a]	Concentration (U/mL)	*Volume (mL)*	*Dose (U)*	Cumulative Dose (U)
1	1000	0.1	100	100
2	1000	0.2	200	300
3	1000	0.4	400	700
4	1000	0.8	800	1500
5	1000	1.6	1600	3100
6	1000	3.2	3200	6300
7	1000	6.4	6400	12,700
8	10,000	1.2	12,000	24,700
9	10,000	2.4	24,000	48,700
10	10,000	4.8	48,000	96,700
11	80,000	1.0	80,000	176,700
12	80,000	2.0	160,000	336,700
13	80,000	4.0	320,000	656,700
14	80,000	8.0	640,000	1,296,700
Observe for 30 min				
15	500,000	0.25	125,000	
16	500,000	0.5	250,000	
17	500,000	1.0	500,000	
18	500,000	2.25	1,125,000	

[a]*The interval between steps is 15 min. (Reproduced from Sullivan TJ.* Current Therapy in Allergy. *St. Louis, Mosby, 1985:57–61, with permission.)*

TABLE A1–6. Parenteral Desensitization Protocol

Injection No.	Benzylpenicillin Concentration (U)	Volume (mL)	Route
1[a,b]	100	0.1	ID
2	100	0.2	SC
3	100	0.4	SC
4	100	0.8	SC
5[b]	1000	0.1	ID
6	1000	0.3	SC
7	1000	0.6	SC
8	10,000	0.1	ID
9	10,000	0.2	SC
10	10,000	0.4	SC
11	10,000	0.8	SC
12[b]	100,000	0.1	ID
13	100,000	0.3	SC
14	100,000	0.6	SC
15[b]	1,000,000	0.1	ID
16	1,000,000	0.2	SC
17	1,000,000	0.2	IM
18	1,000,000	0.4	IM
19		Continuous IV infusion at 1,000,000 U/h	

[a]Administer doses at intervals of not less than 20 min.
[b]Observe and record skin wheal-and-flare response.
From Weiss ME, Adkinson NF. Immediate hypersensitivity reaction to penicillin and related antibiotics. Clin Allergy 1988; 18:515–540, with permission.

Appendix 2

▶ DRUG-INDUCED HEMATOLOGIC DISORDERS

TABLE A2–1. Drugs Associated With Aplastic Anemia

Acetazolamide	Felbamate	Phenothiazines
Aspirin	Furosemide	Phenytoin
Captopril	Gold salts	Propylthiouracil
Carbamazepine	Indomethacin	Quinacrine
Chloramphenicol	Interferon-α	Quinidine
Chloroquine	Methimazole	Sulfonamides
Chlorothiazide	Oxyphenbutazone	Sulfonylureas
Chlorpromazine	Penicillamine	Sulindac
Dapsone	Pentoxifylline	Ticlopidine
Diclofenac	Phenobarbital	

TABLE A2–2. Drugs Associated With Agranulocytosis

Acetaminophen	Flucytosine	Penicillamine
Acetazolamide	Fosphenytoin	Pentazocine
Allopurinol	Furosemide	Phenothiazines
p-Aminosalicylic acid	Ganciclovir	Phenytoin
Benzodiazepines	Gentamicin	Primidone
β-Lactam antibiotics	Gold salts	Procainamide
Brompheniramine	Griseofulvin	Propranolol
Captopril	Hydralazine	Propylthiouracil
Carbamazepine	Hydroxychloroquine	Pyrimethamine
Chloramphenicol	Imipenem–cilastatin	Quinine
Chloropropamide	Imipramine	Rifampin
Cimetidine	Isoniazid	Streptomycin
Clindamycin	Levodopa	Sulfonamides
Clomipramine	Lincomycin	Sulfonylureas
Clozapine	Meprobamate	Thiazide diuretics
Colchicine	Methazolamide	Ticlopidine
Dapsone	Methimazole	Tocainide
Desipramine	Methyldopa	Tolbutamide
Doxycycline	Metronidazole	Vancomycin
Ethacrynic acid	Nitrofurantoin	Zidovudine
Ethosuximide	NSAIDs	

TABLE A2–3. Drugs Associated With Hemolytic Anemia

Acetaminophen	Levodopa	Procainamide
α-Interferon	Mefenamic acid	Quinidine
p-Aminosalicylic acid	Melphalan	Quinine
β-Lactam antibiotics	Methadone	Rifampin
Chlopropamide	Methyldopa	Sulfonamides
Chlorpromazine	Methysergide	Streptomycin
Hydralazine	NSAIDs	Tacrolimus
Hydrochlorothiazide	Nomifensine	Tetracycline
Imipenem-cilastatin	Omeprazole	Tolbutamide
Isoniazid	Probenecid	Triamterene

TABLE A2–4. Drugs Associated With Oxidative Hemolysis

Ascorbic acid	Menadiol	Salazosulfapyridine
Benzocaine	Methylene blue	Sulfacetamide
Chloramphenicol	Nalidixic acid	Sulfamethoxazole
Chloroquine	Nitrofurantoin	Sulfanilamide
Dapsone	Nitrofurazone	Sulfapyridine
Diazoxide	NSAIDs	
Furazolindone	Phenazopyridine	

TABLE A2–5. Drugs Associated With Megaloblastic Anemia

p-Aminosalicylate	Hydroxyurea	Phenytoin
Azathioprine	6-Mercaptopurine	Primidone
Chloramphenicol	Metformin	Pyrimethamine
Colchicine	Methotrexate	Sulfasalazine
Cyclophosphamide	Neomycin	Triamterene
Cytarabine	Nitrofurantoin	Trimethoprim
5-Fluorodeoxyuridine	Oral contraceptives	Vinblastine
5-Fluorouracil	Phenobarbital	

TABLE A2–6. Drugs Associated With Thrombocytopenia

Abciximab	Disopyramide	NSAIDs
Acetazolamide	Fluconazole	Penicillin
Allopurinol	Furosemide	Phenothiazines
Aminoglutethimide	Ganciclovir	Phenytoin
Amphotericin B	Gold salts	Procainamide
Amrinone	Heparin	Quinidine
β-Lactam antibiotics	Hydrochlorothiazide	Quinine
Carbamazepine	Hydroxychloroquine	Rifabutin
Chlorothiazide	Imipenem-cilastatin	Rifampin
Cimetidine	Interferon	Sulfonamide antibiotics
Colchicine	Isoniazid	Sulfonylureas
Desipramine	Low-molecular-weight heparin	Ticlopidine
Diazepam	Meclofenamate	Trimethoprim
Didanosine	Milrinone	Valproic acid
Digitoxin	Morphine	Vancomycin

Appendix 3

DRUG-INDUCED LIVER DISEASE

TABLE A3–1. An Approach to Evaluating a Suspected Hepatotoxic Reaction

Step 1	Does the sex or age of the patient increase his or her risk? Does the patient's occupation increase his or her risk? Does the patient's recreational drug use increase his or her risk? Is the patient using any herbal remedies, tonics, or teas that increase risk? Is the patient's diet deficient in vitamins or micronutrients? Is the patient's diet excessive in vitamins or micronutrients? Is the patient pregnant? Does the patient have diabetes mellitus?
Step 2	Is there a temporal relationship between the drug and the onset of disease?
Step 3	Is there supporting literature for this type of reaction? Is the clinical evidence consistent with the presentations in the literature? What is the statistical risk for the reaction, and for progression to fulminant failure?
Step 4	Is this a common reaction associated with this drug? Have all more common causes (viruses, alcohol) been ruled out?
Step 5	What happened when the drug was discontinued?
Step 6	Is rechallenge with the drug possible? If so, what happened?
Classifying a Lesion Established as a Case of Hepatotoxicity	
Step 7	What are the biopsy results? What are the CT, MRI, and/or ultrasound results? What is the pattern of enzyme elevation? Is there evidence of recovery or is cirrhosis dominating the clinical outcome?

TABLE A3–2. Environmental Hepatic Toxins[a]

Toxin	Group Associated With Exposure
Arsenic	Chemical, construction, agricultural workers
Carbon tetrachloride	Chemical plant workers, laboratory technicians
Copper	Plumbers, copper foundry workers
Dimethylformanide	Chemical plant workers, laboratory technicians
2,4-Dichlorophenoxyacetic acid	Horticulturalists, gardening enthusiasts
Fluorine	Chemical plant workers, laboratory technicians
Toluene	Chemical and agricultural workers, laboratory technicians
Trichloroethylene	Printers, dye workers, cleaners, laboratory technicians
Vinyl chloride	Plastics plant workers

[a]A partial list of environmental toxins that can cause liver injury. At lower exposure rates, these compounds may also predispose the patient to liver injury from a drug.

TABLE A3–3. Herbal Remedies Associated With a Relatively High Incidence of Hepatotoxicty

Aminita	Grease wood	Skullcap
Comfrey	Margosa oil	Yerba
Germander	Mistletoe	
Gordolobo	Pennyroyal (squawmint)	

TABLE A3–4. Relative Patterns of Hepatic Enzyme Elevation Versus Type of Hepatic Lesion

Enzyme	Abbreviation(s)	Necrotic	Cholestatic	Chronic
Alkaline phosphatase	Alk Phos, AP	↑	↑↑↑	↑
5′-Nucleotidase	5-NC, 5NC	↑	↑↑↑	↑
γ-Glutamyltransferase	GGT, GGTP	↑	↑↑↑	↑↑
Aspartamine transferase	AST, SGOT	↑↑↑	↑	↑↑
Alanine transferase	ALT, SGPT	↑↑↑	↑	↑↑
Lactate dehydrogenase	LDH	↑↑↑	↑	↑

↑, <100% of normal; ↑↑, >100% of normal; ↑↑↑, >200% above normal.

Appendix 4

▶ DRUG-INDUCED PULMONARY DISORDERS

TABLE A4–1. Drugs That Induce Apnea

Central Nervous System Depression	
Narcotic analgesics	F[a]
Barbiturates	F
Benzodiazepines	F
Other sedatives and hypnotics	I
Tricyclic antidepressants	R
Phenothiazines	R
Ketamine	R
Promazine	R
Anesthetics	R
Antihistamines	R
Alcohol	I
Fenfluramine	R
L-Dopa	R
Oxygen	R
Respiratory Muscle Dysfunction	
Aminoglycoside antibiotics	I
Polymyxin antibiotics	I
Neuromuscular blockers	I
Quinine	R
Digitalis	R
Myopathy	
Corticosteroids	F
Diuretics	I
Aminocaproic acid	R
Clofibrate	R

[a]Relative frequency of reactions: F, frequent; I, infrequent; R, rare.

TABLE A4–2. Drugs That Induce Bronchospasm

Drug	Frequency	Drug	Frequency
Anaphylaxis (IgE-Mediated)		**Anaphylactoid Mast Cell Degranulation**	
Penicillins	F[a]	Narcotic analgesics	I
Sulfonamides	F	Ethylenediamine	R
Serum	F	Iodinated-radiocontrast media	F
Cephalosporins	F	Platinum	R
Bromelin	R	Local anesthetics	I
Cimetidine	R	Steroidal anesthetics	I
Papain	F	Iron–dextran complex	I
Pancreatic extract	I	Pancuronium bromide	R
Psyllium	I	Benzalkonium chloride	I
Subtilase	I	**Pharmacologic Effect**	
Tetracyclines	I	β-Adrenergic receptor blockers	I–F
Allergen extracts	I	Cholinergic stimulants	I
L-Aspariginase	F	Anticholinesterases	R
Pyrazolone analgesics	I	α-Adrenergic agonists	R
Direct Airway Irritation		Ethylenediamine tetraacetic acid (EDTA)	R
Acetate	R	**Unknown Mechanisms**	
Bisulfite	F	ACE inhibitors	I
Cromolyn	R	Anticholinergics	R
Smoke	F	Hydrocortisone	R
N-Acetylcysteine	F	Isoproterenol	R
Inhaled steroids	I	Monosodium glutamate	I
Precipitating IgG Antibodies		Piperazine	R
α-Methyldopa	R	Tartrazine	R
Carbamazepine	R	Sulfinpyrazone	R
Spiramycin	R	Zinostatin	R
Cyclooxygenase Inhibition		Losartan	R
Aspirin/NSAIDs	F		
Phenylbutazone	I		
Acetaminophen	R		

[a]Relative frequency of reactions: F, frequent; I, infrequent; R, rare.

TABLE A4–3. Drugs That Induce Pulmonary Edema

Drug	Frequency
Cardiogenic Pulmonary Edema	
Excessive intravenous fluids	F[a]
Blood and plasma transfusions	F
Corticosteroids	F
Phenylbutazone	R
Sodium diatrizoate	R
Hypertonic intrathecal saline	R
β_2-Adrenergic agonists	I
Noncardiogenic Pulmonary Edema	
Heroin	F
Methadone	I
Morphine	I
Oxygen	I
Propoxyphene	R
Ethchlorvynol	R
Chlordiazepoxide	R
Salicylate	R
Hydrochlorothiazide	R
Triamterene + hydrochlorothiazide	R
Leukoagglutinin reactions	R
Iron–dextran complex	R
Methotrexate	R
Cytosine arabinoside	R
Nitrofurantoin	R
Dextran 40	R
Fluorescein	R
Amitriptyline	R
Colchicine	R
Nitrogen mustard	R
Epinephrine	R
Metaraminol	R
Bleomycin	R
Iodide	R
Cyclophosphamide	R
VM-26	R

[a]Relative frequency of reactions: F, frequent; I, infrequent; R, rare.

TABLE A4–4. Drugs That Induce Pulmonary Infiltrates With Eosinophilia (Loeffler's Syndrome)

Nitrofurantoin	F[a]	Tetracycline	R
para-Aminosalicylic acid	F	Procarbazine	R
Sulfonamides	I	Cromolyn	R
Penicillins	I	Niridazole	R
Methotrexate	I	Gold salts	R
Imipramine	I	Chlorpromazine	R
Chlorpropamide	R	Naproxen	R
Carbamazepine	R	Sulindac	R
Phenytoin	R	Ibuprofen	R
Mephenesin	R		

[a]Relative frequency of reactions: F, frequent; I, infrequent; R, rare.

TABLE A4–5. Drugs That Induce Pneumonitis and/or Fibrosis

Oxygen	F[a]	Chlorambucil	R
Radiation	F	Melphalan	R
Bleomycin	F	Lomustine and semustine	R
Busulfan	F	Zinostatin	R
Carmustine	F	Procarbazine	R
Hexamethonium	F	Teniposide	R
Paraquat	F	Sulfasalazine	R
Amiodarone	F	Phenytoin	R
Mecamylamine	I	Gold salts	R
Pentolinium	I	Pindolol	R
Cyclophosphamide	I	Imipramine	R
Practolol	I	Penicillamine	R
Methotrexate	I	Phenylbutazone	R
Mitomycin	I	Chlorphentermine	R
Nitrofurantoin	I	Fenfluramine	R
Methysergide	I		
Azathioprine, 6-mercaptopurine	R		

[a]Relative frequency of reactions: F, frequent; I, infrequent; R, rare.

TABLE A4–6. Drugs That May Induce Pleural Effusions and Fibrosis

Idiopathic	
Methysergide	F[a]
Practolol	F
Pindolol	R
Methotrexate	R
Nitrofurantoin	R
Owing to Drug-induced Lupus Syndrome	
Procainamide	F
Hydralazine	F
Isoniazid	R
Phenytoin	R
Mephenytoin	R
Griseofulvin	R
Trimethadione	R
Sulfonamides	R
Phenylbutazone	R
Streptomycin	R
Ethosuximide	R
Tetracycline	R
Pseudolymphoma Syndrome	
Cyclosporine	R
Phenytoin	R

[a]Relative frequency of reactions: F, frequent; I, infrequent; R, rare.

Appendix 5

▶ DRUG-INDUCED SKIN DISORDERS

TABLE A5–1. Selected Drugs Associated With Maculopapular Eruptions

Allopurinol	Nitrofurantoin
Barbiturates	Ofloxacin
Benzodiazepines	Penicillamine
Captopril	Penicillins
Carbamazepine	Phenothiazines
Chloramphenicol	Phenylbutazone
Ciprofloxacin	Phenytoin
Enalapril	Piroxicam
Erythromycin	Pyrazolon derivatives
Ethionamide	Rifampin
Etoposide	Streptomycin
Gold salts	Sulfonamides (includes sulfonylureas and thiazides)
Hydantoin derivatives	Sulindac
Ibuprofen	Tetracyclines
Indomethacin	Tolmentin
Isoniazid	

TABLE A5–2. Selected Drugs Associated With Urticaria, Angioedema, and Anaphylaxis

Acetylsalicylic acid	Insulin	Opiates
Amitriptyline	Interleukin-2	Penicillins
Bisacodyl	Iodinated radiocontrast media	Ranitidine
Cyclophosphamide	Mannitol	Senna
Gold	Mesna	Sulfonamides
Granulocyte colony-stimulating factor	Metoclopramide	Sulindac
Heparin	Naproxen	Tolmentin
Ibuprofen	Nizatidine	
Indomethacin	Omeprazole	

TABLE A5–3. Selected Drugs Associated With Fixed-drug Eruptions

Barbiturates	Gold	Phenothiazines
Carbamazepine	Griseofulvin	Phenylbutazone
Dapsone	Hydralazine	Quinidine
Digoxin	Hydroxyurea	Sulfasalazine
Diphenhydramine	Ibuprofen	Sulfonamides
Disulfiram	Ipecac	Sulindac
Epinephrine	Metronidazole	Tetracyclines
Erythromycin	Phenolphthalien	Trimethoprim

TABLE A5–4. Selected Drugs Associated With Photosensitivity Reactions

Amiodarone	Ketoprofen	Quinidine
Barbiturates	Mitomycin C	Simvastatin
Benzodiazepines	Naproxen	Sulfonamides
Carbamazepine	Oral contraceptives	Sulfonylureas
Chlorothiazide	Phenylbutazone	Sulindac
Chlorpromazine	Piroxicam	Tetracyclines
Dacarbazine	Promethazine	Thiazides
5-Fluorouracil	Protryptyline	
Furosemide	Psoralens	

TABLE A5–5. Selected Drugs Associated With Alopecia

Anticonvulsants	Etretinate	Mitoxantrone
Busulfan	Granulocyte colony-stimulating factor	Oral contraceptives
Carbamazepine	Heparin	Propranolol
Clofibrate	Hydantoin derivatives	Tricyclic antidepressants
Colchicine	Hydroxyurea	Valproate sodium
Cyclophosphamide	Interferon-α	Vitamin A, high dose
Doxorubicin	Isotretinoin	Warfarin
Ethionamide	Methotrexate	

TABLE A5–6. Selected Drugs Associated With Vasculitis

Allopurinol	Ibuprofen	Piroxicam
Anticoagulants	Indomethacin	Propylthiouracil
Cimetidine	Penicillins	Quinine
Fluoxetine	Phenylbutazone	Sulfonamides
Hydralazine	Phenytoin	Thiazides

TABLE A5–7. Heavy Metal-Induced Hyperpigmentation

Agent	Color	Region Involved	Special Features
Mercury	Gray-brown, slate green	Skin folds (topical), gingival pigmentation (systemic)	Caused by deposition of metallic granules and increased melanin production; formerly used in bleaching agents
Silver	Slate gray, blue-gray	Sun-exposed areas, mucosa, sclerae, nails	Silver granule deposition that activates melanin production; occurs months to years after ingestion
Bismuth	Blue-gray	Skin, conjunctiva, oral and vaginal mucosa, black line along gingival margin	Deposition of metallic granules or interaction with bacteria in mouth; more common with parenteral use
Arsenic	Brown, bronze	Trunk, "raindrop"-shaped hyperkeratotic papulonodular lesions; palms, soles	Activates enzymes that form melanin and deposit in skin; used systemically for psoriasis and as a health tonic; pigmentation appears 1–20 years after exposure
Gold	Blue-gray	Periorbital, generalized chrysiasis, sun-exposed areas	Caused by deposition of metallic particles in epidermis, occurs months to years after exposure and is permanent

TABLE A5–8. Chemotherapeutic Agents Associated With Hyperpigmentation

Agent	Color	Region Involved	Special Features
Busulfan	Brown	Face, forearms, chest, trunk, hands	Accelerates melanin formation by enzymes; incidence more frequent in dark-skinned patients; resolves on discontinuation
Bleomycin	Brown	Linear bands on chest, back	Incidence 8–20%; reversible on discontinuation
Doxorubicin	Black-brown	Tongue, palms, soles, nails	Increased incidence in dark-skinned patients; reversible on discontinuation
Mechlorethamine (topical)	Brown	Areas of contact	Toxic effect on keratinocytes; increased melanocytes; some aggregation

TABLE A5–9. Selected Drugs Associated With Acute Generalized Exanthemous Pustulosis

Acetaminophen	Cotrimazole	Mercury
Acetazolamide	Diltiazem	Methoxalen (plus PUVA)
Allopurinol	Doxycycline	Metronidazole
Amoxacillin	Enalapril	Nifedipine
Amphotericin	Erythromycin	Phenytoin
Ampicillin	Furosemide	Pyrimethamine
β-Lactam penicillins	Gentamicin	Quinidine
Carbamazepine	Griseofulvin	Quinolones
Cephalosporins	Hydroxychloroquine	Streptomycin
Chloramphenicol	Imipenem	Sulfonamides
Chloroquine	Isoniazid	Terbinafine
Clindamycin	Itraconazole	Tetracycline
Clobazam	Macrolides	Vancomycin

TABLE A5–10. Selected Drugs Associated With Drug Rash With Eosinophilia and Systemic Symptoms

Allopurinol	Diltiazem	Phenytoin
Atenolol	Isoniazid	Ranitidine
Captopril	Mexiletine	Sulfasalazine
Carbamazepine	Minocycline	Sulfonamides
Chlorpropramide	Phenobarbital	Thalidomide
Dapsone	Phenylbutazone	Zalcitabine

TABLE A5–11. Selected Drugs Associated With Drug-Induced SLE

Most Common	Good Evidence	
Hydralazine	Atenolol	Minocycline
Procainamide	Carbamazepine	Penicillamine
Quinidine	Chlorpromazine	Phenytoin
	Isoniazid	Sulfasalazine
	Methyldopa	Thiazides

TABLE A5–12. Selected Drugs Associated with Erythema Multiforme/ Stevens–Johnson Syndrome

Acetaminophen	Macrolides	Propranolol
Allopurinol	Methazolamide	Quinolones
Carbamazepine	Penicillins	Sulfadiazine
Cephalosporins	Phenobarbital	Sulfonamides
Cotrimoxazole	Phenylbutazone	Thiazides
Ibuprofen	Phenytoin	Valproic acid

TABLE A5–13. Selected Drugs Associated With Toxic Epidermal Necrolysis (TEN)

Allopurinol	Lamotrigine	Quinolones
Barbiturates	Macrolides	Sulfonamides
Carbamazepine	Penicillins	Sulindac
Chloramphenicol	Phenylbutazone	Tolmentin
Ibuprofen	Phenytoin	Valproic acid
Indomethacin	Quinine	

Appendix 6

▶ DRUG-INDUCED RENAL DISEASE

TABLE A6–1. Drug-Induced Renal Structural–Functional Alterations and Examples

Pseudo Renal Failure
- Corticosteroids
- Trimethoprim
- Cimetidine

Hemodynamically Mediated Renal Failure
- Nonsteroidal anti-inflammatory drugs
- Angiotensin converting enzyme inhibitors

Renal Vasculitis, Thrombosis, and Cholesterol Emboli

Vasculitis and thrombosis
- Mitomycin C
- Methamphetamines

Cholesterol emboli
- Warfarin
- Thrombolytic agents

Glomerular Disease

Nephrotic syndrome
- Gold
- Nonsteroidal anti-inflammatory drugs

Glomerulonephritis
- Hydralazine
- Cytokine therapy

Tubular Epithelial Cell Damage

Osmotic nephrosis
- Mannitol
- Intravenous immunoglobulin

Acute tubular necrosis
- Aminoglycoside antibiotics
- Radiographic contrast media

Interstitial Nephritis

Acute allergic
- Methicillin
- Nonsteroidal anti-inflammatory drugs

Chronic
- Cyclosporine
- Lithium

Papillary necrosis
- Combined phenacetin, aspirin, and caffeine analgesics

Obstructive Nephropathy

Intratubular
- Acyclovir
- Sulfadiazine

Lower urinary tract
- Tricyclic antidepressants

Nephrolithiasis
- Triamterene
- Indinavir

TABLE A6–2. Drugs That Interfere With the Jaffé Measurement of Creatinine and Can Falsely Increase the Serum Creatinine Concentration

Cefoxitin
Cephalothin
Cefazolin
Cefotaxime
Flucytosine
Methyldopa

TABLE A6–3. Drugs That Can Cause Tubular Necrosis

Higher Incidence	Lower Incidence
Acetaminophen (overdose)	Amoxapine
Aminoglycosides	Carboplatin
Amphotericin B	Cyclosporine
Cisplatin	Low-molecular-weight dextran
Radiographic contrast agents	Mannitol
Streptozocin	Methoxyflurane anesthesia
	NSAIDs
	Tetracycline

TABLE A6–4. Potential Risk Factors for Aminoglycoside Nephrotoxicity

A. Related to aminoglycoside dosing:
- Large total cumulative dose
- Prolonged therapy
- High 1-h postdose concentration
- Trough concentration exceeding 2 mg/L
- Recent previous aminoglycoside therapy

B. Related to synergistic nephrotoxicity. Aminoglycosides in combination with:
- Cyclosporine
- Amphotericin B
- Vancomycin
- Diuretics

C. Related to predisposing conditions in the patient:
- Preexisting renal insufficiency
- Increased age
- Poor nutrition
- Shock
- Gram-negative bacteremia
- Liver disease
- Hypoalbuminemia
- Obstructive jaundice
- Dehydration
- Potassium or magnesium deficiencies

TABLE A6–5. Considerations for Use of Newer, Lower Osmolar Radiocontrast Agents Compared to Older, Higher Osmolar Ionic Radiocontrast Agents

Advantages:
- Less histamine release with fewer allergic or hemodynamic adverse effects
- Less nephrotoxicity (30–50% decreased incidence in patients with preexisting nondiabetic or diabetic renal insufficiency)

Disadvantage:
- Greater than 10-fold higher cost

TABLE A6–6. Commonly Used Drugs That Cause Allergic Interstitial Nephritis

Antibiotics
- Acyclovir
- Aminoglycosides
- Amphotericin B
- Aztreonam
- Cephalosporins
- Ciprofloxacin
- Erythromycin
- Ethambutol
- Penicillins
- Polymyxin B
- Rifampin
- Sulfonamides
- Tetracyclines
- Trimethoprim-sulfamethoxazole
- Vancomycin

Neuropsychiatric
- Carbamazepine
- Lithium
- Phenobarbital
- Phenytoin
- Valproic acid

Nonsteroidal anti-inflammatory drugs

Diuretics
- Acetazolamide
- Amiloride
- Chlorthalidone
- Furosemide
- Triamterene
- Thiazides

Miscellaneous
- Acetaminophen
- Allopurinol
- Interferon-α
- Aspirin
- Captopril
- Cimetidine
- Clofibrate
- Cyclosporine
- Glyburide
- Gold
- Methyldopa
- *p*-Aminosalicylic acid
- Phenylpropanolamine
- Propylthiouracil
- Radiographic contrast media
- Ranitidine
- Sulfinpyrazone
- Warfarin sodium

TABLE A3.6. Drugs that May Induce Pleural Effusions and Fibrosis

Idiopathic	
Methysergide	F[a]
Pindolol	R
Methotrexate	R
Nitrofurantoin	R
Due to Drug-Induced Lupus Syndrome	
Procainamide	F
Hydralazine	F
Isoniazid	R
Phenytoin	R
Mephenytoin	R
Griseofulvin	R
Trimethadione	R
Sulfonamides	R
Phenylbutazone	R
Streptomycin	R
Ethosuximide	R
Tetracycline	R
Pseudolymphoma Syndrome	
Cyclosporine	R
Phenytoin	R

[a]Relative frequency of reactions: F, frequent; I, infrequent; R, rare.

INDEX

Note: Page numbers followed by *f* refer to illustrations; page numbers followed by *t* refer to tables.

A

Index

B

C

D

F

H

I

M

N

O

P

Q